Handbook of
PHYSICAL MEDICINE
AND
REHABILITATION

D1553285

Handbook of
PHYSICAL MEDICINE
AND
REHABILITATION

Randall L. Braddom, M.D., M.S.
Professor
Department of Physical Medicine and Rehabilitation
Indiana University School of Medicine
Indianapolis, Indiana

SAUNDERS
An Imprint of Elsevier
Philadelphia   London   New York   St. Louis   Sydney   Toronto

Saunders
An Imprint of Elsevier Inc.
The Curtis Center
Independence Square West
Philadelphia, Pennsylvania 19106-3399

ISBN 0-7216-9448-9

Printed in the United States of America
Last digit is the print number: 9 8 7 6 5 4 3 2 1

*This book is dedicated to my parents,
Audy L. and Ruth J. (Williams) Braddom. As I
get older, it is becoming clearer to me just how
wise and intelligent they really are.*

PREFACE

In the late 1930s a group of physicians interested in the new field of Physical Medicine decided that a book should be written that would instruct both medical students and practitioners. The man selected to write that book was Frank H. Krusen, M.D., then of the Mayo Clinic. The book, *Physical Medicine*, was published by W. B. Saunders of Philadelphia in 1941. Future editions of the original textbook were "edited," rather than being written by a single author. A direct descendant of that work is *Physical Medicine and Rehabilitation*, now in its second edition.

One of the interesting things about Krusen's book is that it was originally conceived as a "handbook" that could be put in the coat pocket, rather than as a large textbook. Krusen was aware that his book and its successive printings and editions did not meet the goal of fitting in the coat pocket (even with wartime restrictions on paper use). In fact, it weighed 5 pounds. As other editors took up the work over the years the book became longer and heavier, and the current version has grown to weigh 12 pounds. Its widespread acceptance indicates that there is a real need for such a large textbook. However, this companion version is designed to finally deliver what was intended from the start: a book that will fit in the lab coat pocket and that contains the practical knowledge needed for use on rounds and in the clinic.

To meet the goal of developing a handbook, we reduced the length of each chapter by selecting out the material most useful on the ward and in the clinic. Long explanations regarding etiology and pathophysiology were removed, and the reader was referred to the textbook for that information. This companion version includes clinical pearls, treatment options, and diagnostic tips.

For assistance in this effort, I recruited the chief resident at Indiana University's Department of Physical Medicine and Rehabilitation, Dr. Andrea Peterson. Dr. Peterson did such a good job that I decided to expand our group to a total of three senior residents and a residency program director. They joined me as Associate Editors and Contributors. What better group to help determine what material was essential on the ward and in the clinic?

The reader should be aware that in no way is this companion version meant to replace the textbook. It is simply a portable extension of it—one that can be used more conveniently on the ward and in the clinic. Those who use only this companion version and do not also refer to the textbook will miss out on many excellent figures, tables, references, and explanations of etiology and pathophysiology that are needed for the development of a well-rounded clinician.

While others have attempted to write "coat-pocket-size" textbooks of Physical Medicine and Rehabilitation, this is the first such book to be based on a full-size textbook. The editor and the associate editors trust that you will find it interesting, stimulating, and informative. It is written in the style of the textbook, a style designed to maximize the learning efficiency of the reader. We know your time is valuable, and we have tried to present the information in such a way that it can be grasped as rapidly as possible. Happy reading!

Randall L. Braddom, M.D.
Editor

CONTENTS

SECTION III
COMMON CLINICAL PROBLEMS IN PHYSICAL MEDICINE AND REHABILITATION

SECTION IV
ISSUES IN SPECIFIC DIAGNOSES IN PHYSICAL MEDICINE AND REHABILITATION

EVALUATION

1

Original Chapter by Lisa A. McPeak, M.D.

Physiatric History and Examination

• The physiatric history and physical examination (H&P) includes the standard H&P but adds an emphasis on functional capacity in both the home and the community.

• The physiatrist determines not only physical deficits but also the functional impact of these deficits.

• Identifying functional problems allows the assignment of functional goals that become the basis for developing a therapeutic management plan.

• The physiatric H&P should identify an individual's impairments, disabilities, and handicaps as defined by the World Health Organization (Table 1–1).

• Table 1–2 lists the major categories involved in the physiatric history and examination.

PHYSIATRIC HISTORY (pp. 3–43)

Introduction (pp. 3–4)

• Listen carefully and try to use the patient's own words. Avoid the temptation to reframe them in your own words.

• The patient is often unable to identify the problem directly, especially if a cognitive or psychosocial component of the problem exists. In these situations, observe the patient during the interview for any implied indication of problems. This involves careful scrutiny of body language, attitude, cooperativeness, and social awareness.

• Obtaining a complete history requires developing rapport with the patient. Collect the history in a professional but caring and empathic manner. Shake hands with the patient (or use another greeting gesture if the patient is unable to shake hands), give an appropriate introduction, and address the patient by the last name. Introduction of the physician to any family or friends present is also important. Be aware of any signs of social or physical discomfort due to either the topic of discussion or pain.

• The physician should act as a facilitator, allowing the patient to speak freely, and should only occasionally ask a question to clarify the topic of discussion.

• If communication or cognitive difficulties are present, the history might need to be taken or confirmed through interviews with family members and friends.

TABLE 1–1 World Health Organization Definitions

1980: Definitions of Impairment, Disability, Handicap

Impairment: Any loss or abnormality of psychological, physiological, or anatomical structure or function

Disability: Any restriction or lack resulting from an impairment of the ability to perform an activity in the manner or within the range considered normal for a human being

Handicap: A disadvantage for a given individual, resulting from an impairment or a disability, that limits or prevents the fulfillment of a role that is normal for that individual

1997: Definitions of Impairment, Activity, and Participation

Impairment: Any loss or abnormality of body structure or of a physiological or psychological function (essentially unchanged from 1980 definition)

Activity: The nature and extent of functioning at the level of the person

Participation: The nature and extent of a person's involvement in life situations in relationship to impairments, activities, health conditions, and contextual factors

From World Health Organization: International Classification of Impairments, Disabilities, and Handicaps, 1980; and International Classification of Impairments, Activities, and Participation, 1997. Geneva, World Health Organization.

TABLE 1–2 Outline of the Physiatric History and Examination

Physiatric History	*Physiatric Examination*
Chief complaint	Functional examination
History of present problem	Mobility activities
Functional history	Activities of daily living
Mobility activities	Household activities
Activities of daily living	Driving
Household activities	Musculoskeletal examination
Community activities	Inspection
Cognition	Palpation
Communication	Joint stability
Vocation	Range of motion
Assistive devices	Contractures
Psychosocial history	Manual muscle testing
Substance abuse	Neurological examination
Family/friend support	Level of consciousness
Living situation	Mental status
Vocational history	Communication
Avocational history	Cranial nerves
Psychiatric history	Sensation
Sexual history	Motor control
Finances	Reflexes
Medications/allergies	General medical examination
Diet	*Summary*
Past medical/surgical history	*Problem List*
Family history	*Management Plan*
Review of systems	*Goals*

Chief Complaint (p. 4)

• The chief complaint in a physiatric history should be transcribed from the patient's own words, whenever possible, and is usually only one or two sentences.
• Unlike the conventional history, it should focus on the functional loss or on the reason for the functional loss. For example, on transfer to an inpatient rehabilitation facility, a patient who has had a stroke often complains of inability to walk or to dress.

History of Present Problem (pp. 4–5)

• In a physiatric setting, identifying the problem involves not only discovering an illness but also uncovering the functional implications. It is really the "history of the present problem" rather than the "history of the present illness."
• Describe the problem in a clear, chronological narrative that lists all of the patient's functional, medical, surgical, physical, and cognitive deficits.
• The history of the present problem should include the functional losses or restrictions that have occurred due to the illness or injury.

Functional History (pp. 5–8)

• Functional losses and restrictions should be well documented.
• Patients should be specifically questioned about their ability to perform all activities necessary to function adequately at home and in the community.
• List both the functional skills prior to and since the recent illness or injury.
• The Functional Independence Measure (Table 1–3) is a scale that describes the assistive levels commonly used for documentation purposes.
• Functional activities usually discussed in the functional history are listed in Table 1–4.

Mobility Activities (pp. 5–7)

• Impairments can result in decreased independence and mobility. Each patient should be questioned about the ability to perform all the mobility activities. Include information about the use of ambulation assistive devices such as crutches and canes and the relative safety of the patient's mobility.
• Bed mobility activities include rolling from one side of the bed to the other, and rolling from a supine to a prone position and back.
• Transitional movements allow the individual to change from one level of mobility to another. For example, transitional movements include going from a supine to a sitting position and then from a sitting to a standing position and back again.
• Sitting is an important functional skill. Sitting balance requires adequate trunk and neck stability or strength and appropriate midline orientation.
• Good standing skills are required prior to functional ambulation. Independent standing requires adequate midline orientation, trunk stability, strength, balance, and adequate bilateral leg stability.
• Walking involves balance, strength, coordination, and midline orientation. Question the individual about walking status on different types of surfaces including those indoors and outdoors, uneven surfaces, and carpets.
• Ask about ascending and descending stairs.

TABLE 1–3 Description of the Levels of Function and Their Scores: Modified from the Functional Independence Measure (FIM)

Level of Function	Score	Definition
Independent		Another person is not required for the activity (NO HELPER).
	7	*Complete independence*—All of the tasks described as making up the activity are performed safely, without modification, assistive devices, or aids, and within a reasonable amount of time.
	6	*Modified independence*—One or more of the following may be true: The activity requires an assistive device, the activity takes more than reasonable time, or there are safety considerations.
Dependent		The patient requires another person for either supervision or physical assistance for the activity to be performed (REQUIRES HELPER).
	5	*Supervision or setup*—Patient requires no more help than standby or cueing without physical contact, or the helper sets up needed items.
	4	*Minimal contact assistance*—Patient requires no more help than touching and expends 75% or more of the effort.
	3	*Moderate assistance*—Patient requires more help than touching and expends 50% to 75% of the effort.
	2	*Maximal assistance*—Patient expends 25% to 50% of the effort.
	1	*Total assistance*—Patient expends less than 25% of the effort.

Adapted from the Guide for the Uniform Data Set for Medical Rehabilitation (Adult FIM), version 4.0. Buffalo, State University of New York, 1993.

• Transfer activities, lower limb management in the wheelchair, wheelchair parts management, and wheelchair propulsion skills are important functional activities. Transfers are performed in different ways on differing surfaces and with or without assistance. The most common types of transfers are the stand pivot or the half-stand pivot transfer, the sliding board transfer, and the lateral lift transfer. Floor to wheelchair transfer ability is also investigated because any patient using a wheelchair for mobility is at risk for falling out of the wheelchair.
• Lower limb management in the wheelchair is an important factor in transfer activities. Wheelchair parts management includes the individual's ability to remove and replace armrests and leg rests and the appropriate use of the wheelchair brakes.

Activities of Daily Living *(p. 7)*
• The history should assess activities of daily living (ADL) including feeding, grooming, dressing, bathing, and toileting activities. All of these tasks can require the use of assistive devices. Table 1–5 lists commonly used assistive devices. (See Chapters 23 and 25 for a detailed discussion of ADL and assistive devices.)

TABLE 1–4 Functional Activities That Should Be Discussed in the Functional History

Mobility activities	Household activities
Bed mobility	Cooking
Transitional movements	Cleaning
Supine to sitting	Lawn work
Sitting to standing	Community activities
Sitting	Driving
Standing	Shopping
Ambulation	Social outings
Stair climbing	Cognition
Wheelchair activities	Communication
Propulsion	Vocational activities
Parts management	
Transfer activities	
Activities of daily living	
Feeding	
Grooming	
Dressing	
Bathing	
Toileting	

TABLE 1–5 Common Activities of Daily Living and Household Assistive Devices

Arm orthoses	Devices for dressing
Utilized to hold equipment	Reacher
Adapted hand orthosis	Button aid
Adapted wrist-hand orthosis	Zipper pull
Universal cuff	Long-handled shoehorn
Utilized to assist movement	Stocking aid
Balanced forearm orthosis	Devices for bathing
Overhead sling suspension orthosis	Bath mitt
Devices for feeding	Long-handled sponge
Adapted utensils	Devices for cooking
Plate guard	Suction scrub brush
Rocker knife	Rocker knife
Adapted cup or cup holder	Adapted cooking utensils
Straw	Suction cutting board
Devices for grooming	Suction bowl holder
Adapted brush and comb	One-handed jar opener
Wash mitt	Reacher
Adapted manual razor	Devices for cleaning
Electric razor	Dust mitt
Adapted toothbrush	Adapted handles for cleaning equipment
Suction denture brush	Reacher

• Independent feeding requires the ability to open food packages before eating and the ability to use utensils correctly.

• Grooming includes all of the hygiene activities normally done each morning.

• Upper body dressing includes donning underwear and a shirt or a dress. Pullover items are easier to don if the patient has adequate over-head shoulder range of motion. Independence in lower body dressing requires enough range of motion to reach the feet to don shoes and socks.

• Bathing requires the ability to get in and out of the bathtub or shower safely, to sit or stand for the activity, and to do the cleansing activity itself.

• Toileting skills include mobility activities such as transferring on and off the toilet, sitting on the toilet, and standing. Assistive devices such as grab bars, elevated toilet seats, and bedside commodes are often required.

Household Activities (pp. 7–8)

• Many individuals consider household activities such as cooking, cleaning, and lawn work essential to their daily routines.

• These household activities usually require the use of both upper limbs. (See Table 1–8 in the Textbook for a list of common household assistive devices.)

Community Activities (p. 8)

• Community activities such as driving, shopping, going to church, or participating in social outings are very important to many individuals.

Cognition (p. 8)

• Cognition is the act or process of knowing. It includes adequate orientation to person, place, time, and situation; good memory skills, judgment, and the capacity for abstract thought.

Communication (p. 8)

• Communication is a process by which information is exchanged among individuals.

• Assess whether communication is primarily accomplished verbally or non-verbally with gestural and written communication. (See Chapters 3 and 50 for further information on communication and aphasia.)

Vocational Activities (p. 8)

• The history should assess the vocation of the individual just prior to the recent injury or illness, some specific information as to the physical and cognitive job requirements, and the individual's ability to perform the job since the injury or illness. (See Chapters 35 and 45 for further information.)

Patient's Own Functional Goals (p. 8)

• Goal attainment depends on patient motivation and cooperation. The history should document the specific wishes or goals of the patient. If the physician fails to ask the patient about goals, it might not be noted that the patient has unrealistic goals.

List of Functional Devices (p. 8)

• During the functional history, many patients report having or needing multiple assistive devices or equipment items. These devices are usually used to improve either mobility skills or ADL and homemaking skills. There are hundreds of such assistive devices (see Table 1–5). (See also Table 1–7 in the Textbook, and Chapter 25.)

Psychosocial History (pp. 8–9)

• The individual with a new impairment often has psychosocial problems related to the impairment and decreased functional skills. If the patient can no longer work, the loss of income places stress on the whole family. If a previously independent individual requires physical assistance from family members, the role of both the patient and family member within the home can be changed, leading to a stressful situation. (See Chapter 4 for further information.)

Substance Abuse (pp. 8–9)
• The patient's history of smoking, alcohol abuse, and illegal drug abuse should be assessed.

Family/Friend Support (p. 9)
• After an illness or injury, many individuals need assistance with functional skills. This assistance is usually obtained from family members and, occasionally, from friends. At the time of admission, a possible primary caregiver and other family members or friends should be identified.

Living Situation (p. 9)
• Document the patient's premorbid living situation. This entails asking questions such as whether the patient lived alone or with family members, the location of the bedroom, the number of steps into the home and into the bedroom, the size of the bathroom, and the type of floor covering.

Vocational History (p. 9)
• The patient's present job description was obtained in the functional history. Documentation of educational level and all previous job positions is necessary for the psychosocial history.

Avocational History (p. 9)
• A short summary of previously enjoyed leisure activities will help all members of the rehabilitation team understand the patient's previous lifestyle and possible future goals.

Psychiatric History (p. 9)
• Psychiatric problems such as depression, anxiety, and suicidal or homicidal ideation can have a major influence on an individual's ability to cooperate with a rehabilitation program.
• Depression is common immediately after a disabling injury.

Sexual History (p. 9)
• Questions concerning sexuality should be presented in such a manner that the patient or caregiver remains sufficiently comfortable to provide accurate answers. Past sexuality problems can become worse after a new illness or injury.
• Erectile dysfunction, ejaculation difficulties, and decreased libido are common in male patients after an injury or illness.

• Female patients can have problems with irregular menses, dysmenorrhea, dyspareunia, or decreased libido. (See Chapter 30 for further information.)

Finances (p. 9)
• Loss of income due to a new illness or injury can cause stress-related problems in the patient and the family.

Medications and Allergies (p. 9)

• A complete list of medications and allergies should be obtained during the history. Any prescription or over-the-counter medications or "home remedies" that the patient takes should be documented.

Diet (pp. 9–10)

• Evaluation of the present diet is necessary to see if it is appropriate for the patient's current condition.
• Bowel problems are very common in patients with new impairments.
• If the patient complains of swallowing or chewing difficulties, a diet modification could be necessary.

Past Medical and Surgical History (pp. 10–11)

• Many medical and surgical problems can affect the patient's present function. Often when individuals have learned to compensate effectively for a previous illness or injury, this ability is lost when a new problem or impairment occurs.

Cardiovascular (p. 10)
• Inquire about cardiac function and whether testing might be necessary prior to exercise prescription. (See Chapter 32 for further information.)
• Note symptoms of intermittent claudication and peripheral vascular disease, as well as any history of old amputations or gangrenous areas.

Pulmonary (p. 10)
• Investigation of previous pulmonary function and testing, and discussion of the present physical status with the patient's primary medical physician, can aid in exercise prescription. (See Chapter 33 for further information.)

Rheumatologic (p. 10)
• An exercise program can exacerbate rheumatologic symptoms. The history should include information concerning the rheumatologic disorder, previous sites of joint involvement, and the present level of disease activity. (See Chapter 36 for further information.)

Neurological (p. 10)
• Ask specifically about congenital neurological problems, seizure disorders, peripheral neuropathies, progressive neurological diseases, spinal cord and other central nervous system diseases, or trauma.
• Questions concentrating on symptoms such as muscular weakness, sensory loss, balance, and coordination are also helpful in assessing the patient's neurological status.

Musculoskeletal (p. 10)
• Document disorders such as congenital muscular problems, progressive muscular diseases, amputations, joint contractures, traumatic injuries, osteoporosis, and previous bone fractures.

Family History (pp. 10–11)
• Ask specific questions concerning family members known to have the same disease as the patient. Enquire about other diseases known to be familial or hereditary.

Review of Systems (pp. 11–12)
• A comprehensive review of systems often uncovers problems not previously noted that can affect the patient's clinical course. (See Table 1-9 in the Textbook.)

Skin (p. 11)
• Skin problems are common in patients with loss of mobility or sensation. Questions concerning rashes and skin pressure areas can help identify these problems.

Gastrointestinal Status (p. 11)
• Trouble swallowing and complaints of coughing during eating activities or the sensation of food "getting stuck" while swallowing can indicate significant problems that need further investigation. Diarrhea, constipation, and bowel incontinence interfere with participation in a physiatric program and can also indicate the presence of a neurogenic bowel.

Genitourinary Status (p. 11)
• Complaints of urinary frequency, polyuria, nocturia, dysuria, hematuria, urgency, and hesitancy can all indicate significant problems such as urinary tract infection, bladder outlet obstruction, kidney stones, and neurogenic bladder. (See Chapter 27 for further information.)

Nutritional Status (pp. 11–12)
• Poor nutrition can be secondary to many different problems ranging from swallowing dysfunction to decreased appetite. Two of the most common causes for a loss of appetite are the use of medications and depression.
• Ascertain recent food and fluid intake to help determine whether the patient is at risk for an overall poor nutritional and hydration status.

Neuromuscular Status (p. 12)
• Specific neurological questions concerning headaches, weakness, numbness, tingling, visual problems, incoordination, disorientation, and memory problems should be asked. Specific musculoskeletal questions about overall muscular endurance, joint and muscular pain or stiffness, abnormal joint motion, muscle atrophy, fasciculation, and spasticity are important.

Physiatric Examination (p. 12)
• The main purpose of the physiatric examination is to confirm or disprove the diagnostic impression formed after obtaining the physiatric history and to identify other impairments or disabilities. The basis for the physiatric examination

is the conventional physical examination as outlined in standard medical diagnosis textbooks.

• Functional skills are emphasized in the physiatric examination. Special attention is paid to the ability to perform activities on request.

• If the individual is unable to follow commands, the physiatrist must use inventive techniques to increase the patient's ability to participate in the evaluation process.

• The physiatric examination also includes a detailed evaluation of the musculoskeletal and neurological systems. The specific impairments that led to the patient's functional deficits should be identified.

Functional Examination (pp. 12–14)

• The functional examination includes evaluation of mobility skills, ADL, household activities, and community activities.

• The examiner should determine the functional skills, the required level of assistance, and the need for assistive devices. A commonly used measure of functionality is the Functional Independence Measure (see Table 1–3).

• For an accurate patient evaluation, it is helpful to have the appropriate assistive device available.

• A full patient assessment during the initial physiatric examination is not always possible due to safety issues and time limitations.

Mobility Activities (pp. 12–13)

• The examination of mobility should proceed methodically, initially evaluating the most basic mobility skills and proceeding to increasingly difficult activities. The most basic mobility activity is bed mobility. Examine whether the patient can roll from side to side, roll from supine to prone, and roll from prone to supine.

• The ability to move from supine to sitting should be observed because it is the most basic transitional movement.

• When examining an individual's ability to sit, it should be noted whether the individual is able to sit up straight in the midline (adequate midline orientation) and whether he or she can sit without back support. If the patient is able to sit in the midline, with or without support, then the sitting balance should be physically challenged. This is commonly done by applying a mild or moderate pressure or push in all directions to see if the individual is able to maintain the seated position.

• The next transitional movement examined is the act of going from the seated to the standing position.

• With the patient in the standing position, evaluate midline orientation.

• Standing balance is evaluated similarly to sitting balance by providing the physical challenge of a pressure or push in all directions (within limits of safety).

• Walking requires adequate standing skills, either with or without an assistive device, and should not be attempted unless the patient is able to demonstrate the required standing skills. Basic aspects of gait should be assessed, including: the individual's ability to maintain midline during walking, with or without an assistive device; the size of the base of stance; the fluidity of lower limb movements throughout all phases of the gait cycle; abnormal lower limb movements; appropriate use of an assistive device, if needed; and upper limb movements. (For further information on gait analysis, see Chapter 5.)

• If the patient can walk safely, the ability to descend and ascend stairs is tested. The number of stairs; the need for either one or two hand rails; and the ability to use an assistive device, if required, are also assessed.

• Individuals using a wheelchair for mobility should be assessed for transfer and wheelchair propulsion skills.

Activities of Daily Living *(p. 13)*

• Observation of ADL might not be possible if the patient requires some assistive devices that are not present during the examination (see Table 1–5).

• Feeding skills include the ability to set up a meal, use utensils or hold finger foods, and use upper limb movement to bring food to the mouth.

• Grooming activities usually include toothbrushing or denture care, washing the face and body at the sink, shaving, and hair-brushing.

• A full bathing and toileting evaluation is difficult to observe during the functional examination process because of patient modesty issues. Observing the individual perform the movement activities required for the transfer, and the upper limb and body motions required for the activities is helpful. Dressing skills should be assessed. Patients should demonstrate their ability to open and close different fasteners such as buttons, zippers, and shoelaces.

Household Activities *(pp. 13–14)*

• During the functional evaluation the physiatrist is unable to test household activities in an environment similar to the home. Asking patients to demonstrate the activities as closely as possible is usually the best option.

Driving *(p. 14)*

• Although driving skills cannot be fully assessed without driving a vehicle, demonstration of how the skill is performed (including proper upper and lower limb use) can be done in the clinic or hospital.

Musculoskeletal Examination *(pp. 14–37)*

• The musculoskeletal examination is a major portion of the total physiatric examination. It requires inspection and palpation, as well as unique tests such as range of motion and manual muscle testing.

Inspection *(p. 14)*

• All muscles, bones, and joints are closely inspected for any abnormality. If a difference is seen in side-to-side muscle symmetry, or if an abnormality is noted in one muscle or muscle group, then objective measures such as limb circumference measurements are appropriate for documentation purposes.

Palpation *(p. 14)*

• Palpate all painful areas. Note the activity that produces the tenderness and the site of the tenderness, and whether referred pain symptoms are present. During the bone and joint examination, each area should be palpated to identify the extent of any deformities, warmth, swelling, and pain with palpation.

Range of Motion *(pp. 14–20)*

• Adequate joint and limb range of motion (ROM) is essential for functional activities.

• The evaluation includes assessment of both active and passive ROM. Passive ROM is assessed by the examiner while the patient is relaxed. Each joint is moved through all planes of motion by the examiner and is measured for the extent of its range. Active ROM is assessed by having the patient perform the maneuvers without the assistance of the examiner.

• Exact measurement of ROM activities is most often performed using a universal goniometer. The measurement scale is in 1-degree intervals, 0 to 180 degrees in half-circle scales and 0 to 180 or 0 to 360 degrees in full-circle scales. (See Chapter 1 in the Textbook for goniometry methodology.)

• Figure 1–1 depicts the three planes of movement. For measuring ROM, the patient moves the joint according to the instructions provided. See the textbook for a description of the 180-degree and 360-degree systems of measurement. For example, Figure 1–2 shows normal shoulder flexion and extension in both systems.

• Figure 1–3 shows an example of how a goniometer can be used to determine hip flexion and knee extension. (Other commonly evaluated joints are depicted in Figs. 1–4 to 1–19 in the Textbook.)

• Spinal ROM is more difficult to measure, and techniques utilizing goniometers, plumb lines, inclinometers, and measuring tapes have been described.

Joint Stability *(p. 20)*

• The stability inherent in each joint depends on its bone integrity, ligamentous and joint capsule connections, and muscle activity.

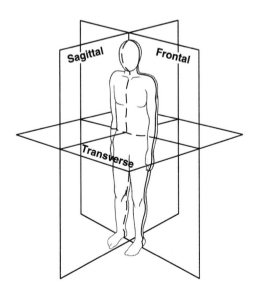

FIGURE 1–1. Three planes of motion.

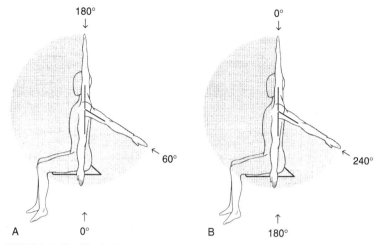

FIGURE 1–2. Shoulder flexion and extension. *A.* 180-degree system. *B.* 360-degree system.

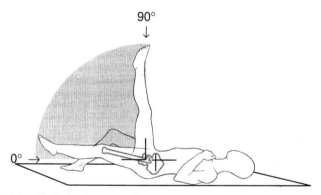

FIGURE 1–3. Hip flexion, knee extension.

Patient Position: Supine or lying on side, knee extended.

Plane of Motion: Sagittal.

Normal ROM: 0 to 90 degrees.

Movements Patient Should Avoid: Arching back.

Goniometer Placement: Axis is centered on lateral leg over greater trochanter, stationary arm remains at 0 degrees. (This is found by drawing a line from the anterior superior iliac spine to the posterior superior iliac spine, and then drawing another line, perpendicular to the first, that goes through the greater trochanter. The last line is 0 degrees.) Movement arm remains parallel to lateral femur.

• Joint stability is evaluated by providing stress to all ranges of motion.
• If joint instability is noted, then a more specific examination of that joint using specialized tests is warranted, such as Lachman's test for ankle stability or McMurray's test for meniscus tear. (See Chapters 39 and 44.)

Contracture (pp. 20–22)
• A contracture causes inability to perform full-joint ROM. It results from either decreased tissue extensibility of soft tissues and muscle or from bony abnormalities.
• Each contracture is evaluated for its possible cause. Placing the joint, soft tissues, and muscles on gentle, prolonged, passive stretch can indicate whether the loss of motion is caused by abnormalities in bone, muscle, or soft tissue.
• Shortening of muscles that cross two or more joints is not a joint contracture, but is often noted during an examination for contractures because shortening of these muscles can lead to ROM abnormalities. Shortening in two joint muscles is particularly likely in the hamstrings and tensor fascia lata.

Manual Muscle Testing (pp. 22–37)
• Manual muscle testing (MMT) is the technique used to document muscle strength. MMT involves the actual test performance as well as muscle strength grading.
• Prior to formal MMT, screening tests for muscle weakness can help identify areas needing specific evaluation. Upper limb strength is screened by having the patient grasp two of the examiner's fingers while the examiner attempts to free the fingers by pulling in all directions. A deep knee bend (squat and rise) screens proximal lower limb strength. Distal lower limb strength is evaluated by having the patient walk on the heels and then the toes. Abdominal strength is screened by observing the patient's ability to go from supine to sitting while the hips and knees are flexed
• Formal MMT requires that the examiner be proficient in the test procedures required to assess each muscle or muscle group. This proficiency requires a working knowledge of muscle function.
• MMT should generally be performed using the "make and break" technique. The patient is asked to "make" the muscle(s) being tested contract and to hold a specific position. The examiner then tries to "break" that muscle contraction by applying pressure.
• MMT requires patient cooperation. Poor patient understanding of the test procedure or poor motivation to participate causes inaccuracies.
• Pain often prevents a full muscle contraction or causes the patient to release the contraction suddenly when resistance is provided. This is called *breakaway weakness*, and it should not be interpreted as true weakness.
• A patient can also either consciously or subconsciously attempt to appear weak by a "ratchety" or inconsistent response to the resistance provided.
• The examiner will generally want to place one hand above and one hand below the joint being affected by the muscle contraction. Avoid placing the hands so that pressure is applied across more than one joint (if possible).
• Patients often try to use other muscles to assist a weak muscle or muscle group, which is called *substitution*. If it is observed, the patient should be counseled on how to avoid contaminating the MMT with substitution.

- At times it is necessary to intentionally place a muscle at a mechanical disadvantage to show a minor degree of weakness. For example, testing elbow extension with the elbow in 90 degrees of flexion rather than full extension can show minor weakness of the triceps muscle.
- MMT can also be quantified by the use of strain gauges, dynamometers, and other apparatus.
- Muscle strength grading was developed to document the results of MMT. The most commonly used system of muscle grading uses numbers (Table 1–6). Words and percentages are sometimes also used to grade muscle strength.
- When describing a muscle that has weakness, the examiner should systematically proceed through the different grades. The patient is asked to contract the muscle while the examiner palpates it. If no movement is palpable in the muscle, it is graded 0 (zero). If muscle contraction is palpable but no joint movement is noted, the muscle is at least grade 1 (trace). Next, the examiner asks the patient to contract the muscle in a gravity-eliminated position. If the patient is able to move the body part through the full ROM, then the muscle has at least grade 2 (poor) strength. The patient is asked to contract the muscle to move the body part against gravity. If the patient can move the body part through the full range of motion against gravity, there is at least grade 3 (fair) strength. The examiner then provides resistance to the muscle activity, and if the patient is able to resist a moderate amount of pressure, the muscle strength is graded as 4 (good). If the patient is able to provide full resistance, the muscle strength is graded as 5 (normal). Grades 0 to 3 (zero to fair) are fairly objective, but both grades 4 and 5 (good to normal) depend on the examiner's subjective interpretation of the amount of resistance.
- See the Textbook for diagrams of common muscles tested, their actions, and their innervations. In the following sections, MMT of multiple muscles is described in a manner that emphasizes function. Functional muscle groups are discussed, with some muscles included in more than one category. The primary muscles involved in the movements are emphasized. Each muscle's peripheral and root level innervation is listed. The innervation listed is the most commonly described innervation, but anatomical variations are common.

TABLE 1-6 Systems of Muscle Strength Grading

Number	Work	Motor Deficit (%)	Definition
5	Normal	0	Complete joint range of motion against gravity with full resistance
4	Good	1–25	Complete joint range of motion against gravity with moderate resistance
3	Fair	26–50	Full joint range of motion against gravity
2	Poor	51–75	Full joint range of motion with gravity eliminated
1	Trace	76–99	Visible palpable or muscle contraction; no joint motion produced
0	Zero	100	No visible or palpable muscle contraction

Adapted from Stillwell GK, deLateur BJ, Fordyce WE, et al: Physiatric Therapeutics in Self-Directed Medical Knowledge Program in Physical Medicine and Rehabilitation, ed 2. Chicago, American Academy of Physical Medicine and Rehabilitation, 1986, p. A1.

SHOULDER MOVEMENTS

Flexion
Deltoid, anterior portion (axillary nerve from posterior cord, C5, C6)
Pectoralis major, clavicular portion (medial and lateral pectoral nerve, C5 to T1)
Biceps brachii (musculocutaneous nerve from lateral cord, C5, C6)
Coracobrachialis (musculocutaneous nerve from lateral cord, C5, C6, C7)

Test. Place shoulder in approximately 90 degrees of flexion with the elbow
flexed. The examiner attempts to move the arm into extension by applying pressure over the distal humeral area. The anterior deltoid mainly produces this
motion, although it is assisted by the other muscles.

Extension
Deltoid, posterior portion (axillary nerve from posterior cord, C5, C6)
Latissimus dorsi (thoracodorsal nerve from posterior cord, C6, C7, C8)
Teres major (lower subscapular nerve from posterior cord, C5, C6)

Test. Place shoulder in approximately 45 degrees of extension with the elbow
extended. The examiner attempts to move the arm into flexion by applying pressure over the distal humeral area.

Abduction
Deltoid, middle portion (axillary nerve from posterior cord, C5, C6)
Supraspinatus (suprascapular nerve from upper trunk, C5, C6)

Test. Place shoulder in approximately 90 degrees of abduction. The examiner
attempts to move the shoulder into adduction by applying pressure over the distal
humeral area.

Adduction
Pectoralis major (medial and lateral pectoral nerve, C5 to T1)
Latissimus dorsi (thoracodorsal nerve from posterior cord, C6, C7, C8)
Teres major (lower subscapular nerve from posterior cord, C5, C6)

Test. Place shoulder at the side. The examiner attempts to pull the arm away
from the side by applying pressure over the distal humeral area.

Internal Rotation (Fig. 1–4)
Subscapularis (upper and lower subscapular nerve from posterior cord, C5, C6)
Pectoralis major (medial and lateral pectoral nerve, C5 to T1)
Latissimus dorsi (thoracodorsal nerve from posterior cord, C6, C7, C8)
Deltoid, anterior portion (axillary nerve from posterior cord, C5, C6)
Teres major (lower subscapular nerve from posterior cord, C5, C6)

Test. Place shoulder in 90 degrees of abduction with full internal rotation and
90 degrees of elbow flexion. The examiner attempts to force the arm into external rotation, applying pressure over the distal forearm.

External Rotation
Infraspinatus (suprascapular nerve from upper trunk, C5, C6)
Teres minor (axillary nerve from posterior cord, C5, C6)
Deltoid, posterior portion (axillary nerve from posterior cord, C5, C6)

Test. Place shoulder in 90 degrees of abduction with full external rotation and
90 degrees of elbow flexion. The examiner attempts to force the arm into internal rotation, applying pressure over the distal forearm.

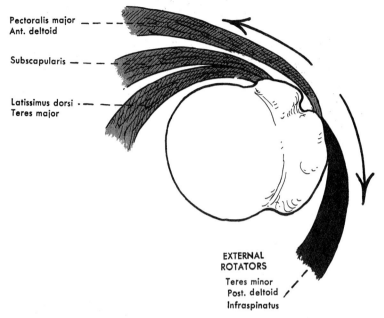

INTERNAL
ROTATORS

Pectoralis major _ _ _ _
Ant. deltoid

Subscapularis _ _ _

Latissimus dorsi · _ _ _
Teres major

EXTERNAL
ROTATORS
Teres minor
Post. deltoid
Infraspinatus

FIGURE 1–4.   Shoulder internal and external rotators. (From Jenkins DB: Hollingshead's Functional Anatomy of the Limbs and Back, ed 6. Philadelphia, WB Saunders, 1998.)

ELBOW MOVEMENTS

Flexion

Biceps brachii (musculocutaneous nerve from lateral cord, C5, C6)
Brachialis (musculocutaneous nerve from lateral cord, C5, C6)
Brachioradialis (radial nerve from posterior cord, C5, C6)

Test. Place elbow in approximately 90 degrees of flexion. The examiner attempts to force the elbow into extension, applying pressure over the distal forearm. Depending on the forearm position, the examiner is able to more specifically test each of the three muscles. In full radioulnar supination, the biceps muscle is the primary elbow flexor, whereas in full radioulnar pronation, the brachialis is the primary flexor. If the forearm is held in 0 degrees of flexion, or neutral position between pronation and supination ("thumbs-up" position), the main muscle of elbow flexion is the brachioradialis.

Extension

Triceps (radial nerve from posterior cord, C6, C7, C8)

Test. Place elbow in a few degrees of elbow flexion. (The number of degrees of elbow flexion can vary from 30 to almost full extension. The elbow is never in a fully extended position, because in that position the patient may be able to stabilize it, and a subtle elbow extension weakness might be missed.) The examiner attempts to force the elbow into flexion, applying pressure over the distal forearm.

RADIOULNAR MOVEMENTS
Pronation
Pronator quadratus (anterior interosseous branch of the median nerve, C7, C8, T1)
Pronator teres (median nerve from lateral cord, C6, C7)

Test. Place elbow in a position of full pronation. The examiner attempts to force the radioulnar joint or forearm into supination, applying pressure at the distal forearm. If the elbow is partially flexed (90 degrees), the pronator teres is primarily tested. If the elbow is held in a position of full flexion, the pronator quadratus is the main pronator muscle.

Supination
Supinator (radial nerve from posterior cord, C5, C6)
Biceps brachii (musculocutaneous nerve from lateral cord, C5, C6)

Test. Because the biceps is tested by elbow flexion (see preceding section, Elbow Movements: Flexion), the arm should be placed in a position to favor the supinator muscle strength. To do this, the elbow is placed in full flexion with the radioulnar joint or forearm in full supination. In this position the biceps is unable to assist in the act of supination. The examiner attempts to force the radioulnar joint or forearm into pronation, applying pressure at the distal forearm.

WRIST MOVEMENTS
Flexion
Flexor carpi radialis (median nerve from lateral cord, C6, C7)
Flexor carpi ulnaris (ulnar nerve from medial cord, C8, T1)

Test. Place the wrist in a neutral position between radial and ulnar deviation and in full flexion, with the fingers extended. The examiner attempts to force the wrist into extension, applying pressure at the midpalm level. To more selectively test the flexor carpi radialis, the patient's wrist is placed in a position of radial deviation and full flexion. The examiner attempts to force the wrist into extension and ulnar deviation. To more selectively test the flexor carpi ulnaris, the patient's wrist is placed in a position of ulnar deviation and full flexion. The examiner attempts to force the wrist into extension and radial deviation.

Extension
Extensor carpi radialis longus (radial nerve from posterior cord, C6, C7)
Extensor carpi radialis brevis (radial nerve from posterior cord, C6, C7)
Extensor carpi ulnaris (radial nerve from posterior cord, C6, C7, C8)

Test. Place the wrist in a neutral position between radial and ulnar deviation and in full extension, with the fingers extended. The examiner attempts to force the wrist into flexion, applying pressure over the dorsum of the hand. To more selectively test the extensor carpi radialis longus, the patient's wrist is placed in a position of radial deviation and full extension. The examiner attempts to force the wrist into flexion and ulnar deviation. To more selectively test the extensor carpi ulnaris, the patient's wrist is placed in a position of ulnar deviation and full extension. The examiner attempts to force the wrist into flexion and radial deviation. It is difficult to position the hand to isolate the extensor carpi radialis brevis because of the midline position of its tendon insertion in the wrist.

THUMB AND DIGIT MOVEMENTS
• Only a few important strength testing movements are discussed; the reader should consult reference texts for additional thumb and digit tests.

Thumb Abduction
Abductor pollicis brevis (median nerve, C8, T1)
Abductor pollicis longus (radial nerve, C6, C7)
Extensor pollicis brevis (radial nerve, C6, C7)

Test. The thumb is placed in abduction and perpendicular to the plane of the palm. The examiner attempts to force the thumb into adduction (toward the palm), applying pressure just above the first metacarpophalangeal joint.

Thumb Opposition
Opponens pollicis (median nerve, C8, T1)
Flexor pollicis brevis (superficial head: median nerve; deep head: ulnar nerve, C8, T1)
Abductor pollicis brevis (median nerve, C8, T1)

Test. The thumb is placed in opposition. The examiner attempts to force the thumb back into anatomical position, applying pressure just above the first metacarpophalangeal joint.

Second to Fifth Digit Flexion
Flexor digitorum superficialis (median nerve, C7, C8, T1)
Flexor digitorum profundus (lateral portion: median nerve; medial portion: ulnar nerve, C8, T1)
Lumbricals (lateral two: median nerve; medial two: ulnar nerve, C8, T1)
Interossei (ulnar nerve, C8, T1)

Test. Because the tendons of the flexor digitorum profundus extend to the distal phalanges, the examiner tests the strength of this muscle by attempting to force each distal phalangeal joint into extension after it is placed in a position of flexion. The tendons of the flexor digitorum superficialis extend to the middle phalanx. The examiner tests both the superficialis and the profundus by attempting to force each middle phalangeal joint into extension after each is placed in a position of flexion. The primary flexors of the metacarpophalangeal joints of the second to fourth digits are the lumbricals and the interossei. The examiner tests these muscles by attempting to force each metacarpophalangeal joint into extension after each is placed in a position of flexion. The primary flexors of the fifth digit metacarpophalangeal joint are the flexors and abductor digiti minimi muscles, and MMT of flexion of this joint evaluates their strength.

Second to Fifth Digit
Extensor digitorum (radial nerve, C6, C7, C8)
Extensor indicis (radial nerve, C7, C8)
Extensor digiti minimi (radial nerve, C6, C7, C8)

Test. The second to fifth digits are placed in extension with the wrist in neutral position between flexion and extension (0 degrees). The examiner attempts to force each finger into flexion by applying a force over each proximal phalanx.

Second to Fourth Digit Abduction, First to Fifth Digit Adduction
Dorsal interossei (ulnar nerve, C8, T1)
Palmar interossei (ulnar nerve, C8, T1)

Test. One method of testing adduction of these digits is to attempt to withdraw a piece of paper that has been placed between the patient's fingers while the patient attempts to retain the paper. Abduction is tested by placing each digit in abduction and attempting to force the digit into adduction. Note that the third digit cannot adduct because movement of this digit to either side is abduction.

Fifth Digit Abduction
Abductor digiti minimi (ulnar nerve, C8, T1)
Flexor digiti minimi (ulnar nerve, C8, T1)

Test. Place the patient's fifth digit in abduction. The examiner attempts to force the digit into adduction by applying pressure just above the metacarpophalangeal joint.

HIP MOVEMENTS
Flexion
Iliacus (femoral nerve, L2, L3, L4)
Psoas (lumbar plexus, L2, L3, L4)
Tensor fascia latae (superior gluteal nerve, L4, L5, S1)
Rectus femoris (femoral nerve, L2, L3, L4)
Pectineus (femoral or obturator nerve, L2, L3)
Adductor longus, brevis, anterior portion of magnus (obturator nerve, L2, L3, L4)

Test. Hip flexion is tested with the patient in both seated and supine positions. With the patient in a sitting position, the hip is placed in flexion by raising the knee. The examiner attempts to force the hip into extension, applying pressure over the distal anterior thigh. With the patient supine, the patient's hip is placed in flexion with the knee extended. The examiner attempts to force the hip into extension, applying pressure over the distal anterior thigh. The primary muscle of flexion is the iliopsoas, especially when resistance is applied.

Extension
Gluteus maximus (inferior gluteal nerve, L5, S1, S2)

Test. With the patient in a prone position, place the hip in extension with the knee flexed to 90 degrees. The examiner attempts to force the hip into flexion, applying pressure over the distal posterior thigh.

Abduction
Gluteus medius (superior gluteal nerve, L4, L5, S1)
Gluteus minimus (superior gluteal nerve, L4, L5, S1)
Tensor fascia latae (superior gluteal nerve, L4, L5, S1)

Test. With the patient in a side-lying position, the hip is placed in abduction. The examiner attempts to force the hip into adduction, applying pressure over the distal lateral thigh. An easier but less accurate test is performed with the patient seated. With the patient in a sitting position, the hips are placed in abduction (knees separated). The examiner attempts to force the hips into adduction, applying pressure over the distal lateral thighs.

Adduction
Adductor brevis (obturator nerve, L2, L3, L4)
Adductor longus (obturator nerve, L2, L3)
Adductor magnus, anterior portion (obturator nerve, L3, L4)
Pectineus (femoral or obturator nerve, L2, L3)

Test. The most accurate method requires the patient to assume a side-lying position. With the patient in a side-lying position, the examiner positions the top leg in abduction and the patient is asked to bring the bottom leg up into adduction to meet the top leg. The examiner attempts to force the bottom leg down into abduction, applying pressure over the distal medial thigh. An easier but less accurate test is performed with the patient in a sitting position. The hips are placed in adduction (knees together). The examiner attempts to force the hips into abduction, applying pressure over the distal medial thigh.

Internal Rotation
Tensor fasciae latae (superior gluteal nerve, L4, L5, S1)
Pectineus (femoral or obturator nerve, L2, L3)
Gluteus minimus, anterior portion (superior gluteal nerve, L4, L5, S1)

Test. The patient is either seated with both knees bent at 90 degrees, or prone with one knee bent at 90 degrees. In either position, the tested hip is placed in internal rotation. The examiner uses one hand to attempt to force the leg into external rotation, applying lateral pressure just above the ankle while stabilizing the knee with the other hand.

External Rotation
Gluteus maximus (inferior gluteal nerve, L5, S1, S2)
Piriformis (nerve to piriformis, S1, S2)
Superior gemelli and obturator internus (nerve to obturator internus, L5, S1, S2)
Inferior gemelli and quadratus femoris (nerve to quadratus femoris, L4, L5, S1)

Test. The patient is either seated with both knees bent at 90 degrees, or prone with one knee bent at 90 degrees. In either position, the tested hip is placed in external rotation. The examiner uses one hand to attempt to force the leg into internal rotation, applying pressure medially just above the ankle while stabilizing the knee with the other hand.

KNEE MOVEMENTS
Flexion
Semitendinosus (tibial portion of sciatic nerve, L5, S1)
Semimembranosus (tibial portion of sciatic nerve, L5, S1)
Biceps femoris (tibial portion of sciatic nerve, L5, S1, S2)

Test. Place the knee in 90 degrees of flexion while the patient is in a seated or prone position. The examiner attempts to force the leg into extension, applying pressure over the posterior tibial surface.

Extension
Quadriceps femoris (femoral nerve, L2, L3, L4)

Test. Place the knee in approximately 30 degrees of flexion while the patient is in a seated or supine position. Full knee extension is avoided because the patient is able to stabilize the knee in that position, and minor quadriceps weakness might be missed. The examiner attempts to force the leg into flexion, applying pressure over the anterior tibial surface.

ANKLE MOVEMENTS
Dorsiflexion
Tibialis anterior (deep peroneal nerve, L4, L5, S1)
Extensor digitorum longus (deep peroneal nerve, L4, L5, S1)
Extensor hallucis longus (deep peroneal nerve, L4, L5, S1)

Test. All of these muscles work together to produce dorsiflexion when the foot is in a neutral position between inversion and eversion. The ankle is placed in dorsiflexion. The examiner attempts to force the ankle into plantar flexion, applying pressure over the dorsum of the foot. To more selectively test the tibialis anterior, the ankle is placed in a position of inversion and full dorsiflexion. The examiner attempts to force the ankle into plantar flexion and eversion. To more selectively test the extensor digitorum longus, the ankle is placed in a position of eversion and full dorsiflexion. The examiner attempts to force the ankle into plantar flexion and inversion.

Plantar Flexion
Gastrocnemius (tibial nerve, S1, S2)
Soleus (tibial nerve, S1, S2)

Test. Place the ankle in plantar flexion. The examiner attempts to force the foot into dorsiflexion, applying pressure over the plantar surface of the foot. To selectively test the gastrocnemius, the knee is extended. To more selectively test the soleus, the knee is flexed to 90 degrees. These muscles are so strong that more functional tests such as standing or walking on toes might show weakness missed during MMT.

Inversion
Tibialis anterior (deep peroneal nerve, L4, L5, S1)
Tibialis posterior (tibial nerve, L5, S1)
Flexor digitorum longus (tibial nerve, L5, S1)
Flexor hallucis longus (tibial nerve, L5, S1, S2)

Test. The tibialis anterior is more selectively tested in a position of inversion and dorsiflexion. The examiner attempts to force the foot into eversion and plantar flexion, applying pressure on the medial surface of the foot. The other three muscles produce plantar flexion and inversion. They are more selectively tested with placement of the foot in inversion and plantar flexion. The examiner attempts to force the foot into eversion and dorsiflexion, applying pressure on the medial surface of the foot.

Eversion
Extensor digitorum longus (deep peroneal nerve, L4, L5, S1)
Peroneus longus (superficial peroneal nerve, L4, L5, S1)
Peroneus brevis (superficial peroneal nerve, L4, L5, S1)

Test. The extensor digitorum longus is more selectively tested in the position of eversion and dorsiflexion. The examiner attempts to force the foot into inversion and plantar flexion, applying pressure over the lateral surface of the foot. The peroneus longus and brevis produce plantar flexion and eversion. They are more selectively tested with placement of the foot in eversion and plantar flexion. The examiner attempts to force the foot into inversion and dorsiflexion, applying pressure over the lateral surface of the foot.

FOOT MOVEMENTS
First Digit Extension
Extensor hallucis longus (deep peroneal nerve, L4, L5, S1)

Test. The first toe is placed in full extension. The examiner attempts to force it into flexion, applying pressure over the dorsum of the first toe.

Second to Fifth Digit Extension
Extensor digitorum longus (deep peroneal nerve, L4, L5, S1)
Extensor digitorum brevis (deep peroneal nerve, L5, S1)

Test. The second to fifth toes are placed in full extension. The examiner attempts to force them into flexion, applying pressure over the dorsum of the toes.

First Digit Flexion
Flexor hallucis longus (tibial nerve, L5, S1, S2)
Flexor hallucis brevis (medial plantar nerve, L5, S1)

Test. The first toe is placed in full flexion. The examiner attempts to force it into extension, applying pressure over the plantar surface of the first toe.

Second to Fifth Digit Flexion
Flexor digitorum longus (tibial nerve, L5, S1)
Flexor digitorum brevis (medial plantar nerve, L5, S1)

Test. The second to fifth toes are placed in full flexion. The examiner attempts to force them into extension, applying pressure over the plantar surface of the toes.

Neurological (pp. 37–43)

• Like the musculoskeletal examination, a complete neurological examination is essential to identify other impairments that help to clarify or confirm a diagnosis.

Level of Consciousness (p. 37)
• A decreased level of consciousness can prevent or seriously limit a patient from participation in a physiatric therapeutic program. Descriptive statements, including such adjectives as *lethargic,* are helpful but are often misinterpreted by others due to the subjectivity of the information. Other subjective but sometimes helpful information includes the length of time and consistency with which an individual is able to attend to a task or to follow commands of the examiner before being unable to respond due to lethargy. This information is an indication not only of an individual's level of consciousness but also of endurance of attentiveness. A commonly used objective scale for an individual with impaired consciousness is the Glasgow Coma Scale (Table 1–7), which assigns a numerical value based on the best eye, motor, and verbal responses. The scale ranges from 3 to 15, with 15 being the best score.

Mental Status (See Also Chapter 49) (pp. 37–38)
• Many mental status examinations are commonly used to document cognitive ability. Usually this can be done in a few minutes. In-depth cognitive assessments and testing procedures often take several hours and should be completed under the direction of a practitioner who is familiar with the specific testing procedures.
• Table 1–8 lists items that can be included in such a short cognitive evaluation. Adequate communication skills are necessary for participation in this type of evaluation. Patients with communication deficits might perform poorly or be unable to participate.
• Orientation is a basic cognitive skill, and severe disorientation often indicates severe cognitive impairments. Orientation is easily tested by asking patients their

TABLE 1–7 Glasgow Coma Scale

Eye opening	
Spontaneous	E 4
To speech	3
To pain	2
Nil	1
Best motor response	
Obeys	M 6
Localizes	5
Withdraws	4
Abnormal flexion	3
Extensor response	2
Nil	1
Verbal response	
Oriented	V 5
Confused conversation	4
Inappropriate words	3
Incomprehensible sounds	2
Nil	1
Coma score (E + M + V) = 3 to 15	

From Jennett B, Teasdale G: Assessment of impaired consciousness. Contemp Neurol 1981; 20:78.

TABLE 1–8 Brief Bedside Mental Status Evaluation

1. Orientation
    Person, place, time, situation
2. Attention span
    Digit retention
3. Memory
    Immediate recall
    Recall at 5- and 10-minute intervals
4. General information
    Remote memory
    Basic intellect
5. Calculation
    Serial 7s
    Simple mathematics
6. Abstract thinking
    Proverb explanation
7. Judgment
    Societal norms

Adapted from Mancall EL: Alpers and Mancall's Essentials of the Neurologic Examination, ed 2. Philadelphia, FA Davis, 1981.

name, the place, the time and date, and the present situation or reason for the physiatric evaluation.

- Attention span can be subjectively documented by noting whether the patient is able to attend to tasks consistently during the history and examination. Digit retention is a more objective test. The patient with an adequate attention span is usually able to recall at least five or six numbers forward and four to five numbers backward.
- Memory depends on the ability of an individual both to store and to retrieve information provided. The examiner provides the patient with three items to remember and asks the patient to immediately recall the items. The patient without immediate recall ability has difficulty with information storage and is unable to remember all three items after a short time, with or without cues. The patient with adequate immediate recall is asked to recall the items at a later time, usually after 5 and 10 minutes. The patient with good storage and retrieval of information is able to recall the items without difficulty. The patient with good storage but poor retrieval of information might require cues to recall some or all of the items. A patient who is unable to recall the items with cues might have information storage difficulties. Documentation of memory ability should include the number of items recalled and whether cues were required.
- Evaluation of general information helps assess the individual's remote memory and basic intellectual skills. The examiner should always take into account the patient's premorbid education and experience level and ask questions that the patient should be able to answer.
- Ask questions concerning common elected officials' names, locations such as state capitals, and local tourist attractions.
- Current events questions are appropriate for an individual who normally follows local or national news.
- Very simple questions concerning holidays are appropriate for the patient who is having difficulty with the preceding questions.
- Calculation is tested by serially sevens and simple addition, subtraction, multiplication, or division problems. Problems with increasing difficulty can be presented if the patient is able to answer simple problems correctly.
- Proverb explanation is commonly used to assess abstract thinking. A patient who has lost abstract thought ability will provide a concrete explanation, missing the basic principle of the proverb. Many individuals will have an educational background that did not involve the use of proverbs; this can affect the patient's ability to answer correctly.
- Judgment, like many of the other mental status activities, depends on the patient's background experience, but simple questions that reflect societal norms are often acceptable. Examples of such questions include what is done if a person smells smoke in a crowded theater, why it is inappropriate to yell "fire" in a theater, or what to do if a stamped and addressed envelope is found on the ground. (See Chapter 4 for further information.)

Communication (pp. 38–39)
- Communication deficits are often noted after an injury or illness. Specific in-depth evaluation of communication is necessary for any such individual, but a short examination at the hospital bedside or in the clinic can help guide the physiatrist in prescribing a more accurate treatment plan. Items often tested in a short communication examination are listed in Table 1–9.

TABLE 1–9 Brief Bedside Communication Evaluation

1. Comprehension
     Verbal, tactile, and gestural commands
     One- and two-step commands
2. Verbal communication
     Name items
     Repeat words or phrases
     Fluency
     Quality
3. Reading
     Written commands
     Matching item with written word
     Reading comprehension
4. Writing
     Personal items
     Write names of items
5. Gestural communication
     Observation

Cranial Nerve Examination (p. 39)

• Evaluation of cranial nerve function is an essential part of the neurological evaluation. A good cranial nerve evaluation can help to identify the lesion site if an individual has a brainstem problem. Table 1–10 lists the cranial nerves, their functions, and common evaluation procedures.

Sensory Examination (pp. 39–42)

• The sensory evaluation can be extensive in the patient with a large number of sensory complaints. It also requires a significant degree of cooperation and subjective response from the patient. All of these facts can make the sensory examination difficult to interpret at times, but if the examination is performed in a systematic manner, valuable information is usually obtained.

• The examiner should be aware of the normal dermatomal and peripheral nerve distribution to ensure completeness of the evaluation (Fig. 1–5). It is usually best to evaluate a normal area first to ensure that the patient understands the sensory examination process.

• The sensory examination is organized to evaluate both superficial and deep somatic sensations along with discriminative sensory functions. The three superficial somatic sensations are touch, superficial pain, and thermal sensations. Touch is easily tested with a wisp of cotton. Superficial pain is assessed by a careful pinprick evaluation, because harshly applied stimuli can draw blood. Usually, the patient is asked to tell the examiner where and when each type of stimulus (cotton wisp or pinprick) is applied. The patient can also be asked to compare each stimulus applied with the sensation felt when the same stimulus is applied to an area of known normal sensation. Thermal sensation is commonly evaluated by the use of test tubes, one with hot water and another with cold water or chipped ice. The patient is asked to relate which test tube is touching a specific skin area. Also, the examiner can test just one thermal sensation (either

TABLE 1–10 Cranial Nerve Examination Techniques

Cranial Nerve	Test
I. Olfactory	Ask patient to smell common substances such as coffee, lemon, vinegar, peppermint, and rose water.
II. Optic	Perform funduscopic evaluation of optic nerve. Acuity testing can be done using standardized acuity charts if available. If charts are not available, then less accurate testing can be done by having the patient read different size newsprint. Visual field testing using the finger confrontation technique can reveal large visual field deficits. Small field deficits may require formal visual testing for diagnosis.
III. Oculomotor IV. Trochlear VI. Abducens	All three nerves are best tested together by checking ocular motility and pupillary reactions. The oculomotor nerve provides innervation to the superior rectus, the inferior rectus, the medial rectus, and the inferior oblique muscles of the eye. The trochlear nerve provides innervation to the superior oblique muscle, whereas the abducens provides innervation to the last eye muscle, the lateral rectus. The pupillary response is checked by flashing light in each eye and looking for an equal and contralateral pupillary contraction.
V. Trigeminal	This provides motor innervation to the masseter and temporal muscles, which are evaluated by asking the patient to clench his or teeth; the examiner then palpates the cheek to feel the muscle contraction. The trigeminal nerve also supplies sensory innervation to the face and is easily evaluated using pinprick, thermal, or light touch sensations. The trigeminal nerve is also evaluated by the corneal reflex (see Table 1–13).
VII. Facial	This provides motor innervation to the muscles of facial expression and taste sensation of the anterior two-thirds of the tongue. The examiner evaluates facial muscle movement by forehead wrinkling, eye closure, lip pursing, smiling, or grimacing. Upper motor neuron lesions do not produce forehead weakness because this muscle is innervated by both sides of the cortex. A lower motor neuron lesion is manifest in weakness of all facial muscles. Taste on the anterior tongue can be tested using sugar or salt.
VIII. Auditory	The cochlear division is tested by using a tuning fork and performing the Rinne and Weber tests. Formal auditory testing is appropriate for the patient with auditory acuity problems. The vestibular portion is evaluated by observing for nystagmus. Caloric testing is appropriate in the patient with impaired consciousness.
IX. Glossopharyngeal	This supplies taste sensation to the posterior two-thirds of the tongue; it can be tested with either salt or sugar. It also supplies sensation to the pharynx and is tested along with the vagus nerve (see below).
X. Vagus	This is the principal motor nerve to the pharynx and larynx. It is examined by watching the patient's soft palate and uvula move when saying "Ah." The gag reflex is tested by stimulating the back of the pharynx. The vagus nerve also provides motor innervation to the diaphragm muscle. Abnormal motion of the diaphragm indicates vagus nerve abnormality.
XI. Spinal accessory	This innervates the trapezius and sternocleidomastoid muscles. It is tested by resisting a shoulder shrug (trapezius) or by resisted head turning to one side (sternocleidomastoid).
XII. Hypoglossal	This innervates the tongue muscles. It is evaluated by tongue protrusion and observation for abnormal tongue movements.

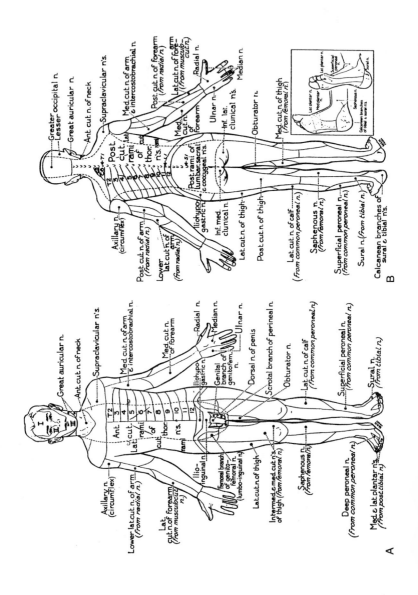

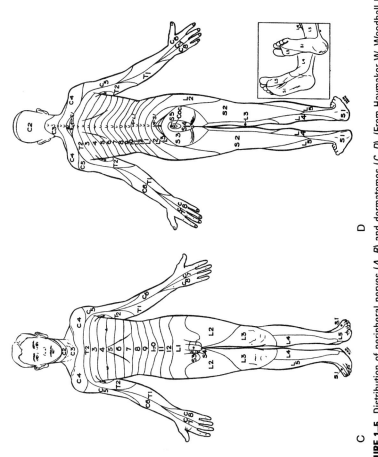

FIGURE 1–5. Distribution of peripheral nerves (A, B) and dermatomes (C, D). (From Haymaker W, Woodhall B: Peripheral Nerve Injuries, Philadelphia, WB Saunders, 1953.)

C

D

31

hot or cold) and request that the patient relate any abnormal sensation it produces in the different areas of the body.
• Proprioception, vibration sense, and deep pain or pressure are all considered to be deep somatic sensations. Proprioception or joint position sensation is evaluated by testing the patient's perception of a distal joint position and motion. Often the great toe in the lower limb and the small joints of the hand in the upper limb are used. Distal to proximal vibratory sensation is also tested in the limbs with a tuning fork with a low frequency and long duration of vibration (128 Hz). Deep pain or pressure is evaluated in each limb by deep palpation of a muscle group or by a firm pinch applied to a muscle tendon.
• Discriminative sensory functions are called *cortical* or *integrative sensations* because an abnormality in these functions usually results from a lesion in the sensory cortex or thalamocortical pathways. These functions include two-point discrimination, cutaneous tactile localization, graphesthesia, and stereognosis. Poor somatic sensation prevents accurate testing of the discriminative functions.
• Two-point discrimination is accurately tested only with a calibrated compass, with both compass points applied simultaneously. A less accurate but often more practical technique uses a paper clip with the two ends separated and measured so the distance between them is known. Common areas for such evaluation include the fingertips (normal separation, 3 to 5 mm), the dorsal surface of the hands and feet (normal separation, 20 to 30 mm), and the trunk (normal separation, 4 to 7 cm). Cutaneous tactile localization is evaluated by asking the patient to close the eyes and to indicate the area that is touched or stimulated with a pinprick by the examiner. The patient should be able to indicate the area accurately over the hands and fingers, and within a few millimeters over the rest of the body.
• Graphesthesia is the ability to recognize numbers or letters traced on the body, often on the palm of the hand.
• Stereognosis is the ability to recognize familiar objects, such as a coin or safety pin, that are placed in the hand. The patient should be able to indicate the type of coin (e.g., nickel or quarter) placed in the hand.
• Sensory extinction or inattention is a discriminative sensation abnormality. It is revealed by simultaneous bilateral presentation of cutaneous stimuli to one area of the body. Extinction is diagnosed if the stimulus on only one side of the body is perceived.

Motor Control (p. 42)
• Motor control depends on adequate muscle strength, balance, coordination, and adequate motor planning of an activity. The presence of involuntary muscle movements can also prevent functional abilities.
• Begin with manual muscle testing (see above), sitting and standing balance (see above), and higher level activities such as tandem walking.
• Poor coordination can prevent independence in many functional skills. Gross motor coordination of the upper limb is evaluated by the finger-to-nose test. Lower limb gross motor coordination is evaluated by the heel, knee-to-shin test. Fine motor coordination is best tested by rapid alternating movements. Hand movements such as hand tapping, rapid pronation and supination of the radioulnar joint or forearm along with hand tapping, and thumb to sequential finger movements evaluate upper extremity fine motor coordination. (The patient

should be directed to touch the thumb to each fingertip in sequence, as quickly as possible.) Foot tapping evaluates fine motor movement in the lower limb. Asking the patient to rapidly repeat "ta" and "pa" evaluates tongue and mouth coordination.

• Document the presence of involuntary motor movements such as spasticity, tremors, chorea, athetosis, ballismus, and dystonia (Table 1–11).

• Apraxia is a loss or impairment in executing complex coordinated movements or in motor planning. The patient with apraxia is often unable to appropriately sequence the motor skills required to perform mobility activities but has adequate strength on formal MMT. Other patients might have difficulty with appropriate object use, such as inappropriate use of feeding utensils during meals and clothing management during dressing skills.

Motor Reflex Examination (pp. 42–43)

• It is important to evaluate all three major types of reflexes.

• Muscle stretch reflex (MSR) evaluation is essential. Each reflex is evaluated for symmetry as compared with the reflex on the opposite side, for hyporeflexic or hyperreflexic activity, and for spreading (reflex contraction noted not only in the muscle tested, but also in adjacent muscles). The MSRs should be observed to make certain that the appropriate response is obtained. Sometimes the opposite response occurs: the so-called *inverted reflex response.* Table 1–12 lists commonly evaluated MSRs.

• Superficial reflex abnormality is noted in many individuals with neurological impairments (Table 1–13). Many abnormal reflexes can be observed after an illness or injury. The Babinski reflex, or abnormal plantar response, is common. The Hoffmann reflex is normal in some individuals, especially in young women.

TABLE 1–11 Definitions of Involuntary Motor Movements

Type	Definition
Spasticity	A state of hypertonicity associated with involuntary quick muscle contraction, increased muscle tone, and increased muscle stretch reflexes
Tremors	Involuntary repetitive movements of a body part or parts, most often in a distal limb. The activity may resemble quivering or trembling. May be seen at rest or in association with movement
Chorea	Involuntary arrhythmic movements that are forcible, rapid, and jerky in quality. Most often the movements are seen in the proximal limbs. They are often incorporated into voluntary movements in an attempt to make them less noticeable.
Ballismus	Unusually violent and flinging motions of the limbs
Athetosis	A condition characterized by the inability to sustain a body part or parts in one position. Most often the distal limbs (fingers, hands, toes) are affected. The movements are relatively slow and fluid in nature
Dystonia	A persistent posturing in one or more of the extremities, trunk, neck, or face

From Adams RD, Victor M: Principles of Neurology, ed 5. New York, McGraw-Hill, 1993. Reproduced with permission of The McGraw-Hill Companies.

TABLE 1–12 Muscle Stretch Reflexes

Reflex	Segmental Level
Biceps	C5, C6
Brachioradialis	C5, C6
Pronator teres	C6, C7
Triceps	C7, C8
Flexor digitorum profundus	C7, C8
Quadriceps (patella)	L2, L3, L4
Semitendinosus and semimembranosus (medial hamstrings)	L5, S1
Gastrocnemius and soleus (Achilles)	S1, S2

- *Primitive reflexes* are abnormal adult reflexes that represent a return to a more infantile level of reflex activity. These abnormal reflexes often result from injury to the frontal cortex, but they are also seen in other disease processes. The *snout, rooting, palmomental,* and *reflex grasp reflexes* are all considered to be primitive reflexes. The snout reflex is a lip-pursing response to a tap either just above or below the mouth. The rooting reflex is a quick contraction of the ipsilateral periorbital muscles toward a brushing tactile stimulus presented to the side of

TABLE 1–13 Important Normal Superficial Reflexes

Reflex	Elicited By	Response	Segmental Level
Corneal	Touching cornea with hair	Contraction of orbicularis oculi	Pons
Pharyngeal	Touching posterior wall of pharynx	Contraction of pharynx	Medulla
Palatal	Touching soft palate	Elevation of palate	Medulla
Scapular	Stroking skin between scapulae	Contraction of scapular muscles	C5–T1
Epigastric	Stroking downward from nipples	Dimpling of epigastrium ipsilaterally	T7–9
Abdominal	Stroking beneath costal margins and above inguinal ligament	Contraction of abdominal muscles in quadrant stimulated	T8–12
Cremasteric	Stroking medial surface of upper thigh	Ipsilateral elevation of testicle	L1, L2
Gluteal	Stroking skin of buttock	Contraction of glutei	L4, L5
Bulbocavernous (male)	Pinching dorsum of glans	Insert gloved finger to palpate anal contraction	S3, S4
Clitorocavernous	Pinching clitoris	Insert gloved finger to palpate anal contraction	S3, S4
Superficial anal	Pricking perineum	Contraction of rectal sphincters	S5, coccygeal

Adapted from Mancall EL: Examination of the nervous system. In Alpers and Mancall's Essentials of the Neurologic Examination, ed 2. Philadelphia, FA Davis, 1993, p. 25.

TABLE 1–14 Rehabilitation Plan

Summary Statement

L.R. is a 32-year-old, right-handed, African-American woman, previously an independent homemaker, with a history of sickle cell disease and left hip fracture treated with open reduction and internal fixation 1 year ago; she is presenting for rehabilitation for paraplegia due to an acute T12 spinal cord injury and compression fracture after a fall 1 week ago. The spine is stable if she wears a thoracic lumbar orthosis when out of bed and when the head of the bed is elevated more than 30 degrees. Physical impairments on examination include flaccid paralysis of the lower limbs, L1 sensory level, poor endurance with upper limb activities, left hip flexion and abduction contracture of 10 degrees each, no clitorocavernous reflex, and no rectal tone. Historically, the patient relates that she has had no bowel movement in 4 days; a Foley catheter is in place, and the only activity she is able to do without assistance is feed herself. Socially, she lives in a second-floor apartment (accessible only by stair climbing) with her husband, who works during the day.

Problem List

REHABILITATION PROBLEMS

1. Functional deficits: Inability to perform any mobility activity, most activities of daily living, or household tasks, and to drive without assistance or assistive devices
2. Flaccid paralysis of lower limbs bilaterally; poor lower limb management skills
3. Poor endurance for upper limb activities
4. Absent sensation below L1 level: High risk for skin pressure areas
5. Left hip flexion and abduction contracture: Possible positioning problem, high risk for left lower limb skin areas due to positioning problems, possible difficulty with limb management
6. Flaccid neurogenic bowel: Poor bowel regulation at present
7. Neurogenic bladder: Needs evaluation for appropriate bladder management
8. Patient and family adjustment to disability
9. Sexuality concerns
10. Discharge planning/living situation: Apartment not wheelchair accessible, equipment needs

MEDICAL/SURGICAL PROBLEMS

1. T12 compression fracture: Stable with appropriate wearing of thoracic lumbar orthosis
2. Sickle cell disease: Stable at present, but will require monitoring
3. Left hip fracture with surgical repair 1 year ago: Surgically healed, but patient has a residual flexion and abduction contracture

Management Plan

1. Physical therapy (PT) to address mobility deficits, concentrating on wheelchair activities, transfer skills, upper extremity endurance for these activities, sitting balance, and tolerance. The physical therapist will instruct patient on lower limb range of motion and management, concentrating on decreasing the left lower limb contractures. All team members will reinforce the skills once patient has received basic instructions from the PT.
2. Occupational therapy (OT) will concentrate on upper limb strengthening and endurance; activities of daily living; and, when it is appropriate, have patient begin homemaking and driving with assistive devices. All team members will reinforce the skills once patient has received basic instructions from the OT.
3. Nursing (RN) to monitor skin and assist patient with bowel and bladder management.
4. The management team (physician, PT, OT, RN, recreational therapist, psychologist, social worker, etc.) presents a patient-specific rehabilitation education program concentrating on prevention of future problems related to accessibility, mobility, skin, bowel, bladder, sexuality, and psychosocial and medical/surgical problems.

Table continued on following page

TABLE 1–14   Rehabilitation Plan—cont'd

5. Community issues such as accessibility, driving, social activities, and difficult psychosocial situations are addressed by the team.
6. Management team emphasis is placed on helping patient identify appropriate discharge placement, including accessible living arrangement, home modifications if needed, special equipment needs, and support systems for financial and psychosocial issues.
7. Management team continues to monitor for lower limb strength and sensory improvements.
8. Management team continues to monitor for emergence of muscle tone in rectal and lower limb muscles.
9. Spinal stability maintained by patient's wearing of the spinal orthosis. Periodic spinal radiographs taken when necessary.
10. Maintain stability of the sickle cell disease with close monitoring of blood count and symptoms. Provide blood transfusions or other treatments as necessary.

Therapeutic precautions: Patient to wear spinal orthosis when out of bed and when head of bed is elevated more than 30 degrees.

Therapeutic setting: Inpatient rehabilitation setting necessary because patient is not safe in or able to return to her previous living arrangement.

Goals

1. Independence with wheelchair mobility skills
2. Independence with activities of daily living
3. Independence with household tasks at a wheelchair level
4. Independence with driving with assistive devices
5. Supervision or independence for community reentry activities
6. Independence with lower limb management and range of motion program
7. Independence with the bladder management program
8. Independence with the bowel management program, or if patient unable to provide own bowel care due to trunk range of motion limit from the spinal orthosis, then independence with ability to instruct another to perform the bowel management program
9. Independence with skin management program
10. Knowledge of sexuality related issues
11. Independence in knowledge about future medical/surgical problems related to spinal cord injury
12. Identify a safe, accessible living situation
13. Obtain necessary equipment
14. Maintain stability of the sickle cell disease
15. Maintain spinal stability

Estimated time of goal attainment: 3 to 4 weeks

Obstacles to goal attainment:

1. Decreased trunk range of motion due to spinal orthosis, which might prevent independence in some activities
2. Left hip contractures might cause positioning and skin and limb management difficulties
3. Poor upper limb endurance might prevent good progress in the rehabilitation program

Time of reassessment of patient's status: 1 week

the mouth. A palmomental reflex is ipsilateral contraction of the chin facial muscles produced by a brisk tactile stimulation of the palm or brisk rotation motion of the thumb. Tactile stimulation of the palm can also produce a reflex grasp. The reflex grasp becomes stronger as the examiner attempts to remove his or her hand, which distinguishes the reflex from a voluntary grasp.

General Medical Examination (p. 43)

• A general medical examination is completed for all patients to rule out problems that might have an impact on progress in a physiatric therapeutic program. The examiner should be familiar with the general medical examination techniques as described in medical diagnosis textbooks.

SUMMARY, PROBLEM LIST, PLAN, AND GOALS
(pp. 43–45)

• After the physiatrist collects baseline patient data by history and examination, the information should be organized into a problem-oriented medical record. A summary of no more than a few sentences identifies the patient's major problems in a narrative form. A typical rehabilitation summary containing the problem list, management plan, and list of goals is seen in Table 1–14.

2

Original Chapter by Dennis J. Matthews, M.D., and Pam Wilson, M.D.

Examination of the Pediatric Patient

• Examination of the child with suspected functional impairment requires an understanding of variations in normal childhood development as well as the ability to perform an assessment for dysfunction. Establishing a diagnostic label is important, but determining the child's functional status is the first step in rehabilitation management. Although the evaluation of the child has many similarities to an adult's evaluation (see Chapter 1), it also has many unique features, as highlighted in this chapter.

DIAGNOSTIC EVALUATIONS (pp. 46–51)

History (pp. 46–47)

• The clinical and developmental history is the basis of an accurate medical and rehabilitation diagnosis.
• The history is generally obtained from the parent or caretaker, but children are generally able to participate in the diagnostic interview by the time they reach school age.
• Make both the child and the parents comfortable.
• It is important to identify the chief complaint quickly, because cooperation is not ensured and because time is limited.
• Develop a functional inventory with an emphasis on the child's development and the impact of the disability or impairment on the child's daily activities.
• Note the child's abilities and compensatory functional solutions as well as limitations.
• Many childhood disabilities reflect prenatal or perinatal problems. Maternal disease or acute illnesses, pregnancy and labor abnormalities, and the family history can help guide the diagnostic examination and investigational studies. The time and type of movements of the fetus should be noted in the record, as should the duration of the pregnancy, the ease or difficulty of labor, and whether any complications occurred during labor and delivery.
• The examiner should record the infant's Apgar scores; any unusual cyanosis or respiratory distress; seizures; and other physical symptoms such as jaundice, anemia, and dysmorphic features. The parents' description of muscle tone and movement can suggest a picture of primary neuromuscular weakness.

• The feeding history can suggest potential neurological abnormalities. The examiner should ask about and record any difficulties with sucking or swallowing, whether the baby is or was breast-fed or bottle-fed, and the volume and frequency of feedings. If feeding difficulties are present, determine the time of onset of the problems, the method of feeding, reasons for changes, the interval between feedings, the amount ingested at each feeding, associated crying, and weight changes.

• The physical growth rate can be plotted on a chart. The child's growth rate should be considered in relation to what is normal for the child, the growth rates of immediate family members, and age-peer growth rates.

• Determine the ages at which major developmental milestones were met; this aids in assessing deviations from normal (Table 2–1). The achievement of major landmarks in gross motor, fine motor, and adaptive skills; in language; and in personal and social behavior should clarify whether the disability is confined primarily to the neuromuscular system or involves deficits in other areas as well.

• Familiarity with the normal landmarks of early childhood development helps in the assessment of the infant and toddler. A more formal assessment of the child's development can be made with the use of standardized developmental evaluations (see Table 2–2 in the Textbook).

• A psychosocial evaluation contributes to the understanding and management of the disabled child. It assesses the child's learning style, probable impediments to learning, and to what degree the child has built on previous learning experiences. It describes the behavioral and cognitive strengths and weaknesses so that specific programs can be implemented both at home and at school. A valuable strategy is to get a description of a typical day's schedule. This information provides insight into the functional impact of the impairment.

• A family history of similar or related problems is helpful. Formal genetic counseling and evaluation is mandatory whenever a familial disease is suspected or known to exist.

TABLE 2–1 Developmental Milestones

Age (mo)	Milestones
1	Lifts head (prone), vocalizes
3	Follows, laughs, smiles, has good head control
5	Plays with feet, reaches for and grasps objects
6	Sits with support
8	Sits without support; equilibrium reflexes present; looks for objects
9	Plays peekaboo, gets to sitting position; parachute reflex present; stranger anxiety
10	Pulls to stand, cruises, babbles
12–14	First words; walks
18	Multiple single words; uses spoon, removes clothes
24	Uses two-word phrases; throws overhand; "terrible twos"
30	Knows full name, puts on clothing
36	Jumps, pedals tricycle, learns nursery rhymes
48	Hops, plays with others

Physical Examination (pp. 47–51)

• Each pediatric examination is tailored to the individual child. The examiner should be familiar with normal and abnormal patterns that can occur at different developmental stages.
• Young children should be examined with the parents present, but parental presence is optional for adolescents.
• Develop a rapport with the child before performing a hands-on examination. This can be achieved by playing with the child, talking with the child, or talking with the parents. During this time the examiner carefully observes the child's every movement and interaction. Even before touching the child the clinician has gained a wealth of information.
• The actual hands-on approach varies from child to child. A flexible approach is recommended that capitalizes on opportunities to evaluate different systems as they present themselves. Young children often are best examined while sitting in a parent's lap, wheras the older child can be examined on the table. Because the child needs to be examined completely, the clothing should be removed. Removing clothing from very young children can be very stressful and should be done gradually. The modesty of older children must be respected.

General Inspection (pp. 47–48)
• The general inspection can reveal abnormalities that need to be more closely evaluated, beginning with the child's appearance. This gives the examiner a sense of how the child interacts with the parents and provides information about the child's general movements, abnormal physical features, and overall general health.
• Evaluation of the skin includes an assessment of the nails and hair. The examiner looks for neurocutaneous lesions and other skin abnormalities. Café au lait spots can indicate neurofibromatosis, whereas white ash leaf spots can point toward a diagnosis of tuberous sclerosis. Port wine stains are flat hemangiomas; when they involve the first branch of the trigeminal nerve they are associated with Sturge-Weber syndrome. Scars, calluses, and abrasions are often indicators of abnormal weight bearing.
• The head, neck, and face are inspected for asymmetries and abnormalities. The size of the head should be measured and recorded. A small head can indicate microcephaly or craniosynostosis. A large head can be the result of hydrocephalus or intracranial mass. It is also important to record the parents' head sizes if familial patterns are suspected. The fontanels should be palpated. The posterior fontanel closes at around 2 months of age and the anterior fontanel at around 12 to 18 months. The ears are evaluated for position and structure. Low-set ears or external anomalies can be associated with genetic diseases. Abnormalities of the neck such as torticollis can be caused by shortening of the sternocleidomastoid or by tumors. Klippel-Feil syndrome typically manifests with a short, broad neck with webbing and reduced range of motion.

Musculoskeletal Assessment (pp. 48–50)
• As with any other part of the pediatric examination, the musculoskeletal evaluation includes observation, palpation, range-of-motion assessment, and functional assessment. Observation focuses on posture, body symmetry, and movement. Palpation should include the skin, muscles, and joints. The muscle

TABLE 2–2 Spinal Abnormalities

Spine Abnormality	Clinical Findings
Scoliosis (idiopathic, congenital, neuromuscular)	Curvature of spine on forward bending Rib humping Shoulder asymmetry Pelvic obliquity
Kyphosis (congenital, Scheuermann's, neuromuscular) Spondylolisthesis	Abnormal posture increases with flexion Loss of lordosis, reduced range of motion Step-off back deformity Gait abnormalities Transverse abdominal creases

examination should evaluate size, bulk, and tone. The joints are palpated to detect tenderness, swelling, synovial thickening, and warmth. Range of motion should be assessed for all major joints and any others in question.

• Assessment of posture and position is part of the spinal evaluation. Evaluation includes having the child stand or sit and bend forward. Any asymmetry most likely indicates a scoliosis, and further evaluation is needed. This generally is done by obtaining a spinal scoliosis series of x-rays. Children should also be evaluated for other spinal pathology (Table 2–2).

• Examination of the lower extremities includes an evaluation of joint range of motion and torsional forces. Most torsional deformities tend to correct spontaneously with growth and development. Evaluation of the foot includes the toes and the three parts of the foot: forefoot, midfoot, and hindfoot. The shoes should be assessed for patterns of wear. A common problem of the forefoot is metatarsus adductus, which is medial deviation of the metatarsal bones.

• Pes planus, or flatfoot, is a common problem but does not cause functional limitations. It is characterized by ligamentous laxity and loss of the medial longitudinal arch.

• Pes cavus is seen in several neuromuscular disorders such as Charcot-Marie-Tooth disease (Fig. 2–1).

• Congenital vertical talus typically manifests with a rocker-bottom foot and can be seen in genetic disorders and myelodysplasia.

• Talipes equinovarus, or clubfoot deformity, can be seen in positional deformities or neuromuscular diseases. The foot classically presents as hindfoot equinus, or plantar flexion of the ankle; hindfoot varus; and forefoot adductus.

• The knee should be evaluated for capsular tightness and joint stability. The child should be assessed for genu varum and genu valgum. A child normally progresses through these stages as the lower extremities mature. Genu varus is common in the 1- to 3-year-old age group, and genu valgus in the 3- to 5-year-old age range. Abnormal bowing of the legs is seen in Blount's disease.

• Tibial torsion can result in either internal or external rotation of the tibia and can be evaluated from the thigh-foot angle (Fig. 2–2).

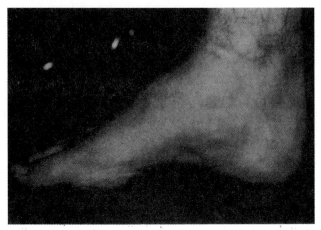

FIGURE 2–1. High-arched foot, or pes cavus, is seen in neuromuscular disorders.

- The hip should be evaluated for torsional forces including femoral anteversion and retroversion. These are best tested with the child prone (see Fig. 2–2). Abduction of the hip should be assessed with the child supine. Asymmetry can indicate hip subluxation, contracture, or spasticity.
- The hips of a newborn should be evaluated for developmental dysplasia. This can be done by using either the Ortolani or the Barlow test. Both tests are done with the infant supine and the hips flexed 90 degrees. In the Ortolani test the examiner attempts to relocate the hips. With the fingers placed over the greater trochanter, the examiner gently abducts the hips. A click or a clunk suggests a hip instability. In the Barlow method, the infant's hips are adducted with the examiner's fingers placed over the medial thigh. The examiner then applies pressure and feels for a posterior click or clunk.
- The upper limb is evaluated for range of motion and function. Common problems identified include brachial plexus injuries, Sprengel's deformity, congenital deformities, and functional limitations. The hand is critical in a child's ability to develop play skills. Hand movement progresses from a very primitive grasp-and-release pattern to a sophisticated ability to manipulate objects.
- Gait should be carefully analyzed and evaluated. Evaluation includes both a stance and a swing phase analysis. Classic abnormal patterns are seen with certain diseases. Children move in the most efficient patterns and are masters of substitution. Movement patterns can indicate weaknesses or asymmetries. Gait generally matures by 7 years of age. Milestones in gait maturation include walking by 15 months, running by 3 years, hopping and walking on the heels by 4 years, and skipping by 6 years. Understanding normal walking and gait facilitates an analysis of gait abnormalities (Table 2–3).
- In-toeing and out-toeing are common gait disturbances evaluated by clinical practitioners. These patterns are seen in torsional deformities of the femur and tibia. The most common cause of in-toeing is related to femoral anteversion; this generally improves with maturation. Functional limitations, frequent

tripping, or lack of hip rotation are reasons to consider surgical or nonsurgical interventions.

Neurological Assessment (pp. 50–51)

• Examination of the neuromuscular system includes testing reflexes and evaluating tone, active motion, coordination, and strength. In children, most of these aspects are assessed simultaneously rather than sequentially.

• Perhaps one of the most critical tools in evaluating neurological development is the evaluation and interpretation of developmental reflexes. The infantile

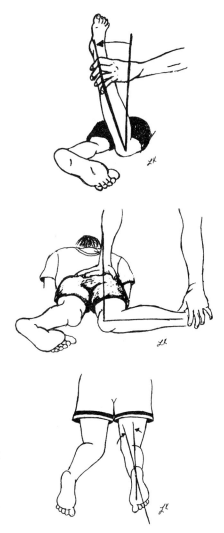

FIGURE 2–2. Evaluation of a child in the prone position allows assessment of the thigh-foot angle and internal and external rotation of the hip. The thigh-foot angle is demonstrated in the lower diagram and ranges from −3 degrees to +20 degrees.

TABLE 2–3 Gait Abnormalities

Gait	Characteristics	Clinical Association
Spastic	Adducted hips Internal rotation of hips Toe walking	Cerebral palsy
Crouched	Weak quadriceps Weak hip extensors Excessive dorsiflexion Hip or knee contractures	Neuromuscular disease Cerebral palsy
Hemiparetic	Posturing of upper extremity Circumduction of hip Inversion of foot	Cerebral palsy Cerebral vascular accident
Waddling (Trendelenburg)	Weakness of hip girdle	Neuromuscular disease
Ataxic	Wide-based gait Coordination problems Poor tandem walking	Cerebellar ataxia Friedreich's ataxia

developmental reflexes are related to various complex functions of the brainstem and spinal cord. Reflexive patterns appear and disappear predictably as the child passes through developmental stages (Table 2–4). This sequencing reflects cortical maturation, and persistence or reoccurrence of abnormal reflexes is a strong indicator of neurological dysfunction. Primitive reflexes are normally and eventually replaced by postural responses that allow the child to adapt to positional changes. The presence of an obligatory tonic neck reflex is abnormal at any age and suggests a central nervous system disorder.

• Muscle tone is the amount of resistance present in muscles through passive range of motion. This tone changes during development and can be affected by activity, alertness, and comfort. A newborn infant is more hypotonic than a toddler. Flexor tone predominates in the first several months of infancy. If true hypotonia persists, it generally indicates an abnormality in the cerebrum, cerebellum, anterior horn cells, peripheral nerves, neuromuscular junction, or

TABLE 2–4 Developmental Reflexes

Reflex	Present at	Disappears by
Rooting	Birth	3 mo
Moro	Birth	4–6 mo
Asymmetrical tonic neck	Birth	6–7 mo
Symmetrical tonic neck	2 mo	6–7 mo
Protective reactions		
Forward	5–6 mo	Persists
Lateral	6–7 mo	Persists
Posterior	9–10 mo	Persists

muscles. Hypertonicity can reflect damage to the cerebrum, brainstem, basal ganglia, or spinal cord. Hypertonicity manifests as either spasticity or rigidity. Severe spasticity and rigidity can present as opisthotonic posturing in the infant.

• Muscle stretch reflexes are easily elicited in children of all ages. A reduction in or absence of reflexes can indicate an anterior horn cell disease, a peripheral neuropathy, or a myopathy. An increase in reflexes is often associated with an upper motor neuron process.

• Strength testing or manual muscle testing can be formally applied in the school-age child. The scoring system is the same as in adults. Testing and scoring are more of a challenge in the younger child. In testing the strength of infants and very young children, reflexive patterns can be useful. Helpful techniques include holding the child under the arms and lifting the child into the air, ventral suspension, checking for age-appropriate head control, and observing the child sitting and standing. The older child can walk, get up off the floor, reach overhead, throw a ball, kick, or skip. Quantitative measurements are generally not required unless specific therapeutic interventions are contemplated.

• Coordination is best assessed by evaluating gross motor and fine motor skills. Impaired coordination is a common sign of a central movement disorder. Specific tests can be done in the older child. Most children are able to walk a straight line, although unsteadily, by age 3 years. Tandem walking is a 5-year-old skill. School-age children can be more formally tested. Subtle symptoms can be seen by evaluating handwriting, drawing, and other higher-level physical skills. The avoidance of organized sports or physical activity can be a clue that coordination problems exist. Ataxia can be evaluated by having the child reach for an object, do the finger-to-nose test, sit or stand, and do tandem walking.

• Sensory evaluation is difficult in young or uncooperative children and has to be age adjusted. A child of 4 to 5 years can interpret joint position, vibration, light touch, temperature, and pain. In the very young child, behavioral responses are the best indicator of sensory awareness. These responses include withdrawing; stopping the activity; and looking, crying, or squirming. A knowledge of infant movement patterns is helpful. For example, withdrawal with isolated spinal reflex activity can be confused with volitional responses.

• The vision examination also must be adapted to the child's ability to cooperate. An infant is able to follow a stimulus with the eyes to midline by 1 month and through 180 degrees by 3 months. Central nervous system dysfunction commonly presents with ocular motor imbalance.

DEVELOPMENTAL ASSESSMENT (pp. 51–53)

• A familiarity with the normal landmarks of early child development is essential to the developmental assessment of the infant and toddler. The assessment includes observing and describing the child's gross motor and fine motor responses, verbal and nonverbal language, personal and social behavior, emotional characteristics, and adaptive skills. A formal assessment of the child's developmental status requires the use of a standardized examination. An interdisciplinary evaluation is particularly helpful when the initial diagnosis is being established or when interventions are being planned for a young child. It can also be used for periodic assessment of developmental progress throughout childhood and adolescence, especially for appropriate educational planning.

• Results of infant tests are best interpreted as a measure of current developmental status relative to a normal peer group. Infant tests rely heavily on motor responses to assess the child's interest and learning. It can be difficult to draw inferences about the child's current or future intellectual ability in the presence of known physical limitations. There is only low correlation between abilities measured on infant tests and later childhood intelligence quotients. Infant test results must be considered provisional and followed by periodic re-evaluation for further diagnostic and prognostic clarification.

• Assessment of preschool and school-age children includes assessment of both physical and intellectual abilities. The chief strength of intelligence tests lies in their correlation with school performance (see Table 2–6 in the Textbook). If appropriately interpreted, the tests reflect the probability of standard academic achievement.

• Most of the standardized intelligence tests rely heavily on language and motor performance. Some disabled children, such as those with central language impairments, significant motor difficulties, or sensory deficits, may need alternative nonverbal and motor-eliminated assessments (see Table 2–7 in the Textbook). Vocabulary tests typically show the strongest correlation with overall intellectual ability and school success.

• The test composite scores, or full-scale scores (IQs), are used to designate a child's overall level of intellectual functioning. On most of these tests, the mean score is 100, which represents average or normal intelligence. Classifications as superior or subaverage typically refer to scores that fall 2 standard deviations above or below the mean. A definition of mental retardation includes three components: (1) subaverage general intelligence, (2) concurrent deficits in adaptive behavior, and (3) developmental delay. Generally, all three criteria must be present to make a formal diagnosis of mental retardation.

• The classification of mild mental retardation (IQ of 55 to 69) encompasses the largest number of children with mental retardation. Generally they show delayed language development as toddlers and weaknesses in the acquisition of pre-academic writing skills. These children generally reach the third- to fifth-grade level academically. If the associated physical handicaps are mild, they can be independent in activities of daily living and achieve relative independence in adulthood.

• Children with moderate mental retardation (IQ of 40 to 54) have a slower rate of developmental attainment. There is also a higher incidence of neurological and physical disabilities. These children are commonly placed in special classes and are primarily taught self-care and practical daily living skills. As adults, many are able to achieve some independence in self-care skills, but they usually continue to need supervision either at home or in group homes and vocationally function primarily in sheltered workshops or protected employment.

• Children with severe mental retardation (IQ of 25 to 39) develop some functional language skills but no formal academic skills. They require intensive programming to master independence in activities of daily living. They need close supervision and supportive care as an adult. Profoundly retarded children (IQ less than 25) have limited language ability and limited potential for acquiring self-care skills. There is also a very high association with severe motor handicaps.

• Several tests have been designed to evaluate visual-motor maturity in children, and to detect delays or impairment in visual-perceptual skills and eye-hand coordination (see Table 2–8 in the Textbook).

• Children with neurological and developmental disabilities sometimes exhibit difficulties in visual-perceptual, perceptual-motor, auditory, kinesthetic, and tactile functioning. A variety of instruments are available to test for these impairments. Achievement tests are designed specifically to evaluate the child's performance in school subject areas such as reading and mathematics (see Table 2–9 in the Textbook). Scores are typically given in terms of school grade equivalence, which can provide an estimate of the child's level of academic skill; as well as standard scores based on age norms. Many are paper-and-pencil tests that penalize handicapped children for their slower pace, poor attention, or difficulty in keeping track of their place on the page.

• A complete assessment of the disabled child must include a description of social and adaptive abilities (see Table 2–10 in the Textbook). It is important to establish the level of achievement in locomotion; communication; and self-care activities such as feeding, dressing, and toileting. It is also important to assess the mode and methods of interaction with family members and peers, and the child's ability to assume increasing levels of responsibility. A number of social adaptive scales have been developed to look at the ages at which children usually achieve such competencies, along with emotional adjustment (see Table 2–10 in the Textbook).

• Care must be taken when arriving at a specific diagnosis on the basis of developmental testing performed early in a child's life. In addition, central nervous system dysfunction is not incompatible with normal intelligence, and the degree to which a child may be intellectually impaired cannot be predicted solely from physical or motor deficits.

SUMMARY (p. 54)

• The pediatric examination shares a common purpose with all physiatric examinations: to ascertain the nature and cause of dysfunction. All the biological, environmental, and developmental factors should be identified. The physiatrist working with the child, family, and rehabilitation team seeks to foster an optimal developmental course so that each child can achieve maximal functional potential.

3

Original Chapter by Paul R. Rao, Ph.D.

Adult Communication Disorders

OVERVIEW OF NORMAL COMMUNICATION PROCESSES (p. 55)

• Speech is just one component in the human repertoire of ways to get a message across. We use facial expression, gesture, tone of voice, writing, singing—in fact, many modes—to communicate a variety of intents.

HEARING (pp. 55–56)

• The human auditory mechanism analyzes sound according to changes in frequency (pitch) and intensity (loudness) over time.
• An audiologist uses an audiometer to measure hearing. Frequencies heard can be tested between 250 and 8000 hertz (Hz). Intensity is measured in decibels (dB) of sound pressure levels (SPLs), and can be tested from 0 to approximately 120 dB (the threshold for pain is around 125 dB).
• The "speech range" extends roughly from 400 to 4000 Hz (4 kHz). Speech contains frequencies below 400 Hz and above 4 kHz, but they are not necessary for nearly perfect intelligibility of routine conversational speech.

VOICE (pp. 57–58)

• Voice is the audible sound produced by phonation, but is only one component of the total speech act. Phonation is sound being made by rapid vocal fold movement excited by the exhaled airstream. Normal voice and speech are produced during the exhalation phase of respiration wherein the vocal folds adduct to constrict the glottis. This momentary interruption of the flow of air from the trachea through the larynx is repeated hundreds of times per second, resulting in phonation. The terms most commonly used in the context of discussing phonation are found in Table 3–1.
• The outcome of speech has three phonological characteristics that are used to describe "voice": pitch, quality, and loudness (see Table 3–1).
• Fundamental frequency (pitch) and intensity (loudness) are two elements of voice and speech that are controlled primarily by the interaction of the respiratory and laryngeal systems. The average fundamental frequency (pitch) for men is around 125 Hz; for women, it is around 200 Hz.

TABLE 3–1 Definitions of Terms Related to Phonation

Voice: Audible sound produced by phonation
Vocal parameters: The elements of voice: pitch, loudness, quality, and flexibility
    Pitch: The perceptual correlate of frequency
    Loudness: The perceptual correlate of intensity
    Quality: The perceptual correlate to complexity
    Flexibility: The perceptual correlate of frequency, intensity, and complexity variations
Dysphonia: Abnormal voice, as judged by the listener, involving either pitch, loudness, quality, flexibility, or combinations thereof
Aphonia: Absence of a definable laryngeal tone. The voice is either severely breathy or whispered
Mute: Unable to phonate and articulate
Vocal folds: Synonymous with vocal cords—shelves of thyroarytenoid muscle covered with mucous membrane and fibroelastic tissue that project into the laryngeal airway
Glottis: The space between and bordered by the vocal folds when the latter are partially or fully abducted
Adduction (of vocal fold): Movement of the vocal folds medially, toward the midline of the laryngeal airway
Abduction (of vocal fold): Movement of the vocal folds laterally, away from the midline of the laryngeal airway

Adapted with permission from Aronson AE: Clinical Voice Disorders. New York, Thieme, 1985, p. 5.

• Voices vary widely by age and sex, and are judged as normal or abnormal on the basis of cultural standards, education, environment, and other similar factors.

SPEECH (p. 57)

• Speech is the motor activity by which the respiratory, laryngeal, and oral structures produce the sound patterns (phonemes) to communicate.
• Speech sounds are divided into vowels and consonants. Vowels are produced with a relatively open vocal tract, with the sound source beginning at the level of the larynx and the differentiation of one vowel from another determined primarily by tongue posture and degree of lip opening. During the classic throat examination, the tongue is down and the mouth is wide open to say "aah," the vowel sound produced in the word "caught." Consonants are produced at varying points along the vocal tract and at varying degrees of constriction, from completely closed for plosive sounds to closely constricted, as in the earlier example, for the /s/ sound. In this context the role of the velopharyngeal (V/P) port should be mentioned: when the V/P port is open and sound is being resonated through the nasal cavity, the nasal consonants /m/, /n/, and /ng/ are produced. This aspect of speech, termed *resonance*, relates to the degree of nasality in the speech.

FLUENCY AND PROSODY (p. 58)

• *Fluency* is the smoothness with which sounds, syllables, words, and phrases are joined together during oral language with lack of hesitations or repetitions.

TABLE 3–2 Definitions and Examples of the Five Dimensions of Language

Dimension	Definition	Example
Phonology	Rules governing the way the sounds of a language are organized	/ks/ sound in English can occur in the middle of a word (bo<u>x</u>er) or the end (boo<u>ks</u>), but never at the beginning.
Semantics	Rules governing the meaning of words and word combinations	Pen = an instrument containing ink and used for writing.
Morphology	Rules governing how words are formed	Grammatical morphemes may change the tense and aspect of sentences (e.g., play<u>s</u>, play<u>ing</u>, play<u>ed</u>).
Syntax	Rules governing how words are combined into larger meaningful units of phrases, clauses, and sentences	"Off the boat got" is *not* a well-formed, grammatical sentence.
Pragmatics	Rules governing the use of language in context	A speaker must be appropriate in initiating a conversation or changing a topic.

The average number of words per minute (wpm), or speaking rate, is 125; however, extremes of normal are seen in relation to a given person's educational, intellectual, and regional status. *Prosody* can also be discussed in the context of rate. Prosody encompasses the rate, rhythm, loudness, and pitch contours that signal stress and therefore carry additional meaning beyond individual speech sounds, words, or sequences of words.

LANGUAGE (pp. 58–59)

• In adults, language can be affected secondary to a host of neurological injuries, including stroke and brain injury. Table 3–2 includes definitions and examples of the five aspects of language.
• Language is *arbitrary* (e.g., the word "drink" is a sign that the community arbitrarily assigned meaning to) and that arbitrariness has implications for the rehabilitation of persons with language impairment.
• There are *levels of language usage*. Adults possess automatic speech such as counting or reflexive language (e.g., profanity) that might not be used to convey a message and can be termed the *automatic* level of language usage. The next level of language usage is *imitation*—simply repeating what is heard. This language is also not typically at the level needed to get a need met. The highest level of language usage, and the one that gets at the functional nature of communication, is the *propositional* level of language. For example, I may be able to recite the days of the week (automatic), or repeat what is said to me (imitative), but neither of these abilities will assist me in getting a need met. The core of communication is to *propositionalize*—to convey a message, a want or need, a joke, and so forth.

TABLE 3–3 Scale of Hearing Impairment

Average Threshold Level (dB)	Suggested Description*
0–25	Normal hearing
26–40	Mild hearing loss
41–55	Moderate hearing loss
56–70	Moderately severe hearing loss
71–90	Severe hearing loss
≥91	Profound hearing loss

* Average threshold level per ANSI-1989 for 0.5, 1, and 2 kHz.
Modified with permission from Yantis P: Puretone Air-Conduction Threshold Testing. In Katz J (ed): Handbook of Clinical Audiology, ed 4. Baltimore, Williams & Wilkins, 1994, pp. 97–108.

ADULT COMMUNICATION DISORDERS (pp. 59–72)

Hearing Impairment (p. 59)

• Hearing impaired is a generic term that refers both to persons who are hard of hearing and those who are deaf. Hearing loss refers to the measured extent, or severity, of hearing impairment. Hearing sensitivity is measured in decibels. The terms generally used to describe the extent of hearing loss are given in Table 3–3. Types of hearing impairment are related to the site of damage or dysfunction and are termed conductive, sensorineural, mixed, and central (Table 3–4).

TABLE 3–4 Definitions of Types of Hearing Loss and Various Causes

Type of Hearing Loss	Definition	Possible Causes
Conductive	Hearing loss resulting from dysfunction of the outer and/or middle ear systems	Occluding cerumen Perforated eardrum Otitis media Otosclerosis
Sensorineural	Hearing impairment resulting from damage/dysfunction of the inner ear (cochlea), or neural fibers of the eighth cranial nerve	Prebycusis Noise-induced Trauma Viral/bacterial illness Ménière's disorder Tumors Hereditary
Mixed	Hearing loss with both conductive and sensorineural components	(See Conductive and Sensorineural)
Central	Hearing impairment resulting from damage or dysfunction of the central auditory pathways; may influence ability to comprehend spoken language, especially in difficult listening situations	Trauma Tumors Vascular damage Demyelinating disease

Voice Disorders (pp. 59–61)

• A voice disorder is said to exist when the quality, pitch, or loudness of the voice, individually or severally, differs from that of other persons of similar age, sex, cultural background, and geographic location.

• Laryngeal disorders have traditionally been classified as either functional or organic, depending on their specific causes. Disorders range from aphonia (no voice) to various dysphonias (disorders of sound quality).

• An otolaryngologist should initially see the person with a voice complaint. Following this the voice evaluation should (1) attempt to determine the cause; (2) describe the current vocal status; and (3) arrive at a communication diagnosis, prognosis, and plan.

• Adult dysphonias that are due to a mass effect are often caused by a faulty phonatory attack (voice misuse or abuse) or substance abuse (smoking and alcohol). The interruption of the smooth approximation of the vocal folds results in a dysphonia. Causes of dysphonias include vocal nodules (a callous formation at the anterior middle third of the vocal folds), laryngitis (an inflammation of the vocal fold mucosa), vocal polyps (fluid-filled sacs that can occur anywhere along the median edge of one or both vocal folds), and contact ulcers (which occur around the area of the arytenoid cartilages).

• Adult dysphonia of neurological origin (excluding dysarthria) may be related to unilateral or bilateral vocal cord paralysis. The folds can be paralyzed in adduction (closed, a life-threatening condition) or in varying stages of abduction (opening). Patients with cords fixed in an adducted position usually require a tracheostomy to maintain a functional airway. They phonate by occluding the stoma and exhaling for speech. In persistent closure due to abductor paralysis, surgical intervention might be indicated to reposition a cord laterally to provide sufficient opening for air. The surgical result, however, often leaves the patient with a breathy voice because the cords are unable to fully approximate. In the case of adductor paralysis (folds in the open position), surgical intervention typically involves either injecting material into a fold to create a mass effect or surgically repositioning a cord to bring it closer to midline.

• Voice disorders of psychosocial origin may need psychological intervention in concert with the SLP voice regimen. The symptoms can range from a variety of dysphonias to complete aphonia.

• A voice disorder can also be one of the first symptoms of laryngeal cancer. Patients with laryngeal cancer may be candidates for a laryngectomy, the total or partial surgical removal of the larynx. A partial laryngectomy might or might not affect vocal quality depending on whether vocal fold tissue has been excised. The postlaryngectomy patient has at least three speaking and several nonspeaking options. The "speaking options" include (1) *tracheoesophageal shunt*; (2) *esophageal voice*, which is produced by oral injection of air into the esophagus followed by a rapid vibrating expulsion; and (3) *an artificial larynx*. Nonspeaking options include writing, complex and simple gestures, communication board, and portable personal computer.

Speech Disorders (pp. 61–64)

Apraxia of Speech (pp. 61–62)

• *Apraxia of speech* (AOS) is a sensorimotor disorder of articulation and prosody that often accompanies Broca's aphasia and can also coexist with dysarthria. The four salient characteristics of AOS are:

Effortful, trial-and-error, groping articulatory movements, and attempts at self-correction

Dysprosody unrelieved by extended periods of normal rhythm, stress, and intonation

Articulatory inconsistency on repeated productions of the same utterance

Obvious difficulty initiating an utterance

• Most experts (but not all) believe that AOS is not due to a language disorder, paralysis, weakness, or incoordination of the speech musculature. Patients with suspected AOS typically have left frontal lesions adjacent to Broca's area. The discriminating behaviors that differentiate AOS from aphasia and dysarthria are the following: relatively spared automatic speech, the absence of any significant motor control problems, and other language modalities that are superior to speech.

Dysarthria (p. 62)

• *Dysarthria* is a collective name for a group of motor speech disorders associated with disturbed neuromuscular control of speech due to central or peripheral nervous system damage. The person with dysarthria is able to understand spoken language, read, write, and use a communication board, book, or device.

DIFFERENTIAL DIAGNOSIS

• Six types of dysarthria can be distinguished on the basis of perceptual characteristics: (1) flaccid, (2) spastic, (3) ataxic, (4) hypokinetic, (5) hyperkinetic, and (6) mixed (see Table 3–7 in the Textbook for a detailed listing).

ASSESSMENT

• Motor speech disorders can be assessed by both perceptual and physiological approaches. The clinician screens hearing and vision and conducts an oral peripheral examination that includes testing alternating motion rates (e.g., rapid repetition of "puh, tuh, kuh"), sequential motor rates (e.g., rapid repetition of "puh, puh, puh"), and prolongation of "aah."

TREATMENT

• The overall goal of dysarthria treatment is enhanced functional communication.

• For anarthria (no speech), a nonverbal communication system may be developed that permits the patient to reliably communicate basic daily living needs.

• For severe dysarthria with the potential for verbal communication, treatment attempts to address three overriding goals, namely: (1) maximization of speech intelligibility, (2) speech efficiency, and (3) functional independence. The general prioritized dysarthria hierarchy of treatment moves through three stages: (1) early, to establish functional verbal skills; (2) middle, to maximize speech intelligibility; and (3) final, to increase the naturalness of speech.

Fluency Disorders (p. 64)

• *Stuttering* is defined as gaps, prolongations, or involuntary repetitions of a sound or syllable that occur during speech production. The most common type of stuttering is developmental dysfluency. Acquired stuttering is fairly rare, and only a few percent begin after age 10 years. Because acquired stuttering is primarily due to brain injury, it has been termed *cortical* or *neurogenic*

TABLE 3–5 Decision Tree for Classifying and Localizing Aphasia after a Left-Sided Cerebrovascular Accident

Impairment and Symptoms	Classification	Localization
Language impairment affecting linguistic components of semantics, syntax, phonology, or pragmatics, or any combination of these	Broca's	MCA, frontal lobe
	Wernicke's	MCA, temporal lobe
	Conduction	MCA, arcuate fasciculus
	Anomic	MCA, angular gyrus
	Global	MCA, multilobes
	Transcortical motor	ACA, prefrontal
	Transcortical sensory	PCA, parieto-occipital
	Isolation	ACA/PCA, watershed area
	Subcortical	Thalamus and basal ganglia
	Alexia with agraphia	PCA, angular gyrus
	Alexia without agraphia	PCA, medial-occipital and splenium of corpus callosum

Abbreviations: MCA, middle cerebral artery; ACA, anterior cerebral artery; PCA, posterior cerebral artery.

stuttering. An additional variety of acquired stuttering that does not fit the above description (except for its relative rarity) is psychogenic stuttering of adult onset.

DIFFERENTIAL DIAGNOSIS
• See page 64 of the Textbook for a description of conditions often confused with neurogenic stuttering.

Aphasia (pp. 64–69)

• *Aphasia involves* an acquired impairment of the language processes underlying receptive and expressive modalities, usually caused by damage to areas of the brain that are primarily responsible for the language function. Aphasia is most common after a left hemisphere stroke.
• The clinician should classify the type of aphasia. There are many classification systems in aphasiology (see Table 3–8 in the Textbook); however, many experts contest the usefulness or even the existence of syndromes.
• Syndromes of aphasia are *not* hard neurological signs but simply suggestive of the presence of brain damage in a particular location of the brain. Table 3–5 summarizes the various aphasia syndromes and suggested localization following a left cerebrovascular accident.
• Three particular discriminating binary language behaviors helpful in classifying aphasia by syndrome are: (1) fluency, (2) comprehension, and (3) repetition. *Fluency* suggests a binary anteroposterior view of the left cortex because nonfluent patients typically have anterior (frontal lobe) lesions, whereas fluent patients typically have posterior (temporal, parietal, or occipital lobe) lesions. *Comprehension* is another binary dimension wherein patients who have suffered strokes in the distribution of the left middle cerebral artery (MCA) can exhibit some degree of deficit in listening comprehension, whereas patients who have

suffered strokes in the left posterior cerebral artery (PCA) exhibit some degree of deficit in reading comprehension. *Repetition* distinguishes patients with MCA infarcts from those with lesions outside the MCA distribution. A left CVA patient who cannot repeat is thus suspected of having a Broca's, Wernicke's, conduction, or global aphasia. The aphasia syndromes listed in Table 3–5 are summarized briefly below.

BROCA'S APHASIA
• Broca's aphasia characteristics:

Nonfluent

Telegraphic speech (like a telegram with the connecting words left out)

Reduced verbal content

Phrase length is generally less than four words

Verbal repertoire is almost exclusively composed of content words (e.g., nouns and verbs), with a notable absence of function words (prepositions and conjunctions)

Functional comprehension is present but patients have trouble following complex grammatical statements

WERNICKE'S APHASIA
• Wernicke's aphasia characteristics:

Fluent with what is termed paragrammatism—speech running on with some semblance of grammatical structure

Phrase length is generally greater than five words and verbal productions are punctuated with paraphasic errors (word substitutions, e.g., pen for pencil)

Poor repetition

Listening comprehension difficulty is a cardinal sign

Secondary language skills of reading and writing are typically also impaired

ANOMIC APHASIA
• Anomic aphasia characteristics:

Striking "loss of words" both orally and in writing

Circumlocute (talk around a word)

Generally have functional reading and listening skills

Fluency and repetition skills are also unremarkable

GLOBAL APHASIA
• Global aphasia characteristics:

Severely impaired in all language modalities, which results in an almost total inability to communicate orally

Fluency, repetition, and comprehension all seriously compromised

CONDUCTION APHASIA
• Conduction aphasia characteristics:

Difficulty repeating a word or phrase back to the examiner

Spontaneous speech relatively fluent with functional comprehension

TRANSCORTICAL MOTOR APHASIA
• Transcortical motor aphasia characteristics:

Fluency and comprehension resembling that of a person with Broca's aphasia, but the repetition skills are spared

Hallmark of this syndrome is adynamia (difficulty initiating speech)

TABLE 3–6 Components of the General Language Assessment

Auditory comprehension	Word identification/discrimination
	Yes/no reliability for personal/general questions
	Ability to follow commands, length and complexity
	Sentence/paragraph level retention and understanding
Visual comprehension	Ability to match symbols/letters
	Word identification skills
	Sentence/paragraph retention and comprehension
	Oral reading
	Functional reading skills
Speech	Social/automatic speech
	Word/sentence repetition
	Confrontation/responsive naming
	Verbal agility, mean length of utterance, fluency rating
	Analysis of form and content
Writing	Biographical information
	Letters, numbers: copying/dictation
	Word/sentence level
	Spontaneous sample

From Porcelli J: Aphasia assessment and treatment. Phys Med Rehabil Clin North Am 1991; 2:487–500. Used by permission.

TRANSCORTICAL SENSORY APHASIA

Relatively rare syndrome is similar to Wernicke's aphasia, save for the retained ability to repeat

ISOLATION SYNDROME

Rare syndrome with severe impairment in all language-processing abilities except for being able to repeat

Assessment (pp. 66–67)

• Table 3–6 summarizes the components of a general language assessment.

Prognosis (p. 67)

• The speech-language pathologist can usually make a best "guestimate" about the odds of recovery based on many factors including age, education, intelligence, handedness, extent of lesion, site of lesion, classification of disorder, memory and attentional deficits, and motivation. Factors that are felt to limit response to aphasia therapy include perseveration and severe auditory comprehension deficit, inability to match objects, unreliable yes/no responses, and jargon and empty speech without self-correction.

Treatment (pp. 67–69)

• Today the focus of treatment is on function!

• Enhance functional capacity by assisting the person with aphasia to change behavior through functional communication treatment.

• Reduce demands of the environment by removing noise in the system (e.g., turning off the TV) and optimizing transmission of signals (e.g., having action pictures in a communication book available).
• Provide assistive devices and alternative methods by determining the menu of core needs and abilities, then training the person with aphasia in the use of alternative communication options to convey wants and needs (the use of Amer-Ind Code is an example of this approach).

Right Hemisphere Communication Disorder (pp. 69–70)

• In an isolated speech and language task, persons with right hemisphere stroke will typically exhibit no difficulty on language and speech tasks done in the laboratory. The patient will break down when the same task is done in a context, however, such as when the individual is required to appreciate the emotion in another's voice, the words on the left side of a newspaper, or the face of a friend or family member. These are the symptoms of a problem that has as its basis the visual-attentional processing mechanism of the right hemisphere.

Traumatic Brain Injury (pp. 70–71)

• Patients who suffer traumatic brain injury can experience a variety of communication disorders including aphasia, anarthria, dysarthria, AOS, and cortical stuttering. The communication problem that is most commonly associated with traumatic brain injury, however, is not based on language, speech, or fluency but on cognition.
• *Cognitive-communication impairments* is the generic term used to refer to the cognitively based communication disorders resulting from deficits in both linguistic and nonlinguistic cognitive processes. This population differs from the language-impaired patients following stroke in that they are typically younger, have lesions that are more diffuse, have a longer recovery period, and often have academic and vocational reentry as significant functional goals. Specific cognitive skills that may be impaired in traumatic brain injury are attention, perception, discrimination, organization, recall, and reasoning/problem solving. Persons with traumatic brain injury can experience impairments in any or all stages of memory from attention and immediate recall to short- and long-term memory. Disturbances in executive functioning can occur even following a mild head injury with normal neuroradiological findings (see Chapter 49).

Dementia (pp. 71–72)

• Dementia is an organic syndrome characterized by decline of memory and other intellectual functions in comparison with the patient's previous level of function. Conditions that can resemble dementia but are clearly distinguishable from it are delirium, psychiatric states, depression, and hearing loss. Dementia is a syndrome that can be due to numerous diseases, infections, toxins, and trauma. Many of the causes of dementia are treatable or reversible.
• The most common cause of dementia is Alzheimer's disease (AD), accounting for 50% to 60% of all patients. Vascular dementias (dementias caused by multiple infarcts or ischemia [MID]) are seen in 20% of demented patients. Alzheimer's dementia and multiple infarct disease co-occur in approximately 15% of the sample, and other conditions such as Pick's disease, Parkinson's

disease, progressive supranuclear palsy, and Creutzfeld-Jakob disease, account for the remainder of the irreversible dementias.

Differential Diagnosis (p. 72)

• The communication problems commonly seen in dementia can be differentiated from those seen in single left or right hemisphere strokes. Factors that help distinguish between aphasia and dementia include memory deficits, anomia, perseveration, dysfluency, jargon, and circumlocution. Additional factors include the cause, course (decline), and constellation of symptoms (decrements in judgment, affect, memory, cognition, and orientation).

Assessment (p. 72)

• Perhaps the most important portion of the assessment is the comprehensive case history obtained from the significant other to determine the type of onset, symptoms, and dysfunctional status of the person with dementia. The clinician should be sensitive to such reversible problems as drug use and depression. A tool commonly used to screen for dementia is the Mini-Mental Status Examination (MMSE), a 30-point screen that examines the patient's orientation, registration, calculation, memory, language, praxis, ability to follow commands, and level of consciousness.

Acknowledgment. Special thanks to Dr. Carmen Brewer, Director of Hearing and Speech at the Washington Hospital Center, for her input on the hearing impairment section of this chapter.

4

Original Chapter by Lance E. Trexler, Ph.D., and David J. Fordyce, Ph.D.

Psychological Perspectives on Rehabilitation: Contemporary Assessment and Intervention Strategies

CONCEPTUALIZING PSYCHOLOGICAL ASPECTS OF REHABILITATION (pp. 75–76)

• Psychological variables significantly influence the rehabilitation process and outcome.

Classification and Terminology in Rehabilitation: Implications for Psychological Assessment and Rehabilitation (p. 76)

• The National Center for Medical Rehabilitiation and Research (NCMRR) model provides a useful model for conceptualizing psychological assessment and intervention in rehabilitation (Table 4–1).

• Psychological assessment seeks to provide insights into the individual characteristics of the patient. For example, the extent to which patients believe or perceive that they have some control over their behavior and that what happens to them is not merely the consequence of luck or fate (referred to as "locus of control" in the psychological literature), has been demonstrated to influence the length of hospitalization and/or outcome in many different medical conditions.

• A variety of psychological tests have been designed to assess emotional "impairments" and functional limitations that have directly resulted from pathophysiological sources or that are a reaction to the resulting neurological impairments.

• The impairments that result from a lesion and the attendant functional limitations and disabilities all interact dynamically in a manner that either facilitates or compromises adaptation. The quality of the interaction is largely determined by psychological and environmental variables.

TABLE 4–1 Terminology in Disability Classification: The National Center for Medical Rehabilitation and Research Model (1993)

Pathophysiology	Interruption or interference with normal physiological and developmental processes or structures
Impairment	Loss or abnormality of cognitive, emotional, physiological, or anatomical structure or function
Functional limitation	Restriction or lack of ability to perform an action in the manner or within the range consistent with the purpose of the organ or organ system
Disability	Inability or limitation in performing tasks, activities, and roles to levels expected within physical and social contexts
Societal limitation	Restriction, attributable to social policy or barriers (structural or attitudinal), which limits fulfillment of roles or denies access to services and opportunities that are associated with full participation in society

PSYCHOLOGICAL ASSESSMENT (pp. 76–84)

Purposes of Psychological Assessment (p. 76)

• Psychological tests are generally constructed to provide objective, reliable, and valid observations about human behavior. However, the results of psychological tests must, by necessity, be integrated with clinical and subjective data, from which clinical interpretation can be provided.

The Nature and Extent of Higher Cortical Impairment (pp. 76–78)

• Because individuals with brain dysfunction, either congenital or acquired, present with an altered capacity and style of learning, a distinctly unique approach to rehabilitation is required. Rehabilitation of the person with brain injury is also unique because reorganization or compensation for neuropsychological impairments is often the goal of the rehabilitation.

• Determining the location and evolution of the lesion, in both the acute and the chronic stages of brain injury, through neuroimaging and neuropsychological studies can be of assistance in choosing appropriate rehabilitation strategies.

• Contemporary research suggests that the best predictors of benefit from post-acute brain injury neuropsychological rehabilitation are measures of insight, awareness, and acceptance.

• The neuropsychological examination should provide information not only about what impairments might exist, but also as to how the rehabilitation staff should address or compensate for the impairments (Table 4–2).

• Brain injury can also result in organic changes in emotional behavior secondary to subtle alterations in the stability of temporolimbic functions. Social interaction and integration are also often impaired secondary to neurobehavioral disorders (Table 4–3).

• Cognitive, neurobehavioral, and emotional reactions to brain injury can, if not properly managed, interact and lead to a spiral of deterioration. The spiral of deterioration often serves to sustain functional impairment of cognitive

TABLE 4–2 Disturbances of Higher Cortical Functions

Functions	Disturbances/Impairments
Motor and sensory	Hemiparesis
	Dyscoordination
	Dyspraxias
	Visual field defects
	Tactile, auditory, and visual sensitivity
Arousal and attention	Cognitive fatigue and poor endurance/sustained attention
	Distractability
	Modality-specific and global attention
Memory	Modality-specific (e.g., auditory, visual) memory
	Short-term working memory
	Prospective memory
	Autobiographical memory
	Episodic-semantic memory
	Procedural-declarative memory
Language and language-related	Dysphasias
	Dysgraphias
	Dyslexias
	Dyscalculias
Perceptual, visuospatial, and visuoconstructive	Agnosias
	Visual and auditory analysis and discrimination
	Hemispatial inattention and neglect
	Visuoconstructive disorders
	Dysprosodias
Executive and metacognitive	Problem-solving and abstraction
	Goal-directed behaviors
	Self-regulation
	Organization
	Monitoring

TABLE 4–3 Partial Taxonomy of Neurobehavioral Disorders and Syndromes

Disorders of Awareness

Anosognosia: Unawareness or denial of illness or consequences of brain lesion

Anosodiaphoria: Lack of emotional reaction to a deficit caused by a brain lesion

Frontal Syndromes

Dorsolateral convexity: Indifference, cognitive slowness, inertia, "pseudo-depression"

Orbitofrontal: Euphoria, hyperkinesia, disinhibition, "pseudo-psychopathic" behavior

Temporolimbic Syndrome

Intensification of affect/ethical/religious feelings, spontaneous episodes of rage, hypergraphia, hypersexuality, and hyposexuality

functions, secondary to depression or anxiety following concussion or mild brain injury, despite the fact that neurologically based cognitive impairments might have resolved.
• Research has demonstrated that cognitive and neurobehavioral impairments following brain injury, and not physical impairments, create disabilities affecting long-term adjustment and social integration.

Emotional Adjustment and Permanent Impairment
(pp. 78–81)

Developmental Stages (p. 78)
• Emotional responses to acutely disabling conditions (e.g., spinal cord injury or stroke) or to the onset of a potentially disfiguring or fatal disease (e.g., cancer) have traditionally been thought to follow a natural course of evolution. It is now clear that such models reflect entrenched biases that are not well supported by empirical findings. Variability in emotional outcomes predominates.

Depression and Disability (pp. 78–79)
• Disturbances in sleep, appetite, arousal, motivation, communication, and affective modulation are common direct consequences of illness and medication. For example, the third leading cause of death among spinal cord–injured patients is suicide.
• Major psychological reactions occur in a minority of acutely impaired individuals. Typically fewer than 30% of those who survive spinal cord injury evidence major emotional distress, either in the acute stages of recovery or over longer periods of adaptation.

Human Resilience and Coping (pp. 79–80)
• Humans typically are fairly resilient in the face of difficult losses or the acquisition of permanent impairments, but significant depression is thought to be an understandable and natural response to loss. The fact that health care professionals commonly overestimate the degree of psychological distress in their patients might reflect this expectation.

Denial (p. 80)
• Denial is a highly dynamic, multifaceted coping process that can be manifested through direct verbal report or inferred from behavior or from the absence of overt expressions of emotional distress. In the case of certain types of brain injury (e.g., nondominant stroke or traumatic head injury), apparent denial is likely to be reflective of impairments in information processing, emotional arousal, or emotional expression. Denial and related phenomena are clearly evident in a variety of other nonneurological situations of loss.
• Many avoidant strategies that disabled individuals employ for coping might be adaptive. Because emotional distress in reaction to loss is not always resolved, strong confrontations of denial might be counterproductive. Seemingly unrealistic expressions of hope can actually reinforce progress through rehabilitation. Denial should be sensitively confronted if it is determined to increase the probability of safety risk or psychosocial failure.

Psychological Forces That Have an Impact on Impairment and Disability
(p. 80)
• Physical and emotional symptom reporting is subject to a number of psychological processes.
• Attention and awareness are dependent on the relative strengths and numbers of competing stimuli. Awareness is also driven by perceptual biases, expectancies, and beliefs.
• Interpretation and labeling of a physiological stimulus is an outcome of a complex psychological process that is dependent on prior experience, current circumstances, and associated cues, goals, and perceived or anticipated consequences.
• Following a medical event, such psychological forces begin to play an increasingly important role, either positively or negatively, in overall level of disability. Such forces can also impede recovery and contribute to more severe and prolonged disability. The more negative outcomes can be particularly prevalent in situations of less severe initial injury or in situations in which physiological healing is nearly always complete (e.g., many back injury or concussion cases).

Social Factors and Rehabilitation *(pp. 80–81)*
• Alterations in social functioning following the onset of impairment can play a major role in concurrent and future adjustment. Social reinforcers can also exert a powerful influence on all aspects of recovery from injury.
• Although social support can ameliorate depression, inappropriate social attention can accentuate suffering or enhance disability, pain, or dependency behaviors. Studies of chronic pain patients have shown a positive relationship between a solicitous spouse responding to pain behavior and patient reports of pain and ratings of disability. Entitlement systems such as worker's compensation insurance and Social Security disability insurance, and the compensatory forces associated with third-party lawsuits, can also influence symptom reporting and general levels of disability. Intervention with patients and families must sort out and selectively guide attributions and interactions that serve to maintain disability.

Types of Psychological Assessment (p. 81)

• Psychological assessment is the integration of personal and medical history and behavioral observations with objectively derived test scores. Psychological testing is therefore one component of a diagnostic process.

The Clinical Interview and Behavioral Observations
(pp. 81–82)

• Meltzer, a psychologist who suffered hypoxic encephalopathy, noted that after extensive inpatient and outpatient therapies, no matter what particular intervention he received, it was the quality of the relationship between him and the therapist that determined the extent to which he benefited from therapy.
• Based on the initial interview and review of the medical records, the psychologist determines which tests are clinically appropriate to administer, depending on the nature of the referral question and the needs of the individual.

Measures of Cognitive, Emotional, and Personality Functioning (p. 81)

Locus of Control Scales (p. 82)
• The extent to which the patient believes that he or she has some control over the impact of illness or disease can significantly influence outcome. Locus of control is easily measured with a brief questionnaire, and the most commonly used is the Multidimensional Health Locus of Control Scale.

Sickness Impact Profile (p. 82)
• The Sickness Impact Profile (SIP) is another behaviorally oriented measure of health status and is commonly used not only to measure the patient's perception of the effects of a given illness on everyday behavior but also to measure the effectiveness of a specific health care program. See Table 4–7 in the Textbook for the types of everyday activities measured by the SIP.

Depression Inventories (p. 82)
• There are a number of self-report screening measures of depression, including the Beck Depression Inventory, the Zung Depression Scale, and the Hamilton Rating Scale.

Minnesota Multiphasic Personality Inventory (p. 82)
• The MMPI is probably the most widely used objective test of personality functioning, although there are some advantages to the more recent Millon Clinical Multiaxial Inventory-II. Recently, the MMPI-2 has been developed, with some clinically important differences from the MMPI. (See Table 4–8 in the Textbook for descriptors of the 14 scales.)

Intelligence and Achievement Tests (pp. 82–83)

• Intelligence tests are useful in rehabilitation for a variety of reasons, and the most commonly used test is the Wechsler Adult Intelligence Scale—Revised (WAIS-R).
• The most comprehensive of the achievement tests is the Woodcock-Johnson Psychoeducational Battery—Revised.
• Another commonly used achievement test is the Peabody Individual Achievement Test—Revised (PIAT-R).

Neuropsychological Tests (pp. 83–84)

Battery versus Individualized Approaches (pp. 83–84)
• The primary impetus for the development of neuropsychological assessment in the United States was to assist in neurological diagnosis. Prior to the development of CT, neuropsychological assessment was targeted at determining whether a brain lesion was present, and, if present, discerning its location and type. This diagnostic approach supported the development of the Halstead-Reitan Neuropsychological Test Battery (HRNTB). In the former Soviet Union, Luria contributed the first organized neuropsychological theory of brain functions and developed examination procedures that emphasize individual differences.

Purpose-Specific Neuropsychological Tests *(p. 84)*

• In the case of brain injury, sequential monitoring of the patient's overall orientation can be quite useful in determining the rate of progress and response to neuropharmacological treatment and in documenting evolution out of post-traumatic or anterograde amnesia.

• Too often patients are unknowingly discharged from the hospital in a state of post-traumatic or anterograde amnesia, often with disastrous results. The Galveston Orientation and Amnesia Scale is a quick and objective measure that is invaluable.

• A variety of scales have been developed for measuring psychosocial and functional adaptation following brain injury and are sometimes used as part of neuropsychological assessment. The most useful include the Katz Adjustment Scale, the Portland Adaptability Inventory, and the Community Integration Questionnaire.

PSYCHOLOGICAL INTERVENTION (pp. 84–87)

• In rehabilitation settings, psychological interventions are typically divided into two broad areas: (1) maximizing general rehabilitation progress, and (2) teaching specific skills to facilitate psychosocial adjustment.

Depressive Symptoms (pp. 84–85)

• Clinical depression or some subclinical depressive symptoms can have a negative impact on participation in rehabilitation and ultimate adjustment. Alterations in sleep or arousal secondary to significant depression can diminish the patient's energy available for rehabilitation. More important, the negative cognitive biases accompanying depression can have an impact on motivation, general activity level, socialization, and reactions to positive feedback.

• Cognitive therapy for depression strives to help the patient become aware of irrational negative perceptual biases and to modify associated information processing styles.

• Various behavioral strategies can also be employed to intervene in depressive symptoms. In fact, most psychological interventions for depression employ a mixture of cognitive and behavioral strategies.

Psychological Treatment of Anxiety (p. 85)

• The onset of serious illness or injury can set the stage for the development of anxiety symptoms. Hemiplegia, amputation, or other impairments affecting physical stability or balance can generate notable fears of falling. Some conditions such as chronic obstructive pulmonary disease or certain cardiac impairments can create chronic anxiety related to doubts about future survival. These interact with the underlying medical state to further compromise function.

• Treatment of anxiety disorders is based on controlled exposure to the feared event or circumstance under conditions that optimize successful function. Teaching skills that modulate the magnitude of such arousal have served as a cornerstone for desensitization strategies. A variety of relaxation techniques are available.

TABLE 4–4 Common Sources of Resistance or Poor Motivation in Rehabilitation

Medical/Physical Factors	Psychological Factors
1. Effects of acute illness	1. Depression, anxiety, fear effects
2. Effects of acute pain	2. Lack of reinforcement/pleasure
3. Lack of sleep/fatigue	3. Denial
4. Medicine effects	4. Efforts at sustaining control
5. Brain injury/delirium effects	5. Limited input into established program/goals
a. Anosognosia	6. Poor understanding of rehabilitation rationale
b. Disorientation/confusion	7. Poor appreciation of progress/gains
c. Agitation	8. Personality conflict with therapist/physician
d. Memory impairment	9. Characterological traits of patient

Interventions with Excessive Chronic Disability (pp. 85–86)

• Specific interventions are required in cases in which excessive disability seems related to faulty attributions or psychosocial contingencies. Supervised progressive physical activity occurs despite the presence of pain behaviors or reports of pain. Rest, analgesics, and social attention are programmed to occur at times that are not pain reinforcing. Attempts are made to intervene in family and vocational arenas to maximize the probability that social forces reinforce independence and function rather than disability (see Chapter 42).

Social Skills Training (p. 86)

• The nature of social interaction in traditional rehabilitation settings commonly offers little preparation for the disabled individual to deal with more natural social environments. Training should be done in regard to disability-specific issues (e.g., incontinence, wheelchair mobility, and forgetfulness) to minimize uncomfortableness on the part of patients and their able-bodied interactional partners.

Resistive or "Unmotivated" Patients (p. 86)

• Seemingly unmotivated, resistive, manipulative, or angry patients are not uncommon to the rehabilitation setting and can serve as a significant source of stress and frustration for staff. Not uncommonly, such behaviors are labeled as reflective of a personality flaw and lead to decisions to terminate services. They often reflect understandable responses to internal and external events (Table 4–4), however, and often offer opportunities for intervention.

Neuropsychological Rehabilitation (pp. 86–87)

• The literature on neuropsychological approaches to brain injury rehabilitation has flourished since the early 1980s. A variety of types of interventions have been developed. In general, neuropsychological treatment of cognitive impairments employs either a theoretical-clinical or a psychometric approach.

• A great variety of studies have addressed the efficacy of interventions for specific cognitive disorders (e.g., using a memory notebook). See the Textbook for more specific information about specific neuropsychological interventions.

• Another neuropsychological intervention can be best described as an organized program of specialized rehabilitation, referred to as "holistic" neuropsychological rehabilitation. A holistic approach to the rehabilitation of the person with acquired brain damage employs a therapeutic milieu with a variety of group therapies emphasizing awareness and emotional acceptance of residual deficits and compensation or remediation of cognitive impairments. Families must be quite involved, particularly from a psychotherapeutic standpoint, and these programs all emphasize a gradual and structured reentry into a target discharge environment, such as a vocational placement.

SUMMARY (p. 88)

• Psychological assessment and treatment are increasingly valuable in all types of physical rehabilitation, from occupational rehabilitation to brain injury rehabilitation. Rehabilitation teams should include, or at least have access to, a psychologist. Rehabilitation clinicians also need to have at least a superficial understanding of the use and limitations of current psychological tests.

5

Original Chapter by Alberto Esquenazi, M.D., and Mukul Talaty, Ph.D.

Gait Analysis: Technology and Clinical Applications

• Gait analysis has evolved into a recognized medical evaluation that is necessary for the appropriate planning of surgery or other therapeutic interventions in the management of spasticity; and for the prescription and optimization of orthotic and prosthetic devices. Other applications include sports analysis, the treatment of many musculoskeletal conditions, and clinical outcomes measurement.

NORMAL HUMAN LOCOMOTION (pp. 94–95)

• Humans are the only animals that characteristically walk upright. The fundamental goal of ambulation is to move from one place to another safely and efficiently. Gait is cyclic and can be characterized by the timing of foot contact with the ground. An entire sequence of functions by one limb is identified as a *gait cycle*. Each gait cycle has two basic components, *stance phase* and *swing phase*. Stance phase describes the duration of foot contact with the ground. Swing phase is the entire period during which the foot is in the air for the purpose of limb advancement. Swing phase can be further divided into three functional subphases: (1) *initial swing,* (2) *mid-swing,* and (3) *terminal swing.* The stance phase can be divided into five subphases: (1) *initial contact,* (2) *loading response,* (3) *mid-stance,* (4) *terminal stance,* and (5) *pre-swing* (Fig. 5–1).
• Alternatively, the stance phase can be divided into three periods according to foot-floor contact patterns. The beginning and the end of the walking stance phase mark the period of *double support,* during which both feet are in contact with the floor, allowing the weight of the body to be transferred from one limb to the other. Using this descriptor, one definition of running is locomotion in which double support is absent. *Single limb support* begins when the opposite foot is lifted from the ground for the swing phase. For normal subjects walking at self-selected comfortable speeds, the normal distribution of the floor contact period during the gait cycle is roughly 60% for stance phase and 40% for swing phase. Approximately 10% of the total cycle is overlap for each double support time. These ratios vary greatly with changes in walking speed (Fig. 5–2 in the Textbook).

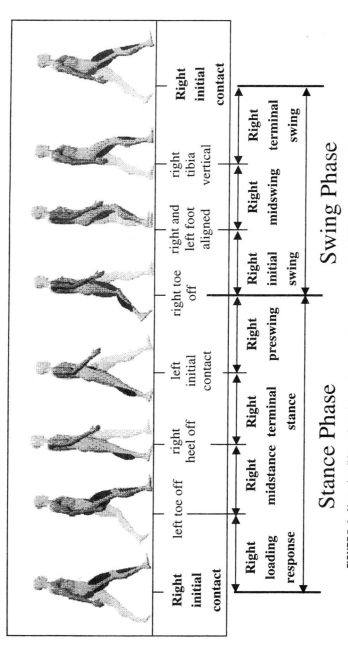

FIGURE 5-1. Normal walking gait cycle terminology with selected lower limb EMG representation. Human figures in the different phases of gait with superimposed primary gait muscles. Muscle shade intensity is roughly proportional to strength of muscle contraction.

TABLE 5–1 Stance Limb Problems

Ankle-Foot Instability	Knee Instability	Hip Instability
Equinus	Excessive flexion (buckling)	Flexion
Varus	Hyperextension	Extension
Equinovarus	Varus	Adduction
Valgus	Valgus	Abduction
Equinovalgus		
Excessive dorsiflexion		
Toe curling		
Hallux hyperextension		

• The *step period* is the time measured from an event in one foot to the next occurrence of the same event in the opposite foot. There are two steps in each stride or gait cycle. The step period is useful for identifying and measuring asymmetry between the two sides of the body in pathological conditions. *Step length* is the maximum distance between the feet in the direction of progression during one step. The *stride period* is defined as the time from an event of one foot until the re-occurrence of the same event for the same foot. *Stride length* is the maximum distance traversed by the same foot in the direction of progression during one stride; it is most often studied as the distance from the initial contact of one foot to the initial contact of the same foot. In most conditions for normal and pathological ambulators, left and right stride measures are equal. The stride period is often time-normalized for the purpose of averaging gait parameters over several strides, both between and within subjects (i.e., the absolute time is transformed to 100%). *Cadence* denotes the number of steps in a period (commonly expressed as steps per minute). Step length, step time, and cadence are fairly symmetrical between legs in normal individuals. The base of support refers to the lateral distance between the feet. It is usually measured as the perpendicular distance between the medial borders or centerlines of the left and right feet.

GAIT DYSFUNCTION (p. 95)

• Because of the complex relationship of multiple body segments, it is difficult to clearly identify the primary cause and compensation (substitution) in a gait deviation. One approach is to look at the different phases of locomotion and identify factors that affect the particular expected functional component. For this functional approach, the stance phase dysfunctions can be categorized into three groups: (1) ankle-foot instability, (2) knee instability, and (3) hip instability (Table 5–1). A brief description of each follows.

Ankle-Foot Instability (p. 95)

• The foot interaction with the ground is inadequate, interfering with the inherent weight-bearing function of the foot. Examples are the abnormal postures of the foot present in such conditions as equinus, equinovarus, ankle valgus with or without equinus, toe flexion, or hallux extension (hitchhiker's great toe).

Inadequate foot-ground interaction may also result from excessive ankle dorsiflexion such as that seen with insufficient plantar flexor strength. This is commonly seen in the patient with neurological sequelae after central nervous system injury.

Knee Instability (p. 95)

• Knee instability refers to flexed, hyperextended, varus, or valgus knee posture. In the sagittal plane, it can be a compensatory response to avoid limb instability like that seen secondary to knee extensor or ankle plantar flexor weakness. Excessive knee hyperextension or valgus or varus knee can also be the result of an inherently unstable joint. An adducted hip or flexed hip can also affect knee stability.

Hip Instability (p. 95)

• Hip instability typically involves hip abductor or extensor weakness or limited hip extension range of motion. Abnormal hip posture can also be a compensation for an abnormal base of support or limb instability. As an example, the patient with knee extensor weakness leans forward to improve knee stability by moving the center of mass anterior to the knee joint.

Swing Phase Deviations (p. 95)

• Swing phase deviations can be divided into those of *impaired limb clearance* and those of *impaired limb advancement.* Impaired limb clearance can result from a drop foot, stiff knee, limited hip flexion, excessive or untimely hip adduction, and/or pelvic drop. Impaired limb advancement can be the result of a flexed knee, limited hip flexion, contralateral hip extension or limitation, or adducted hips.

QUANTITATIVE GAIT ANALYSIS (pp. 95–100)

• Informal visual analysis of gait is routinely performed by clinicians. This sometimes casual observation can be more useful, although with many limitations, if performed in a careful and systematic manner. It can yield good descriptive information, especially when slow-motion video technology is used.
• The four primary components of quantitative gait analysis that can be recorded are as follows: (1) kinetics (analysis of forces that produce motion); (2) poly-EMG or dynamic EMG (analysis of muscle activity); (3) kinematics (analysis of motion and resulting temporal and stride measures); and (4) energetics (analysis of metabolic or mechanical energy).

Kinetics (pp. 96–97)

• Kinetic analysis deals with the forces produced during walking. For our purposes, as long as gravity is present, there is a reaction force when the body interacts with the ground. The ground reaction force (GRF) is a reflection of body weight and acceleration. This force can be resolved into a convenient set of directions such as vertical, anteroposterior (AP), and mediolateral. The AP shear forces are sometimes referred to as propulsion and braking forces. Friction is responsible for the generation of shear forces. The forces in all three directions, measured by the force plates together, make up the total force (see Fig. 5–3 in the Textbook).

• A force plate is a sophisticated scale that can measure vertical (downward) force, similar to the body weight registered on a scale, as well as shear forces.

• A force is transmitted from the floor to the foot, then passed on up to all other body segments. The product of the magnitude of the GRF under each foot and its location with respect to a given joint center (e.g., ankle, knee, or hip) are major factors that determine the torque or moments produced by the external force about that joint. This moment is a measure of the joint rotational tendency (flexion/extension, ab-/adduction, internal/external rotation) produced by the external force. Internal forces, generated primarily by muscles, ligaments, and the geometry of the joint articulation (bony contact), act to control the rotation of the joints caused by this external force. For example, the GRF, when positioned anterior to the knee, produces a moment that tends to drive the knee into extension and must be countered and controlled by muscle force (e.g., knee flexors/extensors).

• Whereas force plates measure the sum or total force acting under the entire foot, it is sometimes useful to measure discrete components of that force acting over specific areas of the foot (the distribution of pressure).

Dynamic Polyelectromyography (pp. 97–99)

• In normal locomotion the body elicits forces from 28 muscles in each lower limb to carefully control the gravitational forces. The end result is a smooth, coordinated, energy-efficient movement pattern. Redundancy exists in the relationship between the muscles and the joints upon which they act.

• The electrical activity of all of the muscles that are capable of producing the target movement needs to be evaluated, not just the electrical activity of a muscle directly spanning a particular segment or joint. EMG recordings provide information about the timing and duration of muscle activation (see Fig. 5–1). Under certain conditions relative to gait can also be determined.

• EMG patterns are highly sensitive to walking speed. For this reason, it is incorrect and potentially misleading to compare the recording of a patient with a slow gait to that of an able-bodied control subject walking at a higher speed with a natural cadence. In addition to timing, amplitude of the EMG signal can provide valuable information for clinical decision making. A particular muscle can be over- or underactive during a given portion of the cycle; such deviations should be carefully correlated with patient kinematics.

Kinematics (pp. 99–100)

• A kinematic analysis considers the patterns of motion, regardless of what forces (external or internal) are producing those motions, and the resulting temporal and spatial parameters.

Temporal and Spatial Descriptive Measures (p. 99)

• Temporospatial measures afford a relatively simple and integrated method of quantifying some useful gait parameters. Temporospatial footfall patterns are the end product of the total integrated locomotor movement. Because gait is periodic, data from a single cycle or, better yet, an average of several cycles can be used to partially characterize a gait pattern.

Motion Analysis *(pp. 99–100)*

• Motion analysis produces a quantitative description of the motion of body segments without regard to the forces that are responsible for generating this motion. However, kinetic quantities such as joint reaction forces and moments are often combined with motion data to give a more complete picture of the coordinated total body movement pattern *and* the forces that are responsible for creating it.

• Video and passive optoelectronic systems utilize retroreflective markers applied to the subject. The markers are illuminated by an external power source and are tracked by the detectors (camera). Near automatic marker identification and digitization is reliable if marker paths do not cross (as can usually be expected for standard marker placements in normal walking). However, conversion into quantitative data can require some manual intervention for marker identification in pathological gait, where increased limb rotation, sudden motions, or crossover of segment paths can occur.

ENERGETICS (p. 100)

• Normal walking requires a relatively low level of metabolic energy consumption during steady state at comfortable walking speeds. Normal gait on level surfaces is most efficient at a walking speed of 1 to 1.3 m/sec, which is equivalent to 60 to 80 m/min or 3 miles/hr. Comfortable walking speed for an individual usually corresponds to minimum energy cost per unit distance. For the human body, the center of mass has been experimentally found to be located 2 cm in front of the second sacral vertebrae (in anatomic position). It has a dynamic nature (meaning that its location changes as the orientation of the body changes) and under certain conditions can even be located outside the body. The position of the center of mass is intimately related to the location of the GRF: simply put, they move in tandem. During walking the center of mass moves in a sinusoidal path with a mean of 5 cm of vertical and horizontal displacement. This displacement of the center of mass requires work, which in turn has an energy cost. The six determinants of gait described by Inman and colleagues (Table 5–2) were identified as the strategies necessary to produce forward pro-

TABLE 5–2 Inman's Six Determinants of Gait

1. **Pelvic rotation in the horizontal plane.** The swinging hip moves forward faster than the stance hip.
2. **Pelvic tilt in the frontal plane.** The pelvis on the side of the swinging leg is lowered. This is controlled by activity in the hip abductors of the stance limb.
3. **Early knee flexion** (15 degrees) during the first part of stance.
4. **Weight transfer from the heel to flat foot** associated with controlled plantar flexion during the first part of stance.
5. **Late knee flexion** (30–40 degrees) during the last part of the stance phase.
6. **Lateral displacement of the pelvis toward the stance limb.** The aim of this determinant is to reduce the displacement of the CM.

gression with the least energy expenditure by minimizing the excursion of the center of mass.

• Sudden acceleration or deceleration of the center of mass increases energy consumption. Running is more efficient than walking, if walking speed is faster than 2 m/sec. Walking on a 10% to 12% incline doubles energy expenditure.

PATHOLOGICAL GAIT (pp. 100–108)

• At the beginning of this chapter, we used an anatomical approach to describe gait deviations. In this section we adopt a more functional approach in describing the various gait deviations likely to be seen and diagnosed clinically.

Abnormal Base of Support (pp. 101–106)

• Base of support is literally the foundation upon which a stable gait pattern is built. An adequate base of support is critical to all aspects of gait. This is particularly true in regard to safety and comfort because it is the foot-floor interaction that transmits the entire weight of the body to the ground and characterizes the GRF interaction with the body. It is the location and magnitude of the GRF in relation to the joints that ultimately determines, in large part, the joint moments that the muscles will have to stabilize and counteract.

Equinus Foot or Ankle (p. 101)

• Equinus foot deformity is often seen after an upper or lower motor neuron injury. This deformity can also be the result of ankle immobilization, fractures, and surgery. The foot and ankle are in a toe-down and, commonly, have a turned-in (varus) position. Toe curling can co-exist. In the resulting pathological gait, limb contact with the ground occurs first with the forefoot. The weight is borne primarily on the anterior and lateral border of the foot and can be concentrated in the area of the fifth metatarsal, resulting in an antalgic gait. Toe flexion can be present, particularly in neurological injuries or cases where a plantar flexion contracture is present. Limited ankle dorsiflexion during mid-stance prevents forward progression of the tibia over the stationary foot, increasing pressure over the metatarsals, promoting ankle instability, and causing knee hyperextension. During the swing phase, sustained plantar flexion of the foot can result in a limb clearance problem unless proximal mechanisms of compensation such as increased hip and knee flexion are used.

Equinovalgus Foot (pp. 101–106)

• The equinovalgus foot can be caused by a number of different problems; these include limited ankle dorsiflexion, particularly in the child or young adult, in whom the subtalar joint can accommodate limited dorsiflexion with valgus posture. Upper or lower motor neuron injury, bony and ligamentous injuries, surgery, and prolonged immobilization with loss of ankle range of motion can all contribute to this deformity. During gait, contact with the ground occurs with the forefoot and weight is borne primarily on the medial aspect of the foot. This position is maintained or worsened during the stance phase and interferes with weight bearing. Antalgic gait can be present if the navicular is overloaded. During the swing phase, sustained plantar flexion of the foot can result in a limb clearance problem unless proximal mechanisms of compensation such as increased hip and knee flexion are used.

Flexion Deformity of the Toes (pp. 106–107)

• The toes might be held in flexion during the swing and stance phases of gait. When wearing shoes, the patient complains of pain at the tips of the toes and also over the dorsum of the phalangeal joints; the pain worsens with weight bearing. Callus formation in these areas is commonly seen. The gait pattern typically shows gradual loading of the affected limb and shortening of the step length and stance time. Likely causes include neurological injuries, a complex regional pain syndrome, prolonged immobilization, and contractures. Clinical examination combined with kinetics and dynamic EMG recordings can be helpful in sorting out the cause of the deformity. In patients with spasticity the recordings likely will demonstrate prolonged or out-of-phase activation of the flexor digitorum longus and flexor hallucis longus, and can demonstrate abnormal co-activation of the gastrocnemius and soleus or lack of activation of the toe extensors.

Hitchhiker's Great Toe (p. 106)

• This deformity is seen in patients with upper motor neuron dysfunction. The great toe is held in extension during stance and often during the swing phase. Equinus and varus posture of the ankle might accompany this deformity. When wearing shoes, the patient commonly complains of pain at the dorsum and the tip of the big toe, as well as under the first metatarsal head during the weight-bearing phase of the gait cycle. During gait, big toe extension can interfere with the weight-bearing phase of locomotion. Overactivation of the extensor hallucis longus and reduction or lack of activation of the flexor hallucis longus often contribute to this deformity.

Joint Instability (p. 107)

Ankle Instability ("Drop-Off" Gait) (p. 107)

• This deviation is caused by excessive and untimely forward progression of the tibia in the mid- to late stance phase. This is usually the result of insufficient calf musculature, which is needed to control the forward progression of the tibia over the stationary foot. In the older literature this clinical picture is referred to as a "weak calf limp." Manual muscle testing of the ankle plantar flexors can be performed by having patients walk on their toes. Obtaining kinetic and kinematic data and dynamic EMG recordings may be necessary to elucidate the biomechanical causes of the problem.

Knee Instability (p. 107)

• Knee instability refers to either knee buckling or hyperextension and typically occurs in early stance phase when knee flexion would normally occur; it is usually due to quadriceps weakness. This weakness can be seen in persons with a lower motor neuron syndrome, other types of knee extensor weakness, or quadriceps tendon rupture. It can also be seen in the early phase of recovery after upper motor neuron injury, when the involved limb is flaccid and weak. A knee flexion deformity further complicates this problem. If knee buckling occurs, the patient might need to use the upper extremities for support. The patient might not produce the normally expected full knee extension in either late swing phase or stance phase, further compromising limb stability. Bilateral knee and hip flexion may be present and can result in a crouched gait. This posture increases energy consumption markedly and results in muscle fatigue and joint pain. The lack of full knee extension in terminal swing limits limb advancement and reduces step length.

Hip Instability *(p. 107)*
• Excessive hip flexion during stance phase is a less common gait deviation. This deformity is characterized by sustained hip flexion that interferes with limb positioning during gait. During the stance phase, excessive hip flexion interferes with contralateral limb advancement and results in a shortened step length. Possible causes include degenerative changes of the hip joint, bony deformities such as heterotopic ossification, knee extensor weakness and ankle plantar flexor posture, hip flexion contractures, and hip flexor spasticity.

Trunk Instability *(p. 107)*
• Trunk instability is an abnormal anterior or lateral lean of the trunk during walking, when the trunk normally is mostly upright. Trunk instability can result from hip extensor weakness, limited hip extension, compensation for knee extensor weakness and ankle plantar flexor posture, and hip flexor spasticity. Hip hiking and contralateral trunk lean can be used to compensate for decreased limb advancement and swing phase clearance problems.

Limb Clearance and Advancement *(pp. 107–108)*

• Limb clearance and advancement occur during the swing phase of gait and are vital precursors to proper limb positioning so that the leg can accept the body weight during the ensuing stance phase. When limb clearance is inadequate, limb advancement is usually compromised. Impaired limb clearance can cause a patient to trip and fall, particularly when walking on uneven, inclined, or carpeted surface. Reduction of limb advancement produces shortening of step length and a reduction in walking speed.

Stiff Knee Gait *(p. 107)*
• Stiff knee gait is most commonly seen in patients with spastic hemiplegia. The use of a locked knee prosthesis for the transfemoral amputee or a locked knee brace by a patient who really needs a knee-ankle-foot orthosis can also cause this gait deviation. In stiff knee gait, the knee and hip maintain an extended attitude in the swing phase instead of flexing up to the normal 60 degrees for the knee and 30 degrees for the hip. Even if the ankle-foot system has an appropriate dorsiflexed position, the lack of adequate limb clearance can result in a foot drag.

Excessive Pelvic Obliquity (Pelvic Drop) *(p. 108)*
• Increased hip adduction can interfere with limb advancement by contacting the contralateral stance leg. In contrast to ipsilateral swing phase hip adductor activity, stance phase hip abductor weakness can compromise both limb clearance and advancement. Normally, hip abductors help counter gravity's pull on the swing side pelvis by producing an abductor moment that helps keep the pelvis level; weakness can allow the pelvis to sag (more obliquity). Imbalance in the abductor and adductor muscle groups is the main cause.

Because many hemiplegic patients use the adductors to compensate for reduced hip flexion in limb advancement, the clinician needs to be certain that elimination or reduction of adductor activities does not result in the patient becoming nonambulatory.

Inadequate Hip Flexion (p. 108)
• Inadequate hip flexion is another cause of abnormal limb clearance. This problem effectively prevents physiological "shortening" of the limb, producing a swing-phase toe drag or early foot contact. The use of compensatory techniques (e.g., hip external rotation or circumduction to promote the use of the adductors to advance the limb) should be attempted. The use of a shoe lift to cause functional lengthening of the contralateral limb can also be done.

Drop Foot (p. 108)
• Drop foot refers to the lack of ankle dorsiflexion during the swing phase, which can result in impairment of limb clearance during swing phase. Compensation for this often includes increased knee and hip flexion (steppage gait), or vaulting up on the toes of the contralateral limb to make it functionally longer. A common cause of drop foot is lack of activation of the tibialis anterior. This can be secondary to a peroneal nerve injury, loss of strength such as that seen in residual polio, spastic imbalance between ankle plantar flexors and dorsiflexors, or out-of-phase activation of the tibialis anterior in the swing phase of locomotion.

SUMMARY (p. 108)

• Gait analysis is a key adjunct to clinical examination and other diagnostic studies in the management of walking and mobility problems. When used appropriately by a clinician who can adequately interpret the data, these tools and methods can provide direct evidence of cause and effect in an otherwise redundant physiological system, a system that can produce a deformity or deviation based on many different muscle and joint interactions or adaptive mechanisms. Gait analysis can also help differentiate primary problems from those that are compensatory in nature. The results of gait analysis can be used to address gait dysfunction treatment, including the prescription of therapeutic exercises, the optimal design and alignment of orthoses, pharmacological treatment (local or intrathecal or systemic), prosthetic alignment optimization, and surgical planning.

6

Original Chapter by Robert D. Rondinelli, M.D., Ph.D.

Practical Aspects of Impairment Rating and Disability Determination

• This chapter attempts to provide the reader with a working vocabulary and conceptual understanding of the processes of impairment rating and disability determination. The chapter is also intended to provide an orientation to the AMA *Guides*.

DEFINITIONS AND TERMINOLOGY (pp. 109–111)

Definitions (pp. 109–110)

• The World Health Organization (WHO) definitions are as follows:

Impairment: "Any loss or abnormality of psychological, physiological, or anatomic structure or function."

Disability: "Any restriction or lack (resulting from an impairment) of ability to perform an activity in the manner or within the range considered normal for a human being."

Handicap: "A disadvantage for a given individual, resulting from an impairment or a disability, that limits or prevents the fulfillment of a role that is normal (depending on age, sex, and social and cultural factors) for that individual."

• The fourth edition of the AMA *Guides* provides the following working definitions for purposes of medical reporting:

Impairment: "The loss, the loss of use, or derangement of any body part, system or function."

Permanent impairment: "Impairment that has become static or well stabilized with or without medical treatment, and is not likely to remit despite medical treatment."

Disability: "A decrease in, or the loss or absence of the capacity of an individual to meet personal, social, or occupational demands or to meet statutory or regulatory requirements."

Permanent disability: "Occurs when the limiting loss or absence of capacity becomes static or well stabilized and is not likely to change in spite of continuing use of medical or rehabilitative measures."

Handicap: "Refers to 'obstacles' to accomplishing life's basic activities that may be overcome only by . . . compensation or accommodation."

- Impairment can be considered in absolute terms, but its relationship to disability and handicap tends to be a relative one. Disability and handicap are perhaps best viewed in the context of performing specific tasks or functions. In terms of employment, for example, if the impaired individual can perform the task or function required of the job without specific accommodation, no disability or handicap exists relative to that function. If the impaired individual can successfully perform only in the presence of specific accommodation, and if that accommodation is provided, again no disability or handicap exists relative to that function. If the impaired individual can successfully perform only in the presence of accommodation, yet the accommodation is not provided, both disability and handicap exist. If the impaired individual cannot successfully perform even in the presence of "reasonable accommodation," a disability exists and a handicap might exist, depending on the degree to which social barriers preclude full accommodation.

Terminology (pp. 110–111)

- Following are some of the terms that commonly appear in the process and procedures of impairment evaluating and reporting:

Aggravation: A circumstance or event that (temporarily or permanently) worsens a preexisting or underlying and susceptible condition.

Apportionment: A determination of percentage of impairment directly attributable to preexisting or resulting conditions and directly contributing to the total impairment rating derived.

Causality: An association between a given cause (an event capable of producing an effect) and an effect (a condition that can result from a specific cause) within a reasonable degree of medical probability. Causality requires determination that:

An event took place.
The claimant experiencing the event has the condition (impairment).
The event could cause the condition (impairment).
It is medically probable that the event caused the condition (impairment).

Diagnosis-related estimates (DREs): Estimates of impairment assigned on the basis of a diagnosis rather than on the basis of findings on physical examination. The AMA *Guides* provide DREs for regional impairments affecting the spine and extremities. The rating physician must choose between the impairment estimate derived by diagnostic and that derived by examination criteria for a specific region. The physician is encouraged to use whichever approach yields the greater estimate.

Ergonomics: The science of matching the job to the worker and the product to the user. An effective match optimizes efficiency, safety, comfort, and ease of use.

Functional capacity assessment (FCA): A generic assessment of an individual's job-related functional abilities, including strength, flexibility, endurance, and overall capability to perform physical work.

Functional capacity evaluation (FCE): A comprehensive assessment of an individual's strength, flexibility, endurance, and job-specific functional abilities. An FCE includes a feasibility assessment of the impaired individual's ability to perform the essential functions of a specific job and could be the most valid predictor of return-to-work potential and restrictions applicable in a given case.

Independent medical evaluation (IME): In cases involving workers' compensation in which either party disputes maximum medical improvement (MMI), an administrative law judge can refer to a separate physician examiner for a second opinion regarding MMI and impairment rating. Some regard an IME as any examination done for evaluation purposes by a physician other than the treating physician.

Job description: A formal listing of the essential functions that constitute a particular job in terms of their specific physical performance requirements.

Job site evaluation (JSE): An on-site analysis of the workplace to determine optimal ergonomic design and to validate specific physical performance requirements of the job. A JSE can be useful in concert with an FCE to determine applicable return-to-work restrictions and to help ensure employer/ employee compliance when necessary.

Maximum medical improvement (MMI): The point at which medically determined impairment resulting from injury becomes stable and no further treatment is reasonably expected to improve the condition. MMI is felt to occur when the following criteria have been satisfied:

The healing period has ended (a minimum documented duration of 6 months since injury onset has been proposed in prior editions of the AMA *Guides*); or
The medical condition has fully resolved; or
No further reasonable progress occurs or is expected to occur toward resolution of the medical condition.

MMI does not preclude the deterioration of a condition that is expected to occur with the passage of time; neither does it preclude allowances for ongoing follow-up or maintenance care.

Medical possibility: Something could occur due to a particular cause (probability of 50% or less).

Medical probability: Something is more likely to occur than not (probability exceeds 50%).

Scheduled loss: Allocation of a specified value for purposes of indemnification to a regional anatomical or functional unit to which an impairment rating can be assigned. The specified value allowed for a given unit can be expressed in terms of weeks or months of lost wages.

Unscheduled loss: Estimated functional loss to the "whole person" for purposes of indemnification and accorded to a physiological system rather than to a regional anatomical or functional unit. The cardiopulmonary, gastrointestinal, and central nervous systems are examples of systems to which an unscheduled loss can apply.

"Waddell's signs": Findings on physical examination that are thought to reflect a "nonorganic" basis of physical complaints and collectively serve to invalidate the examination itself. Five markers are described:

1. Tenderness that is provoked by superficial palpation and/or that is nonanatomical in distribution
2. Pain on simulated provocation by axial loading or sham rotation of the spine
3. Inconsistency of findings with patient distraction
4. Regional weakness or sensory loss
5. Overreaction to the examination

Work hardening: A work-oriented treatment program, delivered in a highly structured environment that simulates the workplace, designed to improve job productivity of an injured or deconditioned worker.

Work simulation: An individually focused work-hardening exercise program that simulates specific components of a specific job for purposes of making a transition to work-ready status and documenting work-ready status.

HISTORICAL DEVELOPMENT OF IMPAIRMENT RATINGS AND DISABILITY DETERMINATIONS (pp. 111–113)

Workers' Compensation (pp. 111–112)

• Workers' compensation is the earliest known disability system, with origins dating at least to Roman times. The United States' system of workers' compensation was created in 1908 under the Federal Employees Compensation Act.

• Workers' compensation in the United States is a federally mandated system of health and disability insurance administered at the state level. Its purpose is to provide benefits to disabled workers for any and all claims of injury or illness arising directly out of employment.

Other Disability Systems (pp. 112–113)

Social Security (p. 112)

• The Social Security Disability Act of 1954, and subsequent establishment of Social Security Disability Income (SSDI) in 1956, provided for a federally administered disability insurance program within the Social Security Administration (SSA) with benefits for individuals who are unable to work because of a disability. The SSA defines disability as the "inability to engage in any substantial gainful activity by reason of any medically determinable physical or mental impairment which can be expected to result in death or has lasted or can be expected to last for a continuous period of not less than 12 months."

• Entitlement is based on the claimant's contributions from prior earnings to Old Age, Survivors and Disability Insurance (OASDI) or by meeting criteria of a "means test." Benefits include a monthly stipend, Medicare supplemental insurance, and coverage for vocational rehabilitation.

• Supplemental Security Income (SSI) provides SSA disability benefits to individuals who meet the SSA definition of disability but who lack evidence of a recent work history. Entitlement is based on financial need according to the means test, and benefits include a monthly stipend, Medicaid insurance supplement, and coverage for vocational rehabilitation.

Department of Veterans Affairs (p. 112)

• The Department of Veterans Affairs (VA) maintains a federally administered disability program available to veterans whose disability is recognized as any condition "which is sufficient to render it impossible for the average person to follow a substantially gainful occupation, but only if it is reasonably certain that such disability will continue throughout the life of the disabled." Service-connected entitlement requires determination that the disability be related to injury or disease incurred during the course of active military duty, whereas non-service-connected entitlement requires determination that the disability was not incurred during the course of active military duty. Benefits awarded to eligible service-connected veterans include a disability pension with monthly financial support, hospitalization and medical care at VA facilities, prosthetic and orthotic devices, durable medical equipment, and home and motor vehicle modifications as necessary and appropriate.

Americans With Disabilities Act (pp. 112–113)
• With the passage of the Americans With Disabilities Act (ADA) in 1990, disabled Americans were guaranteed equal rights to employment opportunities, transportation, and public access. The ADA defines disability as "a physical or mental impairment that substantially limits one or more of the major life activities of such individual, a record of such impairment or being regarded as such an impairment." Although it is broad and somewhat imprecise, this definition is narrowed under Title 1 of ADA (Employment) to recognize employment as a major life activity, and views disability within the context of performance of the "essential functions" of an employment position with or without "reasonable accommodation." Reasonable accommodation can include structural modifications at the work site to improve accessibility, availability of modified duty options, and acquisition of adaptive equipment or devices to enable an otherwise qualified worker with a disability to perform the essential functions of the job. Accommodations exempted under ADA include those that would pose "undue hardship" to the employer in terms of cost or feasibility of implementation, or those that would pose a "direct threat" to the health and safety of the disabled individual and/or co-workers.

Impairment Rating Systems (p. 113)

Early Systems (p. 113)
• The earliest attempts at medical impairment rating systems were anatomically based and regional in scope, with emphasis on the musculoskeletal system.

The AMA Guides (p. 113)
• In 1956, the AMA created an ad hoc committee to address medical impairment rating practices, and this resulted in 13 separate publications in the JAMA from 1958 to 1970. These publications were subsequently compiled into the AMA *Guides,* the first edition of which was published in 1971. By 1981, an advisory panel had been formed to update and revise the *Guides,* and four subsequent revisions appeared from 1984 through 1993.

APPLICATION OF THE AMA *GUIDES* (MUSCULOSKELETAL SYSTEM) (pp. 113–116)
General Consideration (p. 113)

• The fourth edition of the AMA *Guides* is a standard reference for evaluating and reporting medical impairment and is the preferred rating system where permitted by law.

Qualitative Impairments (p. 113)

• Qualitative impairments are anatomically based and belong to discrete, mutually exclusive categories that can only be measured in descriptive terms. Examples of qualitative impairments pertaining to the extremities and recognized by the AMA *Guides* include amputation, joint ankylosis, sensory change (present versus absent), and cosmetic disfigurement (present versus absent).

Quantitative Impairments (p. 113)

• Quantitative impairments are also anatomically based. They are measured according to continuous scales (interval or ratio) whose units represent fixed values, the ordering of which reflects a uniform and consistent increase in magnitude. The AMA *Guides* recognizes loss of motion (in degrees) in each cardinal plane of function for a given joint as representing quantitative impairment relative to the normally accepted range of motion for that joint.

Diagnosis-Based Impairments (p. 113)

• The fourth edition of the AMA *Guides* has advanced a diagnosis-related estimate (DRE) as an alternative approach to impairment rating. It is categorical in nature, less dependent on findings during physical examination, and emphasizes the key elements of history of injury and corroborative, objective findings on diagnostic testing. Where applicable, the DRE model has advantages of simplicity and ease of determination, and it is perhaps less biased in terms of the concrete rating guidelines provided.

Shortcomings and Pitfalls (pp. 113–114)

• Any person who uses the AMA *Guides* should recognize the following key shortcomings:
• First and foremost, the process whereby functional loss is inferred and extrapolated from anatomically determined impairment might not be valid. More specific and objective determinations concerning normal functioning of an organ system and the impact of impairments on an organ system are needed.
• Second, concerns abound with regard to the validity and reliability of the impairment measures conventionally in use. For example, surface inclinometry is the adopted procedure of choice for determining spinal mobility, according to the AMA *Guides*. However, the degree to which surface inclinometry reflects underlying spinal mobility has been questioned.
• The role of pain in disability determinations has been dealt with extensively. Simply stated, pain as a phenomenon is entirely subjective and cannot be measured directly. Consequently, pain behavior or complaints should not serve as the only basis for ratable impairment determination in the absence of corroborative objective criteria.

Extremities as Regional Units (pp. 114–115)

The Hand and Upper Extremity (p. 115)
• The AMA *Guides* has adopted a system for evaluating hand and upper extremity impairment that is divided for purposes of separate evaluation into five regional units: thumb, finger, wrist, elbow, and shoulder.

• Qualitative impairments are as follows: Total loss of motion or sensation within a regional unit or ankylosis/malposition that precludes functional use of same is equated to total functional loss, as would result from amputation of that unit. Ankylosis of a unit or subunit in optimal functional position is considered the least impairment of that unit.

• Estimates of impairment resulting from peripheral nerve dysfunction involve losses attributable to sensory deficits, pain, or weakness. Sensory loss estimates are equated to 50% of comparable functional loss due to amputation.

• Quantitative impairment in terms of restricted ROM for a given member is presented in tabular form as a percentage loss of the normative range for that member. Estimates of ROM are determined goniometrically, using procedures illustrated in the AMA *Guides*. The AMA *Guides* specifies that active ROM determination takes precedence over passive ROM whenever possible, and ROM estimates are rounded to the nearest 10 degrees.

• In some cases, categorical (i.e., diagnosis-based) losses due to joint instability, implants, or other connective tissue disorders not covered in the preceding discussion are ratable according to the appropriate tables of the AMA *Guides*.

The Lower Extremity (pp. 114–115)

• The lower extremity is considered in terms of five regional units: hip, knee, ankle, foot, and toes. Qualitative impairments for amputation and ankylosis are recognized, and tabular references for these are provided. Losses due to peripheral nerve dysfunction affecting the lower extremities and attributable to sensory deficits, pain, or weakness are treated in similar fashion as those affecting the upper extremity. In addition, categorical impairment estimates according to limb-length discrepancies, gait "derangements," and muscle atrophy are separately recognized and tabulated.

Diagnosis-Based Estimates (p. 115)

• The AMA *Guides* separately recognizes diagnosis-based categories of impairment of the lower extremity, including fractures of the regional units, endoprosthetic replacement of the hip or knee, and major skin grafting procedures. Separate reference tables are provided. The examiner is encouraged to use diagnosis-based ratings as an alternative to (*never* in addition to) anatomically based ratings for each specific impairment.

Spine as Regional Units (p. 115)

Qualitative Impairments and Diagnosis-Related Estimates (p. 115)

• The AMA *Guides* has developed the DRE approach to the assessment of impairments of the spine in an attempt to recognize and differentiate clinical findings due to illness or injury from those that accompany the normal aging process. The DRE or *injury model* recognizes specific diagnostic categories for which diagnosis-based ratings can be derived (e.g., vertebral body compression graded according to severity; fracture of vertebral posterior elements or transverse processes; loss of motion segment integrity; cauda equina syndrome; and paraplegia). The spine is treated as three regional units (cervicothoracic, thoracolumbar, and lumbosacral) for which maximal impairment estimates of 35%, 20%, and 75%, respectively, can be derived. Eight categories of gradation of severity are developed that are applicable to recognized disorders of each regional unit; categorical differentiators for each emphasize objective and reproducible evidence of neurological dysfunction or loss of structural integrity.

Quantitative Impairments and Inclinometry (p. 115)
• The traditional, anatomically based approach to impairment rating of the spine is termed the *range of motion model,* and the AMA *Guides* currently recommends its use "only if the Injury Model is not applicable, or if more clinical data are needed." Under this model the three regions of the spine are cervical, thoracic, and lumbar, for which maximal ratings for loss of motion are 80%, 40%, and 90%, respectively. All impairment ratings are rendered to the whole person.

Impairments Due to Specific Spine Disorders (p. 115)
• In situations where the range-of-motion model is being applied, four categories of diagnoses (separate from the DRE model) are recognized including fractures, intervertebral disk or soft tissue, spondylolysis/spondylolisthesis (unoperated), and spinal stenosis/segmental instability/spondylolisthesis (operated). In contrast to the DRE model, this option enables the examiner to take into account surgical interventions and multiple operative procedures in developing the final impairment rating.

Combining Impairments and Whole Person Ratings
(pp. 115–116)
• Impairment ratings derived independently for each regional unit or subunit of the spine and extremities are expressed in terms of scheduled values for each unit (exceptions being the unscheduled expressions of whole person ratings derived by the DRE model or other diagnosis-based ratings described earlier). It is possible for the examiner to combine these scheduled and unscheduled ratings to achieve a single cumulative impairment rating for the whole person according to a *combined values chart* provided by the AMA *Guides.*

IMPAIRMENT AND DISABILITY REPORT WRITING
(p. 116)
• Disability-examining physicians must be thoroughly familiar with the rules, jurisdictional requirements, and nuances applicable to the particular system and locale in which they are working.
• A number of risk factors for *delayed recovery* syndromes have been described and are important items to address in the IME patient history. These risk factors are:

Occupational
Time off work
Low job satisfaction
Patient perception of mismatch between physical capacity and job demands
Lack of modified duty options

Psychosocial
Poor English proficiency
Disabled spouse
Anger toward system
Ongoing or prior litigation/compensation
Disability convictions by patient or physician

Medical
Prior history of injury
History of substance abuse
Poor cardiovascular fitness

• The history serves as an important screening tool to identify patients as high risk, and should address these items inclusively.

PHYSICIAN RESPONSIBILITIES/REPORTING REQUIREMENTS (pp. 116–123)

IME (p. 116)

• In cases involving a dispute between the claimant and the insurer concerning MMI determination or impairment rating derived, a physician examiner unfamiliar with the case can accept a referral from an administrative law judge or other official. The physician should review the case records, examine the claimant independently, and render a second opinion concerning the findings. In some cases, additional testing and treatment is authorized to be undertaken by the examiner to satisfy an MMI determination.

MMI Determination (pp. 116–119)

• The physician examiner is typically required to complete a physician's initial report, supplemental interim reports, and a maximal medical improvement form at the time of case disposition. Reporting requirements vary by state, but they are generally similar and must include an estimate of when MMI occurred or is expected to occur.

Impairment Rating, Causality, and Apportionment (pp. 119–121)

• The physician examiner must determine the nature and degree of physical impairment, if any, and express the impairment in terms of functional loss to the unit or to the whole person.
• The physician examiner might be asked to render a medical opinion "within reasonable certainty" as to causality of a specific impairment. A direct or "proximate" causal relationship is thought to exist if a medical probability exists that the impairment is a direct result of reported illness or injury.
• In cases involving preexisting conditions and/or recurrent injury, apportionment is necessary and involves the physician's best estimate of the relative contributions of preexisting or resulting conditions to the impairment rating that is ultimately derived.

Disability Determination/Return-to-Work Restrictions
(pp. 121–123)

• The AMA *Guides* recognizes that disability benefits, in terms of wage-loss compensation for work-related impairment, are independent of the impaired individual's capacity to work and are formulated in terms of expected long-term negative financial impact of a given impairment category. Indemnification schedules exist and vary by individual states with stipulations of the maximum number of weeks of average lost wages payable for loss of use of body parts.

• During the initial, interim, and MMI phases of reporting, the physician examiner is asked to complete a work status report.

• *FCE* is a comprehensive assessment of the individual's strength, flexibility, endurance, and safety in performing job-specific activities, and it is perhaps the most valid predictor of appropriate restrictions to activity during various points of recovery and at MMI.

• A *job description* is commonly available from the employer and can provide a useful list of the essential functions of the job in question for purposes of assessing functional capacities and addressing specific restrictions that can apply.

• *Job site evaluation* can be carried out by a specially trained therapist to validate the essential functions listed in the job description with respect to critical physical demands and relative amounts of time spent performing specific activities of each essential function. In some cases ergonomic analysis can be useful to quantify physical demands relative to observed physical capacities, and to enable specific recommendations for reasonable accommodation in terms of job redesign or workplace modification.

LEGAL, ETHICAL, AND OTHER CONSIDERATIONS
(pp. 123–124)

• Because of the medicolegal nature of many, if not most, workers' compensation referrals, the physician examiner can regularly expect to serve as an expert witness and to undergo deposition and courtroom testimony. The physician can be expected to testify with respect to even minute details of a specific case, often months or years after completion of the IME.

7

Original Chapter by Andrew D. Bronstein, M.D.,
Shane E. Macaulay, M.D., and Andrew J. Cole, M.D.

Neurological and Musculoskeletal Imaging Studies

- Multiple imaging modalities are available to help in making a neurological or musculoskeletal diagnosis.

IMAGING MODALITIES (pp. 125–128)

Plain Radiography and Its Variants (Stress Radiography, Arthrography, Myelography, Discography, Fluoroscopy, and Videofluoroscopy) (pp. 125–126)

- Five different types of tissues can be imaged with plain radiography: (1) gas; (2) fat; (3) soft tissue/water; (4) bone; and (5) metal (e.g., metals, barium, and iodinated contrast material).
- Stress radiography is a procedure in which stress is placed on a given joint to assess for any change in joint width or alignment caused by ligamentous laxity or disruption, usually in comparison to the asymptomatic normal side.
- Arthrography is a procedure in which iodinated contrast material or air (or both) is instilled into a joint before plain radiographs are obtained.
- Tenography involves injection of iodinated contrast material into a tendon sheath to assess for tendon pathology or rupture of a ligament and abnormal communication with an adjacent joint space.
- Myelography is plain radiography performed after instillation of iodinated contrast material into the thecal sac. Although myelography has largely been supplanted by magnetic resonance imaging (MRI), there are some advantages of myelography over MRI. Myelography and postmyelography computed tomography (CT) better show bony detail and subtle impressions on the nerve roots. Myelography also allows imaging of the lumbar spine in the upright weight-bearing position as well as in flexion and extension. The risks of myelography include hemorrhage, infection/meningitis, drug reaction, nerve damage, and cerebrospinal fluid (CSF) leak/spinal headache, but these risks can be minimized with careful technique.
- Discography is a procedure in which plain radiography is performed after instillation of iodinated contrast material into the intervertebral disk spaces. Suspected symptomatic disks are injected along with a "control" disk. The most

important aspect of discography is whether pressurization of the disk space during injection reproduces the location and quality of the patient's symptoms. Unequivocal concordant symptoms during the injection correlate with that disk being the pain generator.

• Fluoroscopy is the real time x-ray visualization of structures and is used during spinal diagnostic and therapeutic procedures and in the instillation of contrast medium for arthrography, myelography, and discography. Fluoroscopy might or might not involve obtaining plain radiographs.

• Videofluoroscopy entails recording fluoroscopic images to study the motion of joints. It can demonstrate dynamic abnormalities during motion, such as in the cervical spine and especially in the atlanto-axialoccipital region. When there is a question of vertebral fusion in a postoperative patient, dynamic video-fluoroscopy can sometimes be helpful.

Computed Tomography (p. 126)

• Contrast between different tissue types is significantly higher with CT than with plain radiography, and there is more precise localization of structures on the cross-sectional imaging. The imaging plane is usually axial or axial oblique, although coronal images of the foot and ankle and sagittal or coronal images of the wrist and elbow can be obtained with variations in patient positioning. CT has a definite advantage over MRI in the imaging of cortical bone. Additionally, CT can better image chondroid and osteoid matrices. The detection of fractures and delineation of positioning of fracture fragments are achieved well with CT, but a fracture tangential to the imaging plane can be missed, in part because of partial voluming artifact.

CT with Contrast Agent Enhancement (p. 126)
• CT with intravenous (IV) contrast agent enhancement is more commonly used for imaging the brain, neck, chest, abdomen, and pelvis. Intravenous contrast medium is rarely used to image the spine or extremities except in the detection of soft tissue tumors or in the evaluation of postoperative spine patients, especially when MRI cannot be performed because of contraindications or artifacts from metal internal fixation devices.

CT-Myelography and Postdiscography CT (p. 126)
• Postmyelography CT is a requisite adjunct to myelography. The bony intervertebral foramina and spondylosis are best seen on axial CT images. Furthermore, intraforaminal or far lateral disk abnormalities can be invisible on the plain film myelogram and are best shown on CT.

Magnetic Resonance Imaging (pp. 126–128)

• Magnetic resonance imaging is the production of cross-sectional images of the body through placement of the imaged body part in a large static magnetic field with a varying magnetic gradient pulsed in such a way as to allow the resonance of hydrogen to be detected. The data obtained are then converted by computer algorithms into cross-sectional images. Table 7–1 describes the relative advantages and disadvantages of MRI versus CT.

TABLE 7–1 Relative Advantages and Disadvantages of MRI and CT

CT	MRI
Advantages	
Rapid acquisition time	Anatomical and pathological information (proton density,
Less sensitive to motion than MRI	T1, T2, chemical shift)
Detection of calcification and	Better tissue contrast than CT
ossification	Direct multiplanar imaging
Less artifact from metallic foreign	No ionizing radiation
bodies or prostheses than MRI	
Good patient tolerance	
Disadvantages	
Anatomical information	More sensitive to motion than CT
predominantly; less pathological	Longer acquisition time than CT, but getting faster
information than with MRI	Lower resolution for cortical bone or calcification than CT
Ionizing radiation	Considerable signal loss from metallic foreign bodies or
Limited imaging planes	prostheses
	Some problems with claustrophobia, although lessened
	with large-bore or open MRI scanners

- Patients with pacemakers, pacemaker wires, implanted electronic devices, ferromagnetic cerebral aneurysm clips, and metal around or within the orbits should not be scanned. Some other metallic devices are contraindications to MRI, and if there is a question of compatibility with the scanner, the consulting radiologist should be contacted before the examination.
- MRI has multiple available imaging planes, including complex imaging planes. Multiple magnetic gradient pulse sequences are also available to accentuate different characteristics of tissues. Standard pulse sequences include T1 weighting, proton density, T2 weighting, short inversion time/inversion recovery (STIR), and fat suppression imaging. The advent of fast spin-echo sequences has shortened imaging times.
- STIR imaging shows additive T1 and T2 characteristics and has a high sensitivity for edema and many types of tumors. There is also suppression of the signal from fat, which causes the fat to appear dark, although some nonfat tissues can be suppressed if they have a short T1.

MRI with Contrast Agent Enhancement (p. 128)
- IV contrast material is useful for assessing for postoperative scar versus recurrent or residual disk extrusion. Gadolinium contrast agents can show a breakdown of the blood-brain barrier with intramedullary or extramedullary intradural tumors.

Nuclear Medicine Studies (p. 128)

- Radionuclide bone scintigraphy is performed after IV injection of a bone-seeking isotope such as ^{99m}Tc-MDP to detect areas of increased bone turnover. Multiple lesions throughout the skeleton can be demonstrated in a single study, but radionuclide scintigraphy often has a low specificity. It can be useful for whole-body screening for bony metastases, but bony metastases in a given area can also be detected with MRI, which has a higher specificity and spatial resolution.

Ultrasound (p. 128)

• Shoulder ultrasound (US) for rotator cuff pathology was initially popular but has become less utilized with the advent of improved shoulder MRI. US does not provide information about bone, the supraspinatus outlet anatomy, the glenoid labrum, or the glenohumeral ligaments.

IMAGING ARTIFACTS (pp. 128–130)

• Imaging artifacts exist in great variety. Some of the most common artifacts are discussed here as they are routinely seen on image interpretation.

Plain Radiography Artifacts (p. 128)

• On plain radiographs, a common artifact is the Mach line, which occurs when a bony edge overlaps another bone. A thin dark line appears just adjacent to the overlapping bone and can be mistaken for a fracture.

CT Artifacts (pp. 128–129)

• The three artifacts seen most commonly with CT are those of partial voluming, streak, and beam hardening. A partial voluming artifact occurs because a CT section has a finite thickness (e.g., 1, 3, 5, or 10 mm). If a structure extends only through a portion of the section, the attenuation is averaged with that of the structure beside it in the section. For this reason, partial voluming is more likely to occur with thicker sections.
• Streak artifact occurs where there is an interface between tissues of very different attenuation (e.g., bone and air), resulting in linear streaks extending along the plane of the interface. This can be seen at the bone-air interface of sinuses or at the interface of a metal prosthesis and bone. A metal prosthesis can result in both beam hardening and streak artifacts.

MRI Artifacts (pp. 129–130)

• Partial voluming can occur with MRI in that there is a finite thickness of tissue sample to make an image and there can be averaging of signal from tissue components within the thickness of the section. This effect can be reduced with thinner section thickness.
• Magic angle artifact is a phenomenon seen on imaging of anisotropic structures that course 55 degrees (the "magic angle") relative to the main magnetic field in the MR scanner.
• Chemical shift artifact is seen because the resonance frequency of hydrogen varies with the structure that the hydrogen is within. The resonance frequency of fat is slightly different from that of water because of the different hydrogen bonds. Consequently, the reconstruction algorithm can position fat slightly dif-

ferently than water-containing structures, leading to artifacts in the frequency encoding direction.
• Motion artifact is usually visible on MR images as blurring or double images. Flow artifact from vessels or CSF can cause artifacts, usually in a line in the phase encoding direction.
• Metal artifact occurs when either microscopic or macroscopic metal fragments cause a localized change in the homogeneity of the magnetic field. This can result in a focus of signal void with an adjacent high-signal-intensity ring. Artifact from metal can be reduced by using T2-weighted fast spin-echo techniques rather than conventional spin-echo techniques.

IMAGING OF THE SPINE (pp. 130–137)

Trauma (p. 130)

• Plain radiography is the best initial screening procedure to use in assessing for fracture. In the cervical spine, a minimum three-view examination (lateral, AP, and open mouth odontoid) should be obtained. If a fracture is seen or suspected, thin-section CT with reformatting or helical CT can better delineate that fracture and can also disclose other associated vertebral fractures not seen on the plain radiographs. MRI can best show any traumatic disk extrusion or spinal cord abnormality if the patient has myelopathic symptoms. Fast spin-echo T2-weighted images with fat suppression can show soft tissue edema or hemorrhage associated with ligamentous tearing in whiplash injuries in the acute setting, but this study is not routinely done in patients without myelopathy or neurological deficit.

Intramedullary Abnormalities (pp. 130–131)

• MRI is the procedure of choice for assessing the intramedullary spinal cord. Six MRI patterns have been defined by their appearance on T1-weighted images, before and after contrast injection, and on T2-weighted images, with a short differential diagnosis for each.
• Intramedullary primary and metastatic neoplasms are well shown on MR T2-weighted images.
• The abnormalities of multiple sclerosis can be located entirely in the cervical spinal cord without brain involvement. Spinal cord multiple sclerosis plaques characteristically are peripherally located, are less than two vertebral segments in length, and occupy less than half the cross-sectional area of the cord.
• MRI can well demonstrate enlargement of the cord from syringomyelia and may demonstrate an associated Chiari I malformation. If a syrinx involves the entire cervical region with no Chiari malformation to explain it, consideration can be given to imaging the rest of the cord because cord tumors located more caudally can be associated with a holocord syrinx.
• Increased T2 signal within the cord can be seen in areas of chronic compression from degenerative disk disease and from spondylosis. The response to surgical or medical treatment is less favorable in patients with increased cord signal than in those without. Improvement in this imaging parameter after surgical treatment is a good prognostic indicator.

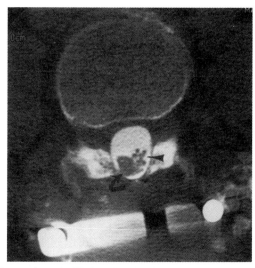

FIGURE 7–1. Postmyelography CT of arachnoiditis following laminectomy, fusion, and dural tear demonstrates clumping of the right-sided roots (*arrow*) with more evenly spaced left-sided roots (*arrowhead*). This clumping was seen just cephalad to the site of dural repair and dural surgical clips.

Intradural Extramedullary Abnormalities (p. 131)

• MRI with IV gadolinium contrast is the most sensitive imaging study for assessing abnormalities within the dural sac, including drop metastases, hematogenous leptomeningeal metastases, meningitis, and arachnoiditis. T2-weighted axial images without contrast can well demonstrate the three different types of arachnoiditis seen on MRI. These include nerve clumping, tumefactive mass-like arachnoiditis, and the "empty sac" sign of the roots being attached to the thecal sac (Fig. 7–1).

Extradural Abnormalities (pp. 131–137)

Degenerative Disk Disease and Spondylosis (pp. 131–134)
• MRI is probably the single best examination to assess the intervertebral disk and surrounding structures; however, plain CT and postmyelography CT can both demonstrate any morphological abnormalities of the disk contour as well. Plain CT or postmyelography CT can show gas within the epidural space from extension through a full-thickness annular tear when the degenerated disk space contains gas (i.e., the "vacuum phenomenon").
• The high incidence of asymptomatic imaging abnormalities in the general population makes it difficult to prove that an imaged abnormality is the pain generator. Discography with pressurization of the disk space may be the most accurate method of determining whether an abnormal-appearing disk is a generator of lower back pain or a generator of pain radiating to the lower extremities in a patient with no MRI evidence of nerve root compression, if

the patient has unequivocal concordant symptoms during pressurization different from a control disk level. However, controversy remains regarding the utility of discography.

• The normal intervertebral disk has a low T1 and high T2 signal, with a lower T2 signal cleft centrally and a surrounding low-signal annulus. With disk degeneration, the T2 signal of the nucleus begins to decrease as the nucleus dehydrates. Once the disk has lost T2 signal, the signal does not return. Loss of the T2 signal can be seen with either intravertebral disk space narrowing or normal disk height, but is more commonly seen with the former.

• Disk herniation is an ambiguous term denoting some form of disk pathology; the pathology can be more precisely described. Other than disk desiccation, there are four stages in the progress of disk herniation:

1. Circumferential bulging of the disk, consistent with weakening of the annulus fibrosis.

2. Protrusion of the disk, in which a focal convexity has a width wider than depth, consistent with a partial-thickness tear through the annulus fibrosis. These partial tears can also show a focus of increased T2 signal that represents fluid or granulation tissue extending through the annular tear. These annular lesions can sometimes appear more like a radial tear; and in some cases more like a partially circumferential tear, shaped like a bucket-handle tear.

3. Extrusion of the disk, in which a focal convexity has a depth greater than the width, consistent with the nucleus extending through a full-thickness tear of the annulus and extending extra-annularly. Other criteria for extrusion that can be used are extension of the nuclear material cephalad and caudad past the levels of the end-plates or visible extension through the annulus and posterior longitudinal ligament.

4. Sequestered or free fragment, in which the extruded disk material is not connected with the native nucleus pulposus. These fragments can be located well cephalad or caudad from the donor site and can extend into the intervertebral foramen. Often these sequestered fragments have different signal characteristics than the native disk.

• Imaging findings of degenerative disk disease must be correlated with clinical history, physical examination findings, and possibly diagnostic injection results; many abnormal imaging findings can be asymptomatic. In 60 asymptomatic patients aged 20 to 50 years old, the patient prevalence of lumbar disk bulge was 20% to 28%. A high prevalence of abnormal findings on cervical MRI of asymptomatic individuals, increasing with age, is also seen.

• Intervertebral disk contour abnormalities can occur anywhere along the circumference of the disk and are usually described by location as central, paracentral, posterior, posterolateral, and far lateral. Posterolateral disk abnormalities can be further described as occurring at the entrance zone, within the foramen, or at the exit zone of the foramen.

Facet Joint Abnormalities (p. 134)

• Facet and pars interarticularis abnormalities can often be seen with plain radiography. Oblique views are necessary to assess for a pars defect (spondylolysis). CT with bone detail is the most accurate means of assessing for a pars defect and can demonstrate any hypertrophic bone formation at the facet or pars contributing to foraminal narrowing. MRI is relatively insensitive to cortical bone defects, and so 30% of cases of lumbar spondylolysis may be undiagnosed if the physician relies on direct visualization of pars interarticularis defects. However, 97% of levels of spondylolysis have been shown to yield one or more secondary MRI signs, including increased sagittal diameter of the spinal canal, wedging of the posterior aspect of the vertebral body, and reactive marrow changes in the pedicle distinct from normal adjacent levels.

• Facet degenerative changes of sclerosis, joint space narrowing, and marginal osteophytosis can be shown on oblique plain radiographs but are optimally demonstrated with CT. MRI is relatively insensitive for demonstrating cortical bone or osteophyte, and shows foraminal narrowing indirectly by effacement of fat around the exiting root.

Spinal Stenosis *(pp. 134–135)*

• Spinal stenosis can be congenital/developmental or acquired. Acquired spinal stenosis can be further classified as central, lateral recess, and foraminal. Central and lateral recess stenosis are usually caused by a combination of disk degeneration, facet hypertrophic change, and ligamentum flavum enlargement. While MRI and CT-myelography can both demonstrate narrowing of the spinal canal, myelography and postmyelographic CT have the additional benefit of showing facet bony detail and end-plate osteophytosis, and allow upright weight-bearing views, which often accentuates the stenosis.

Nerve Roots *(p. 135)*

• Visualization of the nerve roots is excellent on MRI, especially on sagittal images of the lumbar region and thin-section axial images of the cervical region. However, cervical myelography can be better at showing subtle impressions on the root sleeves that are difficult to discern on MRI. Furthermore, postmyelography CT affords a more accurate measurement of the foraminal caliber than MRI, because cervical foraminal narrowing is often accentuated by the pulse sequences used with MRI.

Postoperative Spine Imaging *(pp. 135–136)*

• Postoperative spine patients with residual or recurrent symptoms have special imaging considerations. Plain radiographs can often demonstrate any hardware positioning or failed fusion. If hardware is present, both CT and MRI have some limitations, as described previously. Flexion and extension plain radiographs can show motion at a failed fusion site. CT can show gas within the disk space (vacuum phenomenon), which is an indicator of movement. If the patient is asked to fully flex and then fully extend before CT, the vacuum phenomenon can develop and can be utilized as a sign of nonfusion. With posterior fusions, if the facet joint remains visible and there is resorption of fusion bone, this is an indicator of nonfusion. Persistent lucency above or below a bone plug or anterior fusion cage also suggests nonfusion if enough time has elapsed since the surgery.

• Recurrent or residual disk extrusion is best assessed with MRI before and after IV contrast agent injection to differentiate extruded disk material from epidural scar or fibrosis. Extruded disk material does not show central enhancement during the first 15 minutes following IV gadolinium administration but may show some central enhancement later.

• Non–contrast-enhanced MRI or myelography/postmyelography CT is usually sufficient for imaging the cervical postoperative patient. Contrast-enhanced MRI sequences are not usually indicated in a cervical postoperative patient because most operations are performed by the anterior approach and there is rarely scar formation in the cervical epidural space. If the patient has had a foraminotomy or surgical complication, then cervical spine MRI with contrast agent enhancement might be a consideration.

Infection (pp. 136–137)
• Classic plain radiographic findings of discitis or osteomyelitis can clinch the diagnosis if disk space narrowing and end-plate loss are shown; however, MRI can demonstrate the disk space narrowing, abnormal disk space signal, end-plate loss, and adjacent changes in the vertebral marrow. There is a decrease in the normal high T1 signal from fatty marrow as well as increased T2 signal in the marrow. Most narrowed disk spaces exhibit low T2 signal because of desiccation, so if the T2 signal within the narrowed disk is increased, discitis is a consideration (Fig. 7–2).

Tumors and Extraspinal Abnormalities (p. 137)
• Non–contrast-enhanced MRI is more sensitive in demonstrating vertebral metastatic disease than is radionuclide bone scan. MRI is especially sensitive (relative to radionuclide bone scan or plain radiography) in demonstrating myeloma involvement. However, bone scintigraphy has the advantage of being able to survey the whole body for metastases.
• In the setting of a primary vertebral tumor, it is imperative to obtain plain radiographs and, possibly, CT scans to assess for chondroid or osteoid matrix. Radionuclide bone scan can be helpful in determining whether the tumor is monostotic or polyostotic.

MUSCLE IMAGING (pp. 137–138)

• Muscle is seen as a soft tissue attenuation on plain radiographs, demarcated by adjacent fat planes. Differentiation of the separate muscles and muscular abnormalities is usually not possible with plain radiography.
• Imaging assessment of muscles includes assessment of position, size, and MR signal intensity. CT can be used to assess for position and often size of the muscles, but except for hemorrhage within a muscle, there is little CT attenuation difference between normal and abnormal muscle. MRI is best for assessing muscle position, size, and pathological changes.
• Muscle position is assessed for evidence of retraction, as with a full-thickness muscle or tendon tear (e.g., the supraspinatus tendon in rotator cuff injury). Anomalous muscles, such as an accessory soleus muscle causing an asymmetry between the calf muscles, should not be confused with a tumor.
• Normal muscle has a low T1 and low to intermediate T2 signal. Increased T1 signal can be seen with old intramuscular hemorrhage or chronic fatty atrophy. On STIR sequences an increased T2 signal within the muscle can be seen with trauma, inflammation, and acute to subacute denervation.
• Muscle trauma can be graded on a spectrum from strain (grade 1) to partial tear (grade 2) to full-thickness tear (grade 3). Muscle strain is characterized by a mild, poorly circumscribed, increased T2 signal and greater increased STIR signal, with an intact muscle and no discrete fluid collections within the muscle. There can be some fluid collection in the fascial planes between muscles or beneath the muscle capsule. A full-thickness tear is characterized by retraction

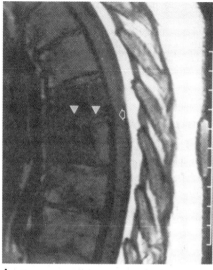

A

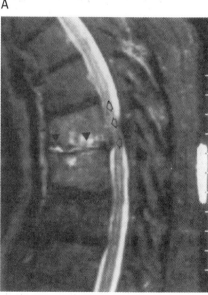

B

FIGURE 7–2. MRI of discitis and osteomyelitis. *A.* Sagittal T1-weighted image at the midline shows decreased signal within the thoracic vertebral bodies adjacent to a narrowed disk space with an irregular end-plate (*arrowheads*). The spinal cord is indented ventrally at the disk clevel (*open arrow*). *B.* Sagittal T2-weighted image obtained through the same area as *A* demonstrates increased T2 signal within the vertebral marrow and disk space with irregular end-plates (*arrowheads*). There is ventral extradural mass effect on the cord at the disk level and posterior to the vertebral body (*open arrows*) consistent with epidural extension of the infection.

of the muscle and free edges, usually with material of increased T2 signal intensity in the gap.
• Acute to subacute denervation of muscle results in a mildly increased T2 signal and more prominently increased STIR signal. Increased muscle signal in the acute to subacute stage changes to fatty atrophy with increased T1 signal and loss of muscle mass in the chronic stage.

NERVE IMAGING (p. 138)

• The larger peripheral nerves can be imaged in cross section on CT when they are surrounded by fat. They are better imaged with MRI, where they have a low T1 signal surrounded by high-signal fat; or with STIR sequences, where they have an intermediate to high signal surrounded by low-signal fat. MRI is excellent for assessing an extrinsic mass effect on nerves (e.g., in the spinoglenoid notch from a suprascapular paralabral cyst or in the brachial plexus from a tumor). Intrinsic abnormalities of the nerves are more difficult to assess on routine MRI unless there is an enlargement of the nerve to indicate the level of abnormality.

TENDON IMAGING (pp. 138–139)

• The tendons can be assessed in imaging studies for position, size, and MR signal intensity. As with muscle, CT can demonstrate tendon position and (to an extent) size, but is unable to show intrinsic abnormalities. The multiplanar capabilities and tissue discrimination available with MRI make it the best imaging modality to assess tendons.
• Tendon position is assessed both in the setting of a complete rupture, where there is retraction; as well as in subluxation or dislocation of an intact tendon, as can be seen with the biceps tendon in a subscapularis tendon tear or transverse ligament tear.

LIGAMENT IMAGING (pp. 139–140)

• Ligaments can be indirectly assessed on plain radiographs by the presence of subluxation or dislocation, or movement with stress maneuvers. The telos stress examination is used to assess the ankle ligaments with posteriorly directed and varus stress. Three-compartment arthrography is utilized to indirectly assess the carpal ligaments for rupture.
• Direct visualization of ligaments is best performed with MRI. Ligaments are assessed for continuity, size, and signal intensity.
• A ligament should be continuous from insertion to insertion, with a smooth linear or curvilinear contour. Waviness of the ligament is consistent with a tear and partial retraction. Some ligaments will have a normal curvature in certain joint positions, and this should be taken into account during assessment (e.g., the posterior cruciate ligament takes a more curvilinear course with the knee in extension and a more linear course with the knee in flexion).

CARTILAGE IMAGING (p. 140)

• Cartilage thickness cannot be directly seen on plain radiographs, although secondary changes of severe chondromalacia such as joint space narrowing, subcortical sclerosis, and cyst formation can be seen. Chondrocalcinosis is probably best detected on plain radiographs. Arthrography can demonstrate the thickness and surface contour of hyaline cartilage, as can postarthrography CT. MRI and MR arthrography best demonstrate cartilage thickness, contour, and any intrinsic signal abnormalities. Fat-suppressed proton-density images show excellent contrast between bone, cartilage, and intra-articular fluid.

BONE IMAGING (pp. 140–141)

• Plain radiography is the initial screening procedure for assessing fractures throughout the body except in the skull, where head CT is the initial procedure of choice. Orthogonal views of the body part of interest are mandatory to exclude a fracture. Some regions require a special view (e.g., a mortise view in the ankle; an oblique view in the hand, wrist, and foot; and an axillary or transscapular view in the shoulder).

• Non–contrast-enhanced CT with or without multiplanar reformatting is utilized to assess the position of fracture fragments in more complex fractures, such as those involving the wrist or ankle-foot. Preoperative assessment of highly comminuted fractures can include CT.

• MRI is insensitive in assessing cortical bone. MRI images mobile hydrogen, and cortical bone has very little mobile hydrogen. MRI does well in assessing bone marrow, as well as bone marrow edema, making it quite sensitive to any fractures or processes that change the normal bone marrow signal.

• MRI is highly sensitive in the detection of reticular infractions (bone bruises); geographic infractions; stress or insufficiency fractures; osteochondral fractures; and, indirectly, macrofractures.

• Assessment for avascular necrosis (AVN) should initially be performed with plain radiography. If the study is negative, then MRI imaging is highly sensitive and specific for AVN.

• Osteochondritis dessecans in its intermediate to severe stages can be well shown on plain radiographs and non–contrast-enhanced CT scans; however, the earliest phase of geographic marrow edema is not visible on plain radiographs, but it is well shown on MR, especially STIR sequences. MR further shows the condition of the cartilage overlying the bony defect and can show if there is loosening, indicated by high T2 signal fluid extending around the lesion or displacement of the osteochondral fragment.

BONE AND SOFT TISSUE TUMORS (pp. 141–142)

• Routine radiography is an absolute requirement in a patient with a suspected bone lesion. If the radiograph is normal and there is focal pain, then MRI is the second imaging study. If the radiograph shows a lesion suspicious for malignancy, MRI is indicated; and if the lesion appears benign on radiographs, CT or MRI is indicated only for preoperative planning. If the lesion is a suspected osteoid osteoma, CT is recommended.

• A whole-body bone scan is useful to assess the entire skeleton to determine whether the lesion is single or multiple. Sometimes bone tumor MR signal can be pathognomonic, such as with an intraosseous lipoma with uniform high T1 fatty signal, or an aneurysmal bone cyst with blood product layering.

• Routine radiography is the first imaging study for suspected soft tissue mass. MRI is usually the second imaging examination recommended, except that CT can be useful for characterizing types of calcification and assessing myositis ossificans, and can possibly be more useful than MRI in areas with motion artifact.

• Certain MR signal characteristics can be helpful in characterizing soft tissue masses, such as high T1 signal fat with a lipoma or liposarcoma, or low signal hemosiderin with pigmented villonodular synovitis (PVNS).

IMAGING OF SPECIFIC BODY REGIONS (pp. 142–147)

Shoulder Imaging (pp. 142–144)

• In the trauma setting, plain radiography is the initial imaging study of choice for the shoulder. Internal rotation and external rotation views, as well as an orthogonal view such as axillary or transscapular view, should be obtained. In the patient with subacute shoulder pain and a question of bursitis or calcific tendinitis of approximately 3 months' duration, the first study recommended is radiography with internal and external rotation views.

Impingement and Rotator Cuff Tears (pp. 142–143)

• Routine MRI is recommended for suspected rotator cuff tear or impingement in patients over the age of 40 years with normal plain radiographs. Direct visualization of the tendons and muscles as well as detection of indirect evidence of rotator cuff tear is available with MRI.

• Assessment of rotator cuff tendon position, thickness, and signal intensity is optimal with MRI. Early impingement results in thickening of the tendon, usually of the supraspinatus. More advanced tendinopathy results in thinning of the tendon. When the rotator cuff abnormality progresses to a partial-thickness tear, there is increased T1, proton-density, and T2 signal intensity within the tendon that reflects a morphological thinning. A full-thickness tear shows through-and-through increased signal; the position of the musculotendinous junction can be identified to determine whether there is any retraction from a full-thickness rotator cuff tear. The proximodistal and AP dimensions of a rotator cuff tear can be estimated.

• Partial and complete rotator cuff tears can be seen on MRI in a significant percentage of asymptomatic individuals, the percentage increasing with age. MRI-evident bone and peritendinous shoulder abnormalities are highly prevalent among asymptomatic individuals, but the prevalence of subacromial spurs, humeral head cysts, subacromial-subdeltoid bursal fluid, and disruption of the peribursal fat plane in each case is closely associated with an increasing severity of MRI-evident rotator cuff abnormalities. US is sometimes used to assess for rotator cuff tear, but it is highly operator dependent and provides less information than MRI.

Glenoid Labral Lesions and Instability (p. 143)

• CT arthrography, MRI, or MR arthrography can be used in suspected cases of labral tear. CT can better show fractures of the bony glenoid. The glenohumeral ligaments are best shown with postarthrography MRI. The abduction–external rotation (ABER) position has been shown to best demonstrate the inferior glenohumeral ligaments.

• The labrum is evaluated for morphology, signal intensity, and position. There is variability in labral morphology, especially at the superior aspect of the anterior labrum. Superior labral anterior to posterior (SLAP) lesions and involvement of the biceps–labral complex are ideally shown following intra-articular contrast agent injection where there is insinuation of the contrast agent between the cartilage and the superior labrum. The axial images can show a Hill-Sachs lesion or Bankhardt lesion of the bony glenoid or labrum if the patient has had a previous anteroinferior humeral dislocation.

Brachial Plexus (pp. 143–144)

• MRI of the brachial plexus can be used to screen for any extrinsic mass compressing or impinging on the brachial plexus. It is also useful to assess for nerve root avulsion with enlargement and tearing of the root sleeve at the intervertebral foramen. However, intrinsic abnormalities of the brachial plexus are more difficult to assess unless there is enlargement of one of the components of the brachial plexus. The components of the brachial plexus are best identified in their relationship to the subclavian artery on sagittal images, which show the nerves in cross section. The development of higher-resolution surface coils might allow better imaging of the intrinsic structure of the nerves of the brachial plexus.

• Impingement on the suprascapular nerve, the first take-off of the brachial plexus, is relatively common and can cause denervation of the infraspinatus and, possibly, supraspinatus muscles. Suprascapular ganglion cysts (paralabral cysts) are well demonstrated on MRI, with high T2/STIR signal intensity. It is thought that most, if not all, suprascapular ganglion cysts are associated with labral tears, but labral tears are often not demonstrated on MRI in these patients.

Elbow Imaging (p. 144)

• Plain radiography in orthogonal planes is the first imaging study that should be obtained in the trauma setting. The posterior fat pad sign or anterior "sail" sign is indirect evidence of a fracture. Fractures in a child's elbow can be more difficult to assess on plain radiographs because of incomplete ossification; MRI can be helpful in these cases.

• Because of its multiplanar capabilities and excellent contrast resolution, MRI is the best modality for assessing the elbow for muscular, ligamentous, or tendinous injuries; bone marrow edema; or osteochondral injury.

• Lateral epicondylitis ("tennis elbow") can manifest with increased T2 signal intensity and thickening of the common extensor tendon. Medial epicondylitis ("Little Leaguer's elbow" in children, medial tendinosis in adults) can manifest with bone marrow edema and medial epicondyle apophyseal separation in children and with increased T2/STIR signal intensity and thickening of the common flexor pronator tendons and muscles in adults.

• MRI can be useful for assessing ulnar nerve abnormalities at the elbow if there is an abnormality of size, signal, or position.

Wrist and Hand Imaging (p. 144)

• In the setting of suspected wrist or hand fracture, preferably three views should be obtained: orthogonal AP and lateral views, and an oblique view. If a scaphoid fracture is suspected, an additional scaphoid view can be obtained that lays out the length of the scaphoid. A carpal tunnel view can be useful in a suspected hook of hamate fracture. Some scaphoid fractures are occult and should be reimaged 7 to 10 days following the initial injury if there is a high suspicion of scaphoid fracture and snuffbox tenderness. The patient should be splinted until the follow-up radiograph. Alternatively, MRI is quite sensitive for occult fractures of the scaphoid and distal radius where there is bone marrow edema and/or intratrabecular hemorrhage early after fracture.

Sacroiliac Joint Imaging (pp. 144–145)

• AP angled and bilateral oblique views of the sacroiliac joints are the standard initial workup. Limited sacroiliac joint CT has proved to be a cost-competitive screening examination that has higher sensitivity for subtle erosive changes of the sacroiliac joints and in the detection of subtle sclerosis.

Hip and Pelvis Imaging (pp. 145–146)

• In the trauma setting, orthogonal plain radiography is the initial imaging study. CT can be considered in the setting of more complex acetabular and pelvic fractures to aid in surgical planning. Fractures, muscle injuries, and soft tissue injuries can be detected with MRI of the pelvis in patients with nonrevealing radiographs after acute trauma.

Avascular Necrosis (p. 146)
• In the setting of unilateral or bilateral hip pain when AVN is suspected clinically, AP pelvis and frog-leg lateral views of the hip or hips are the most appropriate imaging study. If there is evidence of AVN on plain films, MRI can be considered to assess for occult AVN in the contralateral hip. If plain radiographs are suspicious but not definite for AVN or if there is a high clinical suspicion of AVN with normal plain radiographs, then MRI is the most sensitive and specific imaging study to assess for AVN.

Painful Prostheses (p. 146)
• If the initial plain radiographs are normal, but there is clinical suspicion of loosening or infection, then joint aspiration with arthrography is considered the most appropriate study. If the plain radiographs are abnormal and consistent with loosening, but infection is suspected, then aspiration, possibly with arthrography, is considered most appropriate. If aspiration is purulent, arthrography is contraindicated because increased pressure within the joint can lead to intravasation and hematogenous seeding of the infection.

Knee Imaging (pp. 146–147)

• In the setting of trauma, the minimum initial examination includes orthogonal AP and lateral views. If there is a high clinical suspicion of fracture or lipohemarthrosis, then further views (e.g., bilateral oblique, sunrise, and/or tunnel-notch) should be considered. Bone bruise or occult stress fracture are best shown with MRI.

Meniscal Injuries (p. 146)
• MRI is the best method of assessing the meniscus in a patient who has not previously undergone surgery. MRI is noninvasive and multiplanar, allowing

assessment of the meniscus. Radial imaging planes can be obtained that give views similar to those seen with knee arthrography.
- In the setting of an operated meniscus, where the morphology can be abnormal and inherent degenerative change extends to the articular surface, knee arthrography or MRI with intra-articular contrast agent injection can be considered to determine whether the fluid extends into a tear in the meniscus. Comparison with previous studies can be helpful in assessing for recurrent tear versus postoperative change. The two best signs of recurrent tear of the postoperative meniscus on routine MRI are (1) a line of abnormal meniscal signal intensity extending to an articular surface on proton-density–weighted images; and (2) fluid extending into a linear area on T2-weighted images.

Knee Ligament Injuries (p. 146)
- The cruciate ligaments, medial collateral ligament, and lateral collateral ligament complex are best shown with multiplanar MRI. Again, the ligaments are assessed for continuity, caliber, and signal intensity. There is a continuum of sprain, partial tear, and full-thickness tear in the setting of ligamentous injury, similar to what is seen in ligaments elsewhere in the body.
- Discontinuity of the anterior cruciate ligament (ACL) on sagittal and axial MRI planes and failure of the fascicles to parallel the Blumensaat line are the most accurate MRI signs of ACL tear (Fig. 7–3). Multiple other indirect signs are good predictors of ACL tear, including disruption of the fascicles, a posterolateral tibial bruise, a buckled posterior cruciate ligament (PCL), a positive PCL line sign, a positive posterior femoral line sign, displacement of the lateral meniscus more than 3.5 mm posteriorly, displacement of the tibia more than 7 mm anteriorly, and a lateral femoral sulcus deeper than 1.5 mm.

Patellofemoral Abnormalities (p. 147)
- Patellofemoral abnormalities are best assessed in the axial and sagittal planes on MRI. Fat-suppressed proton-density MRI shows excellent contrast between the articular cartilage, bone, and any joint fluid. Grading of chondromalacia is most accurate on axial MRI. Additionally, MRI can demonstrate patella baja/alta and the patellar position within the trochlear groove.

Ankle and Foot Imaging (p. 147)
- A three-view plain radiography that includes AP, lateral, and mortise views is the most appropriate in patients with suspected ankle injury meeting Ottawa rules. Fluoroscopy with stress views may be necessary to assess for Lisfranc fracture dislocations.
- Chronic ankle instability can be detected with a telos stress examination using posteriorly directed or varus stress, although MR arthrography is more accurate and sensitive in the detection of anterior talofibular ligament tears.
- MRI of the ankle or foot provides excellent delineation of ligaments, tendons, and any abnormal bone marrow signal to indicate AVN or a bone bruise/stress fracture.
- The Achilles tendon is ideally shown with MRI in the sagittal and axial planes. MRI can be helpful in differentiating partial tears from tendinitis or peritenonitis. The tendon is assessed for continuity, caliber, and signal intensity as elsewhere in the body.

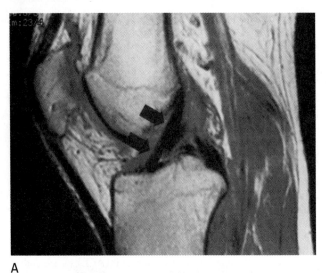

A

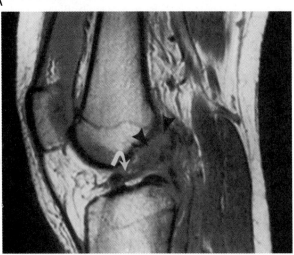

B

FIGURE 7–3. MRI appearance of anterior cruciate ligament tear. *A.* Sagittal proton-density image of the knee demonstrates a normal intact anterior cruciate ligament (*arrows*) with uniform low signal, sharp linear contour anteriorly, and continuous extension from the femur to the tibia. *B.* Sagittal proton-density image demonstrates disruption of the anterior cruciate ligament with loss of the normal low-signal fascicles and intermediate-signal material in the expected location of the ligament (*arrowheads*). The distal stump of the ligament is folded downward (*curved arrow*).

SUMMARY (pp. 147–148)

• Knowledge of the strengths and weaknesses of the multiple imaging modalities available can help the treating physician decide on the optimal imaging study in a given clinical situation for a specific anatomical site. Good communication between the referring physician and the consulting radiologist aids in selecting the most appropriate imaging study or studies and additionally helps in the interpretation of the study.

8

Original Chapter by Carl V. Granger, M.D., Margaret Kelly-Hayes, Ed.D., R.N., C.R.R.N., Mark Johnston, Ph.D., Anne Deutsch, M.S., R.N., C.R.R.N., Susan Braun, M.L.S., O.T.R., and Roger C. Fiedler, Ph.D.

Quality and Outcome Measures for Medical Rehabilitation

- Because an important purpose of medical rehabilitation is to improve the functional status of patients, reliable and valid methods of functional assessment are necessary.

DEFINITION OF FUNCTIONAL ASSESSMENT
(pp. 151–153)

- A *functional assessment* evaluates an individual's abilities and limitations. The essence of it is the measurement of an individual's use of the variety of skills included in performing tasks necessary to daily living, leisure activities, vocational pursuits, social interactions, and other required behaviors.

MEASUREMENT STANDARDS AND PRINCIPLES OF SCALING (pp. 153–155)

- Experts have repeatedly warned that functional assessment scales and procedures now in common use have distinct failings. The empirical properties of scales (e.g., basic validity, reliability, scaling characteristics, and standardization) have been insufficiently developed.

Validity and Related Guidelines (p. 154)

- Validity is the extent to which a test measures what it is intended to measure. Scales of human function or performance may be quite broad or robust across diagnoses, but they still cannot be assumed to have universal or unlimited validity. Content validity, predictive validity, and construct validity are three types of validity that have stood the test of time.

Guidelines for Reliability and Scaling (pp. 154–155)

- Functional assessment tools must have more than external validity characteristics, such as predictive validity; they must also have internal validity characteristics, such as reliability and internal homogeneity of the dimensional structure.

Guidelines for Clinical Application of Scales (p. 155)

• Although measurement standards are based in science and apply most directly to researchers and developers of scales, they also have important implications for clinical practice. Users of measures should read the technical manual or relevant available documentation. They need to understand the scientific basis for the inferences they make from their clinical assessments.

Guidelines for Program Evaluation, Quality Improvement, and Group Applications (p. 155)

• Formal measures are often applied at a group or systems level rather than at the level of individual patients. Group applications include program evaluation, quality improvement, ongoing utilization review, and policymaking by government and managed-care organizations.

EXISTING ADULT FUNCTIONAL ASSESSMENT SCALES (p. 156)

Activities of Daily Living (ADL) Scales (p. 156)

• Activities of daily living refer to those basic skills that one must possess in order to care for oneself independently. Instruments that assess ADL usually assess abilities in self-care (e.g., eating, bathing, grooming, and dressing); transfers; continence; and, in most cases, locomotion. ADL scales are usually hierarchical in arrangement. They include easier activities such as eating, and more difficult tasks such as climbing stairs. The Functional Independence Measure (FIM) and the Patient Evaluation and Conference System (PECS) are examples of scales that include the domains of functional communication and social cognition. Information is collected by observing actual performance, rather than capacity as demonstrated in an artificial setting (e.g., during therapy).
• Table 8–2 in the Textbook describes selected ADL scales that are currently in use in rehabilitation and that meet adequate validity and reliability standards.

Instrumental Activities of Daily Living (IADL) Scales (p. 156)

• The ability to accomplish activities related to maintaining one's living environment is tested using IADL scales. These tasks can include using a telephone, shopping, preparing meals, and managing money. Developing and restoring these skills are often part of a rehabilitation program, but the skills are difficult to evaluate until the individual returns home. (See Table 8–3 in the Textbook for a description of three IADL scales utilized in rehabilitation services.)

Quality of Life Scales (p. 156)

• Quality of life scales denote a wide range of capabilities, symptoms, and psychosocial characteristics that describe functional ability and satisfaction with life. Components of quality of life include social roles and interactions, functional performance, intellectual functioning, perceptions, and subjective health. Indicators can include standards of living and general satisfaction with life.

PROGRAM EVALUATION AND CONTINUOUS QUALITY IMPROVEMENT (pp. 156–163)

Definition (pp. 156–159)

• Quality assessment and quality improvement are "ongoing activities designed to objectively and systematically evaluate the quality of patient care and services, pursue opportunities to improve patient care and services, and resolve identified problems." The directives for achieving quality health care through program evaluation from CARF, the Joint Commission on Accreditation of Healthcare Organizations (Joint Commission or JCAHO), state health departments, and other agencies have been a major stimulus for documentation of outcomes in medical rehabilitation.

Elements of Program Evaluation (p. 159)

• The elements of program evaluation include a description of the purpose of the program (mission statement), program structure, program goals, program objectives, methods of applying measures, and utilization of outcome data in various reports and communications.

Performance Measurement Systems (p. 160)

• The medical rehabilitation industry has been interested in comparing facility data with national comparison data since the 1980s, and many programs subscribe to national performance measurement systems.
• The largest measurement system is the Uniform Data System for Medical Rehabilitation. Medirisk, now Care Data, offered the Formations Clinical Outcomes System, which maintained a database for inpatient medical rehabilitation programs. The Patient Evaluation Conference System (PECS), developed by Richard Harvey and associates at Marianjoy Hospital, has been used by dozens of rehabilitation programs. The PECS provides a comprehensive assessment and is used to organize communication and set goals in the rehabilitation team conference, as well as to evaluate the rehabilitation program.

Uniform Data System for Medical Rehabilitation (pp. 160–163)

• The FIM instrument (Fig. 8–1) and the Uniform Data Set for Medical Rehabilitation are widely used in rehabilitation. A nonprofit organization known as the Uniform Data System for Medical Rehabilitation (UDSMR) was established on the campus of the State University of New York at Buffalo to serve as a repository for information about medical rehabilitation. This data set is now used on a regular basis in more than 70% of the medical rehabilitation facilities across the United States as well as in seven other countries.

FIM™ instrument

L **E** **V** **E** **L** **S**	7 Complete Independence (Timely, Safely) 6 Modified Independence (Device)	**NO HELPER**	
	Modified Dependence 5 Supervision (Subject = 100%+) 4 Minimal Assist (Subject = 75%+) 3 Moderate Assist (Subject = 50%+) **Complete Dependence** 2 Maximal Assist (Subject =25%+) 1 Total Assist (Subject = less than 25%)	**HELPER**	

	ADMISSION	DISCHARGE	FOLLOW-UP
Self-Care A. Eating B. Grooming C. Bathing D. Dressing - Upper Body E. Dressing - Lower Body F. Toileting	☐ ☐ ☐ ☐ ☐ ☐	☐ ☐ ☐ ☐ ☐ ☐	☐ ☐ ☐ ☐ ☐ ☐
Sphincter Control G. Bladder Management H. Bowel Management	☐ ☐	☐ ☐	☐ ☐
Transfers I. Bed, Chair, Wheelchair J. Toilet K. Tub, Shower	☐ ☐ ☐	☐ ☐ ☐	☐ ☐ ☐

Locomotion
L. Walk/Wheelchair
M. Stairs
	☐ W Walk
	   C Wheelchair
	   B Both
	☐
		☐ W Walk
		   C Wheelchair
		   B Both
		☐
			☐ W Walk
			   C Wheelchair
			   B Both
			☐

Motor Subtotal Score	☐	☐	☐

Communication
N. Comprehension
O. Expression
	☐ A Auditory
	   V Visual
	   B Both
	☐ V Vocal
	   N Nonvocal
	   B Both
		☐ A Auditory
		   V Visual
		   B Both
		☐ V Vocal
		   N Nonvocal
		   B Both
			☐ A Auditory
			   V Visual
			   B Both
			☐ V Vocal
			   N Nonvocal
			   B Both

Social Cognition P. Social Interaction Q. Problem Solving R. Memory	☐ ☐ ☐	☐ ☐ ☐	☐ ☐ ☐
Cognitive Subtotal Score	☐	☐	☐
TOTAL FIM Score	☐	☐	☐

NOTE: Leave no blanks. Enter 1 if patient not testable due to risk

FIGURE 8–1. FIM instrument. (From Uniform Data System for Medical Rehabilitation: Guide for the Uniform Data Set for Medical Rehabilitation [including the FIM instrument], Version 5.1. Buffalo, State University of New York at Buffalo, 1997.)

• The data set includes admission, discharge, and follow-up FIM scores, as well as demographic, diagnostic, financial, and length-of-stay variables.
• The WeeFIM instrument is a measure of functional abilities and the need for assistance that is associated with levels of disability in children 6 months to 7 years of age.

Notice: Except as otherwise indicated, all copyrights, service marks, and trademarks associated with UDSMR, FIM, WeeFIM, and LIFEware belong to Uniform

Data System for Medical Rehabilitation, a division of UB Foundation Activities, Inc. ORYX is a trademark belonging to the Joint Commission on Accreditation of Healthcare Organizations. Penn Ability Systems is a registered trademark and PAS is a trademark belonging to the Trustees of the University of Pennsylvania.

9

Original Chapter by Richard T. Katz, M.D., Michael M. Priebe, M.D., and Denise I. Campagnolo, M.D., Ph.D.

Research in Physical Medicine and Rehabilitation

- As recently delineated in the supplement on research published by the *American Journal of Physical Medicine and Rehabilitation,* there are several key reasons why physiatrists must concentrate on research. We have enjoyed an unprecedented growth in the number of specialists in physical medicine and rehabilitation, and this wealth of new physiatrists requires a solid research base on which to practice.

- For physical medicine and rehabilitation to thrive as a specialty, we must develop a clear presence in medical schools, where academic physiatrists are carrying out research and education in contact with peers in other specialties. Physiatric research must demonstrate that the treatments we offer are clinically effective and cost effective, so they will be covered in an age of unrelenting fiscal restraint.

- Finally, research is critical for improving the day-to-day practice of medicine. The skills of clinical research are core knowledge for the improvement of clinical care and should be part of the repertoire for every physician, starting with the residency.

- Since this book is designed to contain only the textbook content that is useful for ready reference on the ward or in the clinic, this very important discussion on research is not presented. Please see the textbook for this important information.

CHAPTER

10

Original Chapter by Daniel Dumitru, M.D., Ph.D.

Electrodiagnostic Medicine I: Basic Aspects

• The electrodiagnostic medicine consultation is the practice of medicine, and as such is predicated on a thorough understanding of the basic science and clinical aspects of nerve and muscle physiology.

PHYSIOLOGICAL FACTORS AFFECTING ACTION POTENTIAL PROPAGATION (pp. 188–191)

• A number of physiological factors have a direct effect on action potential propagation. The most important factor readily amenable to change is a limb's surface temperature. Physiological variables beyond the control of the clinician include the subject's sex, age, height, and digit circumference.

Sex (p. 188)

• A slight increase in the antidromic sensory nerve action potential amplitudes, for both the median and ulnar nerves recorded from the digits, has been noted in women. Also, women demonstrate a greater nerve conduction velocity for upper and lower limb nerves than men. Both of these differences, however, are eliminated when limb length and digit circumference are considered.

Age (pp. 188–190)

• The conduction velocity demonstrates a consistent decline approximating 1 to 2 m/sec per decade. The duration of the sensory nerve action potential (SNAP) is about 10% to 15% longer in 40- to 60-year-olds and 20% longer in 70- to 88-year-olds than in persons 18 to 25 years old. Compared with the 18- to 25-year-old group, the SNAP's amplitude is one-half and one-third, respectively, for the age groups 40 to 60 years and 70 to 88 years old. The distal sensory latencies reveal a similar prolongation with age.
• The newborn's motor nerve conduction velocities are about half of adult values, which are reached by 3 to 5 years of age.

Digit Circumference (p. 190)

• Females consistently demonstrate significantly higher antidromic SNAP amplitudes for the median and ulnar nerves recorded from the second and fifth digits. Because men have significantly larger finger circumferences than women, this appears to explain the difference in SNAP amplitudes.

Height (p. 190)

• Several investigations have documented slower nerve conduction velocities in taller compared with shorter individuals with respect to lower limb nerve conductions. This difference is found to be independent of the limb's temperature or the subject's age. The cause of the difference is unknown, but distal nerve tapering or an abrupt change in axon diameter has been speculated to account for this finding.

Temperature (pp. 190–191)

• As the temperature of the nerve is lowered, the amount of current required to generate an action potential increases. This decreased excitability is a direct temperature effect on the nerve's action potential–generating mechanism at the nodes of Ranvier, not a result of membrane resistance changes. In addition to excitability, the morphology of an action potential is profoundly affected by a drop in temperature.
• The action potential's amplitude, rise time, and fall time all increase as the nerve's temperature declines.
• With every 1 °C drop in temperature, there is typically a 2.4 m/sec decrease in the conduction velocity. Correction factors utilizing subcutaneous and intramuscular readings are equally correct, but it is more convenient and less painful to use surface measurements.
• A cool limb, irrespective of the ambient room temperature, can result in latencies, NCVs, and amplitudes that are not in the "normal" range.

WAVEFORM MORPHOLOGY GENERATION (p. 191)

• See the description in the Textbook.

NERVE AND MUSCLE WAVEFORM MORPHOLOGIES AND CHARACTERISTICS (pp. 191–199)

Nerve Potentials (pp. 191–193)

Sensory Nerve Action Potentials (pp. 191–193)
CLINICAL RECORDINGS
• SNAPs can be obtained with either antidromic or orthodromic techniques. The term antidromic implies that the induced neural impulse propagates along the nerve in a direction opposite to its physiological direction.

SNAP MORPHOLOGY
• Antidromic and orthodromic bipolar SNAP waveform recordings will typically be biphasic rather than triphasic.

• At interelectrode separations of greater than 40 mm, the biphasic potential's negative peak amplitude will no longer grow, but the terminal positive phase will enlarge slightly and may change its morphology. Recording distances less than 40 mm result in the amplitude of the potential declining and the peak latency shortening.

Muscle Potentials (pp. 193–199)

Needle Insertional Activity (p. 193)
NORMAL INSERTIONAL ACTIVITY
• Placing a needle (monopolar or standard concentric) recording electrode into healthy muscle tissue and advancing it in quick but short intervals results in brief bursts of electrical potentials; this is referred to as insertional activity. The observed electrical activity is believed to result from the needle electrode mechanically depolarizing the muscle fibers surrounding its leading edge as it pierces and pushes aside the tissue.

DECREASED INSERTIONAL ACTIVITY
• Muscle that has been replaced by fibrous tissue, or that is otherwise electrically inexcitable, is no longer capable of electrical activity. Consequently, the needle electrode is incapable of mechanically depolarizing this tissue. The result is that few, if any, electrical potentials will be detected following needle movement.

INCREASED INSERTIONAL ACTIVITY
• Practitioners have noted that insertional activity may appear to persist following needle movement cessation. This finding has led to the term "increased insertional activity." In disease states where the muscle is no longer connected to its nerve or the muscle membrane is inherently unstable from primary muscle pathology, the increased insertional activity completes a temporal continuum from the previously normal insertional activity to the development of sustained membrane instability potentials.

End-Plate Potentials (pp. 193–194)
MINIATURE END-PLATE POTENTIALS (MEPPS)
• An active electrode located in the end-plate region can record two distinct potentials. One of the potentials that can be observed is a short duration (0.5 to 2 msec), small (10 to 50 μV), irregularly occurring (once every 5 sec per axon terminal), monophasic negative waveform (Fig. 10–1). These potentials represent the random release of acetylcholine vesicles. Clinically, multiple MEPPs are usually observed with an intramuscular recording electrode, and the sound is referred to as end-plate noise or "seashell murmur."

END-PLATE SPIKES
• A second potential that can be detected with an active electrode placed in the end-plate region is relatively short in duration (3 to 4 msec), of moderate amplitude (100 to 200 μV), irregularly firing, and biphasic with an initial negative deflection. The biphasic potential has an initial negative phase, produced when a current sink originates in the vicinity of the active electrode and then propagates away (see Fig. 10–8 in the Textbook). Triphasic end-plate spikes may also occur if the active electrode induces an action potential in the terminal axon but the electrode's recording surface is some distance from the end-plate. End-plate

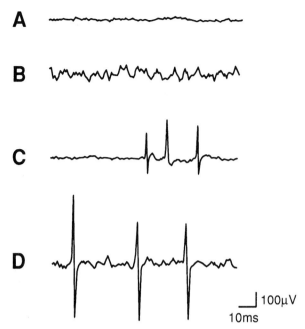

FIGURE 10–1. *A.* Monopolar needle located in a healthy muscle at rest. *B.* Slight needle movement positions the electrode in an end-plate region with the recording of multiple miniature end-plate potentials of a negative spike configuration. *C.* Repositioning the needle electrode to a slightly different region primarily records biphasic, initially negative end-plate spikes. *D.* Advancing the needle electrode slightly permits the simultaneous recording of both potentials noted individually in *B* and *C.* (From Dumitru D: Electrodiagnostic Medicine. Philadelphia, Hanley & Belfus, 1995, p. 220.)

spikes and MEPPs are commonly observed together because they arise from the same region (see Fig. 10–1).

Single Muscle Fiber (p. 194)
• The single muscle fiber's extracellular waveform morphology, like nerve tissue, depends on the characteristics of the muscle's intracellular action potential. A muscle's action potential is approximately 4 to 20 times longer than a nerve's, due in particular to the prolonged repolarization process. A triphasic waveform with a small terminal phase can be seen when recording from an extracellular active electrode placed adjacent to a propagating single muscle fiber action potential at some distance from the end-plate region.

Motor Unit Potential Morphology (pp. 194–198)
ANATOMY
• One anterior horn cell gives rise to a peripheral axon that splits into multiple terminal axons, each of which innervates a single muscle fiber. The anterior horn cell, its axon, and all the single muscle fibers supplied by that nerve are referred

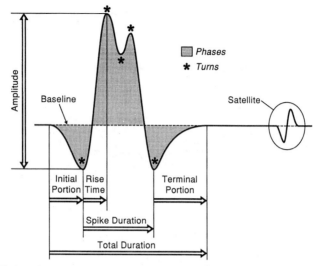

FIGURE 10–2. A motor unit action potential is depicted with various morphological aspects measured. (From Dumitru D: Electrodiagnostic Medicine. Philadelphia, Hanley & Belfus, 1995, p. 53.)

to as a motor unit. The electrical activity from all of these muscle fibers summates to produce a motor unit action potential (MUAP).

• The muscle fibers of a single motor unit are randomly distributed in an oval territory 4 to 6 mm in circumference. The random distribution implies that the single muscle fibers may be in groups of different numbers or singly arranged within the 4 to 6 mm area. Five to ten or more different motor units may share this area.

AMPLITUDE/RISE TIME

• The morphology of an MUAP can be described in terms of its *amplitude* (maximum peak-to-peak CRT trace displacement), *rise time* (temporal aspect of a potential's peak), *duration* (departure from and return to baseline), and number of *phases* (baseline crossings plus one) (Fig. 10–2).

DURATION

• The MUAP's duration depends on (1) the shortest and longest lengths of terminal axons from the point they separate from the parent nerve to the end-plate; and (2) the conduction velocities of the terminal axons and muscle fibers, with respect to the recording electrode, and the muscle fiber length (see Fig. 10–2). A MUAP's duration is the most sensitive clinical parameter in diagnosing disease.

PHASES

• As previously stated, the single muscle fiber usually has a triphasic appearance when recorded outside of the end-plate zone and away from the tendinous insertion. The voltages from all of the single muscle fibers belonging to one motor unit summate to yield a MUAP that is also usually triphasic (positive-negative-positive). This voltage summation does not always produce a smooth result, and small serrations or *turns* can occasionally be seen as part of a MUAP's major phase (see Fig. 10–2). The number of *phases* is defined as the number of CRT trace baseline crossings plus one. Normal MUAPs are considered to have four or fewer phases. MUAPs with five or more phases are called *polyphasic potentials.* Recordings of multiple MUAPs from normal muscle tissue can have between 12% (concentric needle) to 35% (monopolar needle) polyphasic potentials, depending on the type of recording electrode used. Slightly different MUAP morphologies can be expected, depending on the exact location of the recording electrode with respect to different single muscle fibers within the motor unit territory.

Compound Muscle Action Potential (pp. 198–199)
• To elicit a CMAP from a particular muscle, the active electrode is located on the skin's surface directly over the muscle's motor point (end-plate region). The end-plate region typically lies midway between the muscle's origin and insertion. The reference electrode is usually placed on or distal to the tendinous insertion of the muscle so as not to record electrical activity from the activated muscle. Stimulating the peripheral nerve innervating the muscle will result in a relatively large, biphasic waveform with an initial negative deflection (see Fig. 10–15 in the Textbook).
• Occasionally a positive deflection can precede the CMAP's negative phase. Relocating the active electrode over the anticipated motor point region will usually remedy the situation.

MUSCLE GENERATORS OF ABNORMAL SPONTANEOUS POTENTIALS (pp. 199–202)

Fibrillation Potentials (pp. 199–200)

• In vitro observations have shown that about 6 days or so after denervation, the muscle fiber's resting membrane potential decreases to a less negative level of −60 mV, compared with the normal value of −80 mV. Additionally, the resting membrane potential begins to oscillate. Because the threshold level for starting the all-or-none self-sustaining action potential is now closer to the new resting membrane potential, the oscillating membrane potential will eventually reach the threshold level. Once threshold is achieved, a propagating action potential is induced in the muscle fiber; this is referred to as a fibrillation potential.
• Fibrillation potentials are simply spontaneous depolarizations of a single muscle fiber; they demonstrate waveform morphologies similar to those of single muscle fibers that are voluntarily activated (see Fig. 10–4 in the Textbook). Fibrillation potentials occur not only spontaneously, but also can be provoked by electrode movement in pathological tissue. Fibrillation potentials are typically short in duration (less than 5 msec), less than 1 mV in amplitude, and fire at rates between 1 and 50 Hz. They have a typical sound likened to a high-pitched tick or "rain on a tin roof" when amplified through a loudspeaker. When the recording electrode is located in the previous end-plate zone of a denervated muscle, fibrillation potentials can be biphasic with an initial positive deflection.

Positive Sharp Waves (pp. 200–201)

• A potential that can be recorded from a single muscle fiber having an unstable muscle membrane potential secondary to denervation or intrinsic disease

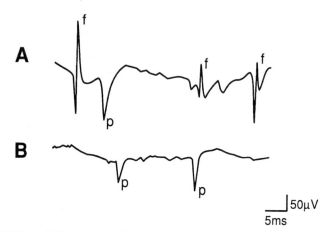

FIGURE 10–3. *A.* Monopolar needle recording of positive sharp waves (*p*) and fibrillation potentials (*f*). *B.* Only positive sharp waves are depicted. (From Dumitru D: Electrodiagnostic Medicine. Philadelphia, Hanley & Belfus, 1995, p. 230.)

typically has a large primary, sharp, positive deflection followed by a small or absent negative potential. These potentials are called positive sharp waves (PSWs) (Fig. 10–3). This waveform is believed to have the same clinical significance as a fibrillation potential in that it is a single muscle fiber discharge. Amplified through a loudspeaker, positive sharp waves have a regularly firing rate (1 to 50 Hz) and a dull thud sound. Their durations are from several milliseconds to 100 msec. Although observed to fire spontaneously, PSWs are more often provoked by electrode movement.

Complex Repetitive Discharge (pp. 201–202)

• A complex repetitive discharge (CRD) is a spontaneously firing group of action potentials (formerly called a bizarre high-frequency discharge or pseudomyotonic discharge). These potentials cannot be observed visually and require a needle-recording electrode to be detected. Morphologically, these potentials are continuous runs of simple or complex spike patterns that regularly repeat at 0.3 to 150 Hz. The repetitive pattern of spike potentials has the same appearance with each firing, and bears the same relationship with its neighboring spikes. A distinct sound likened to heavy machinery or an idling motorcycle is produced by the firing of CRDs. In addition to the sound and repetitive pattern, a hallmark of these waveforms is that they start and stop abruptly.

Myotonic Discharges (p. 202)

• The phenomenon of delayed muscle relaxation following muscle contraction is referred to as myotonia or action myotonia. The finding of delayed muscle relaxation after reflex activation, or after being induced by striking the muscle belly with a reflex hammer, is called percussion myotonia. Clinical myotonia is usually accentuated by energetic muscle activity following a period of rest. Con-

tinued muscle contraction lessens the myotonia and is known as the "warmup." It is believed that cooling the muscle accentuates myotonia, but this finding has been objectively documented only in paramyotonia congenita.
• Myotonic discharges may present in one of two waveform types (see Fig. 10–19 in the Textbook). The myotonic potential induced by needle electrode insertion usually assumes a morphology similar to that of a PSW. It is believed that the needle movement induces a repetitive firing of the unstable membranes of multiple single muscle fibers. This is because the recording needle is thought to have damaged that portion of the muscle fiber with which it is in contact. Myotonic potentials may also appear as a series of rapidly firing triphasic single muscle fiber potentials following muscle contraction. Regardless of the waveform type, the hallmark of myotonia is a waxing and waning in both frequency and amplitude. The myotonic discharge has a characteristic sound likened to a dive bomber and easily recognized. Amplitudes range from $10\,\mu V$ to $1\,mV$ and firing rates from $20\,Hz$ to $100\,Hz$.
• Myotonic discharges can occur with or without clinical myotonia. The observation of these potentials requires needle movement or muscle contraction. These potentials persist after nerve block, neuromuscular block, or frank denervation. This suggests that their site of origin is the muscle membrane itself. Although the exact mechanism of myotonic discharge production remains unclear, it is proposed that decreased chloride conductance is responsible at least in part for the findings in myotonia congenita. In addition to the syndromes noted above, myotonic discharges can also be detected at times in acid maltase deficiency and polymyositis.

NEURAL GENERATORS OF ABNORMAL SPONTANEOUS POTENTIALS (pp. 202–204)

Fasciculation Potentials (pp. 202–203)

• The visible spontaneous contraction of a portion of muscle is referred to as a fasciculation. When these contractions are observed with an intramuscular needle-recording electrode, they are called fasciculation potentials. A fasciculation potential is the electrically summated voltage of depolarizing muscle fibers belonging to all or part of one motor unit. Occasionally fasciculation potentials may only be documented with needle electromyography because they lie too deep in muscle to be seen.
• Fasciculations have a discharge rate (1 Hz to many per minute) that is irregular. They are not under voluntary control, nor are they influenced by mild contraction of the agonist or antagonist muscles. The site of origin of fasciculation potentials remains unclear, although it appears that the spontaneous discharge may arise from the anterior horn cell, or along the entire peripheral nerve (particularly the terminal portion), and at times within the muscle itself.
• Fasciculation potentials occur in normal subjects and in patients with a variety of diseases. Typical diseases in which fasciculation potentials may be found include motor neuron disorders, radiculopathies, entrapment neuropathies, and cervical spondylotic myelopathy. Fasciculation potentials have also been described in metabolic disturbances including tetany, thyrotoxicosis, and anticholinesterase overdose. There is no reliable way to categorize whether fasciculation potentials indicate a disease state just by considering their inherent characteristics based on routine needle electromyography.

Myokymic Discharge (p. 203)

• Myokymia is a readily observable vermicular ("bag of live worms") or rippling movement of the skin. It is usually associated with myokymic discharges. The myokymic discharge consists of bursts of normal-appearing motor units with interburst silent intervals. Typically the firing rate is 0.1 to 10 Hz in a semirhythmic pattern. Two to ten potentials within a single burst may fire at 20 to 150 Hz. These potentials are not affected by voluntary contraction (see Fig. 10–21 in the Textbook).

Continuous Muscle Fiber Activity (pp. 203–204)

• A number of relatively rare syndromes producing continuous muscle fiber activity associated with muscle stiffness have been reported. Portions of both the central and peripheral nervous system have been implicated in generating the sustained firing of motor units. One syndrome with continuous muscle fiber activity is known as "stiff-man syndrome." The motor unit discharges in this condition are believed to have a central origin because they are abolished or attenuated by peripheral nerve block, neuromuscular block, spinal block, general anesthesia, and sleep.

• A "peripheral" form originating in the peripheral motor axon is referred to as Isaac's syndrome or neuromyotonia.

Cramps (p. 204)

• A sustained and possibly painful muscle contraction of multiple motor units lasting seconds or minutes may appear in normal individuals or in specific disease states. In healthy subjects, a cramp usually occurs in the calf muscles or other lower extremity muscles following exercise, abnormal positioning, or maintaining a fixed position for a prolonged time. Cramps may also be induced by hyponatremia, hypocalcemia, vitamin deficiency, or ischemia. They also occur in early motor neuron disease and in peripheral neuropathies.

• A needle-recording electrode placed into a cramping muscle shows multiple motor units firing synchronously at between 40 and 60 Hz and occasionally reaching 200 to 300 Hz. A large portion of the muscle is simultaneously involved in a cramp, as opposed to the asynchronous excitation of motor units during voluntary activation. Cramps are believed to arise from a peripheral portion of the motor unit.

Multiplet Discharges (p. 204)

• A clinical syndrome manifested by spontaneous muscle twitching, cramps, and carpopedal spasm is known as tetany. This entity usually results from peripheral and/or central nervous system irritability associated with systemic alkalosis, hypocalcemia, hyperkalemia, hypomagnesemia, or local ischemia. Clinically one may induce tetany by tapping the facial nerve (Chvostek's sign), by tapping the peroneal nerve at the fibular head (peroneal sign), or by inducing limb ischemia (Trousseau's sign).

• In the above conditions, characteristic MUAPs may be observed. A single MUAP may fire rather rapidly with an interdischarge interval of 2 to 20 msec. If the motor unit fires twice, it is referred to as a doublet; if three times, it is called a triplet; and if more than three times, it is called a multiplet (see Fig. 10–24 in the Textbook). These potentials can be seen following voluntary contraction or can be observed to result spontaneously from the induction maneuvers noted above (Chvostek's sign or Trousseau's sign), in which MUAPs may fire in long trains or short bursts of 5 to 30 Hz (tetany). MUAPs with an interdischarge interval of 20 to 80 msec are called paired discharges but can arise in similar states, as previously described.

NERVE INJURY CLASSIFICATION (pp. 204–206)

• Peripheral nerve injury is one of the most common types of pathology likely to be encountered during an electrodiagnostic medicine classification.

Seddon's Classification (pp. 205–206)

• The degree to which a nerve is damaged has obvious implications with respect to its present function and potential for recovery. Seddon's classification considers neural injury from the perspective of a combination of functional status and histological appearance. In Seddon's scheme there are three degrees or stages of injury to consider: (1) *neurapraxia,* (2) *axonotmesis,* and (3) *neurotmesis.*

Neurapraxia *(p. 205)*
• The term *neurapraxia* is used to designate a mild degree of neural insult that results in blockage of impulse conduction across the affected segment. It is also acceptable to designate this type of neural insult simply as *conduction block.* The most important aspect of conduction block is its reversibility.

Axonotmesis *(p. 206)*
• The second degree of neural insult in Seddon's classification is *axonotmesis,* a specific type of nerve injury in which only the axon is physically disrupted, with preservation of the enveloping endoneurial and other supporting connective tissue structures (perineurium and epineurium). Compression of a profound nature or traction on the nerve are typical lesion etiologies. Once the axon has been disrupted, the characteristic changes of Wallerian degeneration occur.

Neurotmesis *(p. 206)*
• The greatest degree of nerve disruption is designated in Seddon's system as *neurotmesis.* This is complete disruption of the axon and all supporting connective tissue structures, including the endoneurium, perineurium, and epineurium, which are no longer in continuity. A neurotmetic lesion has a poor prognosis for complete functional recovery. Surgical reapproximation of the nerve ends will likely be required. Surgery does not guarantee proper endoneurial tube alignment, but at least it improves the chances that axonal growth will occur across the injury site.

Sunderland's Classification (p. 206)

• A second popular and somewhat more detailed classification is that proposed and subsequently modified by Sunderland. This classification of nerve injury is based on the results of trauma with respect to the axon and its supporting connective tissue structures. Basically, Sunderland's classification is divided into five types of injury, based exclusively on which connective tissue components are disrupted (see Fig. 10–25 in the Textbook). Type 1 injury corresponds to Seddon's designation of neurapraxia. Seddon's axonotmesis is subdivided by Sunderland into three forms of neural insult (types 2 to 4). A type 2 injury involves loss of axonal continuity with preservation of all supporting neural structures, including the endoneurium (closely corresponding to Seddon's axonotmesis). Type 3 and 4 injuries result in progressively more neural disruption. Sunderland's type 5 injury corresponds to Seddon's neurotmesis (complete neural disruption).

INSTRUMENTATION (pp. 206–211)

• An electrodiagnostic instrument comprises many separate components. The most important of these are the electrodes, amplifier, filters, speaker, analog-to-digital (A/D) converter, CRT, and stimulator (see Fig. 10–26 in the Textbook).

Electrodes (pp. 206–207)

• The two basic types of electrodes are surface and needle. Surface electrodes are manufactured in various sizes and shapes for conformity to the body part under investigation. Well-secured electrodes minimize movement artifact that could contaminate the desired signal. Commercially available disposable self-adhering electrodes are now available and eliminate the need for tape.
• Two basic types of needle recording electrodes are commonly used, monopolar and concentric. The monopolar needle is a solid stainless steel shaft coated completely with Teflon except for the bare metal tip. It is this bare metal tip that acts at the recording surface. The needle is typically 12 to 75 mm long and 0.3 to 0.5 mm in diameter, with a recording surface of 0.15 to 0.6 mm². Separate reference and ground electrodes are required. The concentric needle electrode is a hollow stainless steel hypodermic needle with a central platinum or nichrome-silver wire about 0.1 mm in diameter, surrounded by epoxy resin acting as an insulating material from the surrounding cannula. The cannula has a similar length and diameter as the monopolar needle. A separate ground is required, but the cannula serves as the reference electrode.
• Both electrodes have advantages and disadvantages, depending on the clinical circumstances. Monopolar needle electrodes have a wider recording territory and a distant reference, thereby making the recording "noisier" with respect to distant activity and interference. On the other hand, the Teflon coating reduces patient discomfort. The concentric needle electrode has the active and reference electrodes close together, making them quieter than monopolar needles. Concentric needle electrodes, compared with monopolar needle electrodes, give the following: smaller potential amplitudes, possibly fewer phases, comparable durations, and less distant activity. The durations of potentials recorded with monopolar and concentric needle electrodes are the same. The quality of disposable needle electrodes has improved, eliminating the need to use nondisposable needle electrodes.
• Single-fiber electrodes are essentially modified concentric needle electrodes. A small, 25-μm recording port is placed opposite the electrode's bevel and

several millimeters from the tip. The uptake area for this electrode is approximately 300 μm (see Fig. 10–27 in the Textbook).

Amplifier (pp. 207–208)

• The size of biological signals is on the order of microvolts or millivolts and thus must be amplified before being analyzed. Amplification is expressed as gain or sensitivity. Gain is a ratio of the signal's output divided by the input. For example, an output of 1 V for an input of 10 mV implies that the amplifier has a gain factor of 100,000 (output/input = 1 V × 0.00001 V = 100,000). Sensitivity is the ratio of the input voltage to the size of deflection on the CRT and is usually measured in centimeters. For example, an amplifier that produces a 1-cm deflection for an input of 10 mV has a sensitivity of 10 mV/cm or 10 mV/division. The sensitivity or gain setting used is important because it can influence the onset latency.

• The standard electromyograph has two amplifiers. Both amplified signals (inverted and noninverted) are then electronically summated, and like signals are canceled. This is the concept of differential amplification. When the same signal is presented to both amplifiers, theoretically there should be no output from the instrument because there is elimination of the same or common signals. For example, 60 Hz interference recorded by the active and reference electrodes is eliminated as a common mode signal. It is impossible to build two amplifiers with identical properties, so common mode rejection can never be perfect. The ratio of the instrument's output when the same signal is presented to both amplifiers is the common mode rejection ratio. This number should exceed 10,000:1.

Filters (pp. 208–210)

• Perhaps the least understood and most ignored aspect of the instrument is the filters. The main purpose of filters is to form a window or bandwidth of frequencies contained within the desired waveform, but excluding those frequencies not comprising the signal of interest ("noise"). Low- and high-frequency filters are used to prevent those frequencies below and above the respective filter settings from being amplified and subsequently presented for display.

• There are no universally agreed-upon filter settings for any electrodiagnostic medicine procedure. Arriving at optimal filter settings is highly empirical. The high- and low-frequency filters are lowered and raised, respectively, until waveform distortions are observed. The goal is to include the major components of the waveforms while eliminating undesired signals or noise. The most important factor is to reproduce all filter settings originally described by those investigators whose normative data are being used. Recommended filter settings can be seen in Table 10–3 in the Textbook.

Sound (p. 210)

• After the biological signal is filtered it is fed to a loudspeaker. It is not uncommon for practitioners to "hear" an abnormality prior to viewing it on the CRT. The instrument must have a relatively good speaker to accurately present the sounds associated with the biological signals.

Analog-to-Digital Conversion (p. 210)

• All of today's commercially available instruments employ the conversion of a real-time analog signal to a digital representation of the recorded waveform. This is accomplished by sampling the potential at a given rate or frequency and assigning a digital representation of the waveform in the computer's memory.

Averager (p. 210)

• Most modern instruments typically have the capacity for averaging multiple responses. The goal of averaging a number of responses is to improve the size of the signal compared to the background noise (i.e., improve the signal-to-noise ratio). Responses can be averaged by taking advantage of the fact that the desired signal can be time-locked to appear in constant time referenced to a delivered electrical stimulus or internal instrument marker.

Stimulator (pp. 210–211)

• Two different types of stimulators are commercially available, constant current and constant voltage. For both types of devices, neural tissue is activated under the cathode (negative pole) while the anode (positive pole) completes the stimulating circuit.

SUMMARY (p. 211)

• Mastering the information provided in this chapter gives the practitioner a firm grasp of the fundamental principles that underpin the electrodiagnostic medicine consultation.

11

Original Chapter by Lawrence R. Robinson, M.D.

Electrodiagnostic Medicine II: Clinical Evaluation and Findings

CLINICAL ASSESSMENT (pp. 213–215)

• The electrodiagnostic medical consultation is a history and physical examination extended by the singular capabilities of electrophysiological testing, which can include nerve conduction studies, needle electromyography (EMG), somatosensory-evoked potentials (SEPs), single-fiber EMG, and other studies. The consultation starts with a directed history and physical examination and uses electrophysiological testing to help distinguish among the possible differential diagnoses in a more sensitive fashion than is possible with clinical examination alone.

• The electrodiagnostic consultation relies greatly on the consultant's history and physical examination and is a dynamic process. The specific methods employed depend on the clinical assessment and are contingent on the outcomes of some of the initial tests. These can change dynamically throughout the consultation.

• Diagnoses should not be made solely on electrophysiological "abnormalities" but must always be made in the context of the patient's clinical presentation.

History (pp. 213–214)

• The history should be initially directed toward the presenting chief complaint. The time since onset of symptoms is extremely important because the electrophysiological findings evolve over time. For instance, a radiculopathy studied 5 days after onset of symptoms is unlikely to show as much electrophysiological evidence of denervation as one studied 21 days after onset of symptoms. Finding out whether symptoms are intermittent or constant is also important because the likelihood of finding abnormalities on the electrophysiological examination is higher in the case of constant symptoms. The distribution of symptoms is also relevant. Although symptoms are usually reported initially in one or two limbs, the examiner should also ask about other limbs. The patient with hand numbness, for example, could have entrapment neuropathy in the upper limbs.

• The examiner should routinely ask about patient medications, thereby eliciting other pertinent diagnoses and uncovering possible toxic exposures. Such questions may also reveal the possibility of anticoagulation (which is critical to know before starting a needle examination). It is also necessary to obtain a history of systemic disease that might contribute to the chief complaint (e.g., a history of diabetes mellitus, extensive alcohol intake, or rheumatologic disease). It is also important to know whether or not the presenting symptoms have occurred in the past so that finding old electrophysiological changes is not confusing.

• Finally, the examiner should always inquire about the family history of similar or congenital diseases. It is occasionally necessary to examine or test potentially affected family members.

Physical Examination (p. 214)

• Whereas the history contributes most significantly to establishing a differential diagnosis, physical examination offers more objective evidence of peripheral nervous system dysfunction. In most cases, the four most important examinations are muscle strength, sensation, muscle stretch reflexes, and provocative signs.

• Sensory testing should be directed at eliciting subtle deficits in sensation. Unlike patients with spinal cord injury, patients with entrapment neuropathies or radiculopathies often have mild or difficult-to-assess sensory losses. Pinprick and light touch sensation in a questionable area should be compared with that of an asymptomatic area (such as the cheek or forehead) or with the same location on the other side if it is not symptomatic. A useful technique is to touch the asymptomatic area first, then the symptomatic area, asking the patient, "If this (asymptomatic) area is 100%, how much is this (symptomatic) area?" Two-point discrimination has been shown to pick up milder deficits in sensation than simple pinprick testing. Testing vibration is useful if particular involvement of large fibers (as in peripheral polyneuropathy) is expected or if the dorsal column pathways are expected to be spared (as in syringomyelia).

• Muscle stretch reflexes (MSRs) are probably the most objective finding in the examination of the peripheral nervous system because they are not easily influenced by patient cooperation or reporting. In addition to the commonly elicited reflexes in the upper limb (i.e., biceps, brachioradialis, and triceps) and lower limb (i.e., knee and ankle), other MSRs should be considered. In the lower limbs, the most common level for radiculopathy is L5. Because the knee jerk largely represents L4 input, and the ankle jerk largely S1 input, it is quite easy to miss reflex changes in an L5 radiculopathy unless the medial hamstring or tibialis posterior reflexes are checked routinely. In the upper limb, C7 is the most common level for radiculopathy. Although the triceps reflex is useful in this regard, the pronator teres reflex (elicited by tapping the neutrally positioned forearm into supination and palpating over the pronator teres) can be useful for detecting C6 or C7 changes.

• Several useful provocative tests can be employed in the physical examination before electrophysiological studies. When considering entrapment neuropathies, Phalen's test is a moderately sensitive and specific test for detecting median nerve compression at the wrist. This is performed by keeping the wrist in sustained flexion for 60 seconds and monitoring for paresthesias. Tinel's sign (originally developed for detecting the most distal site of peripheral nerve regeneration) is sensitive but not very specific. When considering the possibility of cervical radiculopathy, the examiner should look for Spurling's sign by bringing the neck into extension and lateral flexion toward the side being tested. If pressure applied to the top of the head elicits pain extending out to the shoulder or beyond, this is a positive test and might indicate the presence of cervical radiculopathy. In the lower limb, straight leg–raising tests or other sciatic stretch maneuvers can provide additional useful information about the presence of a lumbosacral radiculopathy.

Differential Diagnosis (pp. 214–215)

• After reviewing the referring physician's request and performing a history and physical examination, the consultant should generate a credible list of differential diagnoses.

Initial Plan (p. 215)

• Based on the list of differential diagnoses, an electrophysiological examination plan should be developed to look for and distinguish between the possibilities listed. This plan could start off with either electromyographic (EMG) or nerve conduction studies (NCS), depending on the differential diagnoses. The initial goal is to get as much pertinent information as possible in the shortest amount of time (and, consequently, at the lowest cost for the patient).

NEEDLE ELECTROMYOGRAPHY (pp. 215–225)
Preparing the Patient (p. 215)

• The patient should get a clear explanation of what is to happen and what the experience is like. Avoid words with strong negative connotations. It is often reassuring, for example, to say "pin" electrode rather than "needle"; electrical "pulse" or "stimulus," as opposed to "shock"; and "uncomfortable" instead of "painful."

Deciding on an Electrode to Use (pp. 215–216)

• The two common types are monopolar and concentric electrodes. Each has advantages, with differences predominantly in recording surface area; price; and, possibly, level of discomfort (see Chapter 10).

Steps of the Needle EMG Examination (pp. 216–224)

• The needle EMG examination for each muscle can usually be divided into four distinct steps: (1) insertional activity; (2) spontaneous activity; (3) examination of motor unit potentials; and (4) assessment of recruitment.

Insertional Activity (p. 216)
• Insertional activity is examined by moving the needle through the muscle briefly and observing the amount and duration of the electrical potentials produced. These potentials are mechanically evoked due to the advancement of the needle. Usually, insertional activity and spontaneous activity should be examined using three or four insertions for each of the four different muscle quadrants. The duration of insertional activity varies from one examiner to another.

After a brief, small movement of the needle, insertional activity usually persists for no more than 300 msec.

• *Decreased insertional activity* means that the usual degree of injury potentials is not elicited. Decreased insertional activity can result from not being in muscle, or from being in a muscle that has fewer viable fibers than normal. Muscles that have become atrophied, been replaced by fat, or become fibrotic have reduced insertional activity.

• *Increased insertional activity* is usually considered to be prolonged muscle membrane activity lasting more than 300 msec after the needle movement stops. Prolonged or increased insertional activity, as an isolated finding, is a "soft" finding. No diagnosis can be made solely on the basis of this "abnormality." One exception is the *syndrome of diffusely abnormal increased insertional activity,* an autosomally dominant inherited syndrome without any clear associated symptomatology. Increased insertional activity can also be seen in association with fibrillations or positive sharp waves, in which cases it supports the impression of either denervation or primary muscle pathological lesions. Some authors argue that increased insertional activity is an early finding after denervation, before sustained positive sharp waves or fibrillations become apparent.

Spontaneous Activity (pp. 216–218)

• Spontaneous activity consists of electrical discharges that are seen without needle movement or voluntary contraction. Some spontaneous activity, recorded near the endplate zone (endplate noise and endplate spikes), is normal.

• Endplate noise (reflecting miniature endplate potentials, or MEPPs) and endplate spikes (reflecting endplate potentials, or EPPs) are normal findings. The endplate zone is a painful area, and staying in this region increases the discomfort of the examination. Second, endplate spikes have short-duration biphasic morphological characteristics that can be mistaken for fibrillation potentials by the inexperienced examiner. Third, if the needle electrode is put into the endplate zone and then pushed through it, the endplate spikes recorded from a distance can assume the morphological characteristics of fibrillation potentials with an initial positivity. It is important to recognize endplate noise and endplate spikes and to withdraw the needle from that area of the muscle quickly and proceed to another area.

• Fibrillation potentials represent abnormal spontaneous single muscle fiber discharges. They are short in duration (usually less than 5 msec) and biphasic, with an initial positivity in almost all instances. Although fibrillation potentials are essentially always abnormal, they are a nonspecific finding. They represent abnormal muscle membrane irritability, which can occur in many disorders. Fibrillation potentials are often seen in denervated muscles. Myopathies can be associated with fibrillation potentials. This is especially common in inflammatory myopathies. They are the least likely to occur in chronic steroid or thyroid myopathies. Direct muscle trauma, intramuscular injections, or intramuscular bleeding have been noted to produce both immediate and chronic fibrillations. Neuromuscular junction disorders, particularly presynaptic disorders (e.g., botulism) or, occasionally, severe postsynaptic defects (e.g., myasthenia gravis), can produce fibrillation potentials. Upper motor neuron lesions (e.g., stroke and spinal cord injury) have also been shown to produce fibrillation potentials. These are usually seen early after onset of the lesion and can be confusing when trying to diagnose a peripheral nerve lesion superimposed on an upper motor neuron disorder.

• Fibrillation potentials, as well as positive sharp waves, are usually graded on a subjective, qualitative scheme. Usually this ranges from 1+ to 4+, with 1+ representing a reproducibly observed fibrillation in an isolated area; and 4+ representing sustained fibrillation potentials, often obscuring the baseline, throughout the muscle. Grading schemes vary somewhat from one laboratory to another.

• Fibrillation potentials decrease in size over time. Large-amplitude fibrillation potentials (greater than $100\,\mu V$) are seen within the first year after onset of denervation, and smaller amplitudes (less than $100\,\mu V$) are seen later. It has been postulated that this relationship reflects muscle fiber atrophy over time, with smaller diameter fibers producing smaller amplitude fibrillations.

• Positive sharp waves represent abnormal single muscle fiber discharges, although they are often evoked by needle movement and may be recorded in a different way (see Chapter 10). Positive sharp waves can be seen in essentially all of the same disorders in which fibrillation potentials are seen. In addition, positive sharp waves can be seen in some cases in which fibrillations are not typically seen. In the autosomally dominant inherited syndrome of diffusely abnormal insertional activity, positive sharp waves are abundant, but fibrillations are not. Early after denervation, particularly when recording with a monopolar electrode, positive sharp waves are much more prominent than fibrillation potentials (fibrillations become more prominent later). In some cases of muscle trauma, positive sharp waves can be seen in isolation without associated fibrillations. Positive sharp waves are thought to have the same pathophysiology as fibrillation potentials and can be graded using the same scheme.

• Complex repetitive discharges (CRDs), formerly known as bizarre high-frequency discharges, probably represent groups of muscle fibers firing in near synchrony (see Chapter 10). CRDs can have any wave shape, with rates varying from 0.3 to 150 Hz. Complex repetitive discharges are a nonspecific finding. They are usually seen in chronic neuropathic or myopathic conditions, but are occasionally seen acutely in inflammatory myopathies. When seen in isolation, CRDs are a nonspecific but usually abnormal finding, similar in diagnostic meaning to positive sharp waves and fibrillations.

• Myotonia is a rarely seen discharge that waxes and wanes in both amplitude and frequency. Its sound, when heard on the electrodiagnostic instrument, has been likened to that of a dive bomber or a revving motorcycle. Myotonia can be seen in a variety of myotonic disorders (e.g., myotonic dystrophy, paramyotonia, or congenital myotonia) but it can also be seen rarely in inflammatory myopathies.

• Fasciculation potentials represent spontaneous discharges of all or of part of a single motor unit. As opposed to a fibrillation potential (in which just a single muscle fiber fires), a fasciculation potential involves multiple muscle fibers of the motor unit. Fasciculations produce enough muscle contraction that they are often visible through the skin on clinical examination. Because a fasciculation potential often involves the discharge of an entire motor unit, a *single* fasciculation potential cannot be distinguished from a *single* voluntary motor unit action potential. It is only by their firing patterns that the two can be distinguished. Fasciculation potentials fire in a *random* pattern that is not under voluntary control.

• Fasciculation potentials can be seen in a variety of neuromuscular disorders. "Benign" fasciculations occur in otherwise healthy individuals in whom there are no other associated signs, symptoms, or electrophysiological abnormalities. They are often seen in healthy people who are stressed, tired, who lack sleep, or who are sensitive to chemicals in the diet (e.g., caffeine). The only reliable judge of the clinical significance of fasciculations is the presence or absence of associated electrodiagnostic findings.

• Myokymia results from groups of motor units firing synchronously in a regular bursting pattern. This can often be seen through the skin surface as a wormlike (or vermicular) movement. When heard over the loudspeaker of the electrodiagnostic instrument, myokymia sounds like a platoon of marching soldiers. Myokymia is a rare finding, but it can be seen in a variety of neurological disorders. It is classified into two distinct groups: facial myokymia and limb myokymia. Facial myokymia has been reported with multiple sclerosis, brainstem neoplasia (pontine gliomas), facial palsy, and hemifacial spasm. Limb myokymia has been reported in radiation plexopathy/neuropathy and in some chronic compression neuropathies, as well as in gold polyneuropathy (patients with rheumatologic disorders treated with gold agents). Knowledge of the association with radiation treatment becomes especially important when trying to identify whether a new brachial plexopathy after radiation treatment for malignancy (e.g., breast cancer) represents a recurrence of tumor or radiation plexopathy. Patients with radiation plexopathy usually have myokymia, upper trunk lesions, and paresthesias, whereas those with recurrent tumor typically have painful lower trunk lesions without myokymia but with Horner's syndrome.

Motor Unit Analysis (pp. 218–223)

• A great deal of information can be obtained from analysis of voluntarily activated motor unit action potentials (MUAPs). This information is more diagnostically specific for neuropathic or myopathic changes than is the assessment of spontaneous activity at rest.

• Theoretically, in neuropathic conditions in which partial denervation and reinnervation has occurred, changes representative of the underlying process of axonal sprouting can be seen (see Fig. 11–1 in the Textbook). Within days after partial denervation, intramuscular axons that remain unaffected send out sprouts, usually emanating from distal nodes of Ranvier or axon terminals, to reinnervate nearby denervated muscle fibers. These sprouts are initially poorly myelinated and conduct slowly. Consequently, in the early phases of reinnervation, motor unit action potentials have increased polyphasicity and duration. This is the direct result of temporal dispersion in these newly formed sprouts, and of poor synchronization of muscle fiber discharges. The neuromuscular junctions at the terminals of these new sprouts are not yet mature and are unreliable with respect to consistently transmitting across the myoneural junction. Unstable MUAPs can be seen with shape and size that vary with repetitive firing. As these sprouts mature, synchronization of muscle fiber discharges improves and the polyphasicity is somewhat reduced. The final status of reinnervated MUAPs is that they are typically large in amplitude, long in duration, and sometimes polyphasic. The increase in amplitude is a result of the increased density of muscle fibers belonging to the same motor unit within the recording area of the tip of the EMG needle.

• Myopathic changes in the MUAP result from loss of individual muscle fibers, impairment to muscle fibers, or temporal dispersion of conduction along muscle fibers. In myopathic conditions, the MUAPs are typically small in amplitude and short in duration. There are fewer muscle fibers from the same motor unit firing within the recording area of the needle electrode. Polyphasicity is increased, although the reasons behind this are not completely understood.

• Neuromuscular junction (NMJ) diseases tend in many ways to mimic the changes seen with myopathy. Because some of the individual muscle fibers in the motor unit cannot fire with the rest of the motor unit, the duration can be shortened and the amplitude reduced. Consequently, NMJ disease should also be considered whenever short-duration, low-amplitude MUAPs are observed. Motor unit variability or instability also increases in NMJ defects as a result of intermittent blocking of NMJ transmission.

• The three most commonly used parameters of MUAPs are amplitude (peak to peak), duration, and number of phases. Amplitude is the easiest parameter to measure but is largely a reflection only of those muscle fibers closest to the tip of the needle. In fact, the high-frequency components of more distant muscle fiber discharges are filtered out during passage through the volume conductor of the body: that is, the intervening tissue acts like a low-pass filter.

• Electromyographers note empirically that amplitude is very dependent on distance from the electrode. An MUAP can be recorded as having a relatively small amplitude or large amplitude, depending on how much effort is put into "focusing" the needle close to the discharging muscle fibers. Typically the needle is moved to obtain the largest amplitude possible for an MUAP, which usually occurs when the potential sound is sharp rather than dull on the electrodiagnostic instrument. This sharp sound comes from the higher amplitude and rapid rise time of the chief spike of the MUAP. Although amplitude is to some extent a reflection of the density of muscle fibers within the MUAP, it is relatively unreliable as compared with other measures because it depends on how much effort is put into "focusing" on the potential.

• Duration from the onset to the end of the motor unit action potential is a better reflection of the number of active muscle fibers within the motor unit (i.e., the motor unit territory). Measurement of mean motor unit duration is the most reliable routine electrophysiological feature to use in distinguishing between "neuropathic" and "myopathic" conditions. It is less dependent on distance from the motor unit because duration is being measured from both the initial and terminal low-frequency components of the potential conducted from distant muscle fibers. A problem with duration, however, is the technical difficulty inherent in its measurement. It is difficult to measure MUAP duration when watching voluntary motor units fly by on a regular sweep speed, except for detecting gross changes. One cannot easily tell where one motor unit starts and another stops when multiple potentials are present, and often baseline noise obscures the start or finish of the motor unit (Fig. 11–1). For an accurate representation of MUAP duration, a trigger and delay line should be used. To reduce random baseline noise, multiple discharges of a motor unit should be combined by averaging. It has been shown repeatedly that mean values for at least 20 different MUAPs must be taken to develop reliable MUAP measures.

• Polyphasicity as an isolated finding is nonspecific and is often overreported and overinterpreted. The phases of a motor unit can be counted as the baseline crossings plus one. When MUAPs have more than five phases, they are termed *polyphasic potentials.* Most normal muscles have at least 10% polyphasic MUAPs, depending on the muscle examined and the type of needle electrode used. Increased polyphasicity can be seen in both neuropathic and myopathic conditions, but it is not specific for either. The electrodiagnostician should be reluctant to make a diagnostic statement solely on the basis of an isolated finding of increased polyphasicity.

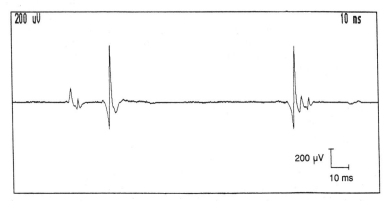

FIGURE 11–1. Two motor unit action potentials (MUAPs) examined during free sweep of the electromyograph. Note that the two potentials superimpose on the right, making it possible to erroneously identify the last potential as a long-duration, polyphasic MUAP.

• Motor unit variability or instability is manifested as a change in amplitude or morphological characteristics of MUAPs during repetitive firing. This is usually due to instability or unreliability in neuromuscular junction (NMJ) transmission, either as a result of a primary defect in the NMJ or as a result of recent reinnervation.

• Several different methods are available to assess voluntary MUAPs during performance of an EMG. The optimal method can vary and depends on the clinical question being asked, the equipment and software available, the experience of the examiner with various techniques, and the probable subtlety of the findings expected.

• The most commonly used method, usually when assessing for possible radiculopathy or entrapment neuropathy, is "semiquantitative." Several MUAPs are examined as they fire during low effort, without a trigger and delay line or any actual quantitative measurement (except possibly for peak-to-peak amplitude of a few of the larger MUAPs). The experienced examiner can notice marked changes in MUAPs, but this method is not sufficient to find more subtle changes.

• An incremental improvement to this method is the employment of a trigger and delay line and a visual examination of several motor units (see Fig. 11–3 in the Textbook).

• Buchthal and colleagues developed traditional quantitative methods in the 1950s. These methods involve recording at least 20 different MUAPs and taking mean values of their measurements. Motor unit potentials are recorded with concentric needle electrodes with wide filter settings (see Fig. 11–4 in the Textbook). The low-frequency filter is set at 2 Hz, rather than 20 Hz, to include the low-frequency initial and terminal phases of the potential (although this makes the baseline less stable). Display sensitivity is set at a consistent level of 100 μV per division. Because duration measurements are dependent on sensitivity of the display, increasing the sensitivity (e.g., to 50 μV/division) produces longer durations, and lower sensitivity (e.g., 200 μV/division) produces shorter durations. During MUAP collection one should not select only the largest MUAPs, but should attempt to collect a representative sampling of all MUAPs near the tip of the needle.

• Reference values have been studied extensively using these methods, and they are available for many different muscles and vary according to age. Mean values are usually given. If a patient's mean value for MUAP duration in a muscle varies by more than 20% from the mean, it is determined to be outside the reference range. The primary role of this type of quantitative analysis is in the evaluation of myopathy.
• Newer, automated techniques allow extraction of single MUAPs from contractions during which several motor units are firing simultaneously.

Recruitment (pp. 223–224)

• Assessment of motor unit recruitment has a number of important purposes. The most important of these is that it can assess whether reduced strength is due to a reduction in the lower motor neuron pool or to poor central effort. In myopathies, recruitment analysis also allows some qualitative assessment regarding how much force is being provided by each motor unit.
• In distinguishing between reductions in the lower motor neuron pool versus poor central drive, the primary feature that should be measured is the rate of motor unit firing. This can be measured in several different ways, but the electromyographer should be facile at rapidly measuring the rate of motor unit firing. For measuring the firing rate of a motor unit, divide 1000 msec by the interpeak interval of two consecutive discharges of an MUAP. For instance, a motor unit whose potentials have an interpeak interval of 100 msec would be firing at 10 Hz (1000/100 = 10). If the sweep speed of the instrument is set at 10 msec/division, a quick way of estimating this is to count the number of divisions between the two motor units and divide the number into 100. If there are 10 divisions between the potentials, the rate would be 10 Hz; 9 divisions would be about 11 Hz; 8 divisions would be 12 Hz; and so on. A second way to estimate firing rates is to count the number of discharges of a given potential on the screen and multiply this number appropriately to arrive at the number that would be expected in 1 sec (1000 msec). If an MUAP fires twice during a 100-msec analysis time, the firing rate is about 20 Hz. The second method is less precise because it does not take into account the possible variable position of the motor units across the screen.
• There are several ways to use the measurement of firing rates to obtain a quantitative estimate of firing patterns. One method is to measure the firing rate of the first recruited motor unit just before the second MUAP starts to fire. This *recruitment frequency* is faster than normal in diseases that reduce the size of the available motor neuron pool. The upper limit of normal for recruitment frequency varies from one muscle to another. In most limb muscles, it is in the range of 12 to 15 Hz; but in the facial muscles, it can be as high as 30 Hz. Consequently, if one MUAP is firing at 20 Hz in a limb muscle, it is likely that the motor neuron pool is reduced (i.e., some axons are not able to fire and others are driven to fire faster to try to provide the requested force).
• There are other alternative methods for measuring recruitment. The recruitment ratio compares the number of motor units firing during a minimal to moderate contraction with their frequencies. A rule of thumb is that (for moderate contraction) the rate of motor units firing, divided by the number of motor units firing, should be less than 5. A number greater than 10 is fairly clear evidence of a loss of motor units. Assessment of the interference pattern looks at how many motor units are firing at maximum voluntary contraction, but it is a more subjective measure. After assessing the firing rate, the recruitment should be

classified as normal or full, central, reduced or discrete, or early. Normal or full recruitment implies that the patient can give a full effort, with many MUAPs firing at normal rates. Central recruitment implies that reduced numbers of motor units are firing but are firing at a normal or slow speed. This is by far the most common "abnormality" in recruitment, but in isolation the finding is completely nondiagnostic. The central pattern of recruitment can be seen in patients with upper motor neuron lesions, pain, or poor voluntary effort. Reduced and discrete recruitment patterns are pathologically significant and imply reduced numbers of rapidly firing motor units. "Reduced" recruitment is less severe than "discrete" recruitment (in which just a few clearly identifiable motor units are firing rapidly, with baseline between them).

• Assessment of recruitment is particularly useful in myopathies. In a myopathy each motor unit is "weak," and it takes more of them, firing faster, to accomplish a task. Consequently, in a myopathy, many MUAPs are activated to provide minimal levels of force. In a severe myopathy, it can be difficult for the patient to fire only a single motor unit because others are recruited quickly at low levels of force.

False-Positive and False-Negative Findings on Needle EMG (pp. 224–225)

• False-positive or false-negative needle EMG findings are common and have many potential causes. False-positive findings are usually related to over-reading of "soft" or subtle changes. The most common examples include over-reading increased insertional activity, mistaking end-plate potentials for fibrillation potentials, overestimating the percentage of polyphasic motor units or over-interpreting the finding of a few polyphasic potentials, and over-reading central or reduced recruitment. False-negative findings are often related to timing. Needle EMG performed too early after the onset of symptoms can produce false-negative results because it often takes 2 to 3 weeks for obvious findings such as positive sharp waves and fibrillations to develop. False-negative findings can also be produced if subtle MUAP changes are missed in a semiquantitative examination.

• Referring physicians usually prefer that the electrodiagnostic medical consultant "under-read" findings.

NERVE CONDUCTION STUDIES (pp. 225–228)

• Nerve conduction studies are a very valuable part of the electrodiagnostic consultation.

Measurement of Compound or Sensory Nerve Action Potentials (pp. 225–226)

• There are usually two measures of nerve action potentials (NAPs): (1) speed of conduction (latency or velocity); and (2) size of the evoked response (amplitude). The speed of conduction for compound nerve action potentials (CNAPs) or sensory nerve action potentials (SNAPs) has traditionally been measured using peak latencies (i.e., the time between onset of stimulation and the peak of the potential). This is technically the easiest latency measurement to make because it is independent of display sensitivity; on older instruments, it was often the only measurement that could be clearly discerned. The peak latency, however, is not always optimal in that it does not represent the arrival of the fastest conducting fibers, and it is affected by interelectrode separation (i.e., overly short active-to-reference separation produces shortened peak latencies). Onset latency, although more difficult to measure (particularly for small potentials or those with noisy baselines), does have the physiological advantage of representing arrival of the fastest conducting fibers and being less influenced by electrode separation.

• Latency and conduction velocity can be affected by a number of physiological and pathological factors, as discussed in Chapter 10. In healthy control subjects, slower conduction can be a result of cold limbs, aging, or increased height. Pathologically, demyelination produces slowing, as does loss of the faster conducting axons.

• Amplitude of the CNAP can be measured (1) from baseline to peak, (2) from initial positive peak to subsequent negative peak if an initial positive peak is present, or (3) from initial negative peak to subsequent positive peak. In the setting of unstable or poorly defined baselines, the peak-to-peak measures are often easier to make, although any subsequent motor volume conducted response makes the later positive phase difficult to measure.

• Amplitude can also be affected by a number of physiological and pathological factors. Cold increases the amplitude of the SNAP when the nerve at the active electrode is cooled. Whenever a prolonged latency or slowed conduction velocity is encountered in the face of a clearly normal or larger than usual amplitude, a cold limb is the probable cause. *Pathological* causes for slowed velocities or prolonged latencies usually produce small amplitudes. Amplitude is also influenced by the distance between the nerve and the recording electrode (i.e., the volume of tissue lying between nerve and electrode). Amplitude declines exponentially with distance from the generator. This explains why subjects with smaller finger circumferences have larger amplitude SNAPs. Aging produces smaller amplitude SNAPs, probably as a result of loss of large myelinated axons.

• The size of the CNAP is roughly proportional to the number of axons depolarizing under the active electrode. Loss of axons reduces the size of the CNAP accordingly. Distal lesions, occurring between the sites of stimulation and recording, drop the amplitude of the CNAP immediately. A reduced amplitude SNAP can be the result of an axonal lesion anywhere distal to the dorsal root ganglion.

Measurement of Compound Muscle Action Potentials
(p. 226)

• Principles of stimulation and recording for motor nerve conduction studies are similar to those used for sensory nerve conduction studies, with several exceptions. The primary difference is that motor nerve conduction studies involve recording a CMAP over muscle rather than recording directly from nerve. Consequently, the distal latency involves not only conduction along the nerve from the point of stimulation but also neuromuscular junction transmission time (approximately 1 msec) and conduction along muscle fibers (approximately 3 to 5 m/sec). Although the onset latency from a distal stimulation site can easily be measured, it cannot be converted into a nerve conduction velocity as it can with the SNAP. To obtain conduction velocities, motor nerves are typically stimulated twice, and the distance between the two stimulation sites is divided by the difference in latency. The neuromuscular junction transmission time and the time for muscle fiber conduction are canceled out in this process.

• Because each axon supplies many muscle fibers (usually hundreds or more), the compound muscle action potential is commonly several hundred times the size of the corresponding nerve action potential. As a consequence, the onset latency of the CMAP is easy to delineate and it, rather than the peak, is usually used for measurement. Amplitudes of the response can be measured either from baseline to peak or from peak to peak, although the baseline-to-peak measurement is more commonly used.

• Although many of the factors that affect sensory nerve conduction studies also affect motor nerve conduction studies, some important differences exist. First, because motor neuron cell bodies reside in the anterior horn of the spinal cord rather than in the dorsal root ganglion, the amplitude of the response is diminished by axon loss at the anterior horn cell or distally (not at the dorsal root ganglion). Second, because the recording is from muscle, neuromuscular junction transmission defects or primary myopathies can reduce the amplitude of the CMAP.

• Occasionally, one may encounter the unusual finding of intact sensory nerve amplitudes with decreased motor amplitudes. It is helpful conceptually to think about areas in the spinal cord or along the peripheral nervous system that could account for these findings. Motor neuron disease or other intraspinal processes (e.g., tumor, syrinx, or carcinomatous meningitis) can reduce CMAP amplitudes; but because these are preganglionic lesions, they do not affect SNAPs. If sufficiently severe, radiculopathies (which almost always occur preganglionically) can result in small motor amplitudes with intact sensory responses. More peripherally, selective motor axonopathies produce a similar discrepancy, although these are relatively rare (e.g., heavy-metal neuropathies, porphyria, and some of demyelinating neuropathies). Neuromuscular junction defects (usually presynaptic) or primary myopathies can also selectively reduce motor amplitudes because the CMAP is recorded over muscle and the SNAP over sensory axons.

• The CMAP and SNAP amplitudes are useful in estimating the degree of axon loss. The degree of axon loss is roughly proportional to the drop in CMAP or SNAP amplitude that is elicited with distal stimulation (assuming that enough time has passed for Wallerian degeneration).

Late Responses (pp. 226–228)

• There are several "late" responses (i.e., those that occur late after the CMAP or M wave) that sometimes provide useful information. These include the F wave, the H wave, and the A wave. The F wave, so named because it was first recorded in foot muscles, is a late response usually recorded from distal muscles. When a motor nerve is stimulated distally, axons are depolarized in both directions: distally (orthodromically) and proximally (antidromically). Whereas the orthodromic volley activates the muscle distally, the antidromic volley proceeds proximally to the anterior horn cell. It is thought that the F wave occurs when a small percentage (3% to 5%) of antidromically activated motor cell bodies discharge and produce orthodromic activation of their motor axons. This is noted as a small-amplitude (approximately 100 to 200 μV) late (approximately 30 msec in the distal upper limb) potential.

• The technique for obtaining F waves is similar to that for motor nerve conduction, with several important differences. First, because the F wave involves such a small percentage of the motor neuron pool, the sensitivity of the recording instrument needs to be greater (e.g., 200 μV/division versus a customary 2 to 5 mV/division for conventional motor studies). Second, because the F wave is a late response, having gone from the distal stimulation site to the spinal cord and back, the sweep speed needs to be slower so that a total of 50 msec (in the upper limbs) or 100 msec (in the lower limbs) can be measured in each sweep. Nerve stimulation for the F wave is typically at the same point in the limb as for distal motor latencies. It is customary practice, however, to turn the stimulating electrode around, with the anode facing distally rather than proximally. The small percentage of axons in the motor neuron pool that are activated for the F wave is not always the same with every stimulation. Consequently, to avoid sampling error, multiple stimulations need to be performed and multiple F waves measured. Some debate exists as to the number of F waves that need to be recorded, but standard practice usually involves 10 to 20 recordings.

• Multiple parameters can be measured in the 10 to 20 or more F waves that are collected. The most widely measured parameter is the minimal latency, which is the shortest latency out of 10 or 20 stimulations. Some advocate using the mean onset latency rather than the minimal latency.

• F-wave measurements usually find their greatest applicability in the assessment of multifocal or diffuse processes, especially those affecting proximal areas of the peripheral nervous system. F waves are particularly helpful in assessing acquired or inherited demyelinating polyneuropathies, which produce multifocal or diffuse slowing of conduction velocity. In Guillain-Barré syndrome (acute inflammatory demyelinating polyradiculoneuropathy) abnormalities in F-wave measures can be the only electrophysiological abnormality early in the disease course. F waves are also useful in the assessment of syringomyelia, in which prolongation or absence of F waves can result from impaired turnaround time (central delay) at the anterior horn cell.

• Although it would seem appealing to use F-wave measurements for the diagnosis of brachial plexopathy or some entrapment neuropathies, they typically are not of significant help in these applications, nor do they offer unique information that cannot be obtained by conventional nerve conduction studies.

• The H wave, unlike the F wave, does involve synaptic transmission at the spinal cord level. The H wave (also known as the H reflex) is in many ways analogous to the muscle stretch reflex. In the case of the muscle stretch reflex, the stretch receptors within the muscle are activated mechanically. But in the case of the H wave, the large-diameter afferent nerve fibers are directly activated electrically (many other fibers are probably activated as well). After the afferent volley reaches the spinal cord, a monosynaptic reflex excites alpha motor neurons and a late response is produced in the muscle. The H wave in adults is most easily elicited in the soleus muscle. In some subjects it can also be recorded from the flexor carpi radialis, foot intrinsic muscles, and the quadriceps. The H wave can be seen in many more muscles in children, especially those younger than 3 years old, possibly because the descending inhibitory pathways are not yet fully myelinated.

• The H wave is recorded using somewhat different techniques than those for F-wave recording. For recording from the soleus muscle, stimulation is performed of the tibial nerve in the popliteal fossa. Although many authors report using a handheld stimulator, we have found it preferable to use a disk electrode taped over the middle of the popliteal fossa with an anode placed anteriorly over the knee, driving the current through the knee. Recording is at a standardized site that is half the distance between the popliteal fossa and the proximal flare of the medial malleolus. As opposed to the F wave, the H wave is largest in amplitude with stimulation levels that are submaximal for the corresponding M wave. The H wave should usually be higher in amplitude than the corresponding M response. Increasing the intensity of stimulation further causes the H wave amplitude to fall. The reason for this decrease in H-wave amplitude with higher levels of stimulation is not clearly known, but probably involves activation of inhibitory phenomena at the spinal cord level.

• Because the H wave depends on a reflex at the spinal cord level, some unique concerns are applicable to obtaining these responses. The patient should be relaxed because even minimal contractions, particularly of the ankle dorsiflexors, markedly reduce the amplitude of the response. Some authors utilize a minimal contraction of the ankle plantar flexors to facilitate the response. Also, there must be ample time between stimuli for the response to recover. Stimulating at rates more than about 0.2 Hz (one every 5 sec) alters the morphological characteristics of the H wave (except for the first one). Stimulation usually involves long-duration pulses, optimally between 0.5 and 1.0 msec, to preferentially activate the type Ia afferent fibers.

• When performing the H-wave studies, a late response is sometimes seen after the M wave, and it might be unclear whether this is an H wave or an F wave. To differentiate the two, one should consider the size, the consistency of the response in latency and shape, and the current required to obtain the response. H waves tend to be large and are usually (but not always) greater in amplitude than the corresponding M wave seen when the H wave is elicited. They tend to be stable with little variability from one stimulation to the next, and they are best elicited at submaximal stimulation intensities and attenuate with higher intensities of stimulation. In contrast, the F wave is small (usually only about 3% to 5% of the M-wave amplitude), variable in morphological characteristics, and best seen with supramaximal stimulation intensities.

• The H-wave latency is dependent on the age of the subject as well as on leg length; hence, reference values have been developed that account for these variables and produce the mean expected latency. It is unusual, however, for a subject to have an H-wave latency that exceeds the mean plus 2 standard deviations (2 SD; 5.5 msec) generated by this calculation, except in severe neuropathies. More commonly, side-to-side differences exceed the reference range. Side-to-side latency differences exceeding 1.2 msec are probably abnormal. H-wave amplitude is dependent on the intensity of stimulation as well as on the level of relaxation. This makes it difficult to compare an H-wave amplitude to absolute reference (normal) values, but side-to-side amplitude comparison has been found useful. When comparing sides, the smaller response should not be less than 40% of the amplitude of the larger response.

• The H wave can be abnormal in a variety of peripheral nervous system lesions. Tibial neuropathy, sciatic neuropathies, and lumbosacral plexopathies can all create abnormalities in the H-wave latency, amplitude, and shape. The most useful application of the H wave is in the detection of S1 radiculopathy. It has been shown that the H wave is more sensitive than needle EMG in the assessment of S1 radiculopathy, probably related to the fact that the H wave can detect conduction block and demyelination, whereas needle EMG can detect only motor axon loss.

- The A wave, formerly termed the *axon reflex,* is a rarely seen late response, usually observed in the setting of a peripheral nervous system lesion. In most cases the A wave is thought to represent aberrant innervation after peripheral nerve injury such that single axons branch to innervate two different groups of muscle fibers. Stimulation distal to the site of the regenerated area of nerve causes depolarization antidromically to the other axon branch. This type of A wave is typically seen only at submaximal stimulation because supramaximal stimulation simultaneously activates both branches and eliminates the A wave. The A wave usually represents an abnormality because it reflects axon branching, although Sunderland has demonstrated axon branching in some normal subjects. The A wave is easily missed in routine clinical nerve conduction studies if the sweep speed is too fast or the sensitivity too low to permit the observation of these small, late responses.

- Another proposed etiology for the A wave is ephaptic transmission. It has been proposed that the A wave might result from the distal activation of an axon in a partially demyelinated nerve. When the volley reaches a demyelinated segment, slower conducting myelinated fibers could ephaptically activate nearby large-diameter faster conducting fibers. This could be seen even in the case of supramaximal stimulation, in which both branches are activated (the refractory period in the faster fiber can already be over by the time the slow fiber is activated at the site of ephaptic transmission). Ephaptically generated A waves have been reported in early cases of Guillain-Barré syndrome.

REPETITIVE STIMULATION STUDIES (pp. 228–230)

Physiological Basis (pp. 228–229)

- Repetitive stimulation studies are most commonly used to search for abnormalities in neuromuscular junction transmission. To understand repetitive stimulation studies, it is first necessary to review the basic synaptic physiology at the neuromuscular junction.

- At the time of synaptic transmission, acetylcholine is released to travel across the neuromuscular junction and reaches receptors at the postsynaptic end-plate. Normally, about three to five times as much acetylcholine is released than is needed to fully activate the postsynaptic membrane. This margin of safety ensures that even though the amount of acetylcholine released during repetitive depolarizations normally progressively decreases, the muscle fiber is still fully activated.

- Stimulation at slow rates (less than 5 Hz) is usually done to detect postsynaptic neuromuscular junction defects. With slow rates of stimulation in normal individuals, a successive decrease occurs in the amount of acetylcholine released. When the safety factor of release is normal, muscle fibers are still fully activated. When the safety margin is less than normal, progressively fewer and fewer muscle fibers are activated during repetitive stimulations at slow rates.

- Fast rates of stimulation (e.g., 20 to 50 Hz) are primarily used to detect presynaptic defects in neuromuscular junction transmission. At these fast rates of stimulation, Ca^{2+} concentrations are progressively increased in the presynaptic terminal and more acetylcholine is released. Presynaptic defects, such as

Lambert-Eaton myasthenic syndrome (LEMS) or botulism, produce marked increments (at least twofold) in the amplitude of the CMAP with high rates of stimulation.

Technical Considerations (p. 229)

• There are a number of important technical variables to keep in mind when performing repetitive stimulation studies. First, because acetylcholinesterase is sensitive to temperature changes, the limb should be adequately warmed before studies are performed. When the limb is too cold (usually under 34 °C), defects in neuromuscular junction transmission can be hidden. Movement artifact is probably the most common technical difficulty in repetitive stimulation studies. This can be reduced by securely taping down all electrodes. Stimulation should be via a block electrode taped to the limb rather than a handheld electrode whenever possible. When performing stimulation distally (e.g., in the hand) it is also advisable to use an arm board to stabilize the limb. Submaximal stimulation can be a potential problem. Using stimuli around the maximal level (rather than supramaximal) can result in intermittent submaximal stimuli and "pseudodecrements" with limb movement during stimulation. To avoid this problem, stimulation intensities should be at least 30% above the maximal level.

• Although distal muscles are usually the least difficult technically to study, they are also usually the least diagnostically sensitive. It is often necessary to perform a progression of studies, starting with the ulnar nerve, which is technically easy to study; then moving proximally to the shoulder (e.g., Erb's point to deltoid or spinal accessory nerve to trapezius); and finally to the facial muscles (nasalis). Facial muscles are the most sensitive for detecting postsynaptic defects of neuromuscular transmission, but technical problems may arise owing to difficulty with stabilization and movement.

• Exercise has a marked effect on repetitive stimulation studies. Immediately after exercise (usually defined as 30 seconds of isometric exercise), a brief period of post-exercise potentiation occurs, acetylcholine release is facilitated, the margin of safety is improved, and initial decrements can be reduced. About 2 to 4 minutes after exercise, there is a period of post-exercise exhaustion. During this period, release of acetylcholine from the presynaptic terminal is reduced and any defects in neuromuscular transmission become more apparent. Consequently, it is customary to perform slow (2 to 3 Hz) repetitive stimulations pre-exercise, immediately post-exercise (during post-exercise facilitation), and then at 1-minute intervals for 4 minutes to look for post-exercise exhaustion (Table 11–1).

Changes in Disease States (pp. 229–230)

• Presynaptic disorders of neuromuscular junction transmission are rare. Lambert-Eaton myasthenic syndrome (LEMS) is an autoimmune disorder that is often, but not always, associated with malignancy or autoimmune disease. Botulism results from exposure to the toxin from the bacterium *Clostridium botulinum*. These disorders have in common a reduced release of acetylcholine from the presynaptic terminal. Myasthenia gravis is an example of a postsynaptic neuromuscular junction disorder. In this disorder not only are the postsynaptic receptors blocked by specific antibodies, but the cleft between the presynaptic

TABLE 11–1 Expected Findings on Single and Repetitive Nerve Stimulation*

	CMAP Amplitude	CMAP after 10 sec Exercise	CMAP after 10 sec Exercise		
			Pre-Exercise	Immediate Post-exercise	2-4 min Post-exercise
Normal	Normal	No change	No change	No change	No change
Presynaptic defect	Very small	Markedly increased	Decrement, 1st to 4th stimulation	Markedly increased initial CMAP amplitude	Decrement similar to pre-exercise
Postsynaptic defect	Normal	No change	Decrement, 1st to 4th stimulation	Less decrement than pre-exercise	Decrement more than pre-exercise

*Recording the CMAP in normal subjects, patients with presynaptic lesions, and patients with postsynaptic lesions.
Abbreviation: CMAP, compound motor action potential.

and postsynaptic terminals is also widened and an increased breakdown of acetylcholine occurs as it crosses the synaptic cleft.

• Presynaptic disorders such as LEMS or botulism are usually characterized by their potentiation with high-frequency stimulation and exercise (see Table 11–1).

• Postsynaptic disorders such as myasthenia gravis usually have a progressive decrement on slow repetitive stimulation studies, which is exacerbated during post-exercise exhaustion. In some cases a decrement can become apparent only during post-exercise exhaustion 2 to 4 minutes after exercise. Postsynaptic disorders also manifest post-exercise facilitation, but this is far less marked than in presynaptic disorders. Repetitive stimulation studies are moderately sensitive for the diagnosis of myasthenia gravis, and most studies suggest that the sensitivity ranges from 60% to 70%. Single fiber EMG studies are probably more than 90% sensitive.

• Abnormalities on repetitive stimulation studies are not entirely specific to neuromuscular junction (NMJ) disorders. After reinnervation, newly developed axon sprouts have immature and unstable NMJs, and can produce a decrement during repetitive stimulation at slow rates. Patients with motor neuron disease, peripheral polyneuropathy, or entrapment neuropathies can have decrements unrelated to any specific neuromuscular junction defect. Similar decrements have also been reported in myopathies.

INTERPRETATION (pp. 230–233)

Normal versus Abnormal (p. 230)

• As with any other type of testing, nerve conduction studies and quantitative measurements on EMG are not always conclusively normal or abnormal. Reference values have been derived for most quantitative measurements, but these do not unequivocally differentiate a healthy subject from one with disease. Reference values provide only the *probability* of a result coming from a healthy subject versus from a patient with disease. It is the finding of multiple "abnormalities" consistent with the clinical presentation that helps to establish a diagnosis.

• The use of 2 SDs to produce reference values at the 97.5 percentile level assumes a normal (Gaussian) distribution to the data. It has been shown, however, that nerve conduction study data (and probably EMG data) do not follow a Gaussian distribution. Consequently, using a mean and 2 SDs to determine reference values is inappropriate and can lead to an increased number of false positives or false negatives. Appropriate adjustments to the data can be made to obtain more reliable reference values; however, these adjustments typically have not been performed in most literature studies.

Principles of Localization (pp. 230–231)

• A number of principles are useful for localizing peripheral nerve lesions based on the electrophysiological examination. Nerve lesions that are very proximal cannot be studied with stimulation both proximal and distal to an entrapment site, making needle EMG the most helpful in their diagnosis and localization. Localization is based on the distribution of the abnormalities determined after examination of the muscles supplied by multiple peripheral nerves, roots, or areas of the plexus. Sciatic neuropathy can be distinguished from peroneal neuropathy, for example, if evidence is found of denervation in muscles supplied by both the peroneal and tibial nerves, with normal findings in the gluteal muscles. Localization is based on finding abnormalities distal to a branch point, with normal findings proximal to that point.

• Although this approach often results in correct localization, there are many instances in which it leads to choosing an erroneous lesion site; for example, even though ulnar nerve entrapment at the elbow usually occurs proximal to the branch to flexor carpi ulnaris, this muscle is usually spared in ulnar neuropathy at the elbow. The fascicles for this muscle are isolated in a relatively protected area of the nerve at the entrapment site.

• The ulnar nerve is not unique with regard to its specific intraneural topography causing potential problems in localization. Cases have been reported of neuropathy of the common peroneal nerve occurring proximal to the popliteal fossa but resulting only in deep peroneal deficits clinically. Sciatic neuropathies, even when they occur near the hip joint, can result in a clinical picture of predominantly peroneal nerve lesions. The fascicular structure within the peroneal division of the sciatic nerve can make it more predisposed to injury than is the tibial division.

• Nerve conduction studies are best at localizing the site of the pathological lesion when demyelination is present. Demyelination causes focal slowing and conduction block. When present, these findings allow precise localization of a focal entrapment. A problem with localizing lesions based on nerve conduction studies arises when there is predominantly axon loss and little demyelination. In such cases, conduction velocity throughout the nerve is mildly slowed because of loss of the faster conducting fibers, but is not focally or markedly slowed. Although a diffuse reduction is seen in CMAP or SNAP amplitude at all sites of stimulation (from axon loss and subsequent Wallerian degeneration), there is no focal drop in amplitude across the lesion site. Conduction block (in which a drop in amplitude of the CMAP is seen in moving from distal to proximal stimulation) is related only to demyelination and neurapraxia, and is not present in axon loss lesions after Wallerian degeneration has occurred (about 7 days after onset).

• Localization of proximal lesions such as radiculopathies or plexopathies is usually best done utilizing needle EMG results and SNAPs. Study of motor nerve conduction studies and recording of CMAPs is less useful in localization because it is usually difficult to stimulate proximal to the site of the lesion. CMAP amplitude, however, is useful for assessing the degree of motor axon loss and for making a prognosis.

• A common problem in proximal localization is in distinguishing between plexus and root lesions. In most cases, only two findings distinguish between these two possibilities. One is the paraspinal needle EMG, which, if abnormal, speaks strongly for a lesion at or proximal to the posterior primary ramus (e.g., a root lesion). However, there are patients with root lesions in whom paraspinal muscles are reportedly normal on EMG. The second is the study of the sensory nerve action potential, assuming that there has been enough time for axonal degeneration after injury. This helps to distinguish between preganglionic and postganglionic (dorsal root ganglion) lesions. Plexopathies are usually expected to have small SNAPs, whereas radiculopathies usually have normal SNAPs. Some cervical radiculopathies occur laterally enough to involve the dorsal root ganglion, however, and result in small-amplitude SNAPs. Moreover, postganglionic lesions (e.g., brachial plexopathies) must have marked axon loss if axonal degeneration is to produce reduction of distal SNAPs. Because there is a wide range of "normal" SNAP amplitudes, a drop in amplitude from 60 to 30 μV, for example, might still leave the SNAP within "normal" limits.

Deducing the Pathophysiology from the Electrophysiological Results (p. 231)

• Whenever possible, it is helpful to provide to the referring physician some indication of the pathophysiology within the peripheral nervous system (e.g., neurapraxia, demyelination, or axon loss).

• Neurapraxia or focal conduction block is seen on nerve conduction studies when a larger amplitude CMAP or SNAP is elicited with stimulation distal to the site of the lesion, as compared to proximally. Purely neurapraxic injuries show no electrophysiological evidence for axon loss (fibrillation potentials or positive sharp waves) or reinnervation.

• Demyelination is best demonstrated by slowing of conduction, often with conduction block. Slowing of conduction can take the form of slowed conduction velocities, prolonged distal latencies, increased temporal dispersion, or prolonged late responses.

• Axon loss lesions are usually demonstrated by evidence of denervation on needle EMG examination as well as by small-amplitude CMAP and SNAP responses with stimulation and recording distal to the site of the lesion. Although needle EMG is a more sensitive indicator for motor axon loss, measurement of CMAP and SNAP amplitude is a better way to quantify the *degree* of axon loss and prognosis.

Timing of Electrophysiological Changes (pp. 231–233)

• The time course of electrodiagnostic changes after onset of a neuropathic lesion should always be kept in mind when planning the electrophysiological examination. Neurapraxia, demyelination, and severe axon loss produce electrophysiological changes immediately if one can perform stimulation both proximal and distal to the lesion. Very proximal lesions, in which it is not possible to access a site both proximal and distal to the lesion, do not immediately produce changes on distal nerve conduction studies or EMG. Distinction between neurapraxia and axonotmesis cannot be made until after Wallerian degeneration has occurred in cases of axonotmesis.

Day 1 after an Axon Loss Lesion
• On needle EMG the only potential abnormality is a change in recruitment, with reduced or discrete recruitment if enough axon loss has occurred. Mild lesions do not produce noticeable changes in recruitment. Nerve conduction studies distal to the site of the lesion are unchanged, but stimulation proximal to a lesion with recording distally might produce a small-amplitude response. Otherwise, nerve conduction studies and EMG are usually unremarkable.

Days 7 to 10
• Seven days after a complete nerve lesion, Wallerian degeneration will have progressed to a point at which stimulation of motor axons elicits no motor responses. Ten days after onset of a complete lesion, SNAPs will be absent as well. Incomplete lesions produce less marked changes, but with similar timing. Seven to ten days after onset, a neurapraxic injury can be distinguished by nerve conduction studies (in which case the distal amplitudes are normal) from an axonotmetic lesion (in which case the distal amplitudes are reduced).

Days 14 to 21
• Two to three weeks after onset of injury, the needle EMG starts to show fibrillation potentials and positive sharp waves. Proximal muscles typically demonstrate these abnormalities before distal ones. Radiculopathies, for example, can show paraspinal abnormalities at days 10 to 14 after onset, but distal limb muscle changes might not be apparent until 3 to 4 weeks after onset. In studies of peripheral nerve lesions in animal models, it has been documented that the longer the segment of nerve left attached to a muscle after section, the longer the interval before the appearance of fibrillation potentials. This has raised the question of the existence of some type of "antifibrillation" trophic factor stored in peripheral nerves, with fibrillations occurring only after it is depleted.
• Fibrillations and positive sharp waves can persist for several months or even many years after a single injury, depending on the extent of reinnervation. Although the presence of positive sharp waves or fibrillations indicates that there has been some denervation, it does not necessarily indicate that there is "active" or "ongoing" loss of axons over time. Fibrillation amplitudes are sometimes helpful in determining the chronology of the lesion. This is because of the fact that the amplitude of fibrillation potentials decreases over time. The presence of fibrillation potentials larger than $100\,\mu V$ indicates an onset less than 1 year ago.

Reinnervation
• The timing and type of electrophysiological changes consequent to reinnervation depend in part on the mechanism of reinnervation. When reinnervation is a result of axonal regrowth from the site of the lesion, as in complete lesions, the appearance of new MUAPs does not occur until motor axons have had suf-

ficient time to grow the distance between the lesion site and the muscle. Nerve regrowth usually occurs at 1 mm/day or 1 inch/month. When these new axons first reach the muscle, they innervate only a few muscle fibers, producing short-duration, small amplitude potentials, sometimes referred to as *nascent potentials*. With time, as more muscle fibers are innervated and join the motor unit, the MUAPs become larger, more polyphasic, and longer in duration.

• Motor unit potential changes also develop when reinnervation occurs by axonal sprouting. Polyphasicity and increased duration develop first as newly formed, poorly demyelinated sprouts supply the recently denervated muscle fibers. As the sprouts mature, large-amplitude, long-duration MUAPs develop and persist indefinitely.

Estimating Prognosis (p. 233)

• Prognosis of a peripheral nerve lesion is related to the pathophysiological problem that has occurred, the time since onset, and the distance between the lesion and the target muscles. Those lesions that have had extensive axon loss are less likely to have recovery of function. Estimation of the extent of axon loss, however, should not be based solely or predominantly on findings during needle EMG because it takes very little axon loss to produce profuse fibrillation potentials and positive sharp waves. The extent of axon loss should be determined chiefly by the distal CMAP amplitude.

• Electrophysiological measures cannot, unfortunately, assess the integrity of supporting structures around the nerve and cannot distinguish axonotmesis from neurotmesis. Neurotmesis (which has complete or nearly complete disruption of supporting structures) carries a much worse prognosis for regeneration than axonotmesis, in which the supporting structures are largely intact. In these cases, careful periodic re-examination of proximal muscles (those expected to be reinnervated first) gives the best information as to ultimate prognosis for full reinnervation.

• Lesions that are predominantly neurapraxic have a much better prognosis because conduction block in these lesions rarely lasts more than a few months. Demyelinating lesions also have a better prognosis than axon loss, but the specific prognosis depends on what intervention is taken (e.g., release of entrapment sites).

• When axon loss is present, it is important to remember that a critical window of time exists for peripheral nerve regeneration, after which the target muscles cannot be reinnervated. This "window" is usually in the range of 18 to 24 months. Because peripheral nerves regenerate roughly at a rate of 1 inch/month, proximal lesions with a great deal of axon loss have a poor chance of reinnervating distal hand or foot muscles. Complete brachial plexus injuries, for example, have very little chance of reinnervating ulnar innervated hand muscles. As a consequence, most neurosurgical interventions in brachial plexus lesions are directed at reinnervating proximal upper limb muscles.

PEDIATRIC EMG (pp. 233–234)

• There are some special points to be considered when performing EMG on pediatric patients. First, the indications for performing EMG in children are substantially different from those for adults, and the indications are changing over time. In the past, pediatric EMG was used to detect changes consistent with such diseases as Duchenne muscular dystrophy or Wernig-Hoffman disease. Now, however, there are well-established gene probes for making these diagnoses. In the evaluation of possible infantile botulism, EMG plays less of a role than it used to because the toxin can now be easily detected in the stool.

• Nevertheless, pediatric EMG is still useful for a number of indications. It is particularly useful for evaluation of possible acute inflammatory demyelinating polyradiculoneuropathy (AIDP or Guillain-Barré syndrome) or the Fisher variant (Fisher syndrome or Miller Fisher syndrome). EMG is often helpful in the assessment of children for myopathies. It should be remembered, however, that many congenital myopathies look about the same on EMG, and that more specific diagnosis requires consideration of the clinical picture and, usually, muscle biopsy.

• Another significant difference between pediatric EMG and that in adults is the reference or "normal" value range. At birth, nerve conduction velocity is about half that of adults because nerves are not yet fully myelinated. As children mature, nerve conduction velocity increases until it essentially reaches the adult range at about 3 years of age. Electromyographers should use age-specific reference values, particularly when assessing for demyelinating neuropathies.

• Perhaps one of the most significant differences between adult and pediatric EMG is the technique. Children simply don't tolerate the procedure as well as adults. Children younger than 6 years generally don't tolerate the procedure, particularly if they have had bad experiences with medical procedures or if the parental anxiety level is high. There are different schools of thought about whether or not sedation should be used for the procedure.

• Finally, another important consideration in performing pediatric electromyography is the difference in the amount of data that can be obtained. Whereas many muscles can be sampled in the adult, looking at both spontaneous activity and voluntary motor unit potentials, the same cannot be said for children. Generally, only a few nerves or muscles can be examined, and muscles can be examined primarily for either spontaneous activity (during sedation) or motor unit action potentials (when awake), but not both.

ELECTRODIAGNOSIS IN THE ELDERLY (p. 234)

• The electrodiagnostic medical consultant needs to be aware of several important changes that occur with aging. Most nerve conduction measures change with age. Latencies become longer, velocities slower, and amplitudes smaller with age. This is not necessarily a linear change with age and some data suggest that nerve conduction remains relatively constant until about age 60, and then declines in the seventh and eighth decades. As a consequence, it is preferable to use age-specific data rather than making linear adjustments for age. These data do not, however, take into account any interactions that can occur between age, temperature, and height.

• Voluntary motor unit action potentials also change with age. Motor units become longer in duration and larger in amplitude as people age. This presumably reflects slow motor neuron loss over time, with consequent reinnervation by distal sprouting. Age-specific normative data should be used when doing quantitative motor unit analysis.

WRITING THE ELECTRODIAGNOSTIC MEDICAL CONSULTATION REPORT (p. 234)

• Guidelines for writing the electrodiagnostic medical consultation report can be found in the American Association for Electrodiagnostic Medicine guidelines for electrodiagnostic laboratories. The report should identify the patient, state the referring problem and indication for the study, and list the findings from the electrophysiological examination. The conclusion should specify whether the study results are normal or abnormal, answer the referring physician's question (e.g., whether or not a specific diagnosis is present), and report any other diagnoses that can have come to light during the clinical or electrophysiological examination. Whenever possible, the pathophysiological basis of the lesion and the prognosis for recovery should be included.

12

Original Chapter by Kathryn A. Stolp-Smith, M.D.

Electrodiagnostic Medicine III: Case Studies

• The ability to perform nerve conduction studies (NCS) and needle electromyography (EMG) in a clinical setting significantly enhances our role as clinicians. Knowledge and skill in clinical neurophysiology allow the clinician a physiological extension and confirmation of the clinical examination. An analytical and sequential thought process; application of medical knowledge of anatomy, physiology, and pathophysiology; and familiarity with electrodiagnostic equipment are necessary to properly perform and interpret NCS and EMG. Clinical neurophysiological studies allow us immediate physiological feedback and confirmation of clinically suspected problems.

• Because this book is designed to present material useful for ready reference in the clinic or on the ward, these cases are not presented here. Please see the textbook for this important information.

TREATMENT TECHNIQUES AND SPECIAL EQUIPMENT

13

Original Chapter by Alberto Esquenazi, M.D.

Upper Limb Amputee Rehabilitation and Prosthetic Restoration

INCIDENCE AND DEMOGRAPHICS (p. 263)

• There are approximately 1,230,000 amputees living in the United States (at all levels of amputation), with approximately 50,000 new amputations performed annually. The ratio of upper limb to lower limb amputation is 1:4.9. The most common causes of upper limb amputation are trauma and cancer, followed by vascular complications of disease. Transradial level is the most common arm amputation (57%). Sixty percent of arm amputees are between the ages of 21 and 64 years, and 10% are younger than 21 years.

• Congenital upper limb deficiency has an incidence of approximately 4.1 per 10,000 live births. The limb deficiencies can be transverse or longitudinal. The term *terminal* is used to describe the fact that the limb has developed normally to a particular level, beyond which no skeletal element exists. In intercalary limb deficiency, a reduction or absence of one or more elements occurs within the long axis of the limb, and in this case normal skeletal elements may be found distal to the affected segments. The most common congenital limb deficiency is the left terminal transverse radial limb deficiency.

LIMB SALVAGE VERSUS AMPUTATION SURGERY
(pp. 263–277)

• The absolute surgical indication for amputation in trauma is ischemia in a limb with unreconstructible vascular injury. Amputation is often ultimately required after multiple surgical procedures. Such surgical procedures also represent a substantial investment of time, money, and emotional energy. Massively crushed or burned muscle and ischemic tissue release myoglobin and cell toxins, which can lead to renal failure, adult respiratory distress syndrome, and death. In addition, the risk of infection, contractures, and nerve injuries that interfere with function needs to be considered. Recent studies show the value of early amputation not only in saving lives, but also in preventing the emotional, marital, and financial disasters and opiate analgesic addictions that can follow desperate attempts at limb salvage.

• The selection of the surgical level of amputation is probably one of the most important decisions that must be made for the amputee. The viability of soft tissue and the amount of skin coverage with adequate sensation usually determine the most distal possible functional level for amputation. After surgery, the patient with an upper limb amputation should ideally be able to use a prosthesis (either body or externally powered) during most of the day. Bony prominences, skin scars, soft tissue traction, shear, and perspiration can complicate prosthesis use. New surgical techniques that permit myocutaneous transfers, skin expansion methods, and bony lengthening procedures are available to optimize the residual limb shape, size, and function. Early prosthetic fitting after arm amputation (1 to 4 months) is imperative if successful prosthetic restoration is to be expected. Once healing has occurred, prevention of scar tissue adhesion formation is critical.

Levels of Amputation (pp. 264–265)

• Finger amputation can occur at the distal interphalangeal, proximal interphalangeal, and metacarpophalangeal levels. Transcarpal amputation and wrist amputation are seen less often because of their limited functional outcome. Multiple finger amputations, including thumb and partial hand amputations and those through the wrist, need to be considered carefully in view of the possible functional and cosmetic implications of prosthesis fitting and restoration. Inappropriate choice of amputation site can result in a prosthesis with disproportional length or width. It can also preclude the use of externally powered devices.
• The transradial amputation is preferred in most cases; it can be performed at three levels (resulting in long, medium, and short residual limbs). The long forearm residual limb is preferred when optimal body-powered prosthetic restoration is the goal. It is the ideal level for the patient who is expected to perform physically demanding work. The medium forearm residual limb is preferred when optimal externally powered prosthetic restoration is the goal. The short transradial amputation level can complicate suspension and limit elbow flexion strength and elbow range of motion. Transradial amputation is the most common level and allows the highest level of functional recovery in the majority of cases.
• The elbow disarticulation has some advantages and disadvantages. The surgical technique permits reduction in surgery time and blood loss; provides improved prosthetic self-suspension while permitting the use of a less encumbering socket; and reduces the rotation of the socket on the residual limb, as compared with the transhumeral level of amputation. Major disadvantages are the marginal cosmetic appearance caused by the necessary external elbow mechanism; and current limitations in technology, which impede the use of externally powered elbow mechanisms at this level of amputation. In the patient for whom bilateral transhumeral amputation is the alternative, the elbow disarticulation is a more desirable level when feasible despite the possible cosmetic problems.
• The transhumeral amputation can be performed at three levels (resulting in long, medium, and short residual limbs). The long arm residual limb (7 to 10 cm from the distal humeral condyle) is preferred for optimal prosthetic restoration.
• The shoulder disarticulation and forequarter amputations are less common, and usually are made necessary as part of the surgical intervention to remove a malignant lesion. Patients with these levels of amputation are the most difficult to fit with a functional prosthesis.

• In regard to surgical techniques, soft tissue handling is especially critical to wound healing and functional outcome in amputation surgery. When tissues are excessively traumatized, the risk of wound failure and infection is high. Flaps should be kept thick, and unnecessary dissection between the skin, subcutaneous, fascial, and muscle planes should be avoided. All bone edges should be rounded, and prominences should be beveled for optimal force transmission during prosthetic use. Split-thickness skin grafts are generally discouraged except as a means to save essential residual limb length and with the understanding that future surgical revision might be necessary. *Myodesis* is the direct suturing of muscle or tendon to bone. This technique is most effective in stabilizing muscles that are needed to counteract strong antagonistic muscular forces. *Myoplasty* involves suturing of muscles to periosteum. Myoplasty does not provide as secure a distal stabilization of the muscle as does myodesis.

• All transected nerves form a neuroma. Nerves should be transected cleanly, allowing the cut end to retract into the soft tissues away from the scar and prosthetic pressure points. The integrity of the peripheral nervous system should be assessed as early as feasible after traumatic amputation because traction injuries often result in temporary or permanent nerve injury that has direct implications for arm function as well as for rehabilitation and prosthetic restoration programs.

The Amputee Rehabilitation Program (p. 265)

• The amputee rehabilitation program should ideally be designed to cover the wide spectrum of care from preamputation to reintegration into the community.

Preamputation Counseling (p. 265)

• During this stage it is essential to develop direct communication involving the patient, the family, and the surgeon regarding the need for amputation and the expected surgical outcome. The clinician should have introductory discussions about phantom limb sensation, prosthetic devices, prosthesis fitting and training, and the timing of these events. When possible, the demonstration of a prosthesis by a trained volunteer with a similar level of amputation and discussion of realistic expected functional outcomes should be arranged. Family involvement throughout this process should be encouraged. For all levels of amputation a "prehabilitation" program should include strengthening exercises for the trunk and remaining upper limb musculature; and range-of-motion exercises for the involved glenohumeral, scapulothoracic, and elbow joints (if present).

Amputation Surgery (pp. 265–266)

• Partial hand amputations should be carefully planned to ensure adequate residual sensation and movement. There is little point in salvaging a partial hand if no metacarpals are present to provide pinch. Prosthetic restoration of the thumb should be attempted before any pollicization procedures or toe transfers are attempted.

• The selection of the level of amputation should take into consideration the amount of space necessary for the appropriate prosthetic components with adequate cosmesis. The transradial amputation has to be a minimum of 5 cm proximal to the distal radius to accommodate an externally powered terminal device. Transhumeral amputations should be performed 7 to 10 cm proximal to the distal humeral condyles to accommodate most of the prosthetic elbows. Longer residual limbs affect the location of the artificial elbow joint center of rotation, which can compromise cosmesis.

Transradial and Transhumeral Amputations (p. 266)
• In the traumatic transradial and transhumeral amputation, it is not uncommon to find a more proximal fracture; a dislocation; or, occasionally, a peripheral nerve injury that can temporarily or permanently interfere with optimal prosthesis fitting and arm motion. Early diagnosis of these problems is needed to ensure inclusion of the necessary appropriate prosthetic modifications and alterations to the rehabilitation program.

Shoulder Disarticulation and Forequarter Amputation (p. 266)
• Shoulder disarticulation is performed in severe electrical injuries, in trauma cases, and in tumor surgery. Prosthetic replacement in these cases is more successful in those who are healthy, young, and male.
• Forequarter amputation is rarely performed, but it may be required in some cases of severe trauma or malignant lesion involving the shoulder. Functional prosthetic use is uncommon after this procedure because suspension is difficult to maintain.

Acute Postamputation Period (p. 266)

• Pain control, maintenance of range of motion and strength, and promotion of wound healing are the goals of this stage, which begins with the surgical closure of the wound and culminates in wound healing. Pain control and residual limb maturation should be pursued aggressively. Immediate application of postoperative plaster of Paris rigid dressing (IPORD) or soft elastic bandage and subsequent pneumatic compression are indicated for edema control. An increasingly popular method of wound protection, swelling control, early shaping and soft tissue shrinking, and return to function is the immediate postoperative prosthesis. Soft compressive dressings or Unna bandages are used in many centers.

Acute Pain Management (p. 266)
• Pain control can be best achieved initially with a patient-controlled analgesia (PCA) system, followed by the use of scheduled parenteral and oral analgesia. A skin desensitization program that includes gentle tapping, massage, soft tissue and scar mobilization, and lubrication is recommended for the patient with a soft or elastic dressing.
• When the patient's condition is medically stable, early mobilization, general endurance, and strengthening exercise are started.

Postoperative Care (pp. 266–267)

• Postoperative edema is common following amputation. If soft dressings are used they should be combined with elastic wrapping to control edema, especially if the patient is a candidate for a prosthesis. The ideal shape of the upper extremity residual limb is cylindrical, not conical. The major complication from elastic wrapping is applying the bandage too tightly at the proximal end in an attempt to improve bandage suspension. This causes congestion, worsens edema, and results in a dumbbell-shaped residual limb. The recommended elastic dressing involves the use of a figure-of-8 wrapping technique that extends over the proximal joint and that is reapplied every 4 to 6 hours.

• The use of an IPORD to control postoperative edema, promote healing, protect the limb from trauma, decrease postoperative pain, desensitize the limb, and allow early mobilization and rehabilitation is the preferred treatment approach for the transradial level. The dressing is made out of plaster of Paris bandages that extend beyond the proximal joint for suspension. An IPORD should be replaced at 1-week intervals. By the time the second dressing is replaced, the prosthesis can be casted and a few days later it can be fitted. If the patient has a fever for which no other apparent cause can be determined, the IPORD should be removed and the wound inspected.

Phantom Limb, Phantom Pain, and Painful Residual Limb (p. 267)

• Phantom limb sensation is the feeling that all or a part of the amputated limb is still present. This sensation is felt by nearly all "acquired" amputees, but is not always bothersome. Phantom sensation usually diminishes over time, and telescoping (the sensation that the phantom hand has moved proximally) commonly occurs. Phantom sensation is not necessarily painful. As many as 70% of amputees perceive phantom pain in the first few months after amputation; however, such pain usually disappears or decreases sufficiently so that it does not interfere with prosthesis fitting and day-to-day activities. Perceived pain intensity is closely related to anxiety level, depression, prosthesis fitting problems, and other personal factors.

• Appropriate management of phantom limb begins by preventing prolonged periods of pain before the amputation because preamputation pain often ends in postoperative phantom pain. Treatment includes prosthetic socket revisions, desensitization techniques, transcutaneous nerve stimulation, neuropharmacological intervention, and the voluntary control of the phantom limb (mental imaging). For severe cases, nerve blocks, steroid injections, and epidural blocks can be useful. Nonsurgical interventions are far more successful than surgical ones.

Joint Contractures (p. 267)

• Joint contractures can occur between the time of amputation and prosthesis fitting. Efforts should be directed at preventing contractures by means of aggressive rehabilitation efforts beginning soon after surgery.

Preprosthetic Rehabilitation (pp. 267–268)

• A preprosthetic rehabilitation program must be initiated as soon as possible. Pain control and residual limb maturation should be promoted during this phase. An IPORD or soft elastic bandages are indicated for edema control. This is also a time for the patient to initiate emotional adaptation to a body image without the artificial limb; and to learn basic skills without a prosthesis, which is essential for the times when the device is not worn. Soft tissue desensitization, early mobilization, improving general endurance, strengthening, avoidance of joint contractures, and emotional counseling are the key goals of this phase.

- Occasionally a patient can become so emotionally disturbed by the limb loss that the result can be a chronic failure to cope. This can have a very negative effect on the rehabilitation outcome.
- The use of the first prosthesis should be implemented as soon as possible in this stage. The early fitting of the prosthetic device is intended to promote prosthesis use for bimanual activities. There is a direct relationship between the time of fitting and long-term prosthetic use. There is a 3- to 6-month window of opportunity for the unilateral upper limb amputee.
- The first prosthesis is intended to promote residual limb maturation and desensitization, to build up wearing tolerance, and to allow the patient to become a functional user. Commonly, this is done with a body-powered or a switch-controlled externally powered prosthesis. Suction suspension or myoelectric control is not practical at this stage because of limb volume fluctuation, which results in the loss of the necessary intimate contact of the socket and electrodes with the soft tissues. When no significant volume fluctuation is noted in the residual limb over a period of 2 months, consideration should be given to proceeding with fitting of the first permanent prosthesis. Serial circumferential measurements of the limb at preestablished locations is the simplest method of determining residual limb size stability.

Prosthesis Fitting and Training (pp. 268–274)

- This task should be accomplished by an expert team of professionals in close communication with the patient. Members of the team ideally should include the surgeon, a physiatrist who devotes time in practice to amputee rehabilitation and prosthetics, a certified prosthetist, an occupational therapist, a physical therapist, a recreational therapist, a psychologist, a social worker, and the patient and family.

Terminal Devices (pp. 268–269)
- The human hand is a very complex anatomical and physiological structure whose functions cannot be replaced by the current level of prosthetic technology. A variety of prosthetic terminal devices are available and include passive, body-powered, and externally powered hooks and hands. They all lack sensory feedback and have limited mobility and dexterity. Prosthetic hands provide a three-jaw chuck pinch and hooks provide the equivalent of lateral or tip pinch. Body-powered terminal devices can be voluntary-opening (most common and practical) or voluntary-closing (most physiological). The voluntary-opening device is maintained in the closed position by rubber bands or tension springs. The patient can open the device by "pulling" with the cable on the harness system in preparation to grasp. Voluntary-closing terminal devices require that the patient close the device by "pulling" with the cable on the harness system to grasp an object. To release, the patient releases the pull on the harness, and a spring in the terminal device opens it. The maximum prehensile force possible is determined by the strength of the individual.

Prosthetic Wrists (p. 269)
- The type of prosthetic wrist most commonly used allows passive pronation and supination. Spring-assisted rotation is available for the bilateral amputee. Quick-disconnect wrists are also available. The friction control permits ease of

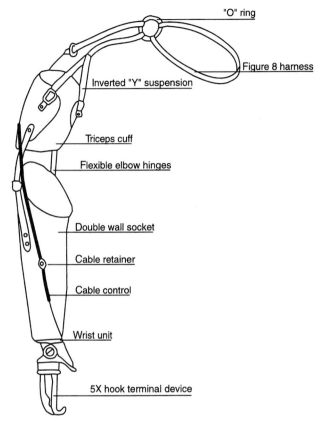

FIGURE 13–1. A body-powered transhumeral prosthesis with components identified.

positioning, but it can rotate when lifting heavy objects. This is particularly problematic when the wearer is carrying a plate or tray. Quick-disconnect wrists permit rapid interchange of different terminal devices. In addition, when it is locked, the quick-disconnect wrist provides a secure control for wrist rotation. A mechanical spring-assisted wrist flexion unit is indispensable for the bilateral upper limb amputee to allow the patient to reach the body's midline for grooming, feeding, hygiene activities, and buttoning of clothing.

Prosthetic Elbows (p. 269)
• The prosthetic elbows available in the treatment of transhumeral amputation have either external or internal joints. These joints can be passive, body-powered, or externally powered (Fig. 13–1). These devices are controlled via mechanical cables, electrical switches, or myoelectric signals. The externally powered systems have digital or proportional control mechanisms. The mechanical elbows have a locking mechanism that is manually applied using the contralateral hand, the chin, or the ipsilateral shoulder via a cable system. Electric

elbows have an electromechanical brake or a switch-controlled lock mechanism to maintain the selected position. The rotation function of the arm (internal/external rotation) is provided through the use of a turntable. This device is useful to provide reach to the body midline. Electric elbows have limited active flexion force. The flexion force across a mechanical elbow is dependent on the wearer's strength, the comfort of the socket fit, and the ability to efficiently transfer the power from the residual limb to the prosthesis.

• For elbow disarticulation, the external elbow joint is indicated in an attempt to maintain the optimal length of the arm. Limited flexion strength and increased maintenance are some of the problems with this type of joint.

Prosthetic Sockets *(pp. 269–271)*

• The key functions of a prosthetic socket include comfortable total contact interface with the residual limb, efficient energy transfer from the residual limb to the prosthetic device, secure suspension, and cosmetic appearance.

• Most upper limb prosthetic sockets have two layers. The first one is closely contoured to the residual limb and the external layer gives the necessary length and shape to the socket. It is to this external layer that the necessary prosthetic components (e.g., elbow and wrist) are attached.

• New flexible plastic materials have made sockets lighter and more comfortable. The inner socket provides total contact with the residual limb and is the interface that provides suction suspension if desired. The outer socket or frame is made of a more rigid material (e.g., thermoplastic or resin) and provides the structural integrity of the socket. When double sockets are used, windows can be cut in the exterior frame to allow muscles to expand during contraction and to improve comfort and sensory feedback.

Suspension Systems *(p. 271)*

• The suspension and control system of a body-powered prosthesis needs to provide suspension, which is the means of securing the prosthetic device to the body; and control. The more secure the suspension system, the more prosthetic control and comfort can be expected by the patient. The upper limb amputee has traditionally been provided with suspension systems that are uncomfortable and that limit mobility. They consist mostly of straps with metal and plastic attachments. The traditional suspension mechanisms (Table 13–1) for the upper limb sockets include a strap that suspends the prosthesis over the shoulder (figure-of-8 harness). The harness is used as a control mechanism to transmit body power to the terminal device and elbow. For the more proximal level amputation, a

TABLE 13–1 Prosthetic Suspension Systems

Harness	Semisuction
Figure-of-8	Hypobaric
Chest strap	Semisuction
Shoulder saddle	Suction
Self-suspension	Full suction
Condylar	Silicone sock
Muenster	
Northwestern	

chest strap or shoulder saddle can be used to further improve suspension. Patients with wrist or elbow disarticulation or transradial amputations can use bony prominences for suspension. The Muenster or condylar suspension is perhaps the best of these. When this type of suspension is used, a figure-of-9 harness can be used for control purposes only. This type of suspension works extremely well with externally powered, myoelectric control prostheses because the patient can be completely free of straps.

• In most cases, a sock is used as an interface between the residual limb and the socket. Using different numbers of sock layers can adjust for the physiological volume changes that occur from day to day. Socks also protect the skin and improve hygiene. The only exceptions are suction sockets, for which direct skin-to-socket contact is required, and socks cannot be used.

Silicone Suction Suspension Application to Upper Limb Body and External Powered Prostheses (pp. 271–273)

• The silicone liner provides improved suspension function by creating a negative atmospheric pressure and an adhesive bond to the skin. The silicone sleeve also improves the socket-residual limb interface by protecting the skin through significant reduction of shear forces and added cushioning. The silicone sleeve provides improved suspension by reducing pistoning and shear, protects the skin, allows for volume adjustment with residual limb girth changes, and improves cosmesis because it reduces or eliminates the need for harness suspension. The system consists of a silicone sleeve with a distal attachment pin that interfaces with a shuttle lock mechanism built into the prosthetic socket (see Figs. 13–5, 13–6, and 13–7 in the Textbook).

• Excessive perspiration and irritation can occur with roll-on silicone sleeve use. Excessive perspiration can be controlled with antiperspirant lotions or Botox injections of the affected skin area to control the focal hyperhidrosis. A contact dermatitis-like reaction can occur even though silicone is a hypoallergenic material. A bland skin protectant agent such as zinc oxide or petrolatum paste (Desitin) can make for rapid resolution of the problem.

• Silicone sleeves are best used by patients who are likely to have problems with skin integrity such as patients who have undergone skin grafting for burns or degloving injuries; those with delicate, insensate skin (e.g., patients with diabetes and scleroderma); or those with adhesive scar tissue. Silicone sleeves afford excellent skin protection and are a good prosthetic suspension system for patients who are very active users, who play sports, or who have short, very sensitive, or delicate residual limbs.

• Individuals who live in areas of the world with warm and humid weather are more likely to develop dermatological problems. These can be minimized by strict hygienic care of the skin and the insert.

Control Mechanisms (p. 273)

• When a body harness is used as a control mechanism for a body-powered prosthesis, the patient needs to be able to produce movements that generate the power requirements to activate the terminal device or elbow. These movements include scapular abduction; chest expansion; shoulder depression, extension, and abduction, and humeral flexion; and elbow flexion and extension. These movements can be difficult to perform if the residual limb is short, painful, or has limited motion; or if the prosthetic socket does not fit well. A poorly adjusted harness decreases the power transmission of the movements.

• Electric switch control mechanisms can be activated with residual limb movements that depress a switch inside the socket. For other cases, a chest strap, waist belt, or figure-of-9 harness can be used. Servo controls that sense tension have been introduced into clinical use.

• Myoelectric controls use the electrical activity generated during a muscle contraction to control the flow of energy from a battery to a motor in the prosthetic device. The control signals come from muscle sites in the amputated limb that still have normal innervation and voluntary control.

Suction Suspension (p. 273)
• For the transhumeral amputee, suction suspension (negative pressure) without the use of straps is the preferred type of suspension. The socket is made small enough and provided with a one-way valve that permits the expulsion of air during donning. The amputee dons the socket using a pull sock or Ace bandage or with a wet fit (using a lubricant liquid or powder).

Shoulder Disarticulation and Forequarter Amputation (p. 273)
• There has been little change in the basic socket design for shoulder disarticulation or forequarter amputation since it was designed, except for the use of lighter materials. Most of the advances in prosthetic design for these levels have occurred with externally powered components. A shoulder joint with a manual lock that provides improvement in the arm control and position is now available.

Cosmetic Covers (pp. 273–274)
• Cosmetic covers can be manufactured for a single digit, for the hand, or to extend to the elbow. They should be considered an integral part of the prosthesis because for many patients the cover is the factor that determines success or failure of prosthetic restoration.

Activity-Specific Devices (p. 274)
• Many devices are commercially available that are designed to permit participation in sports (e.g., golf, fishing, or skiing) or in such activities as construction, cooking, archery, and photography.

Prosthetic Prescription (p. 274)
• The prosthetic prescription should be carefully prepared to satisfy the needs and desires of the patient, using a team approach. The prescription should clearly spell out the components, control system, suspension, materials, and any special features that might be required.

Prosthetic Training (pp. 274–275)

• A new amputee, or an experienced one who receives a prosthetic device that has different components, should participate in prosthetic training. In most cases, this program should be a coordinated effort among the occupational, physical, and recreational therapists and the prosthetist, with frequent physiatric input (kinesiotherapists are also used at some centers). A review and practice of the use of the prosthesis for bimanual activities (e.g., grooming, dressing, feeding, driving, sports, work, and recreation activities) should always be included in the training process.

Special Considerations for the Bilateral Upper Limb Amputee (p. 275)
• For the bilateral upper limb amputee, training should promote the development of a dominant prosthesis and skills for independent donning. Alternative techniques for putting on the prosthesis are often required. These might include using the bed for setup and suspending the prosthetic devices from special wall hooks or frames. The prosthesis should have a wrist rotation and flexion device that permits access to the body midline.
• For bathing activities, the patient with bilateral upper limb amputations ideally should have a modified shower with wall brushes and liquid soap dispensers. In some cases, simplified shower prostheses (devices that are waterproof) are a medical necessity because they allow the patient to perform this activity independently (see Fig. 13–10 in the Textbook).

Reintegration into the Community (pp. 275–276)

• Reintegration into the community is best done gradually over a few weeks or months. When possible, the use of "day" rehabilitation programs, in which the patient participates in rehabilitation 6 hours a day, 5 days a week (returning home evenings and weekends), is a good system to foster community reintegration.
• The patient can return to work when safety concerns are met. Initially, modified or restricted work should be provided, but the patient should not be discouraged from returning to the premorbid work level if it is safe to do so.

Functional Outcomes (pp. 275–276)
• Realistic goals for the majority of unilateral transradial or transhumeral amputees include independence in all activities of daily living, most household activities, driving, and work. Some restrictions should be imposed in relationship to handling delicate, heavy, or voluminous objects. The typical patient with a transradial amputation can be expected to lift 20 to 30 lb unless the residual limb is very short or sensitive. The typical patient with a transhumeral amputation can be expected to lift 10 to 15 lb unless the residual limb is very short or sensitive.
• For the bilateral transhumeral amputee, realistic goals include independence in most activities of daily living after assisted donning; some household activities; driving with a spin ring; and most types of sedentary work, with environmental modifications.

Long-Term Follow-up (p. 276)

• The patient who has successfully completed a rehabilitation program should be seen for follow-up by a minimum of two of the team members at least every 3 months for the first 18 months. After this, the patient should be seen at least every 6 months to ensure adequate prosthetic fit and function and to assess the need for maintenance and the overall medical condition and functional level of the patient. When the patient's condition is stable it may be necessary to replace a prosthesis or parts of it every 18 months to 3 years (for body-powered devices) and every 2 to 4 years (for myoelectric prostheses).

Neuromas (p. 276)
• Neuroma is the formation of scar tissue around the distal end of the severed nerve. As previously mentioned, every time a nerve is cut it forms a neuroma.

Good surgical technique results in the neuroma being buried under large soft tissue masses that serve to protect it from irritation. At times, because of limited soft tissue coverage or very large neuroma formation with compression of the nerve, adhesion of the tissues, or complications from the surgical technique, a neuroma may become symptomatic. This results in pain that can be perceived at the site of the neuroma and that radiates distally to the end of the residual limb (or, at times, into the phantom limb). A painful neuroma is palpable most of the time, and pressure over it reproduces the symptoms. Desensitization techniques; prosthetic modifications; and, at times, use of flexible materials with windowed frame construction to decrease pressure over the neuroma may help. Injection of the neuroma with a mixture of long- and short-acting local anesthetics and a corticosteroid should reduce the scar tissue pressure on the nerve and produce symptomatic improvement. Surgical removal of the neuroma, with careful retraction of the nerve prior to cutting it, should be reserved for those cases in which all other interventions have failed and in which the tissues allow repositioning of the neuroma to a less pressure-exposed location.

Support Groups (p. 276)
• Support groups provide information, peer counseling, and motivation for many patients and their families. These groups ideally should constitute one more component of the comprehensive rehabilitation approach to the patient with an amputation. Patients who have recently sustained an amputation benefit from contact with experienced amputees; at the same time, the veteran amputee enjoys serving as a resource.

Dermatological Problems (p. 276)
• The skin of a patient who wears a prosthesis is subject to much abuse. Most prosthetic sockets prevent appropriate air circulation, thereby trapping perspiration moisture. This can result in a variety of problems such as hyperhidrosis, folliculitis, allergic dermatitis, and even skin breakdown where adherent scars are present. Poor hygiene is commonly the cause of some of these problems, and for this reason the patient should be trained in the proper washing technique for the residual limb, silicone liners, socks, and the socket and its interfaces. A daily routine of washing the skin and the internal wall of the socket with a mild soap might suffice. It can be necessary at times to use concentrated antiperspirants; bacteriostatic or bactericidal soaps; and, in some cases, antibiotics. Topical antibiotics or steroids should not generally be used if the prosthesis has silicone components as part of the socket materials that are in direct contact with the skin. Contact dermatitis can often occur because of this.

Care of the Nonamputated Upper Limb (pp. 276–277)

• There is a high incidence of overuse injuries to the soft tissues, tendon-muscle complex, and joints of the remaining limb. The more proximal the amputation, the more prevalent the problems. A program of education to avoid overuse and promote habilitation, aggressive early management of injuries, and preventative care of the limb with avoidance of potentially injurious activities should be implemented.

PEDIATRIC LIMB DEFICIENCY AND AMPUTATION REHABILITATION (p. 277)

• The pediatric patient can have an acquired or congenital limb deficiency. The child with a congenital limb deficiency has no sense of loss and does not have to go through the psychological adjustment process. The prosthesis is perceived as an aid rather than as a replacement. If the device cannot serve in this role it will be discarded. These children try to engage in the same types of activities as other children. Their only limitations are usually those imposed by adults. In contrast, the child with an acquired limb deficiency goes through the natural readjustment process of limb loss. How well they are able to adjust has a direct impact on their acceptance of an artificial limb.

• Some special considerations should be made for the pediatric patient with upper limb deficiency or amputation. Three specific points to consider in this population are: (1) normal growth and development, which will necessitate regular prosthetic adjustments or replacements; (2) bony overgrowth; and (3) the more rigorous use that the device will be subjected to. It can be expected that a prosthesis (socket only, or all of it) will need to be replaced yearly in the first 5 years of life; every 18 months from 5 to 12 years of age; and every 2 years until age 21 years. To address growth problems, multilayered sockets (onion sockets) for body-powered devices can be used. These allow removal of one layer at a time to accommodate growth. This results in gradual enlargement of the socket to coincide with periods of growth. Length adjustment is also important, although it is not as critical as with lower limb prostheses. This can be adjusted by adding material at the wrist or elbow sites when necessary. Harnesses and cables need to be adjusted for length and replaced more often. For bony overgrowth, surgery with bony capping may be necessary. Regularly required socket replacements can make myoelectric devices less practical for this population because of their cost. Terminal devices and elbows might need to be replaced regularly.

• Parental counseling and support are integral components in the rehabilitation of the pediatric amputee. The prosthetic fitting for the pediatric patient with upper limb deficiency or the pediatric amputee should be initiated at 3 to 9 months of age. This should coincide with sitting and the initiation of bimanual activities. The use of a passive mitten, hand, or inactive hook or California Amputee Pediatric Project (CAPP) terminal device and a preflexed fixed elbow is indicated at this stage. The terminal device can be activated at ages 18 to 24 months and the elbow at ages 36 to 48 months. Myoelectric devices have been used at these young ages with good results. For very proximal upper limb deficiency, use of the feet should be encouraged.

SUMMARY (p. 277)

• The rehabilitation process for the patient with an upper limb amputation is best accomplished when the patient is able to work in a close cooperative relationship with a comprehensive, multidisciplinary, specialized treatment team. The team members should be ready and able to assist the patient throughout the rehabilitation program, from preamputation to community reintegration.

14

Original Chapter by Ellen I. Leonard, M.D., Robert D. McAnelly, M.D.,
Maria Lomba, M.D., and Virgil W. Faulkner, C.P.O.

Lower Limb Prostheses

• The types of amputation by level are partial foot, Syme, transtibial (below-knee), knee disarticulation (through-knee), transcondylar/supracondylar, transfemoral (above-knee), hip disarticulation, transpelvic (hemipelvectomy), and translumbar (hemicorporectomy). There are 358,000 persons with major amputations living in the United States, yielding a rate of 1.7 major amputations per 1000 persons. Of the major amputations, 91,000 were upper limb, 92,000 were transfemoral, 113,000 were transtibial, 22,000 were partial foot, 36,000 were bilateral lower limb, and 4000 were combined lower and upper limb amputations. An estimated 205,000 persons use an artificial leg or foot.

• Vascular disease and infection account for 70% of all amputations; trauma, 22%; tumor, 5%; and congenital deformity, 3%. The largest number of amputations for disease occurs in the 61- to 70-year age group; for trauma, the 21- to 30-year age group; and for tumor, the 11- to 20-year age group. Male amputees outnumber female amputees in the disease group 2.1:1; in trauma, 7.2:1; in tumor, 1.3:1; and in congenital deformity, 1.5:1. The ratio of lower to upper limb amputations was 11:1. The distribution of lower limb amputations by level is Syme, 3%; transtibial, 59%; knee disarticulation, 1%; transfemoral, 35%; and hip disarticulation, 2%.

• Vascular diseases requiring amputation include diabetes mellitus, arteriosclerosis, and Buerger's disease. Diabetic patients not only experience vascular compromise but also suffer motor, sensory, and autonomic neuropathy, all of which lead to ulceration.

• Advances in chemotherapy and radiation therapy with better tumor staging now make it possible, in many cases, to perform segmental limb resection with wide local excision of the tumor. Post-tumor amputee patients who have received doxorubicin (Adriamycin) require cardiac screening before prosthesis fitting. Amputees on chemotherapy have residual limb volume fluctuation, and it is important to coordinate prosthetic and chemotherapy programs. Transfemoral socket fit and gait training should be done when the patient is feeling well, usually before chemotherapy. The permanent prosthesis should not be prescribed until 6 weeks after termination of chemotherapy (with resolution of transient edema) (see Chapter 57).

• All combinations of congenital limb deficiency occur, including missing intermediate parts. For example, the thigh or upper arm can be missing, whereas the other parts of the limb can be present but malformed. If a malformed part is nonfunctional, surgical options might have to be considered for amputation or reconstruction.

PREOPERATIVE MANAGEMENT (pp. 280–283)

Psychological Aspects (p. 280)

• Preoperative counseling by the rehabilitation team, and peer counseling by other amputees, facilitate recovery. Preoperative therapy includes range-of-motion exercise, strengthening, and ambulation with an assistive device. A new amputee typically experiences depression, especially if unaware of the prosthetic options for future function and ambulation.

Surgical Decisions and Level of Amputation (pp. 280–281)

• The rule of amputation is to save as much of the limb as possible, consistent with satisfactory healing and function. This rule demands a thoughtful accounting of advantages and disadvantages. The cost of limb salvage can be high: increased morbidity may occasion multiple operations, which can be financially and psychosocially ruinous. It is often better to choose early amputation and prosthetic fitting over limb salvage of questionable functional benefit. It is difficult to select the optimum level of amputation based on clinical assessment of tissue viability. Criteria such as poor skin edge bleeding during surgery and absence of pulses do not always correlate with failure to heal. Many noninvasive vascular studies are available to determine level of amputation. Adequate nutrition and immunocompetence, as measured by albumin and total lymphocyte counts, also contribute to healing.

• Preamputation arteriography in peripheral vascular disease is of limited value for amputation level selection because distal vessels are not commonly detected. Occlusion of both the deep and superficial femoral vessels indicates a poor prognosis for healing in transtibial amputation.

• Doppler-determined ankle blood pressure measurements are of little value in assessing partial foot amputation viability, probably due to arteriovenous shunting that results in artificially elevated ankle blood pressures. However, thigh blood pressure measurements above 70 mm Hg, and possibly between 50 and 70 mm Hg, are predictive of success in transtibial amputation surgery.

• Skin blood flow technique can be the most accurate measurement to assess skin viability, particularly around the knee joint, but it is not as reliable in assessing regional blood flow. Absolute skin perfusion pressure is also valuable. Healing occurs in 90% of patients with skin perfusion calf pressure greater than 30 mm Hg, and in 67% with skin perfusion pressure from 20 to 30 mm Hg.

• Transcutaneous oxygen pressure ($TcPO_2$) is easy to measure but difficult to interpret. $TcPO_2$ levels greater than 35 mm Hg at the calf predict that a transtibial amputation will heal, but values below this are not predictive. Adding 100% oxygen inhalation to the test improves test reliability dramatically: Successful healing is predicted with a rate of change of 9 mm Hg/min on switching to 100% oxygen from room air, or with a rise in $TcPO_2$ of at least 10 mm Hg after 10 minutes of 100% oxygen inhalation compared with room air values.

• Preoperative noninvasive vascular studies, so that the level selected is at the edge of tissue viability, are crucial in preserving limb length. If limb infection

is present, then the limb blood flow should be evaluated to assess whether healing will occur.
• Proper surgical technique requires suturing of cut muscles to each other and to the periosteum at the end of the cut bone (myoplasty) or to the bone itself (myodesis). The surgeon should taper the muscle mass to reduce distal bulk.

Residual Limb Management (pp. 281–282)

• A postoperative plaster of Paris or fiberglass rigid dressing prevents edema, protects from trauma, and decreases postoperative pain. Postoperative edema occurs within a few minutes, so immediate replacement of the dressing is necessary. Once they are removed for inspection or suture removal, rigid dressings must be replaced within minutes to prevent recurrence of edema.
• The removable rigid dressing (RRD) for the transtibial amputee consists of a plaster of Paris or fiberglass cast suspended by a stockinet and supracondylar cuff; it is adjusted by adding or removing socks to maintain compression. The RRD provides good edema control with the advantage of allowing daily inspection.
• When a rigid dressing is not being used, cotton-elastic bandages can be wrapped around the residual limb if the patient is physically and mentally able to learn the wrapping technique. Poorly applied elastic bandages also can cause circumferential constriction with distal edema. Double-length 4-inch bandages should be used for the transtibial limb, and double-length 6-inch bandages for the transfemoral limb.
• Elastic shrinker socks are easy to apply and provide uniform compression but are more expensive than elastic bandages. The amputee should wear a shrinkage device 24 hours/day except for bathing or when ventilating an open sore for short periods during the day. A shrinkage device for the nonprosthesis candidate helps control pain and edema and facilitates healing. The shrinkage device can be discontinued after fitting the definitive prosthesis if the amputee wears the prosthesis regularly. The shrinkage device can be used overnight if edema is an ongoing problem.
• A contracture is easy to prevent but difficult to correct. The amputee should not lie on an overly soft mattress or use a pillow under the back or thigh; nor should the head of the bed be elevated. All of these practices lead to hip flexion contractures. The amputee should not place a pillow between the legs because this creates a hip abduction contracture. A transtibial amputee should not lie with the residual limb hanging over the edge of the bed, with a pillow placed under the knee, or with the knees flexed; and must not sit in a wheelchair with the knee flexed, because these positions lead to knee flexion contractures. The transtibial amputee should sit with the knee extended on a board under the wheelchair cushion and a towel wrapped over the board. Crutch walking with or without a prosthesis promotes good range of motion and, when feasible, is preferred over wheelchair mobility. Amputees should lie prone for 15 minutes three times a day to help prevent hip flexion contractures. The amputee who cannot lie prone should lie supine and actively extend the residual limb while flexing the contralateral hip (this is, essentially, a Thomas test maneuver).

Preprosthetic Training (p. 282)

• Preprosthetic training includes active range-of-motion exercises, positioning, muscle strengthening, skin care, wheelchair mobility, transfers, ambulation with assistive devices, self-care, and patient and family education.

Immediate Postoperative and Early Prosthetic Training
(pp. 282–283)

• The immediate postoperative weight bearing required by this technique has lost popularity owing to concerns over wound healing, but it is still common practice for pediatric and clean post-traumatic amputees. A pylon and foot are attached to the rigid dressing for immediate postoperative weight bearing. It should be noted that patients should never be fully weight bearing on this type of socket. At 10 to 14 days after surgery, a preparatory prosthesis is provided if the wound has closed. If the wound has not closed, a new rigid dressing should be applied for 10 additional days. Others recommend waiting at least 21 days postoperatively before fitting or using a temporary prosthesis.

Gait Training (p. 283)

• Training for an efficient, cosmetically acceptable gait begins with the parallel bars and includes training in sit-to-stand transfers, balance, knee control, lateral weight shifting, and forward progression. Balancing techniques are taught first, with progression to limited weight bearing. The amputee should use open hands to avoid pulling up on the bars.
• Advanced gait training progresses through gait aids (e.g., walker, crutches, and canes) to ramps; curbs; stairs; clearing obstacles; and, if indicated, falling safety and floor-to-standing transfers. In stair climbing and ramp walking, the amputee ascends by leading with the sound foot and descends by leading with the prosthesis ("Up with the good, down with the bad").

THE PROSTHESIS (p. 283)

• All limb prostheses consist of a suspension device, a socket, rigid components, and a terminal device (foot). Some also include artificial joints. Most amputees require a prosthetic sheath and socks over the residual limb.

Preparatory/Temporary Prosthesis (p. 283)

• Even when a patient's potential success at using a prosthesis is uncertain, a preparatory prosthesis should be provided as a trial. The preparatory or temporary prosthesis is usually uncosmetic but is used during the period of residual limb shrinkage. The amputee uses the preparatory prosthesis until maximal shrinkage has been attained, usually 3 to 6 months post-surgery. When the ply of socks reaches 10 to 15 because of residual limb shrinkage, the amputee should be given a new socket to prevent pistoning.

Definitive/Permanent Prosthesis (p. 283)

• The definitive or permanent prosthesis is cosmetically finished. Its fit, alignment, and components are chosen based on the amputee's experience with the preparatory prosthesis. A test or check socket is usually made to test fit just before fabricating the definitive socket. The definitive prosthesis typically requires replacement about every 3 years in adults.

PARTIAL FOOT AMPUTATIONS (pp. 283–284)

Surgical Procedures (p. 283)

• The most common types of foot amputation are: (1) transmetatarsal, (2) Lisfranc, and (3) Chopart (see Fig. 14–5 in the Textbook). In transmetatarsal amputation, the surgeon sections the metatarsals transversely, usually just proximal to the metatarsal heads, and bevels them inferiorly.

• The Lisfranc amputation is a tarsometatarsal disarticulation. The Chopart amputation is a disarticulation at the midtarsal joint through the talonavicular and calcaneocuboid joints (see Fig. 14–5 in the Textbook). In both of these procedures, the remaining foot often develops a significant equinovarus deformity resulting in excessive anterior weight bearing with breakdown.

• The Boyd amputation consists of excision of all tarsals except the calcaneus. The Boyd amputation is rarely performed in the adult because of residual limb length problems, but is more commonly performed in the pediatric congenital amputee.

Prosthetic and Orthotic Prescription (pp. 283–284)

• For patients with toe amputation, wool, sponge rubber, or foam should be inserted in the shoe to serve as a spacer and to prevent toe deformity. For an amputated great toe, a long steel spring shank, a metatarsal pad, and a rocker sole improve function. The transmetatarsal amputation requires a custom-molded insole and toe filler. The stiff insole should prevent shoe hyperextension proximal to the natural toe break.

• For the Lisfranc or Chopart amputee, a modified shoe or molded plastic socket, or a combination of the two, should be provided. Modern slipper-type prostheses terminate at the ankle joint.

• The Boyd amputation is fitted as a Syme amputation but it requires a contralateral shoe lift in adults because of leg length discrepancy.

SYME AMPUTATION (p. 284)

Surgical Procedures (p. 284)

• Syme amputation is an ankle disarticulation for destructive and infective lesions of the foot that cannot be treated with a transmetatarsal amputation. The main advantage is that, if successful, the patient can walk on the Syme residual limb without a prosthesis, at least for short distances. Syme amputation prostheses are uncosmetic because of the inability to match the shape of the contralateral leg.

Prosthetic Prescription (p. 284)

• The Syme prosthesis usually has a removable medial window that allows the patient to push the residual limb into the socket (Fig. 14–1). The prosthesis gives excellent function. The prosthetic heel should be soft to accommodate lack of ankle motion. Feet for the Syme amputee include all of the SACH-type (solid ankle cushion heel) feet as well as some energy-storing feet.

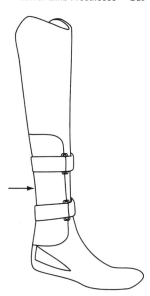

FIGURE 14–1. Syme-type prosthesis with medial opening socket. (From Cestaro JM: The Illustrated Guide to Orthotics and Prosthetics. Alexandria, VA, National Office of Orthotics and Prosthetics, 1992, p. 234.)

TRANSTIBIAL (BELOW-KNEE) AMPUTATION
(pp. 284–290)

Surgical Procedures (p. 284)

• Transtibial amputation is usually performed at the junction of the upper and middle third of the tibia (see Fig. 14–7 in the Textbook). Some advocate a longer residual limb to provide a longer lever arm and more efficient gait, but this is harder to fit. A long posterior flap meets a shorter anterior flap to allow the gastrocnemius-soleus muscles to form the distal soft tissue. Transtibial residual limbs as short as 2.5 inches can be successfully fitted with a prosthesis.

Prosthetic Prescription (pp. 284–289)

Foot-Ankle Assemblies (pp. 284–286)
• Prosthetic feet are classified into five types: (1) the SACH foot, (2) the single-axis foot, (3) the multi-axis foot, (4) the solid ankle flexible keel foot, and (5) the energy-storing foot. SACH is an acronym for solid ankle cushion heel. The SACH foot has a cushioned heel that compresses during heel-strike, simulating plantar flexion, and has a rigid anterior keel to roll over during late stance (Fig. 14–2). It is light, durable, inexpensive, and is most often prescribed for juvenile and geriatric amputees.
• The single-axis foot has a single mechanical axis for plantar flexion and dorsiflexion motion limited by anterior and posterior bumpers; this allows quicker foot flat, which results in a more stable knee (see Fig. 14–9 in the Textbook). The single-axis foot is heavier and less durable than the SACH foot. The single-axis foot has some biomechanical advantages in gait over the SACH. It is most often used in transfemoral prostheses, and seldom in transtibial prostheses.

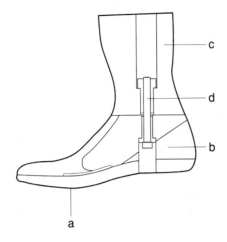

FIGURE 14–2. SACH (*solid ankle cushion heel*) foot. The plastic cover (*a*) is over a wooden core. The heel wedge (*b*) is elastic. The foot is attached to the wooden ankle block (*c*) by a bolt (*d*). (Courtesy of Otto Bock Orthopadische Industrie GmbH and Co.)

• Multi-axis feet (e.g., the Greissinger, Endolite Multiflex, and stationary attachment flexible endoskeleton [SAFE] II) allow dorsiflexion, plantar flexion, inversion, eversion, and transverse rotation (see Fig. 14–10 in the Textbook). Multi-axis feet are good for walking on uneven ground or for an excessively scarred and sensitive residual limb, because of better shock absorption. They are heavier, less durable, and more costly than SACH feet.

• Energy-storing feet (dynamic response feet) store and release energy as the limb is weighted and unweighted, giving a "springy" feeling (see Fig. 14–12 in the Textbook). Examples include the Seattle foot, Seattle Light, Carbon Copy II, Carbon Copy II Light, Carbon Copy III, Quantum Foot, Flex Walk, Flex Foot, and Springlite. Energy-storing feet result in a higher self-selected walking speed and are indicated for the more active amputee.

SHANKS: EXOSKELETAL ("CRUSTACEAN") VERSUS ENDOSKELETAL (MODULAR)

• The two basic designs for the shank are (1) the exoskeletal ("crustacean") and (2) the endoskeletal (modular). The exoskeletal system has a hard outer plastic shell. It is very durable, but does not allow alignment changes in the finished prosthesis. The endoskeletal system has a pylon covered by contoured, soft foam. The endoskeletal system is generally lighter and more cosmetic, and can be more easily accessed for adjustment and component change-out.

Socket Construction (pp. 286–287)
"PATELLAR TENDON-BEARING SOCKET" TOTAL SURFACE WEIGHT-BEARING SOCKET

• The conventional total-contact "patellar tendon-bearing" (PTB) socket is characterized by a bar in the anterior wall designed to apply pressure to the patellar tendon. The trimline extends anteriorly to the midpatella level, can extend mediolaterally to the femoral condyles, and extends posteriorly to below the level of the PTB bar. Pressure-sensitive areas include the tibial crest, tubercle and condyles, the fibular head, the distal tibia and fibula, and the hamstring tendons. Pressure-tolerant areas include the patellar tendon, the pretibial muscles, the gastrocnemius-soleus muscles, the popliteal fossa, the lateral flat aspect of the fibula, and the medial tibial flare (Fig. 14–3). The PTB socket is a total-contact socket because the distal part of the residual limb is in contact with the socket with minimal end-weight bearing.

Bent Knee or Kneeling Prosthesis and Bypass Prosthesis (pp. 287–288)
• The bypass prosthesis receives all pressure from the thigh, ischium, and gluteus, and bypasses the tibia. If the bypass is due to severe knee flexion contracture, it is called a *bent knee* or *kneeling prosthesis.* Protruding external knee hinges are necessary. The biomechanics are the same as for the transfemoral prosthesis, with poorer cosmesis.

SOFT AND HARD SOCKETS
• A plastic socket without an insert is a *hard socket,* and when fitted with an insert it is a *soft socket.* An insert provides extra protection for the residual limb but reduces the intimate contact between limb and prosthesis. It is often fabricated from polyethylene foam, although a silicone gel insert better protects the sensitive residual limb. Inserts should be prescribed when peripheral vascular disease, extensive scarring, or reduced subcutaneous tissue is present. Inserts are almost always prescribed for transtibial prostheses.

FLEXIBLE SOCKET
• Flexible sockets provide a softer, thermoplastic material for weight transmission. Note that the term *flexible* refers to the socket material and not to the socket shape.

Suspension (pp. 288–289)
FLEXIBLE ATTACHMENT
• The supracondylar cuff is a simple cuff or strap fitted just above the femoral condyles to suspend the prosthesis during swing phase (see Fig. 14–15 in the Textbook). It can have a Velcro or buckle closure. A waist belt and elastic strap can be added for extra security.

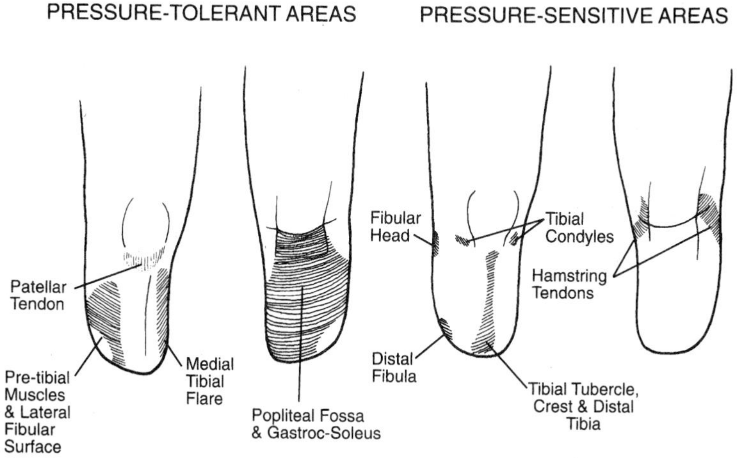

PRESSURE-TOLERANT AREAS   PRESSURE-SENSITIVE AREAS

Patellar Tendon

Medial Tibial Flare

Pre-tibial Muscles & Lateral Fibular Surface

Popliteal Fossa & Gastroc-Soleus

Fibular Head

Tibial Condyles

Hamstring Tendons

Distal Fibula

Tibial Tubercle, Crest & Distal Tibia

FIGURE 14–3. Pressure-tolerant and pressure-sensitive areas of the PTB socket. (Courtesy of the University of Texas Health Science Center at San Antonio.)

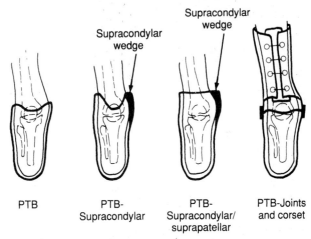

FIGURE 14–4. Examples of the variations of the PTB socket design. (From Karacoloff LA, Hammersley CS, Schneider FJ: Lower Extremity Amputation. Gaithersburg, MD, Aspen Publishers, 1986, p. 27.)

• Neoprene or rubber suspension sleeves provide excellent suspension, fitting snugly over the proximal prosthesis and several inches up on the thigh (see Fig. 14–16 in the Textbook). Sleeves should not be used for very short residual limbs or for amputees who need added knee stability with proximal trim lines. Perspiration and hygiene problems can occur, especially in hot, humid climates, and kneeling shortens the life of the sleeve.

• The silicone suction suspension system (3S, ICEROSS, ALPS) is a thin-walled, highly compliant, closed-end insert or liner of silicone (see Fig. 14–17 in the Textbook). The amputee rolls the silicone liner onto the bare residual limb, then attaches it to the socket by a shuttle lock system. The amputee pushes the residual limb into the prosthesis until a click (or clicks) is heard. The amputee pushes a button to doff the socket. The liner provides friction suspension and absorbs moderate impact and shear forces on the residual limb.

BRIM CONTOUR

Supracondylar. The patellar tendon-bearing socket with supracondylar wedge (PTB-SC) extends its mediolateral trimlines above the femoral condyles for suspension (Fig. 14–4). A wedge is either built into the liner or is completely separate, and is positioned above and over the medial femoral condyle. The PTB-SC provides extra mediolateral support and is helpful for short residual limbs and in overweight amputees.

Supracondylar/Suprapatellar. The patellar tendon-bearing socket with supracondylar/suprapatellar trimline (PTB-SC/SP) is a PTB-SC socket with suprapatellar trimlines (see Fig. 14–6). The alternative name, from France, is *prothèse tibiale supracondylien* (PTS). The suprapatellar trimline helps suspend the prosthesis and increases socket wall support of the expected stance phase varus moment; it is helpful for short residual limbs and for controlling genu recurvatum.

THIGH CORSET
- The patellar tendon-bearing socket with joints and corset (PTB w/J&C) adds a femoral corset to decrease residual limb weight bearing by 40% to 60%. It gives less knee control and worsens gait and is therefore the socket suspension of last resort (see Fig. 14–6). It provides control of significantly lax collateral knee ligaments and protects the knee from varus stresses during stance. It also provides additional mediolateral support for the patient with a short residual limb. The PTB w/J&C relieves weight on a residual limb with poor pressure tolerance, and it is often used for amputees involved in heavy manual labor.

Transtibial Prosthetic Care (p. 289)
- The amputee should be taught to adjust the prosthetic socks so that the patellar tendon bar is over the midpoint of the patellar tendon. The insert should be donned before the prosthesis is donned.

Gait Deviations: Static and Dynamic Analysis (pp. 289–290)

Fit and Alignment (pp. 289–290)
- Aligning the PTB socket to hold the knee in 5 to 10 degrees of flexion increases the weight-bearing surface. During mid-stance there should be a slight varus moment at the knee, pushing the knee laterally. The socket applies a counterposing force to the medial femoral condyle and the lateral fibular shaft. The foot is set medial to the socket center. Moving the foot medially increases the varus moment. Moving the foot laterally decreases the moment but can create a valgus moment, resulting in pressure over sensitive areas.
- Pistoning should be checked by marking the posterior brim of the socket against the sock while the amputee is standing. Pistoning of more than $1/4$ inch indicates inadequate suspension or loose socket.

Gait Analysis (p. 290)
- Table 14–1 lists gait problems, causes, and solutions in the transtibial amputee.

Energy Expenditure (p. 290)

- The average measured gait velocity of the vascular transtibial amputee is decreased 44%, with oxygen consumption increased 33% per distance walked. The gait velocity of the traumatic transtibial amputee is decreased only 11%, with oxygen consumption increased 7% per distance walked, as compared with normal subjects without vascular disease. Longer residual limbs have lower oxygen requirements than short residual limbs, ranging from 10% to 40% increased oxygen requirement per distance walked.

KNEE DISARTICULATION (THROUGH-KNEE AMPUTATION) (pp. 290–291)
Surgical Procedures (p. 290)

- Knee disarticulation is removal of the tibia and fibula at the knee. Knee disarticulation provides the capacity for partial end-weight bearing.

TABLE 14–1 Gait Analysis of the Transtibial Amputee

Problem	Cause	Solution
Delayed, abrupt, and limited knee flexion after heel-strike	Heel wedge is too soft; foot is too far anterior	Stiffen heel wedge; move foot posterior
Extended knee throughout stance phase	Too much plantar flexion	Dorsiflex foot
Toe stays off floor after heel-strike	Heel wedge too stiff; foot too anterior, too much dorsiflexion	Soften heel wedge; move foot posterior; plantar flex foot
"Hill-climbing" sensation toward end of stance phase	Foot too anterior, too much plantar flexion	Move foot posterior, dorsiflex foot
High pressure against patella throughout most of stance phase; heel is off floor when patient stands	Foot too plantar flexed	Dorsiflex foot
Knee too forcefully and rapidly flexed after heel strike; high pressure against anterodistal tibia at heel-strike and/or prolonged discomfort at this point	Heel wedge too stiff; foot too far posterior; foot too dorsiflexed	Soften heel; move foot anterior; plantar flex foot
Hips level, but prosthesis seems short	Foot too far posterior, foot too dorsiflexed	Move foot anterior; plantar flex foot
Drop-off at end of stance phase	Foot too far posterior	Move foot anterior
Toe off of floor as patient stands or knee flexed too much	Foot too dorsiflexed	Plantar flex foot
Valgus moment at knee (knockkneed) during stance phase; excessive pressure on distomedial limb and proximolateral surface of knee	Foot too outset	Inset foot
Excessive varus moment at knee (bowlegged) during stance phase (a varus moment at the knee should occur in stance phase but should never be excessive); the distolateral residual limb is painful	Mediolateral dimension of socket too large; foot too inset	Fit of socket should be checked; outset foot

Courtesy of Northwestern University Prosthetic-Orthotic Center, Chicago.

Prosthetic Prescription (pp. 290–291)

• The socket is usually a modified quadrilateral socket with some ischial weight bearing, and a soft socket liner with supracondylar buildups to provide suspension. Proximal socket trimlines prevent socket rotation on the limb, although ischial weight bearing is not an absolute requirement if the femoral condyles provide suspension. The problem in prosthetic fitting of a knee disarticulation is that the prosthetic knee's center of rotation needs to go through the distal residual limb. Fitting a knee unit distal to the residual limb has caused problems in the past, but the four-bar polycentric knee has helped to solve the problem (see Fig. 14–19 in the Textbook).
• The average measured gait velocity for the traumatic through-knee amputee is decreased 24%, with oxygen consumption increased 53% per distance walked.

TRANSCONDYLAR/SUPRACONDYLAR AMPUTATION
(p. 291)

Surgical Procedures and Prosthetic Prescription (p. 291)

• In the transcondylar and supracondylar amputation, a conventional single-axis knee unit almost fits distal to the residual limb, although the prosthetic thigh is still slightly longer than the normal thigh.

TRANSFEMORAL (ABOVE-KNEE) AMPUTATION
(pp. 291–298)

Surgical Procedures (p. 291)

• Transfemoral amputation is usually performed with equal anterior and posterior length flaps. This amputation does not tolerate total end-weight bearing.
• With myoplasty or myodesis, the hamstrings are able to assist in hip extension and thereby stabilize the prosthetic knee. Myoplasty produces a smoother, more rounded cylindrical residual limb, although best results appear to be with myodesis or bony attachment.

Prosthetic Prescription (pp. 292–293) (Fig. 14–5)

• The residual limb should be at least 8.5 to 13.6 cm in length, measured from the groin, to fit a transfemoral prosthesis; but no absolute measurement is prescriptive because success is dependent on soft tissue volume.

Foot-Ankle Assemblies (p. 292)

• Compared with a transtibial amputee, a transfemoral amputee needs softer plantar flexion to enhance knee stability. The single-axis foot offers more knee stability than the SACH foot but is also heavier. If an SACH foot is used, a softer heel is necessary. Energy-storing feet should also be considered. An ankle unit torque-absorber can be used to reduce transverse friction forces for the short residual limb.

Shanks (p. 292)

• The choice between an endoskeletal (modular) and an exoskeletal (crustacean) shank is similar to that for the transtibial amputee. The hard shell of the exoskele-

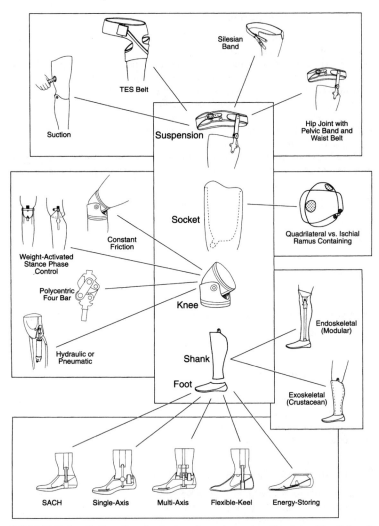

FIGURE 14–5. Prosthetic options for the transfemoral amputee. (Courtesy of the University of Texas Health Science Center at San Antonio.)

tal system is more durable, whereas the endoskeletal system is lighter, more cosmetic, and allows easier prosthetic adjustment.

Knee Units (p. 292)
• Knee units are either single axis or polycentric. They are also either mechanical or fluid controlled. All knee units, except for the hydraulic stance control units such as the Mauch S-N-S, attempt to keep the knee flexion-extension fixed at one angle (without relative motion) throughout the stance phase.

Mechanical Knee Units (pp. 292–293)
• Conventional constant-friction single-axis knees are light, durable, and inexpensive. Single-axis knees rely on alignment for stability and work best at one speed. Excessive heel rise in early swing phase, as well as terminal swing impact in late swing phase, can occur at faster cadences. These problems can be corrected by manually adjusting the constant friction unit, which can only be set for one optimum cadence. The amputee must prevent knee buckling by activating the hip extensors. The debilitated amputee or amputee with a short residual limb cannot adequately contract the hip extensors, and requires a knee that is set posterior to the trochanter-knee-ankle (TKA) line (see Fig. 14–21 in the Textbook). This alignment has the disadvantage of causing difficulty in flexion of the knee for swing phase, which causes increased energy expenditure compared to other knee units.
• A manual-locking knee provides maximum stability for the debilitated or elderly amputee, but this is accompanied by the worst gait efficiency and increased energy consumption. This knee is typically reserved for those with weakness and for those who are likely to sustain severe injuries if they fall.
• The weight-activated stance control knee (*limited slip* or, formerly, *SAFETY knee*) can provide stable stance for up to 20 degrees of knee flexion by producing friction when weight increases during stance (see Fig. 14–22 in the Textbook). This knee design is for amputees with weak hip extensors or for geriatric amputees. The stance control is not automatic, and the amputee must be able to initiate and maintain control of the knee.

HYDRAULIC- AND PNEUMATIC-CONTROL (FLUID-CONTROL) KNEE UNITS
• Both hydraulic and pneumatic control (fluid-control) knee units are cadence-responsive through cadence-dependent resistance. Pneumatic units are air-filled and are lighter in weight, but they cannot support the heavier or more athletic amputee as well as the hydraulic units can. Fluid-control knees are helpful for the active amputee who varies cadence and who can tolerate the extra weight and expense.

Sockets (pp. 293–294)

• An adjustable hinged socket for the temporary prosthesis is an option that allows adjustment for edema reduction. The choice for socket shape in the definitive prosthesis is between the traditional quadrilateral socket and the newer ischial containment socket.

Socket Shape (pp. 293–294)
QUADRILATERAL SOCKET
• The traditional quadrilateral socket has a flat, horizontal posterior shelf on which the ischial tuberosity and gluteal muscles rest. There is an inward bulge over the femoral triangle and a channel for the rectus femoris. The femoral triangle bulge keeps the ischial tuberosity on the posterior shelf. Medially, there is an anterior channel for the adductor longus tendon.

ISCHIAL CONTAINMENT SOCKET
• The ischial containment socket (Narrow M-L socket) has a posterior wall that is 0.75 to 1.25 inches proximal to the ischial level and is contoured to support the ischium and gluteal muscles. Compared with the quadrilateral socket, the ischial containment socket gives mediolateral control, or "bony lock," at the

minor expense of increased anteroposterior movement, and has a narrow mediolateral dimension and wide anteroposterior dimension at the level of the ischial
ramus. The ischial containment socket gives more energy-efficient ambulation
at high speeds for the active amputee, and is helpful for the short residual limb
or weak gluteus medius.

Socket Materials: Laminated versus Flexible (p. 294)
• The choice in materials is between the traditional rigid plastic-laminate socket
and a flexible thermoplastic socket. The soft, flexible socket is often translucent
or transparent and is more comfortable. It gives better total contact; enables one
to better sense external objects through the socket; and feels cooler, with better
heat dissipation. Flexible sockets can be more rapidly fabricated and modified,
but they are also more expensive. They are especially beneficial for the patient
with scarring of the residual limb; and because of better adherence, they provide
better suction suspension. The frames usually do not permit a hip joint and pelvic
band to be attached.

Suspension (pp. 294–295)

• Suspension systems for the transfemoral amputee include suction or partial
suction, total elastic suspension (TES) belt, Silesian band, hip joint with pelvic
band and waist belt, silicone suction suspension system, and hypobaric silicone
suction system.

Suction (p. 294)
• The amputee usually dons a total suction prosthesis while standing. It requires
that a pull sock or elastic bandage cover the residual limb. The sock or bandage
is passed through the valve hole and is used to pull the limb into the socket.
Alternatively, a wet fit can be used. The wet fit procedure uses a gel that turns
into a liquid or powder after the prosthesis is donned. A one-way valve placed
in the valve hole seals the socket by allowing air to escape but not to enter. Total
suction is the best suspension biomechanically, but it requires minimal volume
fluctuation of the residual limb, good hand strength and dexterity, good balance,
and good skin tissue integrity.
• Any socket that has a suction valve but requires the user to wear prosthetic
socks is called "partial suction."

No Suction (pp. 294–295)
• The TES belt is a neoprene belt attached to the prosthesis and pulled around
the waist, providing a relatively cosmetic auxiliary suspension. The Silesian belt
is a soft belt that encircles the pelvis and is attached proximally to the posterolateral aspect of the socket wall, and to the proximal anterior wall at the midline.
The hip joint with pelvic band and waist belt gives excellent mediolateral stability for the frail amputee or for the amputee with a short residual limb, but it
is bulky, heavy, constricting, and cumbersome. Placement of these suspension
mechanisms over bypass graft surgery sites and use in pregnant women are
contraindicated.

Gait Deviations: Static and Dynamic Analysis (pp. 295–296)

Fit and Alignment (pp. 295–296)

• For the quadrilateral socket, the ischium should rest on the posterior shelf, with firm but not excessive pressure between the tuberosity and socket. Insufficient pressure indicates the use of too many plies of socks or a palpable adductor roll, whereas excessive pressure indicates insufficient ply.

• For the ischial containment socket, the pubic ramus should be identified where it exits the medial wall. As the patient takes the weight off of the residual limb, he or she should check to see that the ischial tuberosity rests inside the ischial pocket or flare.

• To allow the amputee to walk with an erect trunk and with a normal stride length, the initial socket flexion is set at 5 degrees of socket flexion plus the amputee's angle of hip flexion contracture. This puts the hamstrings on stretch, giving the amputee greater stance control.

• The TKA line is a line drawn in the sagittal plane through the greater trochanter and mid-ankle (see Fig. 14–21 in the Textbook). If the knee joint is on this line, the knee is in *intermediate alignment.* If it is anterior to this line, it is said to be in *voluntary alignment* because the amputee must actively extend the hip during stance to prevent knee buckling. If the knee is posterior to this line, the knee is in maximum stability and is said to be in *involuntary alignment.*

Gait Analysis (p. 296)

• Table 14–2 lists gait problems and causes in the transfemoral amputee.

Energy Expenditure (pp. 296–298)

• The average measured gait velocity for the vascular transfemoral amputee is decreased by 55%, with oxygen consumption increased by 87%. The average measured gait velocity for the traumatic transfemoral amputee is decreased by 35%, with oxygen consumption increased by 33%. Individual energy expenditure per distance walked increases with a shorter residual limb or with age. The energy expended in walking with a prosthesis is usually less than that in walking with crutches and without a prosthesis. As a rule of thumb, if a patient can ambulate without the prosthesis and with crutches, he or she has the strength and endurance to ambulate with a prosthesis.

HIP DISARTICULATION AND TRANSPELVIC AMPUTATION (HEMIPELVECTOMY) (pp. 298–299)

Surgical Procedures (p. 298)

• A true hip disarticulation involves removal of the entire femur; in practice, however, the proximal femur is usually left to provide prosthetic stabilization and to avoid an uncosmetic cavity. Transpelvic amputation is the surgical removal of the lower limb and part or all of the ileum. These surgical procedures are usually done for malignant tumor, major trauma, or uncontrolled infection.

TABLE 14-2 Gait Analysis of the Transfemoral Amputee

Problem and Characteristics	Prosthetic Causes	Amputee Causes
Lateral bending of trunk: excessive bending occurs laterally from midline, generally to prosthetic side	• Prosthesis can be too short • Improperly shaped lateral wall may fail to provide adequate support for femur • High medial wall may cause amputee to lean away to minimize discomfort • Prosthesis aligned in abduction may cause wide-based gait, resulting in this defect	• Amputee may not have adequate balance • Amputee may have abduction contracture • Residual limb may be oversensitive and painful • Very short residual limb may fail to provide a sufficient lever arm for pelvis • Defect may be due to habit pattern • Patient may have abduction contracture • Defect may be due to habit pattern
Abducted gait: very wide-based gait with prosthesis held away from midline at all times	• Prosthesis may be too long • Too much adduction may have been built into prosthesis • High medial wall may cause amputee to hold prosthesis away to avoid ramus pressure • Improperly shaped lateral wall can fail to provide adequate support for femur • Pelvic band may be positioned too far away from patient's body	

Gait Deviation	Cause
Circumducted gait: prosthesis swings laterally in wide area during swing phase	• Prosthesis may be too long • Prosthesis may have too much alignment stability or friction in knee, making it difficult to bend knee in swing-through
Vaulting: rising on toe of sound foot permits amputee to swing prosthesis through with little knee flexion	• Prosthesis may be too long • Socket suspension may be inadequate • Excessive stability in alignment or some limitation of knee flexion, such as knee lock or strong extension aid, may cause this deficit • Amputee may have abduction contracture of residual limb • Patient may lack confidence for flexing prosthetic knee because of muscle weakness or fear of stubbing toe • Defect may be due to habit pattern • Vaulting is fairly common habit pattern • Fear of stubbing toe may cause this defect • Residual limb discomfort may be a factor • Amputee may be using more power than necessary to force knee into flexion
Uneven heel rise: prosthetic heel rises quite markedly and rapidly when knee is flexed at beginning of swing phase	• Knee joint may have insufficient friction • Extension aid may be inadequate
Terminal swing impact: rapid forward movement of shin piece allows knee to reach maximum extension with too much force before heel-strike	• Knee friction is insufficient • Knee extension aid may be too strong • Amputee may try to assure himself or herself that knee is in full extension by deliberately and forcibly extending the residual limb • Amputee may have hip extensor weakness • Severe hip flexion contracture may cause instability
Instability of the prosthetic knee creating a danger of falling	• Knee joint may be too far ahead of trochanter-knee-ankle (TKA) line • Insufficient initial flexion may have been built into socket • Plantar flexion resistance may be too great, causing knee to buckle at heel-strike • Failure to limit dorsiflexion can lead to incomplete knee control

Table continued on following page

TABLE 14-2 Gait Analysis of the Transfemoral Amputee—cont'd

Problem and Characteristics	Prosthetic Causes	Amputee Causes
Medial or lateral whips: whips best observed when patient walks away from observer; a medial whip is present when heel travels medially on initial flexion at beginning of swing phase; a lateral whip exists when heel moves laterally	• Lateral whips may result from excessive internal rotation of prosthetic knee • Medial whips may result from excessive external rotation of knee • Socket may fit too tightly, thus reflecting residual limb rotation • Excessive valgus or "knock" in prosthetic knee may contribute to this defect • Badly aligned toe break in a conventional foot may cause twisting on toe-off	None
Drop-off at end of stance phase; downward movement of trunk as body moves forward over prosthesis	• Limitation of dorsiflexion of prosthetic foot is inadequate • Heel of SACH-type foot may be too short, or toe break of a conventional foot may be too far posterior • Socket may have been placed too far anterior in relation to foot	None
Extensive trunk extension: amputee creates an active lumbar lordosis during stance phase	• Improperly shaped posterior wall may cause forward rotation of pelvis to avoid full weight bearing on ischium • Insufficient initial flexion may have been built into socket	• Amputee may have hip flexor tightness • Amputee may have weak hip extensors and may be substituting with lumbar erector spinae muscle; abdominal muscles may be weak • Defect may be due to habit pattern • Amputee may be moving shoulders backward in an effort to obtain better balance • Weak abdominal muscles may contribute to this defect

Courtesy of Northwestern University Prosthetic-Orthotic Center, Chicago.

Prosthetic Prescription (p. 299)

• The hip disarticulation amputee bears weight in the socket through the ischial tuberosity and gluteal muscles, whereas the transpelvic amputee bears weight on the soft tissue and lower rib cage. The hip disarticulation socket usually has good contact just above the iliac crest inside the socket rim, though reduced-trimline socket designs are available for young, active amputees (see Fig. 14–27 in the Textbook). Velcro socket closures secure the socket to the torso to prevent pistoning.

• The older Canadian-type exoskeletal hip disarticulation prosthesis has been replaced by the lightweight and ultralight endoskeletal prosthesis. Hip joint mechanisms for the hip disarticulation and transpelvic amputee are similar. The free hip joint has a posterior bumper extension stop and an anterior flexion stop, but allows no abduction or rotation. The hip joint is made to be stable by placing it anteriorly. A hip extension assist and lockable or four-bar polycentric hip joint are options.

• Most of the knee units used with the transfemoral prosthesis can also be used with the hip disarticulation or transpelvic prosthesis, as most prosthetic feet.

• The average measured gait velocity for the surgical hip disarticulation amputee is decreased by 41%, with oxygen consumption increased by 60% per distance walked. The average measured gait velocity for the surgical transpelvic amputee is decreased by 50%, with oxygen consumption increased by 93% per distance walked. Most young men abandon these prostheses in favor of crutch-walking, whereas 50% of women retain their prosthesis for cosmesis.

BILATERAL TRANSTIBIAL, TRANSFEMORAL, OR TRANSTIBIAL AND TRANSFEMORAL AMPUTATION (p. 300)

Prosthetic Prescription (p. 300)

• For the bilateral amputee, as for the unilateral amputee, as much of the limb should be saved as will satisfactorily heal and be functional. For the bilateral hip disarticulation amputee, a molded jacket or bucket socket might be necessary to maintain sitting. If the bilateral hip disarticulation is from pressure ulcers related to spinal cord injury, the socket should be open-ended to relieve pressure over insensate areas, and should distribute weight over the chest wall without compromising respiration. A walking prosthesis is rarely indicated for the bilateral hip disarticulation amputee owing to excessive energy costs.

• Bilateral transfemoral amputees are sometimes limited functional ambulators, but those in the geriatric population rarely ambulate. Lightweight or ultralight componentry should be used. Most dysvascular bilateral transfemoral amputees lack the cardiopulmonary reserve to ambulate. Wheelchairs for bilateral transfemoral amputees and other proximal amputees require anti-tip devices and/or offset rear axles to maintain rolling stability.

• Healthy bilateral transtibial amputees rarely require assistive devices, although the dysvascular amputee can require a cane. Bilateral transtibial amputees are generally better ambulators than unilateral transtibial amputees.

• The combination transfemoral-transtibial amputee obviously has less function than a bilateral transtibial amputee or a unilateral transfemoral amputee, but has more function than a bilateral transfemoral amputee.

PROBLEMS OF AMPUTEES AND THEIR TREATMENT
(pp. 300–302)

Skin Problems (p. 300)

• Skin lesions of the residual limb can expand rapidly, so early intervention is required, particularly for diabetic patients. Daily residual limb and socket washing is mandatory. In adults, split-thickness skin grafts cannot tolerate pressure, particularly over bony prominences, and require socket modifications.

Choke Syndrome (p. 300)

• Lack of total contact with proximal restriction results in distal edema called *choke syndrome*. The distal, strangulated residual limb becomes darkened with hemosiderin. Treatment might involve adding a distal pad, improving suspension, or changing sockets.

• Verrucous hyperplasia is a wart-like skin overgrowth, usually of the distal residual limb, resulting from inadequate external compression and edema; it can be reversed with total contact within the socket.

Skin Infection (p. 300)

• Folliculitis is a hair-root infection resulting from poor hygiene, sweating, poor socket fit, or pistoning. It is important to clean the area with antiseptic cleanser, to keep it dry, and to consider administration of oral antibiotics. Treat boils and abscesses with limited prosthetic use.

• Tinea corporis and tinea cruris mainly result from sweating. They can be confirmed through culture or microscopy and are treated by topical or oral fungicides as well as by good residual limb and socket hygiene.

• Excessive residual limb sweating can be controlled with cornstarch or unscented talc, but astringents and rubbing alcohol should be avoided. Antiperspirants or iontophoresis with copper sulfate or formalin might also be helpful.

Contact Dermatitis (p. 300)

• Allergic contact dermatitis can arise from topical medications or from agents used in prosthetic manufacture. Eczema can appear acutely, with small blisters; and later, with scaling and erythema. Topical corticosteroids should be applied, and the offending agent should be identified and removed.

Bone Problems (pp. 300–301)

• Symptomatic bone spurs can arise from bone from which the periosteum was incorrectly stripped during surgery or trauma. Bone pain can also result from a hypermobile fibula that is left longer than the tibia. If a balanced myodesis was not performed in the transfemoral amputation, the femur can extrude through the muscle and present subcutaneously. If prosthetic adjustments, such as a flexible socket, are inadequate for the extruded femur, surgical intervention might be needed. If the amputee has severe hip joint arthritis, total hip arthroplasty is an option.

Pain (p. 301)

• Incisional pain should subside with healing, although shear forces on an adherent scar can be painful. Deep massage helps prevent scar adhesions. Intermittent claudication pain in parts of the residual limb can be experienced by the amputee. Remember that not all residual limb pain is the result of a poorly fitting prosthesis.

Neuromas (p. 301)

• Every severed nerve develops a pressure-sensitive neuroma. The surgeon should sever nerves proximally to avoid socket pressure. Palpating directly over the neuroma typically elicits lancinating pain. The treatment for neuromas is socket adjustment. Direct injection of local anesthetic, with or without steroids, is helpful and aids in making the diagnosis. Neurolysis with phenol can be tried after multiple anesthetic injections have failed. If conservative measures fail, surgery to move the neuroma to a deeper or more proximal site should be considered.

Phantom Pain and Phantom Sensation (p. 301)

• Patients with acquired amputation typically have the sensation of the amputated part, or "phantom sensation," which usually diminishes with time. Occasionally, new amputees have such a dramatic phantom sensation that they transfer out of bed in a darkened room at night and fall when the phantom limb fails to support them.

• Phantom pain can accompany the phantom sensation, localizing in the phantom limb rather than in the residual limb. The longer a person has pain in a limb before it is amputated, the more likely he or she is to have phantom pain. Phantom pain usually diminishes with time, and chronic phantom pain is rare. Occasionally, medical intervention is required, although tricyclic antidepressants, mexiletine, anticonvulsants, capsaicin, propranolol, and chlorpromazine offer some limited benefit. Ambulation on a temporary prosthesis can help alleviate phantom pain. Transcutaneous electrical stimulation over the tibial nerve in the popliteal fossa and lumbar paravertebral sympathetic block at the L2 level should be considered if the phantom pain is burning and of a character similar to that of "reflex sympathetic dystrophy" (complex regional pain syndrome).

Contractures (p. 301)

• Maintaining the residual limb in extension is necessary to prevent flexion contractures. For severe knee flexion contractures beyond 25 degrees in an amputation without vascular disease, hamstring lengthening with posterior knee capsule release or a bent-knee prosthesis should be considered. Less severe contractures can be treated with stretching, either with or without simultaneous ultrasound. When a contracture is less than 10 degrees, the patient should be encouraged to walk as much as is tolerated because this might further reduce the contracture. More than 15 degrees of hip flexion contracture in the transfemoral amputee requires marked compensatory lumbar lordosis. Hip flexion contractures up to 25 degrees can be accommodated in the short transfemoral amputee with resulting loss of hip extensor power, but contractures are more difficult to accommodate for longer residual limbs. Hip flexion contractures result in knee instability and poor cosmesis, and often require that the prosthesis have a lockable knee. Contractures in children can lead to scoliosis.

Psychosocial Adjustments (p. 301)

• Amputees can develop a sense of inferiority, inadequacy, or repulsiveness. They should be encouraged to discuss problems openly. Their sexual identity and body image are altered, and phantom pain can occur with orgasm. Some amputees need psychological counseling. The clinician should also remember never to refer to the residual limb as a "stump." New amputees often benefit from positive visits from "peer" amputees.

Activities of Daily Living and Vocational Adjustments
(pp. 301–302)

• Trousers are put on the prosthesis before the prosthesis itself is donned. Shoe heel height cannot be changed unless foot wedges are used or unless an adjustable foot or second foot is available for the prosthesis. Driving a car can require moving the gas or brake pedal for the unilateral amputee, or installing hand controls for the bilateral amputee.
• The team should be aware of how much lifting, bending, climbing, and carrying of heavy objects is necessary in the patient's job, both for prosthetic training and for prosthetic prescription. Fine balance while standing can also be a job requirement to be addressed. Cosmesis can also be a significant part of the requirement.

Recreational Activities (p. 302)

• The transfemoral amputee with a mechanical knee must run with a hop-skip pattern, but with a hydraulic knee the person can run with a more normal motion. Recreational opportunities for the amputee are endless.

PEDIATRIC AMPUTEE (pp. 302–307)

• Approximately 3% of new amputees are in the first decade of life and 7% are in the second decade.

Differences between Adult and Pediatric Amputees
(p. 302)

• Major pediatric amputee concerns include skill development, growth, and psychosocial issues. Just as for adults, all possible functional residual limb length should be preserved. A contraindication to lower limb amputation is severe upper limb deformities that make lower limb prehension necessary.
• *Pediatric bony overgrowth* refers to pressure-related periosteal appositional growth, not epiphyseal growth. Bony overgrowth is a problem of the skeletally immature, particularly after mid-shaft amputation of the fibula or tibia. It occurs often enough in acquired amputations to require residual limb revision about 10% of the time, and it also can occur in congenital amputation. To preserve the

epiphysis, amputations should be done through a joint rather than through a bone.
• Leg length discrepancy from epiphyseal growth asymmetries can be substantial in the pediatric amputee. The epiphyseal plates about the knee give the greatest contribution to growth, with the distal femoral plate contributing 70% to femoral growth lengthening and the proximal tibial plate contributing 56% of tibial growth lengthening. Some residual limbs, such as a short transtibial limb, can be improved by skeletal lengthening.
• Unlike the case in adults, pediatric split-thickness skin grafts provide good residual limb coverage, even on end-bearing surfaces, and surgical incisions tolerate more tension. Symptomatic neuromas are rarely a problem in children, and socket modifications can usually relieve neuroma pain. Phantom limb pain is less frequent and of shorter duration in children. Knee and hip flexion contractures in children can largely be ignored and the affected limb fitted for conventional alignment because those contractures usually stretch out with walking and growth.

Classification of Congenital Deformity (p. 302)

• A transverse deficiency has no distal skeletal elements; all others are longitudinal deficiencies. The transverse level is named after the segment beyond which no bony elements exist. Digital buds do not count. Longitudinal level names the bones affected, and indicates whether the bones are partly or totally affected.
• Congenital limb deformities can be genetic or environmental. Embryologically, the limbs appear at about day 26 and are completely formed during the first 8 weeks of gestation. An estimated 1 of every 2000 human births has limb malformations, primarily from unknown etiologies.
• Congenital limb deficiencies outnumber acquired amputations 1.6:1. Forty-one percent are unilateral upper limb amputees, 40% are unilateral lower limb amputees, and 19% are multiple limb amputees. Boys outnumbered girls 2.1:1 for acquired amputations and 1.5:1 for both congenital unilateral lower limb and multiple limb deficiencies. Girls outnumbered boys 1.1:1 for congenital unilateral upper limb deficiencies.

Corrective Surgery: Surgical Possibilities (p. 303)

• Reasons for corrective surgery include bony overgrowth, better prosthetic fit, leg-length discrepancy, severe contracture, unstable joints, feet in a non–weight-bearing position, limb malrotation, severe neurological anesthesia, polydactyly, and cosmesis. Surgery can be indicated to change a congenital anomaly to an amputation. The family can offer valuable insight into the potential effects of surgery. Surgery for congenital deformity should be planned, if possible, so that all surgical procedures can be carried out in one stage. Surgery for limb lengthening should be preceded by calculating the mature predicted discrepancy. Surgery done as early as 1 year of age provides early fitting and adaptation. Joint disarticulation is preferred over the long shaft of bones to preserve normal bone growth, to prevent bony overgrowth, and for distal end-bearing. The Ilizarov device increases length, epiphysiodesis stunts bone growth, osteotomy corrects malalignment, and joint fusion improves stability.

Prostheses (p. 303)

• Several specialists—physicians, prosthetists, therapists, and social workers—are necessary to fully meet the needs of the pediatric amputee.

Timing of Prosthetic Fitting (p. 303)
• Children generally do not need a lower limb prosthesis until they are ready to stand. Most children sit at about 6 months, crawl on all fours at about 8 to 9 months, and walk at about 1 year. Children are ready for a lower limb prosthesis between 9 and 12 months for standing. Some, however, fit pediatric transfemoral amputees at 6 months of age to promote a symmetrical sitting posture. A child with a high-level amputation is often fitted with a locked knee joint once he or she appears to be ready to ambulate. At age 3 years, the child can usually handle a constant friction knee joint with an extension strap. Children tolerate immediate postoperative fitting. Crutches can be tried at about 4.5 years of age.

Pediatric Prosthetic Components (pp. 303–304)
• Flexible thermoplastic transfemoral sockets within a rigid frame allow for some growth. Children are active and have prominent fat, and often require auxiliary suspension such as waist belts, bilateral shoulder suspension, elastic sleeves, or the silicone suction suspension system. Suction is more difficult to achieve because of growth. Alignment must be age-specific because toddlers ambulate with legs externally rotated, abducted, and flexed. The prosthesis must adjust to the child's rapidly changing needs and challenges (e.g., to the prosthetically destructive teenager). Most prefer the greater durability of exoskeletal construction, unless the patient feels that cosmesis is a high priority.
• Many common adult components, such as feet and mechanical knee joints, are also available in pediatric sizes. A good first non-locking knee unit around age 3 years is a constant friction hinge using an elastic extension aid to help prevent buckling. The active child and teenager are likely to want a hydraulic knee for activities, and will test prosthetic durability to the maximum.

Growth Considerations (pp. 304–307)

• Children require a new lower limb prosthesis at least annually up to age 5 years, biannually until age 12 years, and every 3 or 4 years until age 21 years. Pediatric prostheses must be altered or replaced depending on the growth rate (or when the prosthesis has become more than 1 cm shorter than the sound limb). Pediatric limbs grow faster longitudinally than circumferentially. Growth can be accommodated by removing distal end pads or liners, extending an endoskeletal pylon, or adding wedges between the foot and exoskeletal shank.

Common Longitudinal Deficiencies (pp. 305–306)
FIBULAR LONGITUDINAL DEFICIENCY, TOTAL/PARTIAL (FIBULAR HEMIMELIA)
• Fibular longitudinal deficiency (formerly known as fibular hemimelia) is the most common congenital deficiency, and is bilateral in 25% of cases (see Fig. 14–32 in the Textbook). It consists of complete or partial absence of the fibula. The clinical picture is that of a shortened tibia with an anteromedial bow, foot equinovalgus deformity, occasionally a shortened femur, and leg length discrepancy. There can be a ball-and-socket ankle joint, fusion of tarsal bones,

absent lateral rays, ankle instability, genu valgum, and abnormal distal tibial epiphysis. Anatomically, there is often a cartilaginous or a fibrous rudimentary fibula. The muscles originating on the fibula, such as the peroneals and flexor hallucis longus, can be deficient.

• The leg length inequality can be severe. The amount of inequality is roughly correlated with the percent of the fibular aplasia. There can also be some correlation with the severity of foot deformity, particularly the number of absent lateral rays. Conservative treatment is indicated if the final shortening is not expected to be greater than 7.5 cm. Most of the treatment is to correct the limb length inequality with considerations of a shoe lift, bracing, contralateral epiphysiodesis (to stunt growth), ipsilateral limb lengthening, or Syme or Boyd amputation. The bow tends to straighten with growth after Syme or Boyd amputation.

PROXIMAL FEMORAL FOCAL DEFICIENCY OR FEMORAL LONGITUDINAL DEFICIENCY, PARTIAL

• Proximal femoral focal deficiency (PFFD) is characterized by partial deficiency of the proximal femur and involves the hip joint (see Fig. 14–33 in the Textbook). It comprises a spectrum of deformities ranging from mild hypoplasia to complete absence of the proximal femur, classified as Aitken class A (mild) through D (severe). The femur is typically short and held in flexion, abduction, and external rotation. Partial fibular absence and foot deformity are often present, with possible tibial shortening, hip and knee flexion contractures, and an unstable knee joint. The incidence is about 1 in 50,000 births. About 10% to 15% are bilateral. Treatment depends on whether PFFD is unilateral or bilateral, if a hip joint is present, the amount of coxa vara, the presence of pseudarthrosis, and the estimated ultimate leg length inequality.

• Bilateral deformities should usually not be treated by amputation unless there is great likelihood the patient can walk with prostheses after bilateral amputations. For bilateral PFFD, the child with symmetrical shortening often is able to ambulate without a prosthesis. If the upper limbs are either absent or severely deformed, both feet must be saved for self-care activities.

• Options for PFFD include special prostheses to lengthen the leg, surgical limb lengthening, surgical correction of the coxa vara and the pseudarthrosis, hip stabilization with an iliofemoral fusion, Syme or Boyd amputation, knee disarticulation and prosthetic fitting, and knee fusion with a van Ness rotationplasty.

TIBIAL LONGITUDINAL DEFICIENCY, TOTAL/PARTIAL (TIBIAL HEMIMELIA)

• Tibial longitudinal deficiency occurs in approximately 1 in 1 million births and is characterized by complete or partial absence of the tibia (see Fig. 14–34 in the Textbook). Clinically, the foot is in severe varus; the leg is shortened; and there can be instability of the knee, ankle, or both. It can occur with PFFD and coxa valga. Associated upper limb deformities include supernumerary digits, partial adactyly (floating thumb), and central aphalangia of the hands ("lobster-claw" hands). Longitudinal tibial deficiency can be part of an inherited autosomal dominant syndrome, and 30% of cases are bilateral. Treatment depends on the anatomical abnormalities.

• The foot and ankle are usually not salvageable, and therefore require a Syme or Boyd amputation. If a proximal tibia and quadriceps mechanism are present, fusing the fibula to the remaining tibia allows the patient to function as a transtibial amputee. With no proximal tibia and no quadriceps mechanism, a knee disarticulation provides a functional amputation.

Training and Treatment Goals (pp. 306–307)

• Most children require minimal training because they adapt quickly and easily to new devices. Play is a primary motivation; thus games with the prosthesis can be useful. Games keep the child's attention while increasing proficiency.
• Toddlers should be encouraged, but not forced, to wear a prosthesis; they will wear a prosthesis if it truly helps them. Remember the milestones of the normal child: heel-to-toe gait at age 2 years, standing on one foot with help at 20 months, and standing on one foot momentarily at 3 years.
• When prostheses are contraindicated in severely impaired multiple amputees, alternative mobility should be provided at approximately 16 months of age. The alternative can be a caster cart, swivel-rocker, or electrically powered cart.

Psychosocial Issues (p. 307)

• Peer counselors make a significant difference in acceptance of the prosthesis. Congenitally limb-deficient children accept their deficiency more readily than do acquired amputees. Children deal with limb loss better if they are adequately prepared. Adolescents, of course, place a high priority on cosmesis. Parents should encourage the child to engage in as much normal physical activity as possible.

CHAPTER

15

Original Chapter by Atul T. Patel, M.D., Laura M. Garber, O.T.R, C.H.T., and John B. Redford, M.D.

Upper Limb Orthotic Devices

• An *orthosis* is any externally applied device used to modify structural and functional characteristics of the neuromuscular skeletal system. The terms "splint" and "brace" are less preferred because they imply mere immobilization and do not suggest either improved function or restoration of mobility.

PRINCIPLES AND INDICATIONS (p. 311)

• The objectives of upper limb orthotic applications can be classified into three major areas: (1) protection, (2) correction, and (3) assistance with function.

1. *Protection:* Provide compressive forces and traction in a controlled manner, thus protecting the impaired joint or body part. Restricting or preventing joint motion allows for corrective alignment and serves to prevent deformity. Stabilize any unstable bony components and promote healing of soft tissues and bones. Traction forces can permit joint motion with decreased compressive forces applied to the joint cartilage.
2. *Correction:* Orthoses help in correcting joint contractures and subluxation of joints or tendons, thus preventing or reducing joint deformities.
3. *Assistance with function:* Orthoses can assist function by compensating for deformity, muscle weakness, or increased muscle tone.

CLASSIFICATION (pp. 311–314)

• We call upper limb orthoses by the joint they cover, the function they provide (e.g., immobilization), the condition they treat, and by their appearance. Other orthoses bear the name of the person who designed them. Most splints are known by their common names, which have evolved over time. Table 15–1 compares the common names of several orthotic devices. The reference numbers in this table refer to references in the Textbook.
• The simplest naming system reports the anatomic region the orthotic device encompasses. A wrist-hand orthosis, for example, is called a WHO. This system, however, fails to define the purpose or function of the orthosis.
• The American Society of Hand Therapists (ASHT) *Splint Classification System* (SCS) provides standard nomenclature for splints based on function. It classifies splints by characteristics (e.g., articular or nonarticular) and

TABLE 15-1 Nomenclature Systems in Current Use

Common Name	ASHT SCS	ISO	McKee and Morgan
Humeral fracture brace	Nonarticular splint-humerus	N/A	Circumferential nonarticular humerus-stabilizing
Tennis elbow splint/brace	Nonarticular splint-proximal forearm	Elbow orthosis (EO)	Circumferential nonarticular proximal forearm strap
Long arm splint	45-degree elbow flexion immobilization; type 1 [1]	Shoulder-elbow-wrist-hand orthosis (SEWHO)	Posterior static elbow/wrist orthosis
Resting hand splint	Index through small finger PIP extension, thumb CMC palmar abduction mobilization; type 3 [16]	Wrist-hand orthosis (WHO)	Volar forearm-based static (or serial static) wrist-hand orthosis
Ulnar deviation splint	Index through small finger MP extension/radial deviation mobilization; type 0 [4]	Hand orthosis (HO)	Circumferential hand-based dynamic traction D2-5 MCP corrective radial deviation orthosis
Kleinert splint	Wrist, MP, PIP, DIP flexion immobilization/extension restriction; type 0 [13]	Wrist-hand orthosis (WHO)	Dorsal forearm-based dynamic MCP-IP protective-flexion and MCP extension-blocking orthosis
Modified Kleinert splint			
Postop flexor tendon splint	Wrist and finger flexion immobilization; type 0 [4]	Wrist-hand orthosis (WHO)	Dorsal forearm-based static MCP-IP protective-flexion and MCP extension blocking orthosis
Duran splint			
Postop flexor tendon splint	Wrist, MP, PIP, DIP extension immobilization/flexion restriction; type 0 [1]	Wrist-hand orthosis (WHO)	Volar/dorsal forearm-based dynamic MCP-IP protective-extension and flexion-blocking orthosis
Postop dynamic extensor tendon splint			
Swan neck splint	Index finger PIP extension restriction; Type 0 [1]	Finger orthosis (FO)	Finger-based static PIP extension-blocking orthosis

Postop MCP arthroplasty splint	Index through small finger MP extension/radial deviation mobilization; type 1 [5]	Wrist-hand-finger orthosis (WHFO)	Dorsal forearm-based dynamic D2-5 MCP assisted extension/radial deviation orthosis
Swanson splint Radial nerve palsy splint	Wrist extension, MP flexion mobilization/MP flexion, wrist extension mobilization; type 0 [5]	Wrist-hand-finger orthosis (WHFO)	Dorsal forearm-based dynamic low-profile wrist and D1-5 MCP assistive-extension orthosis
Ulnar nerve palsy splint	Ring though small finger MP extension restriction; type 0 [2]	Hand-finger orthosis (HFO)	Circumferential hand-based dynamic joint-aligned coil-spring D4-5 MCP assistive- flexion orthosis
Median nerve palsy splint	Index through small finger MCP flexion mobilization and thumb CMC opposition mobilization; type 0 [5]	Hand-finger orthosis (HFO)	Circumferential hand-based dynamic joint-aligned coil-spring D2-5 MCP assistive-flexion and thumb assistive-opposition orthosis
Flail arm splint	Not classified	Shoulder-elbow-wrist-hand orthosis (SEWHO)	Not classified
Dynamic finger flexion splint, forearm-based	Index through small finger MP flexion mobilization; type 3 [7]	Wrist-hand-finger orthosis (WHFO)	Volar hand-based dynamic MCP corrective-flexion orthosis
Dynamic finger final flexion splint, hand-based	Index through small finger flexion mobilization; type 0 [12]	Wrist-hand-finger orthosis (WHFO)	Volar forearm-based dynamic MCP, PIP, DIP corrective-flexion orthosis
Dynamic finger extension splint, forearm-based	Index through small PIP and DIP extension mobilization; type 2 [13]	Wrist-hand-finger orthosis (WHFO)	Volar forearm-based dynamic MP, PIP, DIP corrective-extension orthosis
Dynamic finger extension splint, hand-based	Index through small finger extension mobilization; type 0 [12]	Wrist-hand-finger orthosis (WHFO)	Circumferential hand-based dynamic D4-5 MCP, PIP, DIP assistive-flexion orthosis
Static progressive splint	Index finger MP flexion mobilization; type 1 [4]	Wrist-hand-finger orthosis (WHFO)	Volar forearm-based static progressive MERiT-screw MCP-flexion orthosis
Dynamic wrist flexion splint	Wrist flexion mobilization; type 0 [1]	Wrist-hand orthosis (WHO)	Dorsal forearm-based dynamic-joint-aligned wrist assistive flexion orthosis
Dynamic wrist extension splint	Wrist extension mobilization; type 0 [1]	Wrist-hand orthosis (WHO)	Dorsal forearm-based dynamic-joint-aligned wrist assistive extension orthosis

Table continued on following page

TABLE 15-1 Nomenclature Systems in Current Use—cont'd

Common Name	ASHT SCS	ISO	McKee and Morgan
RIC tenodesis splint	Not classified	Functional orthosis (FO)	Volar forearm-based tenodesis wrist-hand orthosis
Elbow flexion splint	Elbow flexion mobilization; type 0 [1]	Elbow-wrist orthosis (EWO)	Posterior dynamic elbow corrective-flexion orthosis
Elbow extension splint	Elbow extension mobilization; type 0 [1]	Elbow-wrist orthosis (EWO)	Anterior serial static elbow corrective-extension orthosis
Dynamic pronation/supination splint	Forearm pronation/supination mobilization; type 2 [3]	Elbow-wrist-hand orthosis (EWHO)	Posterior forearm-based dynamic radius/ulna corrective pronation/supination orthosis
Wrist splint, carpal tunnel splint	Wrist extension immobilization; type 0 [1]	Wrist orthosis (WO)	Volar forearm-based static wrist orthosis
Thumb spica splint	Thumb MP extension immobilization; type 2 [3]	Wrist-thumb orthosis (WHFO)	Volar forearm-based static wrist-thumb orthosis
Mallet finger splint, DIP extension splint, Stax splint	Index finger DIP extension immobilization; type 0 [3]	Finger orthosis (FO)	Volar finger-based static DIP-flexion-blocking orthosis
Capener splint	PIP extension mobilization; type 0 [1]	Finger orthosis (FO)	Three-point finger-based dynamic joint-aligned coil-spring PIP corrective-extension orthosis
Figure-of-8 harness	Nonarticular splint-axilla	Shoulder orthosis (SO)	Figure-of-8 nonarticular axilla orthosis
Airplane splint	Shoulder abduction immobilization; type 3 [4]	Shoulder-elbow-wrist-hand orthosis (SEWHO)	Lateral trunk-based static shoulder-elbow-wrist orthosis
Gunslinger splint	Not classified	Shoulder-elbow-wrist-hand orthosis (SEWHO)	Not classified
Mobile arm support			
Orthosis sugar tong splint	Elbow extension immobilization; type 3 [4]	Shoulder-elbow-wrist-hand orthosis (SEWHO)	Bivalved static elbow orthosis

location of body part covered. A humeral fracture brace, for example, is identified as a nonarticular splint-humerus (see Table 15–1). It also identifies the direction of the force applied, and whether the splint is for mobilization, immobilization, or restriction.

DESIGN CATEGORIES (pp. 314–316)

• Orthotic devices can be classified by the support or forces provided to improve motion or function. Categories of splint design are as follows:

Nonarticular: This type of splint provides support to a body part without crossing any joint and protects a bone or body part. For example, a humeral fracture splint provides circumferential support to the upper arm during fracture healing.

Static: This type of splint provides static support to hold a joint or joints stationary. For example, a volar wrist splint for acute carpal tunnel syndrome reduces motions and rests injured tissues (Fig. 15–1). Static splints can be used to protect healing structures, to decrease or prevent deformity, and to reduce tone in spastic muscles.

Serial static: This splint is also static but is periodically changed to alter the joint angle at which the splint is positioned.

Static motion blocking: This type of splint permits motion in one direction but blocks motion in another. For example, a swan neck splint is designed to allow flexion but to block hyperextension of the proximal interphalangeal (PIP) joint.

Static progressive: This type of splinting is the one most commonly used for regaining joint motion. Unlike the serial static splint, the orthosis is not remolded to increase joint motion; rather, it uses a static line of pull that is tightened periodically to increase tissue length. One such device is similar in principle to a tuning screw on a guitar.

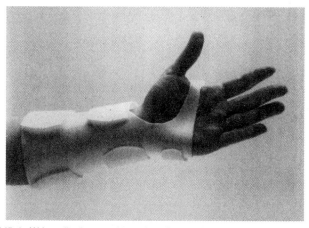

FIGURE 15–1. Wrist splint for carpal tunnel syndrome with the wrist in a position of 0 to 5 degrees of extension; distal palmar crease left free to allow for MCP motion.

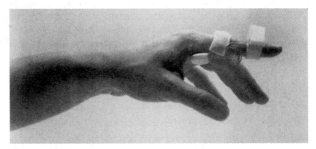

FIGURE 15–2. Capener splint for increasing extension in the PIP joint of the finger.

Dynamic: This type of splint provides an elastic force to regain motion. An example of such an orthosis is a Capener splint, which uses a spring coil assist to increase extension in a PIP joint with a mild contracture (Fig. 15–2).

Dynamic motion blocking: This type of splint allows certain motions but blocks others. It utilizes a passive, elastic line of pull in the desired direction but permits active motion in the opposite direction. An example is a Kleinert postoperative splint for flexor tendon repairs (see Figs. 15–5 and 15–6 in the Textbook).

Dynamic traction splints: This type of splint offers traction to a joint while allowing controlled motion. An example is a splint for an intra-articular fracture, which gives constant longitudinal traction while the joint is gently flexed and extended.

Tenodesis: This type of splint facilitates function in a hand that has lost motion due to nervous system injury. An example is a Rehabilitation Institute of Chicago (RIC) tenodesis splint (Fig. 15–3), which assists the patient with a C6 spinal cord injury to achieve a functional pinch. Active extension of the wrist produces, through tenodesis action, controlled passive flexion of the fingers against a static thumb post.

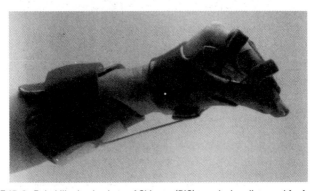

FIGURE 15–3. Rehabilitation Institute of Chicago (RIC) tenodesis splint, used for functional pinch during activities of daily living (ADL).

Continuous passive motion (CPM) orthoses: These are electrically powered devices that mechanically move joints through a desired range of motion. This keeps the joints supple and maintains articular, ligamentous, and tendinous structure mobility during the healing phases following injury or surgery.

Adaptive/functional usage: These devices promote functional use of the upper limb with impairment due to weakness, paralysis, or loss of a body part. An example is the universal cuff, which encompasses the hand and holds various small items such as a fork, a pen, or a toothbrush (see Fig. 15–8 in the Textbook).

BIOMECHANICAL CONSIDERATIONS (pp. 316–317)

• When increasing joint range of motion with splinting, the angle of pull needs to be perpendicular to the bony axis that is being mobilized.

• Wrist position is an important consideration in the design of a splint. Power grasp is most effectively achieved when the wrist is extended slightly. When writing, most right-handed individuals extend the wrist; however, many left-handed individuals place their wrists in slight flexion.

• To maintain tissue length through static positioning, one needs to consider the ligamentous structures involved, the anatomic angle of pull on structures, and the positions that may produce deformity. For example, when the hand is made nonfunctional after a dorsal burn, the metacarpophalangeal (MCP) joints tend toward hyperextension.

• The improvement in range of motion is directly proportional to the length of time a joint is held at its end range. This principle is used with static progressive splinting, as noted previously.

• The therapist should be sure to fabricate it in a position that enhances prehension and does not force the thumb into a position of extension and radial abduction. This position causes the rest of the arm to compensate for poor thumb positioning. To decrease the stresses on the hand and thumb, built-up pens and pencils can be used for improved function, especially with a thumb spica splint.

• Splints designed to encompass the hand must preserve both longitudinal and transverse arches. The distal palmar crease must not be blocked if full MCP flexion is desired (see Fig. 15–1).

• In designing dynamic or static progressive hand splints to improve digital flexion, the direction of pull should be toward the scaphoid bone on the palmar surface to mimic the angle noted in the healthy hand. The angle of pull across the palm is oblique, not straight down toward the wrist. This is most apparent when the fingers are flexed individually and less pronounced when flexed all at once.

• The mobility of the ulnar two digits is critical to the power grasp of the hand. The radial three digits are used for pinch and prehension.

• Active and passive range-of-motion measurements need to be assessed to determine the mechanics of the joint. Joint torque angle measurements can be used to determine whether (1) a splint is needed, (2) conservative treatment would be beneficial, or (3) surgery is indicated. Torque angle measurement assesses what occurs at the joint as the force is applied at a given distance from the joint axis.

DIAGNOSTIC CATEGORIES AND SPLINT EXAMPLES
(pp. 317–324)

Musculoskeletal Conditions (pp. 317–319)

Tendinitis, Tenosynovitis, and Enthesopathy (pp. 317–318)
• Tendinitis, tenosynovitis, and enthesopathy can all result from excessive repetitive movement. In the upper limb the wrist extensor tendons are commonly affected. DeQuervain's tenosynovitis, involving the abductor pollicis longus and extensor pollicis brevis muscles, is also common. The goal of splints for these conditions is to immobilize the affected structures in order to facilitate healing and decrease inflammation. The forearm-based thumb spica splint immobilizes the wrist, the carpometacarpal joint, and the MCP joint of the thumb (see Fig. 15–1 in the Textbook).
• Lateral epicondylitis is the most common enthesopathy of the upper limb. It can be treated by a tennis elbow orthosis. This is a forearm band that changes the lever arm against which the wrist extensors pull; in essence, it puts the origin of the extensor muscles at rest and decreases microtrauma from overuse (see Chapter 38).
• Trigger finger describes a snapping sensation in the volar surface of the digits on release of grasp. It is usually a result of trauma to the flexor tendon sheath of the fingers or thumb, producing thickened tendinous sheaths and restriction of motion. In advanced trigger finger the digit can become "locked" in flexion. The goal in this condition is to halt the repetitive motion temporarily to allow for healing. This is usually achieved by immobilization, but patients should have functional use of the hand while the affected digit is immobilized.

Sprains (p. 318)
• Sprains require joint immobilization in a position of function to allow for healing as well as functional use. Common sprains include dislocation of the IP and MCP joints caused by hyperextension injuries, something often seen in sports injuries (see Chapter 44). For a first- or second-degree ligamentous tear, the goal is to protect and rest the area by applying functional splinting. The goal for a third-degree tear is to fully immobilize and approximate the ligaments.
• Common splints used for digital sprains are finger extension splints that hold the PIP joint in extension but allow flexion of the distal interphalangeal (DIP) joint. This action keeps the oblique retinacular ligament and the terminal extensor tendon lengthened, preventing boutonnière deformities during healing. Ulnar collateral ligamentous injuries at the MCP joint of the thumb are treated with a hand-based thumb spica splint, producing immobilization during the healing phase (see Fig. 15–10 in the Textbook). Wrist splints that place the wrist in slight extension are used for wrist sprains. For mild sprains, splints with no spline (metal bar insert) permit some motion but avoid creating significant stiffness. They also keep available range to about 40 degrees of total motion (see Fig. 15–13 in the Textbook). Elbow neoprene sleeves are helpful for mild sprains at the elbow because they limit the extremes of range but permit limited function.

Fractures (pp. 318–319)
• Most major fractures need total immobilization, requiring casting and/or surgical intervention. Some fractures, however, do not need total immobilization and can be treated with orthotic devices (see Fig. 15–14 in the Textbook).

These devices should immobilize the body part or the joint sufficient to promote healing while also optimizing function. An example of such an orthotic device is the humeral fracture brace that holds healing bony parts in alignment.

Arthritis (p. 319)

• Osteoarthritis is the most common disease affecting the joints in the upper limb. Joint diseases of the hand and wrist have the most significant impact upon function. Chronic inflammation often exposes these digital joints to further risk of deformity and injury. Orthotic devices can provide functional positioning to prevent further deformity and loss of use in arthritic diseases as well as protecting the joints from further injury.

Rheumatoid Arthritis (p. 319)

• Rheumatoid arthritis is a chronic inflammatory disease that primarily affects synovial joints. The joints most commonly affected in the upper limb are the wrist, MCP, and PIP joints. Deformities include subluxation and ulnar deviation at the MCP joints, subluxation and radial deviation at the wrist, and swan-neck deformity and boutonnière deformity of the fingers. These deformities usually progress, especially if no attempt is made to rest and protect the affected joints from overuse.

• Several options are available for splinting the rheumatoid hand. Ulnar deviation splints that pull the MCP joints toward radial deviation and increase the functional use of the hand are now lightweight and permit full MCP joint motion in flexion and extension. Wrist splints that provide light support for the wrist are usually tolerated very well (see Fig. 15–13 in the Textbook). Swan neck and boutonnière splints can be made from thermoplastics, but are often bulky and cosmetically unpleasing. Very thin Siris Silver Ring Splints are now available for digital deformities (Fig. 15–4). Made of sterling silver, these splints are cos-

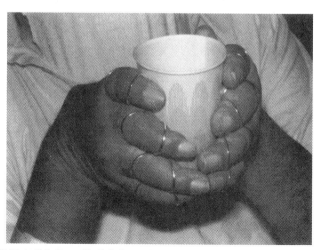

FIGURE 15–4. Siris Swan Neck Splints, which greatly enhance function of the digits for activities of daily living. The patient is holding a cup with the aid of these splints. (Courtesy of Silver Ring Splint Company.)

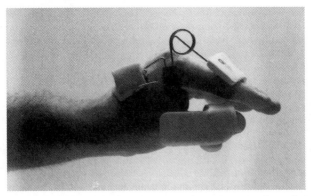

FIGURE 15–5. LMB MP Flexion Spring with Dynamic Thumb Abduction Spring Splint. Used for median nerve palsy to provide opposition of the thumb and flexion of the MCP joints.

metically similar to jewelry; they provide excellent improvement in function and are well tolerated. The swan neck splint allows for flexion of the digit but blocks hyperextension. The boutonnière splint holds the DIP or PIP joint in extension.

Osteoarthritis (p. 319)
• Osteoarthritis, the most common form of arthritis, is primarily a disease of cartilage, not of the synovium. In the upper limb, it most commonly involves the carpometacarpal (CMC) joint of the thumb. A thumb spica hand-based (see Fig. 15–10 in the Textbook) or forearm-based (see Fig. 15–1 in the Textbook) splint can be prescribed for CMC joint osteoarthritis. By limiting motion at the base of the thumb, the splint decreases pain, especially with pinching-type activities.

Neuromuscular Conditions (pp. 319–322)

Nerve Injuries (pp. 319–321)
• In a peripheral nerve injury, the level of injury determines the extent of deficit incurred. For example, in a distal median nerve injury, the type of deformity incurred is usually described as a simian hand and the function most affected is thumb abduction and opposition (see Fig. 15–17 in the Textbook). Distal median nerve palsy splints assist in flexion of all the MCP joints and thumb palmar abduction. The splint usually has a spring coil design holding the MCP joints in slight flexion but permitting MCP extension (Fig. 15–5). This splint also has a portion to position the thumb in palmar abduction.
• With radial nerve injuries distal to the humeral spiral groove, the most common presenting condition is wrist drop and finger drop. The goal of an orthotic device is to enhance wrist and finger extension. A radial nerve palsy splint is forearm based with an outrigger that holds the wrist, fingers, and thumb in extension and allows for flexion of the digits (see Fig. 15–19 in the Textbook).
• With a proximal ulnar nerve injury, the patient has what is called a "benediction hand," featuring hyperextension of the fourth and fifth MCP joints and

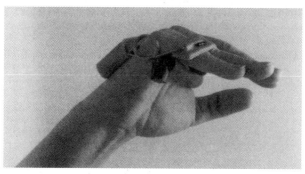

FIGURE 15–6. Ulnar nerve splint. Allows extension but blocks hyperextension of the MCP joints of the ring and small fingers.

flexion of the PIP joints due to the loss of balance between the extrinsic and intrinsic hand muscles. An ulnar nerve palsy splint holds the MCP joints of the fourth and fifth fingers in slight flexion by a spring coil or figure-of-8 splint design. The spring coil design assists MCP flexion and permits extension of the MCP joints but blocks hyperextension (Fig. 15–6).

• Incomplete nerve injuries, such as carpal tunnel syndrome, can be caused by compression or overuse. The purpose of the splint is to immobilize the wrist to minimize overuse of the tendons. The splint is molded to the patient from a thermoplastic that offers excellent conformity to hold the wrist in 0 to 5 degrees of extension. Its common name, wrist cock-up splint, is misleading and should be avoided because this name implies that the wrist should be placed in extension (see Fig. 15–1). The patient should be instructed to reduce stresses at the wrist and to wear the splint all night. Often the patient is instructed to wear it as much as possible during the day as well.

• A word of caution is in order for many prefabricated wrist splints: Many of these splints have a metal spline formed to hold the wrist at a 45-degree angle of extension (see Fig. 15–21 in the Textbook). This angle far exceeds the recommended 0 to 5 degrees of extension.

• Long arm splints hold the elbow in 45 degrees of flexion, the forearm in neutral, and the wrist in 0 to 5 degrees of extension with thumb and fingers free; these splints are helpful with cubital tunnel syndrome (compression of the ulnar nerve at the elbow).

• In patients with multiple nerve injuries or brachial plexopathy with essentially a flail arm, the goal with orthotic devices is to provide some functional use. One type of orthosis is in the form of an exoskeleton on the arm, similar to a prosthesis. This device uses a shoulder harness with scapular activation to produce elbow function, similar to scapular action in an above-elbow prosthesis.

Brain Injury and Stroke *(p. 321)*

• Orthotic devices should be designed to prevent deformities and to help adjust muscle tone. Resting and positioning orthotic devices are also necessary to

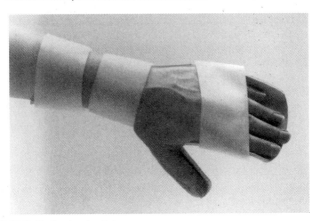

FIGURE 15–7. Resting hand splint.

prevent such complications as distal edema, joint subluxation, and contracture formation. In upper limb paralysis, a resting hand splint is commonly used to position the wrist in slight extension, the MCP joints in slight flexion, and the IP joints in extension. The thumb is supported in a position between palmar and radial abduction. Full support of the first CMC joint prevents ligamentous stresses on the thumb, especially in the insensate hand (Fig. 15–7).

• A mobile arm support can be used to enhance function for patients with proximal upper limb weakness, especially when the weakness is profound and the outlook for recovery is guarded. A mobile arm support is particularly helpful when performing such ADL (activities of daily living) tasks as eating and grooming.

• Many types of slings are available for patients with decreased tone of the upper limb (see Fig. 15–23 in the Textbook). Decreased tone can result in shoulder subluxation, and slings can help reduce subluxation. But an overhead sling device can help increase the function of weakened shoulder and scapular musculature.

Spinal Cord Injury (pp. 321–322)

• With spinal cord injury at C1 to C3 level, the goal is to prevent contractures and hold the wrist and digits in a position of function with a resting hand splint (see Fig. 15–7). In a C4 level injury, the goal is to use the available shoulder strength, providing a mobile arm support to enhance function as previously described. In a C5 level injury, the goal is to statically position the wrist in extension with a ratchet-type hinged orthotic device to hold devices. An orthotic device for a C6 tetraplegic patient can enhance finger flexion using a tenodesis flexion effect from wrist extension. For example, an RIC tenodesis splint molded from thermoplastic materials has several positioning components (see Fig. 15–3). When the patient extends the wrist, the fingers are pulled toward the thumb post. This produces a three-point pinch, allowing the patient to grasp. When the patient flexes the wrist, the fingers extend passively, releasing the object. This custom-made thermoplastic tenodesis device is mainly used in training and practice. If a patient finds the device useful, a light metal custom-made tenodesis orthosis achieves better functional restoration.

Other Injuries (pp. 322–324)

Post-Surgical and Post-Injury Orthosis (pp. 322–323)

• Often the type of surgical procedure or injury level dictates the type of splint used, so that the splints cannot be used interchangeably. For flexor tendon repair, the Kleinert and Duran are common. The Kleinert splint (see Figs. 15–5 and 15–6 in the Textbook) features dynamic traction into flexion but allows active digit extension within the constraints of the splint; the Duran splint statically positions the wrist and MCP joints in flexion and the IP joints in extension (see Fig. 15–27 in the Textbook).

• The form of extensor tendon repair splints depends on the level of injury. A mallet finger injury can require only a Stax splint—a static splint holding the DIP joint in full extension. A more proximal injury, however, needs a splint that holds the wrist statically in extension with dynamic extension of MCP and IP joints. Such a splint permits active flexion of the MCP joints within the constraints of the splint to an angle of approximately 30 degrees. Injuries to the thumb flexor or extensor tendons require more specific splinting.

• Postoperative joint replacements for the PIP, DIP, or the MCP joints of the hand require very specific splints that promote healing or encapsulation of the joints while preserving ROM during the healing phases (see Fig. 15–30 in the Textbook).

Burns (pp. 323–324)

• Burn patients typically prefer an adducted and flexed position of the upper limbs to maintain comfort, but this preference can lead to loss of functional range of motion. The splint prevents contractures and deformities. This is especially important when the patient cannot voluntarily maintain the range or when soft tissues underlying the skin are exposed. With tendon exposure, the splint plays a more protective role. It is important to monitor these patients frequently and reassess the needs for splinting.

• After burn injuries, body parts should be positioned to prevent the tendency toward known deformities. For example, in burns of the dorsal surface of the hand, the wrist is kept in slight extension, the MCP joints in 60 to 70 degrees of flexion, the PIP and DIP joints in full extension, and the thumb between radial abduction and extension (see Fig. 15–9 in the Textbook). To combat a tendency for shoulder adduction deformity after axillary burns, the shoulder should be held in abduction with an airplane splint. The tendency toward hypertrophic scarring after a burn is addressed with a selection of compression garments, elastomer molds, facial splints, shell splints, and silicone gel sheeting.

SPECIAL CONSIDERATIONS (p. 324)

• It is important to ask about the patient's goals for splinting and function before choosing a splint design (Table 15–2). This will maximize compliance in the use of the splint.

TABLE 15–2 Points to Consider for Optimization of Splint Use

Material thickness	Use thinner materials for finger splints and thicker materials for forearm and elbow splints
	Note: Thinner materials cool faster, decreasing working time
Function	Consider patient's goals and functional needs
Patient input	Elicit patient's ideas, preferences, and goals
Cosmesis	Consider patient's age, occupation, and other factors
Color	Allow color choices to increase to improve cosmesis
Wearing schedule	Tailor wearing schedule to meet the goals of the splint
Design	Consider goals as well as biomechanics when choosing factors such as whether a splint should be static, static progressive, or dynamic

• Cosmesis is important, and patients should have every opportunity to assist in choosing design and appearance. Low-temperature thermoplastic materials are now available in a wide range of colors. The person's age or occupation may be factors. Adolescents should be encouraged to "decorate" their splints if they so desire.

• Comfort is also important. The thinner the materials used and the more care the therapist takes in making a close, comfortable fit, the better the acceptance of the splint. Stockinet worn under splints also helps, particularly with perspiration in warmer weather.

• The wearing schedule depends on the goals you have for the splint and the patient's tolerance for wear. Static stretch should be perceived as mild, and it should never awaken the patient at night. In a patient with both flexion and extension splinting needs, the flexion splint can be worn 1 hour on, 2 hours off during the day, and the extension splint can be worn at night. Patients tolerate the splint better and spend more daytime with the splint off so they can do hand exercises.

• A resting hand splint for positioning is often indicated when edema is present. But a splint can also induce edema—the result of an inflammatory response caused by an overly aggressive stretch—particularly in a patient with increased tone. Splint design needs to address this possibility. Structures sometimes change in length because of joint contracture, in which case splint tension must be decreased.

• Splint prescriptions should explain the diagnosis or problem to be addressed. A description of the function or motion desired helps to alleviate confusion (see Table 15–1).

ORTHOTIC MATERIALS (pp. 324–325)

• Most splinting materials are low-temperature thermoplastics (see Table 15–3 in the Textbook). Many are known by their trademark names. Low-temperature thermoplastics become soft and pliable when exposed to relatively low temperatures. High-temperature thermoplastics are more durable but require oven heating (up to 350°F) and placement over a mold to achieve the desired shape.

SUMMARY (p. 325)

• The most important principle in prescription of orthotic devices is gaining cooperation of the patient. Through attention and concern by the physician and therapist, the patient must see the benefit of the orthosis. It also must fit comfortably and be cosmetically appealing.

16

Original Chapter by William J. Hennessey, M.D.,
and Ernest W. Johnson, M.D.

Lower Limb Orthoses

• An orthosis is a device attached or applied to the external surface of the body to improve function, restrict or enforce motion, or support a body segment. Lower limb orthoses are indicated to assist gait, reduce pain, decrease weight bearing, control movement, and minimize progression of a deformity. Lower limb orthoses assist nonambulatory patients with transfer and mobility skills and assist ambulatory patients in becoming safe walkers.

PRINCIPLES OF LOWER LIMB ORTHOSES (p. 326)

• Table 16–1 outlines the common principles of lower limb orthoses. Most orthoses use a three-point system to ensure proper positioning of the limb within the orthosis. For example, a knee that has a tendency to hyperextend, or "back knee," can be treated with a knee orthosis that applies force posterior to the knee but also applies forces anteriorly along the leg and the thigh.

TERMINOLOGY FOR LOWER LIMB ORTHOSES
(pp. 326–327)

• *Orthotic* is the adjective derived from the noun *orthosis*. An orthosis can be referred to as an orthotic device. The term *extremity* specifically refers to the foot. The term *leg* should be used to refer to the portion of the lower limb between the knee and ankle joints. The *thigh* is located between the hip and knee joints. *Lower limb* refers to the thigh, leg, and foot.
• Pathological abnormalities regarding angulation require correct use of the Latin-derived terminology including the use of the suffix of "-us" at the ankle, "-um" at the knee, and "-a" at the hip. Varus and valgus deformities of the foot are described for both the hindfoot and forefoot (e.g., hindfoot valgus or forefoot varus). A bow-legged condition is correctly referred to as genu varum. Deformity at the hip is referred to as coxa valga and coxa vara.
• Lower limb orthoses are commonly referred to with abbreviations. Standard orthotic nomenclature uses the first letter of each joint the orthosis crosses from proximal to distal. It then lists the first letter of the limb to which it is affixed (e.g., "f" for foot). Lastly, the letter "o" is used to signify it is an ortho-

TABLE 16–1 Principles of Lower Limb Orthoses

1. Use only as indicated and for as long as necessary.
2. Allow joint movement wherever possible and appropriate.
3. Orthoses should be functional throughout all phases of gait.
4. Orthotic ankle joint should be centered over tip of medial malleolus.
5. Orthotic knee joint should be centered over prominence of medial femoral condyle.
6. Orthotic hip joint should be in a position that allows patient to sit upright at 90 degrees.
7. Patient compliance will be enhanced if orthosis is comfortable, cosmetic, and functional.

sis. Thus, AFO designates an ankle-foot orthosis. KAFO means knee-ankle-foot orthosis. HKAFO means hip-knee-ankle-foot orthosis.
• The orthotic literature uses variable medical terminology, which can make it difficult to understand the literature. The calcaneus is commonly referred to as the os calcis. A plantar flexion deformity is referred to as an equinus deformity. Torsion and rotation have incorrectly been used interchangeably. Torsion refers to twisting of a portion of a limb. Rotation of a limb occurs only at a joint. Pronation has been referred to as inrolling, whereas supination has been referred to as outrolling. An orthosis is not put on and taken off but rather is donned and doffed. Checkout means an examination of the patient after the orthosis is fitted.

SHOES (p. 327)

• The normal foot does not require support from shoes. The sole should be pliable so as not to interfere with the normal biomechanics of the foot. A practical way of ensuring that a shoe is of adequate length is to determine whether the index finger can be placed between the tip of the great toe and the toe box. The presence of calluses indicates areas of friction from poorly fitting (loose) shoes. The presence of corns indicates areas of friction over bony prominences, most often caused by tight-fitting shoes. Leather shoes are good choices for all types of activity. They are durable, allow ventilation, and mold to the feet with time. A good pair of shoes can eliminate the need for foot orthoses and should be considered before orthotic prescription.

Shoe Parts (p. 327)

• Two types of dress shoes are commonly worn, the Blucher and the Bal. A Blucher shoe is recommended for patients requiring an orthosis because there is more room to don and doff the shoe and the orthosis, owing to the open throat.
• A shoe with a welt should be recommended to patients. A welt is a narrow strip of leather used to unite the upper part of the shoe, the inner sole, and the outer sole of a shoe by means of stitching. The welt design allows the orthotist to disassemble the shoe for modifications more easily than with other types of shoes.

FOOT ORTHOSES (pp. 327–328)

• Foot orthoses (FOs) range from arch supports found at a local pharmacy or athletic store to customized orthoses fabricated by an orthotist. FOs affect the ground reactive forces acting on the joints of the lower limb. They also have an effect on rotational components of gait.

• Mild conditions can be treated with over-the-counter orthoses. More severe problems require customized orthoses. These are available in three types. A soft type is most commonly used in over-the-counter orthoses. Orthotists usually provide semirigid orthoses, which provide more support than the soft type but are still shock absorbing. A rigid orthosis is indicated only for a problem that requires aggressive bracing to control the deformity.

• To make a custom foot orthosis, the subtalar joint should be placed in a neutral position before casting. This position minimizes abnormalities related to foot and ankle rotation (e.g., hyperpronation) and it is also the position in which the foot functions best. The cast is a negative mold from which a positive mold can be made. The positive mold can be modified to increase the effectiveness of the orthosis. The custom orthosis is obtained by heating and form-fitting (often by use of a vacuum) the plastic to the positive mold.

COMMON FOOT CONDITIONS (pp. 328–331)

Pes Planus (Flat Foot) (p. 328)

• Symptomatic relief of pain is obtained by controlling excess pronation of the foot. Pronation of the foot can be defined as a rotation of the foot in the longitudinal axis resulting in a lowering of the medial aspect of the foot. Pronation is also referred to as inrolling. Pronation and abduction of the foot occur at the subtalar joint. Foot pronation is a component of eversion. Eversion involves pronation and abduction (at the subtalar joint) and dorsiflexion (at the ankle joint). The key to controlling excess pronation is controlling the calcaneus to keep the subtalar joint in a neutral position.

• Pes planus can be due to abnormalities such as excessive internal torsion of the tibia (which results in pronation of the foot) or malalignment of the calcaneus. It is the interaction between the tibia and the foot at the subtalar joint that allows pathology outside the foot to cause inrolling of the foot (see Fig. 16–2 in the Textbook).

• The reduction of pronation is accomplished by maintaining the calcaneus and the subtalar joint in correct alignment. The subtalar joint should be in a neutral position during the custom molding process. The orthosis should extend beyond the metatarsal heads to provide better leverage for control of the deformity. A custom-made foot orthosis designed to prevent hyperpronation is also referred to as a UCBL orthosis (or UCB), denoting the University of California Biomechanics Laboratory.

• Some cases of pes planus are due to ligamentous laxity within the foot. For these cases, a medial longitudinal arch support can be helpful for alleviating pain. Initial use of an arch that is too high can cause discomfort. The height of the arch can be increased as necessary as the foot develops a tolerance for the inlay. A Thomas heel extension (Fig. 16–1) can also offer medial support, particularly for heavier individuals. A most practical piece of advice for runners who have hyperpronation/pes planus is to purchase a pair of running shoes with a firm medial heel counter as well as shoes with a wide last at the shank.

Pes Cavus (High-Arched Foot) (pp. 328–329)

• A typical complication of pes cavus is excess pressure along the heel and metatarsal head areas, which can lead to pain. This can be prevented by making

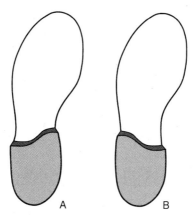

FIGURE 16–1. *A.* Thomas heel. *B.* Reverse Thomas heel.

the height of the longitudinal support just high enough to fill in the space between the shank of the shoe and the arch of the foot to distribute weight more effectively (Fig. 16–2). Weight should also be evenly distributed over the metatarsal heads. The lift is extended just to the metatarsal head area to help distribute and alleviate pressure over the metatarsal weight-bearing area. Because there is no tendency to pronate as in pes planus, the high point of the arch is located at the talonavicular joint. If the tibia is externally rotated, this can give the appearance of an elevated arch as the foot supinates and the lateral aspect of the foot assumes additional weight-bearing responsibility. In these cases, a

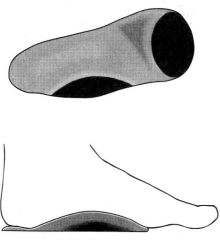

FIGURE 16–2. Pes cavus orthosis. (Modified from Diveley RL: Foot Appliances and Shoe Alterations: Orthopaedic Appliances Atlas. Ann Arbor, MI, Edward Brothers, 1952, p. 464.)

foot orthosis is custom molded with the subtalar joint in a neutral position to prevent excess supination from occurring.

Forefoot Pain (Metatarsalgia) (p. 329)

• Relief of pain in the forefoot is accomplished by distributing the weight-bearing forces to an area proximal to the metatarsal heads. This can be done by either internal or external modification. A metatarsal pad (also referred to as a "cookie") can be placed inside the shoe just posterior to the second, third, and fourth metatarsal heads. It should also be just posterior to the lateral aspect of the first metatarsal head and medial to the fifth metatarsal head. A metatarsal bar (see Fig. 16–6 in the Textbook) is recommended for cases in which the foot is too sensitive to tolerate a pad inside the shoe. Prevention of forefoot pain should also be emphasized to patients. Patients should avoid shoes with high heels or pointed toes, which place excess stress on the metatarsal heads.

Heel Pain (pp. 329–330)

• The painful area can be alleviated by using an orthosis to help distribute weight. Rubber heel pads can be applied inside the shoe to offer relief in cases of minor discomfort. A calcaneal bar is recommended for cases in which the foot is too sensitive to tolerate a pad inside the shoe and the heel pain is associated with a chronic condition.
• A common cause of heel pain along the anteromedial calcaneus is plantar fasciitis. Pain occurs at the attachment site of the fascia along the medial aspect of the heel. Point tenderness is located over the anteromedial calcaneus. It is common in people who hyperpronate their feet, thereby placing excess stress on the medial longitudinal arch. A custom-made orthosis with the subtalar joint in a neutral position (such as that described for pes planus) helps prevent excessive inrolling from occurring and reduces the stress placed along the proximal arch. A custom-made orthosis is indicated for cases in which conservative treatment has failed.
• Plantar fasciitis is also common in patients with high arches. For these patients, the medial longitudinal arch undergoes marked stress during weight bearing. This can be treated with either an elevated arch support or a heel well that helps distribute pressure along the medial longitudinal arch.
• Spurs are commonly mistaken as the source of heel pain. Heel spurs related to plantar fasciitis are the result of mechanical stress acting through the plantar fascia onto its origin at the calcaneus and are not the source of the pain. Inferior heel spurs are related to advancing age and are not painful in nature.
• Heel lifts help some causes of Achilles pain by decreasing the amount of stretch placed on the Achilles tendon (by keeping the ankle joint plantar flexed). A heel lift can be used to treat Achilles enthesitis, an inflammatory reaction at the insertion of the tendon into the periosteum of the calcaneus.

Toe Pain (p. 330)

• The goal of orthotic intervention in toe pain is to decrease pain by immobilization. This is done by extending the steel shank forward to reduce the mobility of the distal joints. A metatarsal bar can also be used for partial immobilization. Common conditions associated with toe pain include hallux rigidus, gout, and arthritis.

Leg Length Discrepancy (p. 330)

• A symptomatic leg length discrepancy should first be evaluated with proper measurement. True leg length is measured from the distal tip of the anterior superior iliac spine to the distal tip of the medial malleolus. Apparent leg length is measured from a midline point such as the pubic symphysis or umbilicus to the distal tip of each malleolus. This can be abnormal in cases in which the true leg length is normal but pelvic obliquity is present secondary to conditions such as scoliosis, pelvic fracture, or muscle imbalance. There is no support in the medical literature for treating low back pain associated with an alleged leg length discrepancy and it is not advised unless there is a traumatic event, such as a femur fracture, resulting in a significant acute onset "leg" (lower limb) length discrepancy.
• Leg length discrepancies less than $\frac{1}{2}$ inch do not need correction. At most, 75% of the leg length discrepancy should be corrected. The first $\frac{1}{2}$ inch of the discrepancy can be managed with a heel pad. Additional correction requires the heel to be built up externally. The sole should also be built up proportionally when the heel is built up externally in order to provide a comfortable, stable gait.

Osteoarthritis of the Knee (pp. 330–331)

• Although osteoarthritis of the knee is not a foot condition, it is mentioned here because pain related to it can be alleviated with foot orthoses. Foot orthoses alter the ground reaction forces affecting the more proximal joints such as the knee, and this relationship should be considered when prescribing a foot orthosis. Lateral heel wedges can be used for conservative treatment of osteoarthritis when medial compartment narrowing results in genu varum. The heel wedges used are $\frac{1}{4}$ inch thick along the lateral border and taper medially.

Pediatric Shoes (p. 331)

• Children's shoes should have a simple design. To facilitate gait, a heel should not be present. Soft soles are recommended to permit the natural development of feet. Tennis shoes are adequate for most children. A high quarter or three-quarter shoe will stay on a child's foot better than a low-cut shoe and is recommended during the first few years of life.
• It is a common misconception that all flat feet need to be treated in children. Flat feet are usual in infants, common in children, and occasionally are found in adults. Flat feet improve over time, in part because of the loss of subcutaneous fat and the reduction of laxity of the joints that occur with growth and the maturation of the gait pattern. Regular shoe size change is necessary in the first few years of life.

ANKLE-FOOT ORTHOSES (pp. 331–338)

• Ankle-foot orthoses (AFOs) are the most commonly prescribed lower limb orthoses. They were formerly known as short leg braces. Metal or plastic AFOs can be used effectively to control ankle motion. Metal AFOs are relatively con-traindicated in children because the weight of the brace can cause external tibial rotation. Plastic AFOs are now more common in all age groups.

• AFOs should provide mediolateral stability as a safety feature. AFOs can also stabilize the knee during gait. They are prescribed for conditions affecting knee stability (e.g., genu recurvatum). An AFO should be considered for conditions affecting the knee, particularly when a concurrent problem exists at the ankle or subtalar joints. A proper AFO prescription considers the biomechanical influ-ence of the orthosis at the foot, ankle, and knee in all planes of movement. It should be remembered that plantar flexion creates a knee extension moment and dorsiflexion creates a knee flexion moment.

Metal AFOs (pp. 331–332)

• The metal AFO comprises a proximal calf band, two uprights, ankle joints, and an attachment to the shoe to anchor the AFO. The posterior metal portion of the calf band should be $1\frac{1}{2}$ to 3 inches wide in order to adequately distribute pressure. The calf band should be 1 inch below the fibular neck to prevent a compressive common peroneal palsy. A leather strap with Velcro is used to close the calf band because this provides ease of closure for patients with only one functional upper limb. Ankle joint motion is controlled by pins or springs inserted into channels (see Figs. 16–9 through 16–11 in the Textbook).

Ankle Stops and Assists (pp. 332–335)

• The ankle joint can be positioned so that it is in a neutral, dorsiflexed, or plantar-flexed position, depending on the gait disturbance. It can be set to permit a partial range of motion or to eliminate a certain motion.

Plantar Stop (Posterior Stop) (pp. 332–333)

• The plantar stop is used to control plantar spasticity or to help incrementally stretch plantar contractures. The plantar stop is most commonly set at 90 degrees. An AFO with a plantar stop at 90 degrees produces a flexion moment at the knee during heel strike. Because the dorsiflexors cannot eccentrically activate to permit the foot to make contact with the ground, the ground reactive force remains posterior to the knee after heel strike, which creates a flexion moment at the knee (and possibly an unstable gait). The proximal portion of the AFO also has an effect on knee stability. The posterior portion of the proximal AFO exerts a forward push on the proximal leg to increase the knee flexion moment after heel strike (Fig. 16–3). The opposite occurs at toe-off, with an extension moment created at the knee. This concept has been used to develop what has been referred to as a plastic ground reaction AFO, with a solid proximal ante-rior tibial closing that provides a greater influence on the knee.

• The posterior stop should be set at the minimal amount of plantar flexion required to clear the foot during swing-through. Plantar flexion creates a knee extension moment at the knee after heel strike. This provides a more stable knee during gait than when the ankle plantar stops are set in any degree of dorsiflexion.

• A balanced decision should be made between providing resistance to plantar flexion to clear the foot during the swing phase of gait and the amount of insta-

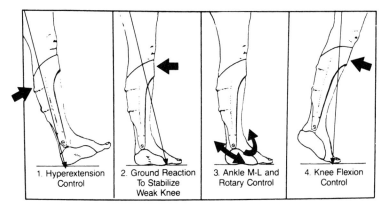

1. Hyperextension Control
2. Ground Reaction To Stabilize Weak Knee
3. Ankle M-L and Rotary Control
4. Knee Flexion Control

FIGURE 16–3. Ground reaction AFO dynamic illustration. Note the effect of the proximal portion of the AFO on the knee throughout gait. (Courtesy of Oregon Orthotic System, Albany, OR.)

bility at the knee during the stance phase of gait. No AFO is effective in reducing the amount of knee flexion to "normal" levels during the stance phase of gait.

Dorsiflexion Stop (Anterior Stop) (pp. 333–334)
• An anterior stop is used to substitute for the function of the gastrocnemius/soleus complex. Because of its effect on the knee it is used in conditions with weak calf muscles or weak quadriceps. Weak calf musculature allows the ankle to enter dorsiflexion. The anterior stop set at 5 degrees of dorsiflexion best substitutes for gastrocnemius/soleus function.
• The earlier the dorsiflexion stop occurs during the stance phase, the greater the extension moment at the knee. This is useful in clinical situations where quadriceps weakness is also present. If the extension moment at the knee is too great for too long, then genu recurvatum ("back knee") can occur. A balance should be obtained such that the extension at the knee is sufficient to stabilize the knee in extension yet prevent genu recurvatum.

Dorsiflexion Assist (Posterior Spring) (p. 334)
• The posterior spring serves two purposes: (1) it substitutes for concentric contraction of dorsiflexors to prevent flaccid foot drop after toe-off; and (2) it substitutes (inadequately) for the eccentric activation of the dorsiflexors after heel strike. The metal dorsiflexion assist ankle joint is also known as a Klenzak ankle joint.

Metal AFO Varus/Valgus Control (pp. 334–335)
• Varus and valgus deformities are associated with rotation at the subtalar joint. A T strap is attached along the side of the shoe distal to the subtalar joint to help minimize the deformity. T straps are also used to help prevent worsening of the deformity. T straps also help distribute pressure properly along the foot during weight bearing.

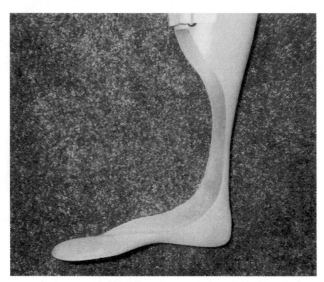

FIGURE 16–4. Custom plastic solid (means no ankle joint although still flexible) AFO with posterior trimline to allow some flexibility with plantar flexion. This is the most commonly prescribed AFO for foot drop.

• T straps are referred to as being either medial or lateral. A medial T strap is sown to the medial aspect of the shoe and the belt is cinched around the lateral upright of the AFO. A medial T strap is used to control a valgus deformity. The opposite is true for a varus deformity, with the T strap being laterally located.

Plastic AFOs (p. 335)

• Plastic AFOs are the most commonly used AFOs because of their cost, cosmesis, light weight, interchangeability with shoes, ability to control varus and valgus deformities, provision of better foot support with the customized foot portion, and ability to achieve what is offered by the metal AFO (Fig. 16–4). Energy consumption is equal to a plastic solid AFO or a metal double upright AFO. Although a plastic orthosis weighs less than its metal counterpart, the weight of the orthosis is not as important as the influence of the ground reactive force created by the presence of the orthosis. The same orthotic principles apply to orthoses made of plastic or metal.

• Plastic AFOs can be prefabricated or custom made. The reasons for prescribing a custom-molded orthosis include long-term need, conformed molding for comfort or insensate feet, placement of the orthosis in a fixed amount of plantar or dorsiflexion, better control of rotational deformities, and further reduction of weight bearing for a tibial fracture or diabetic plantar ulcer.

• Some practical advice should be offered to the patient regarding the use of a plastic AFO. If changing shoes, it is best to have another pair with a similar heel height to prevent altering the biomechanical effects at the foot, ankle, and knee. Tennis shoes are most accommodating for donning and doffing of the AFO.

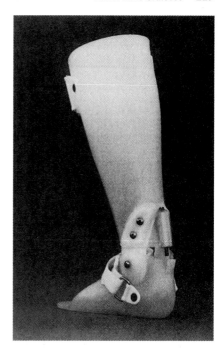

FIGURE 16–5. Elite midline posterior stop articulated AFO. Note the use of a plastic ankle joint to further decrease weight. Plastic ankle joints are more common in children (and lightweight individuals). The use of a plantar stop with ankle joints is recommended for an active lightweight patient with plantar spasticity (e.g., a child with cerebral palsy).

Plastic AFO Components (pp. 335–336)

• The foot component of the AFO should extend beyond the metatarsal heads. The footplate can be extended beyond the toes to reduce the spasticity aggravated by toe flexion. The shape and molding of the foot portion influence the biomechanics of more proximal joints.

• The ankle and subtalar joints can be made more stable under four circumstances: (1) the trim line extends more anteriorly at the ankle level (a trim line is the anterior border of the plastic AFO), (2) the plastic material is thicker, (3) carbon inserts are placed along the medial and lateral aspects of the ankle joint, and (4) corrugations are made within the posterior leaf of the AFO.

• Plastic AFOs can also be hinged at the ankle (Fig. 16–5). Ankle hinges allow full or partial ankle motion, which can permit a more natural gait. They should be considered when complete restriction of ankle motion is not required. Plastic ankle joints are light and are a good choice for children. Metal ankle joints are preferred for adults, particularly heavy adults. Newer designs have a single midline posterior rod/spring mechanism.

• The leg component should encompass three quarters of the leg and should be padded along its internal surface. The proximal extent should end 1 inch below the fibular neck to prevent a compressive common peroneal nerve palsy.

To Hinge or Not to Hinge (p. 336)

• Unfortunately, there is no medical research available on this topic to provide general guidelines. The authors recommend that a plastic AFO for foot drop not be hinged. This keeps the orthosis narrower to accommodate shoe wear, and needs less maintenance. Some movement at the ankle can still be achieved by making the AFO flexible with a posterior trim line. The authors recommend a hinged AFO for the active patient with plantar spasticity who would take advantage of some of the range of motion permitted at the ankle (e.g., a child with cerebral palsy or a young adult with a traumatic brain injury).

The Solid Plastic AFO (p. 336)
• The solid plastic AFO is the most commonly prescribed plastic AFO (see Fig. 16–4). It can be made to serve several purposes. A solid AFO can still be flexible enough to allow some ankle motion, and it should be flexible with a posterior trim line for the treatment of a foot drop. A solid AFO should be truly solid (not flexible) for the treatment of plantar spasticity.
• Solid AFOs set at 90 degrees are commonly used for foot drop. Less obvious but equally important is the solid AFO's ability to treat conditions affecting the knee. Again, it should be remembered that plantar flexion creates knee extension and dorsiflexion creates knee flexion at heel strike.

Plastic AFO Varus/Valgus Control (p. 336)
• The goal of orthotic intervention is to alter the ground reactive forces with custom molding to help maintain proper alignment of the lower limb by "building up" selected portions of the AFO. Some orthotists believe that an orthosis should be firm ("not conforming") in order to control a deformity. Pressure points should be present in expected areas at follow-up visits if the orthosis is serving its purpose.

Patellar Tendon-Bearing AFOs (pp. 336–337)

• A patellar tendon-bearing (PTB) AFO uses the patellar tendon and the tibial condyles to partially relieve weight-bearing stress on skeletal structures distally with more weight bearing distributed along the medial tibial condyle. PTB is a misnomer for this orthosis because only about 10% of the weight is distributed along the patellar tendon and the medial tibial condyle.
• PTB AFOs are often prescribed for diabetic ulcerations of the foot, tibial fractures, relief of the weight-bearing surface in painful heel conditions (e.g., calcaneal fractures), postoperative ankle fusions, and avascular necrosis of the foot or ankle. The orthoses are made of plastic and so are lightweight and highly durable. They are bivalved and fit snugly with the use of Velcro straps or buckles similar to those of ski boots (see Fig. 16–18 in the Textbook). A custom-molded PTB AFO can reduce weight bearing in the affected foot by up to 50%.
• The solid plastic orthosis makes contact with the ground before the reactive force is absorbed significantly by the foot and then distributes this force more proximally along the leg. Compared with a prefabricated AFO, a custom-made PTB AFO more effectively distributes pressure over a greater surface contact area for maximal weight-bearing reduction. Additional weight-bearing reduction is obtained by eliminating ankle movement and when a rocker bottom is directly incorporated into the plastic orthosis.

Checkout (p. 338)

• The patient should be examined after fitting and use of the orthosis. The first and most obvious form of a checkout is to verify that the gait pattern is improved with the orthosis in comparison to without the orthosis. The orthotic ankle joint should coincide with the tip of the medial malleolus. The patient is to be checked for ease of donning and doffing the orthosis, and while it is off, observed for areas of skin breakdown.

KNEE-ANKLE-FOOT ORTHOSES (pp. 338–341)

• Knee-ankle-foot orthoses (KAFOs) were formerly referred to as long leg braces. The components are the same as those of an AFO but also include knee joints, thigh uprights, and a proximal thigh band. Various knee joints and knee locks are available for a variety of conditions. KAFOs are used in patients with severe knee extensor and hamstring weakness, structural knee instability, and knee flexion spasticity. The purpose of the KAFO is to provide stability at the knee, ankle, and subtalar joints during ambulation. They are most commonly prescribed bilaterally for patients with spinal cord injuries and unilaterally for patients with polio. There is a common misconception that patients with a complete femoral neuropathy (i.e., no quadriceps function) should have their knees braced. From a functional anatomical standpoint, it should be kept in mind that there are three stabilizers to the knee: the quadriceps, the hamstrings (via eccentric activation at heel strike), and the plantar flexors (plantar flexion creates a knee extension moment).
• KAFOs can be prescribed for functional ambulation or exercise (or both). The benefits of exercise to the patient requiring bilateral KAFOs include preventing lower limb contractures, enhancing cardiovascular fitness, maintaining upper body strength for activities of daily living, delaying the development of osteoporosis, and fewer medical complications such as deep venous thromboses.
• The use of KAFOs often complements the use of a wheelchair for ambulation. The proprioceptive level is a reliable indicator of which spinal cord–injured patients can achieve ambulation status. It is helpful to have sensation and proprioception in the lower limbs in order to ambulate safely with KAFOs. The level of the spinal cord injury is also important in predicting the ability to ambulate. Adult spinal cord–injured patients with lesions at or above T12 generally are not functional ambulators because of the metabolic cost involved. Children have a higher center of gravity and can have a functional gait with a higher spinal cord lesion. Muscle function is a predictor of the quality of ambulation. Good trunk control and upper body strength are needed in order to ambulate with KAFOs because these devices are used in combination with ambulation aids (e.g., walkers and Lofstrand forearm orthoses).
• Some paraplegic patients, such as those with lower lumbar lesions with some knee extensor strength, are able to ambulate without KAFOs. Ambulation in these patients can often be accomplished with the use of bilateral plastic ground reaction AFOs with the ankles fixed in 10 to 15 degrees of plantar flexion.

Knee Joints (pp. 338–340)

• There are three basic types of knee joints.
• The straight set knee joint provides rotation about a single axis (Fig. 16–6). It allows free flexion but prevents hyperextension. It is often used in combination with a drop lock, which keeps the knee in extension throughout all phases of gait for further stability.

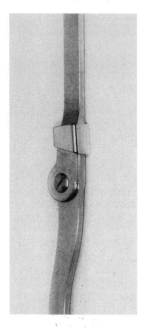

FIGURE 16–6. Straight-set knee with drop lock. (Courtesy of USMC, Pasadena.)

• The polycentric knee joint uses a double-axis system to simulate the flexion-extension movements of the femur and tibia at the knee joint (see Fig. 16–20 in the Textbook). Although this concept is theoretically sound, the polycentric knee joint has not proved to be advantageous over the straight set knee joint and it is less commonly used. It also adds bulk to the orthosis. It is most commonly used in sport knee orthoses.

• The third type of knee joint is the posterior offset knee joint (see Fig. 16–21 in the Textbook). It is prescribed for patients with weak knee extensors and some hip extensor strength. It allows free flexion and extension of the knee during the swing phase of gait and helps keep the *orthotic* ground reactive force in front of the knee axis for stability during stance. The center of gravity is normally posterior to the knee at heel strike, creating a flexion moment at the knee, which requires knee extensor muscle contraction to counteract this force. The offset knee joint component of the KAFO helps place the ground reactive force anterior to the orthotic knee joint, creating an extension moment at the knee during stance to compensate for the weak knee extensors. The offset knee joint should have a hyperextension stop to help prevent genu recurvatum.

Knee Locks (pp. 340–341)

• Knee locks are used to provide complete stability at the knee. There are four common types of knee locks; these are discussed in order of their frequency of use, beginning with the most commonly used.

• The ratchet lock has recently become the most commonly prescribed knee lock (see Fig. 16–23 in the Textbook). The ratchet lock has a catching mechanism that operates in 12-degree increments. As the user rises from a seated to a standing position, if there is a tendency for the knee to become unstable and flex, the ratchet lock prevents that movement and keeps the gains made toward extension. Once the patient is standing with the knees extended, knee flexion is achieved by pressing down on a release lever.

• Before the development of the ratchet lock, the drop lock (ring lock) was used most commonly in both the medial and lateral uprights of the KAFO (see Fig. 16–19 in the Textbook). The drop lock can "settle" after ambulation and might be difficult to pull up to unlock the knee. The disadvantage of the drop lock in comparison with the ratchet lock is that there is no locking mechanism until full knee extension is obtained. Consequently, a patient's knee can collapse into flexion when not sufficiently extended to activate the drop lock.

• The bail lock (also called the Swiss, French, Schweitzer, or pawl lock) provides an easy method of simultaneously unlocking the medial and lateral knee joints of a KAFO (see Figs. 16–24 and 16–25 in the Textbook). Lifting up the bail posteriorly releases the knee joint to permit flexion, allowing the patient to sit down. The patient can also catch the bail on the edge of a chair to release the lock mechanism to permit sitting.

• The dial lock (formerly known as a turn buckle) is used to stabilize the knee in varying amounts of flexion (see Fig. 16–26 in the Textbook). It can be adjusted in 6-degree increments and is more precise for the management of a knee with a flexion contracture than a KAFO with ratchet locks. Its uses include helping prevent progression of a flexion contracture or assisting with the gradual reduction of a flexion contracture.

The Thigh Component of a KAFO (p. 341)

• The thigh band needs to be wide enough to adequately distribute the pressure of the ground reactive force transmitted through the knee axis. A partial plastic thigh shell can provide a greater contact area and decrease high-pressure areas if properly fitted.

KNEE ORTHOSES (pp. 342–344)

Swedish Knee Cage (p. 342)

• The knee orthosis (KO) known as a Swedish knee cage (Fig. 16–7) is used to control minor to moderate genu recurvatum caused by ligamentous or capsular laxity. It should be prescribed only in an articulated form. The articulated version allows full knee flexion and prevents hyperextension. The articulated version is recommended for the treatment of genu recurvatum.

• Genu recurvatum can also be controlled with a solid plastic AFO that resists plantar flexion. This can be used in cases where pathology also affects the ankle or subtalar joints. The more rigid the AFO, the greater the flexion moment at the knee during heel strike (which counters the extension moment of the recurvatum).

Osteoarthritis Knee Orthoses (pp. 342–343)

• The same orthotic three-point principle that has been applied for years in the Swedish knee cage for genu recurvatum has recently also been applied to

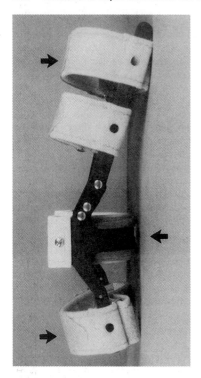

FIGURE 16–7. The articulated Swedish knee cage, which uses a three-point system to control genu recurvatum.

osteoarthritis of the knee, more commonly with medial compartment narrowing (see Fig. 16–29 in the Textbook). The limiting factor regarding this knee orthotic prescription is the patient's weight. A morbidly obese patient with an abundance of fatty tissue around the knee will not support the knee orthosis adequately.

Sport Knee Orthoses (pp. 343–344)

• There is an increasing abundance of sport orthoses on the market. There is also a lack of definitive research regarding their role in sports. Prophylactic knee bracing attempts to prevent or reduce the severity of knee injuries. There is currently no evidence to support the use or cost benefit of these orthoses. Some studies have found that the use of these orthoses actually increased the number of athletes with knee injuries. It is theorized that knee-braced players can put themselves in compromising positions because of over-reliance on the orthosis and that this can contribute directly to the increasing injury rates observed.

• Rehabilitative knee bracing is used to allow protected motion within defined limits. It is useful for postoperative and conservative management of knee injuries.

• Functional knee bracing is designed to assist or provide stability for the unstable knee. Knee braces are used most commonly to stabilize a laterally subluxing patella or an anterior cruciate ligament-deficient knee. Their use

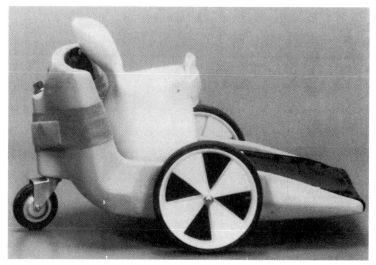

FIGURE 16–8. Caster cart. This is an initial mobility aid for the disabled child. The child uses it as a "pre-wheelchair device." The deep seat bucket stabilizes the seated ataxic child while permitting free use of the upper limbs for ambulation. (Courtesy of the Hugh MacMillan Rehabilitation Center, Toronto.)

has been shown to be effective only at loads much lower than those placed on the knee during athletic participation. Functional knee bracing can possibly play a role in the treatment of pathological laxity by possibly decreasing the frequency of unstable episodes.

PEDIATRIC ORTHOSES (pp. 344–347)

Caster Cart (p. 344)

• The disabled child should identify early with motion so that ambulatory skills can progress naturally. Without familiarity with motion, disabled children lack the desire to ambulate once placed in a parapodium or reciprocating gait orthosis.

• The caster cart (Fig. 16–8) is used for children with a developmental delay in ambulatory skills, and it serves as an initial mobility aid. It is most often prescribed for children with spina bifida. Most children are upright and cruising by 10 months. Children with paraplegia should be fitted for a caster cart once they have obtained enough upper limb strength and trunk balance to propel themselves.

Standing Frame (pp. 344–345)

• The use of a standing frame (see Fig. 16–32 in the Textbook) typically follows successful use of a caster cart. The age range for initial use is usually 8 to 15 months. Children can continue to use their caster carts during this time. Children who are pulling themselves up along furniture are typically ready for a

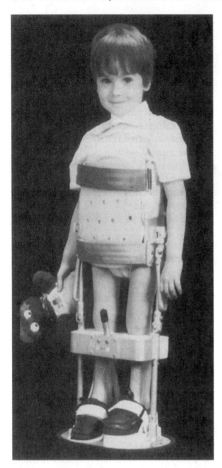

FIGURE 16–9. Parapodium. Note the lift on the left leg to compensate for a leg length discrepancy and the wide abdominal support pad to assist in upright posture. (Courtesy of the Hugh MacMillan Rehabilitation Center, Toronto.)

standing frame. The standing frame helps balance the body in space and allows free use of the upper limbs for participation in activities. Children with thoracic level lesions need AFOs to provide good ankle and foot support in the standing frame or parapodium.

Parapodium (p. 345)

• The parapodium was also referred to in the past as a swivel orthosis (Fig. 16–9). Before children are given a parapodium, they should first demonstrate adequate use of a standing frame and exhibit a desire to ambulate. A child who has not used a standing frame will likely be unable or unwilling to ambulate with a parapodium.

• A parapodium is an appropriate prescription for children who are unlikely to become functional walkers owing to the severity of their impairment. It often complements wheelchair use. It is most commonly prescribed for children between $2\frac{1}{2}$ and 5 years of age.

• A parapodium allows crutchless gait. Ambulation occurs by the child pivoting the hips and using "body English" to swivel one side of the oval-based stand forward and then repeating the same event for the other side. Its design is similar to the standing frame, but it has hip and knee joints.

Reciprocating Gait Orthosis (pp. 345–347)

• The reciprocating gait orthosis (RGO) can also be referred to as a bilateral hip-knee-ankle-foot orthosis (HKAFO). The purpose of the RGO is to provide contralateral hip extension with ipsilateral hip flexion. The RGO is appropriate for children who have used the standing frame, developed good trunk control and coordination, can safely stand, and are mentally prepared for ambulation.
• Spinal cord injury level is not a very reliable predictor of ambulation capability for children. As children with spinal cord injuries grow taller, they might experience more difficulty walking as their center of gravity becomes lower.
• The RGO is prescribed most commonly for children ages 3 to 6 years. Gait is initiated with unilateral hip flexion and can be assisted by swaying the trunk when hip flexion is inadequate. This type of gait pattern can also be considered to be a form of physical therapy because hip extension occurs passively with each step, helping to reduce flexion contractures.
• Crutches are used with the RGO to provide a control mechanism, taking advantage of the forward momentum to produce small propulsive forces when needed. This also is a disadvantage of this orthosis (compared with the parapodium) because the upper limbs are not free for other activities.
• The hip joints of the RGO have hip flexion and abduction capabilities upon release of the locking mechanisms (see Fig. 16–35 in the Textbook). It is recommended that one hip joint have abduction capability to permit catheterization and to allow sitting in a hip-flexed and abducted position.

AMBULATION AIDS (pp. 347–348)

• The purpose of using ambulation aids (Fig. 16–10) is to increase the area of support for patients who have difficulty maintaining their center of gravity safely over their own support area. Ambulation aids improve balance, redistribute and extend the weight-bearing area, reduce lower limb pain, provide small propulsive forces, and provide sensory feedback. They should be considered an extension of the upper limb. Their proper use requires adequate upper limb strength and coordination. A supervised period of training is recommended after prescription of an aid.
• The type of aid needed depends on how much balance and weight-bearing assistance is needed. The body weight transmission for a unilateral cane opposite the affected side is 20% to 25%. It is 40% to 50% with the use of a forearm or arm cane. Body weight transmission with bilateral crutches is estimated at up to 80%.

Canes (pp. 347–348)

Prescription. Measure the tip of the cane to the level of the greater trochanter with the patient in an upright position to determine the proper cane length. The elbow should be flexed approximately 20 degrees, which is a desirable elbow position for all ambulation aids. Canes are made of wood or aluminum.

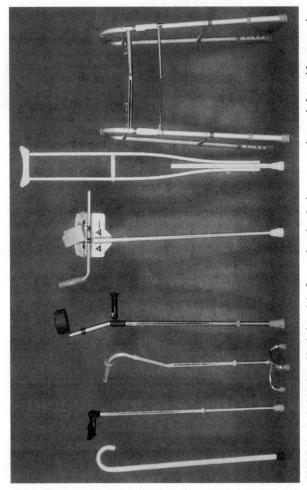

FIGURE 16–10. Ambulation aids. *Left to right*: C cane, functional grip cane, quad cane, Lofstrand forearm orthosis, platform forearm orthosis, crutch, and walker.

• There are three common types of canes (see Fig. 16–10). The C cane is most commonly used. It is also known as a crook top cane, straight cane, or J cane. A functional grip cane offers the patient a grip that can be more comfortable than with the C cane. A quad cane provides an increased area of support compared with the other canes. Quad canes also come in narrow- and wide-based forms for different degrees of support.

• A cane is used on the side opposite the supporting lower limb. It is advanced with the opposite lower limb, and is usually held on the patient's unaffected side to lessen the force exerted on a hip with pathology. The load is increased by four times the body weight on the stance side during gait because of the gravitational forces and the gluteus medius-minimus force exerted across the weight-bearing hip. The cane helps decrease the force generated across the affected hip joint by decreasing the work of the gluteus medius-minimus complex.

• Patients should be instructed on how to ascend and descend stairs. The phrase "up with the good and down with the bad" serves as an easy reminder. The patient should always have the "good" lower limb assume the first full weight-bearing step on level surfaces.

Walker (p. 348)

Prescription

1. Place the front of the walker 12 inches in front of the patient (the walker should partially surround the patient).
2. Determine the proper height of the walker by having the patient stand upright with the shoulders relaxed and the elbows flexed 20 degrees.

• A walker provides maximum support for the patient but also necessitates a slow gait. It is useful for hemiplegic and ataxic patients. Wheels can be added to the front legs to facilitate movement of the walker for those who lack coordination in the upper limbs.

Visual Impairment Cane (p. 348)

Prescription

1. Instruct the patient to flex the shoulder until the upper limb is parallel with the floor.
2. Measure the distance from the hand to the floor. That is the proper length.

• A visual impairment cane should be lightweight, flexible, and easily collapsible. The distal inches of the cane are red.

Crutches (p. 348)

Prescription

1. *Crutch length:* Measure the distance from the anterior axillary fold to a point 6 inches lateral to the fifth toe with the patient standing with the shoulders relaxed.
2. *Handpiece:* Measure with the patient's elbow flexed 30 degrees, the wrist in maximal extension, and the fingers forming a fist. This is measured *after* the total crutch height is determined with the crutch 3 inches lateral to the foot.

• A crutch is defined as a device that provides support from the axilla to the floor. Although there are different types of crutches and canes, they can all be referred to as orthoses because they are applied to the external surface of the body to improve function.

• The patient should be able to raise the body 1 to 2 inches by complete elbow extension. It needs to be emphasized to the patient that crutches are not designed to be rests for body support.

Nonaxillary Crutches (p. 348)

• Nonaxillary crutches are more appropriately called forearm or arm canes, or forearm or arm orthoses.

FOREARM ORTHOSES (pp. 348–351)
Lofstrand Forearm Orthosis (p. 348)

Prescription. Measure the handpiece as described above for crutches, with the patient standing upright and the elbow in 20 degrees of flexion.

• The proximal portion of the orthosis is also angled at 20 degrees to provide for a comfortable, stable fit. It is often made of tubular aluminum. It provides less support than crutches for ambulation, but is sufficient for many patients. Lofstrand forearm orthoses are most often used bilaterally.

Wooden Forearm Orthosis (Kenny Stick) (pp. 348–349)

• Another forearm orthosis option is the Kenny stick (see Fig. 16–37 in the Textbook). It was designed for polio patients who had satisfactory proximal upper limb musculature but were weak distally and unable to effectively hold and control the orthosis. Its advantage over the Lofstrand orthosis is the presence of a closed leather band. This assures the patient (more so than the Lofstrand forearm orthosis does) that he or she will not drop the ambulation aid.

Platform Forearm Orthosis (p. 349)

Prescription. Have the patient stand upright with the shoulders relaxed and the elbows flexed 90 degrees. The distance from the ground to the forearm rest is the proper length.

• This orthosis is helpful for patients with painful wrist and hand conditions as well as for those with elbow contractures.

Triceps Weakness Orthoses (Arm Orthoses) (p. 349)

• These orthoses, also known as triceps weakness crutches, were originally developed for polio patients. The metal version is known as a Warm Spring crutch or Everett crutch. The wooden version is known as a Canadian crutch. These crutches resemble the "axillary" crutches in style, but end proximally with a cuff at the mid-arm level.

Crutch Tips and Hand Grips (p. 349)

• The purpose of crutch tips is to absorb shock and prevent slippage. Crutches are only as safe as the quality of their crutch tips. Handgrips are used to reduce pressure on the hands and are also safety features because they help prevent slippage.

Crutch Gaits (p. 349)

• Strength, balance, coordination, and walking surface all have an effect on which crutch gait should be used under different circumstances. Each patient should be comfortable with more than one type of crutch gait.
• The four-point crutch gait follows the sequence: left crutch→right foot→ right crutch→left foot→repeat. Its advantage is stability. At least three points are always in contact with the ground.
• The three-point crutch gait follows the sequence: both crutches and the weaker lower limb "good" lower limb→repeat. The advantage of the three-point gait is that all weight bearing on the affected lower limb is eliminated. This gait is commonly used by patients with lower limb fractures or amputations. It is also known as the non–weight-bearing gait. The patient should have good balance to perform this gait.
• The alternate two-point crutch gait follows the sequence: left crutch and right foot→right crutch and left foot→repeat. This gait pattern provides stability and is useful for ataxic patients and with decreased lower limb weight-bearing capabilities. It is faster than the four-point gait and provides some weight-bearing relief to both lower limbs.
• Gait can also be classified as swing-through, swing-to, and drag-to. The swing-through pattern sequence is: both crutches→advancement of both lower limbs past the crutches. It is very energy consuming and its use requires functional abdominal muscles. The swing-through gait is the fastest gait (even faster than able body walking). The swing-to gait sequence is: both crutches→advancement of both lower limbs almost to the crutch level. There are alternate and simultaneous forms of drag to gait. The alternate sequence is: left crutch→right crutch→drag to crutch level. The simultaneous sequence is: both crutches→ drag to crutch level. These are useful as initial gait patterns for paraplegic patients. They can advance to another gait pattern. These patterns provide stability during gait but are slow and laborious methods of ambulation.

Prescription (pp. 349–351)

• A medical diagnosis with delineation of the impairment and any resulting disability should be made before an orthotic prescription is written. The orthotic goals should be documented for the orthotist. An AFO prescription should include the type of ankle (e.g., rigid, flexible, or jointed) and the position of the ankle (e.g., neutral, dorsiflexed, or plantar-flexed). If the ankle is jointed, the range of motion should be specified. In the case of a compressive peroneal nerve palsy, for example, the physical impairment would be a flaccid foot drop. The ankle should be flexible and held in a neutral position with a plastic AFO set at 90 degrees. Figure 16–11 is a sample prescription form.

SUMMARY (p. 351)

• An appropriate lower limb orthotic prescription requires a thorough biomechanical analysis of gait and a knowledge of the available orthotic components available to treat specific conditions. The prescribing physician should maintain

LOWER LIMB ORTHOTIC PRESCRIPTION

NAME: _____ AGE: _____

DIAGNOSIS: _____

ORTHOTIC GOALS:_____

JUSTIFICATION: _____

ORTHOTIC COMPANY:_____

REFERRING PHYSICIAN: _____

❏ FO   ❏ AFO   ❏ KAFO   ❏ HKAFO   ❏ KO

❏ Right   ❏ Left   ❏ Bilateral

❏ Custom

❏ Plastic   ❏ Metal   ❏ Combination

ANKLE TYPE:	❏ Solid (flexible)	❏ Solid (rigid)	❏ Hinged: __ dorsi-assist

ANKLE TYPE: ❏ Solid (flexible)   ❏ Solid (rigid)   ❏ Hinged: __ dorsi-assist
                                                              __ dorsi-stop
ANKLE ROM: ❏ Plantar flexion   _____ degrees   __ plantar stop

              ❏ Dorsiflexion   _____ degrees

              ❏ Neutral (90°)

KNEE TYPE: ❏ Straight set   ❏ Posterior offset   ❏ Polycentric

KNEE LOCKS: ❏ Two per knee joint   ❏ One per knee joint

KNEE LOCK TYPE: ❏ Drop lock   ❏ Bail lock   ❏ Dial lock   ❏ Ratchet lock   ❏ Fan lock

HIP JOINTS with drop locks: ❏ Standard   ❏ Abduction

MISCELLANEOUS: _____

_____   _____
Physician Name   Date

FIGURE 16–11. Lower limb orthotic prescription sheet.

a close working relationship with the certified orthotist to make certain that the patient is receiving the best orthotic options available.
• Patient complaints about orthoses usually are related to cosmesis, comfort, clothing soiling or damage, weight, and difficulty with donning and doffing.

17

Original Chapter by Steven V. Fisher, M.D., and Robert B. Winter, M.D.

Spinal Orthoses in Rehabilitation

CLINICAL USE OF SPINAL ORTHOSES (pp. 353–363)

• There are four primary objectives for the application of a spinal orthosis: (1) controlling the position of the spine by the use of external forces; (2) applying corrective forces to abnormal curvatures; (3) aiding spinal stability when soft tissues cannot adequately perform their stabilizer role; and (4) restricting spinal segment movement after acute trauma or surgery to protect against further injury. In the case of traumatic spinal injury, the most important objective is the protection of the spinal cord and nerve roots. In other words, the goal of an orthosis is to control the position of the spine by the application of an external force for protection, immobilization, support, or correction of a deformity.

• Spinal orthoses can also have negative effects, including axial muscle atrophy secondary to reduced muscle activity. The control of motion by the orthosis also promotes contractures of the immobilized part. Moreover, psychological dependency on the orthosis can occur.

Cervical Orthoses (pp. 353–359)

• Proper prescription of a cervical orthosis requires knowledge of the general principles of bracing and the biomechanics of the cervical spine (see Chapter 37), as well as an understanding of the indications and limitations of specific cervical orthoses. All spinal orthoses utilize the principle of a three-point pressure system. The corrective component of force is ideally located midway between the opposing forces. The effectiveness of a cervical orthosis is determined by its ability to resist not only gross motion, but intersegmental motion as well (Table 17–1).

• The biomechanical consequences of the spinal orthosis are dependent on the points of application, the direction and magnitude of the force applied by the device, the tightness with which the device is worn, and the amount of force the patient exerts against it. The patient's body habitus also plays a significant role in the effectiveness of the orthosis. Spinal trauma produces unpredictable instability at times; hence a given orthosis must be tested to ensure its effectiveness. In order to judge the effectiveness of an orthosis on a particular patient, a clinician must take radiographs in different positions while the patient is wearing the orthosis.

TABLE 17–1 Normal Cervical Motion from Occiput to First Thoracic Vertebra and the Effects of Cervical Orthoses

	Mean of Normal Motion (%)		
	Flexion/Extension	Lateral Bending	Rotation
Normal*	100.0	100.0	100.0
Soft collar*	74.2	92.3	82.6
Philadelphia collar	28.9	66.4	43.7
SOMI brace	27.7	65.6	33.6
Four-poster brace	20.6	45.9	27.1
Yale cervicothoracic brace	12.8	50.5	18.2
Halo device*	4.0	4.0	1.0
Halo device†	11.7	8.4	2.4
Minerva body jacket‡	14.0	15.5	0

* Data from Johnson RM, Hart DL, Simmons EF, et al: Cervical orthoses: A study comparing their effectiveness in restricting cervical motion in normal subjects. J Bone Joint Surg [Am] 1977; 59:332.
† Data from Lysell E: Motion in the cervical spine, thesis. Acta Orthop Scand Suppl 1969; 123.
‡ Data from Maiman D, Millington P, Novak S, et al: The effects of the thermoplastic Minerva body jacket on cervical spine motion. Neurosurgery 1989; 25:363–368.

- The cervical spine is the most mobile part of the entire spine and has multiple planes of motion. Moreover, little body surface area is available for adequate contact of the orthosis. Adequate contact of the orthosis on the bony structures of the skull and thorax is anatomically difficult. The occiput is rounded and the chin can easily be lifted away from the mandibular support by extending the upper cervical spine. Additionally, the shoulders and clavicle are mobile. Any strong force that acts on the head or over the clavicles is unpleasant for the patient. The chin becomes tender rather easily with undue pressure, especially in males who need to shave, and complications such as skin breakdown and local pain may develop.
- Cervical orthoses can be categorized in several different ways. Some arrange cervical appliances into four basic designs: (1) cervical collars, (2) poster appliances, (3) cervicothoracic orthoses, and (4) halo devices. Probably the most widely used orthoses are the soft and hard collars, Philadelphia orthosis, SOMI (sternal-occipital-mandibular immobilizer) orthosis, poster orthosis (two or four), Yale-type cervicothoracic orthosis, thermoplastic Minerva body jacket (TMBJ), and halo jacket or vest.
- There are several basic types of cervical collars. The soft cervical collar (Fig. 17–1) is made of foam rubber covered by stockinet. This device is low in cost, easy to fabricate, and well tolerated by most patients. It does not restrict cervical motion in any plane (see Table 17–1). It provides warmth and psychological comfort but no support. It probably serves only as a reminder to hold the neck relatively still.
- The hard collar is made of a rigid polyethylene. It can have an optional occipital and mandibular support. The hard collar without the mandibular and cervical support does not significantly immobilize the cervical spine. With the two supports, it gives more restriction in flexion and extension, but it is not truly effective. It does not limit lateral bending or rotation. It does not contact the

thorax. It can press on the clavicles, creating areas of high pressure with subsequent discomfort.

• The Philadelphia ("collar") orthosis (Fig. 17–2) is made of plastizote reinforced with anterior and posterior plastic struts. This orthosis has a molded mandibular and occipital support. The anterior and posterior caudal aspects of the brace extend onto the upper thorax. The Philadelphia orthosis does restrict cervical spine motion, particularly in flexion and extension (see Table 17–1). This is probably because of the better fit at the occiput and chin, as well as the improved contact on the upper thorax. However, the Philadelphia orthosis is relatively ineffective in controlling rotation and lateral bending (see Table 17–1). Depending on the prominence of the clavicles of the individual wearer, the Philadelphia orthosis may be quite uncomfortable.

• The Jobst Vertebrace is constructed from a high-density polyethylene. It provides full contact along its costal end to the sternum and it closely cups the mandible. A radiological study of 10 normal volunteers showed that this orthosis functioned as well as, or better than, the Yale (see below) and Philadelphia orthoses. The investigators concluded that it was a good orthotic choice for use in emergency transport situations. It does not, however, appear to be comfortable enough for long-term rehabilitation use. The Miami J, NecLoc, and Aspen are other, newer orthoses that were initially designed for emergency extrication purposes. However, the Miami J, the Aspen, and the NecLoc are probably comfortable enough to be used in the rehabilitation phase of management.

• The four-poster brace (Fig. 17–3) represents the first true cervical thoracic orthosis discussed here. It has a molded mandibular and occipital support with

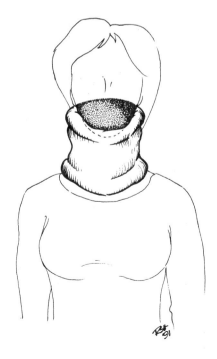

FIGURE 17–1. Soft collar.

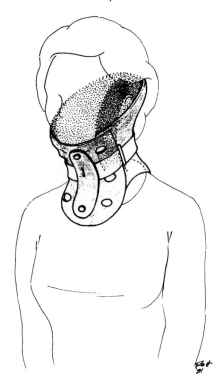

FIGURE 17–2. Philadelphia collar.

adjustable struts attaching to anterior and posterior padded thoracic plates. The Guilford brace (see Fig. 17–4 in the Textbook) is a two-poster brace with a front and back strut connecting the anterior and posterior thoracic plates to the chin and occipital piece. These orthoses are relatively effective in limiting range of motion in flexion and extension (see Table 17–1).

• Another true cervical thoracic brace is the Yale orthosis (see Fig. 17–5 in the Textbook). This cervicothoracic orthosis was originally a modified Philadelphia collar with molded plastizote reinforced with plastic struts. It extends down onto the anterior and posterior thorax, with strapping beneath the axilla. The occipital piece can extend higher on the skull than does the original Philadelphia orthosis. The increased contact on the body surface at the occiput and onto the thorax improves the stability that this brace offers (see Table 17–1).

• The SOMI orthosis (see Fig. 17–6 in the Textbook) is also a cervicothoracic orthosis. It has a rigid anterior plastic chest piece and shoulder straps. The occipital piece is attached with two posters, which run anteriorly. The mandibular piece has a single poster, which also attaches anteriorly. These posts are made of rigid aluminum. The SOMI brace is well tolerated. This brace can be applied without moving the patient from the supine position. It is supplied with an optional headpiece that snaps onto the occipital rest and passes around the forehead. This allows removal of the mandibular support while eating. It is relatively effective in restricting flexion-extension (see Table 17–1).

• It is known that no cervical orthosis totally immobilizes the cervical spine. There is a recognized "snaking" of the cervical spine, with some segments moving into flexion and others into extension, especially when forced flexion-extension is attempted against the orthosis.

• In the United States, the halo brace (Fig. 17–4) has become the most commonly used method of treating cervical fractures or dislocations. There are basically two types of halo orthotic devices currently used to control neck motion: (1) the halo cast and (2) halo vest. The halo component is the same on each type and consists of a rigid metal or graphite ring attached to the skull with four fixation pins: two anteriorly, usually in the frontal region; and two posteriorly in the parieto-occipital area. The ring is bolted to four posters that run down onto either a rigid polyethylene vest or a plaster cast, both of which extend to about the umbilicus. If further intimate contact on the thorax is needed, a body cast is fabricated distally with contact onto the pelvis.

• Lind and colleagues found that the maximal cervical motion in the halo apparatus was 70% of the normal motion and that most of this motion occurred in the upper cervical spine area. Because most motion occurs in the upper cervical spine, it is not surprising that upper cervical spine injuries commonly require surgical intervention as well as halo immobilization. Rehabilitation exercises did not cause any greater movement to the spine than did daily motion and activity.

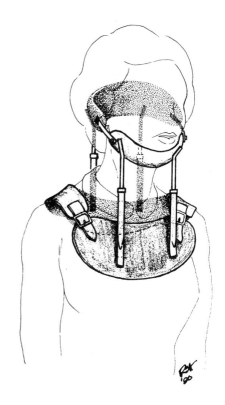

FIGURE 17–3. Four-poster collar.

• The original Minerva molded-type orthosis (see Fig. 17–8 in the Textbook) contacts the head or thorax but not any better than the more traditional Philadelphia or four-poster. The newer design of the Minerva body jacket (TMBJ) (see Fig. 17–9 in the Textbook) runs down the thorax to a level similar to that of the halo vest and provides significant contact on the head with its circumferential forehead adaptation. It is noninvasive—an advantage over the halo device whose pins inherently present the risk of infection and slippage.

• Pringle stated that both the Minerva and the halo vest are far superior to other cervical thoracic orthoses, and are the treatment of choice in the ambulatory management of the unstable cervical spine. Additionally, there is literature that supports the use of the Minerva vest in preference to the halo vest in children of preschool age. The Minerva vest provided necessary stabilization and yet was lighter and more comfortable, thereby allowing mobilization of the patient for rehabilitation with satisfactory stabilization of the cervical spine.

• There is very little published on the management of upper thoracic fractures. The typical thoracic orthosis, such as the Jewett hyperextension device or the chairback brace with sternal pad, provides immobilization up to the level of T6 and is therefore of no value in the upper thoracic spine. The ribs act as support struts in the thorax, but many times there are associated rib fractures that reduce the desired stability. Surgical stabilization can also be required. Other orthoses can be utilized for attempted posture control if the spinal cord is not in jeopardy of compromise. Upper thoracic fractures require either a halo cast to the pelvis or a Milwaukee-type orthosis (e.g., cervicothoracolumbosacral orthosis, CTLSO) if surgery is not selected.

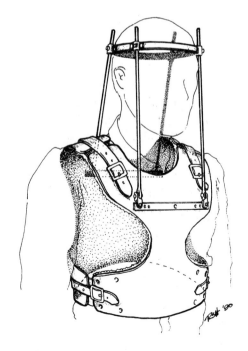

FIGURE 17–4. Halo device/vest.

Thoracolumbosacral Orthoses (pp. 359–363)

- As with cervical orthoses, proper prescription of a thoracolumbar orthosis (TLO) requires knowledge of the general principles of bracing and the biomechanics of the thoracic and lumbar spine, as well as an understanding of the indications and limitations of specific thoracic and lumbar orthoses.
- As in the cervical spine, the range of motion of each spinal segment is directly related to the anatomy of the region. In the thoracic spinal column, the facets are primarily oriented in the horizontal plane. The rib cage plays a great role in enhancing the stiffness of the thoracic spine. Rotation and lateral bending are the predominant movements possible: about 6 degrees of lateral bending at each segment, and 8 to 9 degrees of axial rotation. There is an average of 4 degrees of flexion and extension in the upper portion and 6 degrees in the middle segments of the thoracic spine. The transitional segments from thoracic to lumbar spine (T10 to T12) have much greater flexion-extension (average 12 degrees). There is also increased lateral bending (average 8 degrees) and less rotation (2 degrees). This is in part because the ribs do not articulate with the sternum in the last segments and the facet joints are in transition from the alignment in the thoracic spine to that of the lumbar spine.
- The lumbar spine has nearly sagittally placed articular processes. Because of the anatomical alignment of the facets, there is between 12 degrees of flexion and 17 degrees of extension, 3 to 6 degrees of lateral bending, and only 1 to 2 degrees of axial rotation at any given level. The greatest flexion-extension, and the least lateral bending and axial rotation, occurs at L5 to S1.
- There is very significant variability in the effectiveness of back braces. Orthotic devices that are well fixed to the chest but inadequately so to the pelvis leave the lumbosacral segments unsupported. Braces such as the chairback brace, which has shorter supports, tend to pull away from the pelvis less, thereby giving more support to the lumbosacral (LS) area. If an orthosis is to be effective, it must supply sufficient pressure over bony prominences to remind the wearer to change position or maintain posture. All braces employ a three-point pressure system. The more contact the brace has with the wearer, the more evenly the pressure is distributed and the better the control achieved.
- Increasing the abdominal pressure by using an orthosis decreases the net force applied to the spine when lifting a weight from the floor. Because the spinal column is attached to the sides of the abdominal and thoracic cavities, the action of the trunk muscles converts the thoracic and abdominal chambers into nearly rigid containers. These containers transmit part of the forces generated in loading the spine when lifting, thereby relieving the load directly on the spine.
- Nachemson and co-workers, however, noted that no LSO significantly raised intragastric pressure. Intra-abdominal pressure increases only with closure of the glottis during muscular activity. The LS support decreases the intradiskal pressure at the lumbar spine by approximately 30%. Nachemson demonstrated that wearing a lumbosacral orthosis reduces disk pressure values during about two-thirds of a set of exercises, and increases pressure during the remaining third.
- Morris and colleagues found that the chairback brace and the LS corset decreased or had no effect on the electrical activity of back muscles.
- A 1994 NIOSH report concluded that there is no scientific evidence that lumbosacral belt wearing is protective to an industrial population on the basis of changes in intra-abdominal pressure and trunk muscle EMG. Some have argued in favor of their proprioceptive efficacy.

• The studies mentioned earlier of thoracic-lumbar orthoses were in large part carried out on normal volunteers. The authors did not take into consideration important complicating factors such as pain, decreased muscular strength, insensate skin, altered biomechanics secondary to trauma and instability, or surgical changes. Because there is significant variability of fit and effectiveness, radiographic analysis of spinal motion is necessary for a given patient to determine the effectiveness of the device in limiting unwanted motion.

• These appliances can be classified as corsets, rigid braces, hyperextension braces, hyperflexion braces, and jackets. All spinal orthoses, with the exception of hyperextension braces, give abdominal support. The ability of these devices to restrict motion has not been measured in as great detail as with the cervical orthoses. The evaluation of effectiveness is therefore more subjective.

• The most commonly prescribed lumbosacral support is the LS corset. In general, a corset is made of canvas with rigid backstays often made of steel. There is adjustable side or back lacing. A corset is a stock item and can usually be fitted by a corsetiere without difficulty. The corset can be lumbosacral (LS) or thoracolumbosacral (TLS). The stays can be either rigid or semirigid. Fidler and Lantz found that a corset significantly reduced spinal motion by as much as two-thirds. The corset gives minimal actual support and its effectiveness might be more related to the discomfort it can produce for patients because it reminds them to maintain adequate posture.

Lumbosacral Orthoses (p. 361)
• The chairback brace is the most popular of the rigid braces. It consists of an anterior corset with midaxillary metal uprights (Fig. 17–5). It can also have two paraspinal uprights and two uprights in the midaxillary line (see Fig. 17–11 in the Textbook). It is designed to control flexion-extension and lateral motion.

• Another commonly prescribed lumbosacral orthosis is the William's back brace, which is used primarily to control extension and lordosis and to give some lateral control (see Fig. 17–12 in the Textbook). It is a specialized orthosis in that it allows free flexion but limits extension, and uses a lever action and abdominal support to reduce lumbar lordosis.

Thoracolumbosacral Orthoses (pp. 361–363)
• There are two major types of thoracolumbosacral orthoses (TLSOs). The more common is the Taylor orthosis, which is constructed to restrict flexion and extension (see Fig. 17–13 in the Textbook). This type of orthosis is relatively ineffective for limiting lumbar spine motion. This orthosis appears to be a poor choice for thoracolumbosacral immobilization. The chairback brace has sternal pad attachments (see Fig. 17–14 in the Textbook) that transmit pressure through the sternum and ribs directly to the spine. This provides better lumbosacral and thoracic immobilization than in a brace that transmits force through the pectoral girdle and is attached to the spinal axis only by muscles and the sternoclavicular joints.

• Molded jackets are made either of plaster of Paris or a thermoplastic material to conform to the contours of the body (Fig. 17–6). If made properly, they become a nearly total-contact type of orthotic device. The pressure distribution is more uniform and more support is provided. The molded TLSO restricts spinal movement better than a corset or chairback brace. A spica attachment to the molded TLSO was best at restricting movement, presumably by partially immobilizing the pelvis. These jackets are used commonly for patients with spinal

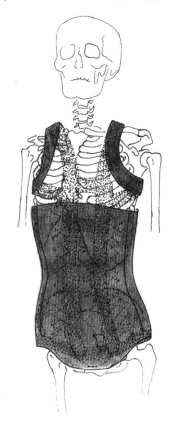

FIGURE 17–5. Chairback lumbosacral orthosis with side lacing attachment to an abdominal apron.

fractures or low back fusions to allow early mobilization and rehabilitation. They also may be of value when there are metastases in vertebrae, to provide support and control pain. Donning and doffing the molded jacket is more difficult than with other orthoses.

• The hyperextension orthosis differs from other devices because it does not have an abdominal apron and does not give abdominal support. This hyperextension brace applies three-point pressure over the sternum and the pubis anteriorly and over the upper lumbar spine posteriorly. This hyperextension orthosis is used to permit the upright position while preventing flexion after a compression fracture of a vertebral body (Fig. 17–7). It is not recommended in the management of compression fractures in osteoporotic elderly patients because it can place excessive hyperextension forces on lower lumbar vertebrae, possibly inducing posterior element fractures or exacerbating a degenerative arthritis condition.

• It should be stressed that orthoses only partially limit rather than immobilize the spine. Spinal orthoses should be considered to be temporary devices. At the same time that the orthotic device is prescribed, a rehabilitation treatment plan

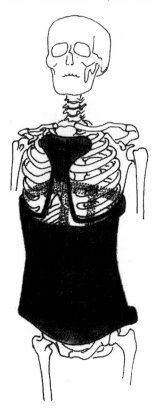

FIGURE 17–6. The custom-molded thermoplastic jacket-type thoracic lumbosacral orthosis.

should be outlined to attempt to rid the patient of the need for the device in the future.

SPINAL ORTHOSES FOR SPINAL DEFORMITY
(pp. 363–368)

Biomechanics (pp. 363–364)

• Scoliosis is a three-dimensional problem. Rotation of vertebrae is an integral component of all structural scolioses. The frontal plane radiograph—both anteroposterior (AP) and posteroanterior (PA)—must be studied, as well as lateral films. However, the physical examination of the patient typically reveals the rotational aspects far better than radiographs. Bracing affects the spinal column itself, but it also affects the physiology of internal organs, playing a role, for example, in pulmonary function.

• The biomechanics of the spine are quite dynamic. A common error is to think only in terms of *passive* forces. Many orthoses, especially the Milwaukee brace (CTLSO), are designed to stimulate *active* corrective forces on the part of the patient. In a well-fitted Milwaukee brace for a right thoracic idiopathic scolio-

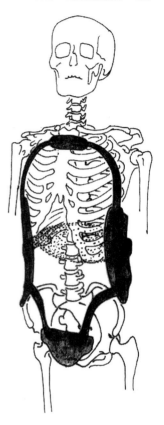

FIGURE 17–7. Jewett hyperextension orthosis restricts spinal flexion by anterior pressure over the sternum and pubic symphysis, and posterior pressure across the lower thoracic/upper lumbar region.

sis, for example, there is a constant force only in the pelvic section. It is a circumferential force, but so mild that pressure sores do not develop and the patient experiences no pressure-related discomfort. The design is such that the patient's neck "floats" within the neck ring; that is, there are usually zero forces anywhere on the neck. The main corrective force pad—the right thoracic pad—is broad, thus distributing the force over a wide area of skin. The patient can, at any time, shift the thorax to the left so that there are zero forces under the pad.

• These concepts of dynamic muscle activity can be carried over into underarm orthoses (TLSOs) if they are carefully designed. The great virtue of the Milwaukee brace is its open design and its lack of circumferential torso constriction. Thus a TLSO can be designed that incorporates a "space" into which the torso can shift. The counterforce opposing the right thoracic pad must therefore be a high axillary padded margin of the TLSO above the space area. Because this high axillary contact point can be an irritant if the patient sags down, the patient will tend to "elongate" and lean the upper thorax to the right, adding to the effectiveness of the right thoracic pad. Lumbar pads, whether in a TLSO or a Milwaukee brace, tend to be much more passive than thoracic pads.

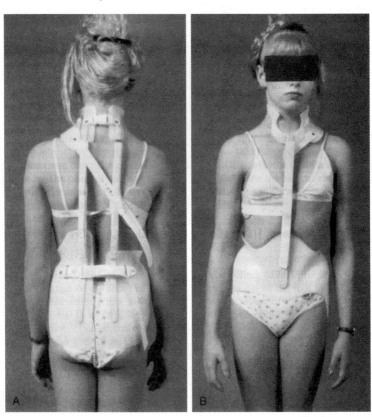

FIGURE 17–8. *A.* Posterior view of a modern Milwaukee brace showing the pelvic section, a lumbar pad, a right thoracic pad, a left trapezius pad, and the new style plastic neck-ring. *B.* Frontal view of the same patient, again showing the pelvic section, the anterior upright, the trapezius pad, and the modern plastic neck-ring, which avoids all dental prob-lems and is much more aesthetically acceptable to the patient.

Types of Orthoses for Spinal Deformities (p. 364)

Milwaukee Brace (p. 364)
• The Milwaukee brace (CTLSO) (Fig. 17–8) was the first to have statistically proven positive results in spinal deformity; it is thus a "gold standard" against which other orthoses can be compared. It consists of a well-molded pelvic section (almost universally made of plastic), two posterior uprights, a single anterior upright, and a neck ring. These components are always made in straight alignment; that is, the pelvic section is level, the uprights are all perfectly ver-tical, and the neck ring is centered over midpelvis.

Thoracolumbosacral Orthosis (p. 364)
• The thoracolumbosacral orthosis (TLSO) reaches only to the axillary level and exerts no corrective action on the upper thoracic spine. It is typically used for

scolioses having their apex at T9 or lower, and for kyphoses having their apex at the thoracolumbar junction.
• There are corrective types designed primarily for adolescents with idiopathic scoliosis and passive TLSOs made with the patient held in a corrected alignment (see Fig. 17–18*A* and *B* in the Textbook). These latter types are most commonly used for neuromuscular deformities.

Lumbosacral Orthosis (p. 364)
• The lumbosacral orthosis (LSO) is a specific design only for lumbar scolioses. It is firmly locked to the pelvis, has a strong force pad against the apex of the lumbar curve, and no thoracic extension on the opposite side. The patient's own active righting reflexes and muscle power do the correction. It is intended only for idiopathic scoliosis patients (see Fig. 17–19*A* and *B*, in the Textbook).

Bracing for Infantile Idiopathic Scoliosis (pp. 364–365)

• Idiopathic infantile scoliosis occurs in children younger than 3 years. Because 80% to 85% of infants with this type of scoliosis have spontaneous resolution of their curvature, it is important to avoid bracing a mild curve that will disappear on its own. Similarly, it is important to aggressively treat those children with progressive curves. If the curve exceeds 20 degrees, the prognosis is poor and treatment is indicated. Although some prefer using serial plaster casts, the author favors the use of the classic Milwaukee brace.
• In many cases, the scoliosis will resolve with a vigorous brace program. The spine is held straight in the brace for a few months; then the brace is gradually removed (the "weaning" process). At times, however, the spine does well as long as the brace is on, but deforms with attempts at weaning. In this case, long-term bracing is necessary until the pubertal growth spurt, at which point the curve usually gets worse despite the brace so surgical fusion typically becomes necessary. Brace failure can also occur; that is, the curve may fail to respond to the brace from the beginning. In that case, serial Risser casts should be used, followed by another brace trial. When all such nonoperative attempts fail, epiphysiodesis and rodding without fusion may be required.

Bracing for Juvenile Idiopathic Scoliosis (p. 365)

• Juvenile idiopathic scoliosis is far more common in North America than is infantile idiopathic scoliosis, and it is more likely to affect females than males. Curves developing after age 3 years, but before puberty onset, are in this category.
• Unlike infantile idiopathic scoliosis, the juvenile type almost never spontaneously resolves. Moreover, because there are several years of growth during which progression can take place, extremely severe curves can develop. In North America, this is the type of idiopathic scoliosis most likely to cause adult cor pulmonale and early death. Because of the very poor prognosis of this scoliosis, and the great desire to avoid fusion at a young age, bracing becomes an extremely important method of management.
• Thoracic curves predominate, although a compensatory lumbar curve can become quite significant. Because of the thoracic curve, and because the rib cage is soft and pliable, it is critical to use a Milwaukee brace rather than any type of TLSO. Early bracing with the correct orthosis is imperative for success.

• Brace treatment should begin when the curve reaches approximately 25 degrees, but curves as high as 60 degrees can still respond to a brace.

• Brace wearing always begins with a full-time (23 hours per day) schedule with subsequent adjustments according to the curve's response. It is not unusual for a child to require 5 to 8 years of full-time brace wearing. This may seem unduly harsh; however, children this age adapt readily, and the alternative of curve progression is unacceptable.

Bracing for Adolescent Idiopathic Scoliosis (pp. 365–366)

• This is the most common diagnosis for which scoliosis bracing is used. The indications for bracing are a growing child with a curve of between 25 and 45 degrees. Below 25 degrees there are too many curves that are nonprogressive to justify treatment, and above 45 degrees bracing is ineffective. The highest-risk child for progression is the premenstral girl with a thoracic curve.

• These adolescent scolioses are associated with a variety of highly standardized curve patterns: single thoracic (almost always to the right); single lumbar (almost always to the left); single thoracolumbar (apex at the thoracolumbar junction); double thoracic (high left thoracic T1 to T5 and low right thoracic T5 to T12); and double major right thoracic and left lumbar.

• As mentioned earlier, curves with an apex at T9 or lower can be managed with a TLSO, but curves with an apex higher than that require a Milwaukee brace. The high left curve T1 to T5 of the double thoracic pattern requires a trapezius pad mounted on a Milwaukee brace. Single lumbar curves do best with the dynamic LSO; low thoracic and thoracolumbar curves, with the TLSO; and higher thoracic curves, with the Milwaukee brace.

Bracing for Scheuermann's Disease (pp. 366–367)

• Scheuermann's disease is a developmental disorder of the disks and vertebral end-plates occurring in adolescents. The etiology is unknown, but there is a strong genetic tendency. Males and females are affected equally. Second only to adolescent idiopathic scoliosis, Scheuermann's disease is the most common diagnosis for which bracing is prescribed. There are two locations of the condition: the classic midthoracic with apex at T7, T8, and T9; and the less common thoracolumbar apex. The latter is more likely to present with pain; the former, to present with deformity.

• The indications for bracing are a growing child with an increasing deformity, pain, or both. The upper limit of normal thoracic kyphosis is 50 degrees.

• For the classic midthoracic disease, the only brace of proven value is the Milwaukee brace. Underarm braces (TLSOs) are the braces of choice for lesions at the thoracolumbar junction. The duration of bracing depends greatly on the time of onset of the problem because bracing to the end of growth is usually necessary. Short-duration programs (e.g., 18 months) have failed. The intensity and duration of bracing are also related to the severity of the disease process because there is a wide spectrum within the diagnosis (see Fig. 17–20 in the Textbook).

Bracing for Neuromuscular Scoliosis (p. 367)

• Most of these children responded well to a brace until the pubertal growth spurt, at which time the curve may increase and surgery may be necessary.

Rarely, if ever, is bracing done to prevent surgery entirely. Virtually all bracing in neuromuscular diseases is achieved with TLSOs. These can be back-opening, front-opening, or bivalved.

• Good brace results are seen in patients with cerebral palsy, myelomeningocele, traumatic paraplegia, and spinal muscular atrophy. Bracing has *not* proved to be of value in patients with Duchenne muscular dystrophy, Friedreich's ataxia, or syringomyelia.

Bracing for Congenital Spine Deformity (pp. 367–368)

• Bracing is of no value in congenital kyphosis or congenital lordosis, but does have limited value in some congenital scolioses. The curvatures most likely to benefit from bracing are the long curves (10 vertebrae or more), which demonstrate considerable flexibility (at least 50% on a supine bending radiograph as compared with an upright radiograph). As with neuromuscular scolioses, the goal of bracing in congenital scoliosis is to control the curve until the adolescent growth spurt, at which time fusion is done. Bracing is also used to control compensatory curves after fusion of the primary congenital scoliosis.

Bracing for Other Scolioses (p. 368)

• In less common scoliotic conditions, a child with a progressive curvature is a candidate for bracing if he or she is at an age when fusion is undesirable or when there is hope that surgery can be prevented. The exceptions are those conditions for which bracing is generally useless: Duchenne muscular dystrophy, congenital kyphosis, and congenital lordosis, as well as dystrophic neurofibromatosis and Marfan's syndrome. These patients typically require surgical fusion. In progressive problems involving loss of respiratory function, the fusion should be done early while there is adequate vital capacity to prevent surgical morbidity and mortality.

18

Original Chapter by Ralph M. Buschbacher, M.D., Judy Atkins, O.T.R., Brian Lay, and Randall L. Braddom, M.D., M.S.

Prescription of Wheelchairs and Seating Systems

• Having the optimal wheelchair and seating system is critical to the habilitation or rehabilitation and ongoing well-being of patients with mobility impairment and many other types of disorders. Because of the myriad brands and types that are now available, the wheelchair user has never had more choices. For the same reason, it has never been more difficult for the practitioner to prescribe a wheelchair.

PURPOSES OF WHEELCHAIRS AND SEATING SYSTEMS (pp. 370–371)

• The five major goals of wheelchair prescription are listed in Table 18–1. With the current emphasis on containing health care costs, the practitioner should prescribe wheelchairs that are the most cost effective, but not necessarily the least expensive ones. The overall expense of a wheelchair includes not only the purchase price, but also the costs of maintenance and repair.

COMMONLY USED WHEELCHAIR TYPES (p. 371)

• The types of wheelchairs now available can be variously categorized in the following ways: adult/pediatric, heavy/moderate/lightweight/ultralight, manually propelled/powered, folding/nonfolding/standup frame, reclining/nonreclining, tilting/nontilting, and metal/composite. Table 18–2 lists the major types of wheelchairs on the market that are commonly prescribed.

MANUAL WHEELCHAIR COMPONENTS (pp. 372–381)

Frames (p. 372)

• The most common type of wheelchair frame in use is the folding type (see Table 18–3 in the Textbook). Rigid wheelchairs are more energy efficient because they have less wasted internal motion during movement; however, they are not as easy to transport as a folding frame type. The rigid chair (see Fig. 18–2 in the Textbook) can have quick-release wheels and a fold-down back to

244

TABLE 18–1 Purposes of Wheelchair and Seating Prescription

1. Maximization of efficient independent mobility
2. Prevention/minimization of deformity or injury
3. Maximization of independent functioning
4. Projection of a healthy, vital, attractive "body image"
5. Minimization of short-term and long-term equipment cost

make it more compact and transportable, but it is still more cumbersome than the folding type. Folding chairs (Fig. 18–1) use a cross-linkage (X-shaped) bar frame assembly. The chair is folded by lifting the center of the seat, which to some extent limits the seating support and cushions that can be fitted to the chair. Because the folding chair has more parts, it is typically heavier than the rigid type, and usually weighs around 27 lb.

• Most wheelchairs are now constructed of aluminum. This makes the chair durable enough for ordinary use, lighter than the steel chair, and available for purchase at a reasonable cost. Even lighter chairs, made of titanium, are available. They are very durable, but are also very expensive. In developing nations, ease of construction and the ready availability of replacement parts are of greatest importance. Wheelchairs in these countries are often constructed of various bicycle parts.

TABLE 18–2 Basic Types of Wheelchairs and Their Characteristics

Wheelchair Type	Characteristics
Rigid frame	Nonfolding; commonly used in institutions; used in sports chairs
X-frame	Common folding wheelchair
User-propelled	User propels chair
Assistant-propelled	Assistant pushes chair; usually large wheels are placed forward (or has four small wheels); commonly used in institutions
Motorized	Various types of battery-powered scooters or chairs available
Standard weight	Usual configuration
Ultra-lightweight	For especially active individuals
Sports chairs	For specific events
Adult chairs	Usual configuration
Pediatric chairs	Various sizes available
Standing frame	Allows user to gain height; motorized and nonmotorized units available
Nonreclining	Usual configuration
Reclining	Useful in patient with hypotension and for pressure relief, though some units increase shear force on sacrum
Nontilting	Usual configuration
Tilting	Useful in high-tone patients, for pressure relief, for pulmonary posture changes

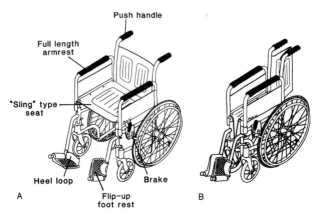

FIGURE 18–1. Folding chair: *A.* Open. *B.* Folded.

Wheels and Tires (pp. 372–374)

• Two basic types of wheels are available: "mag" wheels and spoked wheels (see Table 18–4 in the Textbook). The most commonly used is the mag wheel. The mag wheel was first made out of magnesium, which is how it got its name. It was also first used in bicycles. Now most mag wheels are actually made out of plastic. Although these wheels are typically heavier than their spoked counterparts, they require virtually no maintenance. Spoked wheels are lighter, but the spokes tend to loosen and must be retightened periodically.

• Three types of tires can be fitted to the wheels (see Table 18–5 in the Textbook): (1) hard rubber, (2) pneumatic, and (3) pneumatic with flat-free inserts.

• Wheels and tires come in several size options, the most common being 24 inches in diameter; 22- and 20-inch wheels are also commonly used to vary the height of the chair.

• Wheel placement is an important consideration in chair construction. Many chairs allow for adjustment of the wheel up and down as well as forward and backward (see Fig. 18–4 in the Textbook). Up and down adjustments are used to vary the height of the chair. This can improve positioning and, in the case of chairs for patients with hemiplegia, allow a user to reach the floor with the "good" foot. Forward and back wheel adjustments alter the stability of the chair. The further forward the wheel is placed, the more easily the chair will tip backward. This can be desirable for a patient with paraplegia who does "wheelies" to negotiate curbs. It is undesirable in the bilateral lower extremity amputee because the lack of forward-placed (leg) weight makes it even easier to tip the chair backward. The wheels also need to be placed posteriorly for some types of reclining or posterior-tilting wheelchairs.

• *Camber* is the angle the wheel makes from the vertical axis. The more the bottom of the wheel is moved outward, the greater its camber and stability. Increasing the camber makes it easier to manually propel the chair; this is especially useful in sports chairs. A greater camber also improves the user's ability to propel the wheelchair at higher speeds, and tightens the turning radius. The tradeoff is a wider chair and greater wear and tear (mainly on the tires, but also on doorways and furniture).

TABLE 18–3 Types of Hand Rims and Their Common Uses, Advantages, and Disadvantages

		Common Uses	Advantages	Disadvantages
Large diameter		Community, institutions	Easy to propel	Less distance per stroke
Small diameter		Active individual, sports	Greater distance per stroke	More force required
Thick		Poor hand grip	Easier to grip	More weight and width
Knobby		Poor hand grip	Easier to push	More weight and width

Hand Rims (p. 374)

• Hand rims are placed slightly lateral to the wheel and are smaller in diameter than the wheel (Table 18–3). The larger the hand rim's diameter, the easier it is to propel the chair, but more arm strokes are required to cover a given distance. Some patients with very poor grip, such as those with quadriplegia, benefit from the attachment of knobby projections to the rim.

Casters (pp. 374–375)

• Casters are the small wheels typically found on the front of the chair (see Table 18–7 in the Textbook). They come in different diameters, widths, and materials. In general, the smaller casters are suited for rapid maneuverability; these are often used on sport chairs. Narrow, hard casters are good on smooth, level surfaces but perform poorly on rough terrain or on outside surfaces. For most purposes an 8-inch diameter caster of relatively wide configuration is optimal.

Seats and Backs (pp. 375–377)

• The seats and backs that are standard on most wheelchairs are referred to as *sling upholstery* or *hammock* style (see Fig. 18–1*A*). They consist of a piece of material that is suspended between the frame posts of the chair and are light-weight and easy to fold. The most common material used for such slings is vinyl, which is inexpensive, durable, and easy to clean, and comes in a number of colors.

• Since sling-type chairs provide little support, a solid seat is often placed on top of them. This solid support can be removed when the chair is folded. Other styles utilize a solid folding seat; however, this adds weight to the chair and cannot easily be modified.

• The seat plane angle is the angle the seat makes with the horizontal. The most common seat plane angles range from 0 to 5 degrees, although in sports applications angles up to 20 degrees may be used. The greater angle creates greater stability but can also cause pressure problems.

Seat Cushions (pp. 375–377)

• A number of more specialized seating surfaces are available (Table 18–4). These include air-cell cushions, which can help prevent local pressure-induced skin breakdown. The pressure in each cell can be individually adjusted to provide proper pressure distribution. Gel and foam are also commonly used materials.

• Pelvic and leg position can be maintained with abductor wedges and the proper cushion.

• Seat backs vary in height, depending on the level of control and mobility that is desired. The higher the back, the more support, and the less freedom of mobility. If the back is too low, it leads to a slumped "sacral seating" posture with a tendency toward development of thoracic kyphosis. If the back is too high, it pushes the scapulae forward. Most wheelchair users require seat backs that come to mid-back or to a level a few inches below the inferior poles of the scapulae. Quadriplegic persons require higher back heights, and paraplegic persons sometimes do well with a lower height.

Reclining Backs (p. 377)

• Persons prone to the development of pressure ulcers or orthostatic hypotension often benefit from the reclining or semireclining posture. Semireclining and reclining chairs are available (see Fig. 18–5A in the Textbook) and come with a variety of release mechanisms, including cable releases and hydraulic units that help hold the weight of the patient. Not all chairs recline equally, and this must be considered when ordering a chair. Simple reclining chairs may create shear stress over the back and sacrum during position changes. In the person at risk for pressure ulcers, special nonshear recliners are indicated.

Tilt-in-Space Seats (p. 377)

• An alternative to the reclining seat back is the tilt or tilt-in-space chair (see Fig. 18–5B in the Textbook), which utilizes a system whereby the entire seat and back are tilted posteriorly as a single unit. Such systems generally utilize a hydraulic cylinder to aid in movement. The advantage of tilt systems is that they do not create shear stress during movement. Like reclining units, they also help with pressure release and orthostasis, and are sometimes used for patients in need of help with pulmonary secretions. They may offer an advantage over the reclining units in patients with tone or spasticity problems, in whom reclining can trigger spasticity.

Footrests/Leg Rests (pp. 377–378)

Fixed and Swing-Away Footrests (p. 377)

• Footrests and leg rests help provide balance and positioning and afford protection to the wheelchair user. They also decrease the load on the buttocks

TABLE 18–4 Types of Cushions and Their Common Uses, Advantages, and Disadvantages

		Common Uses	Advantages	Disadvantages
Foam		General use	Good stability, low cost	Pressure relief not optimal
Coated, contoured foam		General use	Excellent stability, cleanability, durability	Heat buildup, expensive
Gel-filled		General use	Good pressure relief, cleanability, heat dissipation	Expensive
Contoured foam with gel insert		When improved pressure distribution needed	Good pressure relief, stability, cleanability, durability	Expensive, heat buildup
Air-filled villous		Optimal pressure relief needed	Excellent pressure relief, cleanability, heat dissipation	Expensive, suboptimal seating stability

From Britell CW: Wheelchair prescription. In Kottke FJ, Lehmann JF (eds): Krusen's Handbook of Physical Medicine and Rehabilitation, ed 4. Philadelphia, WB Saunders, 1990, pp. 548–563.

and thigh. Swing-away footrests (Fig. 18–6*A* in the Textbook) are used most commonly. They allow the footrest to be moved out of the way, which makes transfers easier because the user can position the chair closer to chairs, beds, or toilets. Removable footrests can also improve the portability of the wheelchair.
• Fixed, or nonremovable, footrests are available as well. They generally make the chair lighter and more rigid but interfere with transfers and portability.

Elevating Footrests (pp. 377–378)
• Elevating footrests (see Fig. 18–6*B* in the Textbook) are available for situations in which the knee cannot or should not be flexed. They can also be used to help minimize dependent edema.

Other Footrests (p. 378)
• In a chair for paraplegic patients, the footrest is generally a single bar that connects the two sides of the chair (see Fig. 18–2*A* in the Textbook). This improves structural rigidity but eliminates the folding option. When more leg and foot control is necessary, the footrest can be ordered with special loops or pads. Heel loops (see Fig. 18–1*A*) are often used instead of the leg rest portion of the unit because they reduce weight. Most footrests can also be flipped up to aid in transfers (see Fig. 18–1*A*).

Armrests/Lap Trays (p. 378)
• Armrests are added to wheelchairs for a number of reasons (Fig. 18–2). They help provide balance and stability by allowing the user to rest the elbows. They also help provide a point of pushoff for weight shifting and pressure release. In addition, they decrease intradiskal pressures. The choice of armrest style can affect the patient's independence level, function, and ability to use certain seating systems.

Fixed Armrests (p. 378)
• The main advantages to fixed armrests are that they are inexpensive and cannot be lost. Their chief disadvantages are that they can make fitting of a seating system more difficult and can also hinder transfers.

Removable Armrests (p. 378)
• Removable armrests make transfers easier. They can generally be adjusted in height or replaced to accommodate growth. Their disadvantage is that they increase the width and weight of the chair.

Wraparound Armrests (p. 378)
• The wraparound armrest design reduces the width of the wheelchair. This is accomplished by attaching the armrest behind the seat back rather than next to the seat. These armrests can generally be moved or detached for transfers.

Desk-Length Armrests (p. 378)
• Both fixed and removable armrests are available in full or desk lengths. Full-length armrests extend from the seat back to the front of the chair. Full-length armrests interfere with the ability to maneuver the chair close to tables and desks. Desk-length armrests extend forward only partially, and allow the user to slide

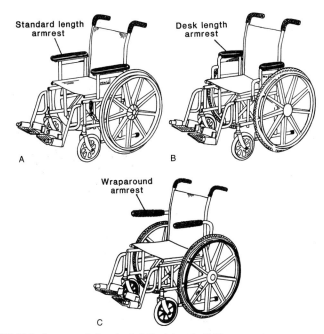

FIGURE 18–2. Armrests. *A.* Standard. *B.* Desk length. *C.* Wraparound.

the knees under a desk. Adjustable-height armrests are available to accommodate individuals of different sizes.

Other Armrests *(p. 378)*
• In addition to the styles described previously, there are swing-away or flip-up armrests. Young persons with paraplegia often prefer chairs with no armrests at all. Persons who need more control of their limbs often require trough-style armrests (see Fig. 18–5A in the Textbook) to hold the forearms in place. In power chairs, one armrest generally has an attached joystick control unit. Hemiplegic individuals often do well with a lap tray instead of regular armrests.

Brakes/Grade Aids (p. 379)

• All wheelchairs are available with wheel locks, commonly known as *brakes* (see Fig. 18–8 in the Textbook). This mechanism is a very important safety feature. Wheel locks are devices that put pressure on the larger wheels or tires to lock them into position. They are installed to prevent unintended rolling of the chair, either on a grade or during transfers. Caster locks can also be used when needed.
• Wheel locks are available in both a lever style and a toggle style. The lever can be set in different notches to provide varying degrees of holding power. This can be an advantage on a steep grade, but its use requires greater control and

strength. Toggle-style brakes are used more commonly. The "power" of the lock is preset, but can be adjusted.

• Grade aids, or "hill holders," are devices that prevent the chair from rolling backward but do not interfere with forward motion. They are useful for persons with poor strength or endurance on inclines, where the chair might roll backward between forward thrusts (see Fig. 18–9 in the Textbook).

Anti-tippers (p. 379)

• Patients at risk of falling backward in the chair often benefit from the addition of anti-tippers (see Fig. 18–10 in the Textbook). These devices can be fixed or removable, and they are capable of being turned. Turning the anti-tipper to the "up" position can help during such maneuvers as negotiating curbs, when the device might interfere. Antitippers are useful for above-knee amputees, who have a more posterior center of gravity. They are generally not used for paraplegic patients who practice "wheelies" to help in climbing curbs. In rare cases, forward facing anti-tippers are necessary.

One-Arm Drive (pp. 379–380)

• Patients who have the ability to propel a wheelchair with one arm only are sometimes given one-arm drive chairs. On these chairs, both propelling rims are on one side. A practical alternative in most hemiplegic patients is to use one hand rim and one foot to properly guide the chair. A motorized chair is also sometimes a more practical solution than the one-arm drive wheelchair.

Hemichair (p. 380)

• Hemiplegic patients are often able to utilize the "good" leg to help propel the chair, but the seat height in a regular chair is too high for their legs to reach the floor effectively. Hemichairs are made lower to the ground and allow the user to propel the chair with the "good" arm and ipsilateral leg.

Stand-up Chairs (p. 381)

• The stand-up design allows the patient to stand within the frame of the chair (see Fig. 18–12 in the Textbook). Patients can benefit from being able to stand for a number of reasons, including having access to more jobs and experiencing an improved psychological outlook. Standing chairs also provide weight-bearing benefits on bone and improved pressure release. They are available in both motorized and manual versions, but have drawbacks of increased weight, width, cost, and complexity.

MOTORIZED WHEELCHAIRS AND SCOOTERS
(pp. 381–382)

• Individuals who do not have the strength or dexterity to efficiently propel a manual wheelchair usually need a motorized wheelchair. Such chairs can provide a high degree of independence, and with modern reclining and tilting models, even severely impaired persons can perform pressure release maneuvers.

• Manual wheelchair use can also hasten the deterioration of the shoulders, so that in the long term the patient may lose function for such critical activities as transfers and activities of daily living. This is becoming an ever more prevalent problem in active paraplegic patients, who typically have a high incidence of shoulder problems and compressive neuropathies.

Direct-Drive Motorized Wheelchairs (p. 381)

• Direct-drive wheelchairs (Fig. 18–3A) are commonly referred to as *power base chairs*. They have a rigid main frame that contains the drive components and provides the base for the required seating system. Direct-drive chairs commonly have four small balloon tires, but some newer models offer larger wheels in the rear. They are durable and suited for rough terrain.

Belt-Driven Motorized Wheelchairs (p. 381)

• Belt-driven wheelchairs (see Fig. 18–3B) usually have large rear tires and small front casters. They are more stable than direct-drive units and are generally capable of reaching greater speeds, but they tend to be less durable. Belt-driven chairs are more versatile than direct-drive versions because the frames are better suited to modification and the addition of different components.

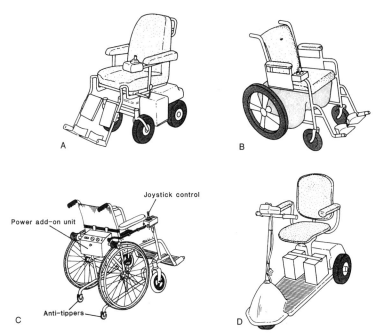

FIGURE 18–3. Power chairs: direct-drive (*A*), belt-drive (*B*), add-on power unit (*C*), and three-wheeled scooter (*D*). (*A, B,* and *D* from Britell CW: Wheelchair prescription. In Kottke FJ, Lehmann JF [eds]: Krusen's Handbook of Physical Medicine and Rehabilitation, ed 4. Philadelphia, WB Saunders, 1990, pp. 548–563.)

Add-on Power Packs (p. 381)

• For individuals requiring a motorized chair that is easily transported, a few add-on power packs are available (see Fig. 18–3C) that convert a manual chair to a motorized chair. These units give the user an advantage in transportability. They are mainly helpful for individuals who use a manual chair most of the time but who occasionally need power assistance for long distance travel or rough terrain.

Motorized Scooters (pp. 381–382)

• Three- and four-wheeled scooters (see Fig. 18–3D) are a good choice of powered mobility for individuals who have the upper body dexterity and strength to manually steer the unit. They are not available with as much "custom fitting" as other wheelchairs and generally do not have as good a seating position. They are more difficult to transfer into and out of than most other motorized chairs. They are optimally used by the person who can ambulate, transfer, and perform most activities of daily living but who lacks the endurance to ambulate for long distances or to use a manual wheelchair. They are also useful in persons who must avoid overuse of their limbs. They are well suited to many patients with rheumatoid arthritis or severe cardiac or degenerative joint disease, and to some patients with multiple sclerosis or motor neuron or neuromuscular junction disease.

• Four-wheeled scooters are available in both rear- and four-wheel drive models. These units are more stable than three-wheeled models, but they are not as compact and are harder to transport. Although they are more stable than three-wheeled scooters, caution is still advised.

Control Systems for Motorized Chairs (p. 382)

• Control systems for motorized wheelchairs can be classified as either proportional (graded response) or nonproportional (on/off). Proportional systems are used most commonly. They require the ability to incrementally control the push or pull of a joystick (see Fig. 18–3C) by the hand, head, or foot. Pushing the joystick further increases the speed of the wheelchair or the angle of a turn. Proportionally operated power chairs are generally fitted with what is known as a *high brake bias*. When there is no input to propel the chair, it brakes automatically.

• Nonproportional systems are used when an individual cannot operate a joystick. They basically have an "on-or-off" type of control. Air-controlled "sip-and-puff" drive controls are nonproportional controls used for individuals with high-level quadriplegia who have the capacity to control their breathing. They are sometimes used even in conjunction with ventilator use.

SPORT WHEELCHAIRS (pp. 382–383)

• Sport wheelchairs have a rigid frame and are usually made of lightweight material such as titanium. They are usually not the primary chair of the user. These chairs are generally expensive, cannot easily be modified, and are of limited use outside their intended sport. Basketball chairs have thin indoor-type wheels with little tread and small casters. Camber is large, and depending on the

type of impairment (usually level of paraplegia), these chairs allow fairly unrestricted upper body mobility.
• Racing chairs (see Fig. 18–14 in the Textbook) are highly specialized. They compress the athlete's body into a compact shape, have a large camber, and have small-diameter hand rims to help get maximum distance from each arm stroke.

ENERGY CONSIDERATIONS IN WHEELCHAIR USE
(p. 383)

• Certain wheelchair modifications and styles affect rolling resistance and energy consumption. Narrower tires have less rolling resistance and are ideal for use on hard, flat surfaces such as those within institutions. They require much more force to propel over uneven surfaces (e.g., gravel) and are not suited for outdoor use. The same holds true for small casters, which are mainly used for maneuverability in sports such as basketball. Weight is obviously another consideration in calculating energy consumption, and for sports applications, very lightweight chairs are available. The energy consumption of wheelchair use is lowest on a flat, hard surface. Carpeting, rough terrain, and even small inclines or slopes greatly increase the energy cost of mobility. This increase can be prohibitive in elderly or debilitated patients. Powered mobility may be a more realistic option in these patient populations.

GENERAL CONSIDERATIONS IN WHEELCHAIR
SELECTION (p. 383)

• When prescribing wheelchairs for adults it is important to note whether the mobility impairment is of adult onset or has existed since birth or childhood. Developmentally disabled adults present with problems of abnormal muscle tone deformity and contractures. Some require custom-molded seating to correct or accommodate these abnormalities.
• Adults with traumatic paraplegia are typically best fitted with high-strength lightweight wheelchairs. High-level quadriplegic persons usually need powered mobility with sophisticated control systems such as chin controls or sip-and-puff systems. Adults with multiple sclerosis often do well with powered scooters, and adults with stroke typically use a hemi-height manual wheelchair that they propel with the "good" arm and leg. Traumatic brain injury patients often initially require a complex wheelchair system, but commonly progress to needing a less sophisticated system or no wheelchair over the course of time.
• The most important prescribing considerations in all cases include the diagnosis, clinical picture, living situation, family involvement, funding, and previous experience of the patient/caregiver with wheelchairs. Table 18–5 shows some indications for powered mobility. The potential disadvantages of powered mobility include relatively high cost, weight, maintenance, lack of physical exercise, limited environmental accessibility, and transportation difficulty.

PEDIATRIC CONSIDERATIONS IN WHEELCHAIR
PRESCRIPTION (pp. 383–385)

• Pediatric patients present with all of the challenges in wheelchair selection seen in adults but with specific additional concerns. These include accommo-

TABLE 18–5 Indications for Powered Mobility

1. Physical limitations not compatible with manual wheelchair mobility
2. Need for increased independence level at school and work
3. To improve self-esteem
4. To increase efficiency of mobility
5. To spare the upper limb joints from premature deterioration

dating the patient's growth, fostering development of self-esteem, and enabling proper interaction with peers and the environment. Children have different needs based on their developmental level and age. They need physical contact and handling (as do adults), and the equipment they use should not limit that physical contact. For example, wheelchair lap trays used in classrooms can sometimes cause peers to keep their distance, and they do not permit the same interaction as occurs at a desk or a table or in a circle on the floor.

Cosmetic Concerns (p. 384)

• Children have very definite ideas about the appearance and color of their equipment. They often reject the traditional chrome frame wheelchair "look." Manufacturers have responded to this concern with brightly colored choices.

Growth Concerns (p. 384)

• Manufacturers offer both manual and power-drive wheelchairs with "growth potential," and decisions should be made on the basis of whether the child can self-propel the chair or will be able to in the future. Some chairs can be expanded in width and depth with modular and expanding frames. Growth of the legs can be accommodated with longer footrest hangers. In general, one should strive to obtain a chair that meets the child's needs for a 5-year period; however, prescribing a chair that is initially too large can be counterproductive because it decreases the child's independence and makes propelling the chair more difficult.

Family Concerns (p. 384)

• Dealing with children requires carefully listening to the parents or primary caregivers regarding function, appearance, and utility of the end product. It is often psychologically difficult for a parent with a very young child to use a device that looks like a wheelchair. The parents are usually still hopeful that the child will learn to sit, have head control, and walk. Although they realize the need for good positioning and proper body alignment to help prevent contractures and added deformity, they often want the seating components fitted into a device that looks more like a stroller. They might also want the capacity to use the seating system as a car seat. Some manufacturers make FDA-approved car seats that interface with a mobility base for transport; these may or may not be the best choice for the child.

Ventilators and Wheelchairs (p. 384)

• Growing numbers of children are ventilator dependent. For these children not only must one choose the best seating system to support function, growth, and positioning needs, but the system must also house and transport the ventilator and other support equipment.

Progressive Disorders (p. 384)

• Functional independence is always a goal in working with children, but for children who have degenerative or progressive disorders, future loss of control has to be considered. Sometimes it is not possible to predict how quickly changes will be required, but the system of choice should be adaptable to those changes when they occur.

Power Chairs (pp. 384–385)

• Power chairs should be considered for children who have adequate intelligence and judgment but lack the necessary muscle control to propel a manual wheelchair. Many 3-year-olds can safely use power chairs, and power has even been successfully used with some 2-year-olds. Powered mobility should be considered in children with a number of diagnoses (e.g., cerebral palsy, muscular dystrophy, hemiplegia, severe arthrogryposis, traumatic quadriplegia, and bronchopulmonary dysplasia). Children with severe juvenile arthritis or cardiac dysfunction often need powered mobility for more freedom of movement. A scooter often meets their needs because a special seating system is typically not needed; however, most children who require powered mobility also require a special seating system for support and control.

TRANSPORTING THE WHEELCHAIR (p. 385)
Manual Wheelchairs (p. 385)

• Manual wheelchairs are easily transported in motor vehicles because of their folding frames. The lifting weight can be lessened by removing the footrests; the armrests; and, on some models, the rear wheels. Trunk lifts are also available for those who lack the strength to put the chair in the trunk by themselves.

Power Wheelchairs (p. 385)

• Power wheelchairs present complex transport problems. Transport of power wheelchairs generally is best done with a van, van lift, and an approved tie-down system. A ramp system can be used instead of a lift, but for safety reasons, the wheelchair has to be pushed or driven up the ramp by someone other than the user. Roof clearance can be increased with an extra top on the vehicle, but because the resultant seating and transfer position is usually too high, the van must often be modified by lowering the floor.

• Adolescents and adults who operate their own vans generally remove the driver's seat so that they can substitute their wheelchair. They use a lift and tie-down so that they can drive while seated in the restrained wheelchair. The tie-down system in these cases is usually an automatic system that can be operated by a driver-controlled button.

Power Add-on Units (p. 385)

• Power add-on systems do not decrease portability because the unit is easily removed. These systems have worked well with many patients and have become popular when used with high-strength lightweight wheelchairs.

Scooters (p. 385)

• Scooters can usually be disassembled for relatively easy transport in a car. They are often too heavy for the user to lift, so trunk lifts are often prescribed.

TRANSPORTING THE WHEELCHAIR USER (p. 385)

• Adults or children who use wheelchairs and seating systems can usually be transferred to the car seat (or child safety seat) and wear a regular seat belt. Sometimes, large children or adults with cognitive problems must be restrained with a vest in combination with the auto seat belt. Persons who must be transported in their wheelchairs require a van with an FDA-approved tie-down system.

Airline Travel (p. 385)

• For air travel, the wheelchair user is advised to call ahead to let the airline know that specific accommodations might be necessary. Most major carriers have aids to assist the traveler in this regard. When power chairs are to be transported, they must have approved batteries, because airlines will not allow some batteries to be transported on board.

Bus Travel (p. 385)

• When traveling by bus, the same general considerations apply as for air travel. The user should call ahead to learn about any specific requirements. Most municipal bus systems now offer wheelchair-accessible facilities. Cities also often provide alternative transport with a van, if necessary, although this usually has to be arranged in advance.

SIZING THE WHEELCHAIR (pp. 385–386)

• Determining the size of the mobility base and seating system components requires careful measurement of the patient. The measurements that should be taken are depicted in Figure 18–4. The thickness of cushions and padding should be taken into consideration and added to the chair's dimensions.

MAINTENANCE AND SAFETY CONSIDERATIONS (p. 386)

• Wheelchairs have many moving parts that must regularly be lubricated, cleaned, and maintained. The user (or caregiver) must make sure that the chair

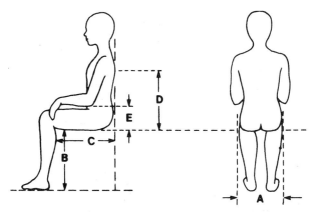

FIGURE 18–4. Standard measurements required for wheelchair dimensions. Seat width: 1 inch wider than the width of the widest part of the buttocks (*A*). Seat height: 2 inches higher than the distance from the bottom of the heel to the popliteal area (*B*). Seat depth: 1 to 2 inches shorter than the distance from the popliteal area to the back of the buttocks (*C*). Back height: 2 inches less (may vary) than the distance from the bottom of the scapulae to the sitting surface (*D*). Armrest height: Distance from bottom of buttocks to elbow (*E*). (From Britell CW: Wheelchair prescription. In Kottke FJ, Lehmann JF [eds]: Krusen's Handbook of Physical Medicine and Rehabilitation, ed 4. Philadelphia, WB Saunders, 1990, pp. 548–563.)

is in proper working order to maximize both durability and safety. Wheelchairs should not be immersed in water because some parts can rust. Power chairs should be taken out of gear when not in use.

SEATING SYSTEMS (pp. 386–388)

• A proper seating system is important for the patient, both in and out of the wheelchair. Proper seating is necessary in the young child who does not yet need a wheelchair for mobility (see Fig. 18–16 in the Textbook). In the elderly, seating is important for general care and to prevent deformity. This section addresses the seating prescription, both as a subset of the wheelchair selection process and as an independent need.

Goals of Seating Systems (pp. 386–387)

• Selection of a seating system is a complex process that requires input from the patient, family, primary caregiver, physician, therapists, vendor, and educator. The team approach can help to ensure a more positive outcome. Goals of seating include the following.

Control Abnormal Tone and Reflexes (p. 386)
• Proper support can help normalize tone and inhibit abnormal reflexes. Abnormal tone and reflexes produce abnormal movement patterns and poor posture,

which in turn contribute to the development of muscle contractures and skeletal deformities. Maintaining proper alignment can help prevent these deformities.

Correct or Accommodate Deformities (p. 386)
• The seating position should help correct or prevent deformities such as hip adduction contractures and ankle plantar flexion contractures. When a deformity cannot be prevented or corrected, it has to be accommodated to prevent its worsening or the development of new compensatory deformities.
• Above all, the seating system should not cause new deformity. One of the problems with the commonly used "hammock" or "sling" wheelchair seat is that it can promote poor posture (see Fig. 18–17 in the Textbook), and it should be avoided in patients at risk for such deformity.

Enhance Function and Improve Control (p. 386)
• Function is enhanced by optimum posture and position. For example, proper support to the head and neck can improve swallowing and decrease the risk of aspiration during eating. Proper alignment and support can also free the upper extremities for self-care activities or for self-propulsion.

Improve Comfort and Improve Sitting Tolerance (p. 386)
• A seating system should provide the necessary support with the least possible restriction of movement. Proper support should provide a secure, stable base and enhance the patient's sitting tolerance.

Provide Pressure Relief and Skin Protection (p. 387)
• The able-bodied child or adult shifts position frequently to redistribute pressure and prevent skin breakdown. Individuals with a lack of sensation or with physical or cognitive limitations are not always capable of such weight shifts, nor do they always understand the need for them. A seating system that equalizes pressure distribution, prevents shear force, and provides proper support decreases the incidence of pressure ulcers.

Facilitate Management and Care (p. 387)
• Seating cannot improve function or control in some patients with very severe neurological impairments. A proper seating system can, however, allow them to be placed in an upright position to improve respiration, digestion, and urinary function. It also allows them to be transported more easily and helps others to do their care and hygiene.

Principles of Seating (pp. 387–388)

• Sitting should provide the necessary support to the body while fostering a comfortable, symmetrical midline posture. Proper sitting position is generally considered to be with the head in midline; trunk erect; hips flexed to 90 degrees; knees at 90 to 100 degrees; and feet in neutral position, with the spine stable and the pelvis level. Seating systems are traditionally grouped into three categories: (1) planar systems, (2) contoured systems, and (3) custom-molded systems.

• *Planar,* also known as *linear seating systems,* are constructed of a support covered with upholstery to provide a relatively flat surface. Possible planar components include seats, seat backs, lateral/head/sternal supports, abductor supports, lap trays, footrests, and cushions. The planar components are generally inexpensive and can readily be modified, repaired, or replaced.

• *Contoured seating systems* are used when patients require a more customized shape to accommodate their bodies. They can be simple or complex. Simple contours can be constructed by using varying densities of foam in the seat cushions to accommodate the body (see Table 18–4). More commonly, however, a more complex design is required. Preformed bases can be obtained with curves to better fit the body. These are then covered with foam or gel to which special add-on pads can be applied, such as lateral supports and thigh abductors. Contoured systems are useful for patients who require mild to moderate support and who are free of severe deformity.

• If more support is necessary, or if the patient's deformity is such that standard seating systems will not fit, a custom-molded seat is needed. Custom-molded systems tend to be used with patients who have more severe deformities and a history of skin breakdown. They are not usually advisable for use in very young children because of their cost and the inability to change the system to accommodate growth. Most of these systems cannot be modified and require replacement if they do not fit properly.

• The covering of the seating system is important. Some patients are allergic to and do not tolerate materials such as latex or neoprene. Incontinence is a problem for some patients, and the material used must be either easily cleaned or impervious to urine. Some coverings can cause increased shear pressure in transfers, which presents a problem in the patient at risk for pressure ulcers.

Prescribing Seating Systems (p. 388)

• Modern technology can enhance the user's potential for independence, but it is not always affordable or practical based on funding restrictions and the environment in which such equipment is to be operated. Clinical assessment should include the following items.

Tone/Spasticity (p. 388)

• Patients presenting with tone or spasticity problems often require special seating considerations such as rolled seats (thinner over the ischial tuberosities to properly position the pelvis), anti-thrust seats, abduction devices, and special back-to-seat angles. They also require parts that are reinforced or made of stronger and more durable materials. Patients with low tone often require lumbar supports to promote spinal extension, tilt mechanisms to improve head and trunk control, or custom headrests. Patients with athetosis may require stabilization of an upper and lower extremity to effectively use the remaining upper extremity functionally.

Contracture (p. 388)

• Knee flexion contractures can affect caster size and the type of footrest that can be used. Hip extension contractures require a more open hip angle and might necessitate a reclining back feature. Assessment of contractures should include whether the patient has a fixed deformity or abnormal posturing.

Impaired Sensation/Body Awareness (p. 388)

• Sensation has a direct impact on positioning, and sensory deficits can impair balance as well as predispose to pressure ulceration. A proper sense of body awareness is important. Patients with perceptual problems, such as hemineglect, often injure themselves in their wheelchairs. They might drag a foot on the floor without realizing that it has fallen from the footrest. Sometimes they injure a hand or arm as it dangles and gets caught in the wheel. Special seating and wheelchair restrictions are needed to prevent these problems.

Skin Integrity (p. 388)

• Tissue integrity should also be assessed. Children and adults with no history of breakdown usually tolerate regular planar seating systems. Clients with current ulcers or a history of previous pressure ulcers require more creative seating and the use of foam, air-cell, or pressure pads.

Other Seating Considerations (p. 388)

• A number of other items should be noted because they can necessitate special seating or wheelchair arrangements. These items include the status of vision and hearing, need for orthoses, presence of deformities, and behavior problems. Textbook Table 18–14 lists some of the more common problems in seating along with their causes and possible solutions.

WHEELCHAIR SAFETY (pp. 388–390)

• Falls and tips are the most common wheelchair accidents. Therefore, it is important to match a person's cognitive capabilities to the type of device being prescribed. Anti-tippers, proper brakes, grade aids, proper axle position, proper seating position, and wheel camber, among others, can all be modified to enhance stability. Special care must be taken when prescribing reclining, tilting, standing, or power chairs.

19

Original Chapter by Barbara J. deLateur, M.D., M.S.

Therapeutic Exercise

THEORETICAL CONSIDERATIONS (pp. 392–401)

- It is common knowledge that strength is somehow related to the ability to lift objects in a gravitational field. It is intuitive that this strength is greater with larger muscles and is also related to the technique of lifting. Scientific research and research-based practice, however, require greater precision of definition.

One- and Ten-Repetition Maxima (p. 392)

- A useful definition is the one-repetition maximum (1 RM); that is, the largest weight that can be lifted once and only once through the full range of motion of a given joint. Another useful definition is the 10 RM; that is, the highest weight that can be lifted through the full range of motion 10 times only. The 10 RM is useful if a set of weights is available but not an isokinetic apparatus or other dynamometer.

Determinants of Strength (pp. 392–393)

Absolute Muscle Strength (p. 392)

- Strength is related to the physiological cross-sectional area of muscle, which is the cross section at the bulkiest part of the muscle for long parallel muscles such as the sartorius. Although figures in the literature vary, a generally accepted value for the absolute muscle strength is $3.6 \, kg/cm^2$ of physiological cross-sectional area. This should be listed technically as $3.6 \, kp/cm^2$ (a kilopond, abbreviated as kp, is the force exerted by the mass of 1 kg in Earth's gravitational field.

Neural or Learning Factors in Strength (pp. 392–393)

- It has been known for almost 40 years that high-force or high-intensity performance could be enhanced without a substantial overall increase in muscle bulk. The improvement in the first 2 weeks of training, in particular, appears to be caused by learning or the ability to recruit or rapidly fire motor units or a combination of these. After this, most of the improvement in high-force intensity is caused by hypertrophy.

CROSS TRAINING

• As currently used, the term *cross-training* means training in one sport to benefit performance in another sport. In the older literature, cross-training meant the extent to which training one limb benefited the opposite limb. This might be of interest, for example, if the untrained side is in a cast. Research shows that there is a learning effect but no hypertrophy in the cross-trained limb musculature.

Endurance, Fatigue, and the Relationship of Endurance to Intensity of Activity (pp. 393–394)

• *Endurance* is the ability to continue a prescribed task in the desired manner. In contrast, *fatigue* can be defined in more than one way. For example, fatigue could be defined as the time elapsed (measured in seconds) in an attempted sustained contraction (or the number of contractions in a dynamic task) until the peak force or torque reaches a specified percentage of the initial force or torque (e.g., the time at which 60% of the initial value is reached). This definition is useful in assessing the response to training or to various therapeutic interventions. A broader definition of fatigue, useful to coaches and others concerned with athletic competition, is any decrement in performance resulting from previous performance.

Absolute Endurance versus Relative Endurance (pp. 394–396)

• Absolute endurance is the time that a subject can sustain a given workload; or, the number of seconds a given force can be held; or, the number of repetitions of a given load. Some examples are the number of seconds that a given bicycle ergometer can be pedaled by a subject at 100 W, the number of seconds a force of 50 N can be held, or the number of times a subject can lift with the right biceps a loaded barbell weighing 10 lb. Note that these activities all have units such as watts, Newtons, and pounds.

Length-Tension Relationships (p. 396)

• Figure 19–1 shows the classic force-velocity relationships, also known as a Blix diagram. A muscle generates the most force at its "resting length." As a practical matter, the resting length, sometimes called the neutral length, of the intact subject could be considered to be at about the midpoint of the joint range or slightly longer.

Leverage Effect (pp. 396–397)

• The site of application as well as the angle of application determines leverage. If the leverage so defined were the only determinant of torque, it would be inferred from Figure 19–2 that the brachioradialis was the strongest of the elbow flexors. However, the force or tension developed by the muscle is, as we have seen, a function of the physiological cross-sectional area of the muscle. The torque developed (the effectiveness of the muscle for producing rotation about the joint) is the net result of muscle size (physiological cross-sectional area) and leverage.

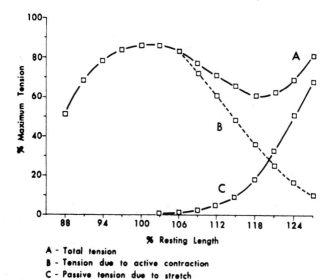

A - Total tension
B - Tension due to active contraction
C - Passive tension due to stretch

FIGURE 19–1. Length-tension diagram for passive stretch of an unstimulated muscle is shown in lower curve *C*. Curve *A*, showing total isometric tension when the muscle was stimulated at various lengths from maximal stretch through moderate shortening, represents the summation of active contraction plus passive tension because of the stretch. Active tension due solely to muscular contraction is obtained by subtracting passive tension (*C*) from total tension (*A*) and is represented by curve *B*. Normal resting length is 100, represented by curve *B*. Normal resting length is 100%. (Redrawn from Schottelius BA, Senay LC: Effect of stimulation-length sequence on shape of length-tension diagram. Am J Physiol 1956; 186:127–130.)

Torque-Velocity Relationships (pp. 397–398)

• Modern isokinetic devices allow easy measurement of torque as it varies throughout the range of motion. They also permit the measurement of such torque-angle curves at varying velocities of contraction. Figure 19–3 shows that one can develop less torque with a fast shortening (concentric) contraction than with a slow shortening contraction, less torque with a slow shortening contraction than with an isometric contraction, less torque with an isometric contraction than with a slow lengthening (eccentric) contraction, and less torque with a slow lengthening contraction than with a rapid lengthening contraction. This relationship has important implications for therapeutic exercise for development of strength and for hypertrophy.

Muscle Fiber and Motor Unit Types (p. 398)

• In the human there appear to be two muscle fiber types, generally designated type I (slow oxidative or SO) and type II (fast-twitch or FT). There is at least one subdivision of fibers into fast glycolytic (FG) and fast oxidative-glycolytic

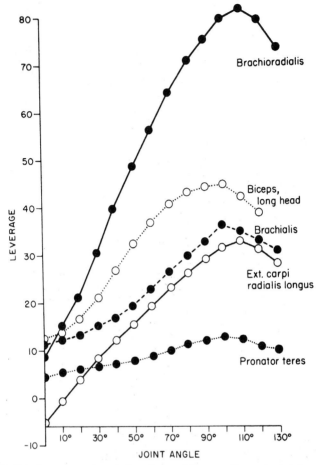

FIGURE 19–2. Leverage curves of elbow flexors; 0 degrees: elbow extended. Leverage is effective lever arm length: $lf \times \sin \alpha$, where lf is the distance from joint axis to site of application of tendon of insertion and α is the angle of insertion of the tendon at that joint angle. (From Brunnstrom S: Clinical Kinesiology, ed 2. Philadelphia, FA Davis, 1966.)

(FOG). The categorization into types I and II is made on the basis of the twitch characteristics (i.e., fast or slow) (Fig. 19–4). The characteristics of the muscle fibers are determined by the type of motor unit (Table 19–1). These characteristics include such things as their metabolic processes and sources of fuel, along with the enzymatic activity, speed of contraction, and rate of fatigue. Descriptions of differences in muscle color and muscle fiber diameter relate more consistently or at least more obviously to animals than to humans, in whom the differences are more subtle. The FOG motor unit, including the muscle fiber, can be thought of as a sort of hybrid that is defined as type II by its FT charac-

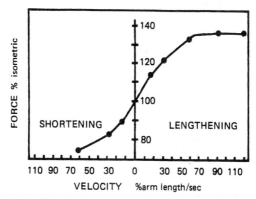

FIGURE 19–3. Relationship of maximal force of human elbow flexor muscles to velocity of contraction. Velocity on abscissa is designated as a percentage of arm length per second. (From Knuttgen HG: Development of muscular strength and endurance. In Knuttgen HG (ed): Neuromuscular Mechanisms for Therapeutic and Conditioning Exercises. Baltimore, University Park Press, 1976, pp. 97–118.)

teristics but retains some of the fatigue resistance associated with the oxidative phosphorylation seen in the type I or SO motor unit types.

The Motor Unit Size Principle (pp. 398–399)

• Henneman first enunciated the size principle, which notes that the smaller motor units have fewer muscle fibers, smaller motor unit action potentials, somewhat smaller cross-sectional areas, and a lower threshold of recruitment. In needle EMG, as motor units are recruited in succession, the smaller motor units

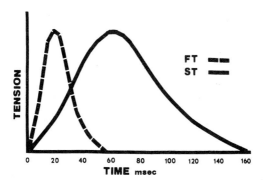

FIGURE 19–4. Twitch characteristics (contraction relaxation curves) of slow twitch (type I) and fast twitch (type II) muscles. (From Ianuzzo CD: The cellular composition of human skeletal muscle. In Knuttgen HG (ed): Neuromuscular Mechanisms for Therapeutic and Conditioning Exercise. Baltimore, University Park Press, 1976, pp. 31–53.)

TABLE 19–1 A Characterization of Skeletal Muscle Fibers Based on Their Metabolic and Mechanical Properties

	Muscle Fiber Characteristics		
	Slow Oxidative (SO)	Fast Glycolytic (FG)	Fast Oxidative-Glycolytic (FOG)
Major source of ATP	Oxidative phosphorylation	Glycolysis	Oxidative phosphorylation
Mitochondria	Numerous	Few	Numerous
Myoglobin content	High	Low	High
Capillarity	Dense	Sparse	Dense
Muscle color	Red	White	Red
Glycogen content	Low	High	Intermediate
Glycolytic enzyme activity	Low	High	Intermediate
Myosin ATPase activity	Low	High	High
Speed of contraction	Slow	Fast	Fast
Rate of fatigue	Slow	Fast	Intermediate
Muscle fiber diameter	Small	Large	Intermediate

Abbreviations: ATP, adenosine triphosphate; ATPase, adenosine triphosphatase.
From Kidd G, Brodie P: The motor unit: A review. Physiotherapy 1980; 66:146–152.

come in first and the larger motor units later. Some later motor units appear smaller because of their distance from the exploring electrode. With the needle adjusted to focus on the motor unit, it becomes much larger. Another way of stating this is that smaller units can be recruited without the larger units, but larger units cannot be recruited without the smaller units. Some variation of the size principle can be seen even among motor units of similar size.

Metabolic Aspects of Exercise (p. 399)

• The point of recruitment of the larger type II fibers depends on the type of exercise. With sustained isometric contractions, type II motor units are brought in at 20% of the MVC; however, if the isometric effort is sustained long enough, type II fibers can be brought in at thresholds somewhat below 20% of MVC. With aerobic exercise, as on a bicycle ergometer, the reliance is on type I motor units below 100% of the maximal aerobic capacity. Beyond this aerobic capacity, both type I and type II are relied on, and the subject will rapidly go into oxygen debt secondary to anaerobic metabolism. However, the threshold for bringing in anaerobic pathways is generally about 70%, although it may be higher in endurance-trained (aerobic-trained) athletes.

Application of Principles to Therapeutic Exercise for Strength, Local Muscle Endurance, and Hypertrophy (pp. 399–401)

Strength (pp. 399–400)
• Muscle performance, including performance on tests of strength, can be enhanced in various ways. These include increases in the amount of weight lifted

(progressive resistance exercise, or PRE); increases in the number of repetitions or sets; increases in both amount of weight and number of repetitions; and increases in the contraction velocity (while keeping the resistance and number of repetitions the same).

Progressive Resistance Exercise (pp. 400–401)

• This type of exercise was described and popularized by T. L. DeLorme, who at the time was a captain in the U.S. Army. It requires the determination, usually once a week, of the 10 RM. At each session, held 3 to 5 days per week, the subject performs 10 repetitions at each of a series of fractions of the 10 RM. In the early stages this was 10 repetitions each at 10%, 20%, 30%, . . . , up to 100% of the 10 RM. Because of the enormous amount of time necessary to train multiple muscles with this technique, a number of modifications of this program were devised and the final form was 10 repetitions each at 50%, 75%, and 100% of the 10 RM. This program has much to recommend it, including the fact that there is a built-in warmup at a lower intensity and the likelihood of fatigue limiting the number of contractions in the final set at 100%. Nevertheless, some workers were concerned about the inability to carry out the full prescribed 10 RM at 100%, and thus the "Oxford technique" was developed. It begins with 10 repetitions at 100% and progresses down in weight to 10 repetitions at 75% and 50% of the 10 RM. The DeLorme technique is probably more effective than the Oxford technique, although the critical study in this regard has not yet been done.

Increasing the Number of Repetitions (p. 401)

• There is essentially 100% transfer-of-training when exercise with relatively high weights and few repetitions is compared with exercise with relatively low weights and more repetitions, as long as the exercise is continued to the point of fatigue. However, two points should be noted. The first is that far more repetitions must be carried out with lower weights than with higher weights to reach the point of fatigue. It is likely that the subject will stop low-weight exercise for reasons other than true muscle fatigue. The amount of mechanical work done will be much greater with the lower weight. Mechanical work is far less relevant to muscle training than is the stimulus of muscle failure (i.e., a short-lasting inability to carry out the task). There may be some circumstances in which the subject should avoid the risk of training that might occur with the higher weights. In general, however, exercising with higher weights to failure is both more effective and more efficient than exercising with lower weights to failure. One can also do multiple sets, continuing to fatigue with each set, with the higher weights.

Other Approaches (p. 401)

• A simple but highly effective technique is to find a relatively high weight, one that can be lifted three to five times before failure (i.e., temporary inability to lift the weight further), and record the number of repetitions. The exercise should be carried out to the point of muscle fatigue or failure each session. The number of repetitions to fatigue is graphed on a daily basis. When the subject can perform some 15 to 20 repetitions, the weight is increased approximately 10% and the process is repeated. A variation on this process, useful when strength begins to reach a plateau, is to do multiple sets during a session, going to fatigue with each set.

CLINICAL AND SPORTS APPLICATIONS (pp. 401–407)

• The practice of sports medicine is characterized by a number of maxims, perhaps one of the most important and useful of which is "Get in shape to play. Do not play to get in shape." Following this single maxim would do more to prevent injury than virtually any other practice.

Are Athletes Born or Made? (pp. 401–402)

• Marked differences between athletes participating in different types of sports can be detected by the casual observer or by the scientist in the human performance laboratory. The weightlifter is heavy and extremely strong. The distance runner is slight of build with very little body fat and relatively low strength but has the ability to continue running, literally for hours. Definite but more subtle changes are observed between the sprinter and the distance runner. Differences in local metabolic capacity of the muscle as well as fiber type differences have been determined by large-needle biopsy. A large study was done to determine the differences in individual athletes of various types. Whereas only minor differences existed for PFK (glycolytic capacity), remarkable differences were found in local muscle oxidative capacity (SDH) and in $\dot{V}_{O_2max}$. The SDH and $\dot{V}_{O_2max}$ of the weight lifters were no greater than those of the untrained men; in fact, the values were slightly less. The endurance-trained athletes had much higher $\dot{V}_{O_2max}$ and local muscle SDH activity than the untrained men or the weight lifters.

• A 5-month training program, with biopsy studies performed before and after training, showed an increase in the ratio of the areas of ST to FT fibers from 0.82 to 1.11. Oxidative capacity increased in both fiber types; anaerobic capacity increased only in the FT fibers. This study indicates the possibility of great enhancement of local muscle metabolic capability (particularly oxidative capacity) with endurance training, and strongly supports the notion of some degree of specificity of training. In human subjects, fiber number does not appear to increase. Regarding the question of whether athletes are born or made, it appears that the genotype sets the rather wide limits, with the actual performance capability determined by the extent and type of training.

Studies on the Specificity of Training (p. 402)

• The exercise literature and clinical experience both strongly support the observation that the poorer the initial condition of the subject (provided that no specific neuromuscular disorder is present), the greater the percentage response to training and the greater the generalizability of the training. Conversely, the more elite the athlete or performer, the greater is the requirement for specific training.

High Weights versus Low Weights: The DeLorme Axiom (pp. 402–404)

• The DeLorme axiom states: "High weight (intensity), low repetition programs build strength; low weight (low intensity) high repetition exercises build endurance. Each of these types of exercise is wholly distinct and wholly incapable of producing the results obtained by the other." In the extreme, this axiom must be true. However, there is a large middle ground in which this axiom is untrue, that is, in which there is a high degree of transferability from relatively low-weight conditions to relatively high-weight conditions as long as the subject goes to the point of fatigue. It should be noted that 50 lb lifted 10 times will have a different training effect from 10 lb lifted 50 times, even though the mechanical work performed by the muscle is the same. What counts is the relative intensity or tax on the muscle.

Isometric versus Isotonic (p. 404)

• In the 1970s, in particular, there was disagreement on the effectiveness of isometric versus isotonic training. Studies have shown that subjects do better on the task on which they had trained. This illustrates the effect of training-to-task. For qualitatively identical tasks, there are comparable results, as long as subjects go to the point of fatigue in training (remember that it will take much longer to go to true muscle fatigue for lower weights). For qualitatively different tasks (or for extreme quantitative differences), the best training for a task is that task itself.

Isokinetic Programs: Strength and Hypertrophy; Specificity of Velocity of Training (pp. 404–406)

• Isokinetic programs require special isokinetic equipment. The type of training and testing involved is not reflective of everyday, nontechnical experience. This is in contrast to isotonic and isometric tasks, in which testing involves the ordinary activity of lifting or holding objects against gravity. Early isokinetic devices involved purely concentric exercise, because knee extension was carried out by the quadriceps (concentric) and knee flexion by the hamstrings (also concentric). In contrast, raising and lowering a weight has both a concentric and an eccentric component. More recent equipment allows either a mixed mode or a purely concentric mode. The preponderance of evidence suggests that if hypertrophy is desired, there should be at least a component of eccentric exercise in the training.

Specificity of Velocity of Training (p. 406)
• If the best training for a task is that task itself, and if the task requires exerting force at high velocities, it would seem advantageous to train at high contraction velocities. The intrinsic shape of the torque-velocity curve (see Fig. 19–3) implies that, regardless of effort, training at high contraction velocities will be less forceful, although the force exerted will gradually, with training, become higher. It appears that the more important variable in developing strength (forceful contractions) is the tension (force) produced in the muscle during training. To the extent that a skill is involved, however, such as throwing a baseball, it is extremely important to practice on the task itself.

Coordination (pp. 406–407)

• The maxim "Practice makes perfect" would be more accurate if restated as "*Perfect* practice makes perfect." Inaccurate practice leads to inaccurate performance, and wrong notes or skills are learned as readily as correct ones. Some extremely complex tasks involving more than one limb should be broken down into simpler tasks and performed slowly enough that the practice is essentially error-free. The simpler tasks should then be brought up to a faster speed, after which combined practice is undertaken at a slow speed. This speed is gradually increased until the combined performance can be carried out at a much faster speed than will be required in recital or concert (in the case of musical performance). This would be appropriate, in the case of pipe organ performance for the training of the lower limbs for a pedal task, because the task of the hands is separated from the pedals. Care must be taken, however, not to develop some techniques that work at slow speeds, or that involve a separation of the limbs that would not be sustainable in faster or combined tasks. Accurate repetitions must be carried out until an engram is generated. A useful definition of an *engram* is a precise automatic performance implying a preprogrammed pattern.

APPLICATIONS TO AGING (pp. 407–409)

Strength Training (p. 407)

• Evidence is accumulating that older people respond favorably to strength training. It has been felt in the past that strength improvement in the elderly was because of learning. However, direct imaging studies have recently shown that the muscles of older people can in fact improve their performance by hypertrophy as well as by learning.

Frailty (pp. 407–408)

• Buchner and Wagner have defined *frailty* as "the state of reduced physiologic reserve associated with increased susceptibility to disability." This is a more inclusive concept and more useful than the popular notion of frailty as thin and weak. Although those who are thin and weak are often frail, many obese people are frail in that they have poor relative strength or strength-to-weight ratio. In either case, because of the loss of reserves, some disruption of their equilibrium by injuries or intercurrent illness might well lead to disability.

Exercise for Fat Reduction (pp. 408–409)

• Evidence is accumulating that the size of the fat cells is regulated in the same way that many things in the body (e.g., oxygen tension, carbon dioxide tension, calcium levels, blood sugar, and temperature) are regulated, and that this "lipostat" is high in some persons and low in others, with all gradations in between. Efforts to reduce fat by restricting caloric intake severely have only a temporary result because the body interprets this restriction as a famine, and mechanisms to defend the fat cell size over the long term are brought into play. The first line of defense is hunger. If this does not succeed in restoring the caloric intake, the next line of defense is energy conservation by decreased production of heat and a strong disinclination to exercise. People who attempt to control their weight without exercise generally have poor long-term results and tend to put on as much or more weight than they took off. In addition, when weight is lost by caloric restriction without exercise, there is some loss of muscle mass as well as fat. When the weight is put back on without exercise, it is mostly fat that is restored. The subject can wind up being more obese, in terms of percentage body fat, than at the start of the program.

- Muscles are the furnaces in which fat is burned. Progressive loss of muscle makes it more and more difficult to burn off even an ordinary intake of calories. The only way to successfully live below a high set-point, that is, to reduce body fat in the face of a high set-point, is by prolonged aerobic exercise.

Reaction Time (p. 409)

- Cross-sectional studies clearly indicate that fitter is faster. In simple reaction time or movement time, although young active subjects are fastest and old sedentary subjects are slowest, old active subjects may be as fast as or slightly faster than young sedentary subjects. This does not, however, establish cause and effect. Perhaps the quickness of some subjects makes their motor activity more pleasurable and reinforcing, and actually promotes their participation in activity, rather than the activity promoting the quickness. More research needs to be done to determine whether putting older subjects on a progressive activity or exercise program will, in fact, improve their reaction time and general quickness.

EQUIPMENT CONSIDERATIONS (pp. 409–411)

- Equipment ranges from simple resistance devices to complex electronic and compression devices available for both resistance and metabolic exercise.

Simple Resistance Training Devices (p. 409)

- These devices fall into two basic categories: elastic resistance devices and free weights. *Elastic resistance* devices, whether they involve tension or compression, have resistance that varies with displacement. Surgical tubing is a commonly used example of an elastic resistance device. It is available in bulk and can be cut to the length needed. It has the advantage of portability, ease of use, low cost, and adaptability to a rather wide range of muscles. Such a device can even be used in the weightless environment of space. A disadvantage is the lack of feedback regarding what is done in precise terms or of the progress being made. With *free weights,* there is a similar advantage of simplicity and versatility for upper extremity use. For the lower limb, adaptations must be made such as the quadriceps boot or DeLorme boot, which is a short bar with circular weights and collar attachments with a metal plate and straps for attaching to the foot. The disadvantage is that numerous weights must be used to adapt to muscles of different strength or to the increasing strength of a given muscle. This greatly restricts the portability of such a device. Progress can be noted by counting repetitions or recording the change in the amount of weight lifted.

Complex Resistance Training Devices (pp. 409–411)

- The past decade has seen the development of a number of complex devices with computerized feedback systems attached. Such devices can be programmed to compare left and right sides, the quadriceps-to-hamstrings strength ratio, and other information considered of interest. Some form of feedback is of great importance, both for its cue value and for its reinforcement or reward value. One need only look at the response to the daily stock market report to see the effect of information feedback about performance.

• Another simple device is the N-K table (see Figs. 19–32 and 19–33 in the Textbook). This has at least two advantages, namely, relative safety and ease of attaching weights. A third advantage is the ability to change the point in the range at which the muscle begins to exert substantial force.

• Recent years have seen the development of accommodating resistance devices that allow concentric and also allow eccentric exercise. With accommodating resistance devices (exemplified by the Cybex, Lido, KinCom, and Biodex) the operator presets a maximum contraction velocity. Accommodating resistance is developed when the subject attempts to accelerate the resistance arm beyond the preset limit. This allows development of different levels of force with concentric and eccentric exercise. The latter appears to be very important for hypertrophy as well as for maximum strength training. In the early phases of strength training, however, it would be safer to use an all-concentric mode.

• Newer devices involving electronic programming and compressors permit the partial counterbalancing of the subject's weight to permit upper body chin-and-dip exercise for subjects whose upper body strength would not otherwise be great enough to permit these rather severe exercises. Such a device is the Gravitron, made by Stairmaster. The subject steps on the platform, turns on the device, and enters his or her accurate body weight, including the weight of the training clothes and shoes. It will be valuable when such devices as these are adapted for persons who use wheelchairs.

Equipment for Metabolic Exercise (p. 411)

• A wide range of equipment is available for metabolic exercise. Some devices are equipped with computers that estimate the number of calories expended based on body weight or typical efficiencies. Arm ergometers range from simple mechanical devices (e.g., the Monark) to more complex electromechanical devices with attached computer software that not only gives caloric readouts but also allows competition with built-in pacers. Depending on the initial state of training of the subject and the intensity of the activity, strength may be increased as well as aerobic capacity. Similarly, for the lower body, one can use a simple bicycle-type attachment to a chair; or one may go to the much more complex devices made by Cybex, Lifecycle, or other devices such as the Wind Trainer. A device that allows simultaneous or separate use of the upper and lower limbs is the Schwinn Airdyne. The lower limbs move in a circular fashion, as with any bicycle, and the upper limbs move in a forward-and-back motion as they move long levers. Resistance is provided by calibrated air-resisting paddles attached to the wheel. As with any wind resistance, the resistance is in proportion to the square of the speed. This type of device allows a very smooth aerobic employment of large numbers of muscles in a reciprocal fashion. As such, it is virtually ideal for burning fat.

• Treadmills allow weight-bearing aerobic activity at precise speeds and grades. The subject can clip an infrared-based pulse meter to the earlobe and monitor the pulse. Speed and grade are varied to bring the heart rate into the desired range.

20

Original Chapter by James W. Atchison, D.O., Scott T. Stoll, D.O., Ph.D., and Ann Cotter, M.D.

Manipulation, Traction, and Massage

MANUAL MEDICINE (pp. 413–425)

Manipulation: Definition and Goal (pp. 413–414)

• The International Federation of Manual Medicine defines *manipulation* as "the use of the hands in the patient management process using instructions and maneuvers to maintain maximal, painless movement of the musculoskeletal system in postural balance."

• The goal of manipulation or manual medicine is to help maintain optimal body mechanics and to improve motion in restricted areas, thus enhancing maximal, pain-free movement in postural balance and optimizing function. This is accomplished by treatments that attempt to restore the mechanical function of a joint and normalize altered reflex patterns, as evidenced by optimum range of motion, body symmetry, and tissue texture.

• The indications for the use of manual medicine: (1) restoration of normality and symmetry at either the disk or facet level; (2) mechanically restoring optimal muscular and myofascial range and ease of motion, thereby restoring function; (3) therapy-induced reduction of afferent signal transmission to the cord, thereby diminishing pain awareness through a gate theory effect; (4) endorphin release, which increases the pain threshold or reduces pain severity; or (5) placebo effect.

History (p. 414)

• Manual medicine dates back to the time of Hippocrates (*fl.* 460–377 BCE), Galen (*fl.* 131–202 CE), and Ambroise Pare (1510–1590 CE). The pioneers of manual medicine include the "bonesetters" of England (Richard Hutton, Wharton Hood, Sir Herbert Baker); Andrew Taylor Still, who founded osteopathic medicine in 1874; and Daniel David Palmer, who founded chiropractic in 1895.

• Still's philosophy stressed wellness and wholeness of the body and included: (1) the unity of the body (i.e., all systems depend on and influence all other systems); (2) the body's natural ability for self-healing; (3) the somatic component of disease; (4) the interrelationship of structure and function; and (5) the use of manipulative therapy.

• Beginning in the 1940s, James Cyriax, a British orthopedic surgeon, published several works related to manipulation, incorporating massage, traction, and injections in the treatment programs.

Nomenclature (p. 415)

• Over the years, the nomenclature for the musculoskeletal pathology or "manipulable lesion" has repeatedly changed. At present, it is labeled "somatic dysfunction"
• *Somatic dysfunction* is defined as impaired or altered function of related components of the somatic (body framework) system; skeletal, arthrodial, and myofascial structures; and related vascular, lymphatic, and neural elements. Somatic dysfunction is manifested as *t*enderness, structural *a*symmetry, altered *r*ange of motion, and *t*issue texture changes (TART). There can be decreased mobility at any point along the physiological range of motion of any joint (see Fig. 20–1 in the Textbook).
• In the United States, manipulation encompasses mobilization techniques—techniques that utilize thrusting (e.g., high-velocity, low-amplitude, or mobilization with impulse) forces (see Figs. 20–2, 20–4, 20–5, and 20–6 in the Textbook) together with many other nonthrusting procedures, as listed in Table 20–1.

Indications and Goals of Treatment (pp. 415–418)

• Manual medicine techniques are potentially useful for treatment of any musculoskeletal problem demonstrating somatic dysfunction. This can include many specific conditions such as acute and chronic cervical pain, thoracic pain, rib pain, functional and mechanical low back pain, chronic low back pain, bulging intervertebral disk, facet syndrome, piriformis syndrome, sciatica, headaches, and sacroiliac syndromes.
• The assessment for somatic dysfunction starts with a history and physical examination that includes a careful neuromusculoskeletal examination. This is followed by a detailed structural evaluation that incorporates observation, palpation, and segmental motion testing (Fig. 20–1). The structural examination requires sophisticated palpatory skills to assess for tenderness, body asymme-

TABLE 20–1 Manual Medicine Techniques

Thrusting
   Mobilization with impulse/high-velocity, low-amplitude
Nonthrusting
   Mobilization without impulse/articulatory technique
   Muscle energy
   Counterstrain
   Functional technique
   Myofascial release
   Soft tissue
   Craniosacral

try, altered range of motion, and tissue texture changes. Greenman's 12-step screen is described in Table 20–2.

• During the structural evaluation, the practitioner tries to determine the relationship of the physiological and anatomical barriers to movement while assessing for potential pathological barriers. The physiological barrier is at the end of normal, active range of motion. The anatomical barrier is at the end of passive motion, and if exceeded, leads to fracture, dislocation, or ligamentous damage. There is a normal feel of increasing resistance as the physiological and anatomical barriers are approached. A pathological barrier limits the usual range of motion or alters the ability of the tissues to perform throughout the usual range of motion, and is evidence of dysfunction.

• A complete structural evaluation of all areas of the body (see Table 20–2) is necessary to establish a diagnosis, to differentiate primary from secondary areas of dysfunction, and to determine the appropriate treatment techniques that can be applied (see Fig. 20–1).

Classification of Manual Medicine Techniques (pp. 418–419)

• Classification regimens include (1) the type of procedure (thrusting or nonthrusting); (2) the type of force utilized (intrinsic or extrinsic); (3) the patient contribution to the force (active or passive); and (4) the type of movement approach to the pathological barrier (direct or indirect). The effects of these different techniques are classified by five basic theoretical models of interaction

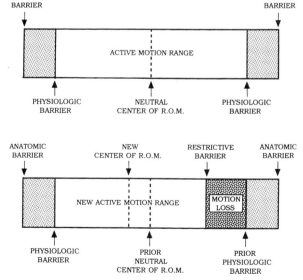

FIGURE 20–1. The diagnostic sequence in manual medicine. The general and/or specific examinations reveal objective changes that help to establish the diagnosis of a specific somatic dysfunction and plan the appropriate treatment. (Modified from Neumann H-D: Introduction to Manual Medicine. Berlin, Springer-Verlag, 1989, p. 14.)

TABLE 20–2 Twelve-Step Screening Examination

Step 1. Gait analysis in multiple directions
Step 2. Observation of static posture and palpable assessment of paired anatomical landmarks
Step 3. Dynamic trunk sidebending
Step 4. Standing flexion test
Step 5. Stork test
Step 6. Seated flexion test
Step 7. Screening test of upper extremities
Step 8. Trunk rotation
Step 9. Trunk sidebending
Step 10. Head and neck mobility
Step 11. Respiration of thoracic cage
Step 12. Lower extremity screening

From Greenman PE: Principles of Manual Medicine, ed 2. Baltimore, Williams & Wilkins, 1996, p. 18.

with the body: (1) postural-structural or biomechanical, (2) neurological, (3) respiratory-circulatory, (4) bioenergy, and (5) behavioral-psychosocial.
• *Extrinsic forces* are applied from the outside of the body and can be provided by gravity, straps and pads, or by another person. The practitioner can use a thrusting, springing, or guiding technique. The patient is usually passively involved with these techniques.
• *Intrinsic forces* occur within a person's body and include muscle forces; respiratory forces; and inherent forces, such as fluctuating body fluid pressures. Patients are considered to be actively involved with these treatments if they are consciously contracting specific muscle groups or performing respiratory sequences.
• The direction of treatment force is related to the barrier concept. *Direct methods* involve moving the patient toward the pathological barrier or in the direction of increasing resistance. Once the barrier has been engaged, a force is applied to move through the pathological barrier toward the normal physiological or anatomical barrier.
• *Indirect methods* involve movement of the patient or segment in the direction of least resistance, away from the pathological barrier. This allows the body's inherent and muscle energy forces to enhance mobility, permitting changes in the relationship between the position of the pathological barrier and the normal physiological barrier. Counterstrain, functional indirect, myofascial release, and craniosacral techniques are most often utilized.

Specific Types of Manual Medicine Techniques
(pp. 420–423)

Mobilization with Impulse (p. 420)
• Mobilization with impulse is more commonly known as the thrust maneuver or the high-velocity/low-amplitude (HVLA) form of manual medicine. This is a direct form of treatment and is commonly prescribed for cervical, thoracic, lumbar, rib, sacroiliac, and extremity dysfunctions. They are commonly performed because they offer the quickest mode of releasing a dysfunctional segment or region. Often, a "crack" or "pop" occurs when a restricted joint is released.

• The following techniques have fewer contraindications and require less training to perform safely, but are more time consuming than HVLA techniques.

Articulatory Technique (p. 420)
• Articulatory technique, or mobilization without impulse, was popularized by Maitland. It is a combination of leverage, patient ventilatory movement, and a fulcrum is used to achieve mobilization of the dysfunctional segment. This is most often done by repeatedly applying a low-velocity/high-amplitude force to engage the barrier directly, then move away from it. This repeated "tapping" on the barrier is designed to move the pathological barrier gently toward the physiological barrier, improving the range of motion.

Muscle Energy Technique (pp. 420–421)
• Introduced by F. L. Mitchell Sr., muscle energy (ME) technique involves the patient's voluntary contraction of muscles (i.e., isometric, concentric, or eccentric) against resistance supplied by the practitioner. An active manual medicine treatment, ME can be applied to most muscle groups in the body as either a direct or indirect technique. The goal is to increase the mobility of hypomobile segments, increase functional range of motion, allow the return of symmetrical motion to affected segments, strengthen weakened muscles, and lengthen contracted or spastic muscles. ME is also believed to have an effect on the nervous system. It is a relatively safe technique, with few contraindications because the patient controls the degree of force applied to the dysfunctional area.
• Dubbed "contract-relax" by physical therapists, this technique can often be learned by patients as part of a home exercise program. The cervical spine and sacroiliac/pelvic regions are more easily and safely treated with ME than with HVLA.

Strain-Counterstrain (p. 421)
• Strain-counterstrain (CS) is a manual medicine technique that attempts to passively place a spinal segment or other joint into its position of greatest comfort or ease. This is an indirect, functional technique developed by Jones. It is aimed at relieving painful dysfunction through a reduction in inappropriate afferent proprioceptor activity. Before using CS treatment, structural evaluation is required to determine the areas of dysfunction and specify the location of Jones's "tender points."
• CS has widespread indications for symptomatic relief, and few contraindications are associated with this passive, indirect technique. If used correctly, CS often allows a patient to begin an active back treatment program earlier than would otherwise be possible, and can even be effectively incorporated into a patient's home treatment program.

Other Functional Techniques (p. 421)
• Other functional techniques also involve the evaluation and treatment of the quality of motion instead of the range of motion. Functional techniques are theoretically a part of the neurological model and can be used in both acute and chronic problems because they are not painful and depend on a release of soft tissue rather than a structural change.

Myofascial Release (p. 421)
• Myofascial release treats the neuromuscular-somatic unit as a whole, combining soft tissue, ME, and craniosacral principles. Each of the techniques uses

a combination of manual traction and twisting maneuvers to achieve tension on the soft tissues, aiming to effect biomechanical and reflex changes.

Craniosacral Therapy (pp. 421–422)
• Craniosacral therapy is a manual medicine technique for diagnosis and treatment of the body by way of the primary respiratory mechanism. It was pioneered by Sutherland, who perceived that the cranial bones undergo subtle cyclical motion about the cranial sutures at a rate of 8 to 12 Hz.
• Craniosacral therapy consists of assessing the amplitude, rate, symmetry, and quality of the primary respiratory mechanism. Craniosacral therapy enjoys more hypothetical than hard scientific support.

Soft Tissue Techniques (p. 422)
• Soft tissue techniques can involve lateral stretching, linear stretching (see Fig. 20–9 in the Textbook), deep pressure (see Fig. 20–10 in the Textbook), traction, or any combination of these, directed at separating the origin and insertion of a muscle. Soft tissue techniques can be used for generalized treatment programs in people with chronic illnesses such as multiple sclerosis, hemiplegia, or any immobility syndrome.

Lymphatic Pump (pp. 422–423)
• The lymphatic pump is a soft tissue technique that utilizes the muscle forces and intrathoracic pressure changes to enhance lymphatic flow. Intermittent compression of the thoracic cage in a rhythmic fashion enhances the return of lymph through the thoracic inlet, which relieves vascular engorgement to allow resumption of normal tissue motion. Other lymphatic techniques can be similarly performed with repetitive movements of the arms or legs. These techniques are often performed distal-to-proximal, similar to the centripetal massage techniques used to relieve edema in the extremities.

Contraindications and Risks (pp. 423–424)
• Mobilization with impulse (HVLA) has the greatest number of absolute contraindications (Table 20–3). Soft tissue, muscle energy, counterstrain, and myofascial release techniques have few contraindications because they have a much lower inherent risk to the patient than HVLA thrusting techniques.
• There are a few general precautions to be followed for all manual medicine techniques for safety and effectiveness. Neck positioning is important, especially in elderly patients. Prolonged neck extension should be avoided because of the risk of potential vertebral artery abnormalities and the possibility of irritating arthritic facet joints or compromising cervical nerve roots.
• Prolonged, extreme neck rotation can be dangerous in patients with carotid artery disease. Many practitioners use an extension-rotation test of the neck to try to determine clinical safety before treatment, but this test has not been validated as a useful screening tool.
• All levels of the spine should be carefully positioned in persons with significant osteoporosis because marked or prolonged flexion can lead to compression fractures (see Chapter 41). Extension should be limited in patients with lumbar stenosis (see Chapter 40). With all techniques, the patient must be kept relaxed and breathing freely to avoid excessive changes in blood pressure, as well as increased intra-abdominal or spinal canal pressure.

TABLE 20–3 Contraindications for High-Velocity Manipulation Techniques

Unstable fractures	Hypermobile joints
Severe osteoporosis	Rheumatoid arthritis
Multiple myeloma	Inflammatory phase of ankylosing spondylitis
Osteomyelitis	Psoriatic arthritis
Primary bone tumors	Reiter's syndrome
Paget's disease	Anticoagulant therapy
Any progressive neurological deficit	Congenital bleeding disorder
Spinal cord tumors	Acquired bleeding disorder
Cauda equina compression	Inadequate physical and spinal examination
Central cervical intervertebral disk herniation	Poor manipulative skills

From Haldeman S: Spinal manipulative therapy in the management of low back pain. *In* Finneson BE (ed): Low Back Pain. Philadelphia, JB Lippincott, 1980, p. 250.

- There are potential side effects that can occur even when manual medicine treatment is successful, including increased autonomic effects (e.g., hypotension, increased menses, and perspiration) and a transient increase in discomfort. Catastrophic outcomes have been reported (e.g., stroke, myelopathy, quadriplegia, cauda equina syndrome, cardiac arrest, and even death), mostly the result of manipulation of the cervical spine with improper technique or misdiagnosis or both. These cases provide the basis for most arguments against the use of manual medicine; however, their frequency is low, at just one case per 1 to 1.5 million manipulations.
- Although some practitioners advocate manipulative procedures in the presence of an acute spondylolisthesis or a disk herniation with radiculopathy, the general guideline is to not use thrusting techniques at that particular level (unless in the hands of a highly trained practitioner). Nonthrusting techniques are typically preferred in these cases and are safely performed at nearby levels with dysfunction.

Using Manual Medicine in Practice (pp. 424–425)

- Greenman has proposed a 12-step examination to screen for structural abnormalities, many of which are already done in a routine physiatric examination (see Table 20–2). Asymmetry of the shoulders, scoliosis, asymmetry at the lumbosacral junction, joint dysfunction in the legs, and leg length differences influence the overall motion, loading, and forces of the spine and the lower extremities. This can lead to impaired functional activities or pain complaints.
- One goal of the musculoskeletal examination is to determine whether there is a structural or pathophysiological abnormality present that is treatable. Somatic dysfunction is just one of many things that must be assessed; if present, it can easily be treated during the same office visit.
- Treatment plans for all types of manual medicine must be developed on an individual basis in relation to the patient's structural diagnosis, the type and location of the somatic dysfunction, the type of manual medicine techniques being performed, and the patient's response to treatment. With each patient visit, the practitioner must re-evaluate these parameters to determine the need for continued manipulative treatment. Clearly, if the patient receives no measurable benefit

after 2 to 4 weeks of treatment (6 to 8 visits), the underlying diagnosis must be reconsidered.

TRACTION (pp. 425–430)
Traction: Definition and Goals (pp. 425–426)

• Traction uses a pulling force to stretch soft tissues and to separate joint surfaces or bone fragments. The force is generally applied through a mechanical pulley system with weights, and stabilization by either a chin strap for the cervical spine (Fig. 20–2) or a pelvic belt for the lumbar spine (Fig. 20–3). The various techniques can be performed in standing, sitting, or lying positions.

History (pp. 426–427)

• Traction can be used in conjunction with other forms of conservative treatment of low back and neck pain to improve symptomatic outcome, but evidence of long-term benefit remains scanty.

Indications and Goals of Treatment (p. 427)

• It is generally held that any condition involving irritation or compression of nerve roots—whether related to trauma, a degenerative process, or compression from the disk—can benefit from a trial of traction. It is most often used for neck or arm pain secondary to cervical nerve root compromise or radiculopathy and low back pain from lumbar radiculopathy.
• Traction has been shown to (1) enlarge intervertebral foramina, (2) separate apophyseal joints, (3) stretch muscles and ligaments, (4) tighten the posterior longitudinal ligament to exert a centripetal force on the adjacent annulus fibrosus, and (5) enlarge the intervertebral space (possibly producing a suction effect on the disk). Traction is theoretically indicated for any condition that could benefit from these anatomical changes.

Types of Traction (pp. 428–429)

• There are several different methods of delivering traction to a patient. These include manual, mechanized, motorized or hydraulic, special tables (see Figs. 20–14 and 20–15 in the Textbook), and inversion methods. All types of treatment, though, must overcome the body's surface resistance to traction, which is equal to about one-half of the weight of the body segment plus the resistance of the involved soft tissues.
• *Continuous* traction uses a low force over a long period, say, 20 to 40 hours. This is hard for many patients to tolerate, and any change in the patient's position can change the direction of the pull. It is often used in spinal traction for the low back, mostly to ensure that a person remains at rest, or for orthopedic uses other than for the spine.
• *Sustained* traction uses force greater than that used in continuous traction, but less than that in intermittent. The pull is maintained for 20 to 60 minutes. This is still difficult to tolerate if too much force is used. Sustained traction is more practical, time-wise, for therapy departments. Sustained traction treatments can be given at varying frequencies, although it is common practice to treat inpatients daily and outpatients three times per week.

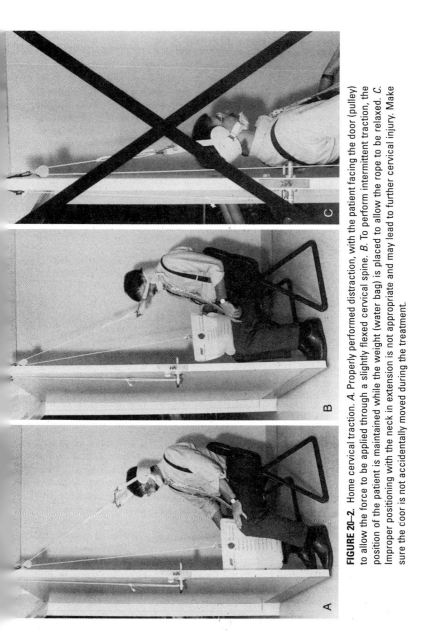

FIGURE 20–2. Home cervical traction. *A.* Properly performed distraction, with the patient facing the door (pulley) to allow the force to be applied through a slightly flexed cervical spine. *B.* To perform intermittent traction, the position of the patient is maintained while the weight (water bag) is placed to allow the rope to be relaxed. *C.* Improper positioning with the neck in extension is not appropriate and may lead to further cervical injury. Make sure the coor is not accidentally moved during the treatment.

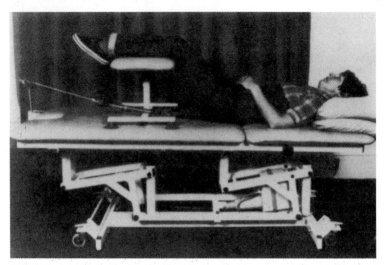

FIGURE 20–3. Motorized lumbar traction with patient in a supine position with hips and knees flexed. The distractive force is directed through the pelvic belt, while the upper belt stabilizes the patient. (From Grieve GP: Mobilisation of the Spine, ed 5. New York, Churchill Livingstone, 1991, p. 261.)

• *Intermittent* traction techniques allow for the use of greater forces, but for a shorter period. The force is gradually increased and decreased during each treatment cycle, and can be administered by pulley or motorized system. The duration can be adjusted, and can be on a timed, rhythmic schedule; or controlled manually by the patient. For a preprogrammed treatment protocol, the time sequences can vary from as little as 7 to 10 seconds of tractive force with a 5-second rest, up to 30 to 60 seconds of tractive force followed by 10 to 15 seconds of rest. The on-off cycle is repeated for 15 to 25 minutes. The patient-controlled protocol is based more on tolerance, with the amount of time with a tractive force and resting variable for each sequence depending on that patient's tolerance. Intermittent traction is used in the cervical region to allow the use of progressively higher forces (up to 50 lb), which increases vertebral separation.

Cervical Traction (pp. 428–429)
• Cervical traction is most commonly administered by a manual force (often with manipulation) or with the use of a head or chin sling by a mechanized or motorized force (see Fig. 20–2). The best clinical relief reportedly occurs between 20 and 30 degrees of cervical flexion. The most common reason clinically for cervical traction to either fail or to exacerbate symptoms is applying the force in extension rather than flexion.
• The optimal force for cervical traction varies depending on the method of delivery. At least 10 lb of force is necessary to counter the effects of gravity on the head, whereas 25 lb of force is necessary to provide straightening of the cervical lordotic curve and the earliest separation of posterior vertebral segments. Several studies have shown that larger forces definitely cause more separation,

but higher forces cannot always be tolerated by patients. When tolerated, the longer a constant force can be applied, the greater the separation.
• The maximum separation occurs anteriorly at C4 to C5 after 25 minutes and posteriorly at C6 to C7 after 20 minutes. The distraction effect is short-lived, because 20 minutes after traction there is no evidence of posterior separation.
• The pulley systems and motorized instruments can be used in either the sitting or the supine position (see Fig. 20–11 in the Textbook).
• When a patient is noted to be benefiting from cervical traction, it can be performed with a home over-the-door unit as long as the correct angle for pull is maintained (see Fig. 20–2). The patient should always be facing the door to which the pulley is attached. There are newer inflatable collar units and supine posterior distraction units that are more expensive than the standard over-the-door units (see Fig. 20–13 in the Textbook). These alternative devices are indicated primarily when the head sling cannot be tolerated because of temporomandibular joint syndrome or headaches. Patients using traction at home should never be alone because someone might need to assist them if any untoward effects arise.

Lumbar Traction (p. 429)

• Lumbar traction that provides vertebral separation requires significantly larger forces than cervical traction to overcome the body's resistance. Pelvic belts (see Fig. 20–3) or the use of gravity by tilting (see Fig. 20–15 in the Textbook) or inversion are necessary to deliver sufficient tractive force to the lumbar spine. Because of the large amount of weight necessary to overcome the body's resistance in this area, either a thoracic or chest belt or a corset is necessary to hold the upper body in place during distraction of the lower body. These chest harnesses are often uncomfortable and can limit breathing and venous return, affecting a patient's cardiovascular status.
• Lumbar traction can be delivered by continuous, sustained, intermittent, or pulsed intermittent methods. Several studies have shown that the larger the force, the greater the vertebral separation; but these high forces (e.g., 300 to 400 lb) have to be delivered intermittently for patients to tolerate them. The use of sustained delivery methods with less weight (e.g., 40, 50, 80, 100, and 132 lb) becomes more effective when surface resistance is reduced by increasing lumbar flexion, using a Scott traction frame or a standing technique.
• Split-traction tables have a mobile half and a stationary half. Because the force necessary to overcome surface resistance is reduced, treatment can be provided with as little as 80 to 150 lb rather than 300 to 400 lb. Optimal treatment frequency and duration have not yet been established.
• The autotraction table allows both sections of the table to move, which induces rotational and side bending forces into the spine. It has been shown that pain relief is quicker with the lumbar spine in flexion, and Colachis and Strohm found that, with the hips flexed to 70 degrees, an angle of pull of 18 degrees provided the greatest vertebral separation.
• The duration of beneficial treatment varies with the amount of force used; but even in studies showing a strong clinical benefit, there is no evidence of residual effect following removal of the tractive force.

Contraindications and Risks (pp. 429–430)

• Absolute contraindications to traction are listed in Table 20–4.

TABLE 20–4 Contraindications to Traction

General	Cervical
Osteomyelitis or discitis	Central intervertebral disk herniation
Primary bone tumor or spinal cord tumor	Hypermobile joints
Unstable fracture	Rheumatoid arthritis
Severe osteoporosis	Carotid or vertebral artery disease
Hypertension	Lumbar
Cardiovascular disease	Pregnancy
Inadequate expertise	Cauda equina compression

- In the cervical region, midline disk herniation is also a contraindication because traction could pull the cord into contact with the disk. Traction should be used with caution in all elderly patients, and should not be used in those with evidence of significant carotid or vertebral artery disease. Most clinicians recommend that no one should have a trial of traction unless x-rays have ruled out instability, infection, and other contraindications. Lumbar traction should be performed with caution in persons with abdominal problems (e.g., peptic ulcer and hiatal or other hernias), aortic aneurysm, or hemorrhoids. Patients with neurogenic bladder related to nerve root entrapment should not receive lumbar traction.
- Inversion traction involves more risk than standard traction because it can increase systolic and diastolic blood pressure; decrease heart rate; and cause persistent blurred vision, persistent headaches, and periorbital/pharyngeal petechiae. Because the center of gravity in adults is at the vertebral level of S2, there is a greater force across the lumbar disks if the patient is hanging upright.
- Traction of any type should be discontinued in those who experience nausea, dizziness, exacerbation of temporomandibular joint dysfunction, or increased pain in the soft tissues of the neck.

Using Traction in Practice (p. 430)

- In clinical practice, traction is used most often for patients who present with signs and symptoms of cervical radiculopathy. It can be used as both a diagnostic and treatment tool because patients with nerve root compression often receive benefit, whereas patients with soft tissue or myofascial pain commonly have an exacerbation of symptoms. The limiting factor for successful cervical traction treatment is often the amount of weight the patient can tolerate. Manual traction during the examination can give an initial indication whether a patient can tolerate cervical traction. Another benefit of cervical traction is that it can potentially be used at home, but initial instruction and testing of a home unit should always be done under the supervision of a physician or physical therapist.
- Aggressive nonoperative low back programs for either soft tissue or radicular symptoms have not typically found lumbar traction necessary, although it can be effective within the framework of a comprehensive treatment program. It has been combined empirically with other modalities such as heat, cold, massage, and electrical treatments; but there are, as yet, no studies proving that such combinations improve clinical outcomes.

MASSAGE (pp. 430–435)

Massage: Definition (p. 430)

- In 1884, Graham defined massage as "a group of procedures which are usually done with the hands, such as friction, kneading, rolling, and percussion of the external tissues of the body in a variety of ways, either with a curative, palliative, or hygienic object in view."

Indications and Goals of Treatment (pp. 431–433)

- There are mechanical, reflex, neurological, and psychological effects of massage. The goals of treatment can include sedation, adhesion reduction (see Figs. 20–9 and 20–10 in the Textbook), fluid mobilization, muscular relaxation, and vascular changes. Massage can be useful with any diagnoses in which mobilization of tissues, relief of muscle hypertonicity, relief of discomfort, or reduction of swelling would benefit the patient.
- Deep continuous stroking of an extremity from distal to proximal compresses the low-pressure vasculature and augments venous return. Edema is alleviated by massage-induced increase in tissue hydrostatic pressure.
- Massage clearly has temporary effects on cutaneous blood flow. This can be readily observed by the hyperemia of the skin after vigorous cutaneous stimulation or the increased prominence of superficial veins. Mechanical stimulation of mast cells in the skin causes release of histamine. Local histamine release causes the triple response of redness, flare, and then wheal formation at the site of cutaneous stimulation. Autonomic neurological reflex changes are also probably involved.
- Massage can be used as a substitute for muscular contractions to augment venous and lymphatic flow in patients who are immobile. Retrograde massage is commonly used to control the edema seen with hemiparesis after stroke or reflex sympathetic dystrophy, or following axillary node dissection.
- Deep massage also has mechanical effects on fascia and connective tissue. Deep friction massage can, for example, be used to treat shoulder hypomobility secondary to myofascial and tendinous restrictions. Deep friction massage can result in an immediate increase in shoulder mobility and decrease in pain by easing fascial restrictions.
- Massage has also been shown to improve myofascial flexibility. Although it does not increase strength, massage can aid in developing strength by enabling more exercise with decreased probability of injury. Massage does not, however, stimulate the metabolism of fat, as health spas once maintained.
- Many massage strokes do not necessarily mobilize fluids, release myofascial restrictions, or initiate reflex neurological effects. These strokes are comforting and relaxing and have their greatest effect on the psychological health of the patient.
- Patients with low back pain, neck pain, fibromyalgia, arthritis, bursitis, tendinitis, fascitis, and even neuromas can benefit from massage techniques. Complications associated with multiple sclerosis; cerebral palsy; hemiplegia; or with spinal cord injury (e.g., spasticity, reflex sympathetic dystrophy, edema, and contracture) can also be significantly improved. Specific techniques for respiratory problems can help persons with respiratory muscle paralysis. Limited use with varicose ulcers, localized draining infections, and following skin grafting has been reported. Light massage with a lubricant can be useful on a recent skin

graft. Deeper massage techniques can be beneficial later after skin grafting to prevent or model scar tissue. Massage can also release deep scar adhesions and contracture following amputations to improve prosthetic fit and comfort.

Types of Massage (pp. 433–435)

• The most commonly accepted types of hand movements used in therapeutic massage are from the Swedish system. The four basic stroke types are called (1) effleurage, (2) petrissage, (3) friction, and (4) tapotement (Fig. 20–4).

Effleurage (p. 433)
• Effleurage, or stroking massage, involves lightly running the hand over the skin. Effleurage is especially effective in assisting return of venous or lymphatic drainage, such as following joint sprains; peripheral muscle strains or bruising; and vascular congestion related to surgery, peripheral vascular disease, or reflex sympathetic dystrophy.

Petrissage (p. 433)
• Petrissage, or compression massage, includes *kneading, picking up, wringing, rolling,* and *shaking.* The common characteristic is the compression of the body's soft tissues between two hands or between the hand and the underlying skeletal tissue. These techniques are designed to mobilize fluid and tissue deposits, as well as to break up tissue and muscle adhesions.

Friction Massage (p. 433)
• Friction massage is performed by applying circular or transverse motions through the fingers, thumb, or the heel of the palm of the hand to a small area of tissue. Deep friction can be uncomfortable and even cause mild bruising, but it is especially effective for soft tissue problems such as tendinitis or fascitis (e.g., lateral epicondylitis, supraspinatus tendinitis, subacromial bursitis, and plantar fascitis) and trigger points as described by Travell.

Tapotement (p. 433)
• Tapotement, or percussion massage, produces stimulation by rhythmic, alternating movements of the hands on the soft tissue of the patient. *Clapping, hacking, vibrations, beating, pounding,* and *tapping* are all types of tapotement massage.
• There are many different styles of massage other than the commonly employed Swedish forms described above. Alternative techniques include acupressure, shiatsu, reflexology, Rolfing and its offshoots, Trager therapy, and lymphatic massage.

Acupressure (pp. 433–434)
• Acupressure is a technique of applying constant, circular friction pressure to specific points for treatment purposes. In acupressure, practitioners use their fingers, thumbs, or hands to stimulate these points by circular friction. Acupressure can be used as a nonpharmacologic technique to (1) control nausea and vomiting related to morning sickness, chemotherapy, spinal anesthesia, or postoperatively; (2) decrease postoperative pain; (3) treat headache and temporomandibular joint pain; or (4) assist with pulmonary rehabilitation.
• See page 434 in the Textbook for additional discussion of Shiatsu, Reflexology, Rolfing, and Trager Psychophysical Integration.

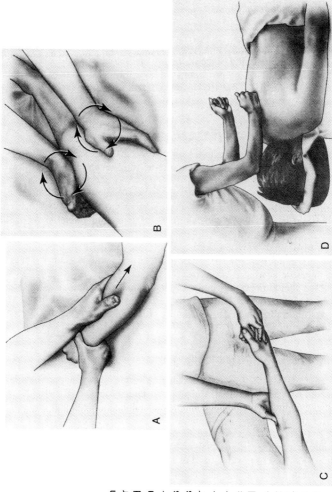

FIGURE 20–4. The common Swedish massage techniques. *A.* Effleurage or gliding strokes cover a large area, and generally go from distal to proximal with light strokes. *B.* Pettrissage or compression involves movement of deeper tissues in a nonlocalized area. *C.* Friction involves the practitioner using the thumb or fingers in a small area to go from superficial tissue to deeper layers. *D.* Tapotement or percussion involves rhythmic alternating movements of the hands and may be used as superficial or deep tissue. (From Loving, JE: Massage Therapy: Theory and Practice. Stamford, CT, McGraw-Hill, 1999, pp. 83, 86, 89, 90. Reproduced with permission of The McGraw-Hill Companies.)

Lymphatic Massage (p. 435)

• Gentle manual pressure is used to encourage lymph flow from obstructed to unobstructed lymph nodal areas. Usually, treatment consists of skin care followed by manual treatment, bandaging, use of compression garments, and exercises aimed at maintaining range of motion and muscle strength and tone. This end reduction in limb volume compares favorably with sequential pneumatic compression, and its popularity in the United States is increasing for postmastectomy arm lymphedema and postinguinal node resection leg lymphedema.

Contraindications and Risks (p. 435)

• There are numerous contraindications to Swedish massage, but the absolute and relative contraindications for acupressure, shiatsu, and reflexology have not been determined.

• Massage should not be performed over areas of malignancy, cellulitis, or lymphangitis. The effects of massage on mobilizing vascular and lymphatic fluid may only serve to disseminate tumor cells or spread infection. Areas of recent trauma or bleeding can re-bleed if massage is applied too soon after injury or surgery. Massage is commonly used to increase elasticity and mobility in scar tissues, but caution should be taken not to disrupt the incision by beginning massage before healing is complete.

• Massage should not be applied over an area of known deep venous thrombosis or over a known atherosclerotic plaque. Deep massage might dislodge venous or arterial thrombi, which can potentially cause pulmonary, cerebral, or peripheral embolic infarcts.

Using Massage in Practice (p. 435)

• Because massage is a passive modality, any massage technique must be supplemented with an active treatment program at the proper time. During the initial stages after a fracture or dislocation, tissue mobilization and soft tissue stretching without joint or bone movement is beneficial. Other diagnoses for which massage is commonly prescribed (e.g., lumbar sprain or strain, cervical sprain or strain, fibrositis or fibromyalgia, supraspinatus tendinitis, and lateral epicondylitis) should have some form of active range-of-motion program started at the time of initial treatment, and should eventually be progressed into a strengthening program when appropriate.

• For a few disorders such as postmastectomy lymphedema, rheumatoid joints, COPD, and headaches, massage can be considered for isolated use. Prescription for treatment should include the diagnosis, area of concentration, goals, precautions, and number of visits necessary for a particular patient complaint.

• The basic principles of massage treatment are as follows: (1) the patient must be comfortable, relaxed and not too cold; (2) the therapist must be comfortable and able to complete the technique without shifting position; (3) the therapist should have clean hands, short nails, and no areas of broken skin; (4) the use of lubricants can facilitate ease of techniques; and (5) the skill of the practitioner lies more in the ability to distribute even pressures throughout the hands rather than in strength.

21

Original Chapter by David C. Weber, M.D., and Allen W. Brown, M.D.

Physical Agent Modalities

- Physical agents can be utilized to produce a therapeutic response in tissue. These agents include heat, cold, water, sound, electricity, and electromagnetic waves. These agents are generally considered adjunctive treatments rather than primary curative interventions.

MODALITY PRESCRIPTION (p. 440)

- The prescription should include the condition/indication, modality, location, intensity, duration, and frequency.
- Most modalities allow only qualitative dosimetry and rely on patient perception of thermal intensity for safety. Duration is usually 20 to 30 minutes, except for ultrasound, which is typically 5 to 10 minutes per site.
- Modality selection (Table 21–1) is influenced by many factors including condition, location, body habitus, co-morbid conditions, age, and gender (e.g., fetal malformations with gravid uterus).

HEAT (pp. 441–443)

- Heat is classified by depth of penetration (e.g., superficial and deep) and form of heat transfer (e.g., conduction, convection, radiation, and evaporation). Superficial heat includes hot packs, heating pads, paraffin baths, fluidotherapy, whirlpool baths, and radiant heat. Deep heating agents (diathermies) include US, shortwave, and microwave.

Physiological Effects of Heat (pp. 441–443)

Hemodynamic (pp. 441–442)
- Localized heating can produce a two- to threefold increase in forearm blood flow following hydrotherapy at 45 °C or with shortwave diathermy. The vasodilation results in ingress of nutrients, leukocytes, and antibodies, and egress of metabolic byproduct and tissue debris. This can facilitate resolution of inflammation. It can also increase bleeding and edema exacerbating acute inflammation. Acute inflammation generally responds unfavorably to heat, whereas chronic inflammatory conditions tend to have favorable response (Table 21–2).

TABLE 21-1 Factors to Consider in Modality Selection

Target tissue
Depth of heating or cooling desired
Intensity of heating or cooling desired
Body habitus (e.g., amount of subcutaneous adipose)
Co-morbid conditions (e.g., cancer, vascular disease, neuropathy)
Specific patient features (e.g., metal implants, pacemaker, cold allergy)
Age (e.g., open epiphyses)
Sex (e.g., pregnant female)

Neuromuscular (p. 442)
• Heating produces a modest increase in nerve conduction velocity. Heat also possibly produces increased firing rates of group IA, IB fibers with a decreased firing rate of group II fibers.

Joint and Connective Tissue (p. 442)
• Heat can result in increased tendon extensibility, especially when used in conjunction with stretching. Decreased joint stiffness and increase in collagenase activity has been reported with the use of heat. Temperature also affects enzymatic activity because collagenase activity can increase fourfold with a temperature increase from 33 °C to 36 °C.

Miscellaneous Effects of Heat (pp. 442–443)
• Analgesia is a major effect of heat, and the postulated mechanisms for analgesia include: (1) cutaneous counterirritant effect; (2) vasodilation with decreased ischemic pain and washout of pain mediators; (3) endorphin response;

TABLE 21-2 Physiological Effects of Heat

Hemodynamic
    Increased blood flow
    Decreased chronic inflammation
    Increased acute inflammation
    Increased edema
    Increased bleeding
Neuromuscular
    ?Increased group Ia fiber firing rates (muscle spindle)
    ?Decreased group II fiber firing rates (muscle spindle)
    ?Increased group Ib fiber firing rates (Golgi tendon organ)
    Increased nerve conduction velocity
Joint and connective tissue
    Increased tendon extensibility
    Increased collagenase activity
    Decreased joint stiffness
Miscellaneous
    Decreased pain
    General relaxation

TABLE 21–3 General Uses of Heat in Physical Medicine

Musculoskeletal conditions (e.g., tendinitis, tenosynovitis, bursitis, capsulitis)
Pain (e.g., neck, low back, myofascial, neuromas, postherpetic neuralgia)
Arthritis
Contracture
Muscle relaxation
Chronic inflammation

(4) alteration of nerve conduction and cell membrane permeability; and (5) general relaxation effect.

General Uses of Heat in Physical Medicine (p. 443)

• The general uses of heat are summarized in Table 21–3. Therapeutic uses include gaining musculoskeletal benefits from analgesia, muscle relaxation, inflammation resolution, increased soft tissue extensibility, and joint stiffness.

General Precautions for the Use of Heat (p. 443)

• Heat can exacerbate acute inflammation and should be avoided in the acute management stage. In vascular disease, increased metabolic demands may exceed arterial supply causing ischemia. Patients with bleeding diatheses respond with increased bleeding. Care must be taken with scars because avascular tissue does not dissipate heat easily.
• Heat should be avoided in patients with impaired sensation, cognition, or communication because these patients' deficits preclude them from reporting pain causing thermal injury.
• Heat should be avoided near malignancy because of potential hyperemia and tumor growth (this does not preclude its use for analgesia in the terminally ill patient).

SUPERFICIAL HEAT (pp. 443–445)

• Superficial agents achieve their maximum temperature in the skin and subcutaneous fat. Superficial heat is used in arthritides, neck and back pain, muscle pain syndromes, and among other musculoskeletal conditions.

Hot Packs (p. 443)

• Commercially available hot packs (e.g., Hydrocollator packs) come in a variety of sizes. They are made of silicon dioxide that is encased in a canvas pack. The pack is immersed in water at 74.3 °C and applied over several layers of insulating towels. The skin must be checked briefly after a few minutes to ensure heating is not excessive. The typical treatment time is 30 minutes. Patient should not lie on the pack because this may cause overheating of the skin and, especially, of bony prominences. Sedation or somnolence is a relative contraindication to hot packs because patients are less likely to notice overheating that can lead to a burn.

Heating Pads (pp. 443–444)

• There are two main types of heating pads, the electric and the circulating-fluid pads. Electric pads may have periodic temperature oscillations and the potential for electric shock (especially when moisture is present). Inspect the insulating material regularly. As with hot packs, the patient should not lie directly on them. Close attention is especially needed for slender or cachectic patients with minimal adipose over bony prominences. Repeated and prolonged exposure can lead to *erythema ab igne,* characterized by reticular pigmentation and telangiectasia.

Radiant Heat (p. 444)

• Infrared heat lamps produce heat by inducing molecular vibration. Main determinants of intensity are distance and angle of delivery. The Inverse Square Law denotes that the intensity of radiation varies inversely with the square of the distance from the source. Maximal radiation is applied when the source is perpendicular to the surface. Typical distances used are 30 to 60 cm. Radiant heat is often preferable in patients who cannot tolerate the weight of heat packs. Precautions include general precautions, light sensitivity, skin drying, and dermal photoaging. There is a potential synergistic effect with UV radiation in terms of photocarcinogenesis.

Fluidotherapy (pp. 444–445)

• Fluidotherapy is a superficial, dry heating modality with convective heating using forced hot air (46.1 °C to 48.9 °C) and a bed of finely divided particles (solid-gas system). Advantages of this fluidization modality include a massaging action and the ability to perform range of motion exercises. The temperature and the level of agitation can be adjusted. Infected wounds should be avoided because of the risk of cross contamination.

Paraffin Baths (p. 445)

• Paraffin baths are done in a mixture of paraffin wax and mineral oil in the ratio of 6:1 to 7:1. The temperature used is 52.2 °C to 54.4 °C. This high temperature can be tolerated because of the low heat conductivity of mixture. A thermometer should be used to monitor the temperature. A thin film on the wall of the tank generally indicates that the temperature is in the safe range. Methods used include dipping, immersion, and brushing. Dipping 7 to 12 times in the paraffin, followed by wrapping in plastic or towels to retain the heat, is a popular technique. Immersion involves a doing a few dips to form a paraffin glove, followed by immersion in the paraffin mixture for 30 minutes. Brushing the paraffin on the skin is used when the area being treated is too difficult to immerse. Children find the brushing technique to be fun and prefer it. Double boilers and tanks are available for home use. Avoid the use of paraffin for heat if there is an open wound or active infection.

DEEP HEAT (pp. 445–449)

• Diathermy refers to several forms of deep heating including shortwave, microwave, and ultrasound. The target tissue being heated is generally muscle, tendon, ligament, or bone (rather than skin or adipose tissue). Therapeutic target temperature is considered to be 40 °C to 45 °C. Thermal pain threshold is approximately 45 °C, and therefore pain perception may be used to monitor the intensity, assuming that the patient has normal sensation and normal cognition. Unfortunately, there is a fine line between therapeutic temperature and the point at which there can be thermal injury.

Ultrasound (pp. 445–448)

• Therapeutic ultrasound (US) uses high-frequency acoustic energy to produce thermal and nonthermal effects in tissue. As waves travel through tissue, energy of the sound wave is lost to absorption, deflection, and beam interference in a process called attenuation. Attenuation of the sound beam increases as frequency increases. Divergence decreases as frequency increases. Beam deflection is the process of reflection, refraction, and scattering. Mismatch of acoustic impedance of any two media leads to an increase in the reflected wave. Because mismatch between air and tissue is high, a coupling agent is needed for the wave to penetrate to deeper tissues (see Fig. 21–5 in the Textbook). Constructive interference of the source and reflected waves generate focal heat at bone-soft tissue interface.

• Ultrasound parameters are listed in Table 21–7 in the Textbook. Clinical US frequency is typically 0.8 to 1.1 MHz. US intensity is measured in watts/cm^2. The usual clinical dose is in the range of 0.5 to 2.0 W/cm^2. Temperatures of up to 46 °C at bone-muscle interface are easily achieved with US.

• US delivery can be in pulsed or continuous form. Pulsed results in less heating, and presumably emphasizes nonthermal effects of US. Nonthermal effects of US include cavitation, media motion, and the formation of standing waves.

• Cavitation is the production of gas bubbles, which can be stable (bubbles oscillate), or unstable (grow and collapse). US can produce platelet aggregation, localized tissue damage, and cell death. Using a stroking technique can minimize these effects, as does using higher frequency, lower intensity, and pulsed delivery mode.

• Media motion includes microstreaming and acoustic streaming. (See the Textbook for further information.)

• Standing waves are produced by superimposition of incident and reflected sound waves and can produce focal heat at tissue interfaces of different densities. Stasis of red blood cells has been seen in vitro. The clinical significance of this and the untoward effects, if any, have yet to be clearly delineated. Stroking technique minimizes standing waves.

• Absorption by the media attenuates the sound wave. The impedance mismatch between transducer, medium, and the tissue should be minimized. Degassed water (allow tap water to stand overnight to remove air bubbles) is useful for irregular surfaces (treatment under water). Mineral oil and standard coupling gels have similar transmissivities. Hydrocortisone phonophoresis agents have significantly lower transmissivity. Encased silicon gel may be used for open wounds, irregular surfaces, and sensitive skin.

• Stroking technique allows for a more even energy distribution and avoids standing wave formation. This minimizes the risk of burns.

• US uses include a variety of musculoskeletal conditions including periarticular inflammatory conditions (e.g., bursitis, capsulitis, epicondylitis, and tendinitis) and chronic inflammatory conditions (e.g., rheumatoid arthritis,

TABLE 21–4 Ultrasound Precautions

General heat precautions	Malignancy
Near brain, eyes, reproductive organs	Skeletal immaturity
Gravid or menstruating uterus	Arthroplasties?
Near pacemaker	Methyl methacrylate or high-density polyethylene?
Near spine, laminectomy sites	

ankylosing spondylitis, nonspecific musculoskeletal pain, low back pain, adhesive capsulitis, and osteoarthritis).
• US precautions are listed in Table 21–4.

Shortwave Diathermy (p. 448)

• Shortwave diathermy (SD) accomplishes deep heating via conversion of electromagnetic energy to thermal energy. Oscillation of high frequency electrical and magnetic fields produces movement of particles with resultant heat generation. The Federal Communications Commission limits the commercially available frequencies for clinical purposes to 13.56 MHz, 27.12 MHz, and 40.68 MHz (with the 27.12 MHz most commonly used).
• SD can be either inductive or capacitive. Inductive applicators involve putting the patient in a magnetic field, which achieves higher temperatures in water-rich tissues than the capacitative method. Capacitative applicators may achieve higher temperatures in water-poor tissues such as bone and fat. Pain perception is used to monitor the intensity. Terrycloth towels are used for spacing and to absorb sweat (which is highly conductive and could result in severe focal heating). The depth of the patient's subcutaneous fat has a significant effect on the resulting temperature distribution.
• Typical SD treatment time is 20 to 30 minutes.
• SD can be used in a variety of musculoskeletal conditions. It is rarely used now in most physical therapy sites.
• Precautions include general heat precautions, and no metal can be in the field (e.g., jewelry, pacemaker, or IUD). Contact lenses, the gravid uterus, and skeletal immaturity are contraindications as well.

Microwave Diathermy (p. 449)

• Microwave diathermy uses electromagnetic energy through conversion as its primary form of heat production. Heat is produced by increasing the kinetic energy of molecules within the microwave field. The two commercially available frequencies are 915 MHz and 2456 MHz. The lower frequency has increased depth of penetration but greater beam dispersion and requires a larger applicator. In general, tissues with high water content absorb greater amounts of energy and are selectively heated. Microwave diathermy has largely been replaced over the past few decades by US and hot packs. Precautions include those for general heat use, as well as avoidance of metal implants, pacemakers, sites of skeletal immaturity, reproductive organs, brain, and fluid-filled cavities.

CRYOTHERAPY (pp. 449–451)

• All forms are superficial cooling agents (see Table 21–10 in the Textbook).

Physiologic Effects of Cold (See Table 21–5) (pp. 449–450)

Hemodynamic (pp. 449–450)
• Application of cold to the skin results in immediate cutaneous vasoconstriction followed by reactive vasodilation. Some have described temperature "hunting," with cycling of vasoconstriction and vasodilation and back again. Cryotherapy moderates inflammation and is more effective in the acute than chronic phase (Table 21–5).

Neuromuscular (p. 450)
• Cold has been shown to temporarily reduce spasticity in patients with hemiplegia and multiple sclerosis; however, increased spasticity has been shown as well in some patients.

Joint and Connective Tissue (p. 450)
• Decreases in intra-articular temperature in inflammatory arthropathies may slow the rate of collagenase activity. Potentially negative effects include decreased tendon extensibility and increased joint stiffness.

Miscellaneous Effects of Cold (p. 450)
• The analgesic effect of cold may be related to reflex muscle relaxation, cutaneous counterirritation, or its slowing of nerve conduction.

TABLE 21–5 Physiological Effects of Cold

Hemodynamic
  Immediate cutaneous vasoconstriction
  Delayed reactive vasodilation
  Decreased acute inflammation
Neuromuscular
  Slowing of conduction velocity
  Conduction block and axonal degeneration with prolonged exposure
  Decreased group Ia fiber firing rates (muscle spindle)
  Decreased group II fiber firing rates (muscle spindle)
  Decreased group Ib fiber firing rates (Golgi tendon organ)
  Decreased muscle stretch reflex amplitudes
  Increased maximal isometric strength
  Decreased muscle fatigue
  Temporarily reduced spasticity
Joint and connective tissue
  Increased joint stiffness
  Decreased tendon extensibility
  Decreased collagenase activity
Miscellaneous
  Decreased pain
  General relaxation

TABLE 21–6 General Uses of Cryotherapy in Physical Medicine

Musculoskeletal conditions (e.g., sprains, strains, tendinitis, tenosynovitis, bursitis, capsulitis)
Myofascial pain
Following certain orthopedic surgeries
Component of spasticity management
Emergent treatment of minor burns

General Uses of Cryotherapy in Physical Medicine (p. 450)
• Cold is most commonly used acutely after musculoskeletal injury to minimize formation of edema and for symptomatic relief in painful soft tissue and articular inflammatory states (Table 21–6).
• Cryotherapy in the form of ice water immersion is advocated as the primary treatment for minor burns.

General Precautions for the Use of Cold (pp. 450–451)

• The most common relative contraindication is cold intolerance (to be distinguished from true cold hypersensitivity, characterized by urticaria and angioedema). A patient with cold intolerance will have muscle guarding and co-contraction, both of which are counterproductive to therapeutic goals (Table 21–7).
• Caution should be exercised near peripheral nerves because peroneal and ulnar palsies have been reported.
• Ischemia can be precipitated by cold induced vasoconstriction in tissues with vascular compromise.
• As with heat, caution must be used in patients with sensory, cognitive, or communication deficits that preclude reporting of pain.
• Other contraindicated disorders include cryoglobulinemia (immune complex precipitation with cold), cryoglobulinemia (hemolysis secondary to cold induced antibody to red blood cells), cold hypersensitivity (urticaria and angioedema), Raynaud's disease (idiopathic arteriolar vasospasm induced by cold), and Raynaud's phenomenon (digital pallor and reactive hyperemia) associated with rheumatological diseases.

TABLE 21–7 General Precautions for the Use of Cold

Cold intolerance	Cryopathies
Cryotherapy-induced neurapraxia/axonotmesis	Cryoglobulinemia
Arterial insufficiency	Paroxysmal cold hemoglobinuria
Impaired sensation	Cold hypersensitivity
Cognitive or communication deficits that preclude reporting of pain	Raynaud's disease/phenomenon

Cryotherapy Agents (p. 451)

Cold Packs (p. 451)
• Cold packs include hydrocollator packs, endothermic reaction packs, and ice packs. Hydrocollator packs are cooled in a freezer to $-12\,°C$ and applied after being wrapped in a moist towel. Endothermic chemical gel packs have separate compartments that, when mixed, undergo endothermic reaction. They are portable and easy to use in the field. Ice packs are easy to use at home and may be applied with elastic bandage or tape. Duration is usually 20 to 30 minutes.

Ice Massage (p. 451)
• Ice massage is the direct application of ice to the skin using gentle stroking motions. It combines the therapeutic effects of cooling with the mechanical effects of massage. Water can be frozen in a paper cup, with the ice exposed by tearing the top rim of the paper off as the ice melts. It is generally used for localized symptoms, and is applied for 5 to 10 minutes per site depending on amount of subcutaneous adipose tissue. There is an initial perception of coolness followed by burning or aching, then hypesthesia and analgesia.

Cold Water Immersion (p. 451)
• This is best suited for circumferential cooling of the limbs, usually at 5 to $13\,°C$. It is often uncomfortable and poorly tolerated. It can be helpful as an emergency treatment for local burns, rapidly lowering the temperature of the skin.

Cryotherapy Compression Units (p. 451)
• Cryotherapy compression units consist of a cuff or boot through which cold water is circulated and can be pneumatically compressed statically or in serial distal to proximal pumping action. These units combine the beneficial effects of cold and compression. They are primarily used after acute musculoskeletal injury with soft tissue swelling and after some surgical procedures. The temperature is typically $45\,°C$ and the pressure is $60\,mm\,Hg$.

Vapocoolant Spray (p. 451)
• Spray-and-stretch methods are used to treat myofascial and musculoskeletal pain syndromes. This can be done using a series of unidirectional applications of Fluori-Methane spray. Begin in the "trigger area" (area of deep myofascial hypersensitivity) and extend the spray to "reference zone" (area of referred pain) while passively stretching the muscle. This is performed parallel to the muscle fibers at approximately 4 inches/second. Wait briefly between applications to help prevent skin freezing.

HYDROTHERAPY (pp. 451–452)

• Hydrotherapy is the external application of water for the treatment of disease. The most commonly used forms are whirlpool baths, Hubbard tank, shower cart, and contrast baths. The primary uses include arthritis, various musculoskeletal conditions, and in the cleansing and debridement of burns and other dermal injuries. Hydrotherapy can loosen adherent dressings to facilitate removal, allows for removal of antimicrobial cream prior to reapplication, and softens eschar to facilitate debridement.

Whirlpool Baths and Hubbard Tanks (p. 452)

• Whirlpool baths and Hubbard tanks control water temperature and agitate it by aeration. Whirlpool baths are typically used for treatment of limb or localized lesion. Because only a part of the body is immersed, greater extremes of temperature can be used without causing a significant change in core temperature. Hubbard Tanks are larger and generally used for whole-body immersion, so neutral temperatures (34 °C to 36 °C) should be used to prevent core temperature fluctuation. An immersed body experiences vertical antigravity force and decreased stress on bones and joints. This, along with therapeutic effects of water temperature, makes hydrotherapy an appropriate adjunctive treatment for cases of degenerative arthritis and acute musculoskeletal injury.

• Truly sterile conditions are not easily achieved in hydrotherapy. Sodium hypochlorite is the most commonly used antibacterial solution. For the Hubbard Tank, NaCl can be added to minimize fluid shifts. (Isotonic saline is 0.9% sodium chloride, or 900 g salt/100 L or 2 pounds of salt per 25 gallons.)

Shower Cart (p. 452)

• This allows for gentle spray during mechanical debridement of large surface area burns and other wound under relatively sterile conditions. The shower cart was developed to lessen the risk of contamination, as well as requiring less water, less space, less maintenance, and less risk of contamination as compared with the Hubbard tank.

Contrast Baths (p. 452)

• Contrast baths consist of alternating immersion of distal limbs in hot (42 °C to 45 °C) then cold (8.5 °C to 12.5 °C) water. The therapeutic effect is believed to be related to cyclic vasoconstriction and vasodilation. A 30-minute session is typically used. Begin with 10 minutes in hot water, followed by alternating 1 minute cold, 4 minutes hot, ending the session with cold to limit swelling. This may be beneficial in the treatment of rheumatological disease, neuropathic pain, or other chronic pain syndromes such as complex regional pain syndrome.

OTHER MODALITIES (pp. 452–455)

Ultraviolet (p. 452)

• The therapeutic use of ultraviolet is almost exclusively dermatological. The most common treatments utilize either UVA or UVB wavelengths. The Minimal Erythema Dose (MED) is the duration of exposure that produces only erythema. Traditionally used in the treatment of psoriasis, it can be efficacious in a number of other disorders. Potential adverse effects of ultraviolet include premature aging of skin, nonmelanoma skin cancers, and cataracts.

Iontophoresis (pp. 452–453)

• Iontophoresis is the migration of charged particles across biological membranes under an imposed electrical field. It is used in physical medicine to deliver medicines directly to soft tissues. It can also be used to deliver medicines systemically when other routes are not practical. The ionic solution to be iontophorized is placed on the electrode of the same polarity. The solution with the medicine is driven with direct current (10 to 30 mA) away from electrode into tissues. The quantity transported is dependent on the local current, duration of treatment, and solution concentration. Iontophoresis is commonly used to treat musculoskeletal conditions and generally well tolerated. Miliarisis has been reported while treating hyperhydrosis.

Phonophoresis (p. 453)

• This uses US to facilitate transdermal migration of topically administered medications. The most common medications are corticosteroids, which are believed to have synergistic anti-inflammatory effect with US. Standard US coupling gel is mixed with hydrocortisone or lidocaine. Proposed indications include osteoarthritis, bursitis, capsulitis, tendinitis, strains, fasciitis, epicondylitis, tenosynovitis, contracture, scar tissue, neuromas, and adhesions. The general US precautions apply.

Low-Energy Laser (p. 453)

• This typically delivers 90 mW and should be distinguished from higher-power lasers used surgically. There are no significant temperature changes, so the effects are likely nonthermal. There is no consensus on the indications or efficacy. It is not currently approved by the FDA for any therapeutic indication.

Interferential Current Therapy (pp. 453–455)

• Interferential current therapy (ICT) utilizes two alternating current signals of slightly different frequencies that are periodically in phase and out of phase (see Figs. 21–10, 21–11, and 21–12 in the Textbook). This periodic interference results in a new wave with cyclical modulation of amplitude producing a "beat frequency." IFC machines typically use medium-frequency currents of approximately 4000 to 5000 Hz, which can pass through tissue more easily than lower frequencies. ICT uses 2, 4, or 6 applicators that can be arranged in the same plane (planar), as in the lumbar region; or in different planes (coplanar), as in the shoulder.
• There are reported benefits of ICT in a variety of musculoskeletal conditions, neurological conditions, and in management of urinary incontinence. It should not be used near implanted stimulators (e.g., pacemakers, intrathecal pumps, and spinal cord stimulators). Vascular responses may occur when stimulation is done near sympathetic ganglia or the carotid sinus. Current concentration can occur near open incisions or abrasions. It should not be used near a gravid uterus. There is potential mechanical stimulation of thromboses with resultant precipitation of emboli. As with heat and cold, caution should be used in patients with sensory, cognitive, and communicative deficits precluding the adequate reporting of pain.

22

Original Chapter by W. Jerry Mysiw, M.D., and Rebecca D. Jackson, M.D.

Electrical Stimulation

PHYSIOLOGICAL EFFECTS OF NEUROMUSCULAR ELECTRICAL STIMULATION (pp. 459–463)

Response of Muscle Fibers to Electrical Stimulation (pp. 460–463)

• Following electrical stimulation of normal, fast-twitch skeletal muscles, a stereotypical series of events occurs resulting in transformation from fast-twitch type IIb fibers to a composition with slow-twitch type I characteristics (see Table 22–2 in the Textbook).

• Within 2 to 4 days of the onset of stimulation, changes in the sarcoplasmic reticulum result in a decrease in calcium sequestration and a reduction in calcium-buffering capacity. This functionally affects contractile properties, increasing the time to peak velocity within the first week. The isotonic twitch characteristics are unaltered during this early stage of transformation.

• Calcium-activated myosin ATPase activity begins to decline by 3 weeks. There are corresponding changes in myosin light chain (LC) patterns. If combined with stretch, there is a synergistic effect of mechanical and electrical forces leading to biochemical changes within 4 days. Asynchronous transformation from fast to slow type myosin subunits can lead to the coexistence of both slow and fast within a single muscle fiber (type IIc fibers).

• By 3 weeks after the onset of stimulation, tropomyosin changes from fast to slow type. Conversion of fiber type is completed within 8 weeks of initiation. This new type I muscle fiber composition is functionally associated with both an increase in resistance to fatigue and a decrease in the maximum velocity of shortening.

• The changes of fiber type are associated with changes in metabolic activity from use of an anaerobic/glycolytic pathway, to the aerobic/Krebs cycle pathway. These changes are also associated with increases in capillary density and oxygen consumption, which might be responsible for the development of increased resistance to fatigue. In addition to the increase in oxidative capacity, there is a suppression of enzymes involved in anaerobic glycogenolysis.

• Several studies have helped to confirm the applicability of some aspects of the data derived from animal models to the effects of electrical stimulation on human muscle in vivo.

• After discontinuation of electrical stimulation, the muscle fiber begins to transform to its prestimulation characteristics in a time course that reflects a "first in, last out" relationship. Within 6 weeks, the former fast-twitch muscle fiber regains its previous contractile behavior with a change in maximum velocity of contraction. A return to an anaerobic metabolic pathway is seen by 12 weeks. Capillary density changes are one of the last features to be modified and may be present for up to several months.

• Stimulation frequency for fiber transformation has also been a subject of intense investigation. If an equal number of stimuli is given per minute (short burst of high-frequency [40 Hz], or continuous low-frequency [10 Hz]), similar histochemical changes are found. Increase in *both* frequency and number of stimuli per minute dramatically affects the phenotypic expression of the muscle fiber.

• Electrical stimulation started within 24 hours of denervation results in a decrease in atrophy and maintenance of oxidative enzyme levels. Later initiation of electrical stimulation (e.g., 28 days postdenervation) retards atrophy and induces a hybrid fiber type with changes suggestive of both type I and type IIb fibers. Histological and biochemical data suggest that denervated muscles exhibit some properties of plasticity independent of neurological input.

WAVES (pp. 463–465)

• Three basic types of waveforms exist: direct current, alternating current, and pulsed current. Direct current is not applicable to FES systems. *Alternating current* refers to an uninterrupted bi-directional flow of charged particles that can be symmetrical or asymmetrical (Fig. 22–1). The pulsed waveforms are the most common waveforms applied for therapeutic purposes.

• A number of studies have been done to explore the impact of different waveforms and stimulation parameters on patient comfort, force of contraction, strengthening effect, and fatigue.

• Both burst-modulated alternating current and asymmetrical biphasic pulsed current appear to induce the most forceful contractions. No consensus exists as to which waveform provides the greatest patient comfort.

• The relationship between current amplitude (mA) and the force of muscle contraction is linear. Stimulation frequencies of 60 to 100 Hz are necessary to produce the most forceful muscle contraction; however, stimulation at these rates results in muscle fatigue and is associated with greater pain.

ELECTRODES (p. 465)

• The choice of an electrode type is based on the goal of the electrical stimulation program and its ease of use for the patient. Available types include surface, epimysial, intramuscular, juxtaneural, nerve cuff, epineural, intraneural, intrafascicular, and intraspinal.

• Surface electrodes remain the most commonly utilized electrode type for most FES therapeutic and functional interventions. Longitudinal placement and larger surface of electrodes produces increase in force of contraction. The larger surface electrodes also appear to cause less discomfort.

• Patient discomfort and lack of precision associated with surface stimulation are somewhat overcome with implanted electrode systems. Epimysial, intramuscular, and nerve cuff electrodes are the most common examples of implanted elec-

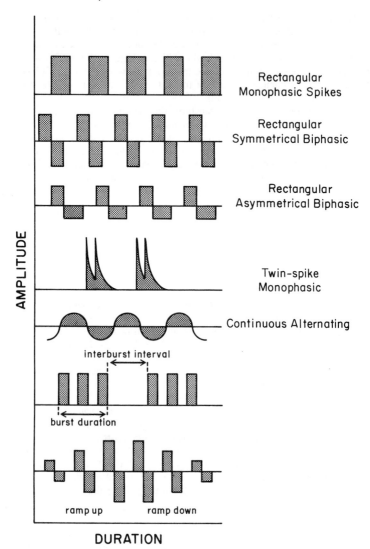

FIGURE 22–1. Diagrammatic representations of waveforms and modulations.

trodes. Use of percutaneous intramuscular electrodes has resulted in local tissue injury at the voltage necessary for maximal muscle contraction. This is somewhat avoided by inserting electrodes into multiple motor points of a muscle, with subsequent sequential or simultaneous stimulation at a lower voltage.

THERAPEUTIC NEUROMUSCULAR ELECTRICAL STIMULATION FOR MUSCLE STRENGTHENING
(pp. 466–471)

Stimulation of Normal Muscle (pp. 466–469)

• No data suggest that the use of neuromuscular electrical stimulation (NMES) in normal healthy muscle results in improvement in strength compared with that achieved by voluntary isometric exercise. Multiple studies have shown that similar gains in isometric muscle strength occur with both exercise regimens. When a combination of the two regimens was compared with either program alone, no significant augmentation was seen. Similarly, NMES can improve the endurance of muscle in sedentary humans, but not beyond the endurance noted in normal active adults.

• Maximal force depends on the degree of type II fiber activation. Selected augmentation of type II muscle fibers by NMES may lead to a greater increase in the overall strength of muscle at submaximal training intensity. Thus, NMES strengthening might offer specific advantages in training certain populations of individuals who have cardiovascular disease or other limitations that preclude training at higher workloads.

• Another potential benefit of NMES in normal muscle is in the prevention of muscle atrophy associated with prolonged immobilization. The benefit of NMES appears to be limited to the period of immobilization. By 12 weeks postsurgery (6 weeks after discontinuation of immobilization), no significant differences are seen between patients, nonexercise control, and NMES groups. NMES could be of greatest benefit in the treatment of individuals who desire a rapid return to maximal performance levels (e.g., elite athletes). It might be of little or no benefit in individuals who can afford delay in return to peak physical activity after the period of immobilization and reconditioning is complete.

• One final application of NMES in normal muscle is to help in evaluating the etiology of weakness in a patient. If a subject is volitionally attempting to maximally contract muscle, direct electrical stimulation of the muscle will not lead to a further increment in muscle force. If, however, the subject is not maximally trying (or if other forces contribute to a drop in volitional muscle force), electrical stimulation will lead to an increase in muscle force.

Stimulation of Myopathic Muscle (p. 469)

• There remains considerable controversy regarding the benefit of electrical stimulation in individuals with neuromuscular disease. When low-frequency electrical stimulation is applied to dystrophic muscle in children with muscular dystrophy, improvements occur in maximal voluntary contraction of the stimulated muscle. If, however, electrical stimulation is initiated after significant strength has already been lost, there appears to be no benefit from treatment. After discontinuation of NMES, strength gains are lost rapidly. It appears that if NMES is to be used for strengthening in neuromuscular disease, it is only of benefit in individuals who have retained more than 15% of normal strength, resulting in only a delay of the inevitable outcome.

Stimulation of Denervated Muscle (pp. 469–470)

• The therapeutic relevance of NMES in denervated muscle is predicated on the ability of the technique to prevent or reduce atrophy and to enhance reinnervation. Denervated muscle appears to have some plasticity, because NMES has been shown to facilitate the transformation from fast-twitch to slow-twitch fiber. This result has been associated with improved maintenance of muscle fiber area and muscle girth for a short time interval until reinnervation occurs. The data are mixed on the effect of initiating NMES late after denervation injury, with some studies demonstrating preservation of muscle fiber using unusually long duration stimulation.

• There are no data to support enhancement of reinnervation. In fact, a number of studies have suggested that stimulation inhibits terminal sprouting and reinnervation. The mechanism for this is unclear and appears to contradict experiments that show an increase in the trophic factor for axonal sprouting.

• In a denervated muscle, long-term NMES might be effective in improving functional outcome by preventing atrophy when reinnervation is expected over a long period, such as after a surgical nerve repair.

Stimulation of Decentralized Muscle (pp. 470–471)

• Electrical stimulation of muscle following CNS injury or SCI can result in reversal of the muscular atrophy associated with the relative immobilization associated with these disorders.

• Applications of NMES after cerebral vascular accident have, in general, been limited to use of NMES as an orthotic assist, rather than as a therapeutic adjunct to strengthening. NMES, however, has been used successfully in the small superficial muscles of the hand and wrist to improve strength and decrease atrophy. Modification of electrical stimulation parameters to achieve muscle fatigability is necessary, especially when spasticity and severe weakness can limit therapeutic gain.

• More attention has been paid to the use of NMES as a modality for rehabilitation of paralyzed muscle following SCI. Electrical stimulation in individuals with chronic SCI results in an increase in the proportion of type I fibers, oxidative capacity, endurance, muscle strength, and contractile properties. But it has no effect on the distribution of fiber sizes or mean fiber area.

• Increases in muscle strength and endurance are most dramatically seen when NMES is combined with resistance training or functional activities. Isometric quadriceps strengthening using NMES to move the knee through a 45-degree arc with increasing resistance has resulted in increases in quadriceps endurance and mass. The development of a functional electrical stimulation cycle ergometry system (FES-CE) has resulted in further therapeutic benefits. The system sequentially stimulates the quadriceps, hamstrings, and gluteal muscles to produce a smooth pedaling motion. Using FES-CE, several investigators have shown increases in thigh circumference, muscle strength and endurance, quadriceps muscle area, and quadriceps muscle protein synthesis rates with no change in whole body protein turnover.

• FES-CE can also affect overall body composition. Individuals with chronic SCI show gains in total lean body mass with a decrease in percent body fat. This has primarily been attributed to gains in the lower extremity lean body mass. Initiation of FES-CE within 3 months of acute SCI has been shown to prevent lower limb muscle atrophy after 3 months of training and to cause muscle hypertrophy after 6 months of training.

ELECTRICAL STIMULATION TO PREVENT COMPLICATIONS OF DISUSE (pp. 471–473)

Cardiovascular Deconditioning (p. 472)

• Within the first 3 months of SCI, a significant decline occurs in aerobic capacity. After discharge from rehabilitation, the workload of a paraplegic individual performing independent activities of daily living (ADL) is insufficient to maintain cardiovascular fitness. This cardiovascular deconditioning is even more pronounced in quadriplegic persons; however, it is not an inevitable consequence of SCI.

• Attention has turned toward the therapeutic use of NEMS as an intervention to improve cardiovascular fitness. Short-term training with FES-CE can produce an increase in both endurance and Vo_{2max}. FES-CE can also result in an improvement in the left ventricular mass of quadriplegic persons.

• A relative increase occurs in Vo_2, pulmonary ventilation, heart rate, and stroke volume following use of FES-CE. Greater increases are noted in paraplegic versus quadriplegic persons. The increase in Vo_2 is thought to be due to augmented blood flow to the exercised muscles. Despite low respiratory efficiency, prolonged training with FES-CE results in increases in blood pressure, heart rate, cardiac output, and Vo_{2max} that are linear with the metabolic demand on the muscle.

• In an attempt to increase the efficiency of cardiovascular training, studies have combined arm crank ergometry with lower extremity FES. Training with these hybrid systems has shown improved increments in Vo_2, minute ventilation, cardiac output, and stroke volume in comparison with arm crank ergometers or FES-CE alone. New approaches include the combination of FES quadriceps extension against 20 lb of resistance with arm crank ergometry at 50 rpm, FES-CE with voluntary arm crank ergometry, or FES-rowing.

• Additional long-term data are necessary to determine whether the short-term improvements in cardiopulmonary fitness can be maintained over long periods and whether they will have a substantial influence on cardiovascular morbidity and mortality.

Osteoporosis (pp. 472–473)

• One prominent metabolic consequence of SCI is a rapidly evolving osteopenia that is a permanent consequence of the injury.

• Recent work has supported a positive effect of FES on bone mass. These increments in bone mass are dependent on achieving a sufficient workload.

• FCE possibly could be of greater benefit in the *prevention* of osteopenia. Early intervention with FES-CE following acute SCI has been reported to significantly slow rates of bone loss and to decrease hypercalciuria. Longer duration studies of continued use of FES-CE will help to define whether NMES is a practical and an effective means of preventing osteopenia and reducing the incidence of fractures.

Deep Venous Thrombosis (p. 473)

• There has been some exploration of the use of NMES to reduce the incidence of thromboembolic disease. NMES of the tibialis anterior and gastrocnemius-soleus muscles in combination with low-dose heparin, in acute SCI, showed a significant decrease in the incidence of DVT in comparison to low-dose heparin alone. Promising results from FES were also seen in a stroke population.

Psychological Effects (p. 473)

• Paraplegic and quadriplegic patients report diminished depression, improved self-image, increased self-esteem, and a greater sense of independence following use of FES-CE. However, some subjects report decreased motivation and increased anger and tension. Individuals with unrealistic expectations showed the fewest psychological benefits. As with regular exercise, FES-CE has been shown to significantly increase beta-endorphin levels.

THERAPEUTIC FUNCTIONAL ELECTRICAL STIMULATION (pp. 473–476)

Urinary Incontinence (pp. 473–474)

• Data clearly suggest that the electrical stimulation of pelvic floor muscles is an important adjunct to the conservative management of stress and motor-urge urinary continence. It has been suggested that this technique is primarily suited for individuals who are not able to voluntarily stop urine flow and who cannot contract the pelvic floor muscles.

• The stimulation systems for the management of bladder incontinence include electrodes implanted into pelvic floor muscles and external electrodes that are primarily intra-anal or intravaginal. The intravaginal electrodes appear to be the most commonly utilized technique.

• Electrical stimulation has also been attempted for the restoration of bladder function after SCI. Sphincter stimulation with an anal plug stimulator did not improve cystometric findings in one study, and most patients in this study did not wish to continue utilizing this technique. Similarly, pudendal nerve stimulation via the penis or clitoris did not improve bladder capacity or incontinence. However, stimulation of the pudendal nerve at twice the bulbocavernosus threshold has been shown to increase bladder capacity.

• Posterior root rhizotomy has been advocated in conjunction with sacral anterior root stimulation as a means of abolishing uninhibited reflex bladder contractions, thereby increasing bladder capacity, restoring bladder compliance to normal, and abolishing reflex contraction of the sphincter. The disadvantages of the posterior root rhizotomy include the loss of reflex erection and reflex ejaculation. The combination of these techniques is useful in that they decrease residual urine volume, improve bladder compliance, improve urinary incontinence, and decrease reflux and hydronephrosis.

Ejaculatory Failure (p. 474)

• Ejaculatory failure is noted in approximately 95% of SCI survivors. Semen retrieval is possible with subcutaneous physostigmine, vas aspiration, vibratory stimulation, and electrostimulation by rectal probe. This technique does not adversely affect sperm motility. Ejaculation via electrostimulation appears to be well tolerated and safe, with minimal autonomic dysreflexia and mild rectal mucosal changes.

Management of Spasticity (p. 475)

• Few studies have attempted to systematically evaluate the therapeutic efficacy of electrical stimulation for the management of spasticity.

• Short-term effects of surface electrical stimulation resulted in improvement that did not persist past 24 hours. An 8-week surface-electrical stimulation protocol in SCI subjects demonstrated a tendency toward increasing spasticity. A 3-month program of FES reduced spasticity and improved gait patterns and velocity in a subject with familial spastic paraplegia.

• Hemiplegic patients receiving surface stimulation and via an implanted peroneal stimulator for 12 months showed a decrease in passive resistance and tonic reflex activity. Electrical stimulation to wrist extensors of hemiplegic individuals also demonstrated a decrease in flexor spasticity. Stimulation has also contributed to a decrease in contractures in persons with chronic hemiplegia, and a prevention of contractures in patients with "subacute" hemiplegia.

• Recent applications of FES in the management of spasticity have documented benefit when FES is used in conjunction with botulinum toxin.

• Electrical stimulation results in a short-term decrease in spasticity that can persist for several hours after a treatment session. There is also evidence that short-term treatment in conjunction with botulinum toxin and long-term treatment decreases spasticity in hemiplegic individuals. The data are less clear regarding the impact of long-term stimulation on SCI survivors.

Upper Limb in Hemiplegia (pp. 475–476)

• The most common application of electrical stimulation in the upper limb in hemiplegia is in the treatment and prevention of shoulder subluxation. It is thought to be a superior option to physical supports because it does not restrict the use of the limb. One study demonstrated that electrical stimulation could reduce existing subluxation by stimulating the supraspinatus and posterior deltoid muscles (see Fig. 22–11 in the Textbook). The results indicate that electrical stimulation was superior to slings and wheelchair arm supports in reducing subluxation; however, there was no reduction of shoulder pain.

• Combining electrical stimulation with voluntary effort can improve functional use of a chronically hemiplegic upper limb. One study assigned subjects to four groups that received electromyographically (EMG) induced electrical stimulation of wrist extensors, low-intensity electrical stimulation of wrist extensors combined with voluntary contractions, proprioceptive neuromuscular facilitation exercises, or no treatment. The results of this study are compelling in that the electrical stimulation appeared to improve the function of chronically hemiparetic upper limbs. Subjects who received the EMG-induced electrical stimulation of wrist extensors demonstrated the greatest improvement, and these gains were retained for 9 months.

Phrenic Nerve Stimulation (p. 476)

• Phrenic nerve stimulation is a valuable adjunct in the care of the patient with chronic ventilatory insufficiency who has a normal phrenic nerve, diaphragm, and lungs. Specifically, this technique is useful in persons with high-level quadriplegia accompanied by respiratory paralysis and central hypoventilation syndromes. It has been estimated that, nationally, 100 SCI survivors would annually meet the criteria for use of a phrenic nerve pacer.

THERAPEUTIC FUNCTIONAL ELECTRICAL STIMULATION AS AN ORTHOTIC DEVICE (pp. 476–477)

Hemiplegic Gait (p. 477)

• NMES has been utilized to improve the gait pattern of hemiplegic individuals. Torque output of the ankle dorsiflexors is increased while spastic reflexes in the plantar flexors are reciprocally decreased. NMES can also be applied to gluteal muscles and/or to the quadriceps muscles to enhance the stance phase of gait. NMES can be utilized to facilitate the swing phase of gait in hemiplegia with stimulation of the sole, dorsum of the foot, or lower posterior thigh to induce the flexion reflex. The greatest role for NMES in the gait of hemiplegic individuals appears to be early during the acute rehabilitation phase of recovery.

FUNCTIONAL NEUROMUSCULAR STIMULATION: CLINICAL APPLICATIONS (pp. 477–480)

Standing and Gait (pp. 477–479)

• FES for gait restoration after SCI has progressed from feasibility studies to the development of a commercially available, FDA-approved ambulation system. Despite considerable progress, a number of barriers remain that continue to render this a cumbersome clinical application of technology. The typical components of the FES system include a power source plus cables, a control mechanism, display and ground, stimulator with cables, and electrodes. FES systems also require a feedback mechanism.
• Because the technology does not yet exist for FES to produce truly functional community ambulation, most FES systems are hybrid systems that concomitantly utilize FES with a mechanical orthosis. The mechanical orthosis permits standing without considerable energy expenditure. Hybrid systems also appear to use less energy than either mechanical orthoses or FES ambulation systems alone. Because FES ambulation systems are unable to meet many of the criteria for a truly functional system, there are relatively few patients who might benefit from existing systems.

Restoration of Upper Limb Function (pp. 479–480)

• The goal of FES in survivors of a high cervical SCI is to provide palmar and lateral prehension grasp and to develop a means to easily change from one type of grasp to the other. Intramuscular and epimysial electrodes have been utilized to stimulate the flexor digitorum superficialis and profundus, flexor pollicis longus, abductor pollicis, flexor pollicis brevis, abductor pollicis brevis, extensor digitorum, and extensor pollicis longus.

ELECTRICAL STIMULATION FOR THE TREATMENT OF SOFT AND HARD TISSUE INJURY (p. 480)

Wound Healing (p. 480)

• A body of scientific evidence has been accumulating to suggest that electrical stimulation can be used to promote the healing of wounds. When electrical stimulation is applied to a wound, a number of biological processes are modified that might lead to enhanced healing with a decrease in fibrotic scarring and better cosmetic results. It appears that electrical stimulation can augment the endogenous chemical factors that initiate the inflammatory stage of healing. Evidence also indicates that electrical stimulation has bacteriostatic and bactericidal properties. The duration of exposure and voltage shows a linear relationship with inhibition of growth of several common wound pathogens.

SUMMARY (pp. 480–481)

• Electrical stimulation is a historical physiatric modality. In addition to rehabilitation medicine, a renewed interest in electrical stimulation has been demonstrated in various fields such as physiology, molecular biology, engineering, neurosurgery, neurology, orthopedics, urology, and plastic surgery. Electrical stimulation appears to have growing importance as a modality in rehabilitation medicine. This is apparent in the increasing number of FDA-approved FES systems available to treat paralysis-related conditions. Continued research is needed to ensure that this technology is maximally utilized.

23

Original Chapter by Keven Caves, B.S.M.E., A.T.P., and Jan C. Galvin, L.L.C.

Computer Assistive Devices and Environmental Controls

• Computers are changing the world for individuals with disabilities, opening up opportunities for independence, community integration, education, and employment. A vast array of computer-related equipment is available to assist individuals with disabilities.

EDUCATION (p. 489)

• Children with disabilities use computers with software programs that are designed to evaluate or develop skills such as reading, spelling, and language. Computers provide a flexible learning and play environment, and can serve as a tool for discovery-oriented activities.
• For high school or college students, *assistive technology labs* provide the support necessary for integration into the world of technology.

DISTANCE LEARNING (p. 489)

• Distance learning is defined as the linking of a teacher and students in several geographic locations via technology. Computers allow students to work at their own pace and revisit courses as often as necessary.

EMPLOYMENT (pp. 489–490)

• The growth in computer technology, in conjunction with the changing nature of commerce and industry, continues to provide opportunities for individuals with disabilities to be productive.
• The growing attraction of telecommuting has many benefits for the disabled worker. Transportation ceases to be an issue, freeing these employees to spend productive hours in familiar surroundings accessing their work on computers at home.

HOME AND COMMUNITY (p. 490)

• Safety and security in the home are major considerations for the individual who is disabled. An environmental control unit (ECU) can be used to manipu-

late and interact with the environment. Accessing one or more electrical devices via switches, voice-activation, remote control, computer interface, and other technological adaptations is possible using the ECU.
• Access to the Internet also brings companionship, albeit virtual, with 24-hour access to the whole world.

TRENDS IN PREVALENCE OF ASSISTIVE TECHNOLOGY DEVICES (pp. 490–491)

• According to the 1990 National Health Interview Survey (NHIS) on Assistive Devices, more than 13.1 million Americans (about 5.3% of the population) use assistive technology devices to accommodate physical impairments.

EVALUATING FOR APPROPRIATE PERSON/DEVICE MATCH (pp. 491–492)

• An evaluation is performed to gather the information necessary to identify the appropriate technology for a given person. A team of individuals including occupational, physical, and speech therapists, as well as engineers, assistive technologists, rehabilitation counselors, nurses, and physicians, often performs these evaluations. An outline for a typical evaluation follows.

Identify Consumer Goals and Tasks (p. 491)

• The first portion of the assessment is used to gather information about the goals of the individual and the need for equipment. It is important to conduct a task analysis of activities (i.e., to look at the components of the activity and determine what actions are required to do it).

Get Comprehensive Information (p. 491)

• Assess the consumer's functional abilities, personal preferences, environmental barriers, and resources, and ascertain product availability (Table 23–1). This information-gathering step is typically ongoing until the final decision is made.

Establish Criteria for a Successful Choice (p. 491)

• Based on the consumer's goals, abilities, and preferences, identify the specific, objective criteria that can be used to judge potential solutions. The major areas of concern are summarized in Table 23–2.

Make a Final Selection (pp. 491–492)

• Apply the criteria to possible solutions and determine which best meets the criteria. Equipment trials utilizing loaner or rental equipment are extremely useful. In lieu of equipment trials, recommendations are made and equipment is procured, set up, and configured. Training and appropriate follow-up are integral parts of the evaluation process.

TABLE 23–1 User's Functional Abilities

User's Functional Abilities	
Disability	Type, severity, age at onset, prognosis
Motor	Strength, endurance, range of motion, fine and gross motor coordination, positioning to use device, type of control that can be operated
Cognitive	Intelligence, judgment, attention span, problem-solving, memory
Communication	Voice quality, pronunciation, speed
Sensory	Vision, hearing, tactile perception
User's Personal Characteristics	
Psychosocial	Interests/activities, personal values, adjustment to disability, coping style, motivation/desire, attitude toward devices, concept of independence
Family and social support	Family, friends, co-workers, neighbors
Environment	
Environmental compatibility	Usable in home, work, play, community; architectural barriers, getting into and out of rooms, access to lighting, kitchen, phones, bath
Resources available	Space, electronics, wiring compatible
Impact on others in environment	Family, housemates, co-workers
Service delivery system	Training provided, follow-up provided, user support services available, installation, timely delivery

From Galvin J, Barnicle K, Perr A: Evaluating and Choosing Assistive Technology. Proceedings of the Technology and People with Disabilities Conference. Northridge, Calif, California State University, 1992.

COMPUTER ADAPTATIONS (pp. 493–495)

• Computer systems consist of hardware (the computer plus the monitor, printer, and other peripherals) and software (programs such as the operating system, or applications such as word processors or Web browsers). A large range of adaptations is now available for individuals with disabilities. This section focuses on personal computer solutions and adaptations (Table 23–3).

TABLE 23–2 Device Selection Evaluation Criteria

Performance	Effectiveness, reliability, durability, safety, comfort
Ease of use	Easy to set up, learn to use, operate, maintain, repair
Aesthetics	Attractive, quiet, well-designed
Cost	Purchase, maintenance, repairs
Convenience	Easy to store, transport
Flexibility	Compatible with other devices, expandable

From Galvin J, Barnicle K, Perr A: Evaluating and Choosing Assistive Technology. Proceedings of the Technology and People with Disabilities Conference. Northridge, Calif, California State University, 1992.

**TABLE 23–3 Common Adapted Computer Input
and Output Hardware and Software**

Alternative computer keyboard	Braille input devices
Braille translation	Braille printers/embossers
Computer keyboard enhancers	CD-ROM
Digitizers	Environmental control unit (ECU)
Expanded keyboards	Facsimile machines
Graphical user interface (GUI)	Keyguards
Keyboard emulators	Large-print software
Magnified CRT displays	Morse code input
Mouse/trackball input	Optical character recognition (OCR)
Refreshable Braille displays	Screen reader software
Signaling systems	Speech synthesizers
Speech recognition	Speech amplification
Telephone amplifiers	Telephone device for the deaf (TDD)
Touch screens	Word prediction software

Positioning (p. 493)

• One of the first areas to evaluate is positioning of the individual and the computer equipment. Ergonomically designed office chairs, footrests, arm supports, and wrist rests can help positioning so that equipment is more easily accessed. Devices such as keyboard trays, copy holders, monitor arms, and printer stands can all help to make access easier. Proper positioning can help prevent computer-related disabilities such as repetitive stress syndromes.

Keyboard Accommodations (p. 493)

• Traditional input devices and methods can be difficult or impossible for persons with disabilities to use. The standard keyboard works very well for people with ten working fingers, but can severely slow down a person who types using a single hand, or even a single finger. Free software packages have been built into both the Macintosh and Windows operating systems that modify the way the keyboard responds. Mini-keyboards are available for individuals whose range or strength is limited. Expanded keyboards can be obtained for individuals who lack fine motor control. Membrane keyboards enable the typist to slide the hand across other keys without causing unwanted keystrokes. Keyboards with different layouts can facilitate typing for one-hand or one-finger typists.

Alternative Access (pp. 493–494)

• Alternative access methods range from selection of characters from scanning arrays, or inputting dots and dashes in Morse code via switches, to using actual voice input. Switches have been designed to capture virtually any movement a person can make to provide input to a computer. Scanning, which involves using a switch to make selections from an array of characters, can allow severely physically disabled persons to use computers.

• Technology such as optical character recognition (OCR), voice input systems, and handwriting recognition can also be used to provide input to computers.

Mouse Substitution and Emulation (p. 494)

• A variety of mouse "pointing" devices have been designed as alternatives to the traditional mouse. For example, a trackball is like an upside-down mouse. The trackball can be set in different positions to improve access, allowing the foot or even the chin to operate it. Another such device is a track pad. There are also inductive or pressure-sensitive tablets that detect movements without any moving parts. Other solutions include digitizers, touch screens, and head pointers.

Keyboard Equivalents (p. 494)

• Many programs have equivalent keystrokes for every mouse command. Built into both the Macintosh and Windows operating systems is MouseKeys, a feature that allows the user to directly control the movement and clicking of the mouse through the keyboard, eliminating the need for a separate mouse altogether.

Output Accommodations (pp. 494–495)

• The monitor and the printer are visual devices, rendering them largely unusable by individuals with visual deficits. Visual limitations can sometimes be accommodated by the use of a larger monitor.

COMMUNICATION TECHNOLOGIES (pp. 495–496)

Augmentative Communication (p. 495)

• Many individuals have difficulty communicating verbally. Computer technology has made possible electronic augmentative or alternative communication systems (AACs). Sophisticated AAC systems offer speech synthesis in appropriate voices and foreign languages. These offer access by touch, pointer, switch, scanning, or even by ocular eye gaze monitors that electronically measure eye movements.

Telecommunications (p. 495)

• Telephone Devices for the Deaf (TDD) enable individuals who are hearing-impaired or speech-impaired to communicate by telephone. The message is typed in on a keyboard and displayed on a screen while being transmitted over the telephone lines. A Braille version is available for individuals who have both severe hearing and visual impairment. Computers with PC/TDD modems are also used as a means of communication. Conversations are typed in and responses are received on the computer screen.

Environmental Controls (pp. 495–496)

• An environmental control system allows an individual with disabilities to independently control the immediate surroundings. These systems typically utilize a set of modules that plug into standard electrical outlets and can be used to operate lights or television, initiate or answer telephone calls, and unlock doors. An ECU can confer a sense of freedom, independence, and security. ECUs can be activated through a range of access strategies, from voice input to touch. ECU technology ranges from the simple, commercially available remote control for switching lights on and off to a fully functional "smart house."

SUMMARY/FUTURE TECHNOLOGIES (pp. 496–497)

• As new technologies and information systems evolve, the needs of all people with all types, degrees, and combinations of disabilities must be kept in mind. As wonderful as these new technologies can potentially be, their use may create new barriers. Computers are rarely, if ever, a solution in and of themselves. We must remember that the computer is a tool; and if that tool is applied appropriately, it can enhance all our lives.

24

Original Chapter by John J. Nicholas, M.D., and Ted A. Lennard, M.D.

Joint and Soft Tissue Injection Techniques

INTRA-ARTICULAR INJECTIONS (pp. 498–500)

Indications (p. 498)

• IA steroids decrease inflammation. Any inflamed joint is a candidate for injection, provided there is no contraindication.

Precautions (pp. 498–499)

• IA steroid injection precautions include avoiding joint infections. The diffusion of a local anesthetic agent into the surrounding tissue can obscure the exact site of the needle tip. There seems to be relatively little advantage to the inclusion of anesthesia for joint or soft tissue injection because it provides at most only temporary relief of symptoms.

• The injection of a joint in a patient who is taking an anticoagulant or who has a bleeding diathesis must be done only after discussion with the managing physician. Adjacent skin infections can be a hazard and should be avoided at sites of IA steroid injection. IA injection in immunocompromised patients should be performed only after consultation with the managing physician. No more than three or four injections should be made in the same joint in any 12-month period to avoid cartilage damage or infection.

Preparations (p. 499)

• Preparations vary in strength, concentration, and duration (Table 24–1). Currently available preparations include the following:

Methylprednisolone acetate (Depo-Medrol, Pharmacia-Upjohn), IA, 40 and 80 mg/mL

Triamcinolone acetonide (Kenalog, Bristol-Myers Squibb), IA, 40 mg/mL

Triamcinolone hexacetonide (Aristospan, Fuzisawa), IA, 20 mg/mL

Betamethasone sodium phosphate and acetate (Celestone Soluspan, Schering), IA, 6 mg/mL

TABLE 24–1 Relative Strengths of Steroids

Duration of Action	Equivalent Glucocorticoid Dose (mg)	Glucocorticoid Potency
Short-acting		
Cortisone	25.0	0.8
Hydrocortisone	20.0	1.0
Prednisone	5.0	4.0
Prednisolone	5.0	4.0
Methylprednisolone	4.0	5.0
Intermediate-acting		
Triamcinolone	4.0	5.0
Long-acting		
Dexamethasone	0.75	30.0
Betamethasone	0.6	25.0

Strength (p. 499)

• The contents of a 1.0-mL vial of any of the above preparations can be injected into a joint. Larger doses have been suggested for larger joints, and smaller doses for smaller joints. A previously unused vial reduces the possibility of contamination. It has not been shown that there are harmful side effects from any dose contained in a single 1.0-mL vial.

Technique (pp. 499–500)

• The "no-touch" technique is strongly recommended. No drapes or sterile room are required, but universal precautions should be observed.
• Select the site of injection through the skin based on bony landmarks, and then outline it with a marker. Clean the area with three swipes of povidone-iodine and one swipe of alcohol. The skin should not be touched with the bare finger after preparation. A 25-gauge needle is used to inject an anesthetic into the epidermis, producing a skin wheal. After waiting 30 to 60 seconds to allow for the anesthetic effect, place a 1.5-inch (3.8-cm), 21-gauge needle on the syringe filled with anesthetic and enter the skin through the wheal. Stop and aspirate every 0.5 cm, and inject another small bolus of anesthetic agent. When the joint has been entered, the hub of the needle should be clasped with a hemostat; the syringe with anesthetic removed; and an aspirating syringe, or series of aspirating and injecting syringes, applied.
• The color and consistency of the synovial fluid are observed and a sample is removed for laboratory analysis. The sample should be evaluated for white blood cell count and polarized light microscopic examination. Evaluation for the presence or absence of crystals and Gram's stain and culture should be performed if indicated. The operator should determine whether there is a normal consistency and viscosity to the fluid by letting a drop of fluid drip from the end of the syringe or by palpating a sample between the fingertips. Normal synovial fluid will stretch approximately 2.5 cm between the fingertips. The WBC count of the fluid can be estimated by attempting to read 0.25-inch print through a

standard test tube of the fluid. If the print can be read, the fluid is probably noninflammatory.

• There are few reported infections following joint injections. Multiple skin punctures are to be avoided. If joint fluid is not readily obtained at the first attempt, the needle should be redirected but not removed or pulled out of the skin.

CHOICE OF SITE (pp. 500–506)

Sternoclavicular Joint (p. 500)

• The site of the injection is the superior aspect of the joint where the clavicle attaches to the sternum. The deposit is made in the subcutaneous tissues adjacent to the joint (see Fig. 24–1*A* in the Textbook).

Acromioclavicular Joint (p. 500)

• The injected steroid is deposited superior to the joint, where the clavicle joins the acromion, medial to the tip of the acromion (see Fig. 24–1*A* in the Textbook).

Long Head of the Biceps Tendons (p. 500)

• The injection is made at the point of maximum palpable tenderness, in the bicipital groove of the humerus (see Fig. 24–1*B* in the Textbook).

Short Head of the Biceps Tendon (p. 500)

• The steroid is injected at the point of greatest tenderness, which is usually on top of the coracoid process (see Fig. 24–1*B* in the Textbook).

Shoulder (p. 500)

• The landmarks are the coracoid process and the head of the humerus (see Fig. 24–1*A* in the Textbook). A site is chosen just lateral to the coracoid process. The joint is entered either between the head of the humerus and the coracoid process or 0.5 cm superior to this site. The steroid preparation is deposited after entering directly perpendicular to the skin.

Subacromial Bursa (p. 501)

• The subacromial bursa lies beneath the tip of the acromion and the steroid is deposited beneath the tip of the acromial process and superior to the head of the humerus (see Fig. 24–1*A* in the Textbook).

Supraspinatus Tendon (Impingement Syndrome) (p. 501)

• The tendon is approached posteriorly and just beneath the acromio-clavicular joint. A tender area will be "discovered" by the point of the needle.

Elbow (p. 501)

• The landmarks are the olecranon process of the ulna, the head of the radius, and the lateral epicondyle. The joint can be entered just anterior to the center of this triangle and posterior to the head of the radius (see Fig. 24–2 in the Textbook).

Olecranon Bursitis (p. 501)

• The olecranon bursa overlies the olecranon process of the ulna. The needle is directed into the most fluctuant part of the bursal sac.

Carpal Joints (p. 501)

• The ulnar and radial styloids are the landmarks for carpal joint injection. A line connecting these two bony landmarks defines the proximal row of carpal bones. Injection should be done at the points of maximal tenderness.

De Quervain's Disease (pp. 501–502)

• The tendons of the extensor pollicis brevis and abductor pollicis longus can be located by palpation (see Fig. 24–3 in the Textbook). The point of injection should be subcutaneous in the area of maximal tenderness. Entering the tendon may cause damage.

Carpometacarpal Joint of the Thumb (p. 502)

• Osteoarthritis at this site usually results in tenderness on palpation. The operator should inject the steroid at the point of tenderness.

Metacarpophalangeal Joint of the Thumb and Fingers (p. 502)

• When the fist is clenched the joint can be palpated just distal to the apex of the knuckle (Fig. 24–1). The joint should be entered at an angle, not directly laterally or directly superiorly, in order to avoid the digital nerve, artery, vein, and the extensor tendon apparatus on the superior aspect of each digit.

Distal Interphalangeal and Proximal Interphalangeal Joints (pp. 502–503)

• Entering these joints with a needle can result in damage. The operator should palpate the bony landmarks in a fashion similar to palpating the bony landmarks of the metacarpophalangeal joints, then deposit the steroid subcutaneously in the area just beyond the apex of the knuckle (see Fig. 24–1).

Carpal Tunnel (p. 503)

• A line connecting the pisiform and trapezoid bones shows the position of the transverse carpal ligament (Fig. 24–2). The median nerve enters the palm just medial to the trapezoid. The injection is made through the transverse carpal lig-

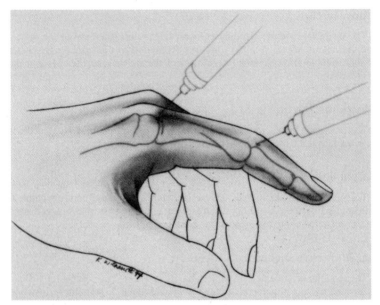

FIGURE 24–1. The metacarpophalangeal joint is more distal than usually thought, just beyond the bony prominence of the distal end of the metacarpal bone (the knuckle).

ament in this area. If paresthesias occur because of the needle being on or near the median nerve, maneuver the needle more laterally and less deep.
• An alternative technique is to enter the skin at a point on the radial side of the palmaris tendon.

Hip Joint (p. 503)

• The hip joint is routinely injected under fluoroscopic guidance and is beyond the scope of this chapter.

Ischial Bursitis (p. 503)

• The ischial tuberosity should be palpated and injection made directly into the point of maximum tenderness.

Greater Trochanteric Bursa (p. 504)

• The bursa is superior to the greater trochanter, which can be palpated (see Fig. 24–6 in the Textbook). Deposit the steroid when the tip of the needle reaches a tender area superior to the greater trochanter.

Sacroiliac Joint (p. 504)

• The sacroiliac joint can be injected at the point of maximal tenderness or it can be injected more certainly under fluoroscopic guidance.

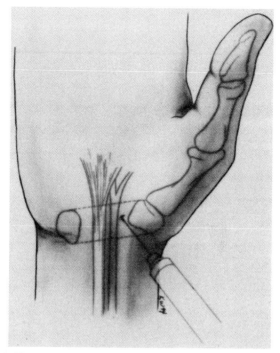

FIGURE 24–2. The boundaries of the carpal tunnel are defined by the pisiform and the trapezoid bones.

Knee Joint (p. 504)

• Outline the patella with a pen and select a site just superior to the superior margin of the patella on the medial aspect. This site should be low enough to allow direction of the needle below the quadriceps tendon (Fig. 24–3). This puts the medication into the suprapatellar pouch, which is contiguous with the synovial cavity.

• An alternative method is performed with the knee flexed. The tibial tubercle and patella are outlined and connected with lines to outline the patellar tendon. The needle can be directed medially or laterally just below the superior margin of the patella toward the knee joint cavity. This is an especially advantageous site when there are osteophytes around the patella or when the patient is very obese. Fluid tends to migrate posteriorly in the flexed knee; therefore it is difficult to obtain fluid with this technique.

"Housemaid's Knee" (p. 504)

• Housemaid's knee is inflammation of the prepatellar bursa, which can be injected at the site of maximal fullness.

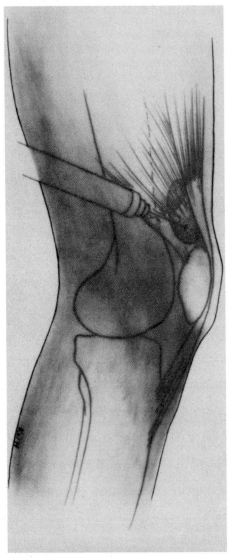

FIGURE 24–3. Palpation of the superior margin of the patella allows the operator to avoid inserting the needle between the patella and the femur.

Anserine Bursa (p. 505)

• The anserine bursa is located, by palpation, distal to the tibial joint line on the medial aspect of the tibia, somewhat posterior. Tenderness to the tip of the needle will indicate the location of the inflamed bursa (see Fig. 24–8 in the Textbook).

Ankle Joint (p. 505)

• The landmarks are the medial and lateral malleoli. A line is drawn 1 cm superior to these two structures outlining the distal end of the tibia (see Fig. 24–9 in the Textbook). With the foot dorsiflexed, the anterior tibial and extensor communis tendons can be readily identified. The dorsalis pedis artery is beneath these structures. Select a site on either the medial or lateral aspect of the joint, and introduce the needle beneath the line at the end of the tibia.

Metatarsophalangeal Joints (p. 505)

• The metatarsophalangeal joints are injected from the dorsal aspect with the foot flexed. The joint is distal to the largest palpable part of the joint. To avoid important structures, the site should not be lateral or superior but between these two planes.

Morton's Neuroma (p. 505)

• The site is determined by palpating the point of maximal tenderness. The preparation is deposited through the skin of the dorsum of the foot into the tender area.

Plantar Fasciitis (p. 506)

• The exact site of inflammation can be determined by palpation. The site is approached from the plantar aspect of the foot and the steroid is deposited midline at the site of maximum tenderness.

COMPLICATIONS (pp. 506–507)

Postinjection Flare (p. 506)

• Postinjection flare occurs after 2–5% of injections and is attributed to the microcrystalline structure of the steroids. Prednisolone acetate and hydrocortisone acetate apparently produce such flares.

Periarticular Calcifications (p. 506)

• Asymptomatic periarticular calcifications in finger joints following injections have been reported, but is rare.

Steroid Arthropathy (pp. 506–507)

• Progressive joint destruction and Charcot-like disorganization has been described after multiple steroid injections. Review of the literature has shown that there is little evidence to support the concept of steroid arthropathy, other than in exceptional cases of multiple injections.

Skin Changes (p. 507)

• Local depigmentation, scarring, and depression of the skin have been described. These changes are not harmful but can be unsightly. Atrophy of the underlying subcutaneous tissues and muscle has also been reported. This can be avoided by using less concentrated preparations. Triamcinolone preparations may cause increased incidence of these complications.

• These lesions are said to remit after a number of years. They are probably unavoidable in a small percentage of patients.

Systemic Effects (p. 507)

• Serum levels can be detected shortly after injection. Suppression of the pituitary-adrenal axis occurs if injections are frequently repeated. Triamcinolone hexacetonide and betamethasone sodium phosphate seem to remain within the joint cavity longer, and their systemic effect is limited because of low serum levels and prolonged release time.

Tendon Rupture (p. 507)

• Tendon rupture, although uncommon, has been reported following injection with IA steroids.

PHONOPHORESIS AND IONTOPHORESIS (pp. 507–508)

• Phonophoresis and iontophoresis have been suggested as substitute techniques for delivering steroid preparations to inflamed soft tissue. The preponderance of current evidence does not substantiate adequate penetration.

LUMBAR INJECTIONS FOR PAIN MANAGEMENT (pp. 508–512)

• Spinal injections are often a useful tool in alleviating pain and identifying pain generators that originate within spinal column.

Lumbosacral Epidural Injections (pp. 508–511)

Midline and Paramedian Approach (p. 508)
• Midline and paramedian epidural steroid injections can be used effectively for pain management when placed at the level of pathology in cases of disk herniations, degenerative disk disease, central stenosis, or compression fractures.
• With the patient prone, the injection interval is marked on the skin under fluoroscopic guidance. This includes the inferior border of the lamina of the upper injection interval and the superior border of the lamina of the lower injection interval. The skin is cleaned, draped, and anesthetized. The operator places a large-bore, blunt spinal needle directly in the lower portion of the injection interval in the midline. Attached to a small-volume glass syringe, the needle is advanced anteriorly to the ligamentum flavum. As the needle is advanced, slight pressure is applied to the syringe. Once the needle tip has been advanced through the ligamentum flavum, immediate loss of resistance will be noted with the syringe (Fig. 24–4). Once the epidural space has been located, careful aspiration is necessary to avoid intrathecal or intravascular injection. Contrast dye can then be injected and observed under fluoroscopy for typical epidural dye patterns (see Fig. 24–11 in the Textbook). Once these patterns are confirmed and the needle is properly placed, a solution of Celestone Soluspan and lidocaine is injected.

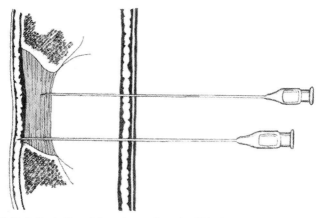

FIGURE 24–4. Illustration of tissue layers through which the needle advances during a paramedian epidural injection. *Top:* needle is located in the ligamentum flavum. *Bottom:* needle is located in the epidural space.

- A paramedian approach is usually more comfortable for the patient and easier for the physician. It differs from the midline approach in needle placement. The needle is placed adjacent to the supraspinous and interspinous ligaments rather than directly in these ligaments. The needle tip is advanced down to the superior edge of the lamina and slowly "walked off" this edge through the ligamentum flavum.

Transforaminal Technique *(pp. 508–510)*
- The transforaminal or selective nerve root block can be performed for disk herniation with or without radiculopathy, foraminal stenosis, or discogenic disease. A greater concentration of medication can be placed at the site of pathology.
- There are unique aspects of the technique when the S1 foramen is injected as compared to the L1 to L5 foramina.
- With the patient prone, the S1 foramen is initially located under fluoroscopy and marked on the skin. The S1 foramen is between the S2 foramen and the L5 to S1 facet joint. The skin is cleaned, draped, and anesthetized. Then a 22-gauge, $3\frac{1}{2}$-inch spinal needle is slowly inserted into the S1 foramen. Usually the initial puncture is made at the inferior aspect of the foramen and the needle is advanced cephalad under fluoroscopic guidance. Lateral views can be helpful to confirm needle depth. When the needle is in the proper location, the inner trocar of the 22-gauge needle is removed and a syringe with nonionic contrast material is attached. After aspiration, the contrast material is injected. The characteristic pattern is of dye flowing along the S1 nerve root (see Fig. 24–12 in the Textbook). Syringes are changed and a mixture of steroid and lidocaine is injected.
- For injections around the lumbar nerve roots, modifications from the S1 injection technique are necessary. Either a posterior or an oblique approach can be used. For an L5 SNRB, landmarks include the L5 transverse process, L5 lamina, and the upper portion of the sacrum. Once proper anesthesia is obtained, a 22-gauge spinal needle can be advanced at the inferomedial portion of the trans-

verse process. The tip of the needle is directed toward the inferior aspect of the pedicle superior to the exiting nerve root. A "safe triangle" in this region includes the base of the pedicle, the outer vertical border of the intervertebral foramen, and the diagonal nerve root and dorsal ganglion. Once the needle is in proper position, contrast agent is injected (see Fig. 24–13 in the Textbook), followed by injection of a solution of steroid and anesthetic.

• A double-needle technique is often used in place of the 22-gauge needle technique. An 18-gauge, 3½-inch needle replaces the 22-gauge needle. The inner trocar is removed and a 23-gauge, 6-inch needle is placed within the 18-gauge needle. The 23-gauge needle is then slowly advanced under fluoroscopic guidance while the 18-gauge needle remains stable between the physician's fingertips. The advancing needle never touches the skin, reducing the risk of infection. The distal tip of the 23-gauge needle can be bent by the physician and reinserted into the 18-gauge needle, allowing the needle to curve into areas that may be difficult to reach.

Caudal Technique (pp. 510–511)
• Caudal epidural injections, mainly performed for disk abnormalities at L4 to L5 and L5 to S1, begin with the patient prone. The operator palpates the sacral cornu and hiatus by locating the coccyx and slowly moving cephalad on the posterior aspect of the coccyx. The skin is then cleaned, draped, and anesthetized. A 3½-inch, 22-gauge spinal needle is directed cephalad through the hiatus at a 30- to 45-degree angle. As the needle advances the bevel should be rotated ventrally until slight contact with bone is made. The needle is then withdrawn several millimeters and advanced at a 5- to 10-degree angle superiorly to the S3 vertebrae (see Fig. 24–6 in the Textbook). The inner trocar of the 22-gauge needle is removed and a syringe containing nonionic contrast material is applied. After aspiration reveals no blood or CSF, the contrast dye is injected and the flow pattern is analyzed under fluoroscopy. If the needle is properly placed, a typical epidural pattern will be observed (see Fig. 24–15 in the Textbook). Improper placement is usually associated with increased resistance. Once the correct dye pattern is confirmed, a steroid-anesthetic solution is injected.

Lumbar Facet Injections (pp. 511–512)

• Lumbar facet injections are indicated when posterior element pain is suspected as the pain generator. This may occur when these joints are the primary source of pathology or in conjunction with discogenic disease. IA injections typically precede medial branch blocks when determining whether the facet joint is the source of pain. Medial branch blocks are commonly done to predict the response to denervation procedures.

Intra-articular Injections (p. 511)
• IA zygoapophyseal joint injections of the lumbar spine are performed with the patient prone and the table tilted obliquely. The z-joints are marked on the skin under fluoroscopic guidance. The patient is cleaned, draped, and anesthetized. A 22-gauge spinal needle is slowly advanced directly into the joint under fluoroscopic guidance. Several needle adjustments may be required before the needle is felt to enter the joint. Usually the joint edge is noted initially and the needle tip can be "walked" into the joint space. If an arthrogram is desired for

needle confirmation, contrast agent can be injected and later aspirated. Dye injection is followed by injection of a steroid-anesthetic solution.
• Often, injection of the L5 to S1 joint from an oblique approach is not possible because of the iliac crest, in which case a direct posterior approach is used. The patient is placed prone and the lower edge of the L5 to S1 joint is noted under fluoroscopy. The needle is advanced and the injection is made using the same technique described above.

Medial Branch Blocks (p. 511)

• Anesthetic injections of the medial branch of the posterior ramus, or medial branch blocks, can be helpful in diagnosing the painful zygoapophyseal joint or in preparation for a denervation procedure. Because a zygoapophyseal joint has dual innervation, two blocks are necessary to anesthetize a single joint (see Fig. 24–17 in the Textbook). To anesthetize the nerve supply to the L4 to L5 zygoapophyseal joint, for example, the L3 medial branch and the L4 medial branch are injected.
• The block is performed under fluoroscopic guidance with the patient prone. Target sites for each block are marked on the skin. The patient is cleaned, draped, and anesthetized. A small-gauge spinal needle is advanced in a superior to inferior approach to the target site. For the L1 to L4 medial branches this site is on the posterior surface of the transverse process at the mamilloaccessory ligament and notch. The target location for the L5 nerve is the interval between the sacral ala and the S1 superior articular process. Contrast material can be injected to rule out vascular uptake. Small volumes of lidocaine or marcaine are then injected at each target site.

Complications (pp. 511–512)

• Lumbar injections have a very low rate of serious complications and are quite safe when proper precautions are observed. Inherent to most needle procedures is transient postinjection soreness, minor swelling, and local tissue bleeding. These symptoms are usually alleviated with ice, limitation of activity, and analgesics. Complications with bleeding can be reduced by taking a good medical history. Aspirin should be discontinued 7 to 10 days before epidural procedures. Anticoagulants and other antiplatelet drugs are also contraindications to epidural procedures. Vasovagal syncope or fainting is relatively common. Venodilator drugs, recent exhaustive exercise, dehydration, hypoglycemia, and aortic stenosis are predisposing factors. Infection is rare.
• Allergic reactions to injected drugs are always a possibility.
• Dural puncture and associated headaches occur after 0.5% to 5% of spinal epidural injections. They are primarily associated with midline or paramedian approaches.
• Other complications are usually related to anesthetic toxicity and include CNS or cardiovascular problems.

Benefits (p. 512)

• Lumbar injections provide considerable pain relief when used in the appropriate clinical setting. They also provide valuable diagnostic information for the spine physician. These injections are generally safe, easy to perform, and carry a low side effect profile. The technical performance of these injections requires proper training, a good knowledge of lumbar gross and radiological anatomy, and the ability to manage any complications resulting from the procedure.

COMMON CLINICAL PROBLEMS IN PHYSICAL MEDICINE AND REHABILITATION

25

Original Chapter by Cristina M. Mix, O.T.R., and Donna Pieper Specht, P.T.

Achieving Functional Independence

- Functional independence is the ability to perform living skills without help. Potential activities include tasks of self-maintenance, mobility, communication, home management, leisure, education, and vocation.

EVALUATION (p. 518)

- Evaluation of performance skills identifies impairments that interfere with a person's achieving the goals of functional independence. Multiple evaluation tools and assessments exist that assist in identifying a person's abilities and limitations. The evaluation begins with an interview to identify the person's interests, premorbid status, and current perception of impairment. Subsequently, physical examination of component areas that can interfere with function is assessed. Examples include range of motion (ROM), strength, tone, sensation, balance, coordination, visual perception, and cognition. Direct observation of functional activities ensures accuracy and shows which areas of limitations are problematic. Throughout the treatment phase of rehabilitation, it is important to measure patient progress. This information provides information about effectiveness and progress. Many outcome-oriented scales exist including the Children's Hospital Rehabilitation Independence Scale (CHRIS pediatric), the Rehabilitation Institute of Chicago Functional Assessment Scale (RICFAS), and the Functional Independence Measures (FIM).

SELF-MAINTENANCE (pp. 518–522)

Feeding (p. 518)

- The process of self-feeding involves range of motion (ROM), coordination, and strength sufficient to scoop and bring the hand to the mouth while grasping a utensil or cup. When coordination is difficult, stabilization of dishes may be needed. Mats made of nonskid materials can be useful. For persons with functional use of just one hand, scoop dishes or plate guards allow food to be stabilized against the raised side. Weighted or swivel utensils may help when hand control is limited. A rocker knife, which is used by pushing the knife down into food and rocking the knife, is appropriate when bilateral upper extremity motor skills are impaired.
- A variety of adapted and built-up utensils are available for use when grasp is impaired, including utensil cuffs, splints with utensil slots, and lightweight cups

333

with adapted handles. A common way to build up handles is to place built-up foam over the utensil (see Fig. 25–1 in the Textbook).

• If ROM is limited for hand-to-mouth activity, long straws, long-handled utensils, sandwich holders, elevated plate setups, mobile arm supports, or suspension slings can be utilized. A mobile arm support is a system that supports the forearm while assisting and maximizing motions in the upper extremity (see Figs. 25–1, 25–2, and 25–3 in the Textbook). For the mobile arm support to be used successfully, a person should exhibit some functional upper-extremity movement in the gravity-eliminated plane. Mechanical feeders are also available.

• Adequate oral motor skills (e.g., sucking, lip closure, and tongue mobility) are necessary for eating. These skills can be facilitated by a variety of feeding tools such as nipples for bottle-drinking, spoons made of sturdy plastic with a shallow bowl, and cups with nose cutouts or spouts.

Dressing (pp. 518–520)

• The person's usual clothing should be used when evaluating and performing dressing training. Dressing requires adequate active ROM, coordination, strength, and gross mobility skills. When providing recommendations for adapted dressing modifications or equipment, it is important to consider developmental age, cognitive abilities, motivation to use the equipment, and its potential to enhance or impede independence.

• There are a variety of modifications that assist with dressing (e.g., loose clothing and minimizing fasteners). When fine motor skills are weak, button aids (a wire loop that hooks around the button and then pulled through the hole), zipper pulls (a loop or a wire hook used to pull the zipper), elastic shoelaces (which do not require repeated ties), and Velcro can be utilized. Modified clothing is now commercially available; but simple, "home-made" modifications can be effective, too. In the case of perceptual or cognitive problems, it can help to label clothes so the person can distinguish front from back. A reacher may be useful for retrieving items of clothing for individuals with limited reach or mobility. Dressing sticks are long sticks with a hook at the end that aid in pulling up pants and socks. Stocking aids have a sock holder and an attached rope; the person puts a stocking over the sock holder, places the holder in front of the foot, and then uses the rope to pull the stocking up.

Grooming and Hygiene (pp. 520–521)

• To perform hygiene and grooming skills, a person must have functional grasp, adequate upper limb ROM, bilateral hand function, fine and gross motor coordination, strength, trunk control, and sitting balance.

• When hand function is limited, several adaptations can be utilized. A utensil cuff is a palmar strap with a slot into which small items such as a toothbrush can be inserted and stabilized. Built-up foam and Velcro straps can be used in conjunction with a toothbrush. A razor or electric shaver, electric toothbrushes, and Water Piks can greatly assist those whose strength and endurance are limited. Soap-on-a-rope and wash mitts assist with face washing. A brush with a suction attachment to the sink will facilitate nail and denture care when bilateral hand function is limited. One can also attach a nail clipper and emery board to a board

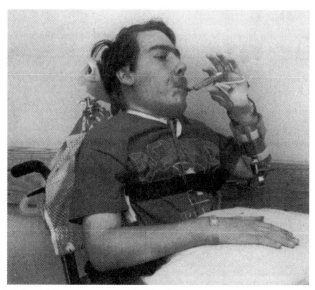

FIGURE 25–1. Mobile arm support used with a long opponens splint and vertical holder to aid in feeding. Mobile arm supports upper extremity function when shoulder or forearm strength is weak. The subject also has a long opponens splint with a utensil and a vertical holder for a spoon for feeding.

backed with Dycem or suction cups to compensate for the strength necessary to pinch or hold a clipper.

• The adaptations discussed consider weak hand strength and incoordination. When shoulder strength is weak, long handles added to grooming tools such as brushes or combs can enhance reach. A mobile arm support or balanced forearm orthosis can also allow one to work in reduced antigravity planes, maximizing motion (Fig. 25–1).

Bowel and Bladder (p. 521)

• An important factor in hygiene is bowel and bladder care. Such care requires adequate upper-extremity ROM, hand function, mobility, endurance, and ability to manage clothes. Therapists work closely with the patient, family, and nurses to discuss possible adaptations and positioning to allow the patient to perform this care. Possible options include reaching aids, commode chairs, raised toilet seats, and potty chairs. To facilitate catheterization, dynamic splints or catheter inserters are helpful, as are labia spreaders for females. Similar equipment is usable for menstrual care. For those using leg bags, there are various adapted leg bag emptiers and catheter clamps, as well as modified strapping for urinary drainage bags. Adapted condom catheter holders can help to secure condom catheters. Bowel care might require use of adapted suppository inserters or digital stimulators. Bowel and bladder care is discussed in detail in Chapters 27 and 28.

Skin Management (p. 521)

• Another aspect of care is skin management, and is especially important for those with impaired sensation. A long-handled mirror allows one to perform skin inspection. Specialized timers provide an auditory reminder to perform weight shifts to assist in preventing pressure sores (beeps occur every 15 minutes as a prompt to perform pressure relief) (see also Chapter 31).

Bathing (pp. 521–522)

• Bathing is a complex activity performed in a potentially dangerous (e.g., slippery) environment that has functional requirements similar to dressing. Various environmental adaptations can assist with bathing (e.g., grab bars, nonskid strips, handheld showerheads, automatic water temperature controls, bath chairs, wheelchair commodes, shower chairs, and inflatable bath beds). Other equipment used to assist those with limited reach or grasp include bath mitts, long-handled brushes with soap holders, soap-on-a-rope, pump dispensers for shampoo, and finger ring brushes for scrubbing the hair.

MOBILITY (pp. 522–527)

• Functional mobility is defined as the ability to move from one position in space (e.g., sitting, lying down, or standing) to another position. Examples include bed mobility, transfers, ambulation, wheelchair mobility, and driving.

Bed Mobility (p. 522)

• Bed mobility includes rolling in bed; scooting up, down, or toward either edge of the bed; and coming to a sitting position at the edge of the bed. Good head control, upper-extremity strength, endurance, and motor planning skills all play a role in efficient bed mobility. Adaptive equipment that can assist with bed mobility includes loops attached along the edge of the bed, overhead trapeze bars, step stools, and electric beds.

Transfers (p. 523)

• A transfer is the act of moving from one position in space to another. The ability to transfer is necessary for anyone who uses a wheelchair. For a person to be independent in daily living tasks, independent transfers must be performed to wheelchair, bed, commode, tub, and vehicle. It is desirable that all wheelchair users be adept at wheelchair-to-floor and floor-to-wheelchair transfers. Sometimes, a small bench can be used as an intermediate step to go halfway between the floor and the wheelchair seat. There are many different ways in which a person can perform a transfer, as described in the following.

Stand-Pivot Transfer (p. 523)

• For persons who can attain standing for short periods, the stand-pivot transfer is the most efficient method. Adequate hip and knee extension and good sitting balance are required. In this transfer, the person rises from a seated to a standing position and pivots to the adjacent chair to sit down. A modification of the stand-pivot transfer is the sit-pivot transfer, in which good sitting balance and upper-extremity strength are used to lift the hips up and across to another chair without standing.

Sliding Board Transfer (p. 523)
• Sliding boards bridge the gap between transferring surfaces. One end of the sliding board is positioned under the buttocks and the opposite end placed on the other surface. Once the board is positioned between the surfaces, the person scoots his or her hips across the board to the new surface.

Wheelchair-to-Floor Transfers (pp. 523–524)
• There are a variety of ways to transfer from the wheelchair to the floor. Using the forward method, the footrests are rotated to the side and the feet placed on the floor. Then, flexing far forward in the wheelchair, the person places both hands on the floor and lowers the body to the floor.
• Pivoting to the floor is another method. With the footrests out of the way, the person scoots to the edge of the wheelchair and pivots the hips so that he or she is sitting on one buttock. Hands are placed on the seat of the wheelchair. Using strong upper extremities, the body is pivoted out of the wheelchair and the knees are lowered to the floor. From the kneeling position facing the wheelchair, the person can then lower the hips to the floor into a side-sitting position.
• Yet another method is used when long leg braces are worn. In this case, the footrests must be removed or rotated to the side, hips are moved to the edge of the wheelchair, and the knees are extended with the heels placed on the floor. Then, placing the hands on the forward-most frame of the wheelchair, the person lowers the hips to the floor. This method requires good upper-extremity strength and long arms for leverage. Children's wheelchairs, with a lower floor-to-seat height, can help some children perform this type of transfer; however, the wheelchair might still be too high for a child to perform this method of transfer.
• The last two methods can be reversed to transfer from the floor back into the wheelchair. The last method is more difficult because very good upper-extremity strength and leverage are important for success.

Ambulation (p. 524)

• A person's level of functional independence can be significantly affected by the ability to ambulate. In order to ambulate, one must have sufficient lower-extremity and trunk strength, balance, coordination, and cognition skills. (See Chapter 5 for a discussion of gait analysis.) If limitations exist in these areas, physical compensations, orthoses, and other assistive ambulation devices can be used to help a person be independent with ambulation.
• Many physical compensations are neither energy- nor time-efficient. Through therapy programs and the use of orthoses and assistive devices, these compensations can be minimized. Many orthoses that support various joints of the lower extremity can help one to compensate for physical limitations. Chapter 16 describes the variety of lower limb orthoses that are available. A person must also be able to don and doff orthotic devices without help for independence to be achieved.
• There are a variety of assistive gait devices. Walkers are considered the most stable devices, followed by crutches and canes, respectively.

Wheelchair Mobility (pp. 524–526)

• For people with limited ambulatory ability, a wheelchair can allow functional independence in the community. Proper positioning in the wheelchair, good sitting tolerance, strength, endurance, and cognitive skills are necessary for appropriate wheelchair use.

• Proper positioning in the wheelchair (described in Chapter 18) is necessary to maintain alertness, increase comfort in and tolerance of the wheelchair, and allow for efficient use of the upper extremities.

• As a result of advances in technology, even persons with significant limitations can be independent in wheelchair mobility. There are many ways to control a power wheelchair. Some examples include using a straw (sip-and-puff), proportional head controller, separate switches for directions, and joysticks. A person must understand the concepts of mobility in order to safely and efficiently drive a power wheelchair. Children as young as $2\frac{1}{2}$ to 3 years can be taught to operate a power wheelchair safely. Physical and occupational therapists are an integral part of the team in helping a person decide which type of wheelchair best meets his or her positioning and mobility needs.

Driving (pp. 526–527)

• Many people with physical limitations can drive with adaptations to the vehicle. Hand controls for driving and braking accommodate diminished upper extremity strength. Levers and knobs can be attached to the controls. Adaptations vary, depending on whether the person will be driving from the wheelchair or from a captain's chair in a van. The adapted vehicle must allow for egress and/or storage of the wheelchair. Companies that specialize in modifications, and some car dealerships can provide information regarding the latest modifications available.

COMMUNICATION (pp. 527–528)

• Patients are often limited in their choice of nonverbal communication tools. The use of communication tools requires adequate fine motor strength, coordination, reach, and grasp.

• Adaptations for writing tools can vary. They include built-up foam, cuffs, or mouthsticks with pens or pencils; hand splints and writing devices that support and compensate for weak hand musculature while positioning and holding writing tools; and weighted pens for controlling coordination of movement for writing. Bookholders, page-turners, mouthsticks, or head sticks can help in handling books. (See Figs. 25–18, 25–19, and 25–20 in the Textbook.)

• Typing can be performed by the use of typing sticks with adapted handles and splints with a slot for a typing stick. If coordination is impaired, keyguards and a key latch can facilitate accuracy. Other accessories include alternative keyboards, adapted switches (e.g., single-switch or sip-and-puff), armrests, mobile arm supports, and overhead slings. For phone use, telephone clip holders, dialing sticks, speakerphones with quick-dial features, and goosenecks to hold the receiver are available. Environmental control units and technology aids are discussed in Chapter 23.

HOME MANAGEMENT (pp. 528–529)

• Home management involves cooking, cleaning, and using tools and appliances. Before providing recommendations, it is important to determine which activities can be done safely with or without adaptations. It is also important to educate and train the individual in energy conservation and work simplification techniques.

• These tasks require gross motor mobility skills and upper-extremity fine and gross motor coordination and strength. When limitations exist, environmental adaptations and assistive devices can be used including reachers, lever-type or extended handle–adapted cooking utensils, cutting boards with suction cups and prongs, and power appliances.

Home Accessibility (p. 529)

• Many adaptations exist for performance of home management skills. Examples include rearranging the furniture, widening doorways, adding a ramp, and construction of a roll-in shower. A thorough home assessment is recommended for persons who may have difficulty functioning within their home environments.

LEISURE SKILLS (pp. 529–530)

• Recreational activities benefit people both physically and emotionally. If the person is in a rehabilitation setting, therapists can facilitate independence in leisure activities through a community reintegration program. Goals can include performance of self-maintenance, mobility skills, and problem solving in a community setting. Exposure to various community activities facilitates comfortable functioning in social settings.

• Information about programs for people with special needs can be obtained from local parks and recreation departments, churches, and national disability-specific organizations.

• Many adaptations exist to compensate for a person's mental limitations and physical disability. These include equipment as well as environmental modifications. Occupational and physical therapists are instrumental in helping individuals access resources, and perform task analysis and identify adaptations for participation in leisure activities.

OCCUPATIONAL ENVIRONMENTS (pp. 530–533)

• Limitations can interfere with a person's ability to perform a job. Public laws exist that have provisions that allow a person with disabilities to enter the work more easily. The Americans with Disabilities Act of 1990 (ADA) provides persons with disabilities with civil rights protection in areas of employment, public services, transportation, public accommodation, and telecommunication. Therapists play a vital role in providing ADA information, task analysis of the person's job, and providing input for environmental and tool adaptations. Assessment should include mobility within the work environment, communication needs, and effective use of all necessary equipment. It is important to recognize that occupations are age specific.

CHAPTER

26

Original Chapter by Stephen F. Noll, M.D., Claire E. Bender, M.D.,
Marge C. Nelson, O.T., Stephanie K. Carlson, M.D., and
Renée J. Andersen, O.T.

Rehabilitation of Patients with Swallowing Disorders

• Dysphagia (difficulty swallowing) can result in loss of enjoyment, aspiration pneumonia, and malnutrition. Dysphagia is a relatively common occurrence in rehabilitation populations.

THE SWALLOWING PROCESS (pp. 535–537)

• Deglutition is typically divided into three phases: oral, pharyngeal, and esophageal (Table 26–1).
• The oral phase prepares the bolus for transit to the pharynx. Preserved lip, tongue, and jaw function is required. Salivation assists the swallowing process. Premature spillage from the oral cavity can result in aspiration or penetration.
• The pharyngeal phase is crucial because impaired laryngeal protection can result in aspiration (Fig. 26–1). Protective mechanisms include epiglottic folding over the laryngeal opening, closure of the vocal cords, and elevation/anterior displacement of the larynx. Normal pharyngeal transit time is about 0.6 seconds. Prolonged or ineffective pharyngeal function results in greater laryngeal exposure to the bolus. There are potential food traps within the pharynx (i.e., the valleculae and pyriform sinuses; see Fig. 26–1 and Fig. 26–3A in the Textbook). Ordinarily, food is cleared from these spaces. The upper esophageal sphincter also serves as a pharyngeal trap. This muscle complex is tonically contracted while other pharyngeal constrictors are at rest. Pharyngeal weakness or incoordination can cause retention in the pharynx and can result in aspiration.
• The esophageal phase lasts 6 to 10 seconds. Peristalsis is responsible for the bolus transport. The lower esophageal sphincter relaxes to allow movement of the bolus distally. Disorders of the esophageal phase are diagnostically problematic because symptoms of this phase can be referred to the pharyngeal region.
• The neurologic organization of deglutition is complex. Peripheral and central systems are involved, including multi-modality sensory input (e.g., taste, pressure, and temperature); cortical, subcortical, and brainstem coordination; and motor output through cranial nerves V, VII, IX, X, and XII.

TABLE 26-1 Stages of Deglutition

	Oral Preparatory/Oral	Pharyngeal	Esophageal
		Stage	
Purpose	Bolus preparation and transport	Bolus transport without aspiration	Bolus transport with limited reflux
Requirements	Mastication and salivation for bolus modification	Tongue elevation to prevent oral regurgitation	Coordinated peristalsis and lower esophageal sphincter relaxation for bolus transport
	Lip closure for bolus containment	Palatal elevation to prevent nasal regurgitation	Cricopharyngeal tonic contraction to prevent pharyngeal regurgitation
	Lingual control for bolus manipulation, positioning, and transport	Laryngeal elevation, folding of epiglottis, and vocal cord adduction to prevent aspiration	Relaxation of lower esophageal sphincter
		Coordinated pharyngeal motility and cricopharyngeal relaxation for bolus transport	
Symptoms	Drooling	Oral/nasal regurgitation	Food sticking
	Pocketing (squirreling)	Food sticking	Heartburn
	Repeated swallowing attempts	Cough or choke	
	Head tilt	Wet, gurgling voice	

341

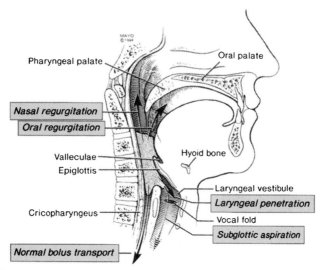

FIGURE 26–1. Pharyngeal phase of swallowing. Without laryngeal protective mechanisms, aspiration can occur. (Reproduced by permission of Mayo Foundation.)

CLINICAL ASSESSMENT (p. 537)

• A clinical or "bedside" evaluation is one method to determine how the swallowing process is impaired and which stages are involved.

History (p. 537)

• Documentation of disease course and specific dysphagia symptoms is imperative, but other information is also important. Examples include dental disorders, recurrent pneumonias, cardiopulmonary disease, previous neck surgery, radiation therapy, and cervical spondylosis. A dietary history should be obtained including types and textures of chosen food.

Examination (p. 537)

• Cranial nerve testing evaluates oral or pharyngeal function. Additional observations include level of alertness, cognitive status, oral secretions, respiratory status, and voice quality. Testing for the gag reflex is helpful, but an absent gag does not imply the inability to swallow safely. Swallowing can be difficult with a rapid respiratory rate. Inadequate respiratory force increases the risk of aspiration. Chest auscultation can uncover lung disease. Palpating for laryngeal excursion helps evaluate this protective mechanism. One final step in evaluation is a feeding assessment with various food textures. The "3-oz water test" compares favorably with the video swallow in identifying aspiration. This test is positive if the patient's voice develops a wet, hoarse quality or if the patient coughs after swallowing 3 oz of water. The bedside evaluation has some predictive capabilities for determining the risk of aspiration but tends to underestimate its occurrence.

Laboratory Data (p. 537)

• Chest radiography can assess for aspiration pneumonia. Where no pathognomonic radiographic sign exists, the presence of infiltrates raises suspicion. Pulse oximetry can be an adjunct to the identification of aspiration when performed before, during, and after a swallow. Other routine laboratory tests can assess nutritional status (e.g., albumin).

TECHNICAL ASSESSMENT OF DYSPHAGIA (pp. 537–545)

Radiographic Imaging (pp. 537–545)

Videofluoroscopy (pp. 537–539)

• Most swallowing disorders are best evaluated with dynamic recorded videofluoroscopy. Although many of the newer imaging methods have been used, videofluoroscopy continues to be the standard. Although this system has some loss of quality when compared with other methods, it is easier to use. Radiation exposure carries attendant risks.

Radiation Risk (pp. 539–540)

• Particular scrutiny must be utilized with the pregnant female. Videofluoroscopy for a swallowing evaluation does not directly irradiate the pelvic region of the patient, so fetal exposure is very minimal. With proper shielding, pregnant support personnel can safely perform these studies.

• The following steps protect both the patient and the operators: minimize radiation duration; use lead shielding; position personnel appropriately; image only the area of interest; and screen for pregnancy. Involved personnel should wear radiation monitor badges.

Equipment (p. 540)

• Fluoroscopy is performed with standard radiographic and fluoroscopic units. A videotape recorder with audio recording capability is adapted to the fluoroscopy unit. A special lightweight mobile chair can be utilized for these studies (see Fig. 26–7 in the Textbook).

Procedural Guidelines (pp. 540–541)

• The examination is facilitated by coordinated consultation between the swallowing therapist and the radiologist. The evaluation team includes the therapist, the fluoroscopist, the radiology technologist, and the patient. A standardized examination protocol is often employed.

Interpretation (p. 541)

• There is a distinct clinical difference between the video-fluoroscopic examination and the routine upper gastrointestinal series. Both examinations evaluate the gastrointestinal tract from the mouth to the small intestine. The videofluoroscopic evaluation of swallowing has both diagnostic and potentially therapeutic capabilities. After aspiration is diagnosed, changes in the texture of the barium meal or variations in head positioning can provide immediate feedback for treatment of a swallowing problem.

• Quantitative evaluation of the pharyngeal transit time (measured during fluoroscopy) can be useful for following the progress of patients with dysphagia and for evaluating the effects of remedial therapy.

Ultrasonography (p. 543)

• Dynamic US examination during swallowing is helpful in the evaluation of tongue and pharyngeal function. The major advantage of US is the delineation of the region of the tongue posterior to the hyoid (Table 26–2; see Fig. 26–13 in the Textbook). US may be used with videofluoroscopy to document aspiration and to further evaluate esophageal activity. Endoluminal US probes allow evaluation of the esophageal wall.

Scintigraphy (p. 544)

• Nuclear medicine techniques are increasingly used in dysphagia. Procedures can assess gastric emptying, gastroesophageal reflux, esophageal motility, airway penetration, and aspiration. Patients can be imaged during and after swallowing radiolabeled thin liquids. Compared with videofluoroscopy, scintigraphy provides more accurate data concerning airway penetration and clearing.

Manometry (p. 545)

• Manometry can be a useful adjunct test, particularly in patients with normal results on barium swallow examinations, patients with motility disorders, and patients with dysfunction of the cricopharyngeus muscle. Pharyngeal manometry measures the intraluminal pressures during swallowing. Simultaneous videofluorography confirms accurate placement of the sensors (see Figs. 26–16 and 26–17 in the Textbook). Manometry may be time consuming and uncomfortable.

Endoscopy (p. 545)

• Fiberoptic endoscopic examination of swallowing (FEES) evaluates the pharyngeal phase of swallowing (see Fig. 26–18 in the Textbook). It can detect premature spillage, laryngeal penetration, tracheal aspiration, and pharyngeal residue. The endoscope is passed transnasally to view the larynx and pharynx. Swallowing is evaluated using food mixed with blue food coloring. Certain patient populations are more amenable to endoscopy. Some authors now advocate using FEES as the primary screening tool for dysphagia and for follow-up, and using videofluoroscopy on a more selective basis. The biggest drawback of FEES is its inability to assess the esophagus.

DYSPHAGIA IN SPECIFIC DISORDERS (pp. 545–550)

• Dysphagia has been reported in multiple types of disorders, and can be classified as neurological or nonneurological (Table 26–2).

Stroke (pp. 545–547)

• Dysphagia is a common impairment after stroke and has been associated with increased mortality, length of hospital stay, and functional impairment (Fig. 26–2). Dysphagia is not limited to brainstem or bilateral infarctions. The most common swallowing impairments associated with stroke are reduced lingual control, reduced pharyngeal peristalsis, and a delayed swallowing reflex. Aspiration is commonly associated with dysphagia in stroke, but it cannot be predicted by stroke location. A post-swallow cough, an absent or abnormal gag reflex, dysphonia, dysarthria, abnormal volitional cough, and voice change after swallow indicate increased risk for aspiration. But aspiration is "silent" in many persons with stroke.

TABLE 26–2 Disorders Associated with Dysphagia

Neurological	Nonneurological
Central nervous system	Structural
Vascular	Cervical osteophytes
Stroke	Goiter
Intracranial hemorrhage	Neoplasm
Motor neuron disorders	Foreign body
Progressive spinal muscular	Congenital anomalies
atrophy	Vascular aneurysm or anomaly
Progressive bulbar palsy	Schatzki's ring
Amyotrophic lateral sclerosis	Zenker's diverticulum
Infantile spinal muscular atrophy	Esophageal webs
Poliomyelitis	Esophageal dysmotility
Degenerative/extrapyramidal	Gastroesophageal reflux
Parkinsonism	Achalasia
Spinocerebellar degeneration	Diffuse esophageal spasm
Olivopontocerebellar atrophy	"Nutcracker" esophagus
Progressive supranuclear palsy	Other gastrointestinal disorders
Huntington's disease	Crohn's disease
Alzheimer's disease	Ulcerative colitis
Adrenoleukodystrophy	Amyloid
Dystonia	Plummer-Vinson syndrome
Tardive dyskinesia	Rheumatologic
Immune-mediated	Scleroderma
Multiple sclerosis	Sjögren's syndrome
Infectious	Systemic lupus erythematosus
Encephalitis/meningitis	Mixed connective tissue disease
Structural	Rheumatoid arthritis
Neoplasm	Infectious
Arnold-Chiari malformation	*Candida*
Syringomyelia, syringobulbia	Herpesvirus
Exogenous	Cytomegalovirus
Traumatic brain injury	Tuberculosis
Drug-induced	Acute pharyngitis
Peripheral nervous system	Retropharyngeal abscess
Guillain-Barré syndrome	Epiglottitis
Sarcoidosis	Human immunodeficiency virus (HIV)
Porphyria	Psychiatric
Myopathy/dystrophy	Globus
Inflammatory myopathy	Skin diseases
(polymyositis, dermatomyositis)	Mucous membrane pemphigoid
Metabolic myopathy (mitochondrial	Epidermolysis bullosa dystrophica
myopathy, dysthyroid myopathy)	Lichen planus
Myotonic dystrophy	Psoriasis
Oculopharyngeal dystrophy	Stevens-Johnson syndrome
Neuromuscular junction	Chronic graft-vs.-host disease
Myasthenia gravis	Metabolic
Eaton-Lambert syndrome	Hypercalcemia
Botulism	Diabetes mellitus
	Treatment-related
	Postoperative head and neck radiation
	Foreign device (tracheostomy tube, nasogastric tube)
	Medication-induced injury

Data from Brin MF, Younger D: Neurologic disorders and aspiration. Otolaryngol Clin North Am 1988; 21:691; Buchholtz D: Neurologic causes of dysphagia. Dysphagia 1987; 1:152; Buchin PJ: Swallowing disorders: Diagnosis and medical treatment. Otolaryngol Clin North Am 1988; 21:663; Jones B, Ravich WJ, Donner MW: Dysphagia in systemic disease. Dysphagia 1993; 8:368; Kosko JR, Moser JD, Erhart N, et al: Differential diagnosis of dysphagia in children. Otolaryngol Clin North Am 1998; 31:435; and Schechter GL: Systemic causes of dysphagia in adults. Otolaryngol Clin North Am 1998; 31:525.

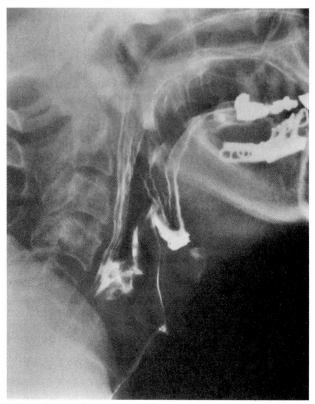

FIGURE 26–2. Tracheal aspiration of barium due to overflow of barium pooled in vallecu-lae in patient who had had a stroke.

- In general, the prognosis for oral feeding after stroke is good, and the risk for aspiration pneumonia decreases over time. Monitoring oral feedings is warranted because of persistent or late-onset dysphagia.

Traumatic Brain Injury (p. 547)

- Dysphagia in the head-injured population is not uncommon. Cognitive impairment, motor control difficulties, drooling and behavioral dysfunction can all be present. Several treatment options exist including oral motor exercises, drug administration (atropine), behavioral programs, and surgical interventions.

Motor Neuron Disease (pp. 547–548)

- Upper and lower motor neuron dysfunction occurs commonly in a significant number of patients with motor neuron disease and results in oral and pharyngeal dysphagia. Because of the progressive nature of this disorder, difficult emotional and ethical issues often arise. Various treatment measures can be used in this disorder, including surgical options such as laryngeal diversion.

Myasthenia Gravis (p. 549)

• Swallowing difficulties in myasthenia gravis are sometimes greater than expected from the symptoms and are not necessarily amenable to pharmacological intervention.

Myotonic Dystrophy (p. 549)

• Although dysphagia is not common in Duchenne muscular dystrophy, the facial and pharyngeal muscular weakness in myotonic dystrophy often results in significant dysphagia.

Nonneurological Disorders (p. 550)

• In addition to the neurological causes, nonneurological causes for dysphagia are important to consider in the rehabilitation setting. The patient with primarily neurological dysphagia might also have a concurrent, nonneurological cause that is aggravating the swallowing process, such as cervical osteophytes (see Fig. 26–12 in the Textbook) or Zenker's diverticulum (see Fig. 26–19 in the Textbook). The presence of pain or difficulties in swallowing solids early in the course of dysphagia raises suspicion of a nonneurological cause.

AGE CONSIDERATIONS IN DYSPHAGIA (pp. 550–551)

Elderly Patients (p. 550)

• Although aging is not a cause of dysphagia, age-related changes can increase the possibility of swallowing problems. These include motor and sensory changes, changes in central and peripheral processes, dentition problems, oral and pharyngeal muscle atrophy, ligamentous laxity, and diminished taste and smell sensitivity.

• Aspiration results from oral phase or combined oropharyngeal phase dysfunction in the elderly as commonly as, if not more commonly than, pharyngeal stage problems alone. Abnormalities include poor bolus containment, dyscoordination, pharyngeal bolus retention, and inadequate laryngeal protection.

• Management of the elderly patient can involve special considerations. From a dietary standpoint, the older patient might routinely take in fewer calories and have secondary deficiencies, particularly vitamin D, calcium, zinc, copper, and chromium. Ethical issues may arise regarding nutrition delivery. For example, a mentally competent patient might not choose to accept enteral feeding despite a risk of aspiration. More difficult decisions arise with end-stage dementia or severe brain injury. Specific goals for treatment help alleviate ethical concerns.

Young Patients (pp. 550–551)

• Swallowing difficulties in children result in similar concerns as adults (i.e., poor nutrition and aspiration). Certain factors, such as anatomical differences, make dysphagia in children unique. Evolution toward the adult configuration begins by age 3 to 4 months and continues until bone growth is complete.

• Differences between the infant and adult are most apparent in the oral phase of swallowing. Suckling consists of a rhythmic compression of the nipple by the tongue and lower jaw against the palate and upper jaw. With development, the oral phase evolves through a series of chewing functions until about age 3 years, and becomes fully coordinated by about age 6 years. The pharyngeal phase in the infant is similar to that of the adult from early on, although the swallow occurs with greater frequency and speed.

• Dysphagia in children can be assessed with videofluoroscopy. Infants less than 6 months are optimally positioned semi-upright with the head in the midline. After 6 months, an increasingly more upright posture is used.

• Difficulties in feeding and swallowing arise from several sources. Prematurity can result in poor coordination of deglutition and ventilation: This can cause prolonged eating times. Because hypoxemia can occur during feeding, pulse oximetry during mealtime can be useful. Neurologically impaired children can exhibit findings such as the bite reflex, tongue thrust, poor trunk control, and slowness in eating. The degree of swallowing difficulty typically parallels the degree of impairment in cerebral palsy, but aspiration can remain clinically hidden.

• As with the adult, gastroesophageal reflux is a common problem. Gastric pH changes with age, and the lowest mean pH occurs in the pediatric age group. This low pH places the child at particular risk for aspiration-induced chemical pneumonitis.

• Congenital structural lesions can interfere with the normal anatomical transport of a bolus. Examples include choanal atresia, cleft lip and palate, craniofacial syndromes, double aortic arch, and aberrant right subclavian artery. With certain structural lesions, prosthetic devices or adapted feeding equipment might be necessary. A Chiari malformation is a structural lesion that can result in neurogenic dysphagia.

COMPLICATIONS OF DYSPHAGIA (pp. 551–553)

Aspiration Pneumonia (p. 551)

• Dysphagia is a major risk factor for aspiration pneumonia, but it usually results in pneumonia only when present with other risk factors (e.g., dependency for feeding, medical comorbidities, or poor oral hygiene). Aspiration typically occurs at the time of eating, but it can also occur at other times. Not every episode of aspiration results in pneumonia. Aspiration results in pneumonia primarily by three mechanisms: chemical injury, bacterial infection, and obstruction (Table 26–3).

• Chemical pneumonitis typically presents with acute dyspnea and hypoxemia. It develops from the burn of gastric acid. The pH and volume of the aspirate seem to be the most important determinants of injury. The natural course of pneumonia is variable. Treatment is supportive, with fluids and ventilation provided as needed. The role of steroids and antibiotics is not clearly defined.

• Bacterial pneumonia typically presents with fever and sputum production. Anaerobes present in oral flora are common pathogens in community-acquired

TABLE 26-3 Classification of Aspiration Pneumonia

Inoculum	Pulmonary Sequelae	Clinical Features	Therapy
Acid	Chemical pneumonitis	Acute dyspnea, tachypnea, tachycardia with or without cyanosis, bronchospasm, fever Sputum: pink, frothy X-ray: infiltrates in one or both lower lobes Hypoxemia	Positive-pressure breathing Intravenous fluids Tracheal suction Corticosteroids
Oropharyngeal bacteria	Bacterial infection	Usually insidious onset Cough, fever, purulent sputum X-ray: infiltrate involving dependent pulmonary segment or lobe, with or without cavitation	Antibiotics
Inert fluids	Mechanical obstruction Reflex airway closure	Acute dyspnea, cyanosis with or without apnea Pulmonary edema	Tracheal suction Intermittent positive pressure breathing with oxygen and isoproterenol
Particulate matter	Mechanical obstruction	Dependent on level of obstruction, ranging from acute apnea and rapid death to irritation chronic cough with or without recurrent infections	Extraction of particulate matter

From Bartlett JG: Aspiration pneumonia. In Baum GL, Wolinsky E (eds.): Textbook of Pulmonary Diseases, ed. 5, vol. 1. Boston, Little, Brown, 1994, p. 593. Reprinted by permission of the publisher.

pneumonia, whereas gram-negative bacilli and *Staphylococcus aureus* become more prominent in hospital-acquired disease.

• Aspiration of food particles can result in airway obstruction. The right main-stem bronchus territory is typically involved, and symptoms include wheezing, coughing, choking, and respiratory distress. The severity of this condition partially depends on the size of the particle aspirated. All caregivers of dysphagic patients should know the Heimlich maneuver. A superimposed bacterial infection is possible.

• In addition to specific treatment for dysphagia, measures to prevent aspiration pneumonia include elevation of the head of the bed, use of H_2-blocking agents or antacids, and decrease in food intake before sleep.

Malnutrition (pp. 552–553)

• Poor nutritional status is a common problem in the acute hospitalized and rehabilitating patient. Presumably, the patient with dysphagia is in a particularly high-risk category for undernutrition.

• When oral intake is insufficient for nutritional needs, enteral feeding is indicated. Options include nasogastric and gastrostomy tubes. The latter provides the nutrition more reliably. The absence of a nasogastric tube facilitates swallowing interventions but does not eliminate the risk of aspiration. Continuous feedings result in the least gastric distention and are useful in patients with poor enteral motility or those requiring hypertonic formulas. Intermittent or bolus feeding is less disruptive to rehabilitation activities and to general daily living.

TREATMENT MENU FOR DYSPHAGIA (pp. 553–557)

Dietary Modification (p. 553)

• Dietary modification is a critical step in a therapeutic feeding program. If oral feedings are appropriate, the type of food needs careful consideration. Although thin liquids can result in less pharyngeal residue, they are often difficult for the neurologic patient to manage. Liquids can be thickened with various agents. The patient or a family member can be instructed in their proper use.

• Food can be modified to pureed, semisolid, or solid consistencies. Pureed consistencies can be used for patients with difficulty chewing or an inability to form a cohesive bolus. As swallowing improves, diets can be advanced. Many centers have "dysphagia diets" as a means for organizing foods. Its benefit is that it links similar foods. Monitoring of the patient with the introduction of each new food type ensures safety. Because many patients are instructed in compensatory techniques, monitoring the patient during mealtime is essential.

• Oral hygiene needs careful consideration because dried secretions can accumulate. Lemon-glycerin, plain swabs, or a damp washcloth can be used to remove the secretions.

Exercise and Facilitation Techniques (pp. 553–555)

• These techniques require that the patient be able to follow directions and participate in a therapy program. The indications for use of the exercises are outlined in Table 26–4.

TABLE 26–4 Indications for Exercises in Patients with Dysphagia

Clinical Diagnosis	Clinical Observation	Exercise/ Technique
Decreased lip range of motion, strength, or coordination	Drooling, facial droop	Lip exercises
Decreased tongue range of motion, strength, or coordination	Inability to propel food from front to back of mouth Food pooling in sulci	Tongue exercises
Decreased jaw range of motion, strength, or coordination	Inability to chew food adequately	Jaw exercises
Weak or absent cough	Nonproductive cough	Respiratory exercises
Increased respiratory rate	Rapid or shallow breathing	Respiratory exercises
Decreased airway protection	Wet or "gurgly" voice Hoarse voice Coughing during the swallow	Vocal cord adduction exercises
Delayed/absent swallow reflex	Decreased laryngeal elevation during swallow Coughing before the swallow	Thermal stimulation
Incomplete contact between tongue base and posterior pharyngeal wall	Pooling in the valleculae	Tongue base retraction exercises

• Exercises designed to facilitate oral motor strength, range of motion, and coordination are best done frequently (e.g., five to ten times per day). Patients and family members can be instructed to perform the exercises between therapy sessions. Examples include smiling, lip pursing, tongue protruding, and yawning. Other exercises are designed to improve laryngeal elevation, respiratory support, and vocal cord adduction.

• Thermal-tactile stimulation is a facilitative technique designed to increase swallow speed. Cold modalities are applied to the anterior facial arch bilaterally. This technique has been found to be of clinical benefit, although long-term results are inconclusive.

• If abnormal oral reflexes (e.g., tongue thrust and bite reflex) are observed, attempts should be made to inhibit them. Techniques include sustained tongue pressure, tongue vibration, upright head positioning, and tongue stretching.

• The gag reflex can be hypoactive or hyperactive. Attempts to normalize the gag reflex are recommended. Facilitation of a hypoactive gag can be achieved by stimulating soft palate. A hyperactive gag can be desensitized by slowly "walking" back on the tongue while applying pressure with a tongue depressor. As the gag reflex becomes less sensitive, the tongue depressor can be advanced farther back in the mouth.

Compensatory Techniques (pp. 555–556)

• Positioning the patient's head and trunk can compensate for swallowing dysfunction (see Table 26–5). The ideal position for most neurologic patients is

TABLE 26–5 Indications for Compensatory Techniques in Patients with Dysphagia

Clinical Diagnosis	Clinical Observations	Compensatory Technique
Delayed swallow reflex	Coughing before the swallow Aspiration	Chin tuck Supraglottic swallow
Decreased pharyngeal peristalsis (unilaterally)	Unilateral pooling in the pharyngeal region Coughing after the swallow	Turning of head to weaker side Tilting of head to stronger side
Decreased pharyngeal peristalsis	Coughing after the swallow	Effortful swallow Double swallow Alternating liquids and swallows
Decreased laryngeal closure	Coughing during or after the swallow	Chin tuck Supraglottic swallow
Decreased opening of cricopharyngeal region	Coughing after the swallow Pooling in the pyriform sinus	Mendelsohn's maneuver Turning of head to weaker side

seated upright with the head in the midline, the trunk erect, and the neck slightly flexed. Pillows and other supports can be used to maintain trunk and extremity support.

• Common postural techniques used to decrease aspiration include tilting the chin down, and turning or tilting the head. The chin tuck narrows the opening of the airway and may widen the vallecular space (Fig. 26–3). It is particularly useful for patients with a delayed pharyngeal swallow, reduced tongue base retraction, or reduced airway closure. Turning the head to the affected side may be beneficial when decreased pharyngeal peristalsis is noted unilaterally. This maneuver helps direct food down the stronger side of the pharynx and also improves upper esophageal sphincter function. Tilting the head toward the stronger side can be of similar benefit. It also helps with unilateral tongue weakness because it directs food toward the stronger side. These techniques can be effective for decreasing or eliminating aspiration in some cases. Videofluoroscopy is useful to determine the effectiveness of these techniques.

• Other compensatory techniques include effortful swallows, double swallows, consistency alteration, supraglottic and supra-supraglottic swallows, and the Mendelsohn maneuver. For the effortful swallow, the patient swallows "hard" in an attempt to help forcefully propel food through the pharynx. For double swallowing, the patient swallows repeatedly. Alternating liquids and solids help to clear any material remaining in the pharyngeal recesses. One or more of these techniques can be can be effective with decreased pharyngeal peristalsis. The supraglottic swallow is designed to close the airway voluntarily. It incorporates closure of the vocal folds along with clearing the airway of any aspirated material. This technique can be with reduced laryngeal closure. The steps of the supraglottic swallow are as follows:

1. Take a portion of food.
2. Chew well.
3. Take a deep breath and hold it.

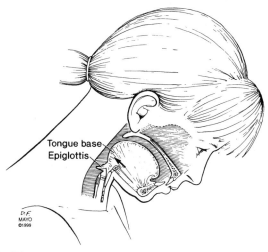

FIGURE 26–3. Chin tuck to protect the airway and prevent aspiration. (Reproduced by permission of Mayo Foundation.)

4. Swallow while holding the breath.
5. Cough immediately after the swallow.
6. Relax and breathe normally.
• The super supraglottic swallow incorporates the supraglottic swallow while the patient performs a Valsalva maneuver. The Mendelsohn maneuver prolongs the opening of the cricopharyngeal region. To perform this maneuver, patients concentrate on the feeling of the Adam's apple rising while they swallow. Next, they are instructed to hold the swallow for 2 to 3 seconds when the pharynx is at its uppermost point. Finally, they are asked to complete the swallow and relax. It is one of the few techniques that may be of assistance in cricopharyngeal disorders.
• Biofeedback techniques also may be of assistance in swallowing retraining. They can be useful for oral motor and facial exercises and for giving the patient feedback on the actual swallow.

Adaptive Equipment (pp. 556–557)

• Numerous devices are available to assist patients who have difficulty with the motor or perceptual components of feeding. Examples include rocker knives, swivel utensils, built-up handles, scoop dishes, nonskid mats, and large-handled cups (see Fig. 26–22 in the Textbook). These devices compensate for decreased upper extremity function (see Chapter 25).

Surgical Procedures (p. 557)

• Operative intervention is another option in the treatment of dysphagia. It is particularly helpful when conservative measures have failed and swallowing difficulties arise from a focal neuromuscular disorder or obstruction.

• A tracheostomy is both a short-term solution for airway protection and a risk factor for aspiration. After tracheostomy, laryngeal elevation is impaired, which increases the risk of aspiration. Aspiration can also be associated with cuff inflation or deflation. The inflated cuff applies a compressive force to the esophagus and may increase resistance to the passage of a food bolus. The deflated cuff allows retained material to pass into the trachea (see Fig. 26–23 in the Textbook).

• Cricopharyngeal myotomy can be indicated for Zenker's diverticulum, cricopharyngeal achalasia, and selected neuromusuclar diseases. Myotomy is not generally recommended for generalized failure of the swallowing process. Botulinium toxin injections have been used to identify patients who will benefit from myotomy.

• Several procedures have been devised for protection of the larynx (e.g., vocal cord augmentation and laryngeal diversion). Microsurgical techniques and miniature electrical stimulation are emerging possibilities.

27

Original Chapter by Diana D. Cardenas, M.D., and
Michael E. Mayo, M.B.B.S.

Management of Bladder Dysfunction

NEUROANATOMY (pp. 561–562)

Receptors (pp. 561–562)

- Cholinergic muscarinic (M_2 and M_3) receptors are active during bladder contraction and are widely distributed in the body of the bladder, trigone, bladder neck, and urethra.
- Adrenergic receptors are concentrated in the trigone, bladder neck, and urethra and are predominantly α_1.
- Norepinephrine containing nerve cells are also found in the paravesical and intramural ganglia. A few authors describe norepinephrine terminals in the striated muscle of the distal sphincter, although most would dispute this. When these cells are active, they have excitatory effects and maintain continence by contraction of the bladder neck and urethral smooth muscle.
- α_2-Adrenergic receptors are found in the bladder neck and also in the body of the bladder. These receptors are inhibitory when activated and can produce relaxation at the bladder neck on initiation of voiding and relax the bladder body to enhance storage (see Fig. 27–1 in the Textbook). In humans, however, the storage role seems to be a minor one.
- Cholinergic nicotinic receptors are found in the striated sphincter muscle.
- The main effector transmitter for contraction of the urethra is norepinephrine, via the α_1 receptors. Smooth muscle relaxation is mediated by acetylcholine and probably by nitric oxide. Prostaglandins, in contrast to their effects on the detrusor, cause a relaxation of the urethral muscle. Serotonin appears to be an antagonist that causes urethral muscle contraction; it might be important in the production of irritable urethral symptoms. The role of estrogens on the lower urinary tract in women is confined to the modification of tissues and receptors, with no apparent direct transmitter effects.
- In the brainstem and spinal cord the various transmitters described above can have a variety of inhibitory and facilitative actions, depending on their site of action. Serotonin might have inhibitory detrusor effects at the midbrain level, and uptake of serotonin might be blocked by tricyclics (which are used in treating nocturnal enuresis). Activation of opiate receptors in the brainstem and sacral spinal cord inhibits voiding. This might partly explain the retention of urine seen with the use of these agents.

Innervation (p. 562)

• The afferent and efferent peripheral pathways include the autonomic through the pelvic (parasympathetic) and hypogastric (sympathetic) nerves, and the somatic through the pudendal nerves (Fig. 27–1).

Central Connections and Control (p. 562)

• The reflex center for the bladder lies in the pons along with the other autonomic centers. There is a reflex with afferent axons originating from the bladder and synapsing on the pudendal nerve nucleus at S2, S3, and S4 that allows inhibition of pelvic floor activity during voiding. Another important reflex is the local segmental innervation of the external sphincter with afferents from the urethra, sphincter, and pelvic floor and efferents in the pudendal nerve. Higher (voluntary) control over the pelvic floor is achieved through afferents that ascend to the sensory cortex. Descending fibers from the motor cortex synapse with the pudendal motor nucleus.

BLADDER FUNCTION (pp. 562–563)

• Urodynamic studies in both intact patients and those with neurological disease have yielded clinical insights into the normal and abnormal function of the lower urinary tract over the course of life.

Infant and Young Child (p. 562)

• Neonates and infants have reflex bladders that empty at approximately 50- to 100-mL volumes. Sometime after the first year of life, the child begins to show some awareness of bladder evacuation and can begin to delay urination for a brief period by contracting the voluntary sphincter. For normal control, the detrusor reflex has to be inhibited by the higher centers at the level of the pontine nucleus. By 5 years of age, approximately 90% of children have normal control. The remaining 10% have a more infantile or immature pattern, with detrusor activity between voluntary voidings that produces frequency, urgency, and occasionally urge incontinence and nocturnal enuresis. Most of these children gradually develop inhibition of the detrusor reflex by the onset of puberty.

Adult (p. 563)

• With bladder filling, there is only a minimal rise in intravesical pressure (accommodation) together with an increase in recruitment of activity in the pelvic floor and voluntary sphincter. Normal voiding is initiated by voluntary relaxation of the pelvic floor with subsequent release of inhibition of the detrusor reflex at the pontine level. The detrusor contraction is maintained steadily throughout voiding, and the pelvic floor remains quiescent.

Elderly (p. 563)

• Frequency, urgency, and incontinence with incomplete emptying are common in the elderly. Urodynamic studies show that many elderly persons have bladder contractions during filling, producing frequency, urgency, and incontinence.

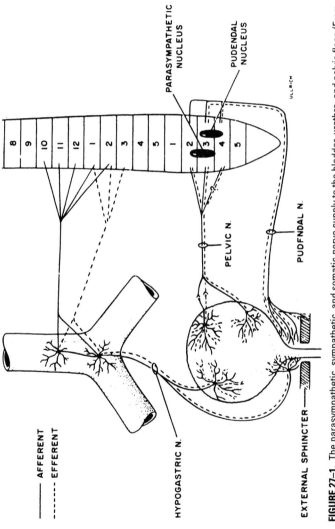

FIGURE 27–1. The parasympathetic, sympathetic, and somatic nerve supply to the bladder, urethra, and pelvic floor. (From Blaivas JG: Management of bladder dysfunction in multiple sclerosis. Neurology 1980; 30(2):12–18.)

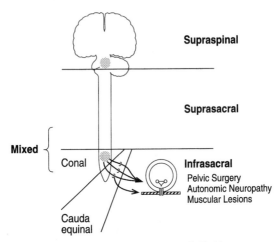

FIGURE 27–2. Anatomical classification of the neurogenic bladder.

CLASSIFICATION (pp. 563–564)

• The neurogenic bladder has been classified in a variety of ways. The first functional classification was based on cystometric findings, and five basic groups were described: (1) reflex, (2) uninhibited, (3) autonomous, (4) motor paralytic, and (5) sensory neurogenic bladders. This system does not take into account the function of the sphincter mechanisms, however, and there are a few patients in whom the detrusor reflex does not return after spinal cord injury above the sacral outflow.

• Later a more anatomical classification system was proposed in which the neurogenic bladder was subdivided into types such as supraspinal, suprasacral spinal, infrasacral, peripheral autonomic, and muscular lesions (Fig. 27–2).

• At the same time, others developed functional classifications, all of which were based on conventional urodynamic evaluations. This was an attempt to categorize the lower urinary tract according to the passive storage ability of the bladder and the activities and coordination of the detrusor and sphincter mechanisms (Table 27–1).

• In practice it is common to use a combination of both anatomical and functional classifications, with any known neurological lesion described in anatomical terms (e.g., supraspinal or suprasacral).

HISTORY AND PHYSICAL EXAMINATION (p. 564)

• The history should help determine whether there were voiding symptoms before the neurological event. The physical examination should assess mental status and confirm the neurological level (if present). The perineal sensation and pelvic floor muscle tone are particularly important in lower spinal cord and peripheral lesions. Reflexes are also important, but the bulbocavernous, cremasteric, and anal reflexes are sometimes difficult to elicit, even in intact persons. The skin of the perineum; state of bladder supports; and, in women,

TABLE 27–1 Functional Classification of the Neurogenic Bladder

Type of Failure	Bladder Factors	Outlet Factors
Failure to store	Hyperreflexia	Denervated pelvic floor
	Decreased compliance	Bladder neck descent
		Intrinsic bladder neck sphincter failure
Failure to empty	Areflexia	Detrusor-sphincter dyssynergia (striated sphincter and bladder neck)
	Hypocontractility	Nonrelaxing voluntary sphincter
		Mechanical obstruction (benign prostatic hypertrophy or stricture)

degree of vaginal support and estrogenization should be assessed. The prostate in males should be evaluated, but size or consistency alone is not a good indicator of obstruction. Lastly, an assessment should be made of the patient's motivation, lifestyle, body habitus, and other physical impairments.

DIAGNOSTIC TESTS (pp. 564–568)

Indications (pp. 564–565)

• The upper tracts need evaluation if there are symptoms suggestive of pyelonephritis or prior history of renal disease. Some neurological conditions such as stroke, Parkinson's disease, and multiple sclerosis rarely or only occasionally cause upper tract involvement. For these conditions, a simple baseline screening test such as renal ultrasonography (US) is sufficient. Conditions such as those involving a complete spinal cord lesion and myelodysplasia need more extensive and regular upper tract surveillance with both structural and functional tests.
• The lower urinary tract evaluation can be quite simple, from urinalysis to urine culture to measurement of postvoid residual. A full urodynamic evaluation might be necessary, however, especially if incomplete bladder emptying, incontinence, recurrent bacteriuria, or upper tract changes are present.
• The bladder findings on urodynamic studies cannot be used to determine the level of neurological lesion. The anatomical level of the neurological lesion can suggest to the clinician the most common pattern of bladder dysfunction, but urodynamic testing should always be performed to confirm this.

Upper Tract Tests (p. 565)

Ultrasonography (p. 565)
• Ultrasonography is a low-risk and relatively low-cost test for routine evaluation of the upper urinary tract. It is not sensitive enough for evaluating acute ureteral obstruction, and in this clinical setting non-contrast-enhanced computed tomography (CT) should be performed.

Plain Radiography of the Urinary Tract—Kidneys, Ureter, and Bladder (KUB) (p. 565)
• A KUB study is often combined with US to identify any possible radiopaque calculi in the ureter or bladder stones not seen on US.

Computed Tomography (p. 565)
• CT is often performed without contrast agent enhancement and has replaced KUB, US, and excretory urography in the evaluation of the upper tracts when acute obstruction from stones is a possibility.

Excretory Urography or Intravenous Pyelography (p. 565)
• The term excretory urography has replaced intravenous pyelography because modern techniques show much more than the collecting system. Renal tomograms obtained 1 to 3 minutes after contrast agent injection should show a clear nephrogram. If the serum creatinine concentration is more than 1.5 mg/dL, or if the patient has insulin-dependent diabetes, intravenous contrast agent administration increases the risk of contrast-related nephropathy. In these cases, alternative studies include US; radioisotope renography; and, possibly, cystoscopy with retrograde pyelography.

Creatinine Clearance Time (p. 565)
• This has been the gold standard for assessing renal function and is said to approximate the glomerular filtration rate, but its accuracy depends on meticulous urine collection. In patients with quadriplegia who have low muscle mass and a 24-hour creatinine excretion of less than 1000 mg, the calculated creatinine clearance time can be too inaccurate to be clinically useful.

Isotope Studies (p. 565)
• The technetium 99m DMSA (dimercaptosuccinic acid) scan is still the best study for both differential function and evaluation of the functioning areas of the renal cortex. The renogram obtained with ^{99m}Tc-MAG 3 (mertiatide) also gives information on urinary tract drainage, as well as a good assessment of differential function. In patients who might have ureteral reflux, these studies should be done with the bladder drained with an indwelling catheter.

Lower Tract Tests (pp. 565–568)

Urinalysis, Culture and Sensitivity Testing (p. 565)
• These tests are done routinely for all patients with neurogenic bladder disease and should be repeated as often as necessary. Bacteriuria should be treated before any invasive test is performed.

Postvoid Residual (pp. 565–566)
• High intravesical pressures can be present in spite of low PVR values. The PVR is simple to determine and clinically useful, when compared with prior recordings and taken in conjunction with the bladder pressure, clinical symptoms, and the appearance of the bladder wall. A catheter insertion has been used for PVR in the past, but there are now simple US machines that can noninvasively obtain the PVR.

Cystography (p. 566)
• This study is usually performed to test for the presence or absence of ureteral reflux, and it also shows the bladder shape and outline. The procedure is usually performed in the radiology department, often with no control over the rate of bladder filling and without any monitoring of intravesical pressure. Significant bacteriuria should be treated before the test is performed. Blood pressure should

be monitored throughout the test in all patients with spinal cord lesions above T6 who are at risk for autonomic dysreflexia.

Cystometrography (p. 566)

• Cystometrography (CMG) is a filling study and gives little information about the voiding phase of bladder function. Although carbon dioxide as a filling medium is convenient with the commercially available apparatus, this type of testing has shown considerable variability, poor reproducibility, and the presence of artifacts due to leakage of CO_2 gas around the catheter. However, the CO_2 CMG is a useful bedside test to monitor the return of a detrusor reflex in the spinal shock phase of spinal cord injury, and to confirm the presence of detrusor hyperreflexia in patients with supraspinal or cerebral insult before pharmacotherapy is started.

• Water CMGs are best obtained with a two-channel catheter, with one channel used for filling and the other for pressure recording. A rectal pressure trace is also helpful in many patients to help distinguish intravesical pressure variations (caused by intra-abdominal transmission) from contractions of the detrusor itself. Reported filling rates vary but are usually in the range of 25 to 60 mL/min. During filling, patients are asked to suppress voiding. Normal values include a capacity of 300 to 600 mL, with an initial sensation of filling at approximately 50% of capacity. The change in volume divided by the rise in baseline pressure during filling (i.e., in the absence of a detrusor contraction) describes the bladder's compliance. This value should be greater than 10 mL/cm H_2O, and 10 to 20 mL/cm H_2O is borderline if the bladder capacity is reduced. Normal persons are able to suppress detrusor contractions during this test. Any detrusor contraction during the test, usually defined as a phasic pressure change of more than 15 cm H_2O, is abnormal. If the patient is neurologically intact, these contractions are referred to as uninhibited. If the patient has a suprasacral or supraspinal lesion, these contractions are called hyperreflexic. The absence of a contraction does not necessarily imply true areflexia in a patient with an infrasacral lesion.

Sphincter Electromyography (p. 566)

• Sphincter electromyography (EMG) can be combined with the CMG or preferably with a full multichannel videourodynamic study. Recordings have been made with a variety of electrodes (e.g., monopolar, coaxial needle, and surface electrodes) from the levator, perianal, or periurethral muscles. Because some authors claim there is a functional dissociation between these muscle groups, periurethral recordings are preferred. The integrated EMG is displayed on the same trace as the bladder pressure. EMG activity gradually increases as bladder capacity is reached during bladder filling, and then becomes silent just before voiding. In complete spinal cord injury, low levels of EMG activity with no recruitment during filling is a common pattern. In these patients, however, as a reflex detrusor contraction occurs, EMG activity in the sphincter can increase rather than decrease. With this detrusor-sphincter dyssynergia, voiding often occurs toward the end of the detrusor contraction because the striated sphincter relaxes more quickly than the smooth muscle of the bladder. This type of sphincter EMG does not display individual motor units and cannot be used for the evaluation of infrasacral denervation of the pelvic floor musculature (for which standard needle EMG is needed).

TABLE 27–2 Urodynamic Definitions

Bladder

Hyperreflexia	Uninhibited contractions of the detrusor during filling due to neurological disease
Hypocontractility	Unsustained contractions causing failure to empty
Areflexia	Absent contractions with attempt to void
Compliance	Change in volume divided by change in baseline pressure with filling (<10 mL/cm H_2O abnormal; 10–20 mL/cm H_2O borderline if capacity reduced)

Outlet

Detrusor-sphincter dyssynergia	
1. At bladder neck	Usually in high quadriplegic patients with autonomic hyperactivity
2. At striated sphincter	Uncoordinated pelvic floor and striated sphincter contraction with detrusor contraction during attempts to void
Nonrelaxing sphincter	Poor voluntary relaxation of voluntary sphincter in patients with areflexia attempting to void by Valsalva's maneuver
Decreased outlet resistance	Incontinence due to damage to the bladder neck or striated sphincter, pelvic floor descent, or denervation

Videourodynamics (pp. 566–567)
• This study is designed to give the maximum information about the filling and voiding phases of lower urinary tract function, and every effort is made to make it as physiological as possible. A videourodynamic study is indicated in the following patients: those with incomplete spinal cord lesions with incontinence who have some ability to void and inhibit voiding voluntarily but empty incompletely; persons with mechanical obstruction (e.g., benign prostatic hyperplasia) with neuropathy; candidates for sphincterotomy, to assess detrusor contraction and the presence or absence of bladder neck obstruction in addition to striated sphincter dyssynergia; those who fail to respond to pharmacotherapy; those who will undergo any surgical procedures such as augmentation, continent diversion, or placement of an artificial sphincter or a suprapubic catheter; patients who have deterioration of the upper tracts; and, finally, patients who relapse regularly with symptomatic bacteriuria. Table 27–2 lists urodynamic terms used to categorize bladder and outlet abnormalities.

Cystoscopy (pp. 567–568)
• The only routine indication for cystoscopy is the presence of a long-term indwelling suprapubic or urethral catheter because there can be a risk of bladder tumor development. Cystoscopy is recommended after 5 years in high-risk patients (e.g., smokers) or after 10 years in those with no risk factors. Cystoscopy should also be performed after excretory urography in patients who have gross or microscopic hematuria that cannot be clearly associated with urinary tract infection (UTI), stones, or trauma. Bladder stones can usually be detected on plain radiographs or US, but persistent infection can be associated with gravel

too small to be detected on imaging studies. Consequently, repeated lower tract infections can be an indication for cystoscopy.

Other Tests (p. 568)

• See the Textbook for descriptions of other less commonly used tests such as long-term monitoring, transrectal or transvaginal ultrasound, urethral pressure profile, and bethanechol stimulation test.

MANAGEMENT (pp. 568–573)
General Principles (p. 568)

• Patient goals are to empty the bladder not more than every 3 to 4 hours, remain continent, sleep without interference from the urinary drainage system, and avoid recurrent UTI or other complications. The following discussion describes specific management approaches (Table 27–3).

Approaches and Rationale (pp. 568–573)

Behavioral Management (pp. 568–569)
TIMED VOIDING
• For patients with hyperreflexia producing urgency or reflex incontinence, a timed voiding program can help by having the patient urinate before the anticipated detrusor contraction. The limitation to this program is that persons with dementia need continual reminding. It is also useful in patients with sphincter weakness because the incontinence is worse when the bladder is full, and timed voiding reduces the amount of urine leakage.

BLADDER STIMULATION
• Various maneuvers have been tried to stimulate the bladder. Stroking or pinching the perineal skin, which is intended to cause reflex stimulation, is rarely effective. Suprapubic tapping or jabbing over the bladder causes a mechanical stretch of the bladder wall and subsequent contraction. Deeper indentation of the bladder with a jabbing technique is the most effective maneuver.

VALSALVA'S AND CREDÉ'S MANEUVERS
• Patients with areflexia and some denervation of the pelvic floor (infrasacral lesions) are able to void by a Valsalva maneuver or straining. This is most effective in women because the paralyzed pelvic floor descends with straining and the bladder neck opens. Over time, however, the pelvic floor descent increases as the paralyzed muscles atrophy and stretch, and the patient complains of worsening stress incontinence. Credé's maneuver, usually performed by an attendant, mechanically pushes urine out of the bladder in patients with quadriplegia. The abdominal wall must be relaxed to allow Credé's maneuver to be effective, and there is a theoretical risk of producing ureteral reflux by the long-term use of this method.

ANAL STRETCH VOIDING
• In patients with paraplegia who have a spastic pelvic floor, effective voiding has been achieved by an anal stretch technique. This technique involves relaxing the pelvic floor by first stretching the anal sphincter and then evacuating by Valsalva's maneuver. It requires transfer onto a toilet for bladder emptying,

TABLE 27–3 Bladder Management Options

Failure to Store	
Bladder factors	
Behavioral	Timed voids
Collecting devices	Diaper, condom catheter, indwelling catheter
CIC	With drugs to lower bladder pressure
Drugs	Anticholinergics, musculotropics, intrathecal baclofen,* calcium channel blockers,* intravesical capsaicin*
Surgery	Augmentation, continent diversion, denervation procedures*
Outlet factors	
Behavioral	Timed voids, pelvic floor exercises
Collecting devices	Diaper, condom catheter, indwelling catheter
Drugs	α-Agonists, imipramine, estrogens
Surgery	Collagen injection, fascial sling, artificial sphincter, Teflon injection*
Failure to Empty	
Bladder factors	
Behavioral	Timed voids, bladder stimulation, Valsalva's and Credé's maneuvers
Collecting devices	Indwelling catheter
CIC	
Drugs	Bethanechol
Surgery	Neurostimulation*
Outlet factors	
Behavioral	Anal stretch void
Collecting devices	Indwelling catheters
CIC	
Drugs	α-Blockers, oral striated muscle relaxant, intrathecal baclofen*
Surgery	Sphincterotomy incision, bladder neck incision, prostate resection, pudendal neurectomy,* stent sphincterotomy*
Failure of Storage and Emptying with Nonusable Urethra	
Surgery	Suprapubic catheter ± bladder neck closure, ileal conduit, continent diversion

Abbreviation: CIC, clean intermittent catheterization.
*Experimental or nonstandard management.

absence of anal sensation, and the ability to generate adequate intra-abdominal pressure. For these reasons it is not widely used.

PELVIC FLOOR EXERCISES
• Pelvic floor exercises are effective only in female patients with stress incontinence caused by pelvic floor descent. Most patients with infrasacral neuropathy need surgery to achieve continence.

Urine Collection Devices (pp. 569–570)
EXTERNAL CONDOM CATHETERS
• External condom catheters are convenient and often the best management for men with tetraplegia who are unable to perform self-catheterization, provided

that any outflow obstruction is adequately treated. Bacteriuria with fever is more common in those who have intermittent catheterization done by an attendant than in those on any other bladder management program, including indwelling catheterization. Problems with skin breakdown and urethral damage can occur if the condom is applied too tightly. There is also an increased risk of UTI because of poor hygiene.

INDWELLING CATHETERS

• Indwelling catheters can be either urethral or suprapubic, and are typically used because other programs have failed or for patient convenience. The combination of sphincterotomy and condom drainage, although ideal for men with tetraplegia, often fails because of inadequate detrusor contractions or penile skin problems. In the past, indwelling catheters had a justifiably bad reputation, but there are recent reports that some patients with indwelling catheters do no worse than those on other methods of management. Good catheter care is still very important. Some of the important aspects of care include monthly catheter changes, copious fluid intake, control of hyperreflexia with medication, sterilization of the collecting bags with bleach, and avoidance of traction on the catheter. The prevalence of squamous cell carcinoma of the bladder associated with an indwelling catheter might be lower than reported. Most centers continue to recommend yearly cystoscopy, cytology, and biopsy, if indicated, when the patient has had an indwelling catheter in place for 10 years or more, and possibly after only 5 years if there are increased risk factors such as smoking.

ADULT DIAPERS AND OTHER PROTECTIVE GARMENTS

• Protective garments have improved considerably over the past few years, and a high-absorbency, gel-impregnated material is now used that allows the lining against the patient's perineal skin to stay dry. Protective garments are commonly used in incontinent demented patients who have adequate bladder emptying.

Clean Intermittent Catheterization (p. 570)

• An intermittent catheter program requires a low-pressure bladder of adequate capacity (greater than 300 mL) and enough outflow resistance to maintain continence with normal daily activities. If the bladder is not sufficiently areflexic and compliant, anticholinergics or musculotropics can be used. If these fail, some form of surgery (e.g., augmentation) can be done to achieve a low pressure reservoir. Men with lesions at C6 and below, and women with lesions at C7 and below, can manage self-catheterization. Patients should restrict fluid intake to maintain an output of not more than 600 mL in the time period chosen. Some patients have enough sensation to be able to catheterize on demand, but most have to do so on a timed schedule. A minimum of three catheterizations per 24 hours is recommended because longer intervals between catheterizations theoretically increase the risk of symptomatic bacteriuria. Most patients wash their catheters with soap and water. If recurrent bacteriuria becomes a problem, sterilization by soaking in Cidex (a glutaral preparation) or boiling the catheters is recommended. Rarely, a completely sterile technique is used.

• The most common problems with self-catheterization are symptomatic bacteriuria, urethral trauma, and incontinence. Occasionally a bladder stone formed on a nidus of hair or lint is found, and patients should be warned to avoid introducing foreign material into the bladder with the catheter. Urethral trauma and catheterization difficulties are usually caused by sphincter spasm. This can be managed by using extra lubrication and local anesthetic urethral gel (lidocaine

2%). Sometimes a curved-tip (coudé) catheter is helpful. Repeated urethral bleeding suggests the presence of a break in the urethral mucosa or a false passage, and using an indwelling urethral catheter for a time might be necessary for this to resolve. Urethroscopy and unroofing of a false passage is occasionally necessary.

Drugs *(pp. 570–571)*
• Bladder management drugs in humans have generally been disappointing. The most effective group of drugs are those that inhibit detrusor activity.

CHOLINERGIC AGENTS
• The detrusor is innervated by cholinergic muscularinic (M_2 and M_3) receptors. Bethanechol, a cholinergic agonist, can be helpful in detrusor areflexia by increasing detrusor activity.

ANTICHOLINERGIC AGENTS
• Anticholinergic agents have been used for many years for suppression of detrusor activity. Propantheline bromide (15 to 30 mg three times a day) is the prototype, and hyoscyamine (0.125 to 0.25 mg three or four times a day) is regaining popularity. Oxybutynin hydrochloride, a more recent preparation, has similar actions when taken at 5 to 10 mg three times a day, but it is effective mostly on the muscle cell membrane (musculotropic) rather than on anticholinergic endings. Imipramine is recommended by several authors for its presumed anticholinergic actions. It is said to be additive in its effectiveness, but not in its side effects, when combined with other agents such as oxybutynin and propantheline. A new agent, tolterodine, in a dose of 2 mg twice daily has anticholinergic activity and fewer troublesome side effects from dry mouth and constipation.

ADRENERGIC ANTAGONISTS
• The α-adrenergic receptor antagonist phenoxybenzamine (10 to 30 mg/day) has α_1- and α_2-blocking actions and has been used for inhibiting smooth muscle activity at the bladder neck and in the prostate. Newer agents with more specific α_1-blocking actions are available (e.g., prazosin, terazosin, and doxazosin). These are typically given in doses of 1 to 20 mg/day as tolerated. These agents have a number of effects: They appear to reduce the irritative symptoms in men with obstruction caused by benign prostatic hyperplasia, and to increase emptying in patients with neurogenic voiding dysfunction. A new, more specific agent, tamsulosin, has been introduced for the treatment of benign prostatic hyperplasia. This agent has fewer vascular effects and rarely causes hypotension. Its effects on the neurogenic bladder have not yet been reported. These agents are effective in control of the vascular manifestations of autonomic dysreflexia, and phenoxybenzamine, with its α_1- and α_2-blocking action, might be better in this regard than the pure α_1-blocking agents.

ADRENERGIC AGONISTS
• Adrenergic agonists have been used to increase urethral resistance in patients with mild stress incontinence. Anecdotally, ephedrine (25 to 75 mg/day) has been effective in children with myelodysplasia, but controlled studies are lacking, and adrenergic agonists are rarely used in adults with bladder neuropathy.

ESTROGENS
• Postmenopausal women often have atrophy of the urethral submucosa, which can lead to stress incontinence. Estrogen administration often restores or main-

tains this tissue and can be helpful in women with a partially denervated pelvic floor and stress incontinence.

MUSCLE RELAXANTS
• Diazepam, dantrolene sodium, and baclofen are commonly used for skeletal muscle spasticity, but have never been shown to be effective in controlled studies in patients with detrusor striated sphincter dyssynergia.

Surgery on the Bladder or Bladder Nerves (pp. 571–572)
TO INCREASE BLADDER CAPACITY
Augmentation. Bladder augmentation is often recommended for patients who have detrusor hyperreflexia or reduced compliance that fails to respond to anticholinergic or musculotropic drugs. The patient must be motivated to continue indefinitely with clean intermittent catheterization and must have adequate outflow resistance. The bladder is opened widely in this procedure, and an opened and reconfigured segment of bowel is sewn in (see Fig. 27–6 in the Textbook).

Continent Diversion. In this procedure, bowel is used not just to increase effective bladder capacity but also to form a continent catheterizable channel that opens onto the abdominal wall. It is particularly useful in women for whom intermittent self-catheterization via the urethra is difficult or impossible because of leg spasticity, body habitus, severe urethral incontinence, or the need to transfer from a wheelchair. Men who are unable to perform intermittent catheterization because of strictures, false passages, or fistulas are also potential candidates.

Denervation Procedures. The denervation technique for bladder hyperreflexia, although theoretically attractive, is not widely used. Operative approaches include sectioning of the sacral nerve roots or interrupting the peripheral nerve supply near the bladder.

TO INCREASE BLADDER CONTRACTION
Electrical Stimulation. Attempts have been made to stimulate detrusor contraction using electrodes driven by an implanted receiver conveying a stimulus generated by an external transmitter. The electrodes have been implanted on the bladder wall, pelvic nerves, sacral roots, and conus. At present, the only site being used clinically is the anterior sacral roots, and most of the reported series come from Europe. To prevent spontaneous hyperreflexic contractions and antidromic reflex contractions, bilateral S2, S3, and S4 dorsal rhizotomies are usually performed. Pelvic floor contraction with anterior root stimulation will still obstruct voiding, and European centers have elected to stimulate intermittently. This leads to intermittent voiding, because the striated pelvic floor muscle relaxes more quickly than the smooth muscle detrusor. One important disadvantage of bilateral S2, S3, and S4 rhizotomies is that reflex erections are abolished; usable erections occurring as a result of sacral root stimulation occur in less than 30% of patients. Bowel evacuation, however, is improved in many patients.

Surgery on the Bladder Outlet (pp. 572–573)
TO INCREASE OUTLET RESISTANCE
• Incontinence due to decreased outlet resistance is relatively uncommon in bladder dysfunction secondary to neurological disease. It is seen in children with myelodysplasia and in women with infrasacral lesions and a denervated pelvic

floor. It can occur in active men with complete denervation, but this is rare. Although α-adrenergic agonists might help minor incontinence, more severe leakage typically requires some form of urethral compressive procedure. The options include injection therapy into the bladder neck and urethra to increase the bulk of tissue under and around the bladder neck muscle, a fascial sling, or an artificial sphincter.

Injection Therapy. Teflon has been used for years in the urethra for certain types of stress incontinence, but its use has recently declined because of the danger of particle migration. Autologous fat and bovine collagen have been tried recently, and one to three injections seem to help some proportion of patients. The procedure has few potential side effects and is especially suitable for elderly and poor-risk patients.

External Compressive Procedures. In the fascial sling procedure, a 2-cm strip of fascia is taken from the anterior rectus abdominis fascia or tensor fascia lata. It is wrapped around the bladder neck and fixed anteriorly to the abdominal fascia or pubic tubercle. Patients who are candidates for this procedure must have compliant low-pressure bladders. They will be unable to void by Valsalva's maneuver after a successful sling procedure and must be willing to perform self-catheterization indefinitely in exchange for being continent.

• The artificial urinary sphincter consists of a cuff, a pressure-regulating balloon, and a control pump. The cuff is usually implanted around the bladder neck in both sexes and, less commonly, around the bulbar urethra in men. The pump in the labia or scrotum allows the patient to open the cuff for voiding. Reinflation of the cuff is automatic and takes about 3 to 5 minutes. Mechanical failure, cuff erosion, and infection can occur with this device. Patients can use Valsalva's maneuver to void and do not have to be on self-catheterization.

TO DECREASE OUTLET RESISTANCE

Sphincterotomy. In male spinal cord–injured patients unable or unwilling to do self-catheterization, the use of a condom catheter is a practical alternative. Because it is unusual to find a lower urinary tract that has adequate detrusor contraction and a coordinated pelvic floor in these patients, some procedure to decrease outflow resistance is usually indicated. The results are poor in patients without adequate detrusor contractions. Preoperative parameters suggested for a good outcome are low volume (less than 200 mL), spontaneous contraction with a quick rise time (less than 20 seconds), adequate amplitude (more than 50 cm H_2O), and an adequate duration of approximately 2 minutes or more. Ablation of the striated sphincter, usually by incision, is the standard procedure. Some patients also have bladder neck obstruction either because of primary hyperactivity (e.g., high quadriplegic patients) or because of total bladder wall hypertrophy (which follows striated sphincter dyssynergia). They need bladder neck ablation either by resection or by incision. The immediate morbidity from sphincterotomy (i.e., bleeding, clot retention, and infection) is relatively high. The long-term results are compromised because of recurrent obstruction from stricture or recurrent dyssynergia.

Other Methods of Decreasing Outflow Resistance. Intrathecal baclofen given for severe spasticity decreases the pudendal reflexes, but the detrusor reflex and contractions are reduced as well. Consequently it cannot be used as a chemical sphincterotomy. Botulinum toxin injected into the striated sphincter has also been used experimentally, but its effects last only a few months.

Urinary Diversion (p. 573)
• The use of any urinary diversion procedure should be restricted to patients with severe urethral problems such as stricture, fistula, periurethral abscess, and intractable incontinence with perineal skin breakdown. The simplest method is to insert a suprapubic catheter and close the bladder neck. If the bladder cannot be preserved because of malignant disease, contracture, or ureteral reflux, a standard bowel conduit is recommended with removal of the bladder in most cases.

MANAGEMENT OF SPECIFIC DISEASES (pp. 573–575)

Diseases of the Brain (pp. 573–574)

Stroke (p. 573)
• After an initial period of areflexia, stroke patients typically have hyperreflexia with frequency and urge incontinence but coordinated voiding and complete emptying (see Chapter 50). Anticholinergics and musculotropics often help ameliorate symptoms without adversely affecting emptying.

Parkinson's Disease (p. 574)
• The prevalence of bladder symptoms in this disease is high (70%) (see Chapter 51). Most have frequency, urgency, and urge incontinence, and 50% complain of difficulty voiding. Evaluation shows hyperreflexia, but the contractions are poorly sustained and result in incomplete emptying. Failure to empty can also be due to bradykinesia secondary to failure of pelvic floor relaxation, the adrenergic effects of levodopa, or the anticholinergic effects of other antiparkinsonian drugs. Treatment is difficult because there is often a combination of incontinence and retention. Intermittent catheterization and detrusor inhibition is often the best choice, but many patients do not have sufficient upper extremity dexterity to do this independently.

Dementia, Brain Tumors, and Trauma (p. 574)
• Dementia, brain tumors, and trauma can all cause hyperreflexia with reflex or urge incontinence with complete emptying. If cognitive impairment is severe, incontinence often persists in spite of detrusor inhibition. Some type of collecting device is appropriate for many of these patients (see Chapter 49).

Diseases of the Brain and Spinal Cord (p. 574)

• Multiple sclerosis is the most common disease in this category, with 90% of patients developing urinary manifestations in the course of the disease (see Chapter 52). The bladder symptoms usually present because of an incomplete spinal cord lesion with hyperreflexia and hypocontractility. In this situation, detrusor inhibition with drugs worsens emptying. Patients with multiple sclerosis and with a predominantly conal lesion have bladder areflexia. Intermittent catheterization is eventually indicated in most patients with multiple sclerosis, but few are able to undertake it because of poor upper extremity strength and coordination.

Diseases of the Spinal Cord (p. 574)

• Injury, tumors, and vascular lesions of the spinal cord cause the majority of suprasacral neurogenic bladder problems (see Chapter 55). The onset and severity of the symptoms varies with the cause of spinal cord dysfunction, but the management discussed here is in relation to spinal cord injury. An indwelling catheter is typically maintained until the patient's medical state is stable and fluid intake can be regulated to achieve a urine output of 1500 to 2000 mL/day. Intermittent sterile catheterization is then started, if possible, by a dedicated catheterization team. The patient should learn self-catheterization when able to do so. A sterile technique is ideal in the hospital, but a clean technique can be used when the patient is discharged home. Maximum allowable bladder volume is 600 mL. In some of these patients, however, retention of interstitial fluid in the lower limbs when the patient is upright, with subsequent mobilization and dumping at night, is commonly a problem. The use of antiembolism stockings such as TED hose, recumbency early in the evening, and an extra catheterization in the middle of the night might all be necessary to manage this.

• In the majority of spinal cord–injured patients, the detrusor reflex returns usually within the first 6 months. Its return is often indicated by episodes of incontinence, but the presence of the detrusor reflex should be confirmed by CMG. Anticholinergics and musculotropics can be given to suppress the reflex and allow intermittent catheterization to continue. Patients with lesions at the level of C7 and below, who are able to do self-catheterization, can continue this in the long term. If the detrusor reflex cannot be suppressed, the patient should consider augmentation, which remains the standard method today for achieving a low-pressure reservoir if medications fail.

• In male patients unable or unwilling to do self-catheterization, and for those who refuse augmentation, sphincterotomy followed by use of an external catheter is probably the best alternative. Some men with quadriplegia end up with an indwelling catheter because of sphincterotomy failure, or inadequate detrusor contractions, or skin breakdown on the penile shaft. Women using intermittent catheterization might be unable to control urinary incontinence with medications and can choose to use an indwelling catheter. A regular long-term urinary tract surveillance program (Table 27–4) should be set up for spinal cord–injured patients who might, with good care, have a near normal life expectancy.

Diseases of the Conus, Cauda Equina, and Peripheral Nerves (p. 575)

• Trauma, disk disease, lumbar stenosis, arachnoiditis, and tumors are some of the mechanical lesions that can affect this region of the spinal canal. The resulting bladder is typically areflexic or noncontractile and insensate. Intermittent catheterization is the initial treatment in all cases. If the pelvic floor is severely paralyzed, patients might be able to void by straining. Men can be helped by α-adrenergic blocking agents to decrease outflow resistance. Women can often empty by straining, but tend to develop severe stress incontinence. These patients can be candidates for a fascial sling or artificial sphincter. Reduced bladder compliance, usually found in patients after radical pelvic surgery, does not respond well to medications. In these cases an augmentation might be indicated, particularly if the outflow resistance is high and the upper tracts begin to dilate.

Diseases of the Spinal Cord and Conus (p. 575)

• Myelodysplasia is the most common disease producing a mixed pattern of bladder dysfunction. Any combination of detrusor and sphincter activity

TABLE 27–4 Routine Urinary Tract Surveillance after Spinal Cord Injury

I. Initial rehabilitation admission
  Urinalysis, initial and as needed
  Urine culture and sensitivity, weekly
  Renal and bladder ultrasound if on IC or condom catheter
  Add KUB in patients with a Foley catheter
  IVP only if US is abnormal
  PVR
  CMG or urodynamics (usually no cystogram at this point)
  CrCl, 24-hr urine
II. Routine evaluations (yearly for the first 5 years and, if stable, every other year thereafter)
  Renal US and KUB for all annual evaluations
  IVP or CT only if indicated by clinical status or US findings
  Urodynamics determined on individual basis (often needed annually for the first few years)
  CrCl, 24-hr urine, annually
  PVR (by portable US or catheter) annually unless indwelling catheter is in place
  Other tests of renal function as needed
III. Cystoscopy
  Generally performed in patients after 10 years of chronic, continuous indwelling
  catheterizations (urethral or suprapubic), or earlier (at 5 years) if at high risk (heavy smoker,
  age >40 years, or history of complicated UTIs) or in any patients with symptoms that warrant
  such a procedure

Abbreviations: IVP, intravenous pyelography; SCI, spinal cord injury; CMG, cystometrography; PVR, postvoid residuals; US, ultrasound; CrCl, creatine clearance; KUB, kidneys, ureters, and bladder, plain film study; CUG, cystourethrogram; UTIs, urinary tract infections; IC, intermittent catheterization.

can be found, but it is most common to have a hyperreflexic or noncompliant bladder, or both, with dyssynergia or a nonrelaxing sphincter. Intermittent catheterization is used initially, along with medication in infancy and childhood. In many cases, reconstructive surgery is necessary early if more conservative measures fail.

MANAGEMENT OF COMPLICATIONS (pp. 575–577)

Bacteriuria (p. 576)

• UTIs are common in patients with neurogenic bladder. In patients with spinal cord disorders, signs and symptoms suggestive of UTI include fever, onset of urinary incontinence, increased spasticity, autonomic dysreflexia, increased sweating, cloudy and odorous urine, malaise, lethargy, or sense of unease. Unexplained signs and symptoms suggestive of UTI in the presence of pyuria warrant empirical therapy for UTI. Absence of pyuria makes the diagnosis of UTI unlikely but does not exclude it.
• Asymptomatic bacteriuria is very common in patients with neurogenic bladder, especially those using intermittent or indwelling catheterization. Most authorities recommend against routine treatment of asymptomatic bacteriuria. However, the presence of significant bacteriuria with urease-producing organisms that are associated with stone formation might warrant treatment.

• The spectrum of uropathogens causing catheter-associated UTI is much broader than that causing uncomplicated UTI. *Escherichia coli* causes the majority of uncomplicated UTIs. *E. coli* and organisms such as species of *Proteus, Klebsiella, Pseudomonas, Serratia, Providencia,* enterococci, and staphylococci are relatively more common in patients with catheter-associated UTI. Polymicrobic bacteriuria is the rule in patients with indwelling catheters.

• Patients with mild to moderate illness can be treated with an oral fluoroquinolone such as ciprofloxacin, norfloxacin, or ofloxacin. This group of antibiotics provides coverage for most expected pathogens, including *Pseudomonas aeruginosa.* Trimethoprim-sulfamethoxazole is another commonly used antibiotic for less ill patients, but it does not provide coverage against *P. aeruginosa.* It is less expensive than the fluoroquinolones and can be used empirically and continued according to the results of susceptibility testing. Amoxicillin, nitrofurantoin, and sulfa drugs are poor choices for empirical therapy because of the high prevalence of resistance to these agents among uropathogens typically involved in complicated UTIs.

• In more seriously ill, hospitalized patients, ampicillin plus gentamicin or imipenem plus cilastatin provides coverage against most expected pathogens, including *P. aeruginosa* and most enterococci. A number of other parenteral antimicrobial agents can also be used. Patients can be switched to oral treatment after clinical improvement. At least 7 to 14 days of therapy is generally recommended, depending on the severity of the infection. There is no convincing evidence that regimens longer than this are beneficial. Patients undergoing effective treatment for UTI with an antibiotic to which the infecting pathogen is susceptible should have definite improvement within 24 to 48 hours. If not, a repeat urine culture and imaging studies (US or CT) are indicated.

• In a patient who has had UTI with high fever or hemodynamic changes suggestive of sepsis, or who is having recurrent symptomatic UTIs, an excretory urogram, cystogram, or urodynamic evaluation might be indicated after successful treatment to look for correctable anatomical or functional abnormalities.

Autonomic Dysreflexia (p. 576)

• Paroxysmal hypertension, sweating, piloerection, headache, and reflex bradycardia are brought on by increased stimulation into and sympathetic output from the isolated spinal cord below a complete lesion. Injuries below T6 are rarely associated with this problem. Afferent stimulation commonly arises in the bladder, and the best treatment is prevention by avoiding overdistention. If symptoms persist when the bladder has been emptied or if the blood pressure is at a dangerously high level, 10 mg of sublingual nifedipine, a calcium channel–blocking agent, can be given and repeated, if necessary, for a total of three doses. Long-term management with phenoxybenzamine (10 to 30 mg/day) has been used to prevent autonomic dysreflexia when all findable causes have been eliminated (see Chapter 55 for further explanation of the treatment of autonomic dysreflexia).

Hypercalciuria and Stones (pp. 576–577)

• Loss of calcium from the bones occurs in all spinal cord–injured patients and is worse in young males. Increased urinary calcium (greater than 200 mg/24 hours) begins about 4 weeks after injury, reaches a maximum at 16 weeks, and can persist for 12 to 18 months. The incidence of bladder stones in the first 9 months in patients on intermittent catheterization is 2.3%. In the presence of an indwelling catheter, and in spite of greater urine output, the prevalence is much higher, at 8.8%. Over the next 10 years upper tract stones are found in 8%, with many of these secondary to infection.

• Bladder stones are effectively treated with electrohydraulic lithotripsy. Small stones and particles can be dissolved by daily bladder irrigations with 30 mL of 10% of hemiacidrin (Renacidin) solution, which is left in the bladder for 30 minutes. Some patients with recurrent stones use this once or twice a week for prophylaxis. In patients who have ureteral reflux, it should be used with caution because of potential nephrotoxicity and absorption of magnesium. Caliceal calculi that are small (less than 1 cm) and asymptomatic can be followed expectantly, but 50% of these patients become symptomatic over 5 years, and half of these will need some sort of invasive procedure. Calculi that are growing or that are located in the renal pelvis should probably be treated before they pass into the ureter and cause obstruction (see Fig. 27–7 in the Textbook). Extracorporeal shock wave lithotripsy (ESWL) is the standard treatment. For large stones (greater than 3 cm diameter), a percutaneous approach is preferred because clearance of fragments is poor if patients are inactive.

• Ureteral stones are potentially dangerous in patients with no renal sensation. These can be managed expectantly if they pass down within 2 to 3 weeks. Obstruction and infection together will require a drainage procedure as an emergency with a percutaneous nephrostomy or a retrograde stent, and this can be followed by an endoscopic removal or ESWL later.

Lower Urinary Tract Changes (p. 577)

• Trabeculation occurs in the majority of patients after spinal cord injury, and in many cases it happens despite appropriate management strategies. Sacculation and diverticula can occur when obstruction and high pressure are severe. If a diverticulum occurs at the ureteral hiatus, ureteral reflux is almost inevitable. Chronic infection of dilated prostatic ducts may be an important source for relapsing UTIs in men.

Ureteral Reflux and Upper Tract Dilation (p. 577)

• Ureteral reflux or high bladder pressure in the absence of reflux can cause upper tract dilation (see Fig. 27–8 in the Textbook). With reflux, or ureteral dilation without reflux, the bladder pressure should be lowered with intermittent catheterization and anticholinergics. If reflux fails to improve but the bladder pressure responds, a surgical procedure to repair the reflux can be considered. If bladder pressures do not improve, the options are to augment the bladder; or, in men, to perform a sphincterotomy and rely on free drainage.

28

Original Chapter by John C. King, M.D., and Steven A. Stiens, M.D., M.S.

Neurogenic Bowel: Dysfunction and Management

- Bowel care capabilities at the time of discharge are not always comparable to other skills that would be expected for a given level of function. Bowel management has been found to be one of the areas of least competence among rehabilitated spinal cord–injured (SCI) persons. Careful training of the patient and attendant care is necessary if satisfactory bowel management results are to be achieved.

EPIDEMIOLOGY (p. 579)

- Neurogenic bowel dysfunction results from autonomic and somatic denervation, and produces fecal incontinence (FI), constipation, and difficulty with evacuation (DWE). These symptoms are common.
- The prevalence of FI and fecal impaction ranges from 0.3% to 5.0% in the general population. The prevalence of DWE ranges from 10% to 50% among the hospitalized or institutionalized elderly. Neurogenic bowel difficulties can be a primary disabling and handicapping feature for patients with SCI, stroke, amyotrophic lateral sclerosis, multiple sclerosis, diabetes mellitus, myelomeningocele, and muscular dystrophy.

IMPACT (pp. 579–580)

- The three primary objectives of the bowel program that apply to all cases are (1) to prevent unplanned bowel movements, (2) to promote efficient and effective bowel care, and (3) to prevent complications.

BOWEL ANATOMY AND FUNCTION (pp. 580–583)

Anatomy: Structure and Innervation (p. 580)

- The colon is the terminal segment of intestine that has been differentiated for fecal formation, storage, and defecation.
- The colon and anorectal mechanisms receive parasympathetic, sympathetic, and somatic innervation and contain the intrinsic enteric nervous system (ENS) between muscular layers and under the mucosa (Fig. 28–1; see Fig. 28–2 in the Textbook).

• The neurogenic bowel is defined as the loss of direct somatic sensory or motor control functions, with or without impaired sympathetic and parasympathetic innervation. However, the intrinsic ENS remains intact with most presenting injuries and illnesses. The most common exceptions are the developmental disorder of Hirschsprung's disease or cases of acquired autonomic neuropathy from diabetes mellitus, which can involve the ENS as well. When intact, the intrinsic ENS continues to integrate and modulate bowel function, even without autonomic and somatic nervous system input, and can be the neurological substrate for bowel habit training.

Physiology: Normal Function (pp. 580–583)

• The colon is a reservoir for food waste. Fecal elimination occurs when colonic pressure exceeds that of the anal sphincter mechanism.
• Other functions of the colon are to reabsorb fluids and gases. The colon also provides an environment for the growth of bacteria needed to assist in digestion, and serves to absorb certain bacterial breakdown products as well.
• The ENS is the key to proper functioning of the entire GI tract. This collection of highly organized neurons is situated in two primary layers, the submu-

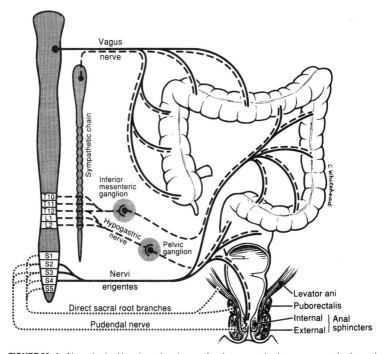

FIGURE 28–1. Neurological levels and pathways for the sympathetic, parasympathetic, and somatic nervous system innervation of the colon and anorectum. Not shown is the enteric nervous system, which travels along the bowel wall from esophagus to internal anal sphincter and forms the final common pathway to control the bowel wall smooth muscle.

cosal (Meissner's) plexus and the intramuscular myenteric (Auerbach's) plexus. The coordination of segment-to-segment function is largely regulated by the ENS and considered by some as a third part of the autonomic nervous system. The ENS also has its own nerve-blood barrier, similar to the CNS.

• The sympathetic and parasympathetic nervous systems seem to modulate the ENS, rather than directly controlling the smooth muscles of the bowel. Sympathetic nervous system stimulation tends to promote the storage function by enhancing anal tone and inhibiting colonic contractions, although little clinical deficit occurs from bilateral sympathectomy. Parasympathetic activity enhances colonic motility, and its loss is often associated with DWE, including impactions and functional obstructions such as Ogilvie's pseudo-obstructive syndrome.

• The normal intact colon wall has a 3 to 6 Hz pattern of slow electrical potential waves with irregularly occurring bursts of spike activity. This spike activity is associated with development of bowel wall tension and with slow peristaltic waves of ring contractions.

• The function of the transverse and ascending colon is largely storage, with propulsion generally retrograde toward the one-way ileocecal valve. Occasionally these proximal traveling colonic waves reverse, especially during a giant migratory contraction (GMC) of the colon. The GMC is associated with mass movement of feces as far as one-third the length of the colon. In the fasting emptied colon, GMCs occur approximately four times per day, but twice or less per day in the normal colon. The origin of the GMCs is poorly understood, but they commonly occur after meals with the gastrocolic response, or due to increased physical activity. The GMC does not seem to be under volitional control.

• The rectum is usually empty until just prior to defecation. Continence is maintained by the anal sphincter mechanism, which consists of the internal anal sphincter (IAS), external anal sphincter (EAS), and the puborectalis muscle. The EAS and puborectalis muscle are the only striated skeletal muscles whose normal resting state is tonic contraction, and these muscles consist mainly of slow-twitch fatigue resistant type I fibers. Anal pressure can be increased volitionally by contracting the EAS and puborectalis muscles. The EAS is physically larger than the internal sphincter, and its contraction is under both reflex and volitional control. Normal baseline reflex action of the anorectal mechanism allows spontaneous stool elimination. The EAS is innervated by the S2 through S4 nerve roots via the pudendal nerve, and the puborectalis muscle is innervated by direct branches from the S1 to S5 roots (see Fig. 28–1).

• Normal defecation begins with reflexes triggered by rectosigmoid distention (Fig. 28–2).

• The external sphincter generally tenses in response to small rectal distentions via a spinal reflex, although reflexive relaxation of the external sphincter occurs in the presence of greater distentions. These spinal cord reflexes are centered in the conus medullaris and are augmented and modulated by higher cortical influences. When cortical control is disrupted, as by SCI, the external sphincter reflexes usually persist and allow spontaneous defecation.

• The "gastrocolonic response" or "gastrocolic reflex" refers to the increased colonic activity (GMCs and mass movements) that occurs in the first 30 to 60 minutes after a meal. This increased colonic activity appears to be modulated both by hormonal effects; from release of peptides from the upper GI tract (e.g., gastrin, motilin, and cholecystokinin), which increase contractility of colonic smooth musculature; and by a reduction in the threshold for spinal cord–mediated vesicovesical reflexes. Upper GI receptor stimulation also results

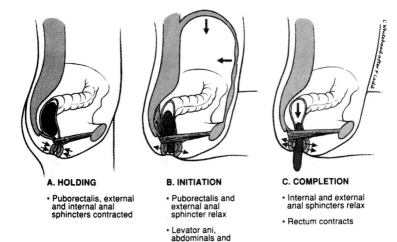

A. HOLDING

- Puborectalis, external and internal anal sphincters contracted

B. INITIATION

- Puborectalis and external anal sphincter relax

- Levator ani, abdominals and diaphragm contract

C. COMPLETION

- Internal and external anal sphincters relax

- Rectum contracts

FIGURE 28–2. *A.* Defecation is prevented by a statically increased tone of the internal anal sphincter and puborectalis, as well as by the mechanical effects of the acute anorectal angle. Dynamic responses of the external anal sphincter and puborectalis to rectal distention reflexes or increased intra-abdominal pressures further impede defecation. *B.* To initiate defecation, the puborectalis muscle and external anal sphincter relax while intra-abdominal pressure is increased by Valsalva's maneuver, which is facilitated by squatting. The levator ani helps reduce the acute anorectal angle to open the distal anal canal to receive the stool bolus. *C.* Intrarectal reflexes result in continued internal anal sphincter relaxation and rectal propulsive contractions, which help expel the bolus through the open canal. (Modified from Shiller LR: Fecal incontinence. In Sleisenger MH, Fordtran JS (eds): Gastrointestinal Disease: Pathophysiology, Diagnosis, Management, ed 4. Philadelphia, WB Saunders, 1989, p. 322.)

in increased activity in the colon, possibly due to reflexively increased parasympathetic efferent activity to the colon. The possibility of a purely ENS-mediated activation exists, although the small bowel and colon motor activities do not seem to be synchronized. In SCI the measured increase in colonic activity after a meal is blunted as compared to normal. The gastrocolonic response is often used therapeutically, even in SCI patients, to enhance bowel evacuation during this 30- to 60-minute postprandial time frame. Occasionally, certain foods can serve as trigger foods that are especially likely to induce bowel evacuation shortly after consumption.

PATHOPHYSIOLOGY: NEUROGENIC BOWEL DYSFUNCTION (pp. 583–586)

Upper Motor Neurogenic Bowel (UMNB) (p. 583)

- Any destructive CNS process above the conus, from SCI to dementia, can lead to the UMNB pattern of dysfunction.
- Spinal cortical sensory pathway deficits lead to decreased ability to sense the urge to defecate.

• Most persons with SCI, however, sense a vague discomfort when excessive rectal or colonic distention occurs.

• Colonic compliance and sphincter tone have been experimentally evaluated in SCI subjects. Recent studies have demonstrated normal colonic compliances in SCI subjects with UMNB. Passive filling of the rectum leads to increases in the resting sphincter tone because of sacral reflexes.

• Internal sphincter relaxation upon rectal distention occurs in persons with SCI as well as in neurologically intact persons. After sufficient rectal distention the external sphincter might completely relax, resulting in expulsion of the fecal bolus. Rectal sphincter dyssynergia does not necessarily correlate with bladder sphincter dyssynergia, but it often results in DWE. The protective vesicorenal reflex, whereby the external sphincter pressure increases in response to increased intra-abdominal pressure, is usually intact. Patients with UMNB also have normal or increased anal sphincter tone, intact anocutaneous (or anal wink) and bulbocavernosus reflexes, a palpable puborectalis muscle sling, and normal anal verge appearance (see Fig. 28–4 in the Textbook).

Lower Motor Neurogenic Bowel (LMNB) (p. 583)

• Polyneuropathy, conus medullaris or cauda equina lesions, pelvic surgery, vaginal delivery, or even chronic straining during defecation can impair the somatic innervation of the anal sphincter mechanism. These conditions can also produce sympathetic and parasympathetic innervation deficits.

• If an isolated pudendal insult has occurred, colonic transit times are normal and FI predominates.

• Colonic sluggishness can occur as a result of loss of parasympathetic supply, adding constipation and DWE to FI difficulties. This is an especially bad combination because the accumulation of a large amount of hard stool that can result from such colonic inertia can overstretch the weakened anal mechanism, resulting in a gaping, patulous, incompetent anal orifice.

• The denervation and atrophy of the EAS leads to loss of the protective vesicorectal reflex, which can result in stool soilage from the increased abdominal pressures associated with everyday activities.

• Rectal distention leads to the expected internal sphincter relaxation, but attenuated or absent external sphincter protective contractions result in FI or fecal smearing whenever boluses are present at the rectum. The presence of a large bolus in the rectal vault can further compromise the rectoanal angulation at the pelvic floor and contribute to paradoxical liquid incontinence around a low (ball-valve effect) impaction.

• Patients with LMNB dysfunction have decreased anal tone due to the smooth muscle internal sphincter. If no tone is found initially upon inserting the examining finger, the examiner should wait up to 15 seconds to allow IAS reflex relaxation to recover and restore tone. Chronic overstretching has probably occurred if tone does not return. The anal-to-buttock contour typically appears flattened and "scalloped" (see Fig. 28–4 in the Textbook) because of atrophy of the pudendal-innervated pelvic floor muscles and EAS. The anocutaneous reflex is absent or decreased (depending on the completeness of the lesion). Likewise, the bulbocavernosus reflex, if present, is weak. The anal canal is shortened (as compared with the normal 2.5- to 4.5-cm length), and the puborectalis muscle ridge may not be palpable. Excessive perineal descent and even rectal prolapse may occur with Valsalva's maneuver.

Evaluation (pp. 583–586)

- The GI history should not only review for cardinal symptoms but should also address the patient's general neuromuscular and GI function.
- A detailed review of the patient's bowel program includes an assessment of fluids, diet, activity, medications, and aspects of bowel care.
- A review of the technique and outcome of bowel care should include a description of schedule, initiation method (chemical or mechanical stimulation), facilitative techniques, time requirements, and characteristics of stool results.
- The history should include premorbid bowel pattern information such as defecation frequency, typical time(s) of the day, associated predefecatory activities, bowel medications and techniques or trigger foods, and stool consistency.
- The presence of GI sensations or pain; warning sensations for defecation; sense of urgency; and ability to prevent stool loss during Valsalva activities such as laughing, sneezing, coughing, or transfers should be noted.
- The physical examination should include the GI system and the associated parts of the musculoskeletal and nervous systems required for independent management of the bowel program.
- The abdomen should be inspected for distention, hernias, and other abnormalities. Percussion and auscultation should precede palpation for masses and tenderness. With the abdomen relaxed, the examiner transabdominally palpates the colon for hard stool. Palpable hard stool should not be present on the right side of the abdomen (ascending colon).
- Physical examination continues with inspection of the anus. The patient should perform a Valsalva maneuver while the examiner observes the anus and perineum for excessive descent.
- Perianal cutaneous sharp stimulation normally results in an externally visible anal sphincter reflexive contraction. This is the anocutaneous reflex, mediated by the inferior hemorrhoidal branch of the pudendal nerve (S2 to S5). This can be checked by tugging perianal hairs or by the application of the sharp edge of a broken cotton swab stick to the perianal skin. The anocutaneous reflex should be checked in all four quadrants because selective (especially side-to-side) deficits can occur. Sensation to pinprick is tested at the same time.
- A gloved lubricated finger should then be inserted through the anus until no pressure is appreciated at the fingertip. The tone and voluntary squeeze strength of the EAS and tone of the IAS should be assessed. The length of the anus, where pressure is sensed, is normally 2.5 to 4.5 cm. The point where the pressure decreases marks the anorectal junction. Along the posterior wall, 1.5 to 2.5 cm from the anal verge, the puborectalis muscular sling can be palpated as a ridge that will push the finger forward as the subject resists defecation. No palpable ridge or push suggests puborectalis atrophy or dysfunction. A shortened length of anal pressure zone suggests EAS muscle atrophy.
- With the examiner's finger in place, the bulbocavernosus reflex can be elicited by rapidly tapping or squeezing the clitoris or glans penis. Multiple random trials are needed to be certain the vesicorectal Valsalva protective reflexes are not occurring at the same time by random chance. The response can be delayed up to a few seconds in pathological conditions. A consistent response to the stimulus indicates an intact bulbocavernosus reflex. Insertion of the finger in the anal canal occasionally triggers IAS relaxation, but more often triggers a tightening squeeze that is efferently equivalent to the bulbocavernosus reflex. If IAS and EAS relaxation occur, the examiner should wait several seconds for tone to be

restored before testing the bulbocavernosus reflex. Ask the patient to volition-ally squeeze the anus before removing the finger ("resist defecation") to check for volitional EAS and puborectalis tone and control.

Diagnostic Testing (p. 586)

• The history and physical examination provide most of the necessary information.
• Additional objective laboratory testing can be helpful when the cause of FI or DWE is obscure; the history appears doubtful; conservative interventions fail; or when surgical interventions are contemplated. (Table 28–2 in the Textbook lists some of the many tests available).
• Basic laboratory tests complement the physical examination. A stool guaiac test is helpful to rule out the presence of blood in the stool. False positives are common after SCI because of hemorrhoids, as well as from anal trauma sec-ondary to bowel care. A flat plate radiograph of the abdomen can be helpful to rule out impaction, megacolon, obstruction, and a perforated viscus.

MANAGEMENT (pp. 586–590)

General Principles (p. 586)

• A bowel program is a comprehensive, individualized, patient-centered treat-ment plan focused on preventing incontinence, achieving effective and efficient colonic evacuation, and preventing the complications of neurogenic bowel dys-function. The subcomponents of a bowel program address diet, fluids, exercise, medications, and scheduled bowel care. Bowel care is the individually devel-oped and prescribed procedure for defecation that is carried out by the patient or the attendant.
• Inability to volitionally inhibit spontaneous defecations leads to incontinence, whereas the inability to adequately empty leads to constipation and impactions. Paradoxically, impactions can result in diarrhea and incontinence.

Disablement and Rehabilitation Models: Methods for Coordinating Efforts of the Interdisciplinary Team
(pp. 586–587)

• The rehabilitation evaluation should be interdisciplinary in approach and include assessment not only of colon and pelvic floor dysfunction, but also of impairments of other organs or systems that could affect rehabilitative strategies to make bowel care independent or prevent unplanned bowel movements.
• The examination should assess reflex function to determine the impairment pattern (UMNB or LMNB) of colonic and pelvic floor dysfunction that is present.
• Disabilities that limit a person's ability to maintain continence and volition-ally defecate must be assessed within the perspective of the entire person. Limitations of functional mobility as well as retained capabilities need to be con-sidered.
• The role performance of the individual that will occur after the acute rehabil-itation process is complete determines the timing and content of the new bowel care schedule. During inpatient rehabilitation, scheduling can be especially dif-ficult because of the time-consuming nature of bowel care. Evening bowel care often allows for more predictable attendance at daily therapies.

• It is crucial to remember that the patient must take a decisive leadership role in designing a bowel program that includes a convenient bowel care schedule.

Dietary Considerations (p. 587)

• Food choices are important when colonic transit time is prolonged, as in SCI (96 hours versus the 30 hours typically found in normal subjects).
• Excessive fluid resorption can result in stool hardening and subsequent constipation. To maintain a more fluid content, stool softeners, both docusate and food fiber, have been used. Fiber increases stool bulk and plasticity, especially in the more physically coarse forms; this also tends to decrease colonic pressures.
• High pressures involved in moving solid feces probably contribute to the 90% incidence of hemorrhoids in Americans and to premature diverticula formation and hemorrhoidal complications in more than 70% of SCI patients. Constant straining at stool can also contribute to peripheral neuropathic deficits in the anal sphincteric musculature. Acceptance of softer stools, from a higher-fiber diet, might help reduce these complications and is often recommended for their treatment.
• A diet that contains at least 15 g of fiber daily is recommended. Increases in the fiber content of the diets of persons with SCI do not decrease colonic transit time but do enhance the rectonal inhibitory reflex. The effects of fiber intake on stool consistency and frequency and efficacy of evacuation should be evaluated in the individual patient. The longer perineal hygiene time required for softer stools might be a deterrent for some and should be discussed with patients. Increases in dietary fiber typically result in increased stool bulk, which can require more frequent bowel care.
• A wide range of "normal" bowel patterns exists. Defecation frequencies vary dramatically in nonimpaired persons, from several times per day to less than once per week. Stool consistencies vary, from liquid to pudding, pasty, semi-solid, soft-formed, medium-formed, and hard-formed. Fully appreciating an individual's premorbid "normal" bowel function is important in the planning and goal setting for a new neurogenic bowel program.

Approaches and Rationale (pp. 587–589)

• Colonic transit time and fecal elimination are enhanced by softer stool; however, if the stool becomes too liquid, the protective angle provided by the puborectalis becomes less effective, and greater EAS pressures are required to maintain continence. Some degree of stool firmness must be tolerated to prevent incontinence. To avoid incontinence upon straining, more firmness (medium-formed) is required for the weaker anal sphincter mechanism of LMNB than for UMNB (semiformed to soft-formed). Bulkier stools can help stimulate the defecatory response more easily in LMNB, although less stimulus is needed in UMNB. The presentation of stool to the rectum, triggering defecation, can be associated with GMC and mass movements more than with the slow accumulation of sufficient rectal stool to trigger reflex defecation, and the GMC might be what is actually habituated.
• The frequency and specific timing of bowel care to induce adequate colonic emptying can be chosen based on previous elimination patterns. Regular bowel emptying is recommended as the primary means for both enhancing elimination and decreasing incontinence between stooling. Adequate emptying is accomplished by (1) making stools easier to move by means of softening, (2) adding

bowel stimulant medication if needed, and (3) triggering the defecatory reflex at consistent desired times to promote habituation.

• Choosing long intervals between elimination allows more fluid reabsorption, resulting in harder stools, which can worsen DWE.

• Chronic oral bowel stimulant medication use has been questioned because of concerns of developing the atonic "cathartic bowel" syndrome. Certain stimulants, especially in the anthraquinone family (e.g., senna, cascara, and aloes), have been shown to damage myenteric neurons with chronic use. It has not been established whether late complications from chronic oral bowel stimulant medications occur in those with neurogenic bowel dysfunction.

• Triggering of defecation can be accomplished by digital stimulation, rectal stimulant medications, enemas, or electrical stimulation. All of these cause reflex relaxation of the IAS, and if strong enough can reflexly relax the EAS as well. This initiates the rectorectal reflex that helps to eliminate any stool that is present. The GMC and mass movement associated with the call to stool for many intact persons often occurs at consistent times, which can be trainable.

• Theoretically, fewer long-term complications will occur if the following are minimized: anorectal overdistention (as with enemas), anal trauma (as by manual disimpaction), and oral stimulant medication use. An accelerating enema volume required for efficacy should be a warning that chronic rectal overdistention might be leading to less responsiveness. Digital stimulation to induce defecatory reflexes should be favored over manual disimpaction because the latter can easily result in inadvertent overstretching of the insensate and more delicate anal mechanisms of the neurogenic bowel. Local rectal stimulant suppositories and mini-enemas with bisacodyl or glycerin do not carry the same risk as oral stimulant medications and do not appear to lead to chronic inflammatory changes of the rectal mucosa.

• One approach to initiating neurogenic bowel training is outlined in Table 28–1.

TABLE 28–1 Protocol for Progressive Steps in Bowel Habituation Program

1. Perform bowel clean-out if stool is present in the rectal vault or palpable proximal to the descending colon, by multiple enemas or oral cathartic.
2. Titrate to soft stool consistency with diet and bulking agents (fiber) and stool softeners (docusate).
3. Trigger defecation with a glycerin suppository or by digital stimulation 20–30 minutes after a meal; 10 minutes later have the patient attempt defecation on toilet, limited to less than 40 minutes, and relieving skin pressure every 10 minutes.
4. If defecation is not initiated, a trial of a bisacodyl suppository PR is initiated.
5. Digital stimulation. Start 20 minutes after suppository placement and repeat every 5 minutes.
6. Timed oral medications. Administer casanthranol-docusate sodium (Peri-Colace), senna (Senokot), or bisacodyl (Dulcolax) tablets timed so that bowel movement would otherwise result 30 minutes to 1 hour after anticipated triggered bowel timing.
7. If defecation occurs in less than 10 minutes after suppository insertion, transition to digital stimulation technique only. Once the patient is well habituated, straining alone may rarely trigger defecations at a desired time.

Note: Steps 1 to 3 are initial interventions and are always followed, with steps 4 to 6 incorporated only as needed. At least 2 weeks' trial with proper technique is pursued before advancing to the next step.

• Bowel function is a very private matter, and patients might be reluctant to seek advice or information despite its major importance to their overall well-being and self-concept. Information should be freely disseminated in order to enhance the development of healthy habits and minimize bowel complications.

• Intrinsic loss of the ENS, or of any segment, including by surgical reanastomosis, can result in loss of the rectoanal inhibitory reflex, causing DWE. Oral laxative abuse can cause dysfunction of the ENS. If bowel training is not accomplishing defecation at the desired times, or if repeated involuntary incontinence occurs, further diagnostic evaluation might be indicated.

• When neurogenic bowel deficits are incomplete and some degree of control and sensation is present, biofeedback might offer a means of enhancing the patient's residual sensory and motor abilities. This typically requires only a few sessions, and most patients improve after just one session.

Surgical Options (p. 589)

• Sacral nerve deficits interfere with the action of the puborectalis, levator ani, and EAS (see Fig. 28–1). The resulting pelvic floor descent impairs the protective puborectalis sling angle and decreases the efficacy of protective EAS contractions. Some patients have benefited from transposition of innervated gracilis, adductor longus, gluteus maximus, or free muscle graft palmaris longus to replace puborectalis function and restore the acute anorectal junction angle that this sling provides.

• Incomplete EAS relaxation during defecation (dyssynergia) results in a functional outlet obstruction and DWE. A prolonged descending colon transit time occurs, which improves with an IAS and partial EAS myotomy. This procedure relieves constipation in 62% of patients but results in FI in 16% and therefore has not become a popular option.

• Stimulation of anterior sacral roots S2, S3, and S4 by transrectal electric stimulation or via a stimulator surgically placed for micturition has been performed. Electrodefecation has been obtainable by sacral root stimulation in up to 50% of patients, but remains unpredictable.

• In clinical scenarios of prolonged bowel care time, recurrent fecal impactions, or poor or intermittent response to rectal medications to initiate bowel care, the options of the antegrade continence enema should be considered. This is an alternative method of orthograde enema delivery that requires the surgical construction of a catheterizable appendicocecostomy stoma. This stoma can be catheterized and infused with 200 to 600 mL of tap water to trigger a propulsive colonic peristalsis and defecation within 10 to 20 minutes.

• Colostomy has been shown to reduce bowel care time, especially when offered to those with chronic DWE. It may be indicated in three general scenarios: (1) when conservative medical measures and training have failed, (2) when intrinsic bowel deficits (e.g., as in Hirschsprung's disease, Chagas' disease, "cathartic colon," and when pressure ulcers or other skin lesions occur that cannot be effectively healed because of frequent soiling), or (3) when recurrent urinary tract seeding by repetitive bowel impactions occurs. Colostomy carries a surgical risk, is cosmetically disfiguring, and is seldom necessary to achieve adequate social continence, but it remains a procedure of last resort for the treatment of FI or DWE.

Complications (pp. 589–590)

• Significant bowel complications requiring medical treatment or lifestyle alterations are reported by 27% of SCI persons by 5 years or greater beyond their injury, even though bowel management was satisfactory during the first 5 years.

• Over 80% of persons with SCI had bowel impactions, and 20% had chronic bowel impaction and DWE problems.

• Hemorrhoids are more symptomatic when patients have intact sensation, but in one study rectal bleeding due to hemorrhoids was reported by 74% of SCI patients. Stool softening is the best preventive and chronic treatment measure, but it should be balanced with the requirement to modulate stool consistency to maintain continence.

• An overstretched patulous noncompetent sphincter associated with rectal prolapse often is the end result of chronic passage of very large hard stools through a weakened anorectal mechanism in LMNB. Overdistention of the weakened neurogenic anal mechanism should be avoided by use of stool softening and gentle care to dilate the sphincter whenever manual disimpaction is required, to minimize trauma to these denervated structures.

• Autonomic dysreflexia occurs in SCI patients with lesions at or above the midthoracic region. FI is a common and potentially dangerous cause of autonomic dysreflexia because of the substantial time that may be required for its clearance (see Chapter 55). If manual disimpaction is required, lubrication with lidocaine gel is recommended to decrease additional nociceptive sensory input from the richly innervated anal region.

• Bloating and abdominal distention are common complaints of patients with neurogenic bowel dysfunction. These complaints can be reduced in SCI patients by increasing the frequency of bowel care. This complaint can be especially severe in those with hyperactive EAS protective responses to rectal distention, which can preclude the passing of flatus. Digital release of flatus might be required, in addition to diet modification to eliminate foods that produce excessive gases. The workup should also include assessment for any contributing aerophagia (air swallowing).

Treatment Outcomes (p. 590)

• Bowel habituation training in children with myelomeningocele by means of suppositories, digital stimulation, or both resulted in 83% of compliant patients having less than one incontinent stool per month. The continence catheter enema, which has a distal rectal balloon to avoid immediate enema expulsion, when used daily or every other day, reduced fecal incontinence to fewer than three episodes per month in children with myelomeningocele.

• Although all complete SCI patients have episodic FI, this is a chronic problem for only 2%. DWE appears to be a progressive problem that develops 5 years or more after SCI.

• Patients with multiple sclerosis, parkinsonism, or muscular dystrophy have also been helped by methods to enhance bowel storage or elimination in the setting of deteriorating neuromuscular and anorectal function. Colostomy can also provide a means of achieving social continence in these patients.

• Patients who develop social bowel continence can venture into public without fear of malodorous embarrassment and unpredictable social disasters that humiliate as well as require substantial clean-up time. When such fears persist, full social and vocational reintegration is impeded.

29

Original Chapter by Richard T. Katz, M.D., Julius P.A. Dewald, P.T., Ph.D., and Brian D. Schmit, Ph.D.

Spasticity

- Occurring in a variety of central nervous system disorders, spastic hypertonia has both diagnostic and therapeutic significance. Diagnostically, it is a hallmark of an upper motor neuron disorder; therapeutically, it represents one of the most important impairments for individuals who care for patients with central nervous system disease.

PATHOPHYSIOLOGY (pp. 592–597)

- Spasticity is "a motor disorder characterized by a velocity-dependent increase in tonic stretch reflexes (muscle tone) with exaggerated tendon jerks, resulting from hyperexcitability of the stretch reflex, as one component of the upper motor neuron syndrome."
- Muscle tone may be characterized as "the sensation of resistance felt as one manipulates a joint through a range of motion, with the subject attempting to relax."

Changes in Passive Muscle Properties (pp. 592–593)

- The passive stiffness of a muscle is one contributor to muscle tone.
- Passive stiffness is defined as the slope of a curve relating joint torque to the angle of joint displacement with the test subject relaxed and without reflex or voluntary activation of relevant muscles.
- Changes in passive stiffness could be mediated by permanent structural changes in the mechanical properties of muscle connective tissues, or could be variable in character.

Neural Mechanisms for Stretch Reflex Hyperactivity (pp. 593–595)

- The basic neural circuit on which to build a framework for understanding spastic hypertonia is the segmental reflex arc. This arc consists of muscle receptors, their central connections with spinal cord neurons, and the motoneuronal output to muscle.
- Presynaptic inhibition is exerted via interneurons which end on primary afferent nerve terminals and which reduce the ability of sensory afferents to

depolarize the postsynaptic membrane (by changing calcium and/or potassium conductances). Exteroceptive (e.g., cutaneous) and interoceptive (e.g., visceral) afferent information can also provide important input into the spinal segmental reflex arc.

• Within this framework, there are two distinct ways in which stretch reflex hyperexcitability could be explained. The first is by selectively increasing motoneuronal excitability, which is reflected as an increased motoneuronal response to a particular level of stretch-evoked synaptic input. The second is by *increasing the amount of excitatory synaptic input elicited by muscle extension.*

Supraspinal Mechanisms (pp. 595–596)

• Descending tracts contribute to spastic muscle hypertonia either via monosynaptic excitatory projections to lower motoneurons (e.g., from the corticospinal tracts), or indirectly by inhibition or facilitation of interneurons within spinal reflex pathways.

• Spasticity can be characterized by a combination of two major disturbances, both mediated by alterations in the balance of descending pathway activity. The first induces an increase in excitability of motoneurons innervating antigravity muscles (which are physiological extensors in the legs, and flexors in the arms); the second changes the patterns of reflex responsiveness of many segmental reflexes, often promoting flexor muscle activity and reduced extensor activity.

Pathways Responsible for Modifications in Descending Control in Spasticity (pp. 595–596)

• Cortex, basal ganglia, and cerebellum all provide important modulation of brainstem structures in normal motor control.

• Selective destruction of corticospinal tracts does not result in spastic hypertonia, but rather hypotonia and loss of fine hand movements.

• Interruption of extrapyramidal fibers is needed before spastic hypertonia develops.

• Lesions of particular premotor cortical sites (i.e., Brodman areas 4 and 6) result in hypotonia followed by hypertonic hemiparesis. Bilateral premotor damage causes spasticity that is more severe.

Upper Motor Neuron Syndrome (pp. 596–597)

• Patients with lesions of cortical, subcortical, and spinal cord structures exhibit a variety of abnormal behaviors beyond those attributable to hypertonia. We use the term *upper motor neuron (UMN) syndrome* to describe such changes.

• Careful study of patients with UMN syndrome reveals that motor difficulties can be divided into abnormal behaviors (positive symptoms) and performance deficits (negative symptoms) (Table 29–1).

• Positive symptoms are easily recognized in disorders of the spinal cord. Symptoms include exaggerated flexion reflexes and a positive Babinski response. Release of reflexes from descending inhibitory control causes flexor or adductor spasms. Flexor spasms may become so severe that a paraplegic person requires the help of restraints in order to remain in a wheelchair. "Scissoring" due to spastic hip adductors can limit a spastic person's ability to ambulate effectively. Clonus, cyclical hyperactivity of antagonistic muscles in response to stretch may become so severe as to prevent functional muscle groups from performing effectively.

TABLE 29–1 Upper Motor Neuron Syndrome

Abnormal Behaviors (Positive Symptoms)	*Performance Deficits (Negative Symptoms)*
Reflex release phenomena	Decreased dexterity
Hyperactive proprioceptive reflexes	Paresis/weakness
Increased resistance to stretch	Fatiguability
Relaxed cutaneous reflexes	
Loss of precise autonomic control	

- Another commonly overlooked component of the UMN syndrome is the loss of precise autonomic control. Loss of UMN modulation of spinal autonomic mechanisms can produce a disorganization of autonomic function below the level of SCI. When spinal cord lesions are above the midthoracic level, seemingly innocuous sensory input can result in a potential hypertensive crisis. This response is one component of autonomic dysreflexia, a gross nonselective "mass response." Disorganization of sympathetic activity below the level of SCI may be responsible for autonomic dysreflexia, but mechanisms other than exaggerated sympathetic outflow may contribute as well.

- Negative symptoms are performance deficits and are more commonly observed in hemiparetic patients than in spinal cord forms of spasticity. Movements are often weak, easily fatigued, and lacking in dexterity. Several physiological factors may contribute to these performance deficits. The loss of orderly recruitment and rate modulation of motoneurons results in inefficient muscle activation, early loss of force, augmented subject effort, and the clinical perception of weakness. High-threshold motor units with rapid rates of adaptation are recruited early, and these "fast twitch" units are poorly suited to maintain sustained muscle contractions.

- Relief of the hypertonic "spastic" components of the UMN syndrome does not necessarily imply enhanced performance. Synergy patterns, flexors spasms, paresis, loss of dexterity, and agonist/antagonist co-contraction are probably more disabling than the hypertonic response to stretch.

QUANTIFICATION OF SPASTIC HYPERTONIA
(pp. 597–601)

- The quantification of spasticity is a challenging problem made even more difficult because measurements tend to be highly observer dependent. In addition, quantification has been hampered by changes in performance caused by training effects, emotional status, and various systemic factors.

- The lack of effective measurement techniques has been quite restrictive because quantification is necessary to evaluate various modes of treatment.

Clinical Scales (p. 597)

- A clinical scale from 0 (normal muscle tone) to 4 (severe spasticity) was first proposed by Ashworth. It offers ease of measurement but may lack temporal and interexaminer reproducibility. A modification of the Ashworth scale that added an additional intermediate grade has high interrater reliability when testing elbow flexors (Table 29–2).

TABLE 29–2   Clinical Scale for Spastic Hypertonia

0
No increase in tone

1
Slight increase in muscle tone, manifested by a catch and release or by minimal resistance at the end of the range of motion when the affected part(s) is moved in flexion or extension

1+
Slight increase in muscle tone, manifested by a catch, followed by minimal resistance throughout the remainder (less than half) of the range of motion

2
More marked increase in muscle tone through most of the range of motion, but affected part(s) easily moved

3
Considerable increase in muscle tone, passive movement difficult

4
Affected part(s) rigid in flexion or extension

From Bohannon RW, Smith MB: Interrater reliability on a modified Ashworth scale of muscle spasticity. Phys Therapy 1987; 67:206–207.

- The *Fugl-Meyer scale* (Table 29–3) is an accurate and objective method of assessing function (but not necessarily spastic hypertonia) in hemiplegic patients, based on the natural progression of functional return. The Fugl-Meyer scale has been demonstrated to have high intratester and intertester reliability, and can be completed in 10 to 20 minutes. Decline of function of the Fugl-Meyer scale has been shown to correlate closely with the severity of spastic tone.

TABLE 29–3   Fugl-Meyer Scale of Functional Return after Hemiplegia

Movement of the shoulder, elbow, forearm, and lower extremity

  I Muscle stretch reflexes can be elicited
  II Volitional movements can be performed within the dynamic flexor/extensor synergies
  III Volitional motion is performed mixing dynamic flexor and extensor synergies
  IV Volitional movements are performed with little or no synergy dependence
  V Normal muscle stretch reflexes

Wrist function—stability, flexion, extension, circumduction
Hand function
Mass flexion, mass extension, five different grasps
Coordination and speed—assess tremor, dysmetria, speed
Finger-to-nose test; heel-to-shin test
Balance
Sit without support
Parachute reaction—nonaffected side, affected side
Stand—supported, unsupported
Stand on nonaffected side, affected side
Sensation—light touch, position sense
Passive joint motion, joint pain

Biomechanical Measures of Spastic Hypertonia
(pp. 598–599)

• Biomechanical measures quantify changes in stretch reflex activity in limbs of spastic patients. They are an extension of the Ashworth scale, in which the clinician applies a stretch to the limb and feels the resistance to stretch.

• Biomechanical measures use a controlled perturbation while quantifying the mechanical response to the movement with torque and position transducers and EMG.

Pendulum Test (pp. 599–600)

• The pendulum test uses gravity for the assessment of spasticity.

• The relaxed limb's impedance to imposed movement reflects the degree of spastic hypertonia in the quadriceps and hamstring muscles and has been evaluated in supine normal and spastic patients.

THERAPEUTIC MANAGEMENT OF SPASTIC HYPERTONIA (pp. 601–613)

• Before treatment for spasticity is initiated, the clinician must address several important questions:

• Does hypertonia exacerbate a functional impairment, or does it threaten to cause disability if left unchecked? Is it causing discomfort? Is it making care of the person by others more difficult?

• Is the disability specifically a result of spastic hypertonia or another motor disorder such as rigidity, muscle "spasms," or weakness? Are several disorders contributing to the disability?

• Is the spastic hypertonia useful to the patient? Is increased lower extremity tone utilized for standing or walking? Is spasticity or disordered motor control the primary detriment to the gait pattern? Is it inappropriate to routinely reduce or inhibit the reflex response to improve functional movement in stroke rehabilitation?

• What are the static (i.e., contracture) and dynamic (reflex) contributions to the problem? How do they affect other areas of function?

• What are the overall functional abilities of the individual—motor, sensory, cognitive, and behavioral? How will these be affected as the goals for treatment of spasticity are achieved?

• Are there other medical issues that might be contributing to the problem? Might these conditions be exacerbated by spasticity treatment?

• How much time has elapsed since the onset of the condition that was the cause of spasticity? What is the prognosis?

• Addressing these questions allows a rational approach to the treatment of spasticity (see Fig. 29–4 in the Textbook).

• Good nursing care can reduce the nociceptive and exteroreceptive stimuli that can exacerbate the patient's hypertonia. The avoidance of noxious stimuli is an important initial management step. This includes such measures as prompt treatment of urinary tract complications (e.g., infections or stones), prevention of pressure sores and contractures, release of tightly wrapped leg bags and clothes, proper bowel and bladder management to prevent fecal impaction and bladder distension, and prophylaxis of deep venous thrombosis. Heterotopic bone has

been suggested as an exacerbant of spasticity, but the prevention of this complication can be difficult.
• Proper bed positioning early after spinal cord injury has been suggested as an important step in the long-term reduction of spastic hypertonia, but this assertion has never been systematically evaluated. A daily stretching program is an integral component of any spasticity management program.

Physical Modalities (pp. 601–603)

• Stretching is probably an essential component for relieving muscle stiffness in spastic patients, although there are few quantitative reports demonstrating spasticity relief following muscle stretch.
• Ranging can reduce the severity of spastic tone for several hours. The reason for the "carry-over" is not completely clear.
• The therapeutic benefit of repeated ranging and stretch is incorporated into the Neurodevelopment Technique of Bobath, and more recently into proprioceptive neuromuscular facilitation.
• The original Bobath technique made use of "reflex inhibitory patterns"—joint positions that stretch the most spastic muscles—with the goal of reducing tone by inhibition of exaggerated reflexes.
• Proprioceptive neuromuscular facilitation also uses stretch in combination with contraction of either the stretched or antagonist muscle, and is often used to improve range of motion.

Cryotherapy (p. 602)
• Topical cold has been reported to decrease muscle stretch reflex excitability, reduce clonus, increase range of motion of the joint, and improve power in the antagonistic muscle group. These effects can be used to facilitate improved motor function for short periods.

Casting and Splinting (p. 602)
• Casting or splinting techniques can improve the range of motion in a joint caused by hypertonic contracture, and positioning the limb in a tonic stretch has been observed to decrease reflex tone.

Biofeedback (pp. 602–603)
• EMG biofeedback may be useful for the treatment of spasticity and associated synergies.
• In general, biofeedback has been used initially to train the subject to relax the spastic extremity, and then to regain active control. Despite great initial enthusiasm, however, biofeedback techniques have not found widespread acceptance.

Electrical Stimulation (p. 603)
• Electrical stimulation of peripheral nerves offers a potential adjunct to traditional rehabilitation therapeutics for patients with paraplegia during standing, walking, and exercise training.
• Cyclical use of electrical stimulation has been shown to decrease upper extremity contractures, improve motor activity in agonist muscles, and reduce tone in antagonistic muscle groups of those with hemiplegia and quadriplegia.
• Stimulation of the sural nerve, a flexor reflex afferent, has resulted in decreased extensor tonus and increased strength of ankle dorsiflexion.

TABLE 29–4 Drug Treatment of Spastic Hypertonia

Agent	Daily Dosage (mg)	Half-Life (hours)	Mechanism of Action
Baclofen	10–80+	3.5	Presynaptic inhibitor by activation of GABA "B" receptor
Diazepam	4–60+	27–37*	Facilitates postsynaptic effects of GABA, resulting in increased presynaptic inhibition
Dantrolene	25–400	8.7	Reduces calcium release, interfering with excitation-contraction coupling in skeletal muscle
Clonidine	0.1–0.4 (po) 0.1–0.3 (patch)** 12–16 (oral)		α-2 adrenergic agonist
Tizanidine	4–36	8.4	α-2 adrenergic agonist

*Half-life of active primary metabolite is significantly longer.
**Patch is changed weekly.

• Peroneal nerve stimulation can suppress ankle clonus in ambulatory patients with hemiplegia via reciprocal inhibition.
• Electrical stimulation has limited but defined applications as an ankle dorsiflexor-assist during hemiplegic gait, and as a hand-opening device in the plegic upper extremity.

Pharmacologic Intervention (pp. 603–608)

Oral Medications (pp. 603–605)
• No medication (Table 29–4) has been uniformly useful in the treatment of spastic hypertonia. Considering the variety of problems associated with spasticity (e.g., flexor spasms in the spinal patient, dystonic posturing in the hemiplegic, and spastic diplegia in the cerebral palsy child), it is unlikely that one agent will be beneficial to all parties. More importantly, all drugs have potentially serious side effects, and these negative features should be carefully weighed when beginning a patient on any drug. Continued use of a drug should be contingent on a clearly beneficial effect.

BACLOFEN
• Baclofen (Lioresal®) is an analog of gamma-aminobutyric acid (GABA), a neurotransmitter involved in presynaptic inhibition.
• Baclofen does not bind to the classical GABA "A" receptor, but rather to a recently discovered and less well-characterized "B" receptor. Agonism at this site inhibits calcium influx into presynaptic terminals and suppresses release of excitatory neurotransmitters. Baclofen inhibits both mono- and polysynaptic reflexes, and also reduces activity of the gamma efferent.
• Baclofen is completely absorbed after oral administration, and is eliminated predominantly by the renal route. Its half-life is approximately 3.5 hours. Baclofen readily crosses the blood-brain barrier, in contrast to GABA.

- Whereas baclofen is probably the drug of choice in spasticity following spinal cord injury, its role in the treatment of spasticity caused by supraspinal injury remains unsettled. It may interfere with attention and memory in elderly and brain-injured patients.
- Baclofen is particularly effective for the flexor spasms with spinal cord lesions. Baclofen may improve bladder control by decreasing hyperreflexive contraction of the external urethral sphincter. It has been shown to be safe and effective in long-term use. Baclofen also has an anxiolytic effect, which probably contributes to its antispasticity actions. Initial adult dosage is approximately 5 mg po, b.i.d., or t.i.d., and may be slowly titrated up toward a recommended maximum dose of 80 mg/day. This "recommended maximum dose" may not, however, be the most effective dose for the patient, and higher doses may be well tolerated by the patient and be additionally therapeutic.
- There is a low incidence of side effects, which include hallucinations, confusion, sedation, hypotonia, and ataxia. Sudden withdrawal of the drug can lead to seizures and hallucinations.
- Safe use of baclofen has not been adequately studied in children, and the Food and Drug Administration (FDA) has not approved its use in this age group. However, physicians have used baclofen in this age group with dosages initiated at 2.5 to 5 mg/day, with maximum dosages of 30 mg (children 2 to 7 years of age) to 60 mg (children 8 years or older).

DIAZEPAM

- Diazepam (Valium) facilitates postsynaptic effects of GABA, resulting in an increase in presynaptic inhibition.
- Diazepam has been a successful treatment for spastic hypertonia in spinal cord injury and is generally well tolerated except for its sedative effect.
- Diazepam is generally unsuitable in patients with brain injury because of deleterious effects on attention and memory. Other side effects include intellectual impairment and reduced motor coordination.
- Evidence of abuse and addiction is rare, but true physiological addiction can occur. Withdrawal symptoms can appear if diazepam is tapered too rapidly.
- Although the potential for overdose exists, the benzodiazepines have an extremely large index of safety. Dosage begins at approximately 2 mg po b.i.d., and may be slowly titrated up to 60 mg or more per day, in divided dosages. Pediatric dosages range from 0.12 to 0.8 mg/kg per day in divided doses.

DANTROLENE SODIUM

- Dantrolene sodium (Dantrium) reduces muscle action potential–induced release of calcium from the sarcoplasmic reticulum, decreasing the force produced by excitation-contraction coupling. Dantrolene is the only drug that intervenes in spastic hypertonia at a "muscular" rather than a segmental reflex level. It reduces the activity of phasic stretch reflexes more than tonic ones. Dantrolene affects fast muscle fibers more than slow muscle fibers and, for unknown reasons, seems to have little effect on smooth and cardiac muscle tissues.
- It is metabolized largely in the liver, and eliminated in urine and bile.
- Its half-life is approximately 8 to 9 hours.
- Dantrolene is preferred for spasticity subsequent to supraspinal injury (e.g., hemiplegia or cerebral palsy), but may be a useful adjunct for the treatment of spasticity after spinal cord injury. It is less likely to cause lethargy or cognitive disturbances than are baclofen or diazepam. Although dantrolene can weaken

muscles, the effects on spastic hypertonia are generally without impairment of motor performance. Its most pronounced effect is possibly the reduction in clonus and muscle spasms resulting from innocuous stimuli.

- Dantrolene is mild to moderately sedative and can cause malaise, nausea and vomiting, dizziness, and diarrhea. The most commonly considered side effect is that of hepatoxicity, which can occur in approximately 1% of patients. Liver function tests should be monitored periodically, and the drug can be tapered or discontinued if enzyme elevations are noted.
- Dosage begins at 25 mg/day and may be slowly increased to 400 mg/day. Higher dosages are occasionally effective and can be tried provided monitoring for hepatotoxicity and other side effects is ensured. Clinical results are not clearly related to dose, however, and may plateau at a dosage of 100 mg/day. Pediatric doses begin at 0.5 mg/kg twice daily, increasing the frequency and dosage until maximum effect is reached. The maximum dosage is generally 3 mg/kg q.i.d. or less than 100 mg q.i.d.

TIZANIDINE

- Tizanidine (Zanaflex) is an imidazoline derivative that has an agonistic action at central α_2-adrenergic receptor sites. Unlike clonidine, it is much less potent in lowering blood pressure.
- It has been shown to be equivalent to baclofen as an antispastic agent (but may be better tolerated) in spastic patients after spinal and supraspinal injury in divided dosages up to 36 mg/day. It has similarly been shown to be equally efficacious and better tolerated than diazepam in patients with chronic hemiplegia. Multiple sclerosis patients have shown significant benefit in several large double-blinded studies.
- Common side effects include dry mouth, somnolence, asthenia, dizziness, headache, and insomnia. Liver function abnormalities have been noted only sporadically; nonetheless, the manufacturer recommends checking liver function tests periodically. Both tizanidine and baclofen are more effective in extensor than flexor musculature.
- The usual initial starting dosage of tizanidine is 4 mg, usually started in the evening. This dosage can be titrated slowly upward in 2-mg increments. The medication is generally prescribed on a t.i.d. schedule. The average daily dosage is 24 mg/day, and the maximum dosage recommended is 36 mg/day. Dosage should be reduced in patients with renal impairment. The half-life of tizanidine is just 2.5 hours, and the clinical effects of the drug peak 1 to 2 hours after each dose, disappearing by 6 hours. Thus even with t.i.d. dosing, it does not remain effective around the clock. It may be used together with baclofen with additive effect.

GABAPENTIN

- Although approved by the FDA only as an antileptic agent, gabapentin (Neurontin) has been shown to be an effective treatment in the treatment of spasticity as well.
- Gabapentin, which is a cyclohexane acetic acid derivative, was synthesized as an analog of GABA. It does not act at any known GABA receptor, and it does not affect the reuptake or degradation of GABA. It is excreted by the kidneys, and has a relatively short half-life of 5 to 7 hours.
- Its common side effects include somnolence, dizziness, ataxia, fatigue, and nystagmus. It has recently been shown to be effective in the treatment of spastic hypertonia secondary to spinal cord injury and multiple sclerosis.

• It is generally necessary to treat with dosages greater than 1200 mg/day in three divided dosages. Maximum recommended dosage per day is 2400 mg, but some use up to 3600 mg/day. Pediatric dosages have not been determined.

BENZODAZEPINES AND DERIVATIVES

• *Ketazolam*, a benzodiazepine, has been shown to be equally effective and less sedating than diazepam in spinal forms of spasticity; it may have a similar pharmacologic action. An additional benefit is that ketazolam can be administered in a single dosage of 30 to 60 mg/day. It is not currently approved for use in the United States.

• *Tetrazepam* (Myolastan), a benzodiazepine derivative, is reported to reduce the tonic component of spastic hypertonia with little effect on tendon hyperreflexia and no influence on muscle strength.

• *Clorazepate*, a benzodiazepine analog that is transformed into desmethyldiazepam (the major metabolite of diazepam), has been shown to be effective in normalizing phasic but not tonic stretch reflexes.

CHLORPROMAZINE AND PHENYTOIN

• Chlorpromazine has been applied to the treatment of hypertonia because of its α-adrenergic blocking effect. Clinical and electrophysiological studies in humans before and after administration of α- and β-blocking agents suggest descending adrenergic and noradrenergic pathways may have important modulatory effects on spastic hypertonia. However, the depression of motor function by phenothiazines is thought to be due largely to their effects on the brainstem reticular formation. A combination of these drugs may be beneficial in the treatment of spastic hypertonia. Neither drug alone is as efficacious as the combination of the two, although chlorpromazine alone was nearly as effective. Phenytoin serum levels did not correlate with therapeutic effect as long as the concentration was above 7 μg/mL. The addition of phenytoin lowered the needed optimally therapeutic dose of chlorpromazine, decreasing its sedative effect. However, because of the danger of tardive dyskinesia, chlorpromazine should not generally be used to treat spasticity.

CLONIDINE

• Clonidine, an α_2-adrenergic agonist, has been used with fair success in patients with spinal cord injury.

• Syncope, hypotension, and nausea and vomiting are the most common side effects.

• Most patients who benefit from the drug note acceptable relief with dosage of 0.1 mg twice a day or less. Clonidine is now available in an adhesive patch (Catapres-TTS) for week-long transdermal delivery. Initial studies have demonstrated favorable results, starting with the 0.1-mg patch and titrating up to the 0.3-mg patch as needed. Adverse effect rates were similar to those reported with oral clonidine.

Intrathecal Medications (pp. 605–606)

• Intrathecal administration of baclofen has been successfully attempted in the treatment of spastic hypertonia related to spinal cord dysfunction and cerebral palsy. A pump can be planted subcutaneously in the abdominal wall, with a catheter surgically placed into the subarachnoid space. In this manner, higher dosages of these medications can be placed near the spinal cord—the desired site for action of the drug—while largely avoiding the central nervous system side effects associated with increased oral intake. The pump can be refilled on a monthly basis by transcutaneous injection. Complications include tube dysfunction (e.g., dislodgement, disconnection, kinkage, and blockage); pump failure; infection; and baclofen overdosage.

• Baclofen is initially infused continuously at $25\,\mu g$/day. The most common side effects are drowsiness, dizziness, nausea, hypotension, headache, and weakness. The dosage is titrated up to an average of 400 to $500\,\mu g$/day or until satisfactory reduction in spasticity has been achieved. Some authors report experience with doses as high as $1500\,\mu g$/day. Although dosages can escalate early in the course of intrathecal baclofen use, it generally reaches a plateau 6 months following implantation. In addition to beneficial effects on limb spasticity, intrathecal baclofen may have a beneficial effect on bladder management. Caution concerning inadvertent overdose should be exercised because reversible coma from baclofen toxicity has been reported. Respiratory depression secondary to accidental intrathecal bolus injection has been reversed upon intravenous administration of $2\,mg$ of physostigmine. The half-life of intrathecal baclofen is approximately 5 hours.

• The administration of 1 to $2\,mg$ of intrathecal morphine has similarly caused a dramatic reduction in spasticity and pain in spinal cord patients. Patients do not seem to develop drug tolerance or lose the beneficial effect of the morphine in long-term follow-up. Despite its efficacy, intrathecal morphine is rarely used.

Nerve Blocks (pp. 606–607)

• Nerve blocks involve the application of a chemical agent to a nerve to impair the function of the nerve, either temporarily or permanently. This can result in improved range of motion, lessening of clonus, increase in speed and dexterity of movement (caused by blockade of inappropriately firing antagonists), improved crawling/sitting/standing in children, and even diminished spasticity in contralateral extremities.

• Commonly used agents include local anesthetics (e.g., lidocaine), phenol, alcohol, and botulinum toxin. Local anesthetics temporarily block conduction by interfering with the increase in permeability to sodium ions that normally occurs when the membrane is depolarized. The effects are short-lived (several hours) and are usually used in the assessment of the potential effect of a longer-acting nerve block or surgical procedure. Ethyl alcohol is also a potent neurolytic agent, but offers no particular advantage over phenol, and has not been as extensively evaluated.

• Aqueous phenol solutions (2% to 7%) are the most commonly used agents to produce chemical neurolysis when applied to a mixed sensorimotor nerve, motor nerve, or its terminal nerve fibers (motor point block). "Motor point" actually refers to electrosensitive sites along a motor branch, but it is not a useful term. Axons destroyed by phenol gradually regenerate, with some increase in fibrous tissue at the site of injection. See Chapter 29 in the Textbook for specific phenol nerve blocks.

• Because both sensory and motor nerve fibers are damaged, mixed sensorimotor nerve blocks with phenol can be associated with burning and discomfort. Dysesthesias, usually lasting 1 to 3 weeks, have been reported in approximately 10% of subjects. Although usually mild, the patient should be advised of this before the block is administered. Dysesthesias do not occur when motor nerves or branches are injected.

Botulinum Toxin Injection (pp. 607–608)
• Botulinum toxin has been used to diminish spasticity and has been evaluated in prospective clinical trials involving patients with multiple sclerosis, cerebral palsy, head injury, spinal cord injury, and stroke. Botulinum toxin was originally developed for clinical use by an ophthalmologist treating disorders such as blepharospasm and strabismus. Its use spread to the treatment of movement disorders such as torticollis and focal dystonias, and most recently to patients with spastic hypertonia.
• Increasing evidence suggests that certain patients, as many as 3%, may develop significant neutralizing antibodies with chronic treatment. This immunoresistance, as well as suboptimal technique, may be two important reasons why some patients are treatment resistant. Available antibody assays may underestimate the true incidence of significant immunoresistance, but certain strategies can be used to minimize this problem, including: (1) The minimal effective dosage should be utilized; (2) treatment sessions should be separated by a period of 3 months; and (3) "booster" injections should be avoided. Patients who develop resistance may benefit from injection with other botulinum toxin serotypes.

Spinal Blocks (p. 608)
• Intrathecal chemical neurolysis is another method of decreasing spastic hypertonia. Spinal root neurolysis may be carried out via spinal administration of 5% to 7% phenol in water or absolute alcohol, but control over affected fibers is rather imprecise. Patients must be carefully immobilized to allow precise layering of the neurolytic material so that damage is limited to the desired spinal roots. Complications of this procedure include urinary and fecal incontinence, paresis, paresthesias, and even death. Complication rates have varied from 1% to 10% in various series of patients. Given the potential complications and the alternatives available, intrathecal neurolysis should rarely, if ever, be necessary.

Surgical Interventions (pp. 608–613)

Orthopedic Procedures (pp. 608–612)
• Surgical procedures are generally reserved for adult patients who have been refractory to more conservative measures (e.g., ranging and/or casting), but have also found widespread use in the pediatric cerebral palsy population. Several considerations should be addressed before surgery is considered:
1. *When was the insult to the central nervous system?* It is important to schedule surgical intervention only when the plastic changes of recovery have more or less plateaued. This may be at least 6 months after a stroke, but 12 to 24 months after a traumatic brain injury.
2. *Are the "spastic" changes dynamic or static in nature? Dynamic* refers to dysfunction that appears with movement such as scissoring of the lower extremities during ambulation in an individual with cerebral palsy. *Static* deformities are fixed contractures, present both at rest and with movement, such as the clenched flexed hand of the hemiplegic upper extremity.
3. *What are the goals of surgery?* Is it to increase function (e.g., hand opening/closing or gait) or simply to increase range of motion to facilitate self-care or nursing care? For example, hip adduction can be lessened to diminish scissoring during gait in a cerebral palsy child, or to facilitate perineal hygiene in a patient with traumatic brain injury.

4. *What is the residual sensory and motor function of the limb in question?* Sensory input is vital to useful function in the upper extremity, and can be assessed with a variety of tools including two-point discrimination. Residual motor function in the upper extremity can be assessed with clinical scales, a vital component of which is the degree of remaining trunk and shoulder stability. A functioning hand and wrist is useless unless one can place them meaningfully, permitting interaction with oneself and the environment. Gait analysis with polyelectromyography is commonly used as an adjunct in planning procedures in the lower extremity. There are occasions when intervention can be rationally performed only after analysis of muscle firing during the gait cycle (see the discussion of stiff knee gait that follows).

5. *What type of procedure will best restore the abnormal forces acting on muscles and joints?* Deforming forces can be eliminated with a tenotomy or neurectomy, redirected with a tendon transfer, diminished with tendon lengthening procedures, or stabilized by a fusion procedure when soft tissue procedures alone would be inadequate (e.g., triple arthrodesis of the foot).

6. *What preexisting complications may interfere with surgery?* Preoperative plain films and bone scans are useful to assess the patient for fractures, dislocations, arthritis, and heterotopic ossification.

• Orthopedic surgery for the upper extremity may be useful in selected spastic patients (see Table 29–9 in the Textbook).

• Table 29–10 in the Textbook lists surgical interventions for the lower extremity.

Neurosurgical Procedures (pp. 612–613)

• Rhizotomies, the interruption of spinal roots, can be performed for the remediation of spasticity in severe cases. Rhizotomies may be categorized as open (requiring laminectomy) or closed, complete or selective, and anterior or posterior.

• Anterior rhizotomies are associated with severe denervation-type atrophy of all innervated muscles, and can place the patient at increased risk of skin breakdown. The recent work in surgical management of spasticity focuses largely around the issue of posterior rhizotomy.

• Radiofrequency rhizotomy utilizes a radiofrequency wave to heat a needle that burns individual dorsal roots localized under fluoroscopy. It can cause significant sensory loss, so is best reserved for patients with complete sensory loss or those who are so impaired that they rely on others for turning and monitoring their skin. Because of the proximity of the cervical roots to the vertebral arteries, radiofrequency rhizotomy is not performed in the cervical area. The reduction of muscle tone usually recurs, but may last for years.

• Selective dorsal rhizotomy (SDR), the neurosurgical ablation of a select proportion of dorsal rootlets, has been most often applied to children with cerebral palsy. Although selective rhizotomy is most often carried out in the lumbosacral roots, success has also been reported for treatment of spasticity and pain in the hemiplegic upper extremity. The term "selective" refers to the sectioning of particular segmental rootlets or fascicles, generally chosen because of their abnormal neurophysiological characteristics. The preferred subjects for this procedure are young children with spastic (not athetoid, ataxic, dystonic, or rigid) cerebral palsy with good motor control and some degree of forward locomotion, whose function is primarily limited because of the spastic hypertonia. However, other forms of spasticity have also been treated with SDR.

• Whereas most surgical series offer favorable outcomes, there is still considerable controversy whether SDR makes a significant contribution to the range of functional motor performance deficits seen in cerebral palsy. Subjective improvements have been noted in range of motion and gait, although difficulties in motor control persist. Intensive therapy appears necessary to maximize long-term functional gains. The most common unwanted postsurgical effects have included hypotonia (usually transitory) and weakness. Sensory changes, bladder dysfunction, and hip subluxation/dislocation have also been reported

• Myelotomy, or severance of tracts in the spinal cord, has been advocated as a treatment modality in the most severe cases of spastic hypertonia. Loss of bowel and bladder function must be considered as possible complications of myelotomy. Sectioning or excision of portions of the cord, or cordotomy and cordectomy, causes severe muscle wasting, frequent voiding difficulties, loss of erectile function, and are rarely practiced.

SUMMARY AND CONCLUSIONS (p. 614)

• Spastic hypertonia is but one component of the upper motor neuron syndrome, whose features also include loss of dexterity, weakness, and fatigability, as well as various reflex release phenomena. The functional impairment due to spasticity must be carefully assessed before any treatment is considered. Therapeutic intervention is best individualized to a particular patient.

• Treatment to ameliorate spastic hypertonia has two basic principles: (1) avoid noxious stimuli, and (2) provide frequent range of motion. Therapeutic exercise, cold, or topical anesthesia may decrease reflex activity for short periods in order to facilitate minimal motor function. Casting and splinting techniques are extremely valuable to extend joint range diminished by hypertonicity.

• Baclofen; diazepam; dantrolene; and, more recently, tizanidine are the most commonly used pharmacologic agents in the treatment of spastic hypertonia.

30

Original Chapter by Diane M.-L. Gilbert, M.D.

Sexuality Issues in Persons with Disabilities

• A virtually universal concern of rehabilitation patients, regardless of their impairment, is the impact their disability has on their sexual function and sexuality.

SEXUAL FUNCTION (pp. 616–634)

Anatomy and Physiology (pp. 616–623)

Normal (pp. 616–617)
• Masters and Johnson have described four phases of sexual response: excitement, plateau, orgasm, and resolution. (For further information, see Table 30–1 and Figs. 30–2 and 30–3 in the Textbook.)
• Educating patients about sexually transmitted diseases and their prevention, and fertility issues such as birth control, should be included with sexuality education.

Excitement or Arousal (pp. 617–621)
• The neurological components of the sexual response are summarized in Figure 30–1. (See Fig. 30–5 in the Textbook for vascular anatomy.)
• Excitement or arousal occurs in response to sexual stimulation caused by either touch (reflexogenic) or imagination (psychogenic).
• The brain is the most important sexual organ in the body, with multiple loci responsible for sexual activity.
• Psychogenic stimuli can be both facilitory or inhibitory, and the degree of tactile stimulation necessary to produce reflex lubrication or erection can be diminished by psychic stimulation.
• Libido is affected by concentrations of neurotransmitters and is decreased by serotonin or stimulated by dopamine.
• Libido is affected by depression and medications affecting the neurotransmitters.
• Reflexogenic erections are those mediated via sensory input elicited by direct stimulation of the genital area via the sensory fibers of the dorsal nerve through the pudendal nerve to the sacral spinal cord. The sacral parasympathetic (S2 to

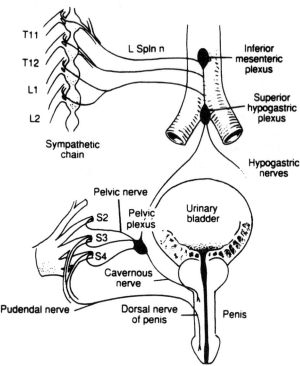

FIGURE 30–1. Summary of neurological sexual anatomy. Parasympathetic innervation: originates in the anterior divisions of spinal roots S2 to S4; preganglionic fibers enter the pelvis as the nervi erigentes or pelvic nerves course in close proximity to the hypogastric vessels, terminating in the pelvic plexus; the cavernous nerve then travels to the corpora, and other fibers to the scrotum and pubis. Sympathetic innervation: T10 to L2 supply the sympathetic fibers to the penis and female genitalia; preganglionic fibers course to the superior hypogastric plexus, join the pelvic plexus via the hypogastric nerves, and travel via the cavernous nerve to the genitalia; postganglionic nerves in the hypogastric nerves travel to the vas deferens, seminal vesicle, ampulla, bladder neck, musculature of the prostate, and blood vessels of the prostate and penis. Somatic innervation: pudendal nerve is formed from the anterior divisions of S2 to S4; it supplies both sensory innervation (to penis, scrotum, and pubis) and motor innervation (to bulbocavernosus, ischiocavernosus, striated urethral sphincter, and perineal muscles). (From Melman A, Christ GJ, Hirsch MS: Anatomy and physiology of the penis. In Bennett AH (ed): Impotence: Diagnosis and Management of Erectile Dysfunction. Philadelphia, WB Saunders, 1994, p. 21.)

S4) response travels via the nervi erigentes to the cavernosal nerves and into the corporal trabeculae by way of autonomic fibers (see Fig. 30–1).
• Psychogenic erections are believed to originate in the cerebral cortex from stimuli passing through the different senses (e.g., visual stimuli like movies, pictures, or fantasizing). The impulses producing psychogenic erection travel through the hypothalamic and thalamic centers to the sympathetic thoracolumbar cord and the parasympathetic sacral cord.

• There is sympathetic discharge to genitals as long as there is no disruption above L2 (T11 to L2).
• There is little evidence to support the role of only *thoracolumbar* sympathetic outflow in erection development.
• Erections are now believed to occur only rarely with complete lower motor neuron lesions.

Plateau (p. 621)
• The plateau phase can be very brief (seconds) or prolonged (minutes) and is described as a pleasurable sense of well being.
• Sexual dysfunctions can occur in this stage. With *anorgasmy* the individual does not progress further than the plateau stage. *Premature ejaculation* refers to emission or ejaculation that is accompanied by loss of erection before or immediately upon penetration.

Ejaculation (pp. 621–622)
• Male ejaculation requires a coordinated series of muscular and neurophysiological events involving the sympathetic, parasympathetic, and somatic nervous supply that cause the constituents of the ejaculate to be deposited in the posterior urethra, then evacuated through the urethra and urethral meatus in an antegrade fashion.
• Sympathetic input to the bladder neck prevents retrograde flow.
• Emission and ejaculation are reflexive and can occur independently, and erection is not an absolute prerequisite.
• Female ejaculation is not as easily a quantifiable response as is the male norm and remains a more controversial subject.

Orgasm (p. 622)
• Orgasm, occurring in the limbic system, is believed to be a cortical experience of "supreme pleasure followed by a feeling of well-being and satiation."
• Orgasm can be experienced separate from ejaculation in those with ejaculatory disorders.
• The waiting period between ejaculations for men is related to the time required to build up seminal ejaculate.
• In women, the muscles involved in orgasm produce a biphasic motor response involving sympathetic contraction of the smooth muscles of the fallopian tubes, uterus, and paraurethral glands of Skene; somatic contraction of striated pelvic floor muscles; perineum; and anal sphincter.

Resolution (p. 622)
• Resolution is the return to the prearousal physiological state, usually occurring over a period of 5 to 15 minutes.

Normal Age-Related Physiological Changes (pp. 622–623)
• These changes occur in women most dramatically at the onset of menopause, when the relative steroid deficit reduces the rapidity and intensity of the physiological sexual response.
• There is a decrease in the frequency of vaginal and uterine contractions during orgasm.
• The vaginal canal becomes thinner and shorter secondary to decreased estrogen.

TABLE 30–1 Normal Age-Related Physiological Changes in Men

Phase	Change
Excitement	Develop erections 2–3 times slower than younger men
	Tactile stimulation may be necessary
	Erection is not as firm, approaches full ridigity only seconds before ejaculation
Plateau	Able to maintain erection for longer period prior to ejaculation
	Less discernible nipple swelling and erection
	Testicular elevation is reduced
Ejaculation/orgasm	Ejaculation lacks the well-defined sense of impending orgasm because accessory organs fail to secrete and create the welling of semen in the prostatic urethra
	One to two expulsive contractions of the urethra occur instead of the usual four major contractions
	Seepage can occur rather than expulsion, which diminishes the sensation through the urethra
Resolution	More rapid detumescence
	Refractory period increases in length (>55 yr ~ 12–24 hr)

Data from Kaiser FE: Sexuality and impotence in the aging man. Clin Geriatr Med 1991; 7:63–71; Schiavi RC, Schreiner-Engel P, Mandeli J, et al: Healthy aging and male sexual function. Am J Psychiatry 1990; 147:766–771; Weiss JN, Mellinger BC: Sexual dysfunction in elderly men. Clin Geriatr Med 1990; 6:185–196; LoPiccolo J: Counseling and therapy for sexual problems in the elderly. Clin Geriatr Med 1991; 7:161–179.

• Lubrication diminishes or takes longer, and non-petroleum-based lubricating jelly can be helpful.
• There is an increased incidence of vulvovaginitis and urethritis, atrophy of the external genitals, changes in the size of the clitoris and labia, and pubic hair loss.
• Prolapse and stress incontinence are also seen in multiparous aging women, but they can be managed well surgically.
• Changes seen in men are summarized in Table 30–1.

Changes with Impairments (pp. 624–634)

• *Sexual dysfunction* can be defined as any sexual behavioral problem that makes sexual expression consistently unsatisfying for the individual or partner (Table 30–2).
• The sudden onset of disability or the more chronic issues of malaise, pain, fatigue, or stress can contribute to decreased libido.
• Sixty percent of all male sexual dysfunction at a performance level is physical in origin, and this dysfunction increases with age.
• Dysfunction is most common in patients with diabetes, circulatory changes, autonomic nervous disorders, venous leakages or arteriovenous shunting, alcoholism; or caused by the effects of medications.
• There is evidence to indicate that it is commonly associated with depression, increased anxiety, and poor self-esteem in affected patients.
• The most common sexual concern for women with or without disabilities is low desire. This must be distinguished from biological sexual drive and lack of

TABLE 30–2 Types of Sexual Dysfunction

Dysfunction	Characteristics
Decreased libido	Decline in sexual drive or desire; may be conscious or subconscious
Decreased vaginal lubrication	Reduction in lubrication fluid in vagina
Delayed orgasm	Prolonged time for orgasm to occur
Anorgasmia	Inability to achieve orgasm
Breast hyperplasia	May adversely affect self-esteem and body image, especially as adolescent
Gynecomastia	Enlargement or excessive development of male breast; may be unilateral or bilateral
Impotence	Inability to achieve or maintain erection sufficient for penetration and intercourse
Priapism	Prolonged, painful erection caused by lack of drainage of corpus cavernosum
Retarded ejaculation	Delayed ejaculation or inability to ejaculate
Retrograde ejaculation	Ejaculation into urinary bladder caused by insufficient tightening of internal urethral neck
Premature ejaculation	When emission/ejaculation is accompanied by loss of erection, before or immediately upon vaginal penetration

Adapted from Seidl A, Bullough B, Haughey B, et al: Understanding the effects of a myocardial infarction on sexual functioning: A basis for sexual counseling. Rehabil Nurs 1991; 16:255–264.

privacy, misinformation, concerns about birth control, lack of sexual skills in the partner, or interruption of the physiological sexual response.

SILDENAFIL (VIAGRA)
• Sildenafil is an orally active, potent, selective inhibitor of cGMP-specific PDE-5, resulting in higher concentrations of cGMP, better vasodilation, and hence an erection that it is easier to get and maintain.
• There has been an 80% rate of improved erections in the studies looking at a general population use.
• It is not an aphrodisiac. The risk of priapism is minimal.
• The primary side effects are autonomic in nature and can include, headache, facial flush, upset stomach, and visual color distortion (a shift toward blue). Other and more severe side effects are possible. Please see manufacturer's description.

Spinal Cord Injury (pp. 625–632)
• Neurological injury can affect either upper motor neurons (e.g., tetraplegia) or lower motor neurons (e.g., cauda equina).
• These lesions usually involve motor and sensory pathways, and the patient has to deal with motor weakness; loss of sensation; and changes in erection or lubrication, ejaculation, orgasm, and fertility.
• Incomplete lesions might spare some sexual function, but genital sensation is lost with injury to the spinal cord above S2.
• Males with complete lower motor neuron disease involving the S2 to S4 segments (i.e., cauda equina) will have poor erectile function because the S2 to S4 reflex is interrupted.

• After SCI, previous erogenous zones may be insensate, which can affect the excitement phase. The demarcation between insensate and sensate skin may become the new erogenous zone.
• Incomplete SCI patients often have erogenous sensation in the perianal area, but cultural attitudes toward anal stimulation can prevent patients from benefiting from this erogenous area.
• Patients must be encouraged to experiment with their bodies to learn and understand the new changes and effectively communicate their needs to their partners.

ACHIEVING ERECTIONS
• Reflexogenic erection can occur with stroking, oral stimulation, vibration, pulling pubic hair, or a full bladder.
• Education by the staff can help prevent uncomfortable or embarrassing situations, such as when a male patient has an erection while a nurse performs a bladder catheterization.
• Psychogenic erections can occur with incomplete lower motor neuron lesions, as previously described.
• Psychogenic erections are typically lost with lesions between T10 and T12, whereas both reflexogenic and psychogenic erections are possible with lesions between L2 and S1.
• Neurogenic causes of ED can be confirmed by testing with vasoactive substances injected into the corpora.
• During the period of spinal shock, which can last from a few hours to several weeks, it is impossible to predict the final sexual impairment status.
• Sexual function might not return for 6 to 24 months; in 80% of patients it does so within 1 year of injury, and in another 5% within 2 years.
• Clinicians should not overlook the possibility of a nonorganic cause (i.e., psychogenic impotence) as the primary cause of erectile dysfunction. Aggressive (especially invasive) intervention should be limited during this period.

TECHNIQUES TO RESTORE ERECTION
• Restoring erection in the SCI male may be accomplished using one of the following four options:

Neuropharmacotherapy: Oral Agents. Oral sildenafil (Viagra), taken as required (not more than once daily), significantly improves the quality of erections and satisfaction with sex life in men with ED caused by SCI between T6 and L5.
• Well-controlled, double-blind studies of yohimbine hydrochloride, an oral α_2-adrenergic blocking agent, have shown it to have only limited efficacy in ED when used singly or in combination with methyltestosterone and a variety of vitamins and caffeine-based stimulants.
• Oral levodopa has also been used, with 55% to 60% of patients reported to achieve rigid erection.

Intracavernous Injection of Vasoactive Substances. Injection into the corpora of papaverine (a nonspecific smooth muscle relaxant producing vasodilation and relaxation of the sinusoidal spaces), a combination of papaverine and phentolamine (an α-adrenergic blocker producing vasodilation), or prostaglandin E_1 produces an erection.

Vacuum Tumescence Constriction Therapy. VTCT refers to the use of external devices that create a vacuum and cause an erection-like state that is maintained by a constricting band (see Fig. 30–6 in the Textbook).

• The flaccid penis is placed in a rigid cylinder. A pump creates the vacuum needed to fill the corpora with blood. A constricting band is placed at the base of the penis, after the cylinder is removed, to prevent blood from leaving the penis (partners may complain of a cold penis) (see Fig. 30–7 in the Textbook). This can maintain an erection for up to 30 minutes. Detumescence follows rapidly after the band is removed.

Penile Prosthesis. Implantable penile prostheses are available in numerous designs, including fixed, semirigid (flexible), or inflatable.
• Semirigid prostheses can be hinged, malleable, or articulated.
• Inflatable penile prostheses can be multicomponent or self-contained (see Fig. 30–8 in the Textbook). With the inflatable prosthesis, the penis is inflated to full erection by means of a pump located in the scrotum. When a valve is opened, the penis deflates. The multicomponents of the inflatable prosthesis make it more difficult and costly to insert than the fixed or flexible rods.
• Indications for these devices in SCI patients include both ED and maintenance of external catheters.
• Their use has recently declined in SCI males. The reason for this decrease is twofold: the frequency of complications (infection and erosions); and the simpler, safer, cost-effective injection and vacuum techniques.

Transcutaneous Agents. Transcutaneous nitroglycerin has been used as topical therapy for ED in SCI patients. It produced an erection sufficient for coitus in 25% of patients in whom papaverine injections had induced rigid erections. Nitroglycerin commonly has side effects, including hypotension and headaches.

Achieving Vaginal Lubrication. Much of what was said in the Achieving Erection section applies to females with respect to vaginal lubrication and engorgement.
• There is both reflexogenic and psychogenic lubrication. Some women with reflexogenic lubrication describe a sensation similar to that of a full bladder, whereas the sensation with psychogenic lubrication is often attenuated.
• Those with complete lesions involving T10 to T12 do not have lubrication and benefit from vaginal lubricants such as saliva, Replens, or K-Y jelly.

Coitus. *Coitus* is defined as intromission and intravaginally sustained erection.
• Studies have show that one-fourth of SCI males who attained an erection were able to achieve successful coitus.
• Although having an erection is important, it is also important that the patients be aware that more than 50% of well-adjusted women do not reach orgasm with vaginal stimulation alone. The "stuffing technique" can be used if the patient or his partner desires vaginal intromission.
• Loss of lubrication in the female patient can interfere with coitus.
• Pelvic floor and adductor muscle spasticity can restrict penile penetration. Premedication with benzodiazepines can help reduce this spasticity.
• Both male and female SCI patients must learn to empty the bladder and bowel before sexual activity and remember to void or catheterize themselves after sexual activity to lessen the chances of urinary tract infection (UTI) and incontinence.

Ejaculation. Failure of synchronous activity involving deposition of ejaculate constituents and antegrade evacuation through the urethra constitutes *retrograde ejaculation* or *ejaculatory failure*. Retrograde ejaculation can be secondary to

an abnormal state (e.g., sympathetic nervous system damage), preventing adequate closure of the bladder neck and leading to retrograde semen flow.
• After sexual activity, males may complain of dry ejaculate (sensation of orgasm with no explusion of semen) or cloudy urine at the time of their next void or catheterization.
• Ejaculatory failure also occurs in up to 90% of patients after transurethral prostatectomy (TURP).
• Ejaculatory failure is seen least often in those with lower lesions or incomplete lesions.

Orgasm. We have previously emphasized the importance of the brain in the experience of orgasm. All the issues discussed in the sexuality section play a vital role in the patient's libido and responsiveness to the sexual experience.
• The brain can work independent of genitalia in the generation of erotic experience, just as the genitalia of SCI patients can work reflexively independent of the brain.
• With SCIs, female orgasms are typically experienced differently than they were premorbidly. They are described as pleasurable feelings of intense excitement or as sudden enhancement of spasticity followed by prolonged relaxation. The extragenital responses during orgasm include headache, warm sensation, physical pleasure, and sexual excitement. It is important to educate the patient that the orgasms are real, just different.
• Orgasm is conveyed in the anterior spinothalamic and pyramidal tracts and can easily be tested in an office setting. A normally appreciated cold stimulus to the clitoris or penis and the ability to voluntarily contract the external anal sphincter indicates intact orgasmic pathways. This allows the patient to know that given the right mental and physical stimuli, he or she could experience orgasm.
• It is important to educate SCI males that pleasurable feelings (orgasm) can occur without ejaculation, because the percentage of successful ejaculation is low.
• Orgasms are practically nonexistent in patients with complete upper motor neuron lesions.
• Persons with complete lower motor neuron injuries occasionally perceive pleasurable sensation lower in the abdomen, pelvis, or thighs.

Autonomic Dysreflexia. All patients with SCIs at or above T4 to T6 are at risk for autonomic dysreflexia.
• To reduce the risk of autonomic dysreflexia, patients are advised to evacuate the bowel and bladder before sexual activity.
• In the event of dysreflexia, the patient should be educated to stop, and to sit up to elevate the head (to help lower blood pressure).
• Medical assistance should be sought if the headache does not subside.
• Prophylactic medication can be used if autonomic dysreflexia is not otherwise manageable.

MALE FERTILITY

• Less than 10% of SCI patients retain the ability to impregnate their partner spontaneously.
• Problems arise from ejaculatory failure, obstruction of genital passages, impairment of spermatogenesis, or a combination of these.

• Techniques to restore ejaculation are usually aimed at restoring fertility. The techniques involve stimulation of the intact neurological center below the SCI through chemical, vibratory, or transrectal electrical ejaculation. These techniques are most successful when the T10 to T11 spinal segments are intact.

• α-adrenergic agonists (e.g., pseudoephrine and imipramine) are used to attempt to convert retrograde ejaculation to anterograde ejaculation. If this is not successful, harvesting and processing of the retrograde ejaculate should be attempted.

• Vibratory stimulation of the glans penis has been used successfully by various groups to collect semen via antegrade and retrograde ejaculation; it is successful in about 50% of SCI males, because it requires an intact reflex arc.

• Transrectal electrical stimulation or electroejaculation involves stimulation of the myelinated preganglionic efferent sympathetic fibers of the hypogastric plexus to obtain seminal emission into the posterior urethra (see Fig. 30–9 in the Textbook). It is currently the most common method used in the United States.

• Electroejaculation is an office- or hospital-based procedure because of the need to monitor for autonomic dysreflexia and the anoscopy performed to evaluate the rectal mucosa.

• Assisted reproductive technologies such as IVF (in vitro fertilization) and GIFT (gamete intrafallopian transfer) have been used to achieve pregnancy.

• Intracytoplasmic sperm injection (ICSI) has revolutionized the treatment of male fertility. High fertilization rates are usually achieved with ICSI independent of semen parameters. Standard sperm retrieval includes microepididymal sperm aspiration, percutaneous sperm aspiration, modified percutaneous sperm aspiration, and testicular sperm extraction.

• Fertility problems can also stem from obstructed passages of the vas deferens, epididymis, and seminiferous tubules, most likely from repeated infections involving the bladder. Duct obstruction can be treated only by surgical resection.

• Spermatogenesis may be impaired, resulting in a decrease in number of sperm, decrease in normal motility, and increase in abnormal morphology. Sperm contact with urine, medication, antisperm antibodies, or raised scrotal temperature may be explanations for the poor semen quality typically seen in patients with SCI.

FEMALE FERTILITY

• Amenorrhea occurs in most women acutely after traumatic SCI, and lasts from 6 months to 1 year. The first ovulation cycle is unpredictable and therefore contraception must be considered from the beginning. There are a number of contraceptive methods that can be used (Table 30–3).

• Although the ability to bear children is usually not affected, pregnancy presents many challenges to the SCI female. Self-care must be heightened to avoid the complications of UTIs, thrombophlebitis, edema of the legs, pressure ulcers, premature labor, and immobilization-induced osteoporosis. Repeated UTIs increase the risk of developing toxemia of pregnancy.

• The uterus is innervated by spinal cord levels T10 to T12; therefore patients with complete lesions above T10 will not appreciate uterine contractions or fetal movement.

TABLE 30-3 Female Fertility and Contraception

Type	Side Effects	Comments
Periodic abstinence or coitus interruptus	None	A woman must be well instructed in her biological rhythms to avoid unplanned pregnancy
Condoms	Decreased effectiveness if properly used Must be reapplied for second sexual activity Taste may be offensive	Ready availability, increased acceptability, increased effectiveness Need dexterity Indwelling catheter may tear condom; therefore, lubricate Protects against sexually transmitted diseases
Foam and sponge	None	Ready availability, increased acceptability, increased effectiveness
Diaphragm/foam	Weakened pelvic muscles may not hold diaphragm in place	Requires dexterity Partner may be trained to insert the diaphragm
Intrauterine device (IUD)	May be unable to feel early signs of pelvic inflammatory disease Manual dexterity is needed to check for placement	Inserted by physician Insertion may be easier with paralysis Teach the patient to look for spotting, irregular periods, increased spasticity, fever, increased or different vaginal discharge
Oral contraceptive pill	Studies of the early use (estrogen, 50–150 µg; progestin) revealed an association with cardiovascular, thromboembolic, cerebrovascular, and thrombophlebitic disease	Most common reason for unplanned pregnancy is improper dosing Need sufficient cognition and reliability as well as the manual dexterity to take pill as required

	Studies of low-dose estrogen (35 μg) and progestin suggest only individual situations of hypertension and thrombophlebitis Both are aggravated by smoking Spinal cord–injured women must be taught the warning signs of thrombophlebitis	Good option for women who do not desire children for a period of years Added benefit of reducing or totally eliminating menstrual bleeding, which can facilitate hygiene
Subdermal hormonal implants (Norplant)	Has not been shown to produce thromboembolic, cerebrovascular, or cardiovascular disease Monitor for hypertension and thrombophlebitis Side effects include irregular vaginal bleeding, changes in weight, and psychic symptoms similar to menopause or premenstrual syndrome	
Medroxyprogesterone acetate (Depo-Provera)	Same as above	Added benefit of reducing or totally eliminating menstrual bleeding, which can facilitate hygiene
Sterilization by tubal ligation or vasectomy	Permanent	Continue to menstruate
Therapeutic abortion		Prior to sexual activity, patient and partner should discuss family planning and options

Data from Bérard EJJ: The sexuality of spinal cord injured women: Physiology and pathophysiology: A review. Paraplegia 1989; 27:99–112; Goddard LR: Sexuality and spinal cord injury. J Neurosci Nurs 1988; 20:240–243.

• Although the discomfort of labor is not felt as in able-bodied women, the onset of labor is typically detected but as a different sensation. The contractions may be stronger, more prolonged, and more frequent, but the duration of labor is shorter than for the non-SCI women.
• Although the abdominal muscles may be paralyzed, the uterus will contract because of hormonal influence.
• Delivery of the fetus may require the use of forceps or episiotomy.
• Cesarean section should be performed for the same indications as in the able-bodied.
• Patients with lesions above T6 are at risk for autonomic dysreflexia during childbirth. The treatment of choice is epidural anesthesia because it allows continuous medication administration. Oral premedication can be tried as an alternative.

Cortical Involvement (p. 632)
• With cortical involvement, one may be required to cope with aphasia (communication); left- or right-sided neglect (disinhibition, impulsivity, poor social interaction); or apraxias (motor planning difficulty). Sexuality and sexual function are related to understanding and communication between the patient and partner, which are affected by these neurological sequelae.
• There is a general decline in sexual activity and libido in both sexes after stroke, but there is little evidence of organic causes for the sexual dysfunction. The comorbidity associated with CVA (e.g., diabetes, hypertension, and cardiac problems) contributes to sexual dysfunction.
• Psychological factors seem to be important in determining changes in sexual life after stroke. These factors may be a result of change in the sex role, dependence on a partner for activities of daily living, or attitudes of partners.
• Impairment of cutaneous sensibility, neurogenic bladder, fatigue, depression, and aphasic disorders have been found to play a role in sexual changes.
• Traumatic brain injury (TBI) patients can suffer cerebral involvement leading to sexual disinhibition, hyposexuality, and hypersexuality (Klüver-Bucy syndrome), in that order of frequency.
• TBI patients may have significant personality changes that adversely affect their relationships and appear to deteriorate over time rather than improve.
• Multiple sclerosis is a chronic illness that affects many aspects of sexuality (often in young adults) (see Chapter 52).

Diabetic Neuropathy (pp. 632–633)
• Peripheral neuropathies such as in diabetes mellitus have many effects on the peripheral somatic and autonomic nervous systems affecting the expression of sexuality.
• Within 5 years of the onset of diabetes mellitus, one-third to one-half of males experience some sexual dysfunction. This is usually impotence secondary to a combination of physiological (neurological and vascular) and psychological factors.
• Oral sildenafil (Viagra) is an effective and well-tolerated treatment for ED in men with diabetes.
• Female diabetic patients experience sexual dysfunction with impaired lubrication, impaired sensation, increased vaginal infections leading to dyspareunia, and changes in sexual desire.

Vascular Disease *(p. 633)*
• Coronary disease resulting in myocardial infarction and peripheral vascular disease leading to amputation have a significant impact on patients and their sexual functioning.
• Viagra has proved to be effective in this population, but once again the precautions are emphasized.
• Medications used for treatment often interfere with libido or sexual function. Sexual dysfunction is one of the main reasons for noncompliance with antihypertensive medication regimens.
• The frequency of sexual activity often decreases dramatically after myocardial infarction or coronary bypass.
• Energy expenditure during sexual activity is similar to that of walking on a treadmill at 3 to 4 miles per hour (i.e., 5 to 6 METS [metabolic equivalents of oxygen consumption]). The amount of energy expenditure during sexual activity has been compared to climbing two flights of stairs at a brisk rate, or climbing 20 steps in 10 seconds.
• It is now recommended that counselors advise patients to use their usual sexual position(s) because these are generally less stressful than learning a new position.

Physical Disfigurement *(pp. 633–634)*
• Physical disfigurement can arise from a variety of conditions including amputations, burns, cancer, and arthritis.
• Genital sexual function is not often affected, but other factors affecting sexuality may be severely affected.
• Oncology patients have multiple issues including body image (as in breast cancer postmastectomy) and mortality.
• Chemotherapy-induced nausea, malaise, or weakness may compromise sexual frequency.
• Patients with an ileostomy or colostomy often have secondary erectile failure because of depression and decreased self-esteem.
• Arthritis is a chronic disease and is associated with decreased sexual function, as are diabetes mellitus, chronic obstructive pulmonary disease, renal disease, increased age, severity of illness, and depression.
• Chronic diseases seen in children (e.g., juvenile rheumatoid arthritis, cystic fibrosis, and myelomeningocele) affect many of the sexuality issues all adolescents face.
• With burn patients, physiological function is usually intact and the concerns are body image, self-esteem, and interpersonal relationships.

Terminal Illness (p. 634)

• When dealing with the terminally ill, physicians do not typically consider the consequences to the patient's sexuality.
• Patients can get mired in the grieving process and not be able to move forward to the enjoyment of their modified sexuality.

SEXUALITY (pp. 634–636)

• Sexuality is a "combination of sex drive, sex acts, and all those aspects of personality concerned with learned communications and relationship patterns . . .

rooted in the human need to relate to others, to receive and share pleasure, to love and to be loved."
• Sexuality is an integral part of a person's psychological makeup and self-concept.

Sexual Development (pp. 634–635)

• Clinicians attempting to assist patients to return to healthy sexual function must be careful not to convey their biases or prejudices to the patient.
• The most common sexual problem in older couples is male erectile difficulties. Disease, drug reactions, and disability can contribute to emotional upset; decreased libido; decreased erectile function; and, consequently, decreased sexual activity.

Factors Affecting Sexuality (pp. 635–636)

Body Image (p. 635)
• Failure to accept one's body as is, in the presence of disability, can lead to feelings not only of shame but also of dissociation from one's body and a perceived loss of control.

Self-Esteem (p. 636)
• Self-esteem, the personal sense of one's inherent worth, is essential to mental health and identity.
• The presence of impairments and physical disabilities can be an assault on one's self-esteem.
• Disabled women more commonly experienced sexual abuse and sexual harassment than nondisabled women, and this can be particularly devastating in view of their already vulnerable self-esteem.
• Some patients react to diminished self-esteem by displaying hypersexuality, apparently seeking assurance or validation from others that they are still attractive. It is important to understand the insecurity that underlies these inappropriate displays so as not to further undermine the patient's self-esteem with negative reactions.
• Assertiveness training has been used successfully to assist with this expression and subsequently has increased patient self-esteem.

Gender Identity (p. 636)
• For disabled patients, gender identity can be compromised by an impairment in their ability to express their assumed gender role. Patients might test their identity by acting out an exaggeration of their assumed gender role. For example, a male who has been raised to value assertiveness, dominance, and strength and then finds himself with quadriplegia is forced to accept a more passive physical role. He may attempt to compensate through verbal abuse of family, therapists, or nursing staff.
• Females, particularly those who value a more traditional feminine role, are much more sensitive to their perceived loss of sexual attractiveness and perceived loss of fertility in defining their female identity.
• For women with cognitive disabilities, particularly if insight and self-awareness are impaired, relationships may be a challenge. Behaviors that promote acceptance by other people have to be learned, and awareness of social subtleties such as eye contact and a sense of personal space may be inadequate.

TABLE 30-4 PLISSIT Model for Sexual Counseling

	Goals	Responsibility	Example	References
P *permission*	Assure the patient that sexuality is a legitimate concern in the rehabilitation process. Provide a positive climate in which patients feel comfortable to ask questions, seek advice, and experiment. Do not expect the patient to initiate the discussion! Open the door with your questions.	Should be addressed by any team member in any discussion.	If sexual history is included as a routine part of *every* intake examination, it signals to the client that sexuality is considered an integral part of rehabilitation. The initial interaction can also serve to set the stage for further discussion and questions. "Being a good listener, attending to and acknowledging spoken or body language, asking leading questions, initiating discussion of sensitive subjects, and making observations about physical manifestations, such as reflex erections in the male client with spinal cord injury." Telling people that their thoughts, feelings, and behaviors are "normal."	The clinician is directed to read general textbooks and review articles.

Table continued on following page

TABLE 30-4 PLISSIT Model for Sexual Counseling—cont'd

	Goals	Responsibility	Example	References
LI *limited information*	Deals with the disability and its implications for sexual health in a general fashion. Used to change relevant attitudes and behavior. Can serve as the means for dispelling general sexual myths relating to breast and genital size, masturbation, oral-genital contact, anal intercourse.	May be provided to the patient in a private, impersonal manner by way of educational material or by any comfortable team member.	This level of information is easily provided during the initial examination. While eliciting the bladder-bowel history or examining the genitalia, one can provide vital information. For example, performing the bulbocavernosus reflex test can be very intimidating or embarrassing for the patient but can be an easy steppingstone to a more in-depth discussion regarding sexual function. Clients should be encouraged to seek out new areas of hypersensitivity. This information should also be provided to family and significant others.	Pamphlets or educational handouts on head injury, stroke, or spinal cord injury. (Sexuality After Spinal Cord Injury: Fact Sheet no 3. National Spinal Cord Injury Association, 1987; Male Reproductive Function After Spinal Cord Injury: Fact Sheet no 10. National Spinal Cord Injury Association, 1988).

SS specific suggestions	Patient and partner are actively assisted by staff to set and reach specific goals to address sexual concerns and dysfunctions.	Rehabilitation team member knowledgeable about sexuality and the particular physical disability affecting the patient.	Therapists can assist patients with positioning for comfortable lovemaking like using the partner for a backboard, sensual ways to undress, techniques of foreplay, the use of fantasy, types of mechanical devices available, how to deal with urinal and bowel mishaps. Pipe-cleaner figures can be useful in demonstrating alternative sexual positions. "You'll have to try it and see" is not good enough. Use peer counseling.	Excellent books and videos depicting different lovemaking options. (Mooney TO, Cole TM, Chilgren RA: Sexual Options for Paraplegics and Quadriplegics. Boston, Little, Brown, 1975; Bregman S: Sexuality and the Spinal Cord Injured Woman. Minneapolis, Sister Kenny Foundation, 1975; Rabin BJ: The Sensuous Wheeler. Long Beach, CA, 1980.)
IT intensive therapy	When is it time to refer? Psychological problems General sexual dysfunction Overall low sexual interest Primary orgasmic dysfunction Vaginismus Primary impotence Ejaculatory incompetence Destructive paraphilias	Requires assistance of a specially trained professional or professional sexual therapist because harm may be done to the patient if a clinician is inexperienced.	"Injury is likely to magnify any sexual difficulties that the patient and the partner have (interpersonal and psychological issues) and these must be overcome before progress can be made."	American Association of Sex Educators, Counselors and Therapists, 435N. Michigan Ave., Suite 1717, Chicago, IL 60611 (312) 644-0828.

Adapted from Annon JS, Robinson CH: Treatment of common male and female sexual concerns. In Ferguson JM, Taylor CB (eds): The Comprehensive Handbook of Behavioral Medicine, Vol 1. New York, SP Medical & Scientific Books, 1980, pp. 273–296.

TABLE 30–5 Sexual Counseling Precautions

1. Do not put persons in conflict with their God.
2. Avoid extreme pressure on the patient to discuss sexuality.
3. Avoid forcing your morality and convictions on the patient.
4. Do not threaten the patient with your own sexuality.
5. Do not make sex an all-or-none sort of experience.
6. Do not assume that once the topic is discussed that you can leave it alone.
7. Do not conclude that there is only one way to convey information.
8. Be sure that the conjoint nature of sexual relationships is held paramount.
9. Do convey the notion that all relationships, including the sexual one, are a matter of compromise.

From Rieve JE: Sexuality and the adult with acquired physical disability. Nurs Clin North Am 1989; 24:265–276. Information compiled by Rieve from Hohmann GW: Sexual dysfunction associated with physical disabilities. Arch Phys Med Rehabil 1975; 56:1, and other sources.

PLISSIT Model (Permission, Limited Information, Specific Suggestions, Intensive Therapy) (pp. 637–638)

• The goals of the patient-clinician interaction should be to develop trusting relationships, support gender identity, maintain body image, and teach socialization. The PLISSIT model provides the basis for addressing sexual issues in a comprehensive manner (Table 30–4).
• Table 30–5 lists precautions that should be followed when counseling patients. The single most important factor in improving sexual relationships between people is communication.

31

Original Chapter by Richard Salcido, M.D., and Robert Goldman, M.D.

Prevention and Management of Pressure Ulcers and Other Chronic Wounds

- The financial burden of chronic wound care is immense. Four basic ulcer types present significant economic burden: pressure ulcers ($3 billion to $6 billion), ischemic/neuropathic ulcers ($3 billion to $5 billion), and venous ulcers (more than $2 billion).

SCOPE OF THE PROBLEM (pp. 645–646)

Definitions (pp. 645–646)

- *Pressure ulcer:* The National Pressure Ulcer Advisory Panel (NPUAP) defines a *pressure ulcer* as an area of unrelieved pressure over a defined area, usually over a bony prominence (e.g., the greater trochanter of the femur, sacrum, or occiput) resulting in ischemia, cell death, and tissue necrosis. Pressure ulcers are associated with impaired sensorium or sensation, poor hygiene or nutrition, and chronic illness.
- *Chronic venous or edematous ulcers of the leg* typically arise above the medial malleolus (the origin of the saphenous vein), but could arise anywhere on the leg or foot dorsum. They are associated with impaired venous return, incompetence of venous perforators, or loss of fascial integrity of the leg (e.g., from trauma) in patients with normal arterial inflow. The cornerstone of treatment is compression.
- *Neuropathic ulcers* are multifactoral but typically follow repetitive trauma to hyposensate distal extremities (e.g., feet), usually on weight-bearing bony prominences (e.g., metatarsal heads). For uncomplicated neuropathic ulcers, the circulation is usually clinically intact. A cornerstone of treatment is mitigating the axial repetitive pressure and shear.
- *Ischemic ulcers* occur on limbs with impaired arterial inflow caused by atherosclerotic disease. Often initiated by minor trauma or shoe pressure on the malleoli, heels, or lateral metatarsal heads, they are typically painful and blanched. Ischemic ulcers are often associated with neuropathy or edema. Healing primarily depends on re-establishing arterial circulation, either medically or surgically.

Epidemiology of Chronic Wounds (p. 646)

• Persons with spinal cord injury (SCI) and associated co-morbidity are at increased risk for the formation of pressure ulcers. The incidence of pressure ulcers in this population ranges from 25% to 66%.
• The incidence of pressure ulcers in acutely hospitalized patients ranges from 2.7% to 29% (prevalence, 3.5% to 69%).
• Patients in critical care units run a higher risk of developing pressure ulcers, as evidenced by 33% incidence and 41% prevalence in this population.
• Pressure ulcers develop or do not develop depending on our ability to handle issues of incontinence, inspection, turning, positioning, range of motion, and nutrition. Variable implementation of these care practices might explain the wide variation in the prevalence of pressure ulcers (e.g., from 2.6% to 24%) in long-term care facilities.

Diabetes Mellitus (p. 646)

• Neuropathy, arteriosclerosis, and microvascular disease combine in diabetes, creating a high risk for chronic wounds of the lower extremities. These foot complications often result in amputation.
• Amputations are 10 times more prevalent among diabetic individuals than in the general population.
• The first major limb amputation for diabetic patients is often followed by a second major amputation, and 28% to 51% have a contralateral amputation within 5 years.

Chronic Venous Disease (p. 646)

• Venous stasis ulcers occur in up to 1% of the population, and it is estimated that 2.5 million Americans suffer from venous ulcers. Only 600,000 per year are treated, however, so it is likely that chronic venous disease is underdiagnosed.
• Intractable ulcers are the most expensive, and 20% to 30% of ulcers present as intractable. Intractable ulcers are those that are present for more than 1 year or those whose area exceeds 10 square centimeters. The cost can approach $10,000 for each of these intractable cases.

WOUND PHYSIOLOGY AND PATHOPHYSIOLOGY
(pp. 646–649)

Definitions (p. 646)

• *Healing:* The Wound Healing Society defines *healing* as complete closing of the integument.
• *Primary intention:* Skin wounds that heal by *primary intention* are similar to incisions that are created by a scalpel blade and then heal rapidly and without complication.
• *Secondary intention:* Secondary intention wounds are large tissue defects that fill by granulation followed by epitheliazation. Wound closure occurs to some extent because of wound contraction.

Process of Normal Healing (p. 647)

• There are four major phases of wound healing: inflammation, provisional matrix formation, repair, and remodeling.
• Normal healing of a wound by primary intention takes 3 to 14 days to complete. The 14-day interval is for deeper, sutured, surgical incisions. The process takes longer for secondary intention wounds.

Pathophysiology of Chronic Wounds (pp. 647–649)

• Chronic wounds appear to be in a chronic inflammatory state synonymous with healing-arrest.
• Five easily identified factors dynamically interact to arrest healing and perpetuate wound status: (1) pathomechanics; (2) reperfusion injury; (3) chronic hypoxia; (4) growth factor derangement, and (5) chronic inflammation.

Pathomechanics (p. 647)

• Pathomechanics implies noxious application of shear (force tangential to the skin surface) and axial pressure (perpendicular to the skin).
• Unrelieved static axial pressure is a critical factor in development of pressure ulcers of the buttocks. Prolonged pressure leads to ulcers if tissue capillary pressure of 32 mm Hg is exceeded. This critical interface pressure is the pressure above which a tissue cannot be loaded for an indefinite period without resulting ulceration. Products aimed at reducing or relieving pressure have tended to use interface pressure as the standard for judging product efficacy.
• *Shear* exacerbates the tendency to ulcerate as a result of axial forces.
• Neuropathic ulcers develop because of both shear and very high transient axial pressure. Repeated noxious pressure causes an inflammatory response with pain, redness, and heat.
• Once ulcers form they are empirically more sensitive to transient or static pressure and shear than is intact skin. Wounds once formed might, in response to pathomechanics, paradoxically get larger.

Reperfusion Injury (p. 648)

• Ischemia from pressure-induced capillary collapse is associated with buildup within the microvasculature of supraoxide free radicals.
• Reperfusion injury can be potentiated by (1) chronic hypoxia, which causes ulceration well below interface pressure and shorter-than-usual ischemic time; and (2) conditions that impair microvessel nitric oxide (NO) production. Such conditions include diabetes, because NO is a potent vasodilator which protects endothelium from reperfusion injury.

Chronic Hypoxia (p. 648)

• Chronic hypoxia results from poor inflow of blood, typically because of arteriosclerotic narrowing proximal to hypoxic skin. If steady-state oxygen is too low, wounds will not heal.

Edema and Impaired Oxygen and Nutrient Exchange (p. 648)

• Edema of the leg is a hallmark of venous stasis disease, and stasis ulceration is the end result of long-standing venous congestion.

• In venous congestion there is breakdown of the ankle pump mechanism.
• Veins can become incompetent because of the presence of old clot or proximal vein occlusion (e.g., from organized deep venous thrombosis, pelvic mass, or fibrosis), which leads to gravity-induced high static pressure and loss of the ankle-pump pressure cycle. The pressure cycle can also be disrupted by traumatic or surgical loss of the fascial envelope, such as from fasciotomies associated with remote compartment syndrome.

Growth Factor Abnormalities (p. 648)
• Growth factor abnormalities can occur in one of four categories: (1) reduced synthesis; (2) increased protein or matrix sequestration; (3) increased breakdown; or (4) insensitivity of target cells.

Chronic Inflammation (pp. 648–649)
• Noxious mechanical stimulation contributes to the clinical persistence of pain, edema, warmth, and redness.
• Inflammation can also result from local infection, which is very common in untreated chronic wounds.
• Wounds that have greater than 10^5 organisms per gram of tissue do not heal.
• Inflammation associated with autoimmunity perpetuates vasculitic ulcers.
• Long-standing skin ulcers are inflamed to a greater or lesser degree by vasculitis, mechanical irritation, or chromic local infection.

Pathophysiological Factors (p. 649)
• The factors that contribute to chronic wound persistence are diverse, interactive, and cumulative, and they affect the whole organism (Table 31–1). These predisposing conditions interact at many levels to promote pathomechanics, reperfusion injury, static hypoxia, and local inflammation; and, speculatively, they may lead to growth factor abnormalities within wounds.

CLINICAL WOUND ASSESSMENT (pp. 649–651)

Wound Area and Volume Assessment (p. 649)

WOUND APPEARANCE
• Color photography dramatically reveals infection, eschar, exudate, complete granulation, and epithelialization.

WOUND OUTLINE
• For lower-extremity ulcers (e.g., ischemic, neuropathic, or venous), a useful, inexpensive technique is drawing outlines on clear plastic with a laundry marker; these drawings then become part of the patient's permanent record. For consistency, one person should do the outlines.

WOUND VOLUME
• For a first approximation of volume, depth and direction of tracks are measured in centimeters and included on the outline.
• For a quantitative measure suitable for careful clinical or research use, volume is assessed by adding a measured amount of saline or moist alginate gel, then removing and measuring the volume of this saline or gel.

TABLE 31–1 Systemic Conditions Associated with Chronic Wounds

Condition	Pathophysiological Effect Related to Wound Healing
Spinal cord injury	Vasomotor instability (>T6 level), insensitivity, denervation atrophy, spasticity, contractures, bowel/bladder alterations
Elderly	Reduced skin elasticity and altered skin microcirculation, co-morbidities, reduced healing rate noted clinically and in animal models
Diabetes	Insensitivity, microangiopathy and altered inflammatory response, foot deformities (intrinsic minus, Charcot), blunted reactive hyperemia, reduced incision breaking strength, and contraction in animal models
Malnutrition	Negative nitrogen balance, cachexia, immunosuppression
Anemia	Local hypoxia
Arteriosclerosis	Local hypoxia
End-stage renal disease	Transient dialysis-related hypoperfusion distal to atherosclerotic plaques, co-morbidities
Steroid medications	Reduced healing rate in animal models, immunosuppression
Transplant recipients	Immunosuppression, co-morbidities
Smoking	Vasoconstriction, increased blood viscosity
Parkinson's disease	Immobility
Osteoporosis	Bony prominences
Upper motor neuron disease	Immobility, contractures, bowel/bladder alterations
Dementia	Immobility, malnutrition, contractures, bowel/bladder alterations
Acutely ill (ICU related)	Hypotension, immobility, bowel/bladder alteration, malnutrition, fever, increased metabolic demands
Noncompliance, abuse and neglect	Multifactoral

Perfusion Assessment (pp. 649–651)

• It is exceedingly rare that large vessel disease contributes to the formation of pressure ulcers of the trunk, occiput, hips, or buttocks. For more distal wounds of the leg and foot, however, perfusion must be assessed because: (1) in the setting of poor perfusion, therapeutic compression might cause pressure necrosis; and (2) perfusion prognosticates wound closure (see also Chapter 56).

MACROCIRCULATION
• Macrocirculation refers to blood flow through named anatomic arteries (e.g., the iliac, femoral, posterior tibial, and plantar).

ANKLE BRACHIAL INDEX AND PULSE VOLUME RECORDING
• Ankle brachial index (ABI) is the ratio of systolic blood pressure of the ankle to that of the arm (brachium). Normal ABI is greater than 0.8.

CONVENTIONAL ANGIOGRAPHY
• Angiography typically involves injecting a radio-opaque dye into the proximal arterial tree. It is typically used before angioplasty or stenting of stenotic arteries.

• Conventional angiography has two important disadvantages: (1) it is less useful for visualizing very distal arteries because dye becomes dilute farther from the site of injection, and it might fail to show distal arteries beyond blockages or stenoses; and (2) nonionic dye-load remains problematic for patients with renal insufficiency, which is not uncommon in the population with significant arteriosclerosis.

MAGNETIC RESONANCE ANGIOGRAPHY (MRA)
• Magnetic resonance angiography (MRA) requires no contrast dye and is superior to conventional angiography in visualizing arteries of the ankle and foot.

MICROCIRCULATION
• Skin microcirculation assessment is being increasingly performed in wound centers, and is recognized as a wound healing benchmark.
• There are three methods to measure skin microcirculation: (1) TcPO2, (2) laser Doppler flow, and (3) vital capillarioscopy.
• Vital capillarioscopy visualizes capillaries.
• Laser Doppler flow measures relative movement of red blood cells through the upper millimeter of living dermis.
• Transcutaneous oxygen is an absolute measure of oxygen tension, and is in essence a "blood gas" of the skin. The normal TcPO2 is greater than 50 mm Hg.
• TcPO2 prognosticates the success of amputation residual limb healing and predicts the healing rate of neuropathic and ischemic ulcers (see Fig. 31–2 in the Textbook).
• The predictive value of TcPO2 is uniquely strong for diabetic individuals, who have distal arterial calcinosis. This makes segmental arterial measurements (i.e., pulse volume recording and ankle brachial index) artefactually high. The surgical literature reports that TcPO2 also prognosticates success of healing incisions of amputation residual limbs. Below the knee, where the disease state is defined as no flow of an artery as assessed by MRA, overlying TcPO2 is 80% sensitive and 83% specific (where TcPO2 measure of "no flow" is set at TcPO2 less than 15 mm Hg).
• TcPO2 is also a measure of integrity of local macrocirculation. As the distalmost capillary bed of the arterial tree, skin microcirculation indirectly assesses flow through upstream arterial feeders. In diabetic patients, upstream feeders are better assessed by TcPO2 than by PVR. Where TcPO2 is normal, healing prognosis is favorable.

Pressure and Shear Assessment (p. 651)

• Although pressure and shear are critical in the pathogenesis of chronic wounds, pressure and shear are not routinely measured in chronic wound practice. Transducers are thick, bulky, rigid, or expensive.

GENERAL PRINCIPLES OF TREATMENT (pp. 651–652)
Debridement (p. 651)

SHARP DEBRIDEMENT
• Sharp debridement is surgical removal of the eschar and any devitalized tissue within it, which is a prerequisite for new tissue growth.
• Surgical debridement is well established as an approach to pressure ulcer care.

• Sharp debridement can be done in the operating room under an anesthetic. Surgical sharp debridement is relatively indiscriminate in the removal of vital and devitalized tissue: Tissue is debrided back to bleeding tissue. To minimize removal of viable tissue, a great deal of clinical skill and judgment is needed. Sharp debridement is contraindicated in those who cannot withstand the loss of blood that can occur during the procedure.

• Less aggressive sharp debridement is commonly performed in the outpatient setting as part of routine wound care, usually with minimal blood loss or pain. Pain is usually not a problem for patients with neuropathic ulcers.

MECHANICAL NONSELECTIVE DEBRIDEMENT

• Mechanical nonselective debridement is accomplished by whirlpool treatments (although, owing to cost, this practice is less popular than in the past); forceful irrigation; or use of wet-to-dry dressings.

• Wet-to-dry dressings involve placing unraveled, moist gauze into the lesion so that all sections of it are touching the dressing, then allowing the dressing to dry. When the dressing is removed, necrotic tissue is removed with it. This is typically done on each shift in the hospital or long-term care setting, or once or twice a day at home. Normal saline solution is commonly used as the wetting agent. Other wetting agents for wet-to-dry dressings include 0.25% acetic acid solution (where pseudomonas is suspected) and dilute povidone-iodine solution or hydrogen peroxide. However, hydrogen peroxide and povidone-iodine are not recommended for long-term use because they are toxic to fibroblasts in vitro.

• Hydrotherapy is typically used for debridement of postsurgical wounds and abscesses in the acute hospital setting. Hydrotherapy performs both irrigation and debridement.

ENZYMATIC DEBRIDEMENT

• Enzymatic debridement uses various chemical agents (e.g., Elase) that act by attacking collagen and liquefying necrotic wound debris without damaging granulation tissue.

• Proteolytic enzymes are used to chemically debride wounds. The action of these enzymes is aimed specifically at necrotic tissue. As a safeguard, enzymatic agents should be removed after 12 to 24 hours.

AUTOLYTIC DEBRIDEMENT

• Proteases and collagenase expressed by wound cells digest eschar in contact with wound fluid. Dressings that maintain a moist wound environment and peri-wound seal (e.g., hydrocolloid) promote autolytic debridement.

Dressings (pp. 651–652)

• In a moist environment, epithelium advances and adjoins without having to digest eschar. The closure rate of wounds is typically twice as fast in a moist environment.

GAUZE DRESSINGS

• Gauze pads and nonadherent gauze (e.g., Telfa) and bulky pads (e.g., ABD pads) might well be considered the foundation of wound care.

• These wound dressings are combined with antibiotic ointments to create a moist environment.

• Antibiotic ointments (e.g., Mupirocin) are especially useful when dressings are changed infrequently, as is the case for venous ulcers under compressive dressings or neuropathic plantar ulcers within casts.
• Bulky pads or antishear pads are especially protective of somewhat transudative wounds in areas subject to excessive friction, such as those over the malleoli or Achilles tendon.

TRANSPARENT ADHESIVE DRESSINGS
• Transparent adhesive dressings (e.g., Tegaderm, OpSite) are semipermeable and occlusive, and are typically indicated for nontransudative stage I or II wounds without necrotic debris.
• Transparent dressings allow gaseous exchange and transfer of water vapor from the skin, and prevent maceration of the healthy skin around the wound. They are not absorptive.
• They reduce the incidence of secondary infection, and they eliminate the risk of traumatic removal.
• They do not work well on diaphoretic patients or in wounds that have significant exudate.

HYDROCOLLOID WAFER DRESSINGS
• Hydrocolloid wafer dressings (e.g., Duoderm) contain hydroactive particles that interact with wound exudate to form a gel.
• These dressings provide absorption of minimal to moderate amounts of exudate and keep the wound surface moist.
• This gel can have fibrolytic properties that enhance wound healing, protect against secondary infection, and insulate the wound from contaminants.
• Hydrocolloid dressings form a seal with peri-wound skin, causing the dressing and skin to move together to minimize shear. This is good for shallow, clean, stage III ulcers in an easily contaminated environment such as the sacrum.
• Hydrocolloid can be applied to clean venous stasis ulcers.

GEL DRESSINGS
• Gel dressings (e.g., NuGel, Vigilon) are available in sheet form; in granules (Intrasite); and as liquid gel (e.g., Curasol).
• All forms of gel dressings, as long as they are not allowed to dehydrate, keep the wound surface moist.
• Some gel dressings provide limited to moderate absorption, some provide insulation, some provide protection against bacterial invasion, and all provide nontraumatic removal.
• Gel dressings provide a moist, nontraumatic environment for clean wounds.
• Some gel dressings are expensive, and gel sheets utilize no adhesive to provide a barrier or prevent shear.

CALCIUM ALGINATE DRESSINGS
• Calcium alginate dressings (e.g., Sorbsan) are semiocclusive, highly absorbent, and easy to use. They are natural, sterile, nonwoven dressings derived from brown seaweed.
• Calcium alginate dressings are extremely effective in treating wet (exudative) wounds and can be used on wounds that are contaminated or infected.
• Dressings need to be frequently changed for very transudative wounds to prevent maceration of fragile epithelium.

DIAGNOSIS AND TREATMENT OF SPECIFIC ULCER TYPES (pp. 652–658)

Pressure Ulcers (pp. 652–654)

Presentation (p. 652)
• Only a patient who can act to relieve a noxious stimulus can prevent pressure ulcers. Patients who are comatose or severely demented, or who are insensate (e.g., spinal cord–injured patients) are at increased risk.
• Spasticity, contractures, incontinence, cachexia, diabetes, and advanced age also increase risk.
• Sites of occurrence vary in different studies and with different diagnoses. The most common sites of pressure ulcer formation are the ischium (28%), the sacrum (17% to 27%), the trochanter (12% to 19%), and the heel (9% to 18%).
• The pressure ulcer staging system is illustrated in Figure 31–1.

Treatment (pp. 652–653)
• The mainstay of pressure ulcer treatment is good medical and nursing care.
• In the long-term care setting or at home, the debilitated or partially dependent patient with a pressure ulcer should be turned every 2 hours and have frequent dressing changes to reduce bacterial count and to keep the wound moist.
• Wound size should be assessed at least weekly, and treatment modified as necessary to maintain healing rate.
• Wounds with necrosis or fibrin must first be debrided (e.g., sharp, mechanical, or enzymatic). Once the wound has been debrided and is granulating, moist dressings (e.g., hydrogel or alginate) are appropriate.
• It is important to seal the wound with surrounding skin. Variable moisture barrier and shear protection is available from hydrocolloid (e.g., Duoderm); or flexible, porous, adhesive gauze (e.g., Coverderm or Medapore).
• In addition to these conservative measures, pressure surface relief is critical.

Pressure Relief (pp. 653–654)
• Table 31–2 describes the selected characteristics as well as the advantages and disadvantages of separate classes of support surfaces.
• Each device can be further described as a pressure-reducing or pressure-relieving device.
• Pressure-relieving devices are those that consistently reduce pressure below capillary closing pressure (32 mm Hg).
• Pressure-reducing devices keep pressures lower than with the standard hospital bed but not consistently below capillary closing pressure.

Uncomplicated Chronic Venous Ulcers (pp. 654–655)

Presentation (p. 654)
• There is usually a history of previous venous ulcer, dependent edema, previous deep venous thrombosis, pelvic surgery or manipulation, vein stripping, vein harvest for coronary artery bypass graft, or leg graft.
• Peripheral pulses are typically intact, although it is sometimes difficult to palpate pulses through edematous skin.

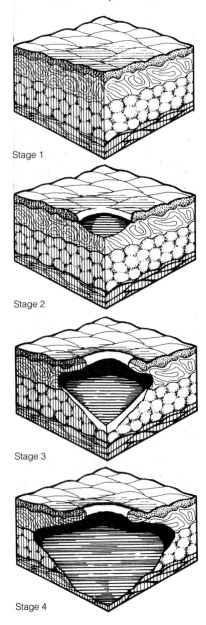

Stage 1

Stage 2

Stage 3

Stage 4

FIGURE 31–1. National Pressure Ulcer Advisory Panel (NPUAP) classification: Identification and staging of pressure ulcers. *Stage 1:* Nonblanchable erythema not resolved in 30 min; epidermis intact; reversible with intervention. *Stage 2:* Partial-thickness loss of skin involving epidermis, possibly into dermis; may appear as blisters with erythema. *Stage 3:* Full-thickness destruction through dermis into subcutaneous tissue. *Stage 4:* Deep tissue destruction through subcutaneous tissue to fascia, muscle, bone, or joint. (Used with permission from the NPUAP.)

TABLE 31–2 Advantages and Disadvantages of Support Surfaces

Surface	Advantages	Disadvantages
Static overlays		
Air	Low maintenance Inexpensive Multipatient use Durable	Can be punctured Requires proper inflation
Gel	Low maintenance Easy to clean Multipatient use Resists puncture	Heavy Expensive Little research
Foam	Lightweight Resists puncture No maintenance	Retains heat Retains moisture Limited life
Water	Readily available in community Easy to clean	Requires heater Transfers are difficult Can leak Heavy Difficult maintenance Procedures difficult
Dynamic overlays	Easy to clean Moisture control Deflates for transfers Reusable pump	Can be damaged by sharp objects Noisy Assembly required Requires power
Replacement mattresses	Reduced staff time Multipatient use Easy to clean Low maintenance	High initial cost May not control moisture Loses effectiveness
Low air loss	Head and foot of bed can be raised Less frequent turning required Pressure relieving Reduces shear and friction Moisture control	Noisy Difficulty with transfers Expensive Requires energy source Restricts mobility Skilled setup required Rental charge
Air-fluidized	Reduces shear and friction Lowest interface pressure Low moisture Less frequent turning required	Expensive Noisy Heavy Dehydration can occur Electrolyte imbalances can occur May cause disorientation Difficulty with transfers Hot

Adapted from Bryant R: Acute and Chronic Wounds: Nursing Management. St Louis, Mosby–Year Book, 1992.

• A well-granulating ulcer with irregular borders positioned about the medial malleolus is typical of saphenous vein dysfunction; however, venous ulcers can be located anywhere on the lower leg, ankle, or edematous foot dorsum.
• Commonly associated with the venous ulcer are lower leg hyperpigmentation and an induration of subcutaneous tissue called lipidermosclerosis. Extensive lipidermosclerosis gives the leg an "inverted wine bottle" appearance (see Fig. 31–5 in the Textbook).
• The differential diagnosis of venous leg ulcers is a long one. If a wound does not respond within 3 months, a biopsy is indicated to rule out malignancy.

Diagnostic Tests (p. 654)
• It is often useful to determine arterial perfusion in anticipation of compression therapy, especially if there is a history of claudication, absent pulses, or other cues of arterial insufficiency.
• Pulse volume recordings are adequate for nondiabetic individuals.
• For diabetic individuals, TcPO2 is determined on nonedematous areas such as the upper leg, foot dorsum, and plantar arch.
• Venous Doppler is useful to rule out acute venous thrombosis.

Treatment (pp. 654–655)
• Compression therapy is the mainstay of treatment for venous or lower extremity edematous ulcers.
• Nonelastic compression, classically the Unna Paste Boot, has been used effectively for more than 100 years to treat venous ulcers. Ambulators obtain the best edema reduction. Unna's boots are wrapped from toe to knee and are commonly left intact for a week or longer, once it is clear that there is no local infection.
• Elastic compression supplies compression of 30 to 40 mm Hg continuously, depending on the elastic compression brand. Brands include Coban (3 M) or Cetapress (Convatec). A middle gauze layer (e.g., Kling) can be wrapped from toe to knee for comfort and to reduce shear. Over-the-counter elastic wraps tend not to supply the adequate compression needed to heal venous ulcers.
• If infection is suspected and is being treated, compression therapy can be used with frequent dressing changes and debridements.
• Most venous ulcers (70% to 80%) close with compression and good wound care.
• Wounds that do not close typically have these characteristics in common: ulcer size greater than 10 cm^2, wound present more than 12 months, and ABI less than 0.8. These hard-to-heal ulcers may need additional measures, depending on the decision of the patient and wound care team. Split-thickness skin grafts have been employed to close intractable venous ulcers.
• Apligraft is FDA-approved as a laboratory-prepared dermal-epidermal construct. This construct is prepared with neonatal human dermal fibroblasts that are cultured in media with bovine type I collagen. Neonatal cells are nonimmunogenic, so tissue sloughing does not occur as would occur with an allograft. Apligraft can increase complete healing of intractable venous ulcers from 25% to 50%. A disadvantage is cost; currently, a 9-cm^2 piece costs $1000. Apligraft should be reserved for venous ulcers that remain open after 24 weeks of conventional treatment.

Compression Stockings (p. 655)
• Once venous ulcers heal, the patient remains at risk for recurrence because the underlying venous or fascial anatomic defect remains.

• Compression must be a lifelong habit. Compression garments, when used as directed, prevent most ulceration recurrences.

• Compression garments come in many sizes, colors, and pressures. Most have the appearance of stiff stockings (e.g., Jobst). Some are segmental and are applied with Velcro straps (e.g., Circ-aide).

• Most patients do well with 20 to 30 mm Hg, whereas some will need 30 to 40 mm Hg garments. Most garments are off-the-shelf and only a few very obese patients, or those with unusual-shaped legs (post-trauma), require custom stockings. Several pairs of stockings should be purchased to allow washing, and stockings should be replaced at 6-month intervals.

Uncomplicated Neuropathic Ulcers (pp. 655–657)

Presentation (p. 655)

• Neuropathic or "insensate" foot ulcers are most often (in the United States) related to diabetes; however, they also occur in the setting of infection (e.g., leprosy), as well as traumatic and congenital sensory neuropathy.

• Neuropathic ulcers commonly affect plantar toes, hallux, or metatarsal heads.

• Neurotrophic osteoarthropathy, or Charcot foot, commonly causes midfoot collapse and plantargrade subluxation of navicular or cuboid, leading to especially problematic neuropathic midfoot ulcers.

• The physical exam of an uncomplicated ulcer typically shows peripheral pulses to be intact, but sensation is diminished or absent in the vicinity of the ulcer as measured by the Simmes 5.07 or 6.10 monofilaments.

• Ulcers most commonly are located on bony prominences of the plantar metatarsals, midfoot, or heel.

• Ulcers might also be associated with digital abnormalities such as claw toes or hallux rigidus.

• Ulcers usually have regular borders and copious surrounding callus (Fig. 31–2).

Diagnostic Tests (p. 656)

• TcPO2 should be used to assess perfusion. Transcutaneous oxygen has value to reveal local macrocirculation.

• TcPO2 should not be assessed over bony prominences or metatarsal heads, but rather at the instep or plantar arch.

Treatment Strategies (p. 656)

• Treatment strategies usually involve "off-weighting" the ulcer, which reduces mechanical irritation, inflammation, and edema; and promotes healing.

• Limited weight bearing must be implemented after a complete physiatric assessment that incorporates inspection, range of motion, muscle testing, and sensory testing. This assessment should also encourage decision making concerning orthoses, assistive devices, weight relief shoes, physical therapy, and facilitate periodic patient education by nursing staff at the clinic and/or in the home.

• Local care of neuropathic ulcers follows general "good wound care" principles. The moist wound environment can be maintained by antibiotic ointments such as Bactroban or Bacitracin. These antibiotic ointments also reduce the bacterial count around an area that is easily contaminated.

• Debridement is also regularly employed. Callus is removed by "saucerization." In this procedure, the rim of the callus is debrided in the manner of an

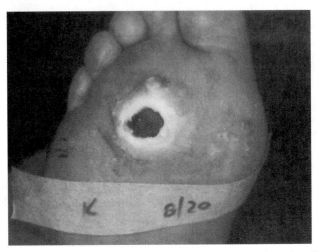

FIGURE 31–2. A neuropathic ulcer in a 56-year-old male with insulin-dependent diabetes and forefoot insensitivity. (His circulation is normal.)

inverted cone, using a scalpel and forceps. Debridements should be done weekly because neuropathic ulcers readily form callus even with very little weight bearing, and a callus paradoxically increases mechanical tension in the wound.
• Regranex, a formulation of rh-PDGF-BB (recombinant platelet-derived growth factor, BB isoform), has been approved by the FDA for healing of non-hypoxic foot ulcers of neuropathic and diabetic etiology.
• Strict non–weight bearing is the cornerstone of treating neuropathic ulcers.
• Sometimes, bevels or reliefs are set in shoe insoles to "off-weight" an area of high pressure and neuropathic ulcer. Although axial pressure may be reduced in the immediate vicinity of the ulcer, shear might be increased. For this reason, "healing shoes" are not recommended.
• Canvas cast boots have specific off-weighted regions that are useful in some situations. Darco forefoot relief shoes are low, with the ulcer set against a raised insole. IPOS heel relief shoes are canvas boots with openings for the commonly ulcerated lateral heel. Heel pain on ambulation can be markedly reduced, and this shoe also helps resolve ulceration in many cases.
• The IPOS forefoot relief shoe has a raised heel with the forefoot "hanging in space." Although it is not clear if shear is eliminated, axial pressure is clearly reduced. After a while, however, the elevation may lead to tendinitis, muscle sprain, or a worsening of pre-existing arthritis.
• Another boot available is the DH walker. By reducing both shear and axial pressure, the DH walker has empirically yielded good results, especially for heel ulcers in some patients who were otherwise without options. However, the DH walker boot significantly reduces step length and gait velocity, and finds limited acceptance.
• A very effective treatment for recalcitrant neuropathic ulcers with good circulation is total contact casting. Pressure is distributed axially by virtue of the custom-contour of the set plaster. There is no shear because there is no space inside the cast in which to move. The disadvantage of the cast is that it is time

and labor intensive. It is best reserved until other, simpler methods are used and the wound plateaus (i.e., healing rate drops to zero). The total contact cast is contraindicated where TcPO2 is less than 35 mm Hg or ABI is less than 0.45 in the affected leg.

Recurrence Prevention (pp. 656–657)
• Neuropathic ulcers often recur in the absence of careful and persistent follow-up.
• Every effort should be made to optimize the shoe prescription.
• After healing, it is often best to let the former wound "mature" (i.e., develop a stronger dermal layer and a thicker epidermal layer). During this maturation process, callus buildup should be kept to a minimum by careful debridements.
• During the period of skin maturation, a shoe prescription can be filled by a certified pedorthist.[1] A pedorthist has been specifically trained and certified in specialty shoes, and is well versed in insole and outsole modifications.
• A typical accommodative shoe prescription is for "orthopedic oxford shoes with high toe box and removable PPT-plastizote insoles." Each element is important. The diabetic foot has claw toes that require space. A two-layer insole allows some "bottoming out," but PPT is a foam without memory, so some resiliency is always maintained.
• If the former wound is at a metatarsal head, the best deweighting strategy is to apply a lift just behind (proximal) to the bony prominence with a cork metatarsal bar. The outsole rocker bottom is modified or rigid, with apex set just behind the metatarsal heads. (Rocker bottoms reduce pressure at the metatarsal heads.) Insoles tend to "bottom out" and should be replaced at 3-month intervals.
• Patient education involves daily inspection of the feet and legs to make sure there are no echymoses or excessive callus, which are harbingers of re-ulceration. Emollients such as lanolin or lac-hydrin help prevent the drying and cracking of skin, especially between toes, that can provide portals for entry of infection.

Ischemic Ulcers (pp. 657–658)
• Ischemic leg ulcers seen in outpatient practice most often occur as mixed disease: neuropathic/ischemic or venous/ischemic.
• Simple ischemic ulcers related to proximal occlusion in patients without co-morbidities should be evaluated for angioplasty or bypass surgery.

Presentation (p. 657)
• Patients may or may not have a history of claudication, because those with diabetes might have peripheral neuropathy and be relatively insensate. Because of their multiple co-morbidities, patients with ischemic ulcers are most often low-level ambulators, who for this reason do not claudicate.
• Ulcers typically occur at areas of trauma or static or transient repeated pressure.
• Static pressure necrosis is most common at the lateral outer heels, which commonly press against the hospital mattress.

1. Contact Pedorthic Footwear Association, 9861 Broken Land Parkway, Suite 255, Columbia, MD, 21046

• A minor or major amputation incision site might not heal and then undergo ischemic change. Ischemic pressure ulcers can also occur at the lateral malleolus.
• Excessively tight shoes can create pressure necrosis at the lateral fifth toe, medial hallux, or medial forefoot at the metatarsal prominence.
• The distal plantar transmetatarsal residuum is a common site for ischemic ulceration, perhaps created and worsened by transient repeated pressure.
• Ischemic ulcers tend to be exceedingly painful for patients without neuropathy, and pain is worsened by leg elevation. Some patients with painful ischemic ulcers are able to sleep only in the sitting position.
• The ischemic ulcer commonly (but not always) has a blanched base, has a "punched out" appearance, is painful to probe, and the area surrounding the ulcer might have a bright or dusky red hue that has been termed ischemic livido.
• The color can be purple or black, signaling the onset of gangrene. The onset of gangrene or cellulitis requires immediate surgical referral.

Assessment (p. 656)
• Vascular studies are critical to establish a prognosis for conservative healing.
• Healing is not likely in the case of a diabetic patient with TcPO2 less than 15 mm Hg.
• Healing requires getting more oxygen to the wound. Because there are nonsurgical protocols for limb rescue that involve inframalleolar perfusion enhancement, MRA of the ankle and foot might be warranted to delineate arteriosclerosis at the ankle and below.

Treatment (pp. 657–658)
• If the wound is truly ischemic, a vascular surgical referral is standard.
• If the surgical consultant concludes that bypass or angioplasty is not indicated, noninvasive methods should be used to save the limb.
• Conservative "good wound care" must be maximized, including liberal use of padding and weight relief strategies such as the DH walker (see the case study described in Fig. 31–8 in the Textbook).
• Other than conventional "good wound care" for limb salvage, few nonsurgical methods have been independently validated.
• Hyperbaric oxygen is not often employed for ischemic ulcers. Hyperbaric oxygen is itself a vasoconstrictor, so it is commonly avoided when there is very distal arteriosclerosis because it could reduce the perfusion of a compromised region.

INFECTION, SURGICAL REPAIR, AND THE TRANSITION FROM OUTPATIENT TO ACUTE INPATIENT MANAGEMENT (pp. 658–660)

Presentation (p. 658)

• All infected ulcer types have a similar presentation: a foul smell, greenish or copious drainage, scant granulation, and dull whitish base (rather than bright red granulation tissue).
• Infected ischemic wounds can present with acute onset of gangrene or eschar of a digit, or cellulitis.

- Cellulitis is an invasion of organisms beyond 1 to 2 cm of the ulcer margin, and is marked by erythema, warmth, swelling, or tenderness.
- Systemic bacteremia often produces symptoms of fever, chills, sweats, nausea, vomiting, or loss of appetite. Signs of bacteremia also include elevated or depressed temperature, elevated white count, change in mental status, or glucose intolerance in patients with diabetes.
- The presence of cellulitis, necrotizing cellulitis, painful fluctuance, or signs of bacteremia are considered limb or life threatening, necessitating an acute hospital admission for intravenous antibiotics and consideration of surgical debridement.

Soft Tissue Infections: Wound Culture, Microbiology, and Antibiotic Therapy (p. 659)

- Because the surfaces of all ulcers are colonized by bacteria, ulcer cultures should not be routinely performed, even for locally infected wounds.
- Cultures can be performed, however, if antiseptic preparation (e.g., Betadine application) precedes local debridement, which exposes a sequestered abscess or fluid collection (which is immediately cultured).
- Surgical debridement under sterile conditions provides the opportunity to aspirate or swab deep tissue from previously unexposed regions, and more reliably isolates causative organisms.
- Clinical infection is almost always polymicrobial, including strict anaerobes and facultative aerobes. Aerobic organisms are usually found in surface swabs, whereas anaerobes are more often isolated from deep tissue or in larger pressure ulcers. Deep tissue isolates reveal *Proteus mirabilis,* group B or D *streptococci, Escherichia coli, Staphylococcus aureus, Pseudomonas aeruginosa, Peptostreptococcus species, Clostridia,* and *Bacteroides fragilis. B. fragilis* is often found in blood cultures associated with clinical sepsis.
- Locally infected wounds are commonly associated with eschar. Eschar should be debrided mechanically, if possible, using acetic acid, Dakin's solution, or dilute Betadine wet-to-dry. If the patient cannot tolerate wet-to-dry dressings, or if wet-to-dry is not feasible from a nursing standpoint, an antibiotic ointment that permeates eschar, such as Silvidine, can be employed.
- Outpatient infections can also be treated with broad-spectrum oral antibiotics that cover gram positives, gram negatives, and anaerobes. Choices for aerobes include cephalexin (Keflex), sulfamethoxazoletrimethoprim (Bactrim), and quinilone (e.g., Ciprofloxicin or Levofloxicin). For anaerobes, choices include metronidazole (Flagyl) and clindamycin (Cleocin). Clindamycin also covers some gram positives and can be used in simple infections as a single agent. Another choice as a single agent is amoxicillin trihydrate-clavulanate potassium (Augmentin). Intravenous antibiotics for inpatient infections are typically best determined in conjunction with infectious disease or internal medicine consultants.

Osteomyelitis (pp. 659–660)

- Osteomyelitis requires a high index of suspicion on initial presentation of ulcers of any etiology. This is especially true if the ulcer occurs over a bony prominence; or is a pressure ulcer stage IV, whether or not tracts to bone are clinically apparent.

• Osteomyelitis is most easily diagnosed in the outpatient setting by imaging studies.

Imaging Studies (p. 659)
• Plain films are positive for osteomyelitis if they show reactive bone formation and periosteal elevation. Plain films are the least expensive imaging study, but have a sensitivity of 78% and specificity of just 50%.
• A combination of the leukocyte count, erythrocyte sedimentation rate, and plain films provided a sensitivity of 89% and specificity of 88%. If all three test results are positive, the positive predictive value of this combination is 69%. If all are negative, the negative predictive value is 96%. The combination is less helpful if only one or two tests are positive.
• Conventional three-phase bone scan is more sensitive for osteomyelitis than plain films, but specificity is still just 50%. Specificity is low because bone scans are poor at differentiating osteomyelitis from soft tissue infection contiguous with bone. Indium leukocyte scanning has been reported to overcome this deficiency, with a sensitivity of 89%. When combined with a three-phase bone scan, the sensitivity of indium white blood cell scanning is 100% and the specificity is 81%. Radionuclide tests, either singly or in combination, have the drawback of not revealing anatomic detail.
• Magnetic resonance imaging (MRI) reveals anatomic detail and is now recognized as an effective tool for diagnosis of osteomyelitis. MRI is extremely sensitive to the presence of marrow edema on the T2-weighted image. An analysis of eleven studies investigating the diagnosis of osteomyelitis by MRI showed a sensitivity of 95% and a specificity of 88%. MRI also offers the advantage of spatial resolution. MRI can highlight sinus tracts to bone abscesses of the long flexor tendons, septic arthritis, periurethral or perirectal fistula, and other soft tissue abnormalities with a single test (see Fig. 31–9 in the Textbook).

Outpatient Treatment of Osteomyelitis (pp. 659–660)
• The advent of home infusion therapy has enabled patients with osteomyelitis to acquire "good wound care" at home. This must be preceded by wound and bone culture, and appropriate antibiotic selection.
• For "aggressive," conservative treatment of osteomyelitis, antibiotics are typically administered to diabetic patients up to 16 weeks, twice as long as for conventional osteomyelitis treatment.
• For recurrent osteomyelitis or an initial presentation of osteomyelitis in an immunosuppressed patient (e.g., a transplant recipient), hyperbaric oxygen therapy is considered in parallel with home antibiotic infusion. An oxygen-rich environment in bone is synergistic with antibiotics, and combining conservative therapies maximizes the opportunity for limb salvage.

Surgical Management (p. 660)

• Surgical repair achieves rapid closure and improves vascularity to promote deep soft tissue healing.
• The health of the entire patient must be considered by the team and the patient. If the surgery is likely to result in prolonged bed rest, this too must be considered. If the pressure defect that led to ulcer in the first place is not corrected, the

ulcer is likely to recur postoperatively. Operative procedures often result in blood loss and prolonged exposure to general anesthesia, which is a relative contraindication for patients with coronary artery disease, ischemic cardiomyopathy, end-stage renal disease, or other high-risk co-morbidities.

Soft Tissue Reconstruction (p. 660)
• Direct closure is the simplest procedure, but there is likely to be excessive tension on the incision and a paucity of soft tissue coverage.
• Direct closure has been advocated for intractable venous ulcers unlikely to generate growth factors.
• Tissue expanders have recently been used to provide more skin surface in selected cases.
• Split-thickness skin grafts can also be used to repair recalcitrant venous ulcers.
• Musculocutaneous flaps are usually the best choice for pressure ulcers of the buttocks in spinal cord–injured patients, or when the concomitant loss of muscle function does not contribute to co-morbidity.
• For ambulatory patients, the choice is less clear because the improved blood supply and reliability of the muscle flap must be balanced against the need to sacrifice functional muscle units.
• Musculocutaneous flaps can help heal osteomyelitis and limit the damage caused by shearing, friction, and pressure.
• Musculocutaneous flaps have a significant recurrence rate in ulceration, with short-term failure rate (most commonly because of suture line dehiscence) from 5% to 36%. The long-term recurrence rate can be as high as 61%.

Orthopedic Surgical Management (p. 660)
• If optimal conservative management has failed to close an otherwise well-vascularized neuropathic ulcer, or if the ulcer heals and then recurs, the orthopedic surgeon should be consulted to evaluate surgical approaches to pressure relief. These include consideration of osteotomies and tendon recessions.

Vascular Surgical Management (p. 660)
• The ischemic ulcers that should be treated surgically are more associated with rest pain and have proximal arterial occlusion with limited collaterals. The potential for bypass surgery or angioplasty should be assessed.

Outpatient Wound Clinic Principles and Logistics
(pp. 660–661)
• Close periodic follow-up of individual patients is a necessity.
• Patients with open wounds typically have co-morbidities that tend to result in limb- or life-threatening infections without close (at least weekly) follow-up. Follow-up by "visiting nurses" is consistent with this principle.
• The clinic often coordinates home care for complex patients needing durable medical equipment and/or having psychosocial issues.
• Teams are made up of visiting nurses, home physical and occupational therapists, vendors, and case managers.
• Other professionals consulted by the wound clinic on- or off-site include nutrition specialists and weight loss and smoking cessation counselors.

• The certified pedorthist has been trained in methods to mitigate noxious foot pressure for patients with previous neuropathic ulcers.

PREVENTION (p. 661)

• Education, inspection, and continued pressure and shear optimization are the keys to preventing the first or recurrent ulcerations.
• In the long-term care setting, assessment by the Braden or Norton index, pressure support selection, and continued good nursing care are critical.
• For chronic venous or edematous ulcers, compression stockings should be used indefinitely.
• All diabetic patients should be screened with the Simmes 5.07 monofilament. Insensitivity to this puts the patient at increased risk for skin breakdown, and orthopedic oxford shoes with high toe box and removable two-layer insoles should be prescribed.
• Skin and nail care must be lifelong for patients at risk for buttock or leg ulcers.
• Emollients (e.g., lanolin, lac-hydrin) prevent cracking of the skin and consequent entry of bacteria.
• In more severe cases, inspection and care of skin and nails is also performed by professionals on routine follow-up. (For additional information, see Chapter 56.)

CONCLUSION (p. 661)

• Prevention and early, aggressive intervention are the cornerstones of outpatient and skilled-care chronic-wound management.

Acknowledgments. Our thanks to the following: NIH K08HD01065-01, NIH HD07425, University of Pennsylvania Research Foundation, and Hartford Foundation 91009-G.

32

Original Chapter by Jonathan R. Moldover, M.D.,
and Matthew N. Bartels, M.D., M.P.H.

Cardiac Rehabilitation

• The two primary goals of any cardiac rehabilitation program are to:
1. Increase the functional capacity of the patient.
2. Change the natural history of the disease in order to reduce morbidity and mortality.

TYPES OF HEART DISEASE (p. 665)

• Physiatrists practicing cardiac rehabilitation encounter a variety of heart disease including post-MI, post-CABG, post-transplant, post-valve replacement surgery, chronic CHF, and life-threatening arrhythmias.

EXERCISE PHYSIOLOGY (pp. 666–668)

AEROBIC CAPACITY

• *Aerobic capacity* is a physiological term used to measure the work capacity of an individual. It is represented by the maximum oxygen consumption ($\dot{V}O_{2max}$), expressed in milliliters of oxygen consumed per kilogram of body weight per minute. The total $\dot{V}O_2$ provides a measure of the increasing metabolic work of the peripheral skeletal muscles, not of the heart itself.
• The $\dot{V}O_2$ is useful as a measure of the physical work being performed.

CARDIAC OUTPUT

• Cardiac output (CO) increases with increasing work.
• In early exercise, CO increases due to augmented stroke volume via the Frank-Starling mechanism.
• In late exercise, CO is increased primarily through an increase in ventricular rate.
• The maximum CO is the primary determinant of the $\dot{V}O_{2max}$.
• The CO has two determinants: the heart rate and the stroke volume (SV).

HEART RATE

• Heart rate (HR) increases in linearly when plotted against the $\dot{V}O_2$ or other measures of physical work (see Fig. 32–2 in the Textbook). HR is limited by a person's age.

• A person's maximum HR can be estimated by subtracting the age in years from 220.

STROKE VOLUME
• Stroke volume represents the quantity of blood pumped with each heartbeat. It increases in a curvilinear fashion (during exercise done in an upright position) until it reaches a plateau at about 40% of the $\dot{V}o_{2max}$ (see Fig. 32–4 in the Textbook). A major determinant of SV is the diastolic filling volume, which is inversely related to the HR.

MYOCARDIAL OXYGEN CONSUMPTION
• The myocardial oxygen consumption ($M\dot{V}o_2$) is the actual oxygen consumption of the heart. The $\dot{V}o_2$ represents the oxygen consumption of the whole body.
• The *anginal threshold* is defined as the point where the myocardial oxygen demand exceeds the ability of the coronary circulation to meet that demand. At the anginal threshold the patient can experience typical anginal chest pain, ischemic changes on the electrocardiogram (ECG), or arrhythmias.
• It has been shown that the HR and systolic blood pressure (BP) correlate well with the actual $M\dot{V}o_2$ and can be used as a clinical guide. The usual measure is the rate pressure product (RPP), which is calculated by multiplying the HR by the systolic BP and dividing the product by 100.
• The linear relationship between the $M\dot{V}o_2$ and the $\dot{V}o_2$ suggests that the relative cardiac stress of various activities can be compared by measuring the $\dot{V}o_2$ produced by the activities.
• Activities performed with the upper extremities as opposed to the lower extremities generate a higher $M\dot{V}o_2$ at the same $\dot{V}o_2$.
• Activities performed supine as opposed to upright generate a higher $M\dot{V}o_2$ at low intensities and a lower $M\dot{V}o_2$ at higher intensities.
• Activities performed under emotional stress, after smoking a cigarette, after eating, or in cold weather all generate a higher $M\dot{V}o_2$ at the same $\dot{V}o_2$ than do activities performed at baseline.
• Activities that have an isometric component generate a higher $M\dot{V}o_2$ than a similar activity at the same $\dot{V}o_2$ without the isometric component (e.g., ambulating while gripping a cane or carrying a briefcase compared with ambulation without anything in the hands).

AEROBIC TRAINING (pp. 668–670)

Principles (p. 668)

INTENSITY
• The *intensity* of aerobic exercise can be defined either in terms of the individual's physiological response (HR or RPP) or in terms of exercise intensity (speed or resistance setting).
• The usual target HR is approximately 85% of the maximum HR achieved during a pretraining exercise tolerance test (ETT). If the individual is very frail or deconditioned, or if the limiting factor on the ETT was a dangerous arrhythmia, an intensity as low as 60% of maximum can be prescribed and a training effect can still be expected.

DURATION
• The duration of each exercise session in the typical aerobic training program is 20 to 30 minutes.

FREQUENCY
• Aerobic training schedules usually involve exercise 3 days a week. Programs involving exercise at lower intensities should be performed at least 5 days a week.

SPECIFICITY
• A key concept in all exercise training is that of specificity of training (see Chapter 19).
• The changes in the cardiac response to exercise apply only to exercise with muscles that have been involved in the training program.

Effects (pp. 668–669)

AEROBIC CAPACITY
• The defining characteristic of a successful aerobic training program is an increase in the aerobic capacity ($\dot{V}O_{2max}$).

CARDIAC OUTPUT
• The maximum CO increases with aerobic training. As with the $\dot{V}O_2$, whereas the CO at maximum exercise increases, the resting and the submaximum CO remain the same.

STROKE VOLUME
• The SV is higher at rest, submaximum work, and maximum work after aerobic training (see Fig. 32–10 in the Textbook). This increase in SV is mostly caused by a combination of increased blood volume and prolonged diastolic filling time.

HEART RATE
• The HR following aerobic training is lower at rest and at any given submaximum workload but remains unchanged at maximum work (see Fig. 32–11 in the Textbook).

MYOCARDIAL OXYGEN CONSUMPTION
• With aerobic training, there is a decrease in the $M\dot{V}O_2$ at rest and at any submaximum workload, but there is no change in the maximum $M\dot{V}O_2$. (see Fig. 32–12 in the Textbook) Pharmacological interventions also have an effect on resting and submaximum, but not maximum $M\dot{V}O_2$
• The maximum level is still determined by the anginal threshold, which is not affected by aerobic conditioning.
• Currently only angioplasty or bypass surgery can raise or eliminate the anginal threshold.

Benefits (pp. 669–670)

• Even though aerobic training does not change the anginal threshold, the change in the cardiac response to exercise is extremely beneficial. The workload that can be tolerated before the anginal threshold is reached increases significantly.
• In addition to the reduced relative stress of specific activities provided by the increased physical work capacity, there is a growing body of evidence that aerobic training has a beneficial effect on the natural history of CAD that can be isolated from other lifestyle alterations.

ASSESSMENT OF CARDIAC FUNCTION (pp. 670–672)

History and Physical Examination (pp. 670–672)

History (pp. 670–671)

• Key issues to address in the history of a patient with cardiac disease are presented in Table 32–1.

TABLE 32–1 Key Issues to Address in the History of a Patient with Cardiac Disease

Key Elements of the History

Family History
Premature CAD (before age 55 yr in first-degree relative)
Family history of familial hypercholesterolemia or hyperlipidemia
Family history of sudden death
Family history of arrhythmias
Family history of Marfan disease
Family history of hypertrophic cardiomyopathy

Social History
Cigarette use, cigar/pipe use
Sedentary lifestyle
Alcohol abuse history

Symptom History
Chest pain: duration, location, character, precipitating and relieving factors, pain radiation
Shortness of breath: duration, precipitating and relieving factors, day or night, position
Dizziness/lightheadedness
Syncope
Presence of nausea/vomiting, anorexia
Cyanosis/pallor
Palpitations
Edema
Cough
Hemoptysis
Fatigue

Functional History
Level of activity prior to cardiac event
Present level of activity
Exercise tolerance level
Level of activity required at home and at work
Level of function, stable or progressively worse
Extent and rate of activities performed

Patient Goals
Vocational plans
Leisure activities
Emotional adaptation to the cardiac condition

Medications
Complete Review of Systems and Past Medical History

• The symptoms discussed in the following require consideration when designing an exercise program.

DYSPNEA
• Shortness of breath (SOB) or dyspnea is often the central symptom in cardiac disease. A complete description of dyspnea should be obtained to help differentiate cardiac and noncardiac causes of dyspnea.
• Among the common causes of exertional dyspnea are congestive heart failure, ischemic cardiac disease, chronic pulmonary disease, and deconditioning.

CHEST PAIN
• Chest pain, tightness, and burning are the classic symptoms of ischemic heart disease.
• Other causes include valvular heart disease, arrhythmia, pleural irritation, chest wall pathology, and musculoskeletal pain.
• Table 32–2 lists symptoms differentiating cardiac versus noncardiac chest pain.

TABLE 32–2 Cardiac vs. Noncardiac Chest Pain by Symptoms

Cardiac Pain Symptoms	Noncardiac Pain Symptoms
Pain Quality	
Constricting/squeezing	Dull aching
Visceral quality	Sharp, stabbing, piercing, knife-like
Burning	Muscular
Heaviness	
Pain Location	
Substernal	Left submammary area, apex of heart
Across precordium	Superficial tissues of the left chest
Neck	Right lower chest
One or both shoulders, arms	Very discrete localization possible
Intrascapular region	
One or both forearms, hands	
Epigastrium	
Pain Duration	
Angina, 2–10 min	Infarction, >20 min to 24 hr
<20 sec	Persistent without change for >24–48 hr
Precipitating and Aggravating Factors	
Exercise, particularly with hurrying	After completion of exercise
Excitement	With specific body positions, chest wall movement, and respiration
Cold temperature exposure	With direct palpation of chest wall
Stressful stimuli	Spontaneous
Postprandially, after heavy meal	Head and neck movement
	During fasting, with cold liquids
Relieving Factors	
Rest	Antacids
Nitroglycerin	Food
	Nonsteroidal analgesia

PALPITATION
• Palpitation is the subjective sensation of an irregular or forceful heartbeat. It is often benign, but can be indicative of serious tachyarrhythmias.

SYNCOPE
• Cardiac syncope is usually abrupt in onset, occurring with little or no warning. Causes of cardiac syncope include aortic stenosis, idiopathic hypertrophic subaortic stenosis (IHSS), primary pulmonary hypertension, ventricular arrhythmias, reentrant arrhythmias, high-degree atrioventricular (AV) block, or sick sinus syndrome.
• Postural syncope can be caused by autonomic dysfunction, neurological disease, vagal stimuli, or psychological stimuli.

EDEMA
• Peripheral edema can be an indication of CHF, postural edema, liver disease, renal disease, or lymphatic obstruction. Edema often impairs the satisfactory use of braces or prostheses.

FATIGUE
• Depression, medications, physical exhaustion, and deconditioning are common noncardiac causes of fatigue.
• Cardiac fatigue, usually seen in severe heart failure, is typically relieved with rest and occasionally presents as a form of atypical angina.

COUGH
• Most causes of cough are related to pulmonary or upper airway irritation. Cardiac cough is often initiated by assuming a recumbent position and relieved by resuming an upright position. Typically, a cardiac cough is nocturnal and episodic, with little or no sputum production.

LIMITATIONS OF THE HISTORY
• The design of a cardiac rehabilitation program cannot be assessed by history alone in patients with known CAD. Cardiac stress testing and other techniques to permit cardiac risk assessment should also be done.
• Table 32–3 lists historical features that can help indicate the overall prognosis.

Physical Examination (p. 671)
• The details of the cardiac examination are described in basic physical examination textbooks. There are specific findings that physiatrists should be aware of in individuals with multiple disabilities.

TABLE 32–3 Historical Data That Indicate Increased Cardiac Risk

Postinfarction angina	History of hypertension, or loss of hypertension
Symptomatic congestive heart failure	Palpitation
Age >70 yr	Syncope
Severe exercise limitation	Fatigue
Diabetes	

EXERCISE TOLERANCE TESTING (pp. 672–679)

• Exercise tolerance testing (ETT) is essential in the exercise design of any cardiac rehabilitation program. It is used to create an individualized exercise prescription, allowing an optimal level of training stimulus without exposing the patient to undue risk.

Electrocardiographic Exercise (pp. 672–678)

Tolerance Testing (pp. 672–675)

• Although more modern tests have taken over the diagnostic role for cardiac ischemia, the exercise stress test is still the most commonly used evaluation technique for determining cardiac risk stratification and functional capacity.

• The contraindications to exercise stress testing are summarized in Table 32–4.

EXERCISE PROTOCOLS

• Exercise protocols are normally designed with 3- to 5-minute stages in order to achieve a steady-state response. The exercise protocol needs to be tailored to the individual patient and should allow testing of patients with very limited cardiac reserve, as well as patients with excellent aerobic conditioning.

TABLE 32–4 Contraindications to Exercise Tolerance Testing

Absolute Cardiac Contraindications to Exercise Testing

1. Unstable angina with recent chest pain
2. Untreated life-threatening cardiac arrhythmias
3. Uncompensated congestive heart failure
4. Advanced atrioventricular block
5. Acute myocarditis or pericarditis
6. Critical aortic stenosis
7. Severe hypertrophic obstructive cardiomyopathy
8. Uncontrolled hypertension
9. Acute myocardial infarction
10. Active endocarditis

Absolute Noncardiac Contraindications to Exercise Testing

1. Acute pulmonary embolus or pulmonary infarction
2. Acute systemic illness

Relative Contraindications

1. Significant pulmonary hypertension
2. Significant arterial hypertension
3. Tachyarrhythmias or bradyarrhythmias
4. Moderate valvular heart disease
5. Myocardial heart disease
6. Electrolyte abnormalities
7. Left main coronary obstruction
8. Hypertrophic cardiomyopathy
9. Psychiatric disease

TREADMILL PROTOCOLS

• The most commonly used treadmill protocol is the Bruce protocol (see Table 32–6 in the Textbook). The Naughton, Weber, and Balke-Ware protocols are sometimes better tolerated by patients with CHF, deconditioning, or other causes of limited exercise tolerance.
• See Table 32–7 in the Textbook for a comparison of the various protocols.

BICYCLE ERGOMETRY AND UPPER EXTREMITY ERGOMETRY

• The most common alternative to treadmill protocols is bicycle ergometry.
• The advantages include better ECG and blood pressure recording, chiefly because the patient's chest and arms remain relatively stable. Bicycle ergometry can also be performed with the patient lying supine.
• Upper extremity ergometry can be used for patients who have orthopedic, vascular, or neurological disabilities and cannot perform the standard treadmill or bicycle test. Typical subjects for this type of testing include patients with amputation, spinal cord injury, arthritis, and recent orthopedic procedures.
• In all forms of exercise testing, it is important that the patient not hold the handrail or handlebars, because an exaggerated cardiac response is caused by the isometric handgrip. This can cause an overestimation in the functional capacity.

PREPARATION FOR STRESS TESTING

• Patients should not eat or have caffeinated beverages for at least 3 hours before a stress test. They should wear comfortable, loose-fitting clothes and comfortable walking shoes.
• The patient is taught how to ambulate on the treadmill or use the ergometer.
• Vital signs and ECGs are taken before the test, at each stage of the test, at the conclusion of the exercise, and during the recovery period.

ECG CRITERIA

• The normal lead placement in cardiac stress testing is the modified 12-lead system.
• The hallmark of ischemia on the exercise cardiogram is ST-segment depression, with ST depressions of 2 mm or more in one lead being a positive test (Fig. 32–1). Not all ST depression is of cardiac origin.
• Other abnormalities can also be seen in patients during exercise stress testing, such as ST elevation, upsloping ST segments, and variation of the R wave amplitude.
• In the absence of a previous MI or Q wave, ST elevation is a marker of high-grade stenosis or coronary vasospasm causing transmural ischemia.
• Upsloping of ST segments is a normal finding in the ECG during maximum exercise.
• The changes in R wave amplitude during exercise are relatively nonspecific.

NON-ECG CRITERIA

• The important data that need to be determined during the stress test include the maximum work capacity, the RPP, and the HR response. The BP in normal exercise increases progressively with increasing workload.
• The failure of systolic BP to increase appropriately can be a sign of ischemia or of left ventricular dysfunction. A fall in the systolic BP with increasing load is an indication for aborting the test. Nonischemic causes of fall in systolic BP in stress testing include cardiomyopathy, cardiac arrhythmias, vasovagal reaction, left ventricular outflow tract obstruction, use of antihypertensive drugs,

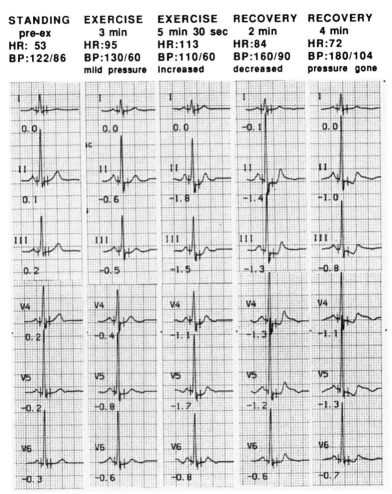

STANDING	EXERCISE	EXERCISE	RECOVERY	RECOVERY
pre-ex	3 min	5 min 30 sec	2 min	4 min
HR: 53	HR:95	HR:113	HR:84	HR:72
BP:122/86	BP:130/60	BP:110/60	BP:160/90	BP:180/104
	mild pressure	increased	decreased	pressure gone

FIGURE 32–1. Electrocardiographic changes of ischemia during exercise testing in a 71-year-old man with exertional chest pain. Progressive ST-segment depression with upsloping contour is noted during exercise. The ST-depression becomes horizontal during recovery with partial T wave inversion. (Courtesy of David Blood, M.D.)

hypovolemia, and prolonged vigorous exercise. The diastolic BP does not change significantly in normal patients during exercise. A rise in diastolic BP in a stress test can be associated with ischemia.

• There should be a gradual decline in the systolic BP after exercise.

• Although chest pain starts after the onset of ST depression in most cases, chest pain can be the only indicator of ischemia in some patients. The presence of pain with no ECG changes is often an indication that nuclear or echocardiographic testing is needed.

• The maximum work capacity can be determined during stress testing and serves as an important prognostic measurement, as well as a target for the maximum work during a rehabilitation program.

• The amount of work performed or the level reached is the best estimate of functional capacity. The time exercised is not as useful because it is dependent on the test protocol used.

• Exercise impairment is determined by comparing the patient's performance to a table of normal levels adjusted for age, which is available in the literature for the specific exercise protocol employed (see Table 32–9 in the Textbook).

ECHOCARDIOGRAPHIC STRESS TESTING

• Exercise echocardiography is one of the more commonly used techniques in exercise testing. The exercise can be performed either on a treadmill or with a bicycle ergometer. Scanning can be done only before and after exercise with treadmill testing, whereas the bicycle allows for continuous monitoring and the detection of transient ischemic changes. This compares favorably with the results of stress ECG.

• The test is particularly useful in situations in which the stress ECG is ambiguous or nondiagnostic, in women (who have a higher likelihood of a false-positive ECG test), and in those having an abnormal resting ECG.

NUCLEAR STRESS TESTING

• Thallium-201 perfusion scintigraphy is widely accepted for the detection of ischemia in CAD. It is more accurate than the use of stress echocardiography alone. The imaging is typically performed in conjunction with a treadmill test. It can also be done with dipyridamole and adenosine pharmacological stress testing.

PHARMACOLOGICAL STRESS TESTING

• The main advantage of the use of these agents for cardiac stress testing is that a patient can be tested regardless of ability to perform adequate levels of exercise.

• *Dipyridamole* has been well studied as a pharmacological agent to induce cardiac stress. It is often used in conjunction with thallium-201 scintigraphy, but is also used with echocardiography. It has been used for detection of CAD, cardiac risk stratification, and perioperative risk evaluation. Dipyridamole causes normal vessels to dilate, but the diseased vascular beds do not have the capacity to further dilate. This phenomenon is described as cardiac steal.

• See the Textbook for use of adenosine and dobutamine as testing agents.

ISOMETRIC HAND GRIP TEST

• This test uses the isometric contraction of the upper extremity with a dynamometer to provide an exercise stress. Typically, the test is performed with the patient squeezing the dynamometer at one-fourth to three-fourths of maximum hand strength for as long as tolerated.

Modifications for the Physically Disabled (p. 678)

• Echocardiographic and nuclear testing increase the sensitivity of testing performed on various exercise devices, partially compensating for the reduced workloads achieved. Exercise devices that have been used successfully include the arm crank ergometer, an adapted Schwinn Airdyne, a supine bicycle ergometer, and a wheelchair ergometer.

Assessment of Cardiac Demands of Activities (pp. 678–679)

• Direct assessment of the cardiac demands of various activities is technically difficult. The use of the RPP or HR gives a reasonable estimate of the relative stress on the coronary circulation by correlation with $M\dot{V}O_2$, and these numbers can be used in conjunction with the patient's stress testing to judge the safety of the activity in relation to the anginal threshold.

• The information obtained in this manner is highly individualized and can be correlated to functional activities through the use of tables of metabolic demands of various self-care, mobility, vocational, and avocational activities (Table 32–5).

• These tables usually express the metabolic demands of the activities in METs (1 MET = approximately $3.5\,mL\,O_2$/kg body weight/min). The use of MET tables can give useful information about the relative metabolic demands of various activities, but they must be used with caution and an awareness of the physiological limitations involved.

CARDIAC REHABILITATION PROGRAMS (pp. 679–684)

Risk Factor Modification (pp. 679–680)

• In addition to exercise training, all cardiac rehabilitation programs should emphasize patient and family education for risk factor reduction and lifestyle modification.

• Risk factor reduction should include smoking cessation, normalizing elevated BP and blood lipids, engaging in a regular aerobic conditioning program, eating a diet low in fat, and stress management.

Primary Prevention Programs (p. 680)

• Programs designed to intervene before the clinical onset of CAD have the greatest opportunity for producing major alterations in the natural history of the disease.

TABLE 32–5 A Typical MET Table

Activity	MET
Lying quietly	1.0
Sitting at ease	1.2–1.6
Sitting writing	1.9–2.2
Standing at ease	1.4–2.0
Walking 1 mph	2.3
Standing, washing, and shaving	2.5–2.6
Standing, dressing, and undressing	2.3–3.3
Light housework	1.7–3.0
Heavy housework	3.0–6.0
Office work	1.3–2.5
Walking 2 mph	3.1
Light industrial work	2.0–5.0
Walking 3 mph	4.3

• The program should consist of identification and modification of risk factors, dietary counseling, stress management training, and instruction in a sustainable exercise regimen. The American Heart Association, in its recent position papers, advocates primary prevention through the institution of exercise programs. Moderate-intensity activities (40% to 60% of maximum $\dot{V}O_2$), performed for 20 to 30 minutes three or four times a week, are sufficient.

Rehabilitation Following Myocardial Infarction (pp. 680–682)

• The rehabilitation program following MI is the classic model for cardiac rehabilitation. It can be divided into four phases: (1) the acute in-hospital phase beginning in the cardiac care unit (CCU); (2) the convalescent phase continuing the program at home until a strong scar has formed on the damaged myocardium; (3) the training phase using aerobic conditioning to increase the patient's physical work capacity; and (4) the maintenance phase, where the gains achieved by training are sustained by regular exercise. Patient education aimed at risk factor reduction and lifestyle modification is included during each of these phases.

ACUTE PHASE
• In the acute phase, the goal is to progress the patient gradually and safely from the initial bed rest of the CCU to a level consistent with most activities of daily living. There is a gradual daily increase in exercise intensity, which progresses as long as there are no arrhythmias, congestive heart failure, or ischemia. Patients are monitored with ECG telemetry during each increase in exercise level. By mobilizing the patient early, deconditioning from excessive bed rest and psychological invalidism are reduced or eliminated. Actual exercise training for a higher work capacity is not a goal of this phase. It is imperative that the educational programs for risk factor modification be introduced at this time.

CONVALESCENT PHASE
• During the convalescent phase, the goal is to maintain early mobilization and to gradually increase the endurance for exercise at the same intensity used at the end of the acute phase program. This is usually walking or bicycling using a target HR taught at the end of the acute phase and known to be within the patient's safe capacity. In an uncomplicated case, this phase lasts for about 6 weeks from the time of the infarction. This allows time for a firm scar to form on the infarcted area, thereby reducing the risk of ventricular aneurysm or wall rupture.

TRAINING PHASE
• This is the actual exercise training program. It begins with a symptom-limited exercise tolerance testing (ETT), with the results being used to determine a target HR for exercise training. The ETT screens out patients with contraindications for exercise training, including dangerous arrhythmias or a drop in BP with increasing exercise intensity.
• If the maximum HR achieved on the ETT is limited only by a relatively benign endpoint such as fatigue, musculoskeletal pain, or angina preceding ECG changes, a target HR as high as 85% of the maximum HR can be used. If the endpoint is a serious arrhythmia or ECG changes without chest pain, a lower target HR should be chosen. Target heart rates as low as 60% of maximum can result in effective training.

• It is critical for patient safety that target heart rates in this population be based on actual ETTs, not tables or equations estimating maximum rates from the patient's age. Monitoring with ECG telemetry is usually used with each upgrading of the exercise prescription, but continuous monitoring is not necessary for each session. The patient can be taught to monitor HR (using the carotid pulse) or to use the Borg scale (Table 32–6).

• The improvements in the cardiac response to exercise that result from aerobic training occur only when the muscles involved with the training are used. It is necessary to individualize each patient's program to include the muscle groups necessary for vocational and avocational goals.

• The usual training program calls for three sessions a week for 6 to 8 weeks. Each session should start with a stretching program, followed by an aerobic program. The aerobic program can use equipment such as treadmills, upper or lower extremity ergometers, Airdynes, rowing machines, walking, running, and calisthenics. Each exercise should have a warm-up period, a training period at target HR, and a cool-down period.

MAINTENANCE PHASE

• The maintenance phase is probably the most important phase of all: if it is neglected, the benefits of the training phase are lost within a few weeks. The minimum requirement is exercise at least twice a week and preferably three times a week for at least 30 minutes. ECG monitoring is not necessary during this phase.

Rehabilitation of the Patient with Angina Pectoris (p. 682)

• Rehabilitation of the patient with stable angina can begin once the medical regimen has been optimized. The exercise program begins with the ETT and then progresses with the training and maintenance programs as outlined above for the post-MI patient.

TABLE 32–6 The Borg Scale of Perceived Exertion

Score	Perceived Exertion
6	Very very light
7	
8	Very light
9	
10	Fairly light
11	
12	Somewhat hard
13	
14	Hard
15	
16	Very hard
17	
18	Very very hard
19	
20	

Rehabilitation Following Bypass Surgery (p. 682)

• In the post-bypass surgery patient, cardiac rehabilitation can provide benefit by several mechanisms (Table 32–7).
• A symptom-limited ETT can be safely performed at 3 to 4 weeks after surgery to determine the level of exercise that a patient can tolerate.
• Cardiac rehabilitation after CABG can be thought of in two phases: the immediate postoperative period, and the later maintenance phase. The in-hospital first phase is usually in the first week or so postoperatively because patients are typically sent home after that time. The initial period can be thought of in three stages: (1) mobilization in the immediate postoperative period; (2) progressive ambulation and daily exercises; and (3) discharge planning and exercise prescription for the maintenance stage.
• Mobilization in the intensive care unit on postoperative day 1 (POD 1) includes sitting upright, active leg exercises, and mobilization out of bed. Only an unstable postoperative course or severe CHF should interfere with this early mobilization. This aggressive early intervention has several benefits, including decreasing the deleterious effects of bed rest such as deep venous thrombosis (DVT), pulmonary embolus (PE), pulmonary complications, and cardiac deconditioning.
• The POD 2 to 5 program should include progressive ambulation and daily exercise. Ambulation begins with supervision for distances of 150 to 200 feet, followed by gradually progressive ambulation until most patients are starting independent ambulation by POD 3. Monitoring with ECG telemetry is usually used during the early mobilization. In the last few days before discharge, the patient and physician should develop a self-monitored home program that allows for gradual progression to previous levels of activity.
• The second stage of a program for the post-CABG patient is conducted at home for the usual patient, or in an inpatient rehabilitation center for the high-risk patient or those who need more intensive interventions and monitoring.
• Each patient can be in one of three types of programs: low, moderate, or high intensity. A low-intensity program is a progressive walking program with energy expenditures in the range of 2 to 4 METs, and a target HR of 65% to 75% of maximum HR. A moderate-intensity program is a progressive walk to walk-jog program from 3.0 to 6.5 METs, with target HR of 70% to 80% of maximum HR. A high-intensity program is a progression from walk-jog to jogging from 5.0 to 8.5 METs, with a target HR of 75% to 85% of maximum HR. For a patient on a β-blocker, the target HR is set at 20 beats per minute above the resting HR. Both objective criteria and patient observation in the postoperative period determine the assignment of patients to a level of exercise. A submaximum stress test

---

TABLE 32–7 Benefits of Cardiac Rehabilitation after Bypass Surgery

Increased ischemic threshold
Improved left ventricular function
Increased coronary collaterals
Ameliorated serum lipids
Decreased serum catecholamines
Decreased platelet aggregation and increased fibrinolysis
Improved psychological status

before discharge is an important way to evaluate physiological response to submaximum effort.

Rehabilitation Following Cardiac Transplantation
(pp. 682–683)

• The transplant itself usually resolves the cardiac disability, but a comprehensive approach to the patient is necessary. Post-transplant, there is a blunted HR response to an incremental exercise test, with peak HR 20% to 25% lower than in age-matched controls. Resting hypertension is common because of the renal effects of cyclosporine, prednisone, and other medications.
• Transplant recipients usually have a 10% to 50% loss of lean body mass from inactivity and high-dose steroids in the perioperative period, with a resultant decrease of maximum work output and $\dot{V}o_{2max}$ by two-thirds. At submaximum exercise levels, perceived exertion, minute ventilation, and the ventilatory equivalent for oxygen are all increased. $\dot{V}o_2$ is the same, however, implying earlier onset of anaerobic metabolism. At maximum effort there is lower work capacity, CO, HR, systolic BP, and $\dot{V}o_2$.
• The cardiac training regimen in transplant patients should address overall conditioning as well as cardiac function. Walking, jogging, cycling, and swimming are commonly used exercises. The initial postoperative period encourages sitting upright, lower extremity exercises, and mobilization from the bed. The patient then starts ambulation, just as with the post-CABG patient. After discharge the patient uses self-monitoring to increase ambulation to 1 mile. The goal of the exercise program is to achieve a pace of 60% to 70% of peak effort for 30 to 60 minutes, three to five times weekly. The Borg level of perceived effort (see Table 32–6) should be maintained at 13 to 14, with activity increasing incrementally to stay at this level.
• Other important aspects of the rehabilitation of cardiac transplant patients include the complicated medical regimen, psychological needs, vocational rehabilitation, and exercises for generalized weakness.
• The outcomes of rehabilitation in the cardiac transplant population have been generally favorable.

Rehabilitation of the Patient with Cardiomyopathy (p. 683)

• Patients with poor left ventricular function have complications and expectations that are different from those of the post-CABG or post-MI population. They are at higher risk of sudden death, and often are emotionally depressed because of their chronic cardiac disability. Exercise in heart failure can cause a drop in ejection fraction, a decrease in SV, and exertional hypotension. Low endurance and fatigue are also a problem. Despite these problems, there is documented benefit from exercise in this patient population.

Rehabilitation of the Patient with Valvular Heart Disease
(pp. 683–684)

• The major problems in patients with valvular heart disease include deconditioning and CHF. The management of the valvular heart disease patient in CHF is essentially as outlined in the section on CHF. A complicating feature is the fact that many of these patients are on anticoagulants postoperatively and need

TABLE 32–8 Patients at High Risk during Cardiac Rehabilitation

Risk of Ischemia

Postoperative angina
Left ventricular ejection fraction <35%
NYHA grade III or IV congestive heart failure
Ventricular tachycardia or fibrillation in the postoperative period
Systolic BP drop of 10 points or more with exercise
Excessive ventricular ectopy with exercise
Incapable of self-monitoring
Myocardial ischemia with exercise

Risk of Arrhythmia

Acute infarction within 6 wk
Active ischemia
Significant left ventricular dysfunction (LVEF <30%)
History of sustained ventricular tachycardia
History of sustained life-threatening supraventricular arrhythmia
History of sudden death, not yet stabilized on medical therapy
Initial therapy of patients with automatic implantable cardioverter defibrillator
Initial therapy of a patient with rate-adaptive cardiac pacemaker

Abbreviations: BP, blood pressure; LVEF, left ventricular ejection fraction.

to be on low-impact exercises to avoid hemarthroses and bruising. The training program is similar to that followed for the post-CABG patient.

CARDIAC ARRHYTHMIAS

• The risk of death from cardiac arrhythmia during rehabilitation exercises is very low. Therefore, it might be prudent to continually monitor only those patients who are at high risk (Table 32–8). For patients with life-threatening arrhythmias, the automatic implantable cardiac defibrillator (AICD) has become a common treatment. The AICD devices are rate sensitive, so it is essential to ensure that this rate is not exceeded during the exercise stress test and that the HR achieved with exercise does not exceed this threshold.

Modifications for the Physically Disabled (p. 684)

• This is an area where physiatrists can take a leadership role, because most existing programs are limited in the ability to compensate for physical impairments. The risk factor modification programs are easily adapted for any patient population. The exercise training can be accomplished with the same adapted equipment described above for modified exercise testing. The same training principles can be applied.

33

Original Chapter by Augusta S. Alba, M.D.

Concepts in Pulmonary Rehabilitation

PRINCIPLES (p. 687)

• *Pulmonary rehabilitation* (PR) is defined as a comprehensive team approach that provides patients with the ability to adapt to their chronic lung disease. It includes medical management, training in coping skills, and exercise reconditioning.

• Candidates for PR should have a decrease in functional capacity caused by pulmonary disease, relative stability of the underlying pulmonary disease, absence of other significant diseases including orthopedic limitations, adequate motivation to undergo a rigorous program, and a pattern of continued improvement.

• When exercise reconditioning is no longer possible in a progressive disorder, mechanical ventilation, partial lung resection, and lung transplants become options in the course of the program.

PRIMARY MODALITIES (pp. 687–697)

General Medical Management (p. 687)

• Pharmacological therapy includes vaccination against influenza and pneumococcal pneumonia, and inhaled quaternary anticholinergic or β_2-agonist bronchodilators, or both. Oral theophylline can improve respiratory muscle endurance and provide ventilatory stimulation. The new leukotriene receptor antagonist (LTRA) zafirlukast has proved valuable in asthma. Persistent airway obstruction may be an indication for a trial of oral or inhaled steroid therapy. If hypoxemia is present, long-term oxygen therapy (LTOT) will improve survival and quality of life. Environmental and occupational pollution must be prevented and eliminated.

Chest Physical Therapy (pp. 687–688)

• A good understanding of pulmonary function tests (Fig. 33–1) and the mechanics and work of breathing in normal and diseased states is essential in pulmonary rehab. Breathing exercises include relaxation techniques for

TEST	OBSTRUCTIVE DISEASE	RESTRICTIVE DISEASE
VC	↔ ↓	↓ ↓
FEV	↓ ↓	↔ ↓
MMF	↓ ↓	↔ ↓
MVV	↓ ↓	↔ ↓
RV	↑ ↑	↓ ↓
FRC	↑ ↑	↓ ↓
TLC	↑ ↑	↓ ↓

FIGURE 33–1. Typical results of disease on ventilatory function. VC, vital capacity; FEV, forced expiratory volume; MMF, midmaximal flow; MVV, maximal voluntary ventilation; RV, residual volume; FRC, functional residual capacity; TLC, total lung capacity.

breathing retraining and respiratory muscle endurance training, consisting of inspiratory resistance training.
• Clearance of secretions is mandatory to reduce the work of breathing and to limit infection and atelectasis. In order for chest physical therapy to be effective, mucoactive medications must be given. These include expectorants, mucolytics, bronchodilators, surfactants, and mucoregulatory agents that reduce the volume of mucus secretion.
• Techniques for clearing secretions are postural drainage, manual or device-induced chest percussion and vibration, device-induced airway oscillation, incentive spirometry, and various measures that improve the ability to cough.
• In a manually assisted cough, the patient's abdomen is compressed while the patient controls the depth of inspiration and the timing of opening and closing of the upper airway. Intermittent positive pressure ventilation (IPPV) or glossopharyngeal breathing (GPB) or both are used, if needed, to increase the depth of inspiration. Similarly, in persons with an upper motor neuron lesion affecting the abdominal muscles (e.g., SCI with a lesion above the midthoracic level), a cough can be produced by electrical stimulation of the abdominal muscles.
• Positive expiratory pressure (PEP) mask therapy followed by "huff coughing" is a useful technique when other methods of raising secretions are not tolerated. Autogenic drainage (AD) is a secretion clearance technique that combines variable tidal breathing at three distinct lung volume levels, controlled expiratory airflow, and huff coughing. The In-exsufflator machine (see Fig. 33–3 in the Textbook) provides a deep inspiration either through a mask or a tracheostomy attachment followed rapidly by a controlled suction. It has been shown to provide highly effective secretion removal.

Exercise Conditioning (pp. 688–689)

• If the cardiovascular, respiratory, and neuromuscular systems have adequate reserve to undergo a program of progressive exercise, skeletal muscles can develop an increased ability to perform aerobic exercise.

• Cardiopulmonary exercise testing is necessary for the selection and evaluation of patients with chronic obstructive pulmonary disease (COPD) for exercise training. Exercise testing is carried out as a baseline measurement and as a measurement of progress. It also helps to define the cause of dyspnea, the need for supplemental oxygen, and the status of the preoperative patient.

• The parameters of inspiratory vital capacity (IVC), forced expiratory volume in 1 second (FEV_1), maximum minute ventilation (VEmax), and maximum oxygen consumption ($\dot{V}O_{2max}$) have the greatest clinical potential for functional assessment of patients because they show the least variability over time in stable COPD patients.

• Types of exercise include lower extremity training on a bicycle ergometer or treadmill, respiratory muscle training using a threshold inspiratory pressure trainer, and unsupported versus supported arm exercise. Ventilatory muscle endurance exercise, muscle rest therapy, and ventilatory support by nasal intermittent positive pressure ventilation (NIPPV) during exercise can also be used.

Exercise in COPD (pp. 689–690)

• The results of exercise in COPD from several studies are summarized in Table 33–2 in the Textbook.

• In COPD, NIPPV during exercise can effectively support ventilation, decrease dyspnea, and prolong endurance time. The results of exercise from several studies are summarized in Table 33–2 in the Textbook. It has been demonstrated that high work rates above pretraining anaerobic threshold (AT) reduce the production of lactate at any given work rate to a considerably greater degree than a low work rate above AT.

• Hypertensive patients who participate in a PR program typically show no change in their hypertension. Medical treatment of the hypertension is necessary.

Exercise in Asthma (p. 690)

• *Moderate asthma* is defined as asthma in which there is no pulmonary impairment during symptom-free intervals.

• *Severe asthma* is defined as asthma with persistent airway obstruction.

• Aerobic training is recommended because it can decrease minute ventilation and hence the tidal volume for any given workload.

Exercise in Cystic Fibrosis (p. 690)

• An estimated 30,000 persons in the United States suffer from cystic fibrosis (CF), which is a hereditary autosomal recessive disorder. The basic defect is one of chloride transport, which produces a viscid mucus that inhibits the capability of the lungs to clear infection. The patient ultimately suffers from severe combined obstructive-restrictive pulmonary disease, which leads to hypoxia, pulmonary hypertension, and death.

• Dornase alfa, or human recombinant deoxyribonuclease (DNase), is an enzyme capable of digesting extracellular DNA. The abnormal viscosity of the CF secretions is caused to a great extent by degenerating neutrophils which produce extracellular DNA. Dornase alfa is used for patients older than 5 years or for those with a forced vital capacity (FVC) greater than 40%.

• Chest physical therapy of all pulmonary segments from one to four times daily is indicated, with increased frequency during exacerbations. Such therapy is rarely available with the necessary frequency in a long-term care setting because patient/staff ratios do not permit it. The person with CF is best cared for in a home setting with personal caregivers who have been trained to deliver the therapy.

Exercise in Disorders of Chest Wall Function (pp. 690–691)

• Ankylosing spondylitis, kyphoscoliosis or scoliosis, pectus excavatum, obesity, the sequelae of thoracoplasty or phrenic nerve crush for the treatment of pulmonary tuberculosis, neuromuscular diseases with weakness of the respiratory bellows mechanism, and superimposed spinal curvatures are all disorders in which respiratory muscle fatigue can be reduced by ventilatory muscle training. Persons with Parkinson's disease show improvement with PR.
• Spinal cord–injured (SCI) patients can benefit from PR techniques. The SCI child as young as three years can learn neck breathing as a form of voluntary respiration. In children with levels as high as C2 with no diaphragmatic function, this technique produces enough tidal volume that the child can spend some time off the respirator.
• Vital capacity (VC) and VE during exercise can be improved even in chronic tetraplegia. The low cervical or incomplete tetraplegic person can perform resistance exercise by pedaling an arm ergometer (AE) for 30 minutes three times a week. Incentive spirometry is a technique in which a patient trains to perform regular deep insufflations by inspiring through a handheld apparatus that gives visual feedback of inspiratory flow. It should be performed for 15 minutes 3 to 5 times a week.
• Glossopharyngeal breathing (GPB) is another technique a patient can use to perform or supplement regular deep insufflations. Air is pumped into lungs by the patient using the tongue as a piston. The ball of the tongue strokes boluses of air at the rate of 100 per minute into the throat. The lips, soft palate, and vocal cords open and close in rhythm during each stroke. The patient usually obtains a full tidal breath by stacking gulps of 60 to 90 mL over a period of 10 to 15 seconds, then exhales. Full inflation of the lungs requires stacking for a period of 30 to 40 seconds. Tetraplegic patients, whose resting $\dot{V}o_2$ is approximately half-normal (150 mL/min), are able to obtain adequate VE by this method if their lungs have no major abnormalities. This enables them to breathe without artificial ventilation for hours. As soon as the oxygen saturation falls to 85% to 90%, the patient will typically ask for mechanical ventilatory assistance. GPB improves vocal volume and the flow of speech, allows the patient to call for help, and provides the deep breath needed for an assisted cough.

Nutrition (pp. 691–692)

• In acute respiratory failure, a fat emulsion (Pulmocare) can be given as 20% to 30% of total daily calories to reduce carbon dioxide production and to provide a volume-concentrated source of calories in the fluid-restricted patient. Dietary fat has a lower level of carbon dioxide production per kilocalorie of energy extracted.

Mechanical Ventilation (pp. 692–696)

• A reduction in the central drive for breathing results in central sleep apnea (CSA). Obstruction at any site in the upper airway produces obstructive sleep apnea (OSA). Both forms of apnea frequently coexist and are generally more severe during sleep, especially during rapid eye movement (REM) sleep, when there is the greatest degree of muscle relaxation. OSA is treated most commonly by continuous positive airway pressure (CPAP) or bilevel positive airway pressure (BIPAP). CSA is treated with mechanical ventilation.

• The physician and the patient should decide jointly what type of mechanical ventilation to use as well as the frequency and duration of its use. The choice of ventilators can be confusing. However, if the basic features of ventilators are kept in mind, the prescription is readily generated.

• Noninvasive artificial ventilation is the use of a ventilator without an endotracheal or tracheostomy tube. There are numerous advantages to a noninvasive approach (Table 33–1). One of the most important is the avoidance of respiratory nosocomial infection.

• Two of the most acceptable forms of noninvasive ventilation for daytime use are mouth intermittent positive-pressure ventilation (MIPPV) with a small mouthpiece held between the teeth (Fig. 33–7 in the Textbook) and the pneumobelt (Fig. 33–8 in the Textbook). The pneumobelt holds a bladder that produces a forced expiration when inflated. This expiration is followed by a passive inspiration. The inspiration may be supplemented by the use of the remaining inspiratory muscles or GPB, or a combination of these. MIPPV can be used at night by using a mouthpiece with a lip seal. The patient can use a rocking bed (Fig. 33–10 in the Textbook) or a chestpiece (Fig. 33–11 in the Textbook) at rest or during sleep. Body ventilators comprise no more than 10% of ventilator usage.

• When a decision has been made to retain a tracheostomy in a ventilator-user, a cuffless tracheostomy tube or a tube with a partially deflated cuff can generally be used. Tubes without a fully inflated cuff require adequate pulmonary compliance and sufficient oropharyngeal strength for functional swallowing and articulation. When a fully inflated cuff must be used, the lowest possible cuff pressure needed to achieve a seal should be used (preferably <15 mm Hg). If the pressure exceeds the critical pressure for perfusion of the tracheal mucosa (25 mm Hg), destruction of the tracheal wall can occur. Ulceration, bleeding, perforation, loss of tracheal cartilage, localized trachiectasis or stenosis, and granulation tissue are potential complications.

• Types of tracheostomy tubes include metal tubes and disposable tubes made of plastic or silicone. Specialized tubes include fenestrated tubes, talking tubes, and tubes for the laryngectomized person. Both pneumatic and electrical devices are available to assist vocalization in the presence of a tracheostomy tube. Speaking valves can be attached to the tracheostomy tube adapter. Currently, the most frequently used valve is the Passy-Muir. When vocalization is not possible, nonvocal communication can be provided by a manual or electronic communication system.

• In cases of advanced COPD, mechanical ventilation via a tracheostomy is often necessary for survival. More controversial, however, is the use of mechanical ventilation to reduce respiratory muscle fatigue.

• Mechanical ventilation in patients with neuromusculoskeletal disorders has been facilitated in the past 15 years by the development of portable volume

TABLE 33–1 Respiratory Assistive Devices: Pros and Cons

Type	Use	Pro	Con
Airway Positive Pressure			
INTERMITTENT POSITIVE-PRESSURE VENTILATION			
Console	Bedside; generally hospital setting, acute care, via tracheostomy	Sophistication (alarms; %O_2)	Stationary; high cost
Compact	Long-term; generally noninvasive	Portability; generally AC/DC; lower cost	Some models bulky
Body Negative Pressure			
Iron lung	Replaces bed; long-term	Reliable; good ventilation	Weight; size; confining
Porta-Lung	Same as iron lung	Same as iron lung	Light weight; relative portability
Poncho (wrap)	In bed; long-term	Same as iron lung	May restrict upper chest expansion
Chest shell (cuirass)	In bed; rarely in wheelchair; long-term	Less confining than iron lung	Restricts upper and lateral chest expansion
Diaphragmatic pacemaker	Long-term; relatively intact phrenic nerve, diaphragm muscle, and lower lobes	Very light weight; easy operation	Surgery; initial cost very high; moves only diaphragm
Body Negative/Positive Pressure			
Rocking bed	Replaces bed; requires healthy lower lobes; "movable abdomen"; long-term	Less confining than iron lung; passive movement of body	Weight; size; moves only diaphragm
Body Positive Pressure			
Pneumobelt	Long-term; generally requires sitting position of at least 45 degrees; "movable abdomen"	Good cosmetic effect	Moves only diaphragm

ventilators and BIPAP used as a ventilator. In the ICU the increased sophistication of console volume ventilators has aided the survival of persons with these disorders.

• The halo brace is frequently used for patients with SCI if surgical stabilization has not been carried out after fracture of the cervical spine. The halo brace permits early patient mobilization and early admission to a rehabilitation setting. Early mobilization helps prevent the pulmonary complications associated with prolonged bed rest and paralysis, the most serious of which are atelectasis and pneumonia.

• Persons with high and midcervical tetraplegia will invariably require mechanical ventilation during the initial hospitalization. Other common neurological disorders in which long-term mechanical ventilation is used include amyotrophic lateral sclerosis (ALS), syringomyelia, multiple sclerosis, muscular dystrophies, and poliomyelitis. The average length of survival in DMD patients is increased by 6 years with respiratory assistance.

• Weaning from mechanical ventilation is an important aspect of PR, both in terms of reduced cost and patient satisfaction. Weaning techniques include CPAP, blow-by systems or T piece, pressure support, and the use of the Passy-Muir ventilator speaking valve. The use of manual and mechanical exsufflation to clear airway secretions and the use of noninvasive positive airway pressure ventilatory assistance by nasal or oral interfaces speed weaning in the patient on tracheal intermittent positive-pressure ventilation. Diaphragmatic strengthening and endurance training can be used to facilitate weaning in the high tetraplegic patient in whom there is only partial involvement of the anterior horn cells of the phrenic nerve at the C3–C5 levels.

• Diaphragmatic pacing (Fig. 33–12 in the Textbook) is a highly sophisticated form of mechanical ventilation. Diaphragmatic pacing is indicated in patients who have damage to the respiratory control centers or their pathways in the brainstem and spinal cord. The pacing system consists of an external transmitter and antenna and implanted electrodes and receiver. The working life expectancy of the receiver is for the lifetime of the patient and batteries last for 2 to 3 weeks.

Oxygen Therapy (p. 697)

• Oxygen therapy with or without mechanical ventilation can be administered on a long-term basis. The physician should provide a prescription to the vendor who furnishes oxygen in the home. The physician must include on the prescription the diagnostic reasons for oxygen, results of blood gas studies, type of delivery system, and specific liter flow for the patient during rest, sleep, and/or exertion. For the hypoxemic patient, oxygen should be administered continuously to improve mortality and morbidity. Oxygen therapy is most easily monitored by pulse oximetry during the different activity conditions of the patient.

• Home oxygen systems include high-pressure compressed gas cylinders in several sizes, transfilling liquid oxygen systems with both a stationary reservoir and a portable device weighing 11 lbs when full, and oxygen concentrators that require an electrical outlet. The liquid oxygen canister can provide up to 9 hours of oxygen at 2 L/min. Methods of conservation include devices that either cause the oxygen to flow only during inspiration (pulse oxygen systems) or that store oxygen during the expiratory phase. Both as a method of conservation and for the cosmetic effect, transtracheal oxygen can be used. Nasal cannulas can be concealed in the eyeglasses.

BIOPSYCHOSOCIAL CONSIDERATIONS (pp. 697–698)

• Biopsychosocial considerations for persons with pulmonary dysfunction include education of the patient and family, psychotherapy, disability evaluation, vocational counseling, and availability of resources. Education must be ongoing in all clinical settings and in the home. Psychotherapy includes the assessment of neurocognition, which can be affected by hypoxemia and hypercapnia, and of the individual's self-concept. Stress management includes cognitive restructuring, progressive relaxation, breathing exercises, and visual imagery. Biofeedback and sexual counseling are additional psychotherapeutic approaches.

SURGICAL APPROACHES TO PULMONARY REHABILITATION (p. 698)

• Lung volume reduction surgery (LVRS), in which 20% to 30% on removal of one or both lungs, is now an option prior to or in lieu of lung transplantation for COPD patients. Areas of the lungs with the most severe lesions (usually the apices) are removed. This results in better respiratory mechanics and relief from severe dyspnea. Improvements in lung function begin to decline in 2 years. The safety, benefits, and cost of this surgery are not clear, and studies are underway to evaluate these issues.

• Single or bilateral lung transplants and heart-lung transplants are available to patients less than 55 to 65 years old, including children. Living donor lobar transplantation is being used in CF. Overall survival rates are between 60% and 65% at 2 years and approximately 40% at 5 years. In selected patients long-term mechanical ventilatory support has not been shown to be a contraindication to lung transplantation. A program of physical training prior to and following surgery expedites postoperative recovery.

LONG-TERM RESULTS OF PULMONARY REHABILITATION (p. 698)

Long-Term Results in Lung Disease (pp. 698–699)

• There is certainty that lower extremity training improves exercise tolerance, and a PR program improves the symptom of dyspnea. Results of PR are somewhat less consistent for the following propositions: that upper extremity training improves arm function; that ventilatory muscle training is of value when there is decreased respiratory muscle strength and dyspnea; that PR improves health-related quality of life and reduces both the number and duration of hospitalizations. Short-term psychosocial interventions have not been shown to be beneficial. Longer-term interventions may be helpful in a setting of a comprehensive PR program. PR might also improve survival.

34

Original Chapter by Ralph M. Buschbacher, M.D.,
and C. Douglas Porter, M.D.

Deconditioning, Conditioning, and the Benefits of Exercise

CONSEQUENCES OF DISUSE (pp. 703–716)

• Bed rest, immobilization, or relative rest is unfortunately necessary in some situations. These include some acute injuries, especially fractures and dislocations; acute myocardial infarction or pulmonary disease; and severe medical or surgical disorders. Yet even when rest is properly prescribed, we should be aware of its deleterious effects. Consequences of such disuse on the body organs and systems are described in the following section and summarized in Table 34–1.

The Musculoskeletal System (pp. 704–710)

• The primary functions of the musculoskeletal system are to support the body, to transport the body, and to use the body to accomplish physical tasks. It is affected by both activity and inactivity, and disorders of the system, in turn, affect the activity level that is possible.

Periarticular Soft Tissues (pp. 706–708)
• Contracture is an abnormal limitation of passive joint range of motion. It is usually caused by a restriction of the periarticular connective tissue, but in more advanced cases also involves tendons, ligaments, muscles, and joints. If not treated, it can lead to bony ankylosis of the joint. Although there are many possible causes of contractures (see Table 34–2 in the textbook), the primary cause is lack of normal joint mobilization.
• A number of conditions predispose patients to contractures. Spasticity, paralysis, or muscle strength imbalance hastens their development. Patients with amputations tend to develop contractures, mainly because of position and strength imbalances.
• In conditions of joint pain and inflammation, the patient tends to position the joint in the least painful position (to minimize intra-articular pressure) (Fig. 34–1).
• Contractures are likely to affect muscles that cross multiple joints because stretching of only one joint or the other may not adequately stretch the entire muscle. Where and how contractures develop depends on the position of the

TABLE 34–1 Major Complications of Immobility by Body System

Musculoskeletal

Muscles
  Atrophy; decreased strength and endurance
  Contracture
  Altered electrical activity/excitation
  Weakened myotendinous junction
  Contractures
  Decreased strength of tendons and ligaments
    and their insertions on bone
Bone
  Osteoporosis
Joints
  Cartilage degeneration
  Fibrofatty tissue infiltration
  Synovial atrophy
  Ankylosis

Cardiovascular

Cardiac (at rest)
  ↑ Heart rate
  ↓ Stroke volume
  Cardiac output unchanged or slightly decreased
  $\dot{V}O_2$ unchanged
  ↓ Cardiac size/volume
  ↓ Left ventricular end-diastolic volume
  Systolic/diastolic blood pressure unchanged
  Arteriovenous oxygen difference unchanged or
    slightly increased
Cardiac (with exercise)
  ↑ Heart rate response to submaximal exercise
  Maximum heart rate unchanged
  ↓ $\dot{V}O_{2max}$
  ↓ Stroke volume (submaximal/maximal)
  ↓ Cardiac output (submaximal/maximal)
  ↑ Arteriovenous oxygen difference
    (submaximal) (maximal is unchanged)
Neurovascular
  Orthostatic intolerance
Fluid balance
  ↓ Plasma volume
  ↓ Total blood volume
  ↓ Red blood cell mass
  Mineral and plasma protein loss (mainly
    isocontent)
Blood coagulation
  ↑ Venous thrombosis
  ↓ Calf blood flow (possible)
  ↑ Blood fibrinogen

Skin

Pressure ulcer
Edema
Subcutaneous bursitis

Body Composition, Metabolism, Nutrition

↓ Lean body mass
↑ Body fat

Minerals
  Nitrogen loss
  Calcium loss
  Phosphorus loss
  Sulfur loss
  Potassium loss

Endocrine

Impaired glucose tolerance
Altered circadian rhythm
Altered temperature and sweating
  response
Altered regulation of parathyroid hormone,
  thyroid hormones, adrenal hormones,
  pituitary hormones, growth hormone,
  androgens, and plasma renin activity

Respiratory

↑ Forced vital capacity
↑ Total lung capacity (slight)
Residual volume unchanged
Functional residual capacity unchanged
↑ Respiratory rate
Vital capacity unchanged (possibly
  decreases in time owing to
  contractures of chest wall)
Maximal minute ventilation unchanged
Possible ventilation/perfusion mismatch
Pulmonary embolism (possible)

Genitourinary

Diuresis
↑ Mineral excretion
Difficulty voiding
↑ Postvoid residual volume (possible)
↑ Urinary tract infection (possible)
↑ Overflow incontinence (possible)
↑ Calculus formation (possible)
↓ Glomerular filtration rate
↓ Ability to concentrate urine

Gastrointestinal

↓ Fluid intake
↓ Appetite
↓ Bowel motility
↓ Gastric secretion
Constipation (possible)

Neurological, Emotional

Compression neuropathies
Sensory deprivation (attention span, altered
  time awareness, hand-to-eye
  coordination, depression, anxiety)
↓ Balance
↓ Coordination
Sleep disturbance
↑ Auditory threshold
↓ Visual acuity

Abbreviations: $\dot{V}O_2$, rate of oxygen consumption; $\dot{V}O_{2max}$, rate of maximum oxygen consumption.

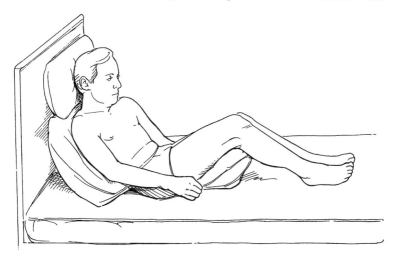

FIGURE 34–1. Common bed position and the areas susceptible to contracture: neck, flexed; soulders, internally rotated; thorax, flexed; arms, flexed; forearms, pronated; fingers, flexed; hips, flexed; knees, flexed; and ankles, plantar flexed.

joint and the length of time that position is maintained (as well as predisposing factors).

• It is commonly believed that contractures can be prevented by daily or twice-daily range-of-motion exercise. This is especially important in the hospitalized patient; in the elderly; and in arthritic joints, which are believed to develop contractures relatively rapidly.

• Once contractures have developed, they are treated with range-of-motion exercise (Table 34–2). Voluntary active range-of-motion exercise is preferred, but in some cases assisted range-of-motion exercise is needed. When stretching a contracted area, it is important to make sure that there is no bony block or other mechanical limitation to motion. It is also important not to be overly aggressive when stretching. If the tissues are torn and damaged during stretching, they are more likely to develop an even thicker connective tissue barrier to normal mobility.

Ligaments and Tendons *(pp. 708–709)*

• Immobilization causes an increase in collagen turnover, a decrease in collagen mass, a decrease in glycosaminoglycan and water content, an increase in soft tissue stiffness, and an alteration in fibroblast function. It is important to continue to stress the tendons and ligaments in all persons, both healthy and ill, and as soon as is clinically feasible in those recovering from injury or surgery.

Bones *(pp. 709–710)*

• Bone is normally in a state of dynamic equilibrium in which the rate of bone formation and resorption is held in balance.

• Lack of stress on the bones leads to a predominance of bone resorption (osteoclastic activity), which decreases bone mass and causes osteoporosis (see

TABLE 34–2 Progression of Treatment of Contractures from Least to Most Aggressive Methods

Proper positioning	Dynamic splinting
Active range-of-motion exercise	Nerve/motor point blocks
Active assisted range-of-motion exercise	Serial casting
Passive range-of-motion exercise	Surgery
Static splinting	

Chapter 41). The rate of loss of bone varies with the type of disuse and by body part, with weight-bearing bones being relatively more affected.

• In addition to generalized osteoporosis, there can also be local bone loss in conditions of partial immobilization, as after casting of fractures. In persons with paralysis, osteoporosis is often severe, and fractures can occur with relatively nontraumatic events such as transfer activities.

• *Immobilization hypercalcemia* is a condition often associated with osteoporosis, especially in adolescent males who have had traumatic injuries. As their bones are resorbed, serum calcium levels rise. They may become symptomatic, usually 2 to 4 weeks after the immobilization began. Signs and symptoms include nausea, vomiting, abdominal pain, lethargy, muscle weakness, and anorexia. If not treated, death can occur. Treatment is with intravenous furosemide and hydration. Etidronate disodium, intravenous pamidronate, and calcitonin can be used as well, especially in refractory cases.

• *Heterotopic ossification* is a condition of bone growth in abnormal locations, usually around joints. It is not caused by immobility, but is generally found in persons who have experienced trauma. The trauma can be neurological (e.g., spinal cord injury) or a direct muscle contusion. It can also be seen in persons immobilized because of other injuries.

Joints *(p. 710)*

• The hyaline cartilage in synovial joints is not supplied by vascular blood flow. It receives its nutrition from the synovial fluid by a regular loading and unloading of pressure, which draws fluid into and out of the cartilage in a process known as imbibition. During immobilization imbibition ceases, and the cartilage is dependent on simple diffusion to obtain nutrients. This diffusion is not adequate to the needs of the cartilage, and the joints begin to deteriorate.

• Immobilization-induced cartilage degeneration affects both the opposing joint surfaces that are in contact with each other and those that are not. These degenerative changes can occur in some joints, not only with cast immobilization, but also when weight bearing is restricted. The cause of the joint changes is believed to be an attempt to repair tissues damaged by inadequate nutrition. In the early stages this degeneration can be reversible to some extent, but later it most likely is not.

The Cardiovascular System *(pp. 710–713)*

Cardiac Deconditioning *(pp. 710–712)*

• Deconditioned persons have a resting tachycardia and an abnormally high heart rate with submaximal exercise. A severely deconditioned person can reach maximal heart rate with a seemingly trivial workload.

DECONDITIONING-INDUCED CHANGES OCCURRING AT REST

• After a period of bed rest, the resting heart rate starts to rise. It is generally believed to rise by about one-half beat per minute each day for the first 3 to 4 weeks of immobilization. Resting stroke volume is decreased for most persons, whereas cardiac output is not changed significantly. Cardiac size falls by up to 11%, and cardiac muscle atrophy may occur. Resting systolic and mean blood pressures are not changed, nor is total peripheral resistance. There is no change in oxygen uptake I $\dot{V}o_2$) at rest and no significant change in the arteriovenous oxygen difference.

DECONDITIONING-INDUCED CHANGES OCCURRING DURING EXERCISE

• After prolonged bed rest the normal heart rate response to exercise is altered. Deconditioning causes a higher heart rate at any given level of submaximal exercise, although maximal heart rate is unchanged or only slightly increased. With this faster heart rate, the diastolic filling period of the cardiac cycle is shortened and myocardial perfusion is decreased. When combined with an increase in the rate-pressure product, this can precipitate angina in the person with pre-existing coronary artery disease.

• After deconditioning there is a decrease in stroke volume (30%) at submaximal and maximal exercise. Cardiac output declines slightly at submaximal exercise and more significantly (26% mean drop) at maximal exercise. In addition, maximal oxygen uptake ($\dot{V}o_{2max}$), an indicator of general aerobic fitness, is reduced (mean, 28% lower), as is the submaximal $\dot{V}o_2$. In the deconditioned person it takes longer for the heart rate to return to the resting state after a period of exercise.

RECOVERY FROM DECONDITIONING

• It is difficult to state the exact rate of recovery from cardiovascular deconditioning because the studies to date have used different patient populations and different methods of enforcing disuse. For most parameters it seems to take at least as long to recover from the disuse as it took to deteriorate.

Hemodynamic and Neurovascular Deconditioning (p. 712)

• The person who has been on prolonged bed rest loses this adaptation and develops an orthostatic intolerance. Blood pools in the legs, venous return drops, stroke volume is diminished, and the systolic blood pressure is not maintained. This may be due, at least in part, to an altered carotid baroreflex or a change in autonomic balance. When a deconditioned person stands up there is an abnormally large increase in heart rate. This is accompanied by the common signs and symptoms of orthostatic hypotension, including a feeling of light-headedness, nausea, dizziness, sweating, pallor, tachycardia, and a drop in systolic blood pressure. In severe cases, syncope or angina can occur.

• Most of the effects of neurovascular deconditioning appear to occur in the first 4 to 7 days of bed rest. After remobilization these effects can take twice as long, or more, to reverse as they took to develop.

Fluid Balance (p. 712)

• When assuming recumbency there is an immediate shift in blood volume to the thorax and a delayed shift of extravascular fluid into the circulation. This causes a compensatory diuresis, which leads to a decreased plasma volume. Plasma volume loss is approximately 10% after 1 week of bed rest and 15% by 4 weeks. It is accompanied by a proportionate loss of plasma proteins. It is unclear what, if any, clinical significance is attached to these changes.

Thrombotic Disease (p. 712)
• Virchow's triad describes the contribution of clot formation, consisting of: (1) factors intrinsic to the blood, (2) blood vessel injury, and (3) stasis of blood flow. Immobility causes stasis because of reduced muscular pumping of the blood out of the venous plexus of the legs, and it can reduce blood flow through the calves. By increasing blood viscosity, immobility also may increase the intrinsic predisposition of the blood to clot. Therefore, disuse is a significant risk factor for developing thrombotic complications.

Prevention and Treatment of the Cardiovascular Complications of Immobility (pp. 712–713)
• Prevention is obviously the best way to deal with cardiovascular deconditioning. Avoiding prolonged bed rest and immobility is important.
• Cardiovascular deconditioning can be reversed by progressively increasing activity and regaining the upright posture (as tolerated). This can be done initially with passive and active range-of-motion exercise in bed and with a tilt table. Later, more aggressive activity is promoted. Deep venous thrombosis (DVT) is obviously associated with bed rest as well as surgery, trauma, and paralysis. It may be prevented with active calf contractions to pump the blood out of the venous plexus of the legs; subcutaneous or low-molecular-weight heparin; intermittent pneumatic compression of the legs; gradient pressure stockings; and, in high-risk patients, with anticoagulation. Proper position, active exercise, and proper leg elevations are also used.

Integumentary System (p. 713)

• Pressure ulcer formation (see also Chapter 31) is a leading health problem in immobilized or bedridden patients. It is a particular problem in persons with insensate skin or mental status deterioration.
• Capillary blood pressure is approximately 30 mm Hg. Sitting can cause a pressure in excess of this amount over the ischial tuberosities, whereas supine lying causes an excess of pressure over the sacrum. Such excess pressures are also found over the heels and occiput (especially in children because of their proportionally greater head size) while supine, and over the greater trochanter while side-lying. These pressures can completely occlude the capillaries; if sustained long enough, they lead to skin necrosis.
• Prevention of pressure ulcers is much more desirable than having to treat them. Proper turning of hospitalized patients, especially those with abnormal sensorium or sensation, the judicious use of a pressure-relieving bed when indicated, proper skin care and toileting, proper seating, and proper nutrition are all important.
• Dependent edema and subcutaneous bursitis can also occur with immobilization. The edema can generally be prevented with adequate mobilization and elevation. In some cases elastic stockings or gloves, pressure gradient compression, or massage may be indicated.
• *Subcutaneous bursitis* is the result of excessive pressure on the bursae. Bursitis is best treated by removing the aggravating pressure, but it can also be treated with nonsteroidal anti-inflammatory agents, percutaneous drainage, and instillation of corticosteroid. In refractory cases, surgical drainage or excision might be necessary.

Body Composition, Metabolic, and Nutritional Changes
(pp. 713–714)

• In addition to the fluid balance changes described earlier, there are a number of metabolic and body composition changes that occur with bed rest or immobilization. There is a decrease in lean body mass and an increase in body fat content.

• The body appears to become less efficient at storing excess calories as fat while on bed rest because the increase in fat percentage is actually less than would be predicted by caloric intake. Bed rest does not cause increased protein breakdown, but if dietary protein is low, total body protein synthesis is decreased. There may be a decrease in basal metabolic rate, probably related to loss of muscle mass. There are a number of changes in body minerals and metabolites seen with immobilization including a loss of nitrogen, calcium, phosphorus, sulfur, sodium, potassium, chloride, magnesium, and zinc.

Endocrine and Receptor Function (pp. 714–715)

• Prolonged bed rest causes a decrease in glucose tolerance. This is primarily caused by changes in peripheral muscle sensitivity to circulating insulin. The glucose intolerance caused by bed rest can, to some extent, be ameliorated with both isotonic and isometric exercise.

Respiratory System (p. 715)

• There are both immediate and long-term consequences of bed rest on the respiratory system. Immediately after assuming a supine or forward-slumped position, the diaphragm and intercostal muscles are restricted in their normal motion and breathing is impaired (an exception could be in spinal cord–injured patients in whom the supine position can place the diaphragm into a biomechanically advantageous position; see Chapter 55). The work of breathing is increased in the slumped or supine position because of increased mechanical resistance. Because of blood pooling in the thorax, there is also an immediate decrease in lung volume and residual volume.

• Although not proven, it is commonly held that if the recumbent position is maintained, gravity-induced changes will occur within the lungs. There is thought to be a pooling of mucus in the lower (dependent) parts of the airway, whereas the upper segments tend to dry out. This is believed to create an environment predisposing to respiratory infection, mucous plugging, and atelectasis. This situation is aggravated by a decrease in respiratory activity and an impaired cough mechanism. In addition, there can also be a mismatch between lung ventilation and perfusion.

• The pulmonary deterioration induced by bed rest can be prevented to a large extent by frequent changes in position, incentive spirometry, deep breathing, coughing, and pulmonary toilet. The only definitive solution to the problem is mobilization.

Genitourinary System (p. 715)

• Genitourinary effects of bed rest and immobility include the increased diuresis and mineral excretion. There are also other changes that are primarily mechanical in nature, including urinary stasis and calculus formation.

• Voiding is more difficult when supine, so patients tend to wait longer before emptying their bladders. There is also a lack of gravity assistance in voiding, and postvoid residual volume may be increased. This predisposes to urinary tract infection and, in severe cases, to overflow incontinence.

Gastrointestinal Tract and Digestion (p. 715)

• Bed rest causes mechanical effects on the gastrointestinal tract similar to those undergone by the genitourinary system. There is an increased risk of constipation because of decreased mobility, decreased peristalsis (possibly caused by an increased adrenergic state), and decreased fluid intake. Gastrointestinal secretion decreases and "heartburn" symptoms increase. There is also a decrease in or loss of appetite, which can lead to impairment of nutrition. The supine position can also interfere with eructation and can increase gastroesophageal reflux.

Neurological System, Emotions, and Intellectual Function (p. 716)

• There are few true neurological sequelae of bed rest that affect either the central or peripheral nervous systems. Instead, there are disorders of coordination, balance, and emotions that may have a component of physiological deterioration as well as a predominant integrative component.
• One potential neurological complication of bed rest is the occurrence of compression neuropathies. Peroneal nerve compression below the fibular head and ulnar nerve compression at the retrocondylar groove are probably the most common such compression neuropathies. They are specifically caused by bed rest rather than immobilization.
• The integrative components of emotions and cognitive function are affected by bed rest and immobilization, most likely caused by sensory deprivation and boredom, and not specifically caused by the lack of mobility. Medications and "ICU (intensive care unit) psychosis" play a role as well in medically ill patients. Affected persons can experience a lowered pain threshold and a decrease in coordination and balance. They can have emotional disturbances such as depression, anxiety, withdrawal, apathy, incontinence, and sleep disturbance, and might even develop paranoia and dementia. Intellectual function is impaired, as is orientation and the perception of time. They can suffer from headache, dizziness, general discomfort, nightmares, and even hallucinations, primarily because of sensory deprivation.

DECONDITIONING AS A REHABILITATION DIAGNOSIS (pp. 716–717)

• There are six basic conditions causing disuse: (1) a sedentary lifestyle that is a result of personal choice; (2) rest that is imposed because of a medical or surgical illness; (3) medical or caregiver "neglect," with a person needlessly restricted from mobility, usually in a hospital or nursing home; (4) immobilization of the body or part of the body by casts or braces, usually after trauma or fracture; (5) disuse because of paralysis or neuromuscular disorder; and (6) disuse caused by weightlessness.

Inpatient Rehabilitation Interactions (pp. 716–717)

• Deconditioned patients are hospitalized with a variety of medical and surgical illnesses, are treated successfully, but are left with residual weakness and other complications of immobility. These residual impairments are often more disabling than the problem for which they were admitted. These patients have what is known as *deconditioning syndrome.* They are unable to function as before, cannot be returned home safely, and require a short inpatient rehabilitation stay to regain their lost independence.

Outpatient Rehabilitation Interactions (p. 717)

• Deconditioning in the outpatient physical medicine and rehabilitation setting centers mainly on persons who have had an injury and who have been off work long enough to develop muscle weakness and inflexibility. This can put them at risk of further injury if they return to work without proper conditioning. Such patients often benefit from a work-conditioning or work-hardening program before return to activity.

THE BENEFICIAL EFFECTS OF EXERCISE (pp. 717–722)
Muscle Strength and Endurance (p. 717)

• Because strength is ultimately proportional to the cross-sectional area of muscle, muscle-building exercise increases the strength available to a person to meet the physical demands of living. Muscular endurance is similarly enhanced by endurance training. The major benefits of exercise are summarized in Table 34–7 in the Textbook. Chapter 19 describes the benefits of exercise in more detail.

Obesity (p. 717)

• *Obesity* is usually defined as a state in which ideal body weight is exceeded by more than 20%. Most obese persons have a long-term battle with their weight. They commonly choose to attack the problem by dieting, even though exercise can be more effective. Regular aerobic exercise helps reduce body weight even while maintaining fat-free weight. It brings about a more sustained weight loss than does dieting alone.

Hypertension (pp. 717–718)

• Aerobic exercise training can be valuable in the treatment of mild-to-moderate essential hypertension. It can cause a decrease of up to 10 mm Hg in blood pressure and appears to lower both systolic and diastolic blood pressures.
• According to the American College of Sports Medicine, in normal healthy adults, aerobic exercise is recommended at 60% to 85% of the maximum heart rate, three or four times per week, for 20 to 60 minutes per session. Because exercise at the upper limit of this level of intensity might actually worsen hypertension, aerobic exercise of more moderate intensity is recommended in the hypertensive patient.
• It has generally been recommended that isometric exercise (approximated by heavy weightlifting) be avoided in the hypertensive population because it

can increase blood pressure both during exercise and for a sustained period afterward.

Cardiovascular Disease (pp. 718–720)

• Aerobic exercise has long been used as part of cardiac rehabilitation in patients who have suffered from myocardial infarction or who have had cardiac surgery. It is also useful in helping prevent the atherosclerosis that causes so much morbidity and mortality in the Western world. It also lowers serum triglycerides and can alter serum cholesterol levels to increase the high-density/low-density lipoprotein (HDL/LDL) ratio.

• In addition to the benefits of reducing atherogenic risk factors, regular aerobic exercise helps to increase the body's aerobic endurance, as demonstrated by a higher $\dot{V}O_{2max}$. There is an increase in maximal cardiac output, an increase in stroke volume for a given level of $\dot{V}O_2$, and an increase in peripheral oxygen extraction. (This peripheral skeletal muscle adaptation has been identified as the primary cause of increased peak aerobic capacity in older patients with coronary artery disease.) Resting heart rate drops. The intensity of the exercise should most likely be moderate; high intensity is not necessarily more beneficial.

• Persons who regularly participate in an aerobic exercise program have an increased life expectancy and a decreased risk of coronary artery disease. They have a decreased heart rate and blood pressure response to submaximal exercise, an increase in $\dot{V}O_{2max}$, a decreased myocardial oxygen demand for a given workload, and decreased angina for a given workload (though anginal threshold for a given myocardial oxygen demand is unchanged). Ideally, exercise should be combined with healthy lifestyle changes and a proper diet. Such risk factor modification has been shown to reverse atherosclerosis to some extent.

Diabetes (p. 720)

• Inactivity causes a decreased peripheral sensitivity to insulin. Conversely, aerobic exercise increases the end-organ cell receptor sensitivity to insulin, primarily in the regions being exercised. This can be an important benefit in those with non-insulin-dependent diabetes mellitus (NIDDM). It may also reduce the other risk factors for diabetes. In insulin-dependent diabetes mellitus (IDDM), exercise has little effect, except that it lowers insulin requirements by utilizing circulating glucose.

Osteoporosis (p. 720)

• As described above, immobility causes a loss of bone mass, primarily in the weight-bearing bones. Conversely, exercise can help to maintain bone mass, and more active elderly women have been shown to have a lower rate of hip and vertebral fractures than their sedentary counterparts.

• The exercises that are most beneficial for maintaining bone mass are walking and running, rather than swimming. The exercise should be combined with adequate calcium intake, proper diet, and treatment of hypoestrogenemia, if appropriate (in young and postmenopausal women).

Sense of Well-Being, Pain Threshold, Sleep, and Immune Function (p. 720)

• Regular aerobic exercise is generally believed to raise the pain threshold, probably by stimulating the release of endogenous opiates. It is useful in conditions such as fibromyalgia, myofascial pain syndrome, chronic pain syndrome, and back pain. It also increases the general sense of well-being and helps to reduce anxiety, depression, and neuroticism.

Exercise in the Older Population (p. 720)

• Exercise earlier in life may help prevent some medical conditions, while later in life it may slow their progression. This can be true for osteoporosis, obesity, coronary artery disease, diabetes, and hypertension. In addition, exercise can increase strength in the elderly. The increase in strength can help prevent falls and other injuries, and exercise appears to improve the quality of life in the elderly. Before prescribing exercise in the older population, a proper screening evaluation is indicated. A proper exercise prescription, tailored to the appropriate activity level, is important as well.

Exercise in Women (pp. 720–721)

• The effect of aerobic exercise on the cardiovascular endurance of women is qualitatively similar to that of men, although women do not seem to be able to attain as high a $\dot{V}O_{2max}$ as men. The reaction of women to strength training is also qualitatively similar to that of men. Because of low levels of testosterone, women are unable to build as much muscle mass as men and thus do not generally attain as great a strength.

• In addition to the physiological effects just described, aerobic exercise can lessen the effects of premenstrual syndrome (PMS) and endometriosis. It also tends to normalize the menstrual cycle, though very heavy endurance exercise can adversely affect the cycle. Exercise in moderation has been shown to be safe for women with routine pregnancies. Although women should probably be counseled not to try to markedly increase their exercise load during pregnancy, moderate exercise is believed to be safe for both mother and fetus and can even improve the process of labor and postlabor recovery. It is important when exercising during pregnancy to avoid dehydration and hyperthermia. Hyperthermia is a teratogen.

Special Issues in the Disabled Population (p. 722)

• Sports are becoming increasingly available to persons with physical impairments. This is especially true for wheelchair athletes having paraplegia. Exercise in wheelchair athletes has been shown to increase $\dot{V}O_{2max}$, decrease cardiovascular disease and respiratory infection, improve self-image, improve psychological function, and decrease time hospitalized. These benefits come at a price: namely, an increase in traumatic and overuse injuries, shoulder pain and degeneration, compression neuropathies, and bladder and skin problems. When done carefully, however, the benefits outweigh the risks in most persons.

35

Original Chapter by Donna Jo Blake, M.D., and Dan D. Scott, M.D.

Employment of Persons with Disabilities

• Disability is a significant public health and social issue. Approximately 54 million noninstitutionalized Americans (almost one person in five) have a mental or physical disability, nearly half of whom can be considered to have a severe disability. And 37.7 million noninstitutionalized Americans (almost one person in seven) have limitations severe enough to prevent them from playing, attending school, working, maintaining a household, or caring for themselves.

DATA: IMPAIRMENT AND DISABILITY (pp. 728–729)

• Impairments caused by chronic disease have become increasingly significant as risk factors of disability. Table 35–1 shows the ranking, by percent of specific conditions, of persons who have functional limitations. Many of the conditions that are significant risk factors for disability are low in prevalence. For example, multiple sclerosis has a low overall prevalence, but is a significant risk factor for disability. Examination of this ranking shows seven out of the top ten disabling conditions to be conditions commonly managed by the physiatrist and the rehabilitation team.

SOCIOECONOMIC EFFECT OF DISABILITY (pp. 729–730)

• Disablement has significant socioeconomic consequences for the individual with disabilities and for society. When a person is unable to participate in his or her social role as a worker or homemaker because of a physical or mental condition, that person is said to have a work disability or a work participation restriction. Work participation restriction results in dependency and loss of productivity for that person. Society, in turn, incurs direct and indirect costs.

DISABILITY-RELATED PROGRAMS AND POLICIES
(pp. 730–731)

Programs (pp. 730–731)

• There is a plethora of disability-related programs and policies. The programs can be characterized as ameliorative or corrective. *Ameliorative programs*

TABLE 35-1 Conditions with Highest Risk of Disability

Chronic Condition	No. of Conditions*	% Causing Activity Limitation	Rank	% Causing Major Activity Limitation	Rank	% Causing Need for Help in Basic Life Activities	Rank
Mental retardation	1202	84.1	1	80.0	1	19.9†	9
Absence of leg(s)†	289	83.3	2	73.1	2	39.0†	2
Lung or bronchial cancer	200	74.8	3	63.5	3	34.5†	4
Multiple sclerosis†	171	70.6	4	63.3	4	40.7†	1
Cerebral palsy†	274	69.7	5	62.2	5	22.8†	8
Blind in both eyes	396	64.5	6	58.8	6	38.1†	3
Partial paralysis in extremity†	578	59.6	7	47.2	7	27.5†	5
Other orthopedic impairments†	316	58.7	8	42.6	8	14.3‡	12
Complete paralysis in extremity†	617	52.7	9	45.5	9	26.1†	6
Rheumatoid arthritis†	1223	51.0	10	39.4	12	14.9†	11
Intervertebral disk disorders†	3987	48.7	11	38.2	14	5.3†	—
Paralysis in other sites (complete/partial)†	247	47.8	12	43.7	10	14.1†	13
Other heart disease disorders§	4708	46.9	13	35.1	15	13.6†	14
Cancer of digestive tract	228	45.3	14	40.3	11	15.9‡	15
Emphysema	2074	43.6	15	29.8	—	9.6†	15
Absence of arm(s)/ hand(s)†	84	43.1	—	39.0	13	4.1‡	—
Cerebrovascular disease†	2599	38.2	—	33.3	—	22.9†	7

* In thousands.
† Conditions frequently managed by physiatrists.
‡ Figure has low statistical reliability or precision (relative standard error >39%).
§ Heart failure (9.8%), valve disorders (15.3%), congenital disorders (15.0%), other ill-defined heart conditions (59.9%).

provide payment for income support and medical care. *Corrective programs* facilitate the individual's ability to return to work and to reduce or remove the disablement.

• Disability-related programs can be categorized into three basic types: (1) cash transfers, (2) medical care programs, and (3) direct service programs (Table 35–2).

VOCATIONAL REHABILITATION (pp. 731–735)

• The objective of vocational rehabilitation is to allow persons with physical disabilities to engage in gainful employment. The Rehabilitation Act of 1973 authorized federal funding for state rehabilitation agencies to provide a variety of services to qualified persons with disabilities. The federal government supplies 80% of the funding for state vocational rehabilitation agencies, whereas the states must provide the remaining 20%.

Traditional Approaches to Vocational Rehabilitation
(pp. 731–734)

• A variety of approaches to vocational rehabilitation have been developed over the years. The traditional approach begins with referral of a person with a disability to a vocational rehabilitation counselor. The person with a disability, a physician, a social worker, or a case manager can also generate this referral. The initial referral includes medical records, documentation of disabilities and capabilities, and neuropsychological testing (if available).

TABLE 35–2 Disability-Related Programs

Type of Program	Specific Programs
Cash transfer	Social insurance: Social Security Disability Insurance
	Private insurance
	Indemnity compensation
	Income support: Supplemental Security
	Income, veterans' pensions, Aid to Families with Dependent Children
Medical care	Medicare
	Private disability insurance
	Veterans' programs
	Workers' compensation
	Tort settlements
	Medicaid
Direct services	Rehabilitation and vocational education
	Veterans' programs
	Services for persons with specific impairments
	General funded programs (e.g., food stamps, developmental disabilities, blind, mentally ill)
	Employment assistance programs (e.g., Comprehensive Employment Training Program)

From Berkowitz M, Hill MA: Disability and the labor market: An overview. In Berkowitz M, Hill MA (eds): Disability and the Labor Market: Economic Problems, Policies, and Programs. New York, ILR Press, 1989, pp. 1–28.

Aptitude Matching versus Work Sample (pp. 732–733)

• Vocational testing is performed to assess the client's level of general intelligence, achievement, aptitudes, interests, and work skills. This type of approach is known as "aptitude matching." When a client's aptitudes match a particular occupation, the counselor undertakes a job search.

• A work sample approach is often used in conjunction with aptitude batteries. The work sample approach measures general characteristics such as size discrimination, multilevel sorting, eye-hand-foot coordination, and dexterity. There is less focus on general intelligence, aptitude, or academic performance. Work samples can also evaluate the type of "work group" in which the client is most skilled.

Sheltered Workshops (p. 733)

• One of the problems with the traditional approach of the vocational rehabilitation agency has been its poor record of success, especially for persons with severe disabilities. As a result of the poor placement record, alternative strategies have been developed for enabling persons with disabilities to obtain gainful employment. These include sheltered workshops, day programs, transitional and supported employment, projects with industry, and independent living center–directed employment. A sheltered workshop is a "public non-profit organization certified by the U.S. Department of Labor to pay 'sub-minimum' wages to persons with diminished earning capacity." There are more than 5000 of these workshops, including Goodwill, Inc., serving approximately 250,000 persons with disabilities. This form of employment serves persons with severe disabilities including limited vision, mental illness, mental retardation, and alcoholism.

Day Programs (p. 733)

• Day programs are meant to provide supervised vocational activity for persons with severe disabilities, usually those with mental retardation or mental illness. These programs are funded by private and corporate sponsors as well as by state and federal agencies. They are not designed as a transition into competitive employment, nor do they allow community integration. They are geared toward providing supervised day activities while the caretakers of these persons work or perform their own daily routines. Activities are performed in facilities that serve only persons with disabilities.

Home-Based Programs (p. 733)

• Home-based programs can be funded by state vocational rehabilitation, insurance carriers, foundations and societies, or by other agencies. The person with a disability can perform a variety of jobs including telephone solicitation, typing, or computer-assisted occupations. Some examples include graphics, accounting, or drafting. Of these programs—sheltered workshops, day programs, and homebound programs—none emphasizes gainful employment in a nonsheltered integrated setting.

Other Programs for Employment (pp. 734–735)

Projects with Industry (p. 734)

• Projects with Industry (PWI) is a federally sponsored collaborative program established by the Vocational Rehabilitation Act. Employers design and provide training projects for specific job skills in cooperation with rehabilitation agencies. The goal of PWI is competitive employment for the participants.

Transitional and Supported Employment (pp. 734–735)
• Transitional and supported employment are two newer strategies for returning disabled persons to competitive, integrated gainful employment. Transitional employment consists of providing the job placement, training, and support services necessary to help persons move into independent or supported employment. Transitional employment is a short-term provision of services for a period not to exceed 18 months, and culminates in an independent or supported employment position.

Independent Living Centers (p. 735)
• The independent living center (ILC) movement has traditionally provided a core of nonvocational services such as housing, independent living skills, advocacy, and peer counseling. Just as supported employment has broadened its scope, so has the ILC movement. Both provide a combination of nonvocational and vocational services to persons with severe disabilities. ILCs often employ workers with disabilities as peer counselors and program administrators. The small business approach of supported employment has been successfully implemented by ILCs to place their clients in competitive community employment. As these two philosophies continue to merge and provide similar services to persons with severe disabilities, cooperative ventures between them will allow persons with severe disabilities to fully achieve their maximum level of independence.

DISINCENTIVES FOR VOCATIONAL REHABILITATION (p. 735)

• Despite changes over the years in public and political policies and attitudes, disincentives to entering "the mainstream" abound for persons with disabilities. In order to become eligible for cash and medical benefits through SSI and SSDI, persons with disabilities must prove that they have total and permanent or long-term disability and must meet strict eligibility criteria. Before meeting those criteria, the individual and the family typically must have suffered a series of indignities including exhausting all personal resources and submitting to significant bureaucratic red tape. "Red tape" means completing substantial paperwork, obtaining medical reports verifying disability, and enduring long waiting periods for commencement of benefits.
• Stereotypes about persons with disabilities being unproductive in society are pervasive. Individuals with disabilities often come to view themselves as totally dependent and unable to work. The government disability entitlement policies state that if you are unable to work, the government will take care of you.
• Employers' attitudes serve as another disincentive. Obstacles to qualified applicants with disabilities who want to participate in the work force include employers' ignorance about the capabilities of a potential employee with a disability, inaccessible work sites, transportation inaccessibility, and discrimination in hiring
• The physiatrist and other physicians can also provide disincentives for persons with disabilities by labeling them as "totally and permanently disabled" or by

restricting their activities. Emphasis should be on the capabilities of persons with disabilities and documentation of their functional abilities, both mental and physical.

INCENTIVES FOR VOCATIONAL REHABILITATION
(pp. 735–737)

• In an effort to overcome disincentives, government policymakers have created incentives for persons with disabilities and for potential employers. These incentives often have a long list of requirements and are very specific in wording in order to prevent abuse.

Incentives for the Individual (p. 736)

• Incentive programs are applicable depending on whether the person with a disability receives SSDI or SSI benefits, or both. SSDI work incentives will be discussed first. Table 35–3 presents a summary of the terminology and abbreviations for easy reference.

TABLE 35–3 Summary of Incentives for the Individual Receiving Benefits to Enter Work Activities

Social Security Disability Insurance (SSDI)	Disability benefits program based on medical disability and a worker's earnings covered by Social Security (Title II—Social Security Act)
Supplemental Security Income (SSI)	Disability benefits program based on medical disability and the amount of income a person receives (Title XVI—Social Security Act)
Trial work period (TWP)	Allows trial return to work to test work ability without affecting benefits (SSDI)
Substantial gainful activity (SGA)	Performance of significant and productive physical or mental work for pay or profit (over $500/mo for nonblind [SSDI and SSI] and $810/mo for blind recipients [SSDI only])
Extended period of eligibility (EPE)	Allows reinstatement of cash benefits without a waiting period if the worker's earnings fall below SGA level within 36 mos after TWP (SSDI)
Impairment-related work expenses (IRWE)	Allows costs for certain items to be deducted from earnings when figuring SGA level (SSI and SSDI)
Earned income exclusion (EIE)	Allows exclusion of a portion of earned income when figuring an individual's monthly benefit (SSI)
Blind work expenses (BWE)	Allows work-related expenses when figuring benefits (SSI)

Incentives for Industry (p. 737)

• Government policymakers have made various attempts to offer tax incentives to business and industry. In the main, these incentives have been directed at making the workplace accessible.

DISABILITY PREVENTION (pp. 737–738)

• With disability ranking as the nation's largest public health problem, it seems reasonable to interface the public health model of prevention with the ICIDH-2 model of disablement. The public health model defines three categories of prevention: primary, secondary, and tertiary.
• Primary prevention is intended for healthy persons, helping them to avoid the onset of a pathological condition. In persons with disabilities, primary prevention comprises efforts toward preventing a worsening of impairments.
• Secondary prevention is aimed at early identification and treatment of a pathological condition and reduction of risk factors for disablement. For persons with disabilities, there are many opportunities for preventing an impairment from limiting one or more activities. The ameliorative and corrective programs discussed above, including vocational rehabilitation strategies, are aimed at reducing activity limitation.
• Tertiary prevention focuses on arresting the progression of a pathological condition and on limiting further disablement. For people with disabilities, tertiary prevention is designed to limit the restriction of a person's participation in some area by the provision of a facilitator or the removal of a barrier. Environmental modifications, provision of services, removal of physical barriers, changes in social attitudes, or reform in legislation and policy are tertiary prevention strategies.

CONCLUSION (p. 738)

• Comprehensive rehabilitation is an intervention directed at human functioning. The desired outcome is to maximize the physical, mental, social, and economic function of the individual with disabilities.
• Vocational rehabilitation is an intervention aimed at preventing an impairment from limiting activities and limiting participation in work. Employment of persons with disabilities supports a better quality of life and promotes function.

ISSUES IN SPECIFIC DIAGNOSES IN PHYSICAL MEDICINE AND REHABILITATION

36

Original Chapter by John J. Nicholas, M.D.

Rehabilitation of Patients with Rheumatological Disorders

• The rheumatic diseases that are most appropriately treated by rehabilitation techniques include rheumatoid arthritis (RA), osteoarthritis (OA), ankylosing spondylitis (AS) and the other spondyloarthropathies, systemic lupus erythematosus (SLE), progressive systemic sclerosis (PSS), polymyositis/dermatomyositis (DM/PMD), and postoperative arthroplasty patients.

EVALUATION OF PATIENTS (p. 745)

Specific Historical Details (p. 745)

• Before prescribing a comprehensive rehabilitation program, the physiatrist must obtain specific information regarding rheumatological patients.

Functional screen: Can the patient perform such ADL tasks as dressing, bathing, feeding, toileting hygiene and transfers, and walking (see Chapter 1)?

Vocational screen: Can the patient get into and out of a car and get into and out of a parking place? Are ergonomic changes required at work, or is a different job necessary (see Chapter 35)?

Physical Examination Techniques (p. 745)

Range-of-Motion Testing. In patients with rheumatic disease the range of motion (ROM) is commonly limited in one or more joints. The examiner should estimate and record the active and passive range of motion of involved joints and determine whether subluxation or dislocation is present. The examiner also records if pain limits motion, or if there is a pain-free limit to the motion. Each joint having limited motion should be compared with its plain radiographs and to the joints on the opposite side. Swollen, deformed, hot, or unstable joints should be noted.

Manual Muscle Testing. The manual muscle test cannot be performed accurately at a joint in which muscle contraction causes pain. The examiner should record whether or not pain is present during muscle contraction and should estimate strength (see Chapter 1). Muscle weakness should be noted, together with a characterization of its distribution as proximal, distal, lateral, or generalized pattern.

The examiner should also take note of medications (e.g., ACS, lovastatin, or hydroxychloroquine) being used that potentially affect muscles.

THERAPEUTIC MODALITIES (pp. 745–747)
Heat and Cold (pp. 745–746)

• Superficial heat is more commonly used than deep heat for treating rheumatic conditions and is considered more beneficial and better tolerated than deep heat.
• Many patients prefer cold to heat. Some patients feel cold is followed by better ROM than hot packs. Trial and patient preference should direct the prescription of heat or cold for rheumatic disease.
• Applications such as moist heat packs, moist heating pads, hot showers, and paraffin baths produce at least temporary diminution in pain and increased ability to move and exercise inflamed joints. There is no scientific evidence to demonstrate that heat improves or increases joint erosions; therefore, superficial heat should be applied before exercising.

Other Modalities for Patients with Rheumatic Disorders (p. 746)

• Various modalities have been tried in the treatment of patients with rheumatic disease, and some scientific evidence supports their efficacy. Nylon spandex compression gloves can be helpful in relieving rheumatoid discomfort, especially in those patients with excessive finger stiffness.
• Topical counterirritant ointments (e.g., capsaicin and trolamine salicylate) have been found to decrease hand and finger pain in patients with OA.
• The use of transcutaneous electronic nerve stimulation (TENS) has been reported for many conditions (see Chapter 22). Improved wrist and hand function with TENS has been reported in RA patients. Unfortunately, application of TENS to hands and wrists is limited by its awkwardness. Selected patients with OA of the knees gain considerable pain relief with application of TENS to the knees.

Relief of Joint Contractures (pp. 746–747)

• Patients with various forms of inflammatory rheumatic diseases or OA can lose full ROM. Historically, such joint contractures have been a great problem, but in contemporary medicine are now commonly relieved by surgical arthroplasty.
• When joint contractures secondary to rheumatic disorders are treated with serial casting or splinting, the results are directly related to the severity of the joint destruction as demonstrated by radiographs (i.e., the better the x-ray appearance, the better the result). Treatment can be provided with various materials (e.g., plaster, fiberglass, plastic). Full cylinder casts, posterior splints, and splints with cuffs have all been used successfully when applied in a position of maximum extension without excessive force and removed for hygiene every day. At the end of 5 to 7 days, the casts or splints are replaced and more extension is noted. The last 10 degrees of extension is typically the most difficult to achieve. The total ROM usually does not change, but the ROM shifts toward the extension limits rather than the flexion limits of joint motion.

APPROACHES TO SPECIFIC RHEUMATIC DISEASES
(pp. 747–753)

Rheumatoid Arthritis (pp. 747–750)

Pain Relief (p. 747)
• The time-honored treatment of joint pain in RA has been application of moist heat. This has been accomplished through various devices including moist heating packs, electric mittens, hot showers, hot water, and spas. It has been demonstrated in normal subjects that hot packs provide heat (lasting for about 15 minutes), to a depth of 1 to 1.5 cm. The frequency of application is guided by cost, custom, and convenience, but should be at least twice daily. Because burns can occur with moist heat, the patient must be tested for sensory deficits before moist heat is used. Additional contraindications to heat are listed in Chapter 21.
• The application of splints, mostly for wrists and knees, has been shown to relieve pain in inflamed RA joints. The chief drawbacks that decrease the use of splints for pain relief are poor cosmesis and inconvenience. Patients often choose to wear them despite these drawbacks. They are particularly helpful during heavy-use activities.

Prevention and Correction of Deformities (pp. 747–748)
• Most deformities in RA are predictable (Table 36–1); however, hand deformities (e.g., swan's neck or boutonnière) are much less predictable.

TABLE 36–1 Predictions of Deformities* in Rheumatoid Arthritis

Joint	Deformity	Position of Splinting
Head and neck	Flexion, rotation	Full extension, cervical spine, chin forward
Dorsal spine	Flexion, chest flat	Full extension
Shoulder	Adduction, internal rotation	90 degrees abduction, neutral rotation
Elbow	Flexion, pronation	90 degrees flexion, 10 degrees supination
Wrist	Palmar flexion	30 degrees dorsiflexion
Thumb	Flexion	Extension, apposition
Finger	Flexion, ulnar deviation	Extension, no lateral deviation
Hips	Flexion, adduction, external rotation	Extension; in line with body; foot pointing upward
Knee	Flexion	Extension
Ankle	Plantar flexion	Right angle to leg
Foot	Valgus, spread of forefoot	No varus or valgus, upward pressure beneath second, third, and fourth metatarsal bones
Toe	Plantar flexion in phalangeal joints, flexion at metatarsophalangeal joints	In line with plantar surface of foot

* The deformities consequent to chronic rheumatoid arthritis have not changed since Dr. Steinbrocker first recorded them, and are thus quite predictable.
From Steinbrocker O: Arthritis in Modern Practice. Philadelphia, WB Saunders, 1947.

- Deformity treatment and prevention require persistent, tedious compliance on the part of the patient. Initially, the application of moist heat to the joints followed by ROM active stretching exercises helps reduce the contracture if the inflammation is relieved or is not too severe. In more severe cases, protective splints should be applied. Spinal and other joint manipulation (see Chapter 20) has not been shown to prevent or correct these deformities.
- Knees and wrist splints are most easily fitted. Several varieties of resting wrist and hand splints are available (see Fig. 36–1 in the Textbook). Molded shoe insoles of materials such as plastizote can be used in combination with "extra-depth" shoes to provide support and spread of pressure. This can relieve pain, extend walking range, and slow progression of deformities such as protruding metatarsal heads.
- Many ADL assistive devices are available to substitute for deformed joints and conserve energy (see Fig. 36–3 in the Textbook and Chapter 25). The concept is that if the patient does not overstress or overuse a joint, and avoids biomechanical torques that excessively bend the wrist and fingers, these deformities can be prevented or limited.

Increasing Strength and Endurance (p. 749)
- Most patients with RA complain of weakness, feel chronically tired, and often do not want to exercise. The clinician can usually demonstrate these deficiencies, which range from diminished $\dot{V}o_{2max}$ to decreased strength on manual muscle testing. There are only minimal changes on microscopic examination of muscles of patients with RA, and even steroid-induced myopathy is amenable to improvement by strengthening exercises.
- Exercise can also be harmful to patients with RA. A patient who has been on a shopping spree or has cleaned the house for guests is a likely candidate for general and specific joint flareups. Many patients know this and often ask for joint injections before undertaking extra work or special activity.
- Because patients complained of weakness and fatigue, several investigators exercised patients with RA and discovered that both strength and endurance can be increased without marked increase in joint pain or signs of inflammation following exercise.
- It is prudent for the physician to try to suppress the inflammation as much as possible before prescribing exercise. The exercise should be performed under careful, controlled conditions, and the patient and the physician should monitor the exercised joints for an increase in joint inflammation. Because long-term follow-up studies are not now available, the patient should be cautioned that moderation must be used.

Psychosocial Counseling (pp. 749–750)
- Patients with RA can be depressed or suffer multiple social problems, mood swings, fatigue, and frustration. Early detection of social and interpersonal problems allows early referral for treatment. Social service or psychological evaluation on a rehabilitation unit can often help such problems. A trial of antidepressants and referral to a psychiatrist might be necessary.
- Patients often find that the physical demands of the workplace exceed their physical capability. Minimal changes in the ergonomics of their workstation, or perhaps something as simple as obtaining a permit to park closer to the workplace, can prolong employment. In general, the employment rate diminishes in direct proportion to the length of time a patient has RA. The physician encoun-

tering a patient with early RA is well advised to evaluate the work situation and suggest that the patient begin training for lighter work immediately.

• Discussion of sexual function in patients with RA is helpful. It is likely that sexual difficulties can arise because of mechanical problems and problems with medication. Mechanical problems related to disease of the hip joint can be treated, if necessary, with total hip arthroplasty. Other difficulties often respond to a change in medication or counseling.

Osteoarthritis (pp. 750–751)

• Patients with OA typically have only one or a few joints involved. The pathological process begins with histological changes and ends in frank destruction of joint cartilage. There is an increase in the density of the bone adjacent to the joint, and bony excrescences (osteophytes) occur at the margins of the joints. Osteoarthritis occurs most commonly in older patients, but it can affect younger ones as well. It is often associated with conditions of previous joint damage, excessive wear, or obesity; and the relationship to exercise and work is probable but not clear.

Shoulders (p. 750)

• Osteoarthritis of the shoulders usually occurs in older patients and can be associated with excessive joint destruction or rotator cuff wear or rupture. Patients should be taught range of motion and isometric exercises to maintain mobility and strengthen the shoulder musculature. Intra-articular steroid injections of the glenohumeral joint can also help. The clinician must be alert to the presence of other shoulder problems (e.g., biceps tendinitis, subdeltoid bursitis, and acromioclavicular arthritis) that can compound or mimic the symptoms of shoulder OA.

Elbows (p. 750)

• Osteoarthritis of the elbow occurs after trauma, joint overuse, or inflammatory joint disease. Injections often provide symptomatic relief (see Chapter 24), and full ROM is not totally necessary. The patient needs only to be able to flex the elbow sufficiently to get the hand to the mouth and face for eating and hygiene. Neoprene elbow sleeves help diminish pain, but should be removed and cleaned often to avoid moisture build-up and fungal growth.

Hip (p. 750)

• Osteoarthritis of the hip is common. Although it can be caused by congenital dislocation, previous infections, or aseptic necrosis, it is generally idiopathic. The pain may be relieved initially by having the patient ambulate with a cane in the contralateral hand. Isometric gluteus medius and gluteus maximus exercises can increase hip pain, so they are not practical for some patients. Steroids are difficult to inject into the joint without fluoroscopic guidance. Most patients now receive total hip arthroplasty for intractable hip OA. Before or after surgery, a shoe lift may be required to correct leg-length discrepancies. Patients who have difficulties performing ADL or ambulation often need admission to a rehabilitation unit or center to maximize their recovery and function.

Knee (pp. 750–751)

• Osteoarthritis of the knee is associated with obesity in women but has not been shown to result from osteochondritis dissecans or athletic activities. Quadriceps muscle strength in patients with OA of the knees has been shown to be consistently weak. Intra-articular steroid injections temporarily diminish pain and may increase the ability to perform exercises, as does the application of a moist heating pad. The use of elastic bandages, neoprene sleeves, or canvas braces can improve proprioception about the knee and diminish arthrogenous muscle inhibition. Many patients note an increased sense of stability and strength and diminished pain with these knee orthoses.

• Use of a cane or crutches helps by relieving some of the weight-bearing stress in the knee. Wearing shoes with soft soles such as those of Vibram diminishes knee pain in many patients with OA of the knees.

• Multiple-angle isometric exercises performed at the knee increase strength throughout the knee ROM and relieve the pain of OA.

Base of the Thumb (p. 751)

• Osteoarthritis of the base of the thumb (carpometacarpal and metacarpophalangeal joints) is a common cause of pain. In this case, a thumb spica that immobilizes these two joints of the thumb can be helpful (Fig. 36–1). Although it is somewhat awkward and interferes with some ADL, it does provide consistent relief of pain.

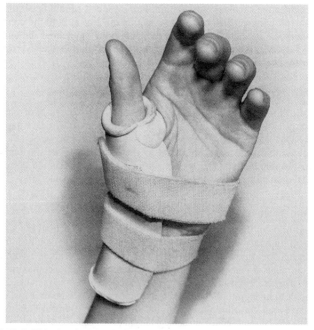

FIGURE 36–1. This thumb spica immobilizes the carpometacarpal and metacarpophalangeal joints of the thumb but still allows fairly dexterous use of the hand.

Cervical Spine (p. 751)
• Osteoarthritis of the cervical spine, which is common in the elderly, can cause symptoms of radiculopathy, caused by osteophytes that impinge on nerve roots; and myelopathy, caused by bony overgrowth that causes spinal cord compression. The x-ray evidence of OA of the cervical spine is common; nevertheless, symptoms of OA are rare. If bony osteophytes can be determined to be a cause of radiculopathy, treatment with a cervical collar or traction with the neck in flexion to hold open the interforaminal spaces can help. Cervical myelopathy from OA usually requires surgical treatment (see Chapter 37).

Lumbosacral Spine and Spinal Stenosis (p. 751)
• Spinal stenosis has been shown to be a common cause of lumbosacral myelopathy and polyradiculopathy, especially involving the L3 and L4 roots. The pain of lumbosacral spinal stenosis is brought on by walking or standing and relieved by sitting or lying. It can occur at night if congestive heart failure is present. Epidural injections and a brace to hold the spine in slight lumbosacral flexion can provide temporary relief. NSAIDs are also helpful in many patients. Exercises have a small part to play in the treatment of this condition, but extension of the spine increases symptoms. If polyradiculopathy is significant and the patient does not wish surgery, a plastic ankle-foot orthosis for foot-drop may help.
• Radiologic OA of the lumbosacral spine is almost universal in middle-aged to elderly persons. Myelopathy and radiculopathy, however, are rare in these patients. Symptoms of back pain in adults at an age when OA is prevalent should be carefully studied to find the exact cause, which may be cancer, infection, osteoporosis, or compression fracture. Osteoarthritis is diagnosed in this age group only by exclusion.

Foot (p. 751)
• Hallux valgus of the great toe and cock-up deformity of digits II-V are the most common expressions of OA in the feet. A deep-toe box shoe (extra depth) with a molded insole to accommodate dropped metatarsal heads is helpful. However, rocker-bottom soles, to compensate for a stiffened great toe (hallux rigidis), often make walking difficult and unstable. Surgical procedures are often helpful for this deformity.

Psoriatic Arthritis (pp. 751–752)

• Psoriatic arthritis occurs in a small subgroup of patients who have psoriasis. The arthritis is characterized by tendonitis, enthesitis, and synovitis of both peripheral and spinal joints in various clinical pictures. The physician should look for psoriatic lesions in all of these patients, and examination of the scalp, anal area, and umbilicus may reveal hidden psoriatic plaques.
• The rehabilitation of psoriasis patients requires detailed attention to the joints most severely involved. Patients with tendonitis and synovitis of the toes should be supplied with high-toe box shoes having soft leather uppers. A heel lift and a longitudinal arch support are helpful for associated plantar fascitis. Intra-articular injections may help individual finger joints and others. Paraffin baths provide moist heat to inflamed fingers for pain relief. Splinting individual proximal or distal interphalangeal joints can relieve pain, but will not prevent deformity in the long run.

• Inflammation and pain in the costochondral joints may require individual injections and the use of superficial heat. If significant spondylitis is present with stiffness and progressive deformity, spinal extension exercises (e.g., walking into the corner with abducted arms and performing push-ups) should be emphasized.

Ankylosing Spondylitis (p. 752)

• Ankylosing spondylitis (AS) is inflammation of the enthesis (the tissue attaching tendons and joint capsules to bone) plus synovitis of the spinal joints. Inflammation of the synovial joints and tendons of the spine heals by ossification, causing the spine to become progressively more rigid and stiff. The spine usually becomes stiff in flexion rather than extension, probably because of the posture of the patient. Inflammation of the uveal tract (iritis) and aortic valve disease also occurs in AS. The condition is similar in some ways to Reiter's syndrome and psoriatic arthritis, but is distinguished because it is predominantly a disease of the spine.

• No studies to date have demonstrated that exercises, braces, or medications preserve the flexibility of the spine or prevent stiffening. The physician's job is to keep the spine as functional as possible, despite gradual stiffening. The physician must make certain that the spine is becoming stiff in extension rather than flexion by measuring the patient at each visit with Schober's test. This is performed by measuring the distance from the patient's occiput to the wall while standing in maximum extension with heels against the wall, and measuring the expansion of the thoracic cage at the third to the fourth intercostal spaces.

• Exercises thought to maintain the erect posture include push-ups and "walking into corners" with the hands on the occiput and the shoulders abducted. The patient must be constantly reminded to attempt to maintain an erect posture and to sleep on a firm mattress with the spine extended as much as possible. Other individual synovial joints can be involved, and NSAIDs, other systemic medication, or intra-articular steroids may be required.

• The physiatrist should assist the patient with AS in the battle to maintain upright posture and not allow the patient to slip into noncompliance with daily exercises. If an arthroplasty is performed, it should be remembered that postoperative heterotopic ossification is more common in patients with AS than in those with RA or OA.

Scleroderma and Progressive Systemic Sclerosis (p. 752)

• Patients with progressive systemic sclerosis (PSS) form excessive amounts of abnormal collagen, which causes thickening of the skin and difficulty moving the joints, especially those of the fingers, shoulders, and knees. Systemic involvement can occur, with the fibrosis affecting the gastrointestinal tract, respiratory tract, cardiovascular system, muscles, and kidneys. Kidney disease is a leading cause of death in patients with PSS. A variant of PSS called the CREST syndrome consists of subcutaneous *c*alcinosis; *R*aynaud's phenomenon; *e*sophageal dysfunction; *s*clerodactyly; and *t*elangiectasia, often of the lips and fingers. These patients usually have less joint restriction.

• The rehabilitation techniques for preventing joint contractures of PSS have been only partially successful but must not be ignored. Patients with myopathy or localized myopathy commonly respond to exercise therapy and decrease of

ACS doses, but the creatine phosphokinase levels must be monitored. Splinting does not typically help finger function; but plaster casts can be used to cover painful ulcers, and patients can be offered finger exercises to maintain strength.
• Speech pathologists and occupational therapists should become involved in treating dysphagia, and can help the patient by determining the appropriate swallowing technique and food consistency (see Chapter 26).

Dermatomyositis/Polymyositis (pp. 752–753)

• Dermatomyositis/polymyositis (DM/PM) is a disease characterized by inflammation of the muscle, with or without a rash. It is divided into five varieties: PM in adults, DM in adults, PM/DM in adults with malignancy, childhood PM/DM, and DM/PM with collagen vascular disease. Regardless of the variety, the physiatrist is faced with a patient who has weakness, usually of the proximal muscles, although distal muscle involvement has been described. Joint disease is rare. Subcutaneous calcinosis occurs commonly in children and can limit joint ROM. Weakness of the respiratory muscles and the muscles of swallowing can result in aspiration pneumonia and subsequent lung dysfunction, which has been negatively linked to survival in this disease. (See Chapters 11, 12, and 48 for further information on myopathy diagnosis.)
• Preserving and increasing muscle strength are main rehabilitation goals. Isometric, resistive, and functional exercises have been shown to be beneficial in DM/PM. It is recommended that exercise be initiated early in the course of DM/PM, preferably within the first 2 years.
• A dilemma commonly occurs when it must be decided whether the patient with increasing weakness has an exacerbation of DM/PM or has steroid myopathy from ACS treatment. The evaluation of serum muscle enzymes, electromyography, muscle biopsy, or a trial of steroids is often required to resolve this dilemma. A trial of increased oral ACS increases strength if active DM/PM is the problem.
• If persistent or chronic weakness cannot be improved, the patient might require fitting with a plastic ankle-foot orthoses to stabilize the knees and ankles and prevent foot-drop (see Chapter 16). In addition, assistive living devices to help with toileting, hygiene, eating, and dressing are often required (see Chapter 25). Wheelchairs or electrically powered wheel carts are helpful in many patients (see Chapter 18). The patient with suspected dysphagia should be referred for a swallowing evaluation and proper dietary precautions taken (see Chapter 26).
• It is still controversial whether or not the physician should extensively test all DM/PM patients for possible malignancy. Adults with a rash are thought most likely to have a malignancy.

Systemic Lupus Erythematosus (p. 753)

• SLE is a systemic immune-mediated disorder, but one of its major manifestations is a mild but painful synovitis that resembles RA. The synovitis results in weakening of tendinous and capsular structures so that the hands demonstrate the deformities characteristic of RA (e.g., ulnar deviation and subluxation of the metacarpophalangeal joints, and boutonnière and swan's neck deformities of the proximal interphalangeal joints). These joint findings are termed nonerosive deforming arthritis or Jaccoud's arthritis and are not RA. If tolerated, lively splints (i.e., powered by springs or rubber bands) to help hold the hands and fingers in place during activities, can be helpful.

- Avascular necrosis occurs with increased frequency in SLE patients independent of treatment with steroids. The knees, hips, shoulders, and other joints are commonly involved. At initial diagnosis, consideration must be given to orthopedic surgery, but the pain can often be relieved by causing less weight to be distributed to the involved joint through the use of a walker, canes, crutches, or other ambulation aids.
- Patients with SLE also have ruptures of the patellar and Achilles tendons, with or without association with ACS. Following repair and diminution of steroid dose, muscle-strengthening exercises must be initiated. Both functional electrical stimulation and biofeedback can help to train patients to once again contract these weak muscles after tendon repair.
- Patients with SLE can also have systemic involvement: wolf-like skin rash, renal failure, central and peripheral nervous system abnormalities, hematological problems (including hemolytic anemia and idiopathic thrombocytopenic purpura), and systemic cutaneous vasculitis. Pleurisy is a common accompaniment of lung disease, and it has been suggested that TENS can help manage the pain of this transient phenomenon.
- SLE patients often have a bland vasculitis of the central nervous system. Psychological testing and counseling are appropriate, and the psychological status must be considered when prescribing exercise or splints because of potential compliance problems.

MAXIMIZING COMPLIANCE WITH TREATMENT
(pp. 753–754)

- It is not yet possible to formulate a definitive list of reasons why patients do not comply with exercise, splint wearing, and other modalities. It has been suggested that the physician or other health professional discuss frankly with all patients whether or not they are compliant, and attempt to discover the specific reasons in each case.

REHABILITATION FOLLOWING ARTHROPLASTY
(pp. 754–756)

Hip Arthroplasty (p. 755)

- Following hip arthroplasty, the physiatrist must determine the weight-bearing status of each patient. With a cemented prosthesis, patients are immediately allowed to bear weight. With an uncemented prosthesis, weight bearing may be limited to touch-down for as long as 8 weeks. Touch-down weight bearing is preferred over non–weight bearing so that the patient may go through the motions of walking without actually bearing significant weight in order to maintain walking reflexes and muscular proprioception. Patients are immediately taught range-of-motion exercises and mild isometric exercises to re-educate muscles that have been inactive and to avoid contractures. Patients are taught to walk with crutches or a walker before going home so that they can maintain weight-bearing status. They generally do not cease use of a walking device until they can walk without a limp or Trendelenburg gait.
- Patients must also be taught precautions in order to avoid dislocating their hip prosthesis. With the standard posterolateral incision (capsular weakness posterior) they must avoid hyperflexion, hyperadduction, and excessive internal rota-

tion or they may lever the head of the femoral component out through the posterior capsule. Patients with anterior incisions must avoid hyperextension. Hip dislocations usually occur shortly after surgery, and this incidence diminishes over time. Patients who have undergone revision commonly are fitted with an abductor brace with an adjustable hip hinge (Newport brace) to limit adduction, internal rotation, and flexion while healing takes place. Conditions associated with increased postoperative dislocation are small femoral head, previous surgery, posterior approach, component malposition, osteotomy of the greater trochanter, a short femoral component, alcoholism, older age, and organic brain disease.

Complications (p. 755)

• Heterotopic ossification may be prevented by low-dose radiation and, possibly, nonsteroidal anti-inflammatory agents. Nerve injuries following hip arthroplasty occur most commonly in the common peroneal in the leg and the ulnar nerve in the hand. Femoral, obturator, lateral femoral cutaneous, brachial plexus, ulnar, axillary, and median nerve injuries have been described. If the leg is lengthened, the sciatic nerve may be damaged. Compartment syndrome and hematomas (potentially curable causes) can also be involved in postoperative neuropathies.
• Deep venous thrombosis following arthroplasty is common and is usually prevented with prophylactic coumadin. Low-molecular-weight heparin and compression stockings have also been advocated.
• Postoperative pain gradually subsides over a few days. If pain persists or there is an acute exacerbation, radiographs should be taken to attempt to discover a dislocation. Signs of inflammation around the wound and drainage should be brought to the attention of the orthopedic surgeon. If superficial infection is suspected, a culture should be obtained and antibiotics started. Deep infections ordinarily are not clinically obvious until after rehabilitation has been completed.
• Leg length discrepancies often appear because of contractures around the hip or because of extremity shortening. The prescription of a shoe lift should be delayed until any contractures have been eliminated.

Knee Arthroplasty (pp. 755–756)

Rehabilitation (pp. 755–756)

• The most difficult rehabilitation problems are obtaining full flexion and extension of the knee. Vigorous passive exercises are prescribed almost immediately postoperatively. Most knee prostheses are now cemented; therefore, partial weight bearing is necessary only when grafting or tendon or muscle tears have occurred and been repaired. Weight bearing is allowed very promptly, and most patients are able to bear weight. An exception is bilateral knee arthroplasties, performed when the patient does not have a good knee. In spite of postoperative pain, patients must be encouraged to flex and extend their knees and utilize their muscles. Sometimes biofeedback or FES may help, but usually the services of a skilled and persistent therapist will suffice.
• The use of passive motion machines postoperatively is quite controversial. Unless the patient utilizes the machine for an unusually long time, no improvement has been demonstrated. Preoperative exercise has not been shown to shorten the length of stay or to decrease the complication rate.

Complications (p. 756)

• Complications following knee arthroplasty have been well described. Peroneal palsy may occur, and surgical exploration may be indicated if direct compression from a hematoma is suspected. Complex regional pain syndrome is rare and requires aggressive treatment. Fractures can occur proximal to the total knee prosthesis, and x-rays are again required for patients who have persistent pain. Deep infections are associated with the use of constrained prostheses, previous surgery, open skin lesions, and rheumatoid arthritis.

• Deep venous thrombosis occurs with alarming frequency following total knee arthroplasty. Anticoagulation with coumadin or heparin is appropriate, and ultrasound Doppler studies should be ordered whenever they seem indicated.

• There are also problems associated with the knee extensor mechanism following knee arthroplasty. Some of these include an unstable patella, a patellar "clunk," or patellar tendon rupture.

Shoulder Arthroplasty (p. 756)

• Complications of shoulder arthroplasty include technical error, instability, rotator cuff tears, heterotopic ossification, loosening, modular component dislocation, sepsis, humeral fracture, and nerve injuries.

• Rehabilitation of the patient with a shoulder arthroplasty should begin on the first postoperative day, and each surgeon probably will recommend his/her own individual protocol. Initial active assisted exercise should be prescribed, avoiding excessive shoulder internal rotation and adduction. Minimal abduction and external rotation is performed until a relatively pain-free arc of motion occurs, and then the activity is extended to approximately 140 degrees of flexion and 40 degrees of external rotation. When nearly full ROM has been achieved, isometric exercises, assistive exercises, and pulley exercises should be employed to strengthen muscles. Weight training is sometimes advised at 12 weeks postoperatively.

37

Original Chapter by Francis P. Lagattuta, M.D., and Frank J. E. Falco, M.D.

Assessment and Treatment of Cervical Spine Disorders

• Many of the conditions that can lead to pain and other associated symptoms in the neck are listed in Table 37–1.

ANATOMY AND BIOMECHANICS (pp. 762–768)

Osseous Structures (pp. 763–765)

• The cervical column is made up of seven vertebrae (Fig. 37–1). The C1 (atlas) and C2 (axis) are considerably different from other vertebrae in the spinal column.

• The lower cervical vertebrae (C3 to C7) have unique articulations called uncovertebral joints, which are also known as joints of Luschka or neurocentral joints (see Fig. 37–4 in the Textbook). They arise from the posterolateral margins of the vertebral bodies and lie anterior to the exiting nerve roots. These joints are not present at birth, but develop by the end of the first decade. These articulations can degenerate by undergoing hypertrophy and calcification with associated disk degeneration. This process can ultimately lead to encroachment on the intervertebral canal, causing nerve root or even spinal cord compression.

Soft Tissue Structures (pp. 765–766)

• Intervertebral disks are located in the cervical spine between the C2 through T1 vertebrae. The intervertebral disks provide shock absorption, accommodate movement, and separate the vertebral bodies to give height to the intervertebral foramina. The disk is made up of the eccentrically located nucleus pulposus and the surrounding annulus fibrosus.

• There are several ligaments found at each vertebral level that give strength and stability to the cervical spine. The transverse, alar, and accessory atlantoaxial ligaments help maintain the integrity of the odontoid and C1 articulation. The anterior (ALL) and posterior longitudinal ligaments (PLL) run along the anterior and posterior surfaces of the vertebrae and disks, providing stability during flexion and extension. The PLL also reinforce the posterior annulus. The

TABLE 37–1 Disorders Affecting the Neck

Mechanical	Tumors
Cervical sprain	Benign tumors
Cervical strain	Osteochondroma
Herniated nucleus pulposus	Osteoid osteoma
Osteoarthritis	Osteoblastoma
Cervical spondylosis	Giant cell tumor
Cervical stenosis	Aneurysmal bone cyst
Rheumatologic	Hemangioma
Ankylosing spondylitis	Eosinophilic granuloma
Reiter's syndrome	Gaucher's disease
Psoriatic arthritis	Malignant tumors
Enteropathic arthritis	Multiple myeloma
Rheumatoid arthritis	Solitary plasmacytoma
Diffuse idiopathic skeletal hyperostosis (DISH)	Chondrosarcoma
Polymyalgia rheumatica (PMR)	Ewing's sarcoma
Fibrositis (fibromyalgia)	Chordoma
Infectious	Lymphoma
Vertebral osteomyelitis	Metastases
Discitis	Extradural tumors
Herpes zoster	Epidural hemangioma
Infective endocarditis	Epidural lipoma
Granulomatous process	Meningioma
Epidural, intradural, and subdural abscesses	Neurofibroma
Retropharyngeal abscess	Lymphoma
Acquired immunodeficiency syndrome (AIDS)	Intradural tumors
Endocrinological and metabolic	Extramedullary, intradural
Osteoporosis	Neurofibroma
Osteomalacia	Meningioma
Parathyroid disease	Ependymoma
Paget's disease	Sarcoma
Pituitary disease	Intramedullary
	Ependymoma
	Astrocytoma
	Arteriovenous malformations
	Syringomyelia

facet capsule ligaments, supraspinous, interspinous, and ligamentum flavum ligaments provide flexion stability. The ligamentum nuchae spans from the occiput to the C7 spinous process and adds support to the posterior neck.

Neural Structures (pp. 766–767)

• The spinal cord begins at the foramen magnum and extends to approximately the L2 vertebral level. The spinal canal is the widest at C3 to C5, and rapidly decreases in size to a small circular lumen throughout the thoracic area.
• The union of the ventral motor and dorsal sensory roots (Fig. 37–2) forms spinal nerves. All of the cervical nerves contain motor and sensory fibers except

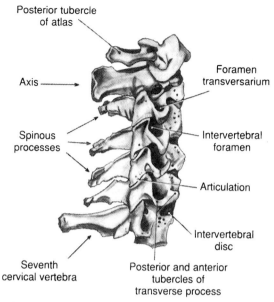

Posterior tubercle
of atlas

Axis

Spinous
processes

Foramen
transversarium

Intervertebral
foramen

Articulation

Intervertebral
disc

Seventh
cervical vertebra

Posterior and anterior
tubercles of
transverse process

FIGURE 37–1. Lateral view of the cervical spine. (From Crafts RC: Textbook of Human Anatomy, ed 2. New York, John Wiley & Sons, 1979. Reprinted by permission of John Wiley & Sons, Inc.)

for the C1 nerve, which has only motor fibers. Cervical spinal nerves exit through the root canals, dividing into anterior and posterior rami. The anterior rami supply the prevertebral and paravertebral muscles and form the brachial plexus to provide innervation for the upper limbs. The posterior rami divide into muscular, cutaneous, and articular branches for the posterior neck structures, including the postvertebral muscles.
• The cervical intervertebral disks receive innervation to the outer third of the annulus anteriorly, posteriorly, and laterally (see Fig. 37–8 in the Textbook). The cervical zygapophyseal joints are innervated by the medial branches from the posterior cervical rami.

Pain Generators (pp. 767–768)

• Many structures in the neck can be potential pain generators.
• Any structure that receives innervation can be a potential pain generator. Injury or compromise of the cervical nerves can cause radicular pain as well as weakness and sensory loss. Nerve injuries can be caused by a disk herniation, an uncovertebral joint impingement, brachial plexopathy, tumor, hematoma, infection, and metabolic or direct trauma. Radicular symptoms include pain into the shoulder and beyond, sensory loss, paresthesias, and weakness. Specific peripheral nerves can be injured, an example being an injury to the occipital nerve producing occipital neuralgia with headaches.

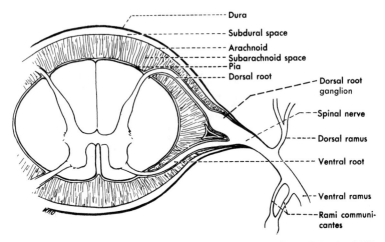

FIGURE 37–2. Formation of spinal nerves from the spinal cord. (From Hollinshead WH, Jenkins DB: Functional Anatomy of the Limbs and Back, ed 5. Philadelphia, WB Saunders, 1981, p. 218.)

HISTORY (pp. 768–769)

Chief Complaint (p. 768)

• Cervical conditions can present with a chief complaint involving the neck or the upper limb. An individual might complain of upper limb pain, numbness, or weakness. The patient can have headaches, visual disturbances, dizziness, or jaw pain. Difficulty in performing activities of daily living, bladder dysfunction, or bowel incontinence can also be the presenting concern.

History of Present Illness (p. 768)

• The history is used to generate a differential diagnosis from a chronological account of the current disorder.
• The onset, duration, origin, and distribution of symptoms, as well as the mechanism of injury, can provide significant clues to the pathophysiology of the disorder.
• Documentation of modifying activities can give additional diagnostic information. For example, the aggravation of neck and upper limb symptoms by lifting, sneezing, and/or coughing typically implies the presence of a disk abnormality.
• The temporal relationship of symptoms also helps identify the cervical condition. For example, neck discomfort that is worse at the end of the day in an elderly individual suggests a degenerative process.

Past Medical History (p. 768)

• Any history of a rheumatological, metabolic, endocrine, or oncological process needs to be investigated as a possible cause of neck pain. Prior cervical surgery (e.g., a fusion) raises important issues such as fusion integrity and stability, as well as work limitations and treatment precautions. The presence of general medical conditions (e.g., diabetes, chronic obstructive pulmonary disease, coronary artery disease, or depression or other mental disorder) needs to be documented because of the potential impact on therapy and recovery.

Social History (pp. 768–769)

• The patient's personal life, childhood experiences, social status, and cultural background all influence treatment and outcome. Use of tobacco can lead to disk degeneration, and has been associated with poor operative outcome. In addition, stressors such as marital difficulties or occupational pressures are detrimental to recovery.

Family/Occupational/Functional History (p. 769)

• The clinician needs to be aware of any family history of diabetes, disability, rheumatological disorders, cancer, neck pain, psychological illness, or fibromyalgia. A family tradition of pain and disability can adversely affect treatment and outcome.
• The current employment status is important information especially in work-related injuries. Knowledge of the individual's job requirements and responsibilities and an understanding of the work environment enable the physician to appropriately determine work status and applicable restrictions.

Review of Organ Systems (p. 769)

• The review of systems should be similar to that for any patient, but certain aspects need to be emphasized in patients with cervical disorders. Bowel and bladder function, difficulty sleeping, psychological problems, extremity weakness, recent weight loss, and night sweats are all important indicators. A previous history of peptic ulcer disease, renal insufficiency, or liver dysfunction is critical information to have before prescribing certain medications.

Pain Diagrams (p. 769)

• The history is often supplemented with pain diagrams that the patient completes after instruction. The visual analog scale (VAS) and pain drawing can provide useful information to the clinician (see Fig. 37–9 in the Textbook).

PHYSICAL EXAMINATION (pp. 769–772)
Observation/Inspection (p. 769)

• Gait, facial expressions, and body language are noted during the evaluation. The neck is inspected for masses (e.g., from adenopathy or goiter, surgical scars, erythema, lesions, or any skin aberrations). The presence of abnormal cervical positioning is recorded (e.g., forward posturing, absent cervical lordosis, kyphosis, or listing).

Range of Motion (p. 769)

• Normal range of motion of the neck is 60 degrees of flexion, 75 degrees of extension, 45 degrees of lateral flexion, and 80 degrees of rotation. The patient with normal neck ROM is able to rest the chin on the chest, look straight up at the ceiling, touch each ear to the shoulder, and tap the chin against each shoulder. Patients accomplishing these movements, without moving the shoulders, have normal range of motion.

• The cervical spine is assessed for both active and passive ROM. The neck should not be forced into a nonphysiological or painful range that can cause an increase in symptomatology. Range-of-motion testing is contraindicated in the presence of spinal instability. The lack of active motion can be secondary to pain or muscle guarding. Decreased active and passive ROM can be secondary to spondylosis or ankylosis.

• Shoulder ROM testing is included in cervical spine evaluations to detect any loss that may affect cervical spine function. Disorders such as adhesive capsulitis, rotator cuff tendonitis, or shoulder impingement often lead to decreased passive and active shoulder range of motion, which leads to altered biomechanics and increased mechanical stress to cervical spine structures.

Neurological Evaluation (pp. 769–772)

• The motor examination can determine the presence of a root, trunk, or peripheral nerve injury when there is involvement of motor fibers. Knowledge of the peripheral nervous system and upper limb innervation patterns allows for localization by eliciting muscle weakness in a root or peripheral nerve distribution (Table 37–2). Neck strength is tested in flexion, extension, and rotation to detect neck weakness that is typically present in myasthenia gravis, myopathy, and some rheumatological conditions.

• Reflex testing is useful in evaluating nerve root function and in localizing the lesion. Although any level of reflex amplitude can be normal, hyporeflexia is consistent with lesions at the root level, plexus, or peripheral nerve. Hyperreflexia is more associated with lesions from the brain to the spinal cord. Hyporeflexia and hyperreflexia can be present together if the lesion involves both the central and peripheral nervous system. Asymmetric hyporeflexia at a

TABLE 37–2 Nerve Root Levels, Peripheral Nerves, and Muscles of the Upper Limb Commonly Evaluated in the Patient with Neck Pain

Nerve Root Level	Nerve	Muscle
C5, C6	Axillary	Deltoid
C5, C6	Musculocutaneous	Biceps brachii
C5, C6	Suprascapular	Supraspinatus
	Suprascapular	Infraspinatus
C7	Radial	Triceps
	Median	Pronator teres
C8, T1	Median	Abductor pollicis brevis
	Ulnar	First dorsal interrossei

specific root level is typical of unilateral radiculopathy, whereas generalized symmetric hyperreflexia with long tract signs is consistent with a myelopathic process.
• When assessing an upper limb reflex, it is important that the correct reflex be elicited and not an inverted reflex. An inverted reflex can occur, for example, if there is a large disk herniation. This could result in elbow flexion rather than extension when checking for the triceps reflex. This often indicates a more serious problem of myelopathy, in addition to a concurrent C7 radiculopathy.
• The reflex examination should include attempts to elicit pathological reflexes, which typically include the Babinski and Hoffmann tests. The presence of these superficial reflexes is suggestive of a central nervous system lesion such as a central cervical disk herniation, cervical spinal stenosis, or other pathology resulting in myelopathy.
• The sensory exam is designed to test the competence of the dorsal roots. Figure 37–3 shows the classic dermatomal pattern of the upper limbs. Pain, tested by pinprick, is usually the last sensory modality to be decreased and is not the most sensitive indication of sensory loss. Although pain testing is more convenient, vibratory and position sense testing are likely to be the first involved in a radiculopathy.

Palpatory Examination (p. 772)

• Palpation of the osseous structures of the anterior aspect of the neck should include the hyoid bone and the thyroid cartilage. The posterior osseous structures of the neck are examined by palpating the occiput, inion, superior nuchal line, mastoid processes, zygapophyseal joints, and the spinous processes. These structures are palpated to identify any painful sites.
• Soft tissue palpation is an important part of the cervical spine examination. The cervical and shoulder musculature are evaluated to identify trigger/tender points that can cause muscular-related referred headache and upper extremity pain patterns. The consistency and size of the thyroid and parotid glands are evaluated to assess for any abnormalities. The greater occipital nerves are commonly affected in flexion/extension injuries, resulting in occipital neuralgia with occipital headaches.

Provocative Maneuvers (p. 772)

• The Spurling test looks for foraminal encroachment on an inflamed cervical nerve root. The patient's head is extended, laterally flexed, and held down for up to 1 minute. The sign is present if there is increased symptomatology into the shoulder and hand in a radicular pattern.
• Lhermitte's sign was first described in patients with multiple sclerosis. It is elicited by briskly flexing the patient's neck. Electric-like pain or shock sensations shooting down through the spine as a result of this maneuver are often indicative of spinal cord pathology. This sign is also positive in some patients with herniated cervical disks.
• The swallowing test assesses the patient's ability to swallow normally on command. Swallowing dysfunction can be secondary to protruding osteophytes, soft tissue swelling from hematomas, infection, or tumors located in the anterior portion of the cervical spine. (See Chapter 26 for more information on swallowing dysfunction.)

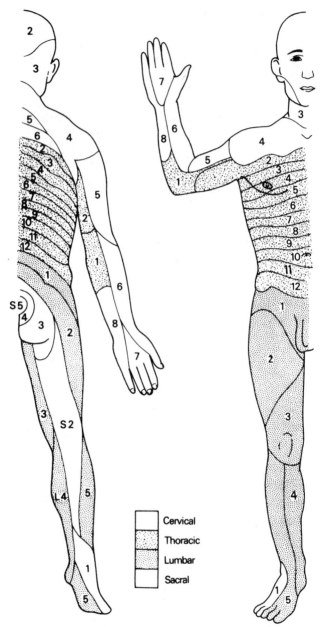

FIGURE 37–3. Dermatomal distribution of the cervical nerve roots. (From Ellis H: Clinical Anatomy: A Revision and Applied Anatomy for Clinical Students, ed 6. London, Blackwell, 1976, p. 205.)

DIAGNOSTIC STUDIES (pp. 772–776)

• Imaging is an important asset in the evaluation and treatment of cervical spine problems. The clinician should remember that imaging techniques evaluate anatomy rather than physiology or function.

• Plain films provide useful information in evaluating the cervical spine for chronic degenerative changes, metastatic disease, infection, spinal deformity, and stability. Cervical spine films in trauma cases typically incorporate seven views, including anterior-posterior (AP), lateral, bilateral obliques, open-mouth, flexion, and extension views. Flexion-extension views can help identify subluxation or cervical spine instability. An open-mouth view is important in evaluating the status of the odontoid process and instability between the first two cervical vertebrae. The AP view helps in the evaluation of the spine for tumors, osteophytes, and fractures. The lateral views check for stability as well as for signs of spondylosis including spurring and disk space narrowing. The oblique views are necessary for evaluating degenerative disk disease and foraminal encroachment by osteophytes of uncovertebral joints or the facet joints.

Computed Tomography (CT)–Myelography (pp. 772–774)

• The CT scan and myelogram individually or in combination continue to be important diagnostic studies in the evaluation of cervical spine problems. The CT scan is particularly helpful when a fracture of the cervical spine is suspected. One advantage of helical or spiral CT over conventional CT scanning is the infinite number of images that can be produced after data acquisition, allowing for a more detailed evaluation of a suspected fracture. A myelogram followed by a CT scan is often the imaging study of choice before cervical surgery for decompression of the spinal cord or nerve root(s). Spinal canal and nerve root compromise is best assessed in this manner; however, CT-myelography is often more expensive and has a higher morbidity than MR imaging. Therefore, CT-myelography is usually not one of the initial diagnostic studies performed to evaluate the cervical spine and typically is reserved for surgical cases.

Magnetic Resonance Imaging (MRI) (pp. 774–775)

• MRI has become the imaging technique of choice in the cervical spine for ruling out a herniated disk. The major strength of the MRI is the definition of soft tissue structures including cervical disks, spinal cord, and cerebrospinal fluid. The MRI is noninvasive and does not expose the patient to radiation.

• Although MRI is widely used and provides useful information, it has some shortcomings. The test is fairly expensive, is not tolerated by claustrophobic patients, requires that a patient cooperate to minimize artifact, and can have false-positive results. The MRI is not as sensitive as the CT scan in evaluating bony structures such as spurs and bony impingements. Individuals with embedded metallic objects such as pacemakers, surgical clips, or prosthetic heart valves cannot be scanned by MR imaging because the powerful magnets can dislodge these items.

• As with any imaging modality or diagnostic test, the MRI has to be interpreted in relation to the patient's symptoms. Many anatomical lesions seen on MRI scans are not functionally important.

Discography (p. 775)

• Cervical discography involves the placement of spinal needles under sterile technique into the cervical intervertebral disks. Once the spinal needles are properly placed within the center of the disk nucleus, contrast material is injected to determine the internal disk architecture and, more importantly, any pain response that is provoked during the injection. The discomfort and invasiveness of this test makes it less desirable than a cervical MRI, which provides most of the anatomical information that a discogram provides. Cervical discography (see Fig. 37–17 in the Textbook) has a role in identifying the symptomatic disk(s), which can be useful in the evaluation of patients with inconclusive diagnostic tests and in the planning of cervical fusions. Large disk herniations and midsagittal spinal canal diameters less than 11 mm are contraindications to discography at any level.

Electrodiagnostic Evaluation (pp. 775–776)

• Nerve conduction studies and electromyography (EMG) provide physiologic information regarding cervical nerve root and peripheral nerve function. Electrodiagnostic studies have the advantage of being relatively inexpensive as well as low in morbidity.
• Acute, subacute, and chronic radicular features can be detected by needle EMG when there is involvement of motor fibers. Abnormal spontaneous potentials and changes in motor unit action potentials in two or more muscles innervated by the same nerve root are highly suggestive of a radiculopathy (Table 37–3).
• Ulnar nerve entrapment, carpal tunnel syndrome, and peripheral neuropathy can be confused with cervical radiculopathy. Electrodiagnostic testing is very helpful in diagnosing these conditions and in separating them out from cervical radiculopathy.
• Somatosensory-evoked potentials (SEPs) are important in evaluating sensory conduction both peripherally and centrally. Lower limb nerve testing, such as of the tibial and peroneal nerves, has been shown to be helpful in diagnosing a myelopathy by assessing spinal cord conduction. Lower limb SEP are more sensitive than upper limb SEP in detecting cervical myelopathy. (See Chapters 10, 11, and 12 for more detailed information on electrodiagnostic testing.)

TREATMENT (pp. 776–782)

Modalities (p. 776)

• Physical modalities should typically be used only in the acute phase of the condition to help with pain control. Once the patient is past the acute phase, modalities are used only on an as-needed basis. (See Chapter 21 for more information on modalities.)

Traction (pp. 776–777)

• Cervical traction can be helpful in relieving symptoms associated with nerve root compression and mild to moderate soft tissue neck injuries. Hot packs, massage, and/or electrical stimulation should be done before traction to help relieve pain and relax the muscles. Cervical traction can be performed using either a heavy weight–intermittent or a light weight–continuous regime in a

TABLE 37–3 Cervicothoracic Stabilization Exercises

	Cervicothoracic Stabilization Levels		
	I Basic	**II Intermediate**	**III Advanced**
Direct cervical stabilization exercises	Cervical active range of motion Cervical isometrics	Cervical gravity Resisted isometrics	Cervical active Range gravity resisted
Indirect cervical stabilization exercises Supine, head supported	Theraband chest press Bilateral arm raise Supported dying bug	Unsupported dying bug	Chest flies Bench press Incline dumbbell press
Sit	Reciprocal arm raise	Swiss ball reciprocal	Swiss ball bilateral
	Unilateral arm raise Bilateral arm raise Seated row Latissimus pulldown	Arm raises Chest press	Shoulder shrugs Supraspinatus raises

Stand	Theraband reciprocal
	Chest press
	Theraband straight
	Arm latissimus
	Pulldown
	Theraband:
	  Chest press
	  Latissimus pulldown
	Standing rowing
	Crossovers
	Triceps press
		Standing rowing
		Biceps pulldown
			Upright row
			Shoulder shrugs
			Supraspinatus raises

Flexed hip–hinge position	0–30 degrees Reciprocal arm raise Unilateral arm raise	30–60 degrees Incline prone flies Reciprocal deltoid raise	60–90 degrees Bilateral anterior Deltoid raises
	Bilateral arm raise Interscapular flies	Cable crossovers Quadruped	Interscapular flies
Prone	Reciprocal arm raise Unilateral arm raise Bilateral arm raise	Head unsupported Swiss ball bilateral Anterior deltoid raises Swiss ball prone Rowing Swiss ball prone flies	Head supported Prone flies Latissimus flies
Supine, head unsupported	Not advised for level I	Partial sit-ups Arm raises	Swiss ball chest flies Swiss ball reciprocal

From Sweeney T, Prentice C, Saal JA, et al: Cervicothoracic muscular stabilizing technique. Phys Med Rehabil 1990; 4:345.From Sweeney T, Prentice C, Saal JA, et al: Cervicothoracic muscular stabilizing technique. Phys Med Rehabil 1990; 4:345.

clinic or home environment. The neck should be positioned in 15 to 20 degrees of flexion rather than extension during traction. The use of light weight–continuous home traction is a cost-effective alternative and gives the patient more autonomy. (See Chapter 20 for more information on traction.)

Cervical Orthoses (p. 777)

• A soft collar is recommended only in acute soft tissue neck injuries and for a short time, not to exceed 3 or 4 days of continued use. When used for radiculopathy management, the wide part of the collar is placed posteriorly and the thin part anteriorly (see Fig. 37–18 in the Textbook). This allows the patient to flex the spine and open the intervertebral foramina while discouraging neck extension. The collar can also be used intermittently for a longer period during certain activities such as sleeping or driving. A Philadelphia collar can be used at night to give more rigid positioning. This helps prevent foraminal narrowing by keeping the neck out of extension. (See Chapter 17 for more information on spinal orthoses.)

Medications (pp. 777–778)

• Nonsteroidal anti-inflammatory drugs (NSAIDs) are the first line of pharmacologic intervention in treating most cervical conditions. They provide pain relief at low doses and reduce inflammation at high doses. Decreasing inflammation is very important when treating cervical radiculopathies.
• Aspirin is not recommended because of the large doses needed for an anti-inflammatory effect, a longer time to action onset, gastrointestinal toxicity, and irreversible binding to cyclo-oxygenase. The traditional NSAIDs have a long history of multiorgan toxicity such as peptic ulcers, renal insufficiency, and hepatic dysfunction. The discovery and recent release of cyclo-oxygenase isomer type 2 (COX 2) NSAID inhibitors provides for the same analgesic/anti-inflammatory properties without as much associated toxicity.
• Oral steroids are used when a potent anti-inflammatory effect is needed in cervical radiculopathy. Treatment with steroids is typically initiated when an inflammatory etiology for the radiculopathy is suspected and there are no contraindications such as the presence of infection or history of peptic ulcer disease. The dosage for prednisone should begin at about 70 mg per day and decrease 10 mg each day for a total course of 280 mg.
• Muscle relaxants, opioids, and antidepressants are other medications that can be helpful for cervical disorders. Muscle relaxants should be used to potentiate the pain-relieving effects of NSAIDs and not necessarily for the reduction of muscle guarding. The only major effect of muscle relaxants in the doses typically used in humans is sedation; they appear to relax muscles by relaxing the patient. Analgesics are a better choice in most cases and are typically of the opioid type. They should be used orally on a scheduled dose basis for a short time. Dependency is a concern with long-term use of these medications, particularly in those with an addiction history such as alcoholism. A narcotic contract between the patient and physician should be used when anticipating long-term consumption. The contract restricts the patient to one pharmacy, prescription by one physician, scheduled use of the medication, no unscheduled refills, and no sharing or selling of medications.

• Tricyclic antidepressants (TCAs) can help decrease pain and improve sleep. Tricyclics appear to decrease pain by affecting Substance P and improve sleep by increasing stage IV (non-REM) sleep.

Manipulation (p. 778)

• Spinal manipulation and mobilization are treatment modalities used to restore normal range of motion and decrease pain. There is no clear explanation of how manipulation works, but some believe that "adjustments" to zygapophyseal joints improve afferent signals from mechanoreceptors to the peripheral and central nervous system. The normalization of afferent impulses results in better muscle tone, decreased muscle guarding, and more effective local tissue metabolism. These physiologic modifications lead to improved range of motion and pain reduction. (See Chapter 20 for further information on manipulation.)

Stabilization (pp. 778–779)

• Cervicothoracic stabilization is a rehabilitation program designed to limit pain, maximize function, and prevent further injury. The stabilization program includes improving cervical spine flexibility, posture re-education, and strengthening. This program emphasizes patient responsibility through active participation. The stabilization program starts within the established pain-free ROM and is then applied outside this ROM as the patient's condition improves. Any soft tissue or joint restriction present is treated using passive ROM, spine mobilization, soft tissue mobilization techniques, self-stretching, and correct posturing.
• The goal of postural training is to teach the patient to maintain a neutral spine position while performing daily activities. These proprioceptive skills are implemented during strengthening exercises designed to help the patient keep the cervical spine in a stable, pain-free, and safe position during strenuous activities.
• Cervicothoracic stabilization requires training and coordination of the muscles in the neck area. The neck and shoulder girdle muscles, especially the scapular muscles, need to be individually strengthened.
• The exercises used for stabilization proceed from the simple to more advanced techniques (see Table 37–3). The patient is instructed to maintain a neutral spine position at all times during stabilization exercises. Advanced exercises challenge the patient to maintain this position during dynamic activities. An engram is achieved through repetition, which eventually enables the patient to stabilize the cervical spine automatically.
• Stabilizing the cervical spine using muscular control and enhanced proprioceptive feedback allows the patient to perform activities safely by balancing forces around the cervical spine.

Functional Restoration (pp. 779–780)

• Functional restoration programs are designed for patients disabled by chronic cervical pain. These medically directed interdisciplinary programs have successfully returned worker's compensation patients with chronic cervical pain to work. These programs typically use an occupational and/or physical therapist, athletic trainer, or nurse to instruct patients in cervical anatomy, biomechanics, pathology, and ergonomics. This accomplishes several goals, including teaching the patient preventive measures against further injury in all activities.

Selective Spinal Injections (pp. 780–781)

• Cervical epidural, selective nerve root (transforaminal), facet, and sympathetic blocks can be used both diagnostically and therapeutically. Cervical epidurals and selective nerve root blocks can be used when there are radicular features associated with a cervical disorder. Cervical sympathetic blocks can be performed when sympathetic mediated pain is suspected, such as in the case of chronic regional pain syndrome (CRPS) types I or II.

• An anesthetic and steroid preparation can be injected into the epidural space (translaminar) or along the nerve root (transforaminal) after precise localization under fluoroscopy with radiopaque contrast. Long-term relief can be expected from the steroid if the pathophysiology is secondary to an intense inflammatory process. Relief typically lasts no longer than the duration of the anesthetic if the problem is secondary to mechanical compression (e.g., foraminal stenosis). Selective nerve root blocks are more precise than the "shotgun" approach of the epidural and can identify the symptomatic root or roots.

• Facet blocks are performed in one of two different ways. Either the intra-articular joint or the medial branch nerves are injected. Those patients who experience pain relief from either intra-articular injections or medial branch blocks are considered to have a facet disorder. These patients often benefit from a medial branch nerve rhizotomy procedure.

• These injection procedures can enhance rehabilitative efforts in two ways. Identification of the pain generator allows for a more specifically designed treatment protocol, and pain relief from the procedure gives a pain-free window of opportunity for more aggressive rehabilitation.

• There are risks involved with performing these procedures, including side effects from the anesthesia, the steroids themselves, and the noniodizing contrast media. Blood clotting parameters should be studied before epidural procedures in anyone suspected of having a bleeding diathesis. There is potential risk of seizures, vertebral artery spasm, and temporary quadriparesis from the anesthetic and respiratory arrest. Proper monitoring and emergency equipment should be present for any complications that might arise so that permanent sequelae do not follow from a temporary complication.

Rhizotomy (pp. 781–782)

• Percutaneous rhizotomy procedures can be done by radiofrequency electro-coagulation (hyperthermia), cryoanalgesia (hypothermia), or chemical neurolysis. As compared to the other techniques, radiofrequency rhizotomy completely destroys the nerve and provides a relatively large denervation area with longer lasting pain relief. Cryoanalgesia procedures provide a shorter period of pain relief because of less complete destruction of the nerve and a smaller area of denervation. One advantage of cryoanalgesia is that there is no risk of neuroma formation, which can occur with the radiofrequency technique. Chemical denervation is typically performed by injecting a sterile phenol preparation on the facet joint nerve. This method of denervation is not as specific as the other two methods because there is little control over injection flow patterns. There is also a risk of potential complications caused by the phenol spreading to nearby structures in the neck during the injection.

• Percutaneous rhizotomies are usually performed in the cervical spine to denervate symptomatic facet joints identified at an earlier time by either intra-articular or medial branch nerve injections. Under fluoroscopic guidance, the facet joint is denervated by destroying the medial branch nerves that supply the joint. Other rhizotomy applications for cervical pain using the radiofrequency electrocoagulation technique include cervical dorsal ganglionotomy, disk annular denervation, and sympathectomy.

Surgery (p. 782)

• Surgical intervention for cervical conditions is typically thought to be indicated when there is neurogenic bowel or bladder dysfunction, deteriorating neurologic function, or intractable pain. Cervical spine surgery results are best in the presence of radicular pain, spinal instability, progressive myelopathy, or upper extremity weakness.

Implantable Devices (p. 782)

• Implantable devices such as a spinal cord stimulator (SCS) and intrathecal drug delivery system (IDDS) are typically used in failed back and neck surgeries, complex regional pain syndromes (CRPS), and chronic painful conditions of benign or malignant origin. The implantable devices are used as a last resort for painful conditions after all other nonsurgical and surgical treatments have failed to provide substantial and long-lasting pain relief.

• Intrathecal drug delivery systems consist of a subcutaneous reservoir pump and catheter that travels from the pump to and into the intrathecal sac. Although SCS is effective primarily in treating limb pain, IDDS is effective in treating both axial and extremity pain using a number of different intrathecal medicines such as morphine, bupivicaine, sulfentanyl, dihydromorphone, and clonidine. At the present time the Food and Drug Administration (FDA) has approved only intrathecal morphine for treating pain in this manner. Potential complications associated with SCS and IDDS include infection, hematoma, seroma, respiratory depression, and paralysis.

COMMON CERVICAL SYNDROMES (pp. 782–787)

Cervical Sprain and Strain (pp. 782–784)

Epidemiology (p. 782)

• Sprain and strain injuries to cervical spine structures are the most commonly encountered cervical disorders. A sprain is an overstretching or tearing of ligaments and/or tendons secondary to joint trauma. A strain is an injury to the muscles. "Whiplash" injuries are the most common causes of cervical sprain and strain. The typical mechanism is a hyperextension injury to the cervical spine from a rear-end motor vehicle collision. Approximately one-third of subjects develop neck pain within 24 hours of the injury. The natural history of whiplash injuries is that 60% get better within the first year, 32% get better in the next year, and 8% have permanent problems.

Pathophysiology (pp. 782–783)

• Whiplash is caused by a hyperextension injury to the cervical spine, typically by a rear-end collision. The impact causes cervical extension followed by flexion with resulting injuries to ligaments, facet joints, and muscle. Other injuries that can occur include nerve root injuries with radicular features, C2 dorsal root ganglia injury resulting in occipital neuralgia, and temporomandibular joint injuries. In rare instances, there can be an injury to the descending portion of the cranial V nerve sensory nucleus resulting in facial sensory disturbances.

Diagnosis (p. 783)

• The history usually includes both neck pain and headaches. Symptoms can also be referred into the upper limbs. The patient typically complains of neck fatigue, stiffness, and pain associated with movement. Other symptoms include dizziness, lightheadedness, difficulty with concentration and memory, unusual skin sensations over the face, blurred vision, difficulty hearing, tinnitus, and other cranial nerve problems.

• The physical exam shows decreased neck ROM with poor quality of movement. Spurling's and Lhermitte's signs are typically negative. Patients often show tenderness to palpation in both the anterior and posterior structures of the neck. Structural defects can occur with dysfunction of cervical facet movement. The neurologic exam is usually normal. Sensation abnormalities in most cases are sclerotomal rather than radicular. Radicular signs are sometimes present early after injury, but usually resolve within the first 2 weeks.

• Plain neck films can show loss of the normal cervical lordotic curvature. MRIs and CT scans are typically normal but can show disk herniations, ligamentous injury, and hemorrhage. Electrodiagnostic studies can help rule out radiculopathy in patients with continued pain and unusual referred limb sensations.

Treatment (pp. 783–784)

• Initial care involves the use of NSAIDs and analgesics to control pain. Tricyclics can also be used to help decrease pain and lessen sleep disturbances. There is usually no need for muscle relaxants when there is sufficient use of analgesics.

• Physical therapy modalities can include mobilization, which can be effective acutely after the injury. Before performing mobilization, the clinician should rule out cervical instability in patients of all ages and vertebral insufficiency in the elderly. Massage, ultrasound, and electrical stimulation are beneficial, as is postural re-education. Orthotic devices should not be used continuously for more than 72 hours because they can delay healing and lead to soft tissue tightening.

• Proper movement patterns need to be re-established within the cervical segments. Stabilization exercises (see Table 37–3) allow the muscles to self-correct the neck into proper position and posture, resulting in decreased pain and trauma to the joints.

• There is a high incidence of facet joint pain in patients with chronic neck pain and headaches. These patients can be identified with facet joint nerve blocks. Although intra-articular steroid injections have been shown not to provide significant relief, rhizotomy of the facet joint nerves in properly identified patients can provide longer relief of symptoms.

Cervical Disk Disorders (pp. 784–785)

Epidemiology (p. 784)

• Internal disk disruption (IDD), herniated nucleus pulposus (HNP), and degenerative disk disease (DDD) are the three general types of cervical disk disorders encountered in clinical practice. Herniated disks are found by MR imaging in 10% of asymptomatic individuals under 40 years old and 5% in those older than 40 years. MRI can identify degenerative disks in 25% of asymptomatic persons under 40 years and nearly 60% in those older than 40 years.

• Cervical radiculopathy is a relatively common consequence of a HNP or because of spurring associated with DDD. A radiculopathy is any sensory, motor, or reflex abnormality secondary to nerve root injury. Job activities and smoking are other factors in addition to abnormal anatomy that predispose to the development of radiculopathy.

Pathophysiology (p. 784)

• *Internal disk disruption* is a term used to describe pathological changes of the internal structure of the disk. IDD is characterized as an abnormality of the nucleus pulposus or annulus fibrosus without any external disk deformation. This disorder is believed to result from either nuclear degradation related to trauma or isolated annular injury from a combination of cervical flexion and rotation movements.

• Intervertebral disk herniations are generally classified into three categories based upon the pathoanatomy. The protruding disk is described as nuclear material that penetrates asymmetrically through the annular fibers without escaping beyond the outside margin of the annulus. If nuclear material extends outside the periphery of the annulus it is called an extruded disk. A sequestered disk is an extruded disk in which a fragment of nuclear material has separated from the rest of the disk and lies in the spinal canal. Disk herniation typically occurs through a weakening of the posterolateral annulus from repetitive stress. Only rarely does herniation occur as a result of a single traumatic incident.

• Cervical radiculopathy can be secondary to mechanical compression or to an intense inflammatory process. Disk degeneration is a normal part of the aging process. Degenerative disk changes on radiographic studies are simply a reflection of the natural aging process and are not necessarily indicative of a symptomatic process.

Diagnosis (pp. 784–785)

• Discogenic pain is typically vague and diffuse in an axial distribution. Pain referred from the disk to the arm is usually in a nondermatomal pattern. Symptoms can vary according to changes in intradiscal pressure. Activities that increase disk pressure (e.g., lifting and Valsalva's maneuver) can intensify symptoms, whereas lying supine can provide relief by decreasing intradiscal pressure. Vibration also has a tendency to exacerbate discogenic pain.

• On physical examination the discogenic patient typically has decreased cervical range of motion. Neurologic examination is usually normal. The pain is made worse by axial compression and better with distraction. Myofascial tender or trigger points are commonly present and palpable.

• Radicular pain is deep, dull, and achy; or sharp, burning, and electric in quality depending on whether there is primarily motor or dorsal root involvement. The pain associated with radiculopathy generally follows a dermatomal or myotomal pattern in the shoulder, arm, and hand. The most common site of cervical radicular pain is the interscapular region, although pain can also radiate to the occiput, shoulder, or arm.

• The radicular patient typically displays decreased cervical range of motion. Pain is usually worse with extension and rotation or during Spurling's maneuver, and improved with neck flexion or abduction of the symptomatic upper limb. There can be decreased sensation to pain, light touch, or vibration. Upper limb weakness can be present when there is significant motor root compromise, but must be differentiated from pain-related weakness. The presence of increased lower extremity reflexes or other upper motor neuron signs suggests the possibility of a myelopathy and needs an aggressive work-up.

• Plain films help evaluate the disk space and vertebral body height, and can reveal degenerative osseous and disk changes. Electrodiagnostic studies are helpful in determining the presence and extent of radiculopathy, as well as peripheral or focal neuropathy. MRI can provide an in-depth anatomical evaluation of the intervertebral disks. Clinical correlation must always be used to interpret the results of diagnostic testing and in particular when using anatomical studies such as imaging techniques.

Treatment (p. 785)

• Conservative treatment is generally the same for discogenic pain with or without radiculopathy. Initially, the patient is placed on NSAIDs for pain control. An oral steroid used in a rapidly tapering dosage schedule provides a powerful anti-inflammatory effect and can be used in treating a radiculopathy that does not initially respond to NSAIDs. In order to avoid gastric and other potential side effects, steroids should not be given concomitantly with NSAIDs or aspirin products. Muscle relaxants can be used as adjuncts to analgesics. Narcotics are used sparingly and only for short periods.

• Physical modalities are initially used for acute pain control and later used on an as-needed basis only. Cervical traction is beneficial in discogenic pain and also with radicular symptoms. Cervical spine range of motion is actively and passively performed to help restore normal function. As the acute episode subsides, the patient is advanced from a passive program to an active stretching and flexibility routine for the cervical spine. Strengthening and stabilization, along with instruction on a home exercise program, comprise the next part of the rehabilitation process. The use of neck education to prevent recurrent episodes is very important.

• Those individuals who progress slowly sometimes require the use of selective spinal injection procedures that can provide enough relief to allow for an aggressive rehabilitation program. Those patients who fail with conservative treatment (including the use of spinal injection procedures) might benefit from surgery. Individuals with neck pain alone and no radicular features typically do not benefit from surgery unless there is instability or a myelopathic process. The best results of cervical disk surgery are in those patients with clear-cut radicular pain.

Cervical Spondylosis and Stenosis (pp. 785–787)

Epidemiology (p. 785)

• Degenerative changes of the cervical spine are very common with advancing age. In asymptomatic individuals under the age of 40 years, 25% have DDD and

4% have foraminal stenosis by MRI. In those over 40 years, almost 60% have DDD and 20% have foraminal stenosis by MRI. Seventy percent of asymptomatic individuals over 70 years have degenerative cervical spine changes in one form or another. Spondylytic changes can result in spinal canal, lateral recess, and foraminal stenosis. The former can result in myelopathy, whereas the latter two can present with radiculopathy.

Pathophysiology (pp. 785–786)
• Intervertebral disks lose hydration and elasticity with age, leading to cracks and fissures. The disk subsequently collapses because of biomechanical incompetence, causing the annulus to bulge outward. The surrounding ligaments also lose their elastic properties and develop traction spurs. Uncovertebral spurring occurs as a result of the degenerative process in which the facet joints lose cartilage, become sclerotic, and develop osteophytes.

Diagnosis (p. 786)
• Cervical spondylosis can cause radicular pain because of nerve root impingement, but it can also cause cervical zygapophyseal joint pain. Patients having only facet joint pain typically have pain confined to the neck and shoulder. The pain is worse at different positions and can interfere with sleep. They do not complain of numbness or weakness in the upper limbs. Those individuals with myelopathic symptoms such as neurogenic bowel and bladder dysfunction need aggressive investigation.
• Physical exam typically shows decreased ROM of the cervical spine, especially with neck extension. The neurologic exam concentrates on detecting long tract signs consistent with myelopathy, as well as signs of radiculopathy. Positive findings for myelopathy include hyperreflexia, Babinski's sign, and weakness at and below the involved levels. Positive signs for radiculopathy are decreased sensation, diminished reflexes, and weakness in a segmental distribution. Spurling's and Lhermitte's signs can both be present in either case.
• Diagnostic testing includes cervical spine films to evaluate the uncovertebral joints, facet joints, foramen, and intervertebral disk spaces. MRI permits evaluation of the spinal canal and foramen in relation to the spinal cord, thecal sac, and nerve roots. SEP responses from lower limb peripheral nerve stimulation are delayed or of low amplitude in the presence of myelopathy. SEP can be performed serially to evaluate the ongoing status of myelopathies. In cases of radicular symptoms, needle EMG can confirm motor nerve root involvement.

Treatment (pp. 786–787)
• The treatment for cervical spondylosis pain that occurs with or without radicular features begins with NSAIDs. Analgesics can also be used in a scheduled manner, but usually only for 6 weeks or less. Tricyclic antidepressants can be used for pain relief and sleep dysfunction.
• Physical therapy modalities in this situation can include a trial of careful traction. Cervical orthoses are typically not helpful. Mobilization, ultrasound, electrical stimulation, and massage can all be very helpful. Extreme mobilization can cause myelopathy and should be closely monitored. The exercise program is the same as for cervical radiculopathy and includes flexibility, strengthening, stabilization, and aerobic conditioning.
• A cervical zygapophyseal intra-articular steroid injection can be helpful in the presence of an active synovitis. The facet injections can be both diagnostic and therapeutic. Mechanical facet pain is better evaluated with facet joint nerve

blocks. Long-term relief can often be accomplished with a rhizotomy procedure. Cervical epidurals might be of benefit in cervical spondylosis, especially if there is an inflammatory component. Epidurals and selective nerve root blocks can be diagnostically and therapeutically helpful in cases of radiculopathy.

• Surgical referral is needed immediately when the clinical evaluation and neurodiagnostic tests are positive for myelopathy.

38

Original Chapter by Jeffrey A. Strakowski, M.D., J. William Wiand, D.O., and Ernest W. Johnson, M.D.

Upper Limb Musculoskeletal Pain Syndromes

SHOULDER PAIN (pp. 792–807)

Rotator Cuff Disease (pp. 792–799)

• Impingement is a term that encompasses a variety of disorders that manifest with anterior shoulder pain. Impingement ordinarily involves pain that occurs through the arc of motion as the arm is raised overhead. Impingement syndrome includes the conditions subacromial and subdeltoid bursitis, as well as rotator cuff tendinitis.

• Many entities other than rotator cuff disease present with pain or decreased range of motion of the shoulder. These entities include adhesive capsulitis, calcific tendinitis, dynamic functional instability, acromioclavicular (AC) degenerative joint disease, glenohumeral joint degenerative disease, tumors of the shoulder girdle and lung apex, crystalline and rheumatoid arthropathies, and cervical radiculopathy.

Stenotic Impingement (pp. 792–793)

• The subacromial impingement syndrome suggests that rotator cuff degeneration and subsequent tears are produced extrinsically by the rigid coracoacromial (CA) arch. Table 38–1 describes the stages of rotator cuff disease progression.

• Partial tears can extend to complete tears with relatively minor trauma. The stages are not discrete but evolve as a continuum over time. Progression can also involve problems with the biceps tendon, subscapularis tendon, subacromial bursa, AC joint, and glenohumeral joint.

• For example, impingement can lead to tendonitis and rupture of the long head of the biceps tendon.

• In addition to the rigid bony structures (e.g., humeral head, anterior third of the acromion, and the AC joint) causing stenotic impingement, it can also be caused by the coracoacromial ligament (CAL). The CAL constitutes the anterior third of the CA arch and contributes to confinement of the tendon in a fixed space.

TABLE 38–1 The Stages of Rotator Cuff Disease

Stage I	Rotator cuff inflammation—edema and hemorrhage
Stage II	Progression to tendinitis—fibrosis and tendinitis
Stage III	Partial or full-thickness tear—tendon degeneration and rupture
Stage IIIA	Tears <1 cm in length
Stage IIIB	Tears >1 cm in length
Stage IV	Multiple tendon tears

Data from Neer CS: Anterior acromioplasty for chronic impingement syndrome in the shoulder. A preliminary report. J Bone Joint Surg Am 1972; 54:41–50.

- Variations in shape and orientation of the acromion significantly affect stenosis and subsequent impingement.
- The main variations are the flat type (type I), the smoothed curve (type II), and the angled curve (hook) (type III).
- Type III acromions are often seen with complete rotator cuff tears (see Fig. 38–2 in the Textbook).

Nonstenotic Impingement (pp. 793–795)
- Rotator cuff disease is not always caused by stenosis. Subdeltoid bursitis is a common cause of anterior shoulder pain. Direct palpation over the subdeltoid bursa to localize the area of tenderness is essential for the diagnosis. It ordinarily responds well to rest, ice, and anti-inflammatory medications. In refractory cases, local injection of a steroid into the subdeltoid bursa might be necessary.
- Subdeltoid adhesions occasionally develop. These typically present as limitation in range of motion and result from repetitive mechanical trauma, chronic bursal inflammation, crystalline disease, and rheumatologic causes. Adhesions are primarily manifested in external rotation and should be suspected when chronicity, loss of motion, and calcific deposits are present.
- Primary glenohumeral instability should also be considered when evaluating rotator cuff disease. Affected individuals are typically younger adults (less than 35 years old) and involved in throwing or repetitive overhead activities. Often dramatic signs of rotator cuff pathology can obscure the more subtle signs of instability. Every effort should be made to identify shoulder instability as a component of the shoulder pathology.
- Anterior shoulder pain and impingement syndrome can also result from adhesive capsulitis at any time during its course. The many other causes of anterior shoulder pain should be excluded before it is attributed to capsulitis.
- The scapular stabilizers are important factors in humeral head control. The muscle groups specifically involved in scapulothoracic instability include the trapezius, rhomboids, and serratus anterior. Deficiencies in the strength or flexibility of these muscles can disrupt the normal scapulohumeral rhythm, leading to excessive stress on the glenohumeral joint. This leads to impingement of the rotator cuff underneath the CA arch, and is an important consideration when designing an exercise program for throwing athletes.
- The intrinsic theory of rotator cuff disease postulates that intrinsic ischemic degenerative changes within the cuff itself lead to tears. There are hypovascular zones in the rotator cuff tendons that are thought to coincide with commonly observed areas of degeneration (e.g., the site of the humeral insertion). These

TABLE 38–2 Conditions with Clinical Appearances Potentially Similar to Primary Rotator Cuff Disease

Acute traumatic bursitis
Instability
Primary acromioclavicular disease
Cervical radiculopathy
Arthritides of the glenohumeral joint
Calcific tendinitis
Adhesive capsulitis

areas may play an important role in the development of tendon degeneration and inability to heal.

- The list of clinical conditions that can resemble primary rotator cuff disease is extensive (Table 38–2). Acute traumatic bursitis usually results from a direct blow to the cuff severe enough to produce hemorrhage and edema. It is a self-limiting condition that resolves with appropriate rest and time.
- With primary AC joint disease a history of previous trauma is usually present in addition to the findings being restricted primarily to the AC joint itself. Physical findings include tenderness and pain reproduced on forcible adduction and internal rotation of the humerus.
- Cervical radiculopathy is discussed elsewhere (see Chapter 37). It can often be distinguished from rotator cuff dysfunction by posterior shoulder pain; by pain extending below the elbow; or by weakness, sensory loss, and reflex changes.
- Calcific tendinitis is thought to represent a separate pathological process. Calcification is seldom seen with degenerative rotator cuff disease, and its radiological demonstration generally precludes the diagnosis of impingement syndrome, although occasionally capsular ruptures into the bursa result in calcification.

Diagnosis (pp. 795–798)
- Age, occupation, avocations, and the presence of systemic disease all can provide clues to the appropriate diagnosis.
- Characteristic signs and symptoms that correlate with the stage of disease are described in Table 38–3. The classic impingement test has been described as a complaint of pain when the examiner flexes the shoulder anteriorly while stabilizing the scapula to prevent scapulothoracic compensation. Internal rotation of the shoulder into this forward flexed position typically accentuates the discomfort.
- An injection of 10 mL of 1% lidocaine directly into the subacromial bursa often eliminates or reduces pain and helps to confirm the diagnosis.

TABLE 38–3 Clinical Stages of Rotator Cuff Disease

Stage I	Minimal pain with activity; no weakness and no loss of motion
Stage II	Marked tendinitis with pain and no loss of motion
Stage III	Pain and weakness (cuff tear)

Data from Hawkins RJ, Kennedy JC: Impingement syndrome in athletes. Am J Sports Med 1980; 8:151–157.

- Stage I disease is common in patients under 25 years of age. Symptoms are commonly a toothache-like discomfort radiating laterally to the middle of the arm. Pain is often induced with flexion and abduction to 90 degrees.
- Stage II disease is most commonly seen in the 25- to 40-year-old age group but can occur at any age. The pain is often worse at night and often limits sleep. It can progress to limit daytime activities that aggravate the discomfort. The tenderness is more severe than in stage I and can secondarily involve the AC joint. Range of motion often becomes painful and difficult at this stage.
- Stage III disease is ordinarily seen in patients older than 40 years and is usually associated with a long history of intermittent or progressive shoulder problems, including the signs and symptoms seen in stages I and II. Symptoms are usually worse with overhead activity and at night. Affected individuals typically exhibit weakness secondary to pain, decreased range of motion, and shoulder stiffness.
- The clinical findings in complete rotator cuff tendon rupture may differ little from the clinical findings of earlier stages; or there may be a dramatic clinical change (e.g., sudden inability to elevate the arm) as a result of an acute event that finally causes rupture. Signs indicative of full-thickness rotator cuff tears include infraspinatus and supraspinatus wasting, tenderness over the greater tuberosity and anterior acromion, AC joint tenderness, painful arc of motion at 90 degrees of abduction or forward flexion, passive range of motion greater than active range of motion, and weakness of abduction and external rotation.
- Plain film evaluation is the first step in radiological imaging of the shoulder. Plain radiography most often yields positive findings in stage III disease. These findings include sclerosis and osteophyte formation on the anteroinferior acromion and greater tuberosity.
- The distance between the acromion and humeral head may be reduced. Osteolysis manifests as demineralization of the distal clavicle and widening of the AC joint. Plain radiography is of limited use in demonstrating abnormal calcifications and soft tissue disease.
- Arthrography is similarly of limited use in evaluating rotator cuff disease. It has good sensitivity only for complete tears or high-grade partial undersurface tears.
- Arthrograms are ordinarily normal in partial-thickness tears or earlier stages of degeneration. Further lowering its sensitivity are situations in which a complete tear is partially fibrosed or healed. Another limitation is the inability to distinguish muscle pathology by arthrography.
- The primary role of radionuclide scintigraphy is in characterizing patterns of disease in patients with known or suspected malignancies or arthritides. Its high sensitivity but low specificity limits its role in the evaluation of monoarticular disease.
- Magnetic resonance imaging (MRI) has become the primary imaging modality of choice. Its 3-dimensional capabilities provide more specific characterization of incomplete tears and afford 3-dimensional characterization of complete tears (see Fig. 38–9 in the Textbook); it also yields important information on the status of muscle groups.

Treatment (pp. 798–799)

- Whereas surgically enlarging the CA space through partial acromioplasty and CAL lysis provides symptomatic relief in some patients, physiatric rehabilitation of the dynamic stabilizers has recently been emphasized as the most effective therapeutic modality. The early rehabilitation techniques employed have the goal of promoting healing and returning the physiological motion and normal scapulothoracic rhythm of the shoulder girdle. The training techniques employed beyond this point must be consistent with the goals and needs of the individual patient.

• Primary prevention should be considered an integral part of the treatment of rotator cuff disease. For example, athletes, particularly those involved in throwing and overhead sports, as well as laborers who incur repetitive shoulder stress, should be instructed in proper warmup techniques, specific strengthening techniques, and the warning signs of early impingement.

• Treatment for stage I rotator cuff disease includes modalities such as ice; alteration of activity; anti-inflammatory medications; therapeutic exercises for strengthening the dynamic stabilizers; and, rarely, the use of intra-articular steroids. Total joint rest is to be avoided in favor of symptom-limited activity and specific therapeutic exercises.

• A technique suggested to correct deficiencies in strength, flexibility, and coordination is proprioceptive neuromuscular facilitation (PNF). This facilitates or inhibits agonist and antagonist muscle groups in a rate-dependent fashion and attempts to redevelop normal scapulohumeral rhythm.

• After symptomatic relief has been obtained, a program of active exercise is initiated with the goal of strengthening both the internal and external shoulder rotators in the nonabducted position.

• The supraspinatus is strengthened by the patient moving the hand from the straight adducted position to abduction at approximately 90 degrees, with the hand in the thumb-down position after the arm is placed in a position of 30 degrees anterior to the straight abducted position.

• The strength and flexibility of all of the muscles involved in the dynamic stabilization of the humerus should be continually assessed as the rehabilitation process progresses. This includes the deltoid and biceps, as well as the rotator cuff and scapulothoracic muscles.

• Selective use of a well-performed, single, intra-articular steroid injection in the subacromial space has been shown to hasten the recovery process by reducing pain and inflammation, allowing more rapid advancement to an exercise program.

• Repeted injections should be avoided because they increase the risk of collagen necrosis, weakness, and possible tendon rupture.

• Current treatment trends limit the role of surgical decompression to symptomatic relief of pain, primarily in elderly patients with more advanced disease.

• Further diagnostic modalities such as MRI, electromyography (EMG), and arthroscopy should be considered in patients with early-stage disease that is refractory to physiatric treatment in order to diagnose and address any unsuspected disorder.

• Conservative treatment protocols for stages II and III disease are the same as for stage I. Surgical decompression is entertained in patients with stage II or III disease that does not respond to appropriate physiatric treatment protocols. In successful surgical decompression, the anterior inferior acromial edge, the undersurface of the AC joint, and the CAL are surgically modified, resulting in reduced pain and improved function.

Bicipital Tendinitis (pp. 799–802)

• Bicipital tendinitis is an inflammation of the long head of the biceps where the tendon passes through the bicipital groove.

• Bicipital tendinitis as a manifestation of repetitive motion disorders occurs most often as an occupational disorder in laborers and others who use regular overhead motions. There can be a spectrum from acute myositis and tenosynovitis to chronic tendinopathy, which may or may not include calcification.

• Although less common, recurrent subluxation can lead to bicipital tendinitis. It is common in throwing athletes. Persons who are most predisposed to this include those with congenitally shallow or posttraumatic bicipital grooves. These medial subluxations can be palpated by the examiner with a finger placed over the bicipital groove.

• Inflammation of the intracapsular portion of the biceps tendon is often seen with associated rotator cuff tendinitis. Its anatomical location close to the supraspinatus and subscapularis tendon predisposes it to the inflammatory and degenerative processes of severe rotator cuff disease. This is particularly true in the elderly, who, after a complete rotator cuff tear, may place undue strain on the bicipital tendon.

• This is the most common cause of a complete bicipital tendon rupture in elderly individuals.

Diagnosis (p. 800)

• Patients often present with anterior shoulder pain and palpable tenderness of the biceps tendon in the bicipital groove. The bicipital groove can be palpated by internally rotating the humerus 30 degrees with the patient supine.

• Other diagnostic tests include pain on straight-arm raising (performed with resisted forward flexion of the shoulder at approximately 80 degrees with the elbow extended) or resisted supination of the forearm (see Fig. 38–12 in the Textbook). On both of these maneuvers, pain is felt in the area of the bicipital groove. Complete ruptures are often apparent on inspection and palpation of the proximally migrated biceps muscle.

Treatment (pp. 800–802)

• The treatment of patients with an intact tendon is physiatric therapy similar to that described for rotator cuff disease. Emphasis is placed on the dynamic stabilizers of the shoulder, with treatment primarily entailing progressive resistance exercises of the internal and external shoulder rotators. Use of a Theraband is a convenient means of achieving this.

• Nonsteroidal anti-inflammatory drugs (NSAIDs), US, heat and cold modalities, and activity modification are also essential components of the treatment plan. The biceps tendon is a dynamic stabilizer of the glenohumeral joint, and therefore, indiscriminate surgical transfer for chronic biceps tendinitis should be avoided.

Biceps Rupture (p. 802)

• In a younger person, violent trauma is ordinarily needed to tear the biceps brachii at the musculotendinous junction, a circumstance often requiring surgical repair. In most cases, particularly in individuals older than 40 years, biceps rupture occurs in the intra-articular area and is often associated with rotator cuff disease.

Instability (pp. 802–804)

- Instability of the shoulder is essentially defined as excessive translation of the humeral head on the glenoid and subsequent labral disease.
- Although instability can be congenital (e.g., Marfan syndrome or Ehlers-Danlos syndrome) it is seen most commonly after trauma or in chronic degenerative fatigue syndromes. The most common dislocation by far is traumatic anterior dislocation with labral injury, the "Bankhart complex" (see Fig. 38–15*B* in the Textbook). Less common, and more often associated with overuse syndromes, are posterior subluxations (so-called Bennett lesions) and multidirectional instability.

Diagnosis (p. 802)

- A thorough medical history is necessary to properly identify the disorder and its cause. A history of trauma, recurrent dislocation, chronic overuse, and multijoint instability can assist in properly identifying the disorder.
- Physical examination in these cases is often insensitive or inaccurate. The dynamic stabilization of this joint and the effects of fatigue are critical elements in the development of instability, which might not be adequately evaluated at rest or under anesthesia.
- The shoulder examination includes visual inspection for gross bony deformity and muscle wasting. The shoulder should be palpated for glenohumeral relationships, coracoclavicular relationships, and AC separation. Range of motion of the shoulder should be tested both actively and passively.
- Specific tests for instability include Lachman's test and the relocation test. To perform Lachman's test, the examiner positions the patient supine on the table and abducts the shoulder to 90 degrees with external rotation. An anterior force is then applied to the humeral head. A positive test is indicated by excessive anterior translation, which can be associated with pain (see Fig. 38–16*A* in the Textbook).
- In the relocation test the patient is positioned supine and the shoulder is abducted and externally rotated. Posterior force is then placed on the humerus to reduce the subluxation of anterior glenohumeral instability (see Fig. 38–16*B* in the Textbook). The most important factor in both tests is patient apprehension when the arm is abducted and externally rotated.
- Plain film evaluation of the shoulder, in internal and external rotation, is complemented by an axillary projection. These views will often show the anterior labral injuries of the Bankhart complex and the notch-like defect on the superior greater tuberosity (Hill-Sachs lesion) characteristic of anterior dislocations. Also evaluated are joint surfaces that provide clues to chronic degenerative glenohumeral disease (see Fig. 38–15 in the Textbook).
- When the initial workup is inconclusive, the next level of testing typically involves arthrography with computed tomography (CT). Increasingly, however, MRI is replacing this invasive procedure.
- MRI allows a noninvasive evaluation of the rotator cuff, impingement, and occasionally nerve palsies.

Treatment (pp. 802–804)

- The initial management for an acute shoulder dislocation is reduction. The mechanism of injury should be identified and the patient evaluated for neurovascular compromise before reduction is initiated. Axillary nerve palsies are common with anterior dislocations. Closed reduction for acute dislocations is often performed in emergency room settings.

• A thorough neurovascular examination should be performed after reduction. The joint is then protected to prevent recurrent dislocation. This is accomplished primarily by activity modification. Younger persons, particularly those less than 20 years old, are more predisposed to redislocation. Immobilization of the shoulder is better tolerated and indicated for a longer period in this group than in more elderly patients.

• Isometric exercises are begun within days following an acute dislocation. The rehabilitation program progresses to include active assisted exercises followed by progressive resistance exercises aimed to strengthen the dynamic stabilizers of the shoulder and scapula. Acute surgical intervention for an initial dislocation is rare unless the dislocation is accompanied by a complete rotator cuff tear.

Hemiplegic Shoulder Pain (pp. 804–805)

• Shoulder pain is a common complication of individuals with hemiplegia.

• The overall function of the shoulder, including stability and flexibility, depends on the musculotendinous sleeve that surrounds it. Impairment of these neuromuscular components in a situation of hemiplegia or tetraplegia greatly disrupts the usual functioning of this poorly balanced joint. There is considerable controversy regarding the precise cause of this common problem, but it most likely is multifactorial.

• Anteroinferior subluxation is the most commonly cited concomitant condition in patients with hemiplegia who have shoulder pain. Although it is seen more often in flaccid shoulders, it is more commonly associated with shoulder pain in conditions with spasticity.

Diagnosis (pp. 804–805)

• The maximal site of tenderness can often be located near the subacromial space. The degree of subluxation should be evaluated.

• The radiographic evaluation is similar to the protocols previously described for rotator cuff disease and instability. Electrodiagnosis can be helpful in ruling out peripheral nerve compromise, radiculopathy, or plexopathy.

Treatment (p. 805)

• The management of patients with hemiplegic shoulder pain is commonly difficult. A primary consideration for treatment should be combating spasticity, if present.

• Strategies should begin with the onset of shoulder plegia with the goal of prevention. Heat and cold modalities can be helpful. Lidocaine or phenol motor point blocks are sometimes indicated in patients with uncontrolled spasticity.

• Proper positioning and range-of-motion exercises should begin early. The shoulder should be positioned in abduction and external rotation while the patient is in bed. Subluxation often occurs in the shoulder that is flaccid. An axillary cushion, attached with a harness bandage, can be used to correct the subluxation while the patient is sitting or standing. A hemisling or wheelchair arm support can also serve this function. An axillary cushion or hemisling can also be used to correct subluxation in patients with spasticity, but caution must be exercised because these devices can increase spasticity or contribute to an elbow flexion contracture.

Adhesive Capsulitis (pp. 805–807)

• Adhesive capsulitis, also referred to as "frozen shoulder," is an abnormality that ordinarily develops gradually with increasing pain and decreasing range of motion. There are three clinical phases in the classic description of adhesive capsulitis: pain, progressive stiffness, and then a phase of gradual improvement with return of motion.
• Stage 1 is clinically similar to early impingement syndrome and is often confused with rotator cuff disease. Shoulder motion is restricted little if at all during this stage. The articular cartilage is normal in this condition.
• Stage 2 is characterized by pain with associated loss of motion in all planes. Arthroscopically, the synovium appears red, thickened, and inflamed.
• Stage 3 is characterized by the transition from inflammatory synovitis to chronic fibrosis.
• There is complete obliteration of the space between the humeral head and glenoid and between the humeral head and biceps tendon.
• Synovitis is not present in stage 4 and shoulder motion is severely limited.

Diagnosis (pp. 805–806)
• An adequate history is essential for evaluation of the painful and stiff shoulder. The differential diagnosis includes hemarthrosis, aseptic necrosis of the humeral head, infection, rotator cuff tears, and anterior capsular tear. The usual history is the insidious onset of a stiff, painful shoulder. The pain is ordinarily poorly localized but often most intense at the posterior and superior aspects of the shoulder.
• Initially the motion limitation might appear secondary to guarding from pain; but eventually, measurable limitation in both active and passive range of motion in different planes is demonstrated. The normal scapulohumeral rhythm is often disrupted in adhesive capsulitis because of excessive compensatory scapular rotation. The addition of accessory muscle strain can lead to additional painful cervical and shoulder musculature. Tenderness over the AC joint and biceps tendon is a common associated finding.
• Radiography is of limited value in diagnosing adhesive capsulitis. The findings are inconsistent and nonspecific.
• Although the diagnosis is ordinarily made clinically it can be confirmed, if in doubt, with arthrography. This can demonstrate loss of the ordinarily loose dependent fold of the joint and a dramatic decrease in the volume of contrast material that can be injected. Subacromial injection of 10 mL of lidocaine can be used to differentiate adhesive capsulitis from rotator cuff disease.
• Arthroscopy is not considered a standard diagnostic procedure for this condition, and its role is limited to the detection of other possible shoulder disorders.

Treatment (pp. 806–807)
• There is some disagreement in the literature regarding the natural course of adhesive capsulitis. Some report it to be a self-limited condition that will improve spontaneously over a 1- to 2-year period. Others think there is a significant subset of patients who, if not adequately treated, will develop persistent symptoms and disability. Either way, aggressive treatment is warranted to accelerate recovery.
• When the diagnosis has been established, the treatment goal is to control pain to facilitate progressive range of motion. NSAIDs, analgesics, heat modalities,

and intensive physical therapy are utilized, with progression to a home exercise program. The emphasis in therapy is on passive stretching of the shoulder capsular contracture in all planes of motion.

• Corticosteroid injections, although popular, have little supportive literature to demonstrate their efficacy. Accurate location of the glenohumeral joint with the injecting needle is a problem when there is a severe contracture. Although one or two steroid injections might have a beneficial effect early in the course of rehabilitation, repeated injections can have an adverse effect on tissue healing and are to be discouraged.

• Codman's exercises are the exercises most often used to improve range of motion. Efficacy can be increased with the use of wrist weights. These exercises can be easily performed by the patient at home after proper instruction.

• Some advocate the use of distention arthrography or infiltration brisement. With this technique, a combination of local anesthetic and saline is injected into the glenohumeral joint to produce hydraulic distention of the capsule and lysis of adhesions. This is ordinarily performed under general anesthesia.

• Manipulation under anesthesia is considered if the patient has made poor progress with the therapy program. The goal is to obtain a range of motion as close to that of the normal opposite shoulder as possible. Physiatric care should begin the day of the procedure, with attention to positioning in bed. The patient is placed in bed with the arm restrained to maintain abduction of 90 degrees and external rotation as far as that obtained during the manipulation.

• For the next few days the arm is maintained above 90 degrees. After this, the arm is allowed down only for short periods, primarily to perform pendulum exercises. During this period the patient should sleep in a sling that maintains the arm in the abducted position, and should participate in a formal daily physical therapy program and a home exercise program.

ELBOW PAIN (pp. 807–809)

Lateral (pp. 807–809)

Lateral Epicondylitis (pp. 807–809)

• Lateral epicondylitis, also known as "tennis elbow," is a common clinical condition. The vast majority of individuals seen with this condition are manual laborers, office workers, or homemakers who engage in repetitive manual activities.

• There is considerable controversy in the literature regarding the precise cause as well as the pathological changes that occur in lateral epicondylitis. A widely accepted belief is that an inflammatory lesion with degeneration occurs at the insertion of the extensor tendons, primarily the extensor carpi radialis brevis (ECRB), with eventual fibrous adherence to the capsule.

• Lateral epicondylitis usually occurs in persons over 35 years of age. Patients often present with a history of chronic activity involving repetitive flexion and extension of the wrist or pronation and supination of the forearm. The onset can be gradual or sudden.

• In tennis players, an incorrect tennis stroke can lead to the development of lateral epicondylitis. Poor technique can place excessive stress on the forearm muscles and tendons and ligaments around the elbow joint. The backhand is the most common stroke that elicits symptoms.

• On examination there is tenderness over the lateral epicondyle, usually at the origin of the ECRB. There is increased pain with resisted wrist extension; the pain is greater with a straight elbow. Pain can be maximally reproduced by having the patient make a fist, pronate the forearm, and radially deviate the wrist while performing this maneuver.

• The middle finger test can also be performed. This involves resisting the extension of the proximal interphalangeal joint of digit 3. This places stress on the extensor digitorum and ECRB. The test is considered positive if pain is elicited over the lateral epicondyle.

• Routine anteroposterior (AP) and lateral radiographs are of little help in evaluating this condition. Oblique views of the lateral epicondyle can show irregularity or punctate calcification around the origin of the ECRB.

• Primary in treatment of this condition is decreasing repetitive stress. Avoidance of painful activities and activity modification, particularly repetitive wrist flexion-extension and forearm pronation-supination, is important.

• Anti-inflammatory medication, heat modalities, US, and ice are useful adjuncts for treatment.

• An injection of cortisone and xylocaine can be helpful for temporary relief and confirmation of the diagnosis. Injection is made directly over the point of maximal tenderness with care not to enter the tendon itself.

• Forearm bands (lateral elbow counterforce braces) have become popular in recent years. The purpose is to prevent full muscular forearm expansion and alleviate tension on the attachment site at the lateral epicondyle.

• Proper exercise is probably the most significant intervention to produce long-term benefit. The authors suggest a technique of using 10 repetitive maximum (10 RM) of the wrist extensors with the elbow flexed to 90 degrees, and then repeated with the elbow extended to 180 degrees. The specific technique is the slow wrist extension followed by slowly allowing the wrist into full flexion (see Fig. 38–21 in the Textbook). The RM weight ordinarily should start at 6 to 10 lb and increase gradually each week. This series of exercises should continue twice daily for 4 to 8 weeks.

• Many operative procedures have been described for this condition. Lateral extensor release is considered by some to be the surgical procedure of choice.

Bone Trauma (p. 809)

• Osteochodritis dissecans of the capitelum is commonly seen in patients younger than 25 years who present with joint pain and occasional locking. Plain films often demonstrate fragmentation of the capitelum associated with an elbow effusion.

• Similarly, a history of trauma, often a direct blow or fall on an extended arm with the elbow locked, can lead to suspicion of an occult radial head fracture. Directly palpable tenderness is noted when the examiner's thumb is placed over the radial head as the forearm is moved through pronation and supination.

• Avulsion of the distal biceps tendon at the elbow is an uncommon injury. It is ordinarily without a prerupture syndrome and it is usually caused by a single, acute event, often a traumatic or heavy lifting episode done with the elbow flexed to 90 degrees.

Medial (pp. 809–810)

Medial Epicondylitis (pp. 809–810)

• Medial epicondylitis, also known as "pitcher's elbow" or "golfer's elbow," develops as a result of a medial stress overload on the flexor musculature and medial collateral ligament (MCL) at the elbow. It is seen often in the skeletally immature, primarily in 9- to 15-year-old boys, as a physeal injury resulting from throwing stresses (Little Leaguer's elbow).

• Critical components of the history include an acute onset or exacerbation of symptoms, which can suggest an MCL tear, epiphyseal fracture, or flexor tendon tear. An insidious onset of medial elbow pain is more typical of medial epicondylitis.

• The specific site of tenderness should be identified on physical examination.

• The characteristic pain can be elicited by stressing the flexor tendons with resisted flexion at the wrist or forced wrist extension. The elbow should be examined for laxity with varus and valgus stress.

• Avulsion fractures and osteochondral defects are often identified on a standard series of AP, lateral, and oblique plain radiographs. Physeal separation in adolescents is difficult to identify and can require comparison views of the noninjured elbow or the use of higher-technology imaging.

• Treatment for this entity is essentially the same as that previously described for lateral epicondylitis, only with the emphasis on the strengthening of the flexor muscles of the forearm.

Medial Collateral Ligament Trauma (p. 810)

• MCL rupture is seen in skeletally mature throwers and is believed to be caused by excessive valgus force on the medial compartment. Flexor and pronator muscle tears, as well as ulnar neuropathy, can also be associated in this condition.

• MCL damage ordinarily is accompanied by a history of chronic and repetitive trauma and pain but it can be the result of acute trauma. Valgus instability is invariably present, and can be tested by gently applying valgus stress to the medial aspect of the elbow while flexing the elbow to 25 degrees and externally rotating the humerus.

• Treatment consists of rest, ice, and a short course of NSAIDs until swelling and inflammation subside. Pain should be resolved and full range of motion should be attained before the individual gradually resumes throwing activities. This might require 6 weeks to 3 months. In patients with MCL injury refractory to treatment beyond 6 months, surgical ligament repair might be considered.

Posterior (pp. 810–811)

Olecranon Bursitis (pp. 810–811)

• Olecranon bursa inflammation is seen very commonly in athletes engaged in contact sports and in laborers. It can present as acute, chronic, or infectious.

• Acute bursitis usually results from a direct blow to or prolonged pressure on the area. Tenderness and distention of the bursa are noted on physical examination. Treatment involves primarily prevention of recurrence and might consist of wearing elbow pads or other appropriate covering, especially in athletes. Aspiration can be considered if the bursa is severely distended and painful. Compression and cold packs can be applied in the first 72 hours.

• After this period, heat can be applied to hasten resorption of the bursal fluid.

• Chronic olecranon bursitis occurs from repeated trauma and results in thickening and fibrosis of the bursal lining. Examination findings are similar to those seen in acute trauma, but fibrous trabeculation of the bursal sac can often be palpated. Aspiration is often indicated and should be followed by a compressive

dressing to minimize the tendency of the bursa to refill. Steroid injections have only limited success in chronic bursitis and are not indicated for acute bursitis because of infection risk. Surgical removal of the bursa is an option in severe refractory or chronic bursitis.
• Septic bursitis is diagnosed with aspiration and culture. It should be suspected in the setting of warmth and erythema. The fluid should be sent for Gram stain, crystal determination, cell count, and culture.
• The most common infectious organism is *Staphylococcus aureus.* Treatment involves appropriate antibiotics.

Triceps Tendinitis *(p. 811)*
• Another common cause of posterior elbow pain is triceps tendinitis. This is seen often in persons who engage in activities requiring rapid elbow extension (e.g., throwers, fly fisherman, and carpenters).
• Triceps tendinitis is managed similarly to the lateral and medial epicondylitides, with the mainstay of treatment involving reduction of inflammation and activity modification.

WRIST (pp. 811–813)
De Quervain's Tenosynovitis (p. 811)

• De Quervain's tenosynovitis involves swelling and palpable tenderness of the abductor pollicis longus (APL) and extensor pollicis brevis (EPB) tendon sheaths at the lateral border of the anatomical snuffbox.
• This disorder is often associated with a history of rapid repetitive movements of occupational and avocational stresses.
• The diagnosis is confirmed by eliciting localized tenderness and by a positive Finkelstein's test (Fig. 38–1). In the absence of a history of predisposing activities, rheumatoid arthritis should be considered with appropriate serologic and rheumatologic testing.
• Treatment focuses on reducing inflammation by means of activity alteration (which can include the use of splinting in severe cases), NSAIDs, and local steroid injection into the tendon sheath. Surgical release of the tendons sheaths is considered in severe cases refractory to treatment.

Acute and Occult Wrist Injuries (pp. 811–813)
Scaphoid Injuries *(pp. 812–813)*
• The scaphoid is the most commonly injured carpal bone.
• A common mechanism of injury involves a direct fall on an outstretched arm with a dorsiflexed wrist.
• The diagnosis of a scaphoid fracture is made from the classic traumatic history described, in the presence of pain and tenderness over its location at the anatomical snuffbox. There is ordinarily little outward visible evidence of this fracture. A plain radiographic series with AP, lateral, and radial and ulnar oblique views should be obtained if this fracture is suspected (see Fig. 38–25*B* in the Textbook). A bone scan should be considered in patients with normal radiographs but in whom there remains a strong clinical suspicion of bone trauma.
• The patient with normal radiographs but a classic history and physical findings should be placed in a short arm-thumb spica cast and re-evaluated in 2

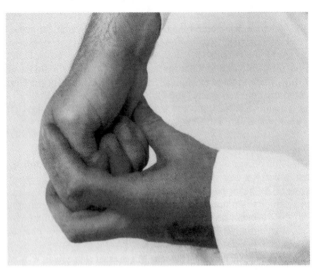

FIGURE 38–1. Finkelstein's test for de Quervain's tenosynovitis. The wrist is forced into ulnar deviation with the thumb flexed and abducted. Pain is exacerbated in a positive test.

weeks. Meticulous follow-up for this condition is imperative because of the high incidence of scaphoid nonunion after fracture.

• Nondisplaced fractures in the distal third, which has an excellent blood supply, often heal within a 6-week period with proper immobilization. Fractures in the middle third are reported to have up to a 30% incidence of nonunion despite adequate immobilization. Nonunion can occur in as many as 90% of patients with fracture in the proximal third of the scaphoid, which has the poorest blood supply. Scaphoid nonunion is associated with a high incidence of the late development of osteoarthritis or carpal collapse. The fracture can be treated with pulsed electromagnetic stimulation to promote healing if it is less than 5 years old and relatively asymptomatic. Surgical intervention is considered in patients with long-lasting symptoms or degenerative carpal changes.

Kienbock's Disease *(p. 813)*
• Kienbock's disease presents as wrist pain with sclerosis and collapse of the lunate secondary to avascular necrosis (see Fig. 38–25C in the Textbook).
• The precise cause of this condition is not well understood, but it is most common in the dominant wrist in 15- to 40-year-old men, most of whom have a history of preceding trauma. Surgical treatment is indicated when satisfactory relief of pain is not obtained with conservative management.

Osteoarthritis of the Carpometacarpal Joint of the Thumb *(p. 813)*
• Another common source of pain about the wrist and hand occurs at the carpal-metacarpal joint of the thumb. It is the most common site of osteoarthritis in the upper limb and commonly the most disabling, particularly in persons older than 60 years.

Scapholunate Advance Collapse (p. 813)

• The most common form of chronic wrist arthritis is scapholunate advance collapse (SLAC). This is a post-traumatic rotary subluxation that causes the scaphoid and lunate to separate and the capitate to migrate proximally. The ensuing impingement and osteoarthritic change can result in neuropathies and extensive arthropathic changes. This entity is readily identified with plain radiography (see Fig. 38–25*B* in the Textbook).

HAND PAIN (pp. 813–815)

Dupuytren's Contracture (p. 813)

• Dupuytren's contracture is a fibrous contracture of the palmar fascia leading to flexion contractures of the fingers. The causative factors are unknown. The condition is more prevalent in men and seen most often in the fifth to seventh decades. It commonly involves the fourth or fifth digit. Thickening of the palmar fascia is the hallmark of this condition.

• Failure to establish the proper diagnosis can lead to inappropriate attempts at progressive stretching, which are typically of no benefit. Continued extensor stress may cause progression of the syndrome. Surgical release is the treatment of choice.

Gamekeeper's (Skier's) Thumb (p. 814)

• Gamekeeper's thumb is characterized by an injury to the ulnar collateral ligament and insertion of the adductor pollicis. It is seen often in skiers and is associated with resultant instability. This condition is identified on physical examination by swelling and tenderness over the metacarpophalangeal joint of the thumb, pain elicited by passive motion, and weakness in pinch. It can occasionally be identified radiographically. Surgical repair is typically the treatment of choice.

Trigger Finger (p. 814)

• Acute or chronic inflammation and flexor tendinitis can result in a disproportion between the flexor tendon and its sheath. Subsequent constriction at the pulley near the level of the metacarpal head is associated with painful snapping of the flexor tendons. This condition is called trigger finger or stenosing tenovaginitis.

• Treatment consists of a local steroid injection.

• Splinting following the injections can also be beneficial. In highly resistant cases, surgery may be needed.

Mallet Finger (p. 814)

• Mallet finger occurs as a result of a tear of the extensor tendon from its attachment on the distal phalanx. This is usually caused by an acute flexion injury when the extensor tendon is taut. In the majority of cases, the tendon itself is torn from the insertion, but a significant percentage sustain a bone avulsion.

• Conservative treatment includes immobilization of the distal phalanx in hyperextension with the middle phalanx in flexion for approximately 6 to 10 weeks. Surgical repair is considered if functional recovery is inadequate.

Raynaud's Phenomenon (p. 814)

• Raynaud's Phenomenon is a vasomotor instability, often triggered by cold or stress, that results in a syndrome of pain, a burning sensation, cyanosis, numbness, and swelling of the upper extremities. Raynaud's phenomenon is ordinarily bilateral and is most often seen in women aged 40 to 50 years. The classic pattern is sudden pallor of the fingers, progressing to cyanosis, and eventually hyperemia with reflex dilation. Although the pattern is most commonly seen alone (primary vascular instability), it occasionally is the first clinical sign of scleroderma, other collagen-vascular disorders, or vasculitides (secondary).

• Management consists of avoidance of precipitating factors such as cold environments and cigarette smoking. Biofeedback can be effective. Medical management with β-blockers or sympathectomies can be considered, but produces inconsistent results.

Heterotopic Ossification (pp. 814–815)

• The abnormal formation of mature lamellar bone in soft tissue is called heterotopic ossification. There are multiple precipitating factors that include neurological insult, burns, direct trauma, surgery, and hereditary disorders. In neurogenic diseases such as spinal cord injury, it typically develops below the level of the lesion. Its development is initiated by a nonspecific inflammatory phase with symptoms generally beginning 1 to 3 months after the inciting event. Osteoid deposition follows the inflammatory phase.

Diagnosis (pp. 814–815)

• In the upper limb, heterotopic ossification is most often seen in the shoulder and elbow. It is generally characterized by swelling; moderate pain; joint limitation; localized warmth and tenderness; and, occasionally, low-grade fever. Alkaline phosphatase levels can be elevated early in this condition. Radiological studies performed early in the course of the disease often are negative, with calcifications appearing later. Bone scanning is more sensitive early in the process.

• The increased uptake of tracer reflects the increased vascularity and ongoing calcium deposition.

Treatment (p. 815)

• Treatment consists of range-of-motion exercises to maintain joint function as the ectopic bone matures. Modalities for pain relief and the use of NSAIDs for their anti-inflammatory effect, with indomethacin being the most studied, are helpful. Etidronate disodium has been extensively described for use early in the course of the disease to minimize eventual ossification. Criteria for its use include early recognition before ossification becoming evident on plain films.

• Although the prophylactic perioperative use of local radiation treatment can be effective for prevention of the process, its indications and uses are complex and controversial and beyond the scope of this discussion.

• Surgical removal in the acute phases before the completion of the ossification process is contraindicated. Aggressive recurrence is likely if surgical intervention is undertaken prematurely. Bone scanning and fractionated alkaline phosphatase levels are helpful to ensure that no active process is ongoing.

COMPLEX REGIONAL PAIN SYNDROME (pp. 815–816)

• Complex regional pain syndrome (CRPS) is a syndrome involving a chronic painful condition of the upper limb associated with neurovascular disturbance and dystrophic changes of the skin and bones. Other names that have been given to this constellation of signs and symptoms include reflex sympathetic dystrophy (RSD), Sudek's atrophy, causalgia, and shoulder-hand syndrome.

• Predisposing conditions include stroke, trauma of any severity, thoracic surgery, cervical radiculopathy, and myocardial infarction. Some cases occur without any known precipitating event. Some believe there is a psychological basis for predisposition to CRPS.

Diagnosis (p. 815)

• The diagnosis is ordinarily made on a clinical basis, primarily from the history and observation and physical signs outlined above. The patient typically reports a burning pain out of proportion to the injury and extending beyond the confines of dermatomal patterns.

• Radiological evaluation can be helpful, but changes might not be seen on plain films until the later stages of the disease (ordinarily after 3 or more months). Triple-phase bone scan can show increased uptake in the involved limb early in the process, possibly reflecting increased blood flow from localized bone turnover caused by sympathetic vasoconstriction.

Treatment (pp. 815–816)

• Graded activities are encouraged to facilitate a "desensitization" of the hypersensitive tissues. Techniques of desensitization include increasingly vigorous massage, Isotoner gloves, contrast baths, TENS, paraffin baths, US, and pneumatic pumps.

• A large majority of patients respond to systemic corticosteroids instituted in the acute phase of the disease. Prednisone is used most commonly, in doses up to 100 mg/day or 1 mg/kg and tapered over 2 weeks. A wide range of drug interventions have been suggested and include NSAIDs, anticonvulsants, tricyclic antidepressants, β-blockers, calcium channel blockers, calcitonin, and even topical capsaicin.

• Early recognition is critical for intervention before the development of trophic changes seen in stages 2 and 3. After this time, the prognosis for satisfactory and complete recovery is poor.

39

Original Chapter by Brian A. Casazza, M.D., Jeffrey L. Young, M.D., M.A.,
and Kirsten K. Rossner, M.S., P.T., A.T.C.

Musculoskeletal Disorders of the Lower Limbs

• The purpose of this chapter is to provide the foundation for assessing a variety of musculoskeletal problems in the lower limbs, with an emphasis on injuries that arise from repetitive musculotendinous overload.

MUSCULOSKELETAL HISTORY (pp. 818–819)

Chronology of the Injury. When did the pain first appear? Was the onset of pain sudden or gradual? Has this happened before? Has the patient just begun an exercise program?

Mechanism of Injury. Was trauma involved? Was the foot planted or in the air at the time of injury? Did the foot invert or evert? Was there a valgus or varus moment at the knee or was there a sense of rotational strain? Did the patient feel or hear a "pop" or a "snap"? Was there a sudden inability to bear full body weight?

Nature of the Pain. Is the pain constant or intermittent? What makes it more tolerable, and what exacerbates it? Is it associated with weight bearing? If so, how soon does the pain occur after beginning activity? Is the pain highly localized or does it radiate to or from another area? Is the pain associated with inflammation?

Injury Inventory. How many other injuries have been sustained? What were the locations? Were they managed nonsurgically or surgically?

Age Considerations. The differential diagnosis of distal Achilles tendon pain in the skeletally immature runner must include calcaneal apophysitis (Sever's disease). In the elderly runner it is much more likely to involve pathological changes within the tendon itself. Hip pain in the young athlete should raise suspicion of a femoral stress fracture or traction apophysitis, whereas the same symptoms in the elderly runner can indicate fracture or symptomatic spinal stenosis.

Exercise Habits. How much does the patient exercise? Has there been a sudden increase in frequency, intensity, or duration of workouts? Does the patient routinely stretch before and after exercising?

Equipment. What type of shoes does the patient use? How often are new pairs purchased and old pairs discarded? Does the patient wear shoe orthotic inserts? When were the inserts originally constructed and for what purpose?

Exercise Environment. Where does the patient typically train? Does the runner train on a level dirt path, on a banked concrete surface, on a treadmill, or on a flat circular track?

Review of Systems. Is there a nonmusculoskeletal process contributing to the current problem? Does the middle-aged tennis club pro who presents with calf pain have signs of vascular claudication? Is the young female runner who presents with pelvic stress fractures amenorrheic and exhibiting signs of disordered body image? What medications are being used? Are anabolic steroids being taken? Has the patient been using narcotics for pain relief?

Function. (How has his injury affected this person's life? Is the patient still working? Is this person still capable of performing all activities of daily living independently?

Coping Skills. Can this person tolerate relative or complete rest? How will this person react if true rest is required for an undetermined amount of time? Are there secondary gain issues at hand, and is there reason to be concerned about this patient developing a chronic pain problem?

PHYSICAL EXAMINATION (pp. 819–822)

- It is critical to adhere to the concept of the kinetic chain and to recognize that biomechanical dysfunction in one body region is capable of causing "injury at a distance." Consequently, it should be routine to examine the low back, hip, knee, and ankle regions in virtually all patients presenting with lower extremity complaints.
- Structures that should be evaluated statically include scoliosis, lumbar spine lordosis, pelvic bony landmarks, genu varum/valgum, femoral and tibial torsion, foot/ankle structure, relative muscle bulk bilaterally, calluses, and visible evidence of inflammation. A gait analysis should be performed to evaluate how these structural problems affect dynamic motion. Often structural abnormalities are compensated for at other sites in the biomechanical chain.
- Coupling the static and dynamic evaluation with the patient's history is imperative. Muscle fatigue might not be immediately evident in the clinic, but can play a significant role in dysfunction.
- For running athletes, video analysis of treadmill running at varying speeds with and without shoes, and with and without orthotic devices, is recommended.
- Foot assessment in non–weight bearing should begin with the identification of callus, and with viewing static forefoot position with the foot in subtalar joint neutral position. A posterior-to-anterior view down the foot will reveal either a varus, neutral, or valgus alignment of the forefoot and rearfoot relative to the horizontal plane. Evaluation of foot motion and relative laxity in the talocrual, subtalar, or midfoot joints, as well as of the first ray, are also important in assessing the non-weight-bearing position.
- The knee is first examined statically. Femoral anteversion, femoral and tibial torsion, patellar position in weight bearing and non–weight bearing, and Q-angle are important measures. The Q-angle (Fig. 39–1) is usually in the range of 10 to 15 degrees and is considered to be excessive if it exceeds 20 degrees. Next the

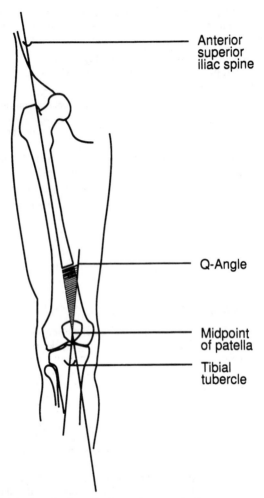

FIGURE 39–1. The Q-angle: the angle formed between the line of pull of the quadriceps and the center line of the patellar tendon (*hatched area*). A line is drawn from the anterior superior iliac spine through midpoint of the patella, and a second line is drawn through the midaxis of the patella to the tibial tubercle for determination.

range of motion in the knee joint, proximal tibiofibula joint, and patellofemoral joint should be assessed. Patellar mobility and tracking should be assessed passively and with an active quadriceps contraction in both non-weight-bearing and weight-bearing positions. The presence of lateral tracking of the patella, patella baja, and patella alta should be noted. Hypermobility of the patella, external tibial torsion, increased Q-angle, femoral neck anteversion, a broad pelvis, and overpronation can combine to form the "malalignment syndrome" that can be associated with medial knee pain. Assessment of the ligaments including the anterior cruciate ligament (ACL), posterior cruciate ligament (PCL), medial collateral ligament (MCL), and lateral collateral ligament (LCL), as well as the menisci, is also indicated. Because nonacute knee dysfunction is often the result of muscular inflexibility, it is important to do a flexibility assessment of the hamstrings, hip rotators, gastrocnemius/soleus complex, and iliotibial band.

- Static measures of the hip in non–weight bearing should include observing for femoral torsion and femoral anteversion/retroversion. Femoral torsion is evaluated by palpating the greater trochanter with one hand and passively rotating the femur internally and externally at the level of the femoral condyles. When the greater trochanter is most easily palpated, the relative position of the femur can be noted by the orientation of the femoral condyles. Weight-bearing assessment should include noting the degree of toe-out, which is directly affected by femoral anteversion/retroversion as well as tibial/malleolar torsion.

- The hip should also be evaluated for the presence of tight flexors, extensors, rotators, and adductors. The Thomas test assesses hip flexor flexibility. For this test the patient lies supine and brings both knees up to the chest. The patient then lowers one knee down to the level of the plinth while continuing to hold the other to the chest. If the leg cannot be brought in line with the plinth, or if the lumbar spine must arch to do so, there is indication of hip flexor restriction. Hamstring flexibility can be measured in the supine position with the hip flexed to 90 degrees while the lower leg is passively extended by the clinician. Tissue restriction is noted at the point where the clinician can no longer extend the lower leg. External/internal rotation of the hip can be evaluated by rotating the hip while the hip and knee are flexed and the patient lies supine. Adductor tightness can be assessed by abducting the patient's leg in the supine position. If the adductors are restricted, the entire body appears to pivot and rotate about the pelvis instead of just the leg abducting. The hip joint capsule can be assessed by placing the hip in flexion in addition to abduction and external rotation. This is called Patrick's test or the FABER test. FABER is an acronym for *f*lexion, *ab*duction, and *e*xternal *r*otation of the hip. The grind test can also be done to assess for the possibility of an arthritic condition. In this test, the patient lies supine with the knee drawn to the chest and flexed while the clinician provides a compressive and rotational force to the femur. This test should not produce discomfort.

- The sacroiliac joint can be a source of pain for a number of reasons. Leg length discrepancies uncompensated for in the lower extremity can place increased shear force through the joint, causing localized pain and surrounding soft tissue spasm. Muscular imbalances can also cause increased sacroiliac joint irritation. Evaluation of the sacroiliac joint should begin with the palpation of the bony landmarks, including the posterior superior iliac spine (PSIS), the anterior superior iliac spine (ASIS), iliac crests, sacral base, inferior lateral angle (of the sacrum), and ischial tuberosities. For a comprehensive evaluation of the sacroiliac joint, bony landmarks should be assessed in non–weight bearing (supine and prone), standing, and sitting. Static asymmetries give only one dimension of possible dysfunction. Further motion testing in standing and sitting should also be incorporated in the evaluation.

- The March test evaluates sacroiliac joint motion relative to the opposite side. The evaluator stands behind the patient and palpates the PSIS with one hand and the sacral base with the other. The patient then draws one knee up to the chest while balancing on the other limb. The relative posterior motion of the PSIS is compared bilaterally, with the restricted joint revealing relatively less range of motion. An additional standing test includes the forward flexion test where the evaluator palpates the PSIS bilaterally and has the patient slowly bend to touch the toes. The evaluator looks for increased motion of one PSIS relative to the other. Often the restricted sacroiliac joint is the one that shows greater range of motion in forward flexion. With the patient sitting with feet supported, the clinician can evaluate the sit-to-slump test. For this test the evaluator palpates the PSIS bilaterally and asks the patient to sit in a neutral pelvic position. The patient is then instructed to alternately "slump" and extend the lower back. Relative movement of each PSIS is compared in all three positions.

• A quick but effective screen of the back incorporates all the observations from the lower body segments because the concept of the kinetic chain must not be forgotten. Lumbosacral spine motion is intimately related to motion at the level of the hip and pelvis. Tightness of lower extremity muscles attaching to the pelvis can interfere with the normally smooth combination of spine flexion–pelvic rotation and spine extension–pelvic derotation (lumbopelvic rhythm) observed during trunk flexion and extension. Approximately 80% to 90% of the motion in the lumbosacral spine should be at L4 to L5 and L5 to S1. Migration of the motion up toward the thoracolumbar junction with altered tone of the paraspinal muscles suggests spinal segment dysfunction.

• A brief neurological examination is recommended regardless of whether or not the patient appears to present with a neurogenic problem. The elderly patient with "hip pain" can have unrecognized spinal stenosis. The young runner with a chronic "hamstring strain" can have an unrecognized S1 radiculopathy. Cutaneous nerve injuries need to be considered as well.

• The person's shoes should be inspected for signs of breakdown. Wearing away of the leather along the distal toecap region can imply subtle anterior tibial weakness. Excessive medial or lateral wear can indicate increased pronation or supination, respectively. As a general rule, pronation control is best achieved with a straight board-lasted shoe having good rearfoot control. Persons predisposed to supination do better with a flexible and curve-lasted shoe.

INJURY ANALYSIS AND REHABILITATION (pp. 822–849)

• Proper rehabilitation requires a thorough understanding of applied anatomy, biomechanics, and the kinetic chain. This section details a "template" for rehabilitation of musculotendinous overload injuries.

Step 1: Establish an Accurate Diagnosis. The vicious circle model for analysis of musculotendinous injury induced by repetitive overload is presented in Figure 39–3 in the Textbook.

• When the musculotendinous unit is subjected to tensile overload, damage occurs at a cellular level. This typically produces symptoms of pain, dysfunction, and instability, which can impair athletic performance.

Step 2: Acute Management. Efforts are directed toward minimizing the effects of inflammation and controlling pain. The PRICE principle (*p*rotection, *r*elative rest, *i*ce, *c*ompression, and *e*levation) is followed. This is usually a period for judicious use of anti-inflammatory medications and pain-relieving modalities.

Step 3: Initial Rehabilitation. This phase continues to focus on promotion of proper healing. Restoration of motion helps to reduce the effects of immobilization, with controlled tensile loading promoting ordered collagen growth and alignment. Identification of correctable biomechanical imbalances is initiated.

Step 4: Correction of Imbalances. Development of symmetric motion and symmetric strength is a twofold goal. When the patient is pain-free, and when nearly full concentric strength has been achieved, it is essential that an eccentric strengthening program be initiated. Closed kinetic chain (CKC) exercises are preferred because they strengthen agonist and antagonist simultaneously via co-contraction, and are more physiological for lower limb sporting activities such as running. One can begin to identify flaws in exercise technique and training practices when the patient is capable of full weight bearing under controlled conditions. Movement patterns that predispose an athlete to injury must be identified and remedied. This includes strengthening of weak musculature, stretching tight tissues, proprioception exercises, and balance training. Alternative aerobic conditioning exercises are encouraged. Other than local icing, treatment modalities are rarely indicated during this phase.

Step 5: Return to Normal Function. Cross-training, aqua training, and the use of alternative conditioning schemes give way to a gradual increase in activity-specific training and eventual resumption of full activity. Endurance performance, power, and agility should be restored to baseline.

Injuries about the Hip (pp. 824–834)

Applied Anatomy and Biomechanics *(pp. 824–825)*
• The mature femoral neck is angled at 120 to 130 degrees to the central axis and is positioned in approximately 15 degrees of anteversion (medial femoral torsion). An increase in the neck-shaft angle is termed *coxa valga,* and a decrease is called *coxa vara.*
• The femoral head receives vascularity from a small artery within the ligamentum teres and through the medial and lateral circumflex arteries, which pierce the capsule. This architecture renders the vascular supply vulnerable to disruption during dislocation.
• Some of the key muscles surrounding the hip joint include the piriformis, gluteus maximus, and gemelli. The piriformis functions as an external rotator. The gluteus maximus functions as a hip and spine extensor and as a hip external rotator. The gemelli function as minor external rotators.

Specific Problems in the Hip Region *(pp. 825–826)*

Piriformis Syndrome. There is the potential for sciatic nerve entrapment beneath the piriformis as the nerve exits the sciatic foramen. Sciatic nerve compression by this muscle leads to complaints of dysesthesias down the posterior thigh and often into the calf or foot. Buttock pain and tenderness through the piriformis can be found. Side-to-side comparisons of piriformis tightness should be made. Electrodiagnostic testing can reveal involvement of tibial and peroneal innervated muscles, with sparing of superior and inferior gluteal nerve-innervated structures and absence of abnormal electromyographic activity in the paraspinal musculature. Magnetic resonance imaging (MRI) can demonstrate injury or edema within the piriformis muscle but is rarely a necessary procedure.
• The clinical symptom complex in piriformis syndrome consists of buttock (and possibly leg) pain and dysesthesias aggravated by sitting or lower limb

exertion. The tissue injury complex includes myotendinous breakdown within the piriformis and possible focal demyelination within the tibial and peroneal divisions of the sciatic nerve. Functional adaptations consist of ambulating with an externally rotated thigh, shortened stride length, and functional limb length shortening.
• Rehabilitation efforts are geared toward stretching of the piriformis and associated external rotators and evaluation of the sacrum and pelvis for other imbalances. Once sacral and pelvic abnormalities have been defined and corrected, strengthening and stabilization exercises should be incorporated into the home exercise program. These include pelvic tilts, minibridges, and hip external rotation strengthening in a variety of positions.

Snapping Hip Syndrome. This is associated with a variety of extra-articular and intra-articular phenomena. The most common cause appears to be the snapping or popping of the iliotibial band (ITB) across the greater trochanter, although involvement of the iliopsoas tendon snapping over the iliopectineal eminence can also be seen. Less commonly, loose bodies, labral tears, and osteochondritis dessicans can be intra-articular sources of the snap. Treatment typically consists of muscle rebalancing with stretching and myofascial release to promote return of muscles and tendons to their normal length. Correction should take only a few weeks. Should symptoms persist despite an adequate stretching program, evaluation of intra-articular pathological changes by computed tomography (CT), MRI, or arthroscopy is recommended.

Trochanteric Bursitis. This is commonly seen in the elderly and manifests as pain in the lateral thigh during ambulation and decreased tolerance for lying on the affected side. The trochanteric bursa lies beneath the tendon of the gluteus maximus and is located posterolateral to the trochanter. Patients can describe a pseudoradicular pattern with the pain extending down the lateral aspect of the lower extremity and into the buttock. The clinical symptoms can be elicited by placing the lower extremity in external rotation and abduction. Direct palpation or deep pressure applied posterior and superior to the greater trochanter will reproduce the pain. Functional adaptations include increased hip external rotation with an altered gait or running pattern. Treatment should be geared toward restoration of flexibility and strength imbalances. Injecting the bursa with corticosteroid and anesthetic can be helpful if the flexibility and conditioning exercises are unsuccessful.

Ischial Bursitis. The ischial bursa lies between the ischial tuberosity and the gluteus maximus. Irritation of this bursa is not common. Classically, *ischial bursitis* occurs with friction and trauma after prolonged sitting on a hard surface. It can also be seen in adolescent runners, often in conjunction with ischial apophysitis. Pain can be aggravated during uphill running. The pain is distributed down the posterior aspect of the thigh and occurs with activation of the hamstring muscles. Initial treatment approaches involve modification of the patient's activity (e.g., a decrease in the duration and frequency of running, or avoidance of prolonged sitting). Ice and nonsteroidal anti-inflammatory drugs (NSAIDs) are helpful in controlling symptoms. Corticosteroid injections can be helpful in cases of persistent pain.

Avascular Necrosis of the Femoral Head. The blood supply to the femoral head is fragile and subject to compromise with hip dislocation or femoral neck fracture. Disruption of this supply can have catastrophic results. Even if initial plain radiographs are negative, there should be a high index of suspicion for *avascular necrosis* (AVN) of the femoral head if the hip is painful with joint loading and no source of pain coming from outside the hip can be identified. Although a bone scan can show a stress reaction within days, MRI scanning is preferable. If the MRI shows evidence of necrosis, immediate surgical consultation and non–weight-bearing status are recommended.

Specific Problems in the Thigh (pp. 826–834)
• The structures of the thigh region are extremely vulnerable both to tensile overload and to direct trauma.

ANTERIOR THIGH
• There are two common mechanisms of anterior thigh injuries: tensile overloading of the musculotendinous unit with induction of a "strain," and high-velocity compressive forces resulting in a "contusion."

Quadriceps Strains. Strain injuries are graded as follows:
1. First degree (mild)—an overstretch with minimal disruption of musculotendinous unit integrity
2. Second degree (moderate)—an actual (although incomplete) muscle tear. There is intramuscular bleeding with hematoma formation, and muscle strength is clearly compromised.
3. Third degree (severe)—a complete rupture. Muscle function is essentially lost. Avulsion injuries are included in this category.

• The rectus femoris is the most commonly strained of the quadriceps group. *Ely's test* (passive flexion of the knee with the patient prone) is useful for isolation of the rectus. A tight rectus induces elevation of the ipsilateral hemipelvis as maximum allowable knee flexion is approached because the hip-flexing component of the rectus femoris is blocked.
• The signs and symptoms of quadriceps strain vary depending on the severity of the injury. Lower-grade injuries might have only pain on deep palpation or passive stretch. Higher-grade injuries are typically accompanied by swelling and discoloration. Total rupture of the muscle typically results in a palpable mass in the zone of muscle injury.
• Functional adaptations that persist when the return to activity is too early include greater reliance on the unaffected leg for upward propulsion in jumping activities, shortened running stride with reduced hip flexion, and reduced running velocity.
• Acute rehabilitation follows the PRICE principle. The role of NSAIDs as modifiers of the inflammatory response to acute injury makes them extremely valuable in the acute management of all first- and most second-degree strains. The early use of NSAIDs in high-degree strains should be weighed carefully because antiplatelet activities can increase local bleeding.
• Initial rehabilitation includes pain-limited stretching to achieve progressive increases in muscle length. The patient should be taught the proper technique and instructed to continue the stretching program on a long-term basis. An example of a combined hip flexor and knee extensor stretch is shown in Figure 39–2. In more chronic or recurrent cases, soft tissue mobilization can be instituted.
• Strengthening should be initiated only after range of motion is pain-free and complete. The progression should be from either isometric or low-resistance

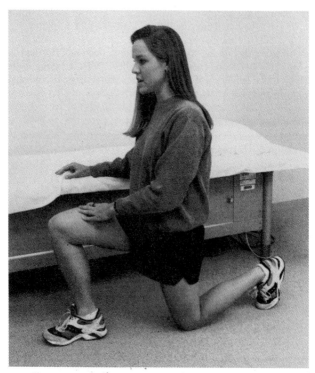

FIGURE 39–2. Stretching of the hip flexors. To obtain additional stretch for the knee extensors, the patient must grab the ankle and increase the knee flexion angle. Note that the spine must maintain a neutral position to avoid the development of lumbar injury.

dynamic contractions to full-range progressive resistance exercises (PREs). Eccentric work against maximal or supramaximal loads should be avoided early in the rehabilitation program to lessen the likelihood of further structural damage. Aerobic conditioning can be maintained initially by upper body ergometry, swimming with a pull buoy between the legs, or via tri-limb exercise with the affected limb kept at rest. When full range of motion is achieved, stationary two-legged bicycling, skiing, or rowing can be attempted. Full-weight-bearing exercises with axial loading of the affected limb (e.g., treadmill or stair climber) are gradually added, with eventual progression to faster-paced activities; agility drills; and, finally, sport-specific training when applicable.

Quadriceps Tendon Rupture. This represents an extreme form of overload to the quadriceps and is often the end result of repeated strain injuries. In contrast to quadriceps strains, which are more common in younger athletes, tendon ruptures tend to occur in older athletes. As with strains, the rectus femoris is the most vulnerable of the quadriceps group. Incomplete tears can be treated conservatively with initial splinting and use of crutches for protected weight bearing. Full rehabilitation and reconditioning of the remaining muscles is required to prevent residual strength deficits. Complete tears require surgical repair.

Quadriceps Contusions. These are characterized by capillary rupture, edema, inflammation, and infiltrative bleeding. The severity of the contusion is proportional to the extent of blood vessel breakdown and muscle crush. Clinical grading of the contusion is related to the available passive, pain-free knee flexion 12 to 24 hours postinjury. Flexion of less than 45 degrees usually indicates a severe injury; 45 to 90 degrees, a moderate injury; and greater than 90 degrees flexion, a mild injury.

- It is important to begin treatment with PRICE as close to the time of injury as possible. The thigh and lower leg should be wrapped or strapped into maximally tolerated knee flexion (see Fig. 39–10 in the Textbook). Crutch walking is advised. As with strains, NSAIDs are used judiciously. Attempted aspiration of the hematoma is not recommended, particularly because blood is usually clotting by the time the physician examines the injury. Corticosteroid and proteolytic enzyme injections probably do more harm than good. Ice is perhaps the only modality that can be used safely. Local heating, soft tissue mobilization, shortwave, and ultrasound have all been implicated in the possible development of the most undesirable complication of a contusion, myositis ossificans traumatica.
- Early rehabilitation focuses on re-establishing normal pain-free range of motion through a progressive stretching program. Aerobic conditioning is started as soon as possible with upper body or tri-limb exercises. As knee flexion returns to normal, isometrics and then CKC strengthening of the knee flexors and extensors are instituted. Criteria for resumption of full activity include minimal thigh tenderness as well as symmetric range of motion and quadriceps strength. If the patient participates in a contact sport, the use of custom-molded protective padding is recommended. A hip spica wrap may also be utilized to limit full motion and provide soft tissue stability. Although recovery from most mild injuries takes less than 2 weeks there is considerable overlap in healing times between mild, moderate, and severe injuries (e.g., a range of 2 to 60 days of disability).

Myositis Ossificans Traumatica. One of the most vexing complications of contusive injuries is *myositis ossificans traumatica* (MOT) or the formation of non-neoplastic cartilage or bone in connective tissue. The quadriceps is the most common site of involvement. Initial symptoms are nonspecific and include local pain, warmth, and tenderness. This usually progresses to a soft tissue swelling, and ultimately to a discrete mass with an associated loss of range of motion at the surrounding joints. MOT develops rapidly and can be evident within 3 weeks on plain films. Even earlier detection is possible with three-phase bone scan or ultrasonography.

- MOT tends to stabilize in size in 3 to 6 months, and there is great likelihood of spontaneous resorption, particularly when the MOT is near the muscle belly and not lying near the tendon.
- Recommended treatment following detection of MOT is adherence to the PRICE principle, with immobilization of the affected area while it is overtly inflamed to facilitate the natural sequence of resorption. Prophylactic use of diphosphonates does not seem warranted because of the low likelihood of a persistent lesion. The use of NSAIDs (e.g., indomethacin) is common among clinicians but has not been conclusively shown to halt the progression of the lesion. Follow-up radiographs showing corticated MOT borders, and "cold" bone scans are useful in determining if the lesion has become "mature." Activity is gradu-

ally increased after maturity has been determined. On rare occasions, surgical excision of a mature MOT lesion is necessary. This should generally be reserved for those patients with pain and loss of range of motion persisting 6 to 12 months after the lesion has matured.

Acute Compartment Syndrome. Far less common than the above entities is an *acute compartment syndrome* of the anterior thigh. Patients present with a palpably tense thigh and exhibit decreased sensation in the front of the thigh, in the saphenous nerve distribution, or in both. They typically also have pain, pallor, and a progressive loss of quadriceps strength. A key symptom is pain that is seemingly disproportionate to the injury. If a compartment syndrome is suspected, surgical consultation should be obtained. Intracompartmental pressure measurements should be made; when the pressure exceeds 40 mm Hg, a fasciotomy is typically necessary.

MEDIAL THIGH

Relevant Anatomy and Biomechanics. The bulk of the medial thigh musculature is composed of the adductor group (see Fig. 39–7 in the Textbook). All the adductor muscles are innervated by the obturator nerve (L2 to L4). The posterior portion of the adductor magnus, in keeping with its role as an accessory hamstring, has tibial innervation as well.

• The adductor muscles function as pelvic stabilizers, femoral rotators, and femoral accelerators during the gait cycle.

Adductor Strain. The most common of the medial thigh injuries is *adductor strain* caused by tensile overload. The adductor longus and magnus are the most commonly affected. High-grade strains can result from sudden femoral abduction in external rotation. Another common mechanism is repetitive forceful adduction.

• The adductor strain clinical symptom complex typically consists of medial thigh and groin pain that is worsened by abduction. Functional adaptations to injury include shortened stride with less crossover, and an attempt to maintain a relatively internally rotated position of the femur (which accentuates the gluteus medius weakness).

• Acute management involves application of the PRICE principle with use of NSAIDs as needed. The patient with a high-degree strain might need crutches because any attempt to advance the femur forward can induce pain. Spica wraps with elastic bandage can be of benefit early on to remind the patient not to suddenly abduct or flex the thigh. If a complete disruption of the adductor longus has occurred, surgical consultation to evaluate the possibility of repair is highly recommended.

• Initial rehabilitation emphasizes establishment of a stretching program for the adductor group, gluteal muscles, and external rotators. Adductor stretching after injury can be quite painful and the stretching should be kept within a pain-free zone.

• Correction of imbalances begins with the stretching outlined above and progresses to more aggressive adductor stretching. Using a partner to help stretch or via a "contract/relax" method (a proprioceptive neuromuscular facilitation technique) helps to achieve greater gains. "Butterfly" stretches can be used for self-stretching of the adductors. Strengthening of all muscles about the hip is necessary. Isometrics and then elastic or rubber tubing for dynamic strengthening can be used early on for adductor strengthening. It can be 1 to 3 weeks postinjury before the patient can safely tolerate higher-resistance weights or aggressive CKC strengthening exercises, particularly in the high-grade adductor strains.

Osteitis Pubis. The diagnosis of *osteitis pubis* should be considered when pain in the groin or symphysis pubis region persists beyond a month. Inflammation in the symphysis pubis generally results from repetitive microtrauma or persistently abnormal mechanics. Runners and cross-country skiers who abruptly increase their mileage (and who have weak gluteal muscles) are particularly prone to this problem. Definitive diagnosis is made with radiographs or bone scan. A bone scan can show findings before radiographs. Typical radiographic findings include periosteal reaction, demineralization, and sclerosis along the pubis, although these might not be present for 2 to 3 weeks.
• The treatment of choice for osteitis pubis is rest for 1 to 2 months with avoidance of lower extremity exercise. Upper extremity conditioning is emphasized, and resumption of a lower extremity rehabilitation and conditioning program is permitted only when there is no tenderness to palpation of the symphysis pubis and hip abduction is pain-free.

POSTERIOR THIGH

Relevant Anatomy and Biomechanics. The bulk of the posterior thigh is comprised of the hamstrings group (see Fig. 39–12 in the Textbook). All hamstrings except the short head of the biceps function as hip extensors and knee flexors. The short head is a knee flexor only. The semimembranosus and semitendinosus are also internal rotators of the flexed knee, whereas the biceps can act as an external rotator. All of these muscles are innervated by the tibial division of the sciatic nerve (L5 to S1) except for the short head of the biceps, which receives peroneal innervation.

Hamstring Strains. These are among the most common of all thigh injuries. The short head of the biceps is the most commonly involved. Injuries are more likely to occur at higher running speeds. The remaining hamstrings, being two-joint muscles, are vulnerable to injury under conditions of extreme hip flexion combined with knee extension. Hurdlers and football punters are at risk for this type of injury mechanism.
• The clinical symptom complex generally consists of pain in the proximal thigh with the onset associated with a popping sensation in the posterior thigh. By the time of examination there might be a palpable mass, presence of ecchymosis, and extreme tenderness over the injured site.
• Functional biomechanical deficits include decreased knee extension, reduced hamstring-to-quadriceps strength ratio (normally about 0.6), and increased hip flexion. The functional adaptations in response to the injury include shortened walking or running stride length.
• Acute management consists of PRICE, cane or crutch walking (especially with the higher-grade injuries), NSAIDs, and gentle passive stretching as tolerated. Isometric and dynamic strengthening begins only when the patient is pain-free. For full stretching of the hamstrings, the hip must be flexed with maintenance of complete knee extension. Stretching should be performed in a supine position, and a towel can be used to facilitate this stretching maneuver (see Fig. 39–13 in the Textbook). Rehabilitation can proceed more rapidly once full muscle length is achieved. Aerobic conditioning exercises applicable during hamstring healing include bicycling without toe clips (which reduce the role of

the hamstrings), upper body ergometry, kayaking, swimming breaststroke, or swimming with a pull buoy between the thighs. Resumption of activity is allowed when motion is restored and is pain-free, strength is at least 90% of the uninjured side, and the hamstrings/quadriceps strength ratio has normalized.

LATERAL THIGH

Relevant Anatomy and Biomechanics. The primary lateral thigh structure most subject to injury is the tensor fascia lata (TFL). It functions as a hip flexor and internal rotator of the hip. It is innervated by the superior gluteal nerve (mainly L5 fibers).

• Tightness of the TFL has been associated with a number of clinical entities including snapping hip (see above), ITB syndrome, patellofemoral pain, and lumbar spine dysfunction. TFL tightness is usually seen in conjunction with gluteal muscle inflexibility and weakness. TFL shortening can be demonstrated using *Ober's test* (Fig. 39–3).

• TFL tightness responds reasonably well to a stretching program, but the appropriate stretching program is difficult for the patient to learn without careful instruction. Stretches can be done initially by simulating the Ober's test position with the help of a therapist, or the patient can perform a self-stretch (see Fig. 39–16 in the Textbook).

Meralgia Paresthetica. This consists of pain and dysesthesias in the lateral thigh typically caused by entrapment of the lateral femoral cutaneous nerve (L2 to L3) underneath the inguinal ligament. Because this nerve is purely sensory, there is no resulting motor deficit. Like many other nerve irritation or entrapment syndromes, the nerve is more vulnerable if "already sick" because of diabetes or other neuropathy-producing condition. Common sources of irritation of this nerve include abdominal distention from pregnancy or obesity, wearing a tight lumbar corset, and sudden hip hyperextension. Treatments include weight reduction, avoidance of binding clothing, local injection of anesthetic agents at the level of the inguinal ligament, and oral medications such as amitriptyline and carbamazepine.

Disorders of the Knee (pp. 834–842)

Applied Anatomy and Biomechanics (pp. 834–836)

• The knee should not be viewed as a simple "hinged joint." The knee actually consists of three joints—the tibiofemoral, the patellofemoral, and the tibiofibular.

• The knee joint is enveloped by an extensive synovial capsule. The capsule is confluent with expansions of the patellar tendon anteriorly, the ITB laterally, and the semimembranosus tendon and the deep fibers of the tibial collateral ligament medially. Laterally the fibular collateral ligament remains separate from the synovium.

• The primary static restraints to tibiofemoral translatory motion are the cruciate ligaments. The ACL functionally prevents forward translation of the tibial plateau relative to the femur and aids in rotational control. The PCL prevents forward translation of the femur on the tibial condyles and provides secondary rotational stability.

• The menisci are cartilaginous structures that assist the motion of the femoral condyles at the tibiofemoral joint. They deepen the articular surfaces, provide a thin layer of lubrication, and assist in shock absorption. The medial meniscus is

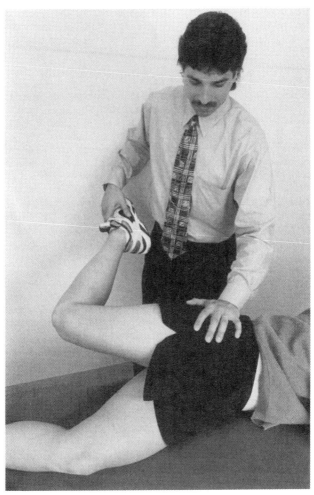

FIGURE 39–3. Ober's test. The patient lies on the untested side, with the lower (untested) leg maintained in mild to moderate hip and knee flexion for stability. The clinician extends and abducts the patient's upper thigh while maintaining the pelvis in a neutral position. The test leg is then slowly lowered.

firmly attached to the medial collateral ligament and the synovial capsule, whereas the lateral meniscus has a less significant bond to the capsule and is separate from the collateral ligament.
• The medial and lateral collateral ligaments control valgus and varus moments acting at the knee and help limit rotation of the tibia.
• The patellofemoral joint is essentially a soft tissue joint under the control of numerous muscular and fascial structures. The patella is the centerpiece of all the static and dynamic stabilizing forces about the patellofemoral joint. These

stabilizing forces, by compressing the patella against the femur, create a patellofemoral joint reaction force (PFJRF). The PFJRF becomes greater with increases in quadriceps tension and with increased knee flexion (see Fig. 39–19 in the Textbook).

Specific Problems in the Knee *(pp. 836–842)*

Patellofemoral Pain Syndrome. This is the most common knee problem in out-patient physical medicine and rehabilitation (PM&R) practice. The differential diagnosis of anterior knee pain includes, but is not restricted to, infrapatellar bursitis, synovial plica, patellar tendinitis, quadriceps tendinitis, Osgood-Schlatter syndrome, osteochondritis dissecans, patellofemoral tracking disorder, and meniscal disorders. Factors that predispose to patellofemoral pain include the presence of patella alta, increased Q-angle, femoral anteversion, and excessive pronation.

• The clinical symptom complex consists of pain, crepitation, and occasionally swelling, all typically worsened by prolonged knee flexion. The "theater sign" might also be present, in which the patient cannot sit for long periods without knee pain. Pain with knee extension should alert the clinician to the possibility of infrapatellar fat pad impingement between the inferior pole of the patella and the femoral condyle.

• The functional adaptation complex consists of knee flexion contracture (loss of terminal extension), lateral patellar tracking, and altered stride to avoid full loading of the knee. The overloaded structures include the patellar tendon and lateral retinaculum, the hip external rotators, the medial longitudinal arch of the foot, and the synovium of the first metatarsophalangeal joint.

• Following acute management, problems with the malalignment syndrome should be corrected. Biomechanical deficits should be minimized by restoring full flexibility and strength of the gastrocnemius-soleus complex, hamstrings, ITB, and VMO. If biomechanical deficits persist after this program, the patient (particularly if a runner) might require the fitting of foot orthotic devices to correct pronation. Taping of the patella to simulate proper patellar alignment accompanied by neuromuscular re-education of the knee musculature (McConnell technique) can also be beneficial.

• A dynamic strengthening exercise for the hip stabilizers and the adductor magnus-VMO complex can be used. (See Figure 39-22 in the Textbook.) A strong adductor magnus-VMO complex is needed to prevent lateral tracking of the patella. Note that the patient is instructed to keep the affected knee over the middle toe to avoid excessive internal rotation of the lower extremity, and to keep the hips level as the knee is flexed. Strengthening of the quadriceps mechanism is typically performed in the last 30 degrees of knee extension.

The ITB Syndrome. The iliotibial band is the extension of the TFL that extends down the lateral leg to insert into Gerdy's tubercle along the lateral tibia. The *ITB syndrome* (also known as the ITB friction syndrome) is associated with painful sensation when the ITB slides back and forth over the lateral femoral condyle as the knee flexes and extends. Risk factors include running on beveled surfaces, limb length discrepancies, tibia vara, foot hyperpronation, and ITB contracture. The Noble compression test is a useful maneuver when an ITB syndrome is suspected. With the patient supine, and after positioning the knee in 90 degrees of flexion, the examiner presses on or just proximal to the lateral epicondyle. The knee is then gradually extended. Pain occurring at about 30 degrees (as the ITB crosses the bony prominence) is a positive finding.

- The functional adaptation complex consists of functional pronation of the foot, external rotation at the hip, internal rotation of the lower leg, and lateral patellar tracking.
- Rehabilitation of ITB syndrome consists of attempts to stretch the ITB, hip flexors, and gluteus maximus. Correction of foot pronation is needed and the runner should either discontinue running or run only on level surfaces. Strengthening of the hip adductors, gluteus maximus, and TFL is emphasized. Symptoms can take 2 to 6 months to resolve. Local injection of a combination of anesthetic agent and corticosteroid placed in the region of the lateral femoral condyle is sometimes helpful.

Pes Anserinus Bursitis. The anserine bursa separates the three conjoined tendons of the pes anserinus (i.e., semitendinosus, sartorius, and gracilis muscles) from the MCL and the tibia. Patients complain of pain inferior to the anteromedial surface of the knee with ascension of stairs. The examiner can reproduce the symptoms by moving the knee in flexion and extension while holding the leg in an internally rotated position. Palpation localizes the pain to the anserine bursa. Steroid injection is typically effective in reducing the inflammatory symptoms. The rehabilitation program should emphasize stretching of the medial hamstring and adductor muscles.

Prepatellar Bursitis. Prepatellar bursitis, colloquially referred to as housemaid's knee, is often the result of frequent kneeling, producing an effusion of the subcutaneous bursa at the anterior surface of the patella. The patient rarely complains of pain unless direct pressure is applied to the bursa. Occupational modifications should include patient education, avoidance of kneeling, and the use of kneepads when pressure must be applied to the patella. The bursal enlargement is reduced with the application of ice.

ACUTE LIGAMENTOUS INJURIES OF THE KNEE
Anterior Cruciate Ligament Injuries. Partial or complete disruption of the ACL can be a disabling event for the athlete or worker. Often the patient describes an audible snap or pop while the lower limb undergoes hyperextension or rotational strain. The injury is painful, and an acute hemarthrosis usually develops in the first few hours following the insult. It is common to damage additional restraints of the knee at the same time.
- Examination should include range of motion testing, palpation for tenderness and effusions, and evaluation of functional limitations. Loss of ACL integrity can be demonstrated with *Lachman's maneuver.* The examiner attempts to introduce anterior tibial translation while the limb is kept in 15 to 20 degrees of knee flexion. Complete tears of the ACL reveal significant anterior tibial translation and a loss of a distinctive end feel. A partial tear will maintain a "soft" end feel, but tibial translation will be greater than on the uninvolved side. The *anterior drawer test,* although technically easier for many clinicians to perform than Lachman's test, has significant limitations. For one, tibial translation will not be appreciated if there is any degree of hamstring activity. For another, an associated meniscal tear can provide a block to tibial motion in this position. Finally, if there is a PCL tear, a false-positive drawer sign can occur. MRI is excellent for visualizing the disrupted ACL, as well as for assessing the presence of other injuries.
- Acute treatment includes aggressive reduction of joint swelling, either via Cryocuff compression or aspiration of the hemarthrosis. Even if surgical reconstruction is planned, early repair within the first 3 weeks is not advisable. An

appropriate "prehabilitation" should be initiated after the injury and continued until the time of surgery or entry into an aggressive nonsurgical rehabilitation program. Gentle passive stretching of the lower extremity musculature, isometric co-contraction of the quadriceps and hamstrings, straight leg raises, and protected weight bearing are encouraged early on. Hyperextension of the knee should be avoided.

• The most common surgical reconstruction is the patellar tendon autograft. Following reconstruction, safe restoration of motion and weight bearing is emphasized. During the immediate postoperative period, passive range of motion is begun. In order to maximize the patient's compliance, it is necessary to provide adequate pain relief. The first step is to control the effusion with compression, ice, and elevation. Electrical stimulation of the quadriceps to help prevent atrophy can be considered. Soft tissue mobilization about the patella should be employed to restore patellar mobility and lessen the chance of adhesion formation.

• It is important to gain full extension at the tibiofemoral joint during the first postoperative week. Weight bearing is done in extension while wearing an immobilizer. Soft tissue mobilization at the origin of the medial and lateral head of the gastrocnemius can also assist in gaining extension.

• Once the swelling is controlled and extension is achieved, the next goal is re-establishment of a normal gait pattern. Crutch walking progresses from two crutches with partial weight bearing to one crutch and then none by the end of the first month. By this time most patients no longer need the knee immobilizer.

• During the weeks that follow, the program emphasizes further increases in range of motion, restoration of baseline strength in both hamstring and quadriceps groups, and progression to functional activities. Cardiovascular efforts are continued on a stationary bike, and the position of the seat should be adjusted to avoid knee hyperextension. With increased muscular control, exercise can be advanced to a cross-country ski machine, stair climber, or slide board. During the second to third month, the rehabilitation program should include unidirectional jogging.

• Agility drills include jumping rope, lateral shuffling around cones, figure-of-8 drills, and carioca. When the quadriceps, hamstrings, and primary movers of the hip show strength that is 90% or better in comparison with the uninvolved limb, and there is no evidence of clinical pivot shifting, the patient can return to full sporting and occupational activities.

• Some patients elect to pursue a nonoperative course. The exercise program is virtually identical to that following surgery, but the use of a functional brace is instituted earlier to protect the tibiofemoral joint and the menisci from potential damage.

Posterior Cruciate Ligament Injuries. Acute tears of the PCL are not as common as ACL injuries. Isolated PCL injury occurs with direct trauma forcing the tibia posteriorly (e.g., when the knee hits a car dashboard during an automobile accident), a fall on a flexed knee, or from knee hyperflexion. Unlike ACL injuries, the patient's symptoms can be vague. Visual inspection typically shows posterior tibial translation with a positive "sag sign." The *reverse Lachman's test* (directing the tibia posteriorly while the knee is in approximately 15 to 20 degrees of flexion) is positive. Roentgenographic examination should be done to exclude a bony avulsion from the tibial insertion of the PCL, which requires immediate surgical fixation. MRI can clearly demonstrate the presence of the PCL injury.

• Treatment of isolated injury to the PCL remains controversial. Most studies have shown good functional outcomes with nonoperative treatment and aggressive rehabilitation. Patients treated conservatively should be monitored for premature tibiofemoral joint degeneration caused by instability. The MCL and the oblique popliteal ligament are commonly injured in conjunction with the PCL, and this may necessitate surgical reconstruction.

• The treatment plan should be congruent with the patient's preinjury lifestyle, functional goals, and motivation for postoperative rehabilitation. Whether or not the patient undergoes surgery, it is essential to reduce the effusion and regain full range of motion as the patient re-establishes neuromuscular control to normalize gait. As strength returns, the patient should begin sport-specific agility drills and be able to return to full activity approximately 2 months postinjury.

Medial Collateral Ligament Injuries. MCL injuries are quite common and are seen in direct trauma or as overuse syndromes.

• Grade I (mild) MCL strains demonstrate pain with palpation, but there is no evidence of valgus instability. Pain and inflammation should be controlled with cryotherapy. The patient should be placed in a locked brace for the first few days and then progressed to a hinge brace. A strengthening and flexibility program should be initiated. Athletes attempting a return to sports can wear the hinged brace for 1 to 2 months following injury.

• Grade II (moderate) injuries to the MCL are characterized by inability to fully extend the knee because of pain and inflammation. There is mild-to-moderate instability when a valgus stress is applied in knee flexion, and there is swelling and hemorrhage. A knee orthosis should restrict the last 20 to 30 degrees of extension for the first week while the effusion is reduced with the application of ice and compression. After the first week, a limited arc of motion (20 to 75 degrees) is permitted. Early mobilization is encouraged within pain-free limits, and range of motion should be regained over a 3- to 4-week period. Near the end of the first month, the patient can be full–weight bearing in a brace that allows full flexion and extension. When pain improves, strengthening of the hip girdle muscles and knee stabilizers is integrated into the rehabilitation program. After 4 to 5 weeks the patient should advance to agility drills and sport-specific activities. Return-to-play criteria include 90% strength or better, minimal or no thigh atrophy, and no inhibition during agility drills.

• Severe grade III MCL tears demonstrate instability to valgus stress in both flexion and extension. Hemarthrosis usually develops within a few hours. Treatment for grade III insufficiency remains controversial. It is essential that the knee be examined to rule out associated meniscal or cruciate ligament damage, which increases the chance that surgical repair is needed. However controversial the decision for surgical care, the development of an appropriate treatment plan should focus on the patient's preinjury demands and motivation to return to biomechanically stressful activities.

Lateral Collateral Ligament Injuries. The treatment program for isolated LCL injuries is similar to the nonoperative approach described for the MCL; however, the vulnerability of the peroneal nerve at the level of the fibular head must be kept in mind.

Meniscal Lesions. These injuries are common in both sport and industry. Injury usually follows forceful rotation of the lower extremity while the foot is firmly placed on the ground. An effusion usually develops within 24 to 48 hours. Damage can range from a small peripheral tear to a larger bucket-handle tear presenting with intense pain. The patient might describe a sensation of giving way or mechanical locking. Clinical examination often reveals tenderness on palpation of the joint line. *McMurray's test* is performed with varying degrees of tibial internal and external rotation combined with valgus or varus moment while the limb is moved from full flexion to extension. The test is positive if a "click" is produced or if pain is reproduced.

• MRI can be used to demonstrate a meniscal tear, but if mechanical symptoms exist, arthroscopy is probably the diagnostic test of choice. Locking can be observed with osteochondral lesions, cruciate ligament rupture, bony avulsions, or meniscal impingement.

• Treatment of meniscal lesions is dependent on the severity of the injury to the meniscus and the possibility of combined damage. In the absence of a locked knee, a period of observation to allow for pain control and reduction of the effusion can help delineate the most appropriate treatment. The presence of associated ligamentous tears or inability to bear weight after 2 to 3 days suggests the need for arthroscopic evaluation. If the swelling goes down and the patient is able to regain full joint motion and full strength, a nonoperative approach can be successful.

• The surgical approach to meniscal tear management has changed significantly in the last 20 years. Total meniscectomy is no longer an acceptable treatment, and efforts are geared toward preserving as much of the cartilage as possible. Preservation of the meniscus reduces the likelihood of degenerative changes.

• For the nonsurgically treated patient, early rehabilitation consists of pain and swelling reduction with institution of hamstring and ITB stretching and short-arc CKC activities. Swimming pool exercise can facilitate recovery and allow the patient to maintain endurance.

• For the surgically treated patient, postoperative rehabilitation depends on the complexity of the repair. Once pain-free range of motion has been established, and there is no joint line tenderness, the patient should return to full weight bearing. Deep squatting should be avoided during the first 6 months.

Osteochondritis Dissecans. This is a lesion of subchondral bone with or without articular cartilage involvement. In the knee, the most common site for a subchondral lesion occurs at the interior portion of the medial femoral condyle. Chondral flaps and chondral loose bodies might also be present. Patients experience intermittent mechanical symptoms with or without pain. An effusion can be present. Radiographs should include a tunnel view to evaluate the intracondylar notch. CT is helpful in evaluating the bony lesions, whereas MRI can provide a more accurate view of the articular cartilage. Treatment is based on the staging of the lesion and the patient's symptoms. Arthroscopic evaluation is indicated when there is separation of the lesion from the femur, mechanical locking, or chronic pain and effusion.

The Leg (pp. 842–843)

Relevant Anatomy and Biomechanics *(pp. 842–843)*

• The tibia and fibula and associated structures make up the leg. All muscles are innervated by the tibial or peroneal nerves. The crural structures are encased in a tight connective tissue fascia, with separation of the muscles of this region into four compartments. The anterior tibial muscle functions as a dorsiflexor and invertor, the posterior tibial muscle as a forefoot flexor and invertor, and the peroneus longus and brevis muscles serve as the only major evertors and provide some plantar flexion as well.

Achilles Tendinitis (Tendinosis). This is perhaps the most common injury of the lower leg. Contributing factors include excessive pronation, supination, tight heel cords, and rearfoot or forefoot varus. Overtraining, a single excessively strenuous workout, and hill running can create this problem as well. It is important to recognize that although the majority of patients feel they have an acute inflammatory problem (tendinitis), they actually have a chronic problem (tendinosis). This can eventually lead to frank rupture of the tendon.

• The clinical symptom complex is pain, located typically 6 to 8 cm proximal to the insertion on the calcaneus, that is worsened by dorsiflexion. The functional adaptation complex includes increased knee flexion and increased pronation (both particularly influenced by the tight gastrocnemius, which crosses both knee and ankle joints).

• The rehabilitation program is initiated with the PRICE principle and anti-inflammatory medications. The tendon is never injected. Heel lifts often provide some relief in early rehabilitation but should not be used indefinitely because this promotes shortening of the heel cord. Reduction in weight-bearing activity is mandatory. These patients are good candidates for aquatic-based conditioning. In chronic cases, additional aggressive soft tissue mobilization to promote an initial inflammatory response, coupled with a controlled passive stretching regime, can help break up scar tissue. As pain is reduced, the patient should go through a gradual program of first concentric and ultimately eccentric strengthening of the plantar flexors. If the pain continues despite all the above measures, an MRI study of the Achilles tendon can help identify previously undetected partial tendon tears, musculotendinous tears, retrocalcaneal bursitis, or stress fractures.

Stress Fractures. A *stress fracture* is defined as a partial or complete fracture of a bone that results from that bony region's inability to withstand a repetitively applied subthreshold and nonviolent mechanical stress. Persons most at risk are those who have asymmetrical limb lengths, who pronate or supinate excessively, or who run on rigid surfaces. The tibia is the most common site (34%), followed by the fibula (24%), metatarsals (20%), and femur (14%). Well-localized pain is a major clinical feature. Stress fracture can also be suggested by pain produced over the suspected fracture site by application of a vibrating tuning fork, or with percussion of the bone away from the affected site. Stress fractures are difficult to detect by routine radiographs early in their course. Bone scans are recommended in cases of increased clinical suspicion when the plain film study is negative.

• During rehabilitation of a stress fracture, the first principle is to have the patient reduce activity to stay below the level of activity that induces symptoms. Running on dry land is prohibited until an adequate amount of time for healing has passed; however, aqua running is a good safe alternative. Healing time is approximately 3 weeks for the fibula, 4 to 8 weeks for the tibia (although considerably longer if the tibial plateau has been affected), and several months (with limited weight bearing) for the neck of the femur.

Compartment Syndromes. In *dynamic compartment syndromes* of the leg, elevated tissue pressure in any of the four compartments transiently reduces the capillary perfusion below the level needed for tissue viability. The anterior compartment is most often affected. Dysesthesias in the distribution of the deep peroneal nerve, foreleg pain, dorsiflexor weakness, and hypoperfusion are common. The syndrome can be confirmed with intracompartmental pressure measurements. Postexertional MRIs can also be of value. Although fasciotomy is often seen as the definitive treatment for this problem, recent evidence suggests that cycling produces lower anterior compartment pressures than does running, implying that for athletes willing to modify their training regimens, an alternative to surgery, with maintenance of fitness, is possible.

Bursal Syndromes of the Foot. The retrocalcaneal, subtendinous bursa lies between the posterior surface of the calcaneus and the tendon of the triceps surae. Inflammation of the bursa can result from training errors, which can create excessive pressure in the heel counter region. Discomfort occurs when the examiner places the thumb and index finger on the anterior edges of the Achilles tendon and applies pressure. Footwear modification is an important first step. Symptoms are controlled with ice and anti-inflammatory medications. When the pain begins to resolve, the patient should stretch the triceps surae complex daily to avoid recurrence. Injections into the bursa are done only with caution because corticosteroids can weaken the Achilles tendon, increasing the risk for tendon rupture.

• *Subcutaneous bursitis,* or Achilles bursitis, involves the bursa lying subcutaneous to the posterior surface of the Achilles tendon. The patient develops midline swelling where the upper edge of the heel counter comes in contact with the heel cord. Subcutaneous bursitis is commonly seen in women who wear high heels that apply direct pressure on the bursa. The mainstay of treatment is to change the patient's shoes. Ice and anti-inflammatory medications can provide symptomatic relief.

Ankle Injuries (pp. 843–847)

Relevant Anatomy and Biomechanics (pp. 843–844)
• The ankle can be described as a hinge joint with a mortise (the tibia and fibula) and tenon (talus). The distal tibia forms the medial malleolus, whereas the fibula, which extends further distally, forms the lateral malleolus. There is approximately 20 degrees of ankle dorsiflexion and 50 degrees of available plantar flexion under normal conditions. The talocrual joint has maximum osteological stability in dorsiflexion and minimal osteological stability in plantar flexion. The subtalar (talocalcaneal) and midtarsal (talonavicular and calcaneocuboid) joints both permit the additional motions of inversion and eversion and influence hindfoot-to-midfoot load transfer.
• The critical ligamentous structures on the lateral side include the posterior talofibular ligament (PTFL), anterior talofibular ligament (ATFL), and the calcaneofibular ligament (CFL) (Fig. 39–3B). On the medial side the deltoid ligament is composed of the anterior tibiotalar, posterior tibiotalar, tibionavicular, and tibiocalcaneal ligaments (Fig. 39–3A). Anterolaterally, between the fibula and the tibia, is the tibiofibular syndesmosis. Given the broadness of the medial malleolus, the angle of the mortise, and the toughness of the deltoid complex, the medial structures provide much greater restriction to extremes of eversion than do the lateral structures to extremes of inversion. Consequently, medial injuries are far less common.

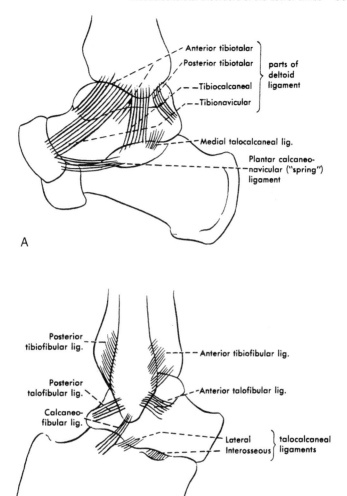

FIGURE 39–3. *A.* Medial ligaments of the ankle. *B.* Lateral ligaments of the ankle. (From Hollinshead WH, Jenkins DB: Functional Anatomy of the Limbs and Back, ed 5. Philadelphia, WB Saunders, 1981.)

Mechanisms of Injury (pp. 844–845)

• Ankle sprains typically occur when the foot and ankle are plantar-flexed. The ATFL is generally the first structure injured with a combined inversion–plantar flexion stress. The CFL is the second structure injured as the inversion stress increases. For the PTFL to become injured, either inversion must continue further or some posterior displacement of the talus must occur. Inversion in neutral dorsiflexion primarily stresses the CFL. The deltoid ligament is injured with eversion stress. Addition of any rotatory stress to the above, or inversion in dorsiflexion leads to syndesmosis injury.

Classes of Injury (pp. 845–846)

Grade I (mild)—minor ligamentous disruption (essentially a stretch) with maintenance of integrity and no signs of instability

Grade II (moderate)—near complete disruption with macroscopic tearing and swelling. There is a moderate amount of functional loss such as difficulty with toe-walking and there is mild or moderate instability.

Grade III (severe)—complete ligamentous rupture with obvious swelling, discoloration, and tenderness. There is significant functional loss with limited range of motion because of swelling, limited weight-bearing tolerance because of pain, and reduced stability because of the ligamentous disruption.

• The mechanism and consequences of the acute ankle injury can be obtained from the history and physical examination. Sensation of a tear or pop with a "rolling over" of the ankle are highly suggestive of an ATFL or CFL tear.

• The examination should be done in a methodical manner. The fibular head region is palpated to detect defects and tenderness suggestive of fracture and to check for irritability over the peroneal nerve. The fibular shaft, distal tibia, fibula, talar dome region, and foot are percussed to identify possible fracture sites. Points of maximal tenderness are commonly elicited over the ATFL and CFL. A complete sensory examination and light percussion over the superficial nerves are important to identify stretch injuries, which can cause superimposed dyesthetic pain. Examination of the injured ankle should be preceded by examination of the uninjured side.

• The *anterior drawer* test is the hallmark test for integrity of the ATFL. The patient's calf muscles should be relaxed and the foot should be in approximately 10 degrees of plantar flexion. The calcaneus is grasped firmly and drawn forward while the tibia is pushed posteriorly with the other hand. Under normal conditions, the translation of the talus is no more than 4 mm. A drawer of more than 8 mm is indicative of at least an ATFL tear.

• The *talar tilt* (inversion) test is more sensitive for CFL tears. With the ankle in neutral, the lower leg is held firmly by one hand while applying an inversion stress to the talus and calcaneus with the other hand. Separation of the surface of the talus from the tibia (i.e., a tilting) is considered a positive test.

• The *clunk test* (side-to-side) is a gross assessment of mortise widening, as when there is a tibiofibular ligament complex injury. Grasping the calcaneus with one hand and surrounding the distal third of the tibia and fibula with the other, the examiner attempts to move the talus from side to side. A "clunk" or "thud" is felt as the talus hits the tibia or fibula. Care must be taken not to allow inversion or eversion to occur during this maneuver or a false-positive result will be obtained.

• The *eversion test* assesses the integrity of the deltoid ligament complex. The lower tibia is grasped in one hand and the heel in the other. If the tibiotalar joint widens medially with eversion stress, the test is positive.

• If a sprain is thought to be grade II or more, radiographs should be obtained to rule out a co-existing fracture. Standard views include an anteroposterior, a lateral, and a "mortise" view. The mortise view is necessary to fully evaluate the talar dome surface as well as to adequately examine the distal tibial and fibular surfaces.

• When examining radiographs of the ankle, it is important to remember the "ring concept." When the mortise is viewed directly, the lateral malleolus, the tibial plafond superiorly, the medial malleolus, and the talus inferiorly form a ring that is held together by the lateral and medial ligaments and the syndesmosis (see Fig. 39–26 in the Textbook). If the ring is deformed on one side (e.g., a distal fibular fracture), one should look for a co-existing injury somewhere else along the ring (e.g., a deltoid ligament injury with widening of the medial mortise).

• There are many types of fractures associated with ankle sprains, and it is beyond the scope of this chapter to discuss them all. The *spiral fracture of the distal fibula* is one of the most common fractures of the ankle region. When seen, the proximal fibula must also be examined because forces might have been transmitted up the interosseous membrane. The *Jones fracture* is a fracture at the base of the fifth metatarsal associated with inversion sprain and pulling of the peroneus brevis. *Osteochondral talar dome fractures* may follow almost any type of ankle injury and should be considered in "slow-healing" cases and where the region over the talus is tender. *Mortise disruption* follows syndesmosis or deltoid ligament injury; the ring of the mortise should immediately be inspected for evidence of bimalleolar (or trimalleolar) fractures. With the exception of the nondisplaced Jones fracture, all of these problems can require surgical consultation.

Ankle Rehabilitation (pp. 846–847)
• Acute treatment of all sprains includes elevating, icing, and compressive wrapping of the injured site. Early mobilization of the sprained but nonfractured ankle is the preferred treatment. The ankle should be protected with elastic support, air stirrup splints, lace-up braces, or plastic-molded supports. Crutches are used only when gait is affected enough to increase the chance of further injury or when pain precludes full weight bearing. Ankle pumping, "writing the alphabet" with the feet, and stretching of the gastrocnemius-soleus complex can all be started during this period. Once the patient is able to bear full weight on the affected ankle, a single-limb balance program should be instituted. The patient begins by balancing on the affected side for 30 to 60 seconds on a hard floor, with progression to other surfaces. During the next phase, strengthening of the evertors, invertors, plantar flexors, and dorsiflexors can be performed dynamically with elastic tubing, and then via heel raises and partial squats. Hip abductor muscle strengthening should be done as well. Balance boards are an essential part of the rehabilitation because these help with proprioceptive retraining and with strengthening. Bicycle exercise is a safe way to maintain or increase endurance without subjecting the ankle to excessive stress. As the patient progresses, more dynamic training is introduced. Functional tests to determine readiness to return to activity include "shuttle runs" and single-leg hopping. In our experience, the majority of sprains treated in this manner are ready to return to activity within 1 to 3 weeks. The use of postrehabilitation bracing is not mandatory, but athletes might elect to use hightop shoes, lace-up braces, or taping for injury prophylaxis.

Foot Injuries (p. 847)

Plantar Fasciitis. This consists of traction-induced microtears of the plantar fascia and its associated structures at the insertion on the calcaneus. Limited ankle dorsiflexion, excessive pronation, and a tight gastrocnemius-soleus complex all increase the chance of developing plantar fasciitis. This subjects other medial support structures, such as the plantar fascia, to increased tensile forces and excessive overload. Plantar fasciitis is usually seen in persons with high or normal arches, but it can also be seen in the person with flat feet.

• Symptoms of plantar fasciitis consist of point tenderness along the medial fascia, inability to run, and a painful first step of the morning. Functional adaptations include attempted inversion to reduce medial structure overload and, in the case of runners, forefoot running with a choppy stride.

• Acute management consists of the PRICE principle and use of anti-inflammatory medications as needed. Ice massage is a particularly useful modality. If the diagnosis is clear, radiographs are not needed. If they are obtained, it is important to realize that heel spurs on the calcaneus are a common radiographic finding (up to 30% of the asymptomatic population) and are likely to represent repetitive plantar ligament traction rather than a site of true pathological changes. Similarly, spurs might not be found in patients with profound symptoms. Consideration is given to steroid injection into the calcaneal attachment, although this is rarely the authors' approach. Arch supports, counterforce taping, and heel pads might be helpful. A structurally rigid shoe insert might alleviate symptoms for an athlete who overpronates, but might exacerbate symptoms for an individual with a rigid high arched foot. The critical measures are stretching of the gastrocnemius-soleus complex, hamstrings, and plantar fascia, together with strengthening of foot intrinsic muscles. Chronic cases can take up to 3 to 4 months to resolve. Formulation of a temporary alternative training program such as rowing, swimming, or aqua running can maintain fitness without delaying resolution of the plantar fasciitis.

Calcaneal Bursitis. This often develops in elderly patients with a calcified spur, subjecting the bursa to trauma after prolonged walking or running. Evaluation of the footwear often reveals poor shock-absorbing capacity. Selecting the appropriate walking or running shoes supplemented with a heel cup is often enough to relieve the symptoms. Restoration of normal flexibility and strengthening of the foot intrinsics can help prevent recurring symptoms.

Morton's Neuroma. This represents the entrapment of interdigital nerves in the foot. The neuromas are most commonly found between the third and second interspaces. Patients complain of an aching forefoot, with at times lancinating foot pain. It is exacerbated by wearing tight shoes, high heels, and athletic activities requiring repetitive forefoot weight bearing. Patients obtain almost immediate relief when they take their shoes off and often prefer to walk barefoot. During physical examination, grasping the foot in one hand and squeezing the metatarsals together reproduces the symptoms. Radiographs or a bone scan should be obtained if there is a question of fracture. Intermediate-to-long-term relief can be obtained with footwear modification (increased width), orthotic inserts, and corticosteroid injection. For those who do not respond to conservative measures, neuroma excision can provide relief.

Common Pediatric Injuries—Traction Apophysitises
(pp. 847–849)

Apophyseal Injuries at the Hip. Five sites in the adolescent hip and pelvis are at particular risk for injury. These sites include the ischium, the anterior superior iliac spine (ASIS), the anterior inferior iliac spine (AIIS), and the lesser trochanter of each femur. The adolescent presents with a dull, aching pain with activity, often with a history of worsening over weeks to months. Pain is accompanied by tenderness at the site of injury. Apophysitis typically does not produce abnormalities on plain films unless an avulsion has occurred.

- Iliac crest apophyseal injuries commonly occur with either sudden or repetitive abdominal contraction opposed by forceful contraction of the tensor fasciae latae and the gluteus medius with a planted leg. A direct blow can also cause injury. This injury, a "hip pointer," can occur in football from a hit from another player or in basketball because of a fall to the hardwood floor. Pain and tenderness are seen at the iliac crest as well as painful active hip abduction.
- ASIS and AIIS apophyseal injuries are usually acute, with a sudden sharp pain in the hip and groin region occurring during sprinting. This is often referred to as "the sprinter's fracture." Distance running can also lead to injuries at these sites; however, these injuries are less acute and often give dull aching pain. Pain and swelling are seen at the site of injury, often with painful active hip flexion and an antalgic gait.
- Sports involving sprinting, jumping, and kicking can lead to apophyseal injury at the lesser trochanter because of the powerful contraction of the iliopsoas against resistance. The patient typically complains of anterior hip pain. Pain can radiate to the groin or flank. Deep palpation of the anterior hip is painful, as is active hip flexion. Passive extension and internal rotation are also painful.
- Ischial apophyseal injury is the most commonly reported apophyseal injury at the hip and pelvis. Injury can be acute with sprinting or hurdling, or chronic with distance runners. Pain is seen in the buttock region, often radiating into the posterior thigh. Tenderness occurs at the ischial tuberosity. Stretching or contraction of the hamstrings elicits discomfort.
- Treatment for each of the hip apophysitises and minimally separated avulsion fractures includes relative rest followed by a progressive restoration of strength and flexibility of the entire hip and pelvic region. Initial treatment should include protected ambulation with crutch walking until the gait pattern is normal. If crutch walking is painful, 2 to 4 days of bed rest might be required in a position of hip flexion and knee flexion. Once gait has normalized (usually 7 to 10 days), gentle stretching and strengthening can begin. By 3 weeks, pain is usually minimal, and more aggressive strengthening can be started. Limited athletic activity can be started by week 4, with a progression to full activity by week 6. Some cases, particularly injury to the lesser trochanter, might take up to 12 weeks for full recovery. Very few patients with these injuries have any residual symptoms beyond 12 weeks.

Osgood-Schlatter Disease. The most common traction apophysitis and one of the most common problems in the adolescent athlete is Osgood-Schlatter disease. The etiology is believed to be microtraumatic with multiple avulsions and healing at the tibial tubercle. The injury, often bilateral, commonly occurs between the ages of 10 to 15 years, with males more often affected. Symptomatic onset often coincides with the beginning of a growth spurt.

- The young athlete complains of pain at the tibial tubercle with running or jumping. Examination typically shows a prominence of the tibial tubercle without a knee effusion. Active knee extension is painful. Weakness of the quadriceps muscle is also common. Plain radiographs can range from a normal appearance to multiple areas of irregular calcification.

• Treatment varies depending on the severity of symptoms. Milder cases often respond to ice, a compressive wrap, or a knee brace. More severe cases might require crutch walking. Immobilization should be avoided. If a compressive wrap or a brace does not alleviate symptoms, a period of rest from sports is recommended. Pain-free straight leg raises should be started almost immediately. Stretching of the quadriceps group is imperative and should be started as soon as tolerated. Pain can persist for months, particularly pain on pressure palpation of the tibial tubercle. Residual deformity at the tibial tubercle persists after symptomatic improvement. Only a very small number of adolescents have symptoms beyond skeletal maturity, and these cases often require surgery for improvement.

Sindig-Larsen-Johansson Syndrome. Sindig-Larsen-Johansson syndrome, though less common than Osgood-Schlatter disease, presents with similar symptomatology. However, pain and tenderness is at the inferior pole of the patella, instead of the tibial tubercle. This condition is most commonly caused by repetitive microtrauma in sports that require frequent kicking, running, and/or jumping. Radiographic findings are similar to those of Osgood-Schlatter, ranging from normal to bony irregularity or avulsion at the distal patella. Treatment and outcome are very similar to those of Osgood-Schlatter disease.

Sever's Disease. This condition usually presents with heel pain in the adolescent athlete. The injury is caused by repetitive microtrauma with resulting inflammatory changes at the calcaneal insertion of the Achilles tendon. Pain occurs during a growth spurt, can be bilateral in up to 60% of the cases, and is almost always associated with sports involving a lot of running. Examination shows tenderness at the Achilles tendon insertion, tightness of the gastrocnemius-soleus complex, and relative weakness of the ankle dorsiflexors. Radiographs or bones scans can be helpful in ruling out other causes of heel pain such as stress fracture, infection, or neoplasm.

• Treatment is similar to other apophysitises. Heel cups or lifts can be helpful while the patient is symptomatic. In cases with significant biomechanical foot abnormalities, orthoses might be necessary. Stretching of the entire gastrocnemius-soleus complex is essential and should be started as early as possible. When the adolescent is asymptomatic, begin dynamic strengthening of the foot-ankle complex with a wobbleboard for dynamic stability. Good athletic shoe fit is imperative, with the addition of an over-the-counter shoe insert if necessary. Most cases resolve within 3 to 6 weeks.

40

Original Chapter by Mehrsheed Sinaki, M.D., M.S.,
and Bahram Mokri, M.D.

Low Back Pain and Disorders of the Lumbar Spine

EPIDEMIOLOGY OF BACK PAIN (pp. 853–854)

• In the industrialized world, low back pain is second only to headache as a cause of pain.

• Some 50% to 80% of adults will have low back pain at some time in their lives. Only 1% of patients with acute low back pain have lumbar radiculopathy. This rate is probably even lower for those with chronic low back pain. Lumbar radiculopathies often occur in patients during the fourth and fifth decades of life.

Risk Factors (pp. 853–854)

Occupational Factors (p. 854)

• Factors such as lifting, pulling and pushing, twisting, slipping, sitting for an extended period, and exposure to prolonged vibration, in isolation or in various combinations, have been attributed to development of low back pain. Persons who view their occupations as boring, repetitious, or dissatisfying might also report a higher rate of low back pain.

Patient-Related Factors (p. 854)

AGE

• The likelihood of developing low back pain gradually increases until approximately 55 years of age.

GENDER

• Men and women have similar risks of low back pain until age 60 years. Thereafter, women are at greater risk, probably because of the development of osteoporosis.

ANTHROPOMETRIC FACTORS

• There is a higher risk of low back pain in very obese persons and, possibly, in tall persons.

POSTURAL FACTORS

• The effect of scoliosis on spine pain is discussed in Chapter 17. The role of other postural changes (e.g., kyphosis, increased or decreased lumbar lordosis, and discrepancy in the length of the lower limbs) in the production of back pain is controversial.

SPINE MOBILITY
• Most subjects with low back pain have at least some limitation of range of motion of the lumbar spine.

MUSCLE STRENGTH
• Several studies have shown decreased strength of abdominal and spinal muscles in patients with low back pain.

SMOKING
• Persons who smoke seem to have an increased likelihood of developing low back pain. Smoking is also known to increase the incidence of osteoporosis.

PSYCHOSOCIAL FACTORS
• Depression, anxiety, hypochondriasis, hysteria, alcoholism, divorce, chronic headaches, and other factors have been reported with higher frequency in patients with chronic low back pain.

Etiology (p. 854)

• Various disease entities can cause low back pain. The causes of low back pain are many, most of which can be categorized according to the classifications provided in Table 40–1.

ANATOMY AND KINESIOLOGY OF THE LUMBAR SPINE (pp. 854–857)

• The vertebrae increase in size distally in the spine. The "shock absorbers" of the spine are the intervertebral disks. The orientation of the facet joints varies at different levels of the spine in order to accommodate spinal movement. Seventy-five percent of lumbar flexion and extension occurs in the lumbosacral joint, 20% at L4 to L5, and the remaining 5% at the other levels.
• The lumbar vertebrae are composed mainly of cancellous bone that is susceptible to collapse under trauma or from osteoporosis. The vertebral body is attached to the neural arch, which is composed of pedicles, superior and inferior facet joints, and the lamina (see Fig. 40–1 in the Textbook). The laminae contribute little to the stability of the spinal column, and unilateral fracture or surgical removal of the laminae (laminectomy) does not cause spinal instability. The posterior longitudinal ligament, along with the anterior longitudinal ligament, helps maintain the axial stability of the vertebral column.
• Intervertebral disks act as cushions between vertebral bodies and are composed of fibrocartilaginous elements. The nucleus pulposus is an ovoid, gelatinous, and paracentrally located middle portion of the disk made of mucoprotein. This is surrounded by a firm, concentric meshwork of collagenous fibers called the *annulus fibrosus.*
• Functionally, the spine is composed of a series of mechanical units. Each unit consists of an anterior segment (two adjacent vertebral bodies and the intervertebral disks between them) and a posterior segment (neural arches). The anterior segment is primarily the weight-bearing and shock-absorbing component, whereas the posterior segment protects the neural structures and directs movements of the units in flexion and extenion.

TABLE 40–1 Causes of Low Back Pain

Cause	Common Diseases
1. Degenerative	Degenerative joint disease (DJD), osteoarthritis, lumbar spondylolysis
	Facet joint disease, facet DJD
	Degenerative spondylolisthesis
	Degenerative disk disease
	Diffuse idiopathic skeletal hyperostosis
2. Inflammatory (noninfectious)	Spondyloarthropathies (ankylosing spondylitis)
	Rheumatoid arthritis
3. Infectious	Pyogenic vertebral spondylitis
	Intervertebral disk infection
	Epidural abscess
4. Metabolic	Osteoporosis or osteopenia
	Paget's disease of bone
5. Neoplastic	Benign
	Spinal (benign bony tumors of spine)
	Intraspinal (meningiomas, neurofibromas, neurilemmomas, low-grade ependymomas)
	Malignant
	Spinal (malignant bony or soft tissue tumors, metastasis)
	Intraspinal (metastasis, high-grade ependymomas, astrocytomas, meningeal carcinomatosis)
6. Traumatic	Fractures or dislocations
	Sprains (lumbar, lumbosacral, sacroiliac)
7. Congenital or developmental	Dysplastic spondylolisthesis
	Scoliosis
8. Musculoskeletal	Acute or chronic lumbar strain
	Mechanical low back pain
	Myofascial pain syndromes
	Fibromyalgia, tension myalgia
	Tension myalgia of the pelvic floor, coccygodynia
	Postural abnormalities, pregnancy
9. Viscerogenic	Upper genitourinary disorders
	Retroperitoneal disorders (often neoplastic)
10. Vascular	Abdominal aortic aneurysm or dissection
	Renal artery thrombosis or dissection
	Stagnation of venous blood (nocturnal back pain of pregnancy)
11. Psychogenic	Compensation neurosis
	Conversion disorder
12. Postoperative and multiply operated-on back	

MUSCLES SUPPORTING THE SPINE AND THEIR FUNCTIONS (p. 857)

Muscle Groups (p. 857)

• Four groups of muscles provide support to the spine: the extensors, the flexors, the lateral flexors, and the rotators of the spine. Normally, the extensors and rotators are the main supportive muscles of the spine. The massive musculo-tendinous bulk over the upper sacral and lower lumbar vertebrae is the origin of the erector spinae muscles, which extend the vertebral column. Deep to the erector spinae lie the semispinalis muscles (see Fig. 40–3 in the Textbook). The interspinal muscles are between spinous processes. The abdominal muscles are the significant flexors and lateral flexors of the trunk and also participate in rotation.

Normal Posture (p. 857)

• In normal posture, the line of gravity passes from C1 to C7 vertebral bodies to T10 and the lumbosacral junction and passes through the common axis of the hip joint or slightly behind it. It passes in front of the sacroiliac articulation and knee joint and then in front of the ankle joint. Any shift from standard align-ment of the spine requires increased muscular activity to maintain posture as close to the line of gravity as possible.

EVALUATION OF THE PATIENT WITH LOW BACK PAIN (pp. 857–862)

Clinical Evaluation (pp. 857–861)

History (pp. 857–858)
• At the very least, the following information should be gathered:

Mode of onset of low back pain (e.g., abrupt or insidious)

Provoking, aggravating, and relieving factors

Effect of cough, sneeze, or strain on the low back pain, especially if these cause pain down the lower limbs

Presence or absence of pain at night and interference with sleep

Course (e.g., date of onset and whether the pain has been progressive, decreas-ing, fluctuating, or episodic)

History of similar or different back or lower limb pains

Associated limb symptoms (e.g., pain, paresthesias, numbness, weakness, atrophy, cramps, or fasciculations)

Presence or absence of urinary frequency, urgency, or retention; bowel or bladder incontinence; or constipation

History of lumbar surgery (e.g., laminectomy or fusion)

Types of previous treatments implemented, medications used, and the effects of these medications on the symptoms

Presence or absence of litigation or compensation issues

Examination (pp. 858–859)
INSPECTION
• Look for deformities, paraspinal spasm, birthmarks, unusual hair growth, listing to one side, corkscrew deformity, decrease or increase in lordosis, presence of scoliosis, muscular atrophy, or asymmetries.

PALPATION AND PERCUSSION

• Determine whether there are tender or trigger points, local tenderness or pain on percussion, spasm, or tightness of the paraspinal muscles. Observe the patient's reaction to pain, whether there is a "touch-me-not" withdrawal to palpation or touch.

RANGE OF MOTION

• Range of motion should be determined for flexion, extension, lateral bending, and rotation. Values for normal range of motion of the lumbar spine are as follows: flexion, 40 degrees; extension, 15 degrees; lateral bending, 30 degrees; lateral rotation, 40 degrees to each side. Some clinicians use as a rule of thumb that spinal flexion is essentially normal if the patient can bring the fingertips to within 6 inches of the floor or less on bending with the knees in full extension.

Tape Measure Method. One method of measuring range of motion was originally described by Schober. This method is a simple and practical way to determine the amount of flexion of the lumbar spine. A line is drawn that connects the "dimples of Venus." Then, two marks are made along a line that perpendicularly bisects the first line. One mark is 5 cm below and the other 10 cm above the point of bisection, with the distance between these two marks being 15 cm. The patient is then asked to bend forward maximally. The measured distance beyond the original 15 cm gives an estimate of the degree of spinal flexion (see Fig. 40–4 in the Textbook).

Inclinometers. This double inclinometer (see Fig. 40–5 in the Textbook) method fails to separate hip motion from spine motion. It is also subject to variability with the subject's effort.

Neurological Examination (pp. 859–861)

• This is a very important part of the evaluation of every patient with low back pain.

GAIT, STATION, AND COORDINATION

• The clinician should look for antalgic gait, foot drop, and functional or hysterical features. The patient should do toe-walking, heel-walking, and tandem gait. It should be determined whether the patient can stand on either foot or can squat and rise.

MUSCLE STRETCH REFLEXES

• An increase, decrease, or absence of muscle stretch reflexes (MSR) should be recorded. Neurologically normal persons can have exaggerated, diminished, or even absent reflexes. A patient's reflexes must be compared with other muscle stretch reflexes, particularly of the corresponding opposite side. Reflex asymmetry, however, is most often significant. The patellar reflex is mainly at the L4 level, and the Achilles reflex is mainly at the S1 level. Although the medial hamstring reflex can be used at times, there is no clinically reliable and easily elicitable MSR for the L5 level.

MUSCLE BULK

• Inspect for muscle atrophy. Comparison of the circumference of the lower limbs, determined with a tape measure, at different levels (such as midcalf level) is sometimes useful.

MUSCLE STRENGTH

• It is important to determine whether muscle weakness is genuine or whether it is a giving-way as the result of pain, functional factors, or poor effort. True weakness causes a muscle to give away smoothly during manual muscle testing. Factitious weakness often gives a jerky type of giving away, referred to as a rachety response to muscle testing. It should be noted whether the distribution of the weakness corresponds to a single root or multiple roots or to a peripheral nerve or plexus, or whether the weakness is of upper motor neuron type.

SENSORY EXAMINATION
• This is the least reliable part of the neurological examination. Asking the patient to outline areas of sensory loss may help orient the examiner and save time. Determine whether the reported sensory changes are consistent and reproducible, and whether they follow anatomical dermatomal patterns. It should be remembered that injured soft tissues can refer a range of sensations that do not represent true sensory changes. These are often referred to as sclerotomal reference sensations.

STRAIGHT-LEG-RAISING TEST
• This test is based on the fact that nerves and nerve roots that are injured typically hurt when tension is applied. The test (also called the Lasègue test) is done with the patient supine in bed or on an examining table. The relaxed lower limb in extension is gently and gradually elevated, and the patient is instructed to inform the examiner when the pain occurs and also to report the location of the pain. If the patient is sitting on an examining table or a chair, gently bringing the knee into extension often produces the same type of pain as does the straight-leg-raising test in a patient with L5 or S1 radiculopathy. Sometimes elevation of the asymptomatic lower extremity causes pain in the symptomatic side ("well-leg" or crossed straight-leg-raising sign). This is often a reliable sign of root irritation. The L4 root can be evaluated by having the patient lie prone and then trying to put the heel on the buttock. This stretches the quadriceps, which stretches the femoral nerve, which puts tension on the L4 root. Many clinicians consider these tests positive only if the pain in the low back or buttock is reported by the patient to extend at least down to the knee.

Diagnostic Studies (pp. 861–862)

Plain Radiography (p. 861)
• Plain radiography is a quick and low cost screening study. It is helpful for detecting fractures, dislocations, degenerative joint disease, spondylolisthesis, narrowing of intervertebral disk space, and many bony diseases and tumors of the spine. Oblique views are helpful for visualizing the neural foramina. Flexion and extension views are useful for studying subluxations and stability.

Radioisotope Bone Scanning (p. 861)
• Radioisotope scanning is a valuable test for screening all or a large part of the skeleton. It is useful for the detection of tumors, particularly bony metastases. Gallium scanning is used if infection is suspected.

CT and MRI (p. 861)
• Both CT and MRI are useful for detecting disk disease, herniated or extruded disk, or tumors (e.g., vertebral, epidural, meningeal, intradural, or cord). Overall, MRI (especially with gadolinium enhancement) is superior to CT. MRI can image the entire lumbar spine in a single scanning session, and shows the soft

tissues better than CT. CT is a better study for defining or demonstrating bony lesions.

Myelography (pp. 861–862)
• The use of CT and, especially, MRI has decreased the use of myelography. This test is, however, still used by many surgeons before a final decision is made regarding lumbar surgery. CT-myelography remains the most accurate imaging method for the diagnosis of disk herniations and extrusions.

Electromyography (p. 862)
• Electrodiagnostic studies are useful for detecting neurogenic changes and denervation, as well as for evaluating the extent of these changes and the level of involvement. Unlike imaging studies, electrodiagnostic studies provide physiological information (see Chapters 10, 11, and 12).

SOME COMMONLY ENCOUNTERED PAINFUL DISORDERS OF THE SPINE (pp. 862–885)
Mechanical Low Back Pain (p. 862)

• *Mechanical low back pain* is a descriptive term commonly used for nondiscogenic back pain that is provoked by physical activity and relieved by rest. This type of pain is often caused by stress or strain to the back muscles, tendons, and ligaments, and is usually attributed to strenuous daily activities, heavy lifting, or prolonged standing or sitting. The pain often progressively worsens during the day. Mechanical low back pain is often a chronic, dull, aching pain of varying intensity that affects the lower spine and might spread to the buttocks.
• Deconditioning and decompensation commonly cause a mechanical type of low back pain. The onset is often insidious, the patients are usually obese and display manifestations of chronic inactivity, and the back and abdominal muscles are weak. Overall, for the management of mechanical low back pain, correction of static or dynamic postural abnormalities is helpful. An exercise program consisting of abdominal and back strengthening exercise is necessary, and patients often improve quickly (see Fig. 40–8 in the Textbook).

Osteoarthritis (p. 862)

• Osteoarthritis, also known as degenerative joint disease, occurs with aging and can begin as early as the third decade of life. If the disease is symptomatic, the associated pain is centered in the lower back. Stiffness is common. Range of motion of the spine may be limited. Pain is often relieved by rest. Hypertrophic changes and spurs can compress nerve roots and cause additional radicular pain. Radiographs, particularly after the early stages, are diagnostic. Improvement and provision of proper static and dynamic posture principles, such as bending one knee during prolonged standing, provide pain relief and decrease the risk of further strain (see Fig. 40–9 in the Textbook). Exercises include abdominal and back muscle strengthening exercises (preferably isometric exercises).

Osteoarthritis of the Facet Joints (pp. 862–866)

• Osteoarthritis of the facet joints results in localized spine pain, often episodic, that sometimes extends to the limb and can mimic radicular pain. The onset of each attack is usually abrupt. Range of motion, especially with extension, is often limited. Pain is increased with activity and relieved by rest. Surgery is rarely indicated. Nonsteroidal anti-inflammatory drugs (NSAIDs) often help, and manipulation can at times give dramatic relief. Some patients may benefit from facet joint injection. Spontaneous improvement is not unusual. Conservative treatment is directed toward reducing hyperextension. Improvement in abdominal muscle strength and isometric contraction of the quadratus lumborum with pelvic tilt exercises place the sacrum in a more vertical position.

• Patients with facet joint pain are instructed to avoid sleeping in the prone position. In general, the objective of exercise is to develop the supportive muscles of the lumbosacral spine. The flexion-based exercises are performed once or twice a day (see Figs. 40–8A through C, in the Textbook). In cases of severe low back pain, application of a lumbosacral support can decrease pain and improve compliance with the exercise program. However, prolonged use of a back support (i.e., more than 3 weeks) is discouraged because muscle disuse can result.

Lumbar Disk Syndrome and Lumbosacral Radiculopathies (pp. 866–871)

• Lumbar disk syndrome is a common cause of acute, chronic, or recurrent low back pain, particularly in young to middle-aged men, but it also occurs in women, older persons, and even adolescents. Disk herniation can occur in the midline, but it often occurs to one side. Pain may be unilateral or bilateral. The cause is usually a flexion injury.

• Different degrees and types of disk herniation can occur. Macnab's classification is useful, and it indeed correlates well with MRI findings.

Bulging Disk. A bulge and convexity of the disk beyond the adjacent vertebral disk margins, but with an intact annulus fibrosus and Sharpey's fibers (Fig. 40–1A).

Prolapsed Disk. The disk herniates posteriorly through an incomplete defect in the annulus fibrosus (see Fig. 40–1B).

Extruded Disk. The disk herniates posteriorly through a complete defect in the annulus fibrosus (see Fig. 40–1C).

Sequestered Disk. Part of the nucleus pulposus is extruded through a complete defect in the annulus fibrosus and has lost continuity with the present nucleus pulposus (see Fig. 40–1D).

• The pain often radiates into the buttock, the posterior thigh, and lateral calf; or to lateral or medial malleoli (in cases of L5 or S1 radiculopathies). The pain radiates to the anterior thigh in L3 or L4 radiculopathies. About 5% to 10% of patients with root lesions do not have associated back pain. In these cases, a mononeuropathy (e.g., sciatica, femoral neuropathy, or obturator neuropathy) or a lumbosacral plexus lesion must be ruled out.

• The most common levels of lumbar disk protrusion, herniation, or extrusion, in decreasing order of frequency, are L5 to S1, L4 to L5, L3 to L4, and L2 to L3. Lower lumbar and S1 radiculopathies are usually a result of degeneration or herniation of intervertebral disks and are usually unilateral. Midline disk protrusion may cause low back pain but no significant radiculopathy. Large midline disk herniations can cause bilateral radiculopathies or cauda equina syndrome

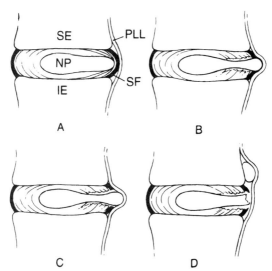

FIGURE 40–1. Classifications of disk herniation. *A.* Bulging annulus fibrosus. *B.* Prolapse. *C.* Extrusion. *D.* Sequestration. IE, inferior end-plate; NP, nucleus pulposus; PLL, posterior longitudinal ligament; SE, superior end-plate; SF, Sharpey's fibers. (From Vanderburgh DF, Kelly WM: Radiographic assessment of discogenic disease of the spine. Neurosurg Clin North Am 1993; 4:13.)

severe enough to produce sphincter problems. Upper lumbar radiculopathies are less commonly caused by disk disease. When upper lumbar radiculopathy is evaluated, other etiologic factors, particularly neoplastic disease, should be ruled out.
• Examination of the back often shows paraspinal muscle spasm, loss of lumbar lordosis, listing of the spine away from the side of root pain, limitation of motions of the lumbar spine with the "corkscrew phenomenon" on flexion and straightening, positive straight-leg-raising test, and, sometimes, crossed straight-leg-raising sign in cases of L5 or S1 radiculopathies. Coughing, sneezing, or straining causes an increase in abdominal pressure leading to distention of epidural and intervertebral veins. These distentions directly compress and put traction on the nerve roots and cause pain, particularly radiation down the involved lower extremity.
• When radiculopathy occurs, several features, including distribution of pain, reflex changes, distribution of weakness, and sensory alterations, provide reliable information that enables the clinician to localize the level of disk protrusion or root irritation.

Laboratory Tests for Lumbosacral Radiculopathies (pp. 868–869)
• MRI has become a major diagnostic tool in the diagnosis of herniated lumbar disks. It is also very useful for demonstrating bone disease, vertebral or epidural intraspinal tumors, scar tissue formations, infections, and even some forms of meningeal disease. Some herniated disks may be missed by MRI.

• CT-myelography is still the most accurate imaging test for documentation of herniated disks. Electromyography is very helpful for localizing the level of involvement, determining whether root involvement is single or multiple, and differentiating a multiple root from a plexus lesion.

Treatment (pp. 869–870)
• Most patients with discogenic low back pain respond to conservative management. The principles of conservative management of back pain are addressed at the end of the chapter.
• Progressive and significant neurological deficits justify early surgical intervention. Large midline disk protrusions with cauda equina syndrome require urgent treatment and decompression. The success of surgical treatment is greatest when there are bona fide objective neurological deficits. However, in many patients with lumbar disk syndrome, the major difficulty is low back pain with only mild, slight, or no evidence of radiculopathy. Most of these patients respond to conservative management. Lumbar laminectomy and discectomy for the sole complaint of low back pain are often unjustified.
• The standard surgical procedure is open laminectomy and discectomy. When there is spondylitic encroachment, facetectomy and foraminectomy may be necessary. Spinal fusion might be needed when there is spinal instability.

MICRODISCECTOMY
• *Microdiscectomy* is a generic term without a specific definition and essentially means the use of an operative microscope to accomplish posterior approaches for removal of a herniated lumbar disk through the smallest possible skin incision. Long-term results from microdiscectomy are not necessarily better than those from standard operation. The recurrence rate after microdiscectomy is higher than that after standard operation. Proponents of this technique argue that this increase possibly is related to earlier return of the patients to higher levels of activity.

PERCUTANEOUS LUMBAR DISCECTOMY
• This technique has been claimed to be effective for treating patients with small to moderate-sized, well-contained disk herniations. A nucleotome is guided into the disk space with precise radiographic control, and the disk material is then aspirated. The claimed advantages are use of local anesthesia, minimal tissue disruption, earlier return to usual activities, and minimizing the possibility of development of epidural fibrosis and scarring. Misplacement of the probe and serious neurological and vascular complications are feared sequelae, and the rate of recurrent symptoms may be higher. The potential for effective treatment with this technique may prove to be limited.

CHEMONUCLEOLYSIS
• Chemonucleolysis is less efficacious than open discectomy. Furthermore, it is associated with a significant incidence of anaphylaxis. The resolution of pain in patients who have chemonucleolysis may be related to prolonged inactivity after the procedure and during convalescence.

Posttraumatic Compression Fracture (p. 871)

• Posttraumatic compression fracture usually results from compressive flexion trauma. It can also occur spontaneously in patients with osteoporosis, osteomalacia, multiple myeloma, hyperparathyroidism, and metastatic cancer. The upper lumbar spine or the middle to lower thoracic spine is most commonly affected. The pain usually acute and is often localized. There may be accompanying paraspinal muscle spasm, and the range of motion of the related level of the spine is limited. Plain radiography, CT, MRI, or bone scanning may be needed to establish the diagnosis.

• Sedative rehabilitative measures (e.g., application of cold for the first 24 to 48 hours, analgesics, and muscle relaxants) are often necessary, especially in the acute phase. The pain can be managed with use of a back support, such as a thoracolumbar support that functions on the basis of three-point contact (see Chapter 17). When therapeutic exercises are to be prescribed, extension rather than flexion exercises should be utilized. Flexion exercises can increase the incidence of vertebral body wedging and compression fractures.

Spondylolysis and Spondylolisthesis (pp. 871–874)

General Considerations (p. 871)
• Spondylolysis refers to a bony defect in the pars interarticularis. Bilateral spondylolysis of the lumbar spine can lead to anterior slipping of the vertebral body on its adjacent vertebra and cause spondylolisthesis. Table 40–2 shows the classification of spondylolisthesis.

Symptoms and Signs (pp. 871–872)
• Spondylolysis or spondylolisthesis may cause back pain. Spondylolisthesis is two to four times more common in males. The pars defect is at L5 in 67% of persons, at L4 in 15% to 30%, and at L3 in 2%. It is rare in the cervical region. In patients with back pain and spondylolisthesis, the back pain is more likely to

TABLE 40–2 Classification of Spondylolisthesis

Type	Criteria
I	*Dysplastic:* The only truly congenital form of spondylolisthesis. The defect is a congenital dysplasia in the superior sacral facet or inferior L5 facet that allows L5 on S1 subluxation.
II	*Isthmic:* Defect (spondylosis) in pars interarticularis; the most common form of spondylolisthesis; typically involves L5 to S1.
	a. Lytic type, probably a fatigue fracture with hereditary predisposition.
	b. Elongated (attenuated) but intact pars, similar to type IIa, but the fatigue fractures have healed, resulting in elongated but intact pars.
	c. Acute fracture or pars due to trauma.
III	*Degenerative:* Secondary to degenerative changes at the disk and facet joints, most frequent at L4 to L5, followed by L3 to L4.
IV	*Traumatic:* Due to fracture of posterior elements other than pars (e.g., fractures of facet joints, lamina, pedicles).
V	*Pathological:* Due to pathological changes in posterior elements as a result of malignancy, primary bone disease, or infection.

From Mokri B, Sinaki M: Painful disorders of the spine and back pain syndromes. In Sinaki M (ed): Basic Clinical Rehabilitation Medicine, ed 2. St Louis, Mosby–Year Book, 1993, pp. 489–502. By permission of Mayo Foundation.

be caused by the pars defect if the patient is younger than 25 years. A pars defect is an uncommon cause of back pain in patients older than 40 years. Spondylolisthesis can also cause compression of nerve roots and lead to radicular pain or neurological deficits in the lower extremities. By narrowing the spinal canal, it can cause pseudoclaudication or compression of the cauda equina and can even lead to sphincter or sexual dysfunction. The lumbar lordosis is often exaggerated in patients with spondylolisthesis, and range of motion of the lumbar spine may be limited. The frequency of pars defects (spondylolysis) in children is about 4.5% (in adolescents it is about 6%), but it increases to 12% in gymnasts. In children, the most common types are dysplastic and isthmic.

Radiographic and Imaging Studies (pp. 872–873)

• The defect in the pars intra-articularis, known as *spondylolysis,* is often visible on lateral lumbosacral radiographs and can be noted as a break in the neck of the "Scottie dog" on oblique views of the lumbar spine. Radioisotope bone scan may show increased activity on one or both sides. Sometimes, single-photon emission computed tomography (SPECT) shows a pars defect that is not apparent on radiographs or bone scans.

• Spondylolisthesis is graded according to Meyerding's classification as grades 1 to 4, depending on the degree of displacement (Fig. 40–2). In advanced cases of displacement, L5 slips completely off S1. Flexion and extension views of the lumbosacral spine are obtained to determine any segmental instability.

Treatment (pp. 873–874)

• In post-traumatic cases of spondylolisthesis, after healing of the fracture and resolution of the pain, provision of immobilization for 10 to 12 weeks with appli-

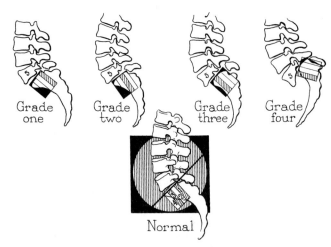

FIGURE 40–2. Meyerding's classification. The degree of subluxation is divided into four groups: grade 1, slipping on the vertebra less than one-fourth the distance of the lumbosacral angle: grade 2, less than half; grade 3, less than three-fourths; and grade 4, more than three-fourths. (From Mokri B, Sinaki M: Painful disorders of the spine and back pain syndromes. In Sinaki M (ed): Basic Clinical Rehabilitation Medicine, ed 2. St. Louis, Mosby–Year Book, 1993, pp. 489–502. By permission of Mayo Foundation.)

cation of a custom-made body jacket is the recommended treatment. In cases of chronic back pain, the patient should be instructed in abdominal muscle strengthening, lumbar flexion exercises, and static and dynamic body mechanics. In cases of persistent pain, the application of a lumbosacral brace or corset is recommended. In children, once the symptoms resolve, normal activities can be resumed, although a return to vigorous spine flexion or hyperextension athletic activities (e.g., football or gymnastics) is controversial.

- For grades 1 and 2 spondylolisthesis and in older patients, nonsurgical treatment is recommended. The physical therapeutic procedures consist of application of heat and massage for reduction of pain and stiffness. Special attention can be given to reducing the tightness of the hip flexors, hamstrings, and Achilles tendons.

- The goals of an exercise program should be reduction of lumbar lordosis through stretching of the lumbar paraspinal muscles and other tight structures and strengthening of the lumbar flexors. Strengthening of abdominal muscles is also of significant benefit. In cases of severe weakness of the abdominal muscles and poor response to strengthening, application of an elastic lumbosacral support can decrease pain until other measures (e.g., weight loss or improvement of posture) contribute to reduction of pain.

- In some cases, severe osteoporosis of the spine occurs with degenerative changes of ligamentous structures and spondylolisthesis. In these instances, a therapeutic exercise program that combines dynamic and static posturing along with isometric strengthening of spinal flexors and extensors without inducing strain on the osteoporotic spine has been shown to be helpful.

- In younger patients or persons who are involved in heavy physical jobs or strenuous sports activities, and when severe symptomatic slips with neurological symptoms or deficits are present, surgical treatment should be considered. Surgical management includes fusion of the unstable segment. Patients with advanced spondylolisthesis beyond grade 2 may need surgical intervention to decrease the symptoms. Adolescents who have spondylolisthesis of grade 2 or more have a greater risk for progression of the defect. In these patients, serial evaluations must be done to monitor the progress of the listhesis. Once patients experience symptoms of spondylolisthesis they should not perform heavy work or participate in high-performance, competitive sports. Segmental fusion results in relief of pain but does not warrant resumption of strenuous activity.

Lumbar Spinal Stenosis (pp. 874–876)

- Stenosis of the lumbar spine may involve the central canal at a single level or multiple levels and may jeopardize the cauda equina. Sometimes the stenosis involves only the lateral recess or root canal at single or multiple levels and jeopardizes one or more nerve roots. At times, a combination of both may be present.

Pathophysiology (p. 875)
- Spinal stenosis can be congenital, developmental, or acquired. Because degenerative joint disease is the most common cause of spinal stenosis, the resulting clinical syndromes occur most commonly after middle age. Degenerative disk disease and narrowing of the intervertebral spaces, spur formation, ligamentous hypertrophy, facet hypertrophy, and subluxation all contribute to the decreased caliber of the central spinal canal, lateral recess, and root canal.

Clinical Manifestations (pp. 875–876)

• Lumbar spinal stenosis clinically manifests as pseudoclaudication (neurogenic claudication), with unilateral or bilateral discomfort in the buttocks, thighs, or legs. Symptoms are produced by standing or walking and are relieved within a few minutes by sitting, lying down, or adopting a posture of flexion at the waist. The symptoms can include pain, numbness or paresthesias, or weakness.

• The anteroposterior diameter of the lumbar spinal canal is increased during flexion. At the same time, as the result of stretching of the posterior aspect of the annulus, particularly in young patients, the bulge of the disk toward the spinal canal is decreased. Lumbar flexion also leads to an increase in the caliber of the intervertebral foramina.

• Patients commonly prefer to walk in a stooped manner rather than with a straight, erect posture, in distinction to patients with vascular claudication. For the former patients, walking uphill (waist-flexion posture) may be easier than walking downhill (straight, erect posture).

• Symptoms are bilateral in more than two-thirds of patients, but a significant asymmetry often exists. The low back pain that is present in two-thirds of patients is typically mild and nondiscogenic.

• An absence or decrease in muscle stretch reflexes is noted in about 50% of patients. Weakness can be detected in about 40% of patients. This is usually mild, unilateral, and often in the distribution of L5 or S1 roots.

• The clinical features of lateral recess syndrome and root claudication are different from those of central canal stenosis. Patients usually report a unilateral intense sciatic pain (L5 or S1 root irritation) that is provoked by standing or walking and is relieved by sitting, lying down, or flexing the lumbar spine.

Differentiation of Vascular Claudication from Neurogenic Claudication (pp. 876–877)

• Some of the factors that are useful for differentiating vascular from neurogenic claudication are listed in Table 40–3.

Laboratory Tests (pp. 876–877)

ELECTROMYOGRAPHY

• Electromyographic abnormalities are noted in more than 90% of patients and are more common than the abnormalities detected on neurological examination. Findings include evidence of denervation in the distribution of a single root or multiple roots, often bilaterally.

PLAIN RADIOGRAPHY

• Most patients have degenerative joint or disk disease with or without spondylolisthesis. In some patients, the lumbar spinal canal appears congenitally narrow.

MELOGRAPHY AND IMAGING STUDIES

• Myelography shows complete or partial obstruction to the flow of contrast at one or more levels. CT and MRI show stenosis of the central canal, lateral recess, root canal, or a combination of these. CT-myelography is a very accurate test for evaluation of stenosis of these regions. Levels of stenosis (in decreasing order of frequency) are L4 to L5 (55%), L3 to L4 (44%), L2 to L3 (26%), L5 to S1 (14%), and T12 to L1 (3%).

TABLE 40-3 Differentiation of Vascular and Neurogenic Claudication

Factor	Neurogenic Claudication (Pseudoclaudication)	Vascular Claudication	Pitfalls and Remarks
Low back pain	Often present	Absent	Sometimes, coincidental degenerative joint disease can be present in patients with vascular claudication
Effect of standing	Provokes symptoms	Does not provoke symptoms	
Direction of radiation of pain in lower limbs	Usually downward	Usually upward	
Sensory symptoms	Present in 66% of patients	Absent	Some patients with vascular claudication can have distal sensory symptoms due to ischemic or diabetic neuropathy
Muscle weakness	Present in more than 40% of patients	Absent	
Reflex changes	Present in about 50% of patients	Absent	In older patients, especially if there is associated neuropathy, reflexes may be decreased or absent
Arterial pulses	Normal	Decreased or absent	In older patients, pulses may be reduced
Arterial bruits	Absent	Often present	
Effect of rest while standing	Does not relieve symptoms	Relieves symptoms	
Walking uphill	Symptoms produced later	Symptoms produced earlier	
Walking downhill	Symptoms produced earlier	Symptoms produced later	
Bicycling (stationary or regular)	Does not provoke symptoms	Provokes symptoms	

From Mokri B, Sinaki M: Lumbar disk syndrome, lumbosacral radiculopathies, lumbar spondylosis and stenosis, spondylolisthesis. In Sinaki M (ed): Basic Clinical Rehabilitation Medicine, ed 2. St Louis, Mosby–Year Book, 1993, pp. 503–513. By permission of Mayo Foundation.

Treatment (p. 877)
- The natural history of pseudoclaudication is not entirely clear. The symptoms of canal stenosis either remain unchanged or gradually worsen. The symptoms of root claudication are thought to either remain unchanged or perhaps gradually improve in some patients, but in an unpredictable time frame. For cases in which progressive neurological deficits occur, surgical decompression should be considered.

CONSERVATIVE MANAGEMENT
- Reduction of lumbar lordosis is effective for reducing lumbar stenosis. Exercises that are aimed at strengthening the abdominal muscles and lumbar flexors are helpful. For patients in whom it is not possible to strengthen the abdominal muscles, or in those with a protuberant abdomen and extensive body weight, an elastic abdominal binder is recommended. Patients should be instructed to avoid exercises that result in hyperextension of the spine. NSAIDs can help in managing the pain.

SURGICAL MANAGEMENT
- When patients are properly selected, decompressive single-level or multilevel laminectomy, with or without foraminotomies, alleviates manifestations of pseudoclaudication in most patients. However, the effect of this surgery on any associated low back pain is often less satisfactory.
- Overall, the more pronounced the degree of spinal canal compromise and neural compression, the better the chance of obtaining a good surgical result. When long-standing and pronounced neurogenic atrophy and weakness have developed, patients may get relief from the leg pain resulting from the pseudoclaudication, but they typically have only a partial or negligible recovery of the muscle weakness and atrophy.

Low Back Pain in Pregnancy (pp. 877–879)

Clinical Manifestations (pp. 878–879)
- Pregnant women commonly have back pains directly related to pregnancy. There are essentially four types of pain: (1) nocturnal back pain, which occurs in more than one-third of patients; (2) low dorsal pain; (3) lumbar pain, which may or may not extend to one or both lower limbs; and (4) sacroiliac region pain. (See Fig. 40–25 in the Textbook.)
- Nocturnal back pain of pregnancy occurs 1 to 2 hours after lying down; it is thought to be related to stagnation of venous blood in the vertebral venous plexus.
- Sacroiliac pain is probably the most common type of back pain in pregnancy. It may be unilateral or bilateral, and may extend to the upper thigh. Normally, the sacroiliac joint moves only minimally. During pregnancy, the production of relaxin (a hormone secreted by the corpus luteum) leads to articular laxity that can result in sacroiliac inflammation, pain, and discomfort.
- The other low dorsal and lumbar pains of pregnancy have mechanical features, are increased by physical activity, and are decreased by rest. The leg pain and radicular symptoms that can accompany the low back pain of pregnancy are commonly caused by the direct pressure of the gravid uterus on components of the lumbosacral plexus.
- The back pain of pregnancy may not disappear with delivery, and in 20% to 25% of cases the pain may linger for some time.

• Other causes of low back pain (e.g., herniated lumbar disk, tumors, and infections) can occur in pregnant women just as in the nonpregnant population. Pregnancy can induce a remission of rheumatoid arthritis, with frequent flareups after delivery.

Prophylaxis (p. 879)

• Options to prevent low back pain include: (1) reducing the load on the spine by appropriate changes in lifestyle and work environment; (2) avoidance of excessive weight gain during pregnancy; and (3) educating the patient regarding proper posture to decrease lumbar lordosis (e.g., proper techniques for lifting, working positions, and resting positions). Pregnancy back supports and exercise instructions for abdominal muscle and pelvic floor contraction, lateral bending, and rotational trunk exercises performed in a standing position may be helpful. Sit-ups requiring a supine position and Valsalva's maneuver should be avoided, particularly after the fourth month of pregnancy.

Treatment (p. 879)

• In most cases, when pregnant women are reassured of the benign nature of the back pain, they find the discomfort tolerable and typically manage the problem symptomatically by rest and modification of their activities. For more bothersome low back pain, application of an abdominal pregnancy support with shoulder suspenders, physical therapy, and massage may help. For pain in the sacroiliac region, a trochanteric belt or a sacroiliac corset may offer reasonably good relief. Nocturnal pain of pregnancy can be difficult to manage. The use of venous support stockings to reduce the dependent edema during the waking hours can help. Acetaminophen is the analgesic of choice for management of low back pain during pregnancy. Nonsteroidal agents are relatively contraindicated, and aspirin can increase the incidence of fetal intracranial hemorrhage in premature infants. Medication for back pain in pregnancy should be used only as a last resort, with the approval of the obstetrician and with the informed consent of the patient.

Paget's Disease (pp. 879–880)

• Paget's disease of bone is a rather common disease, particularly in elderly patients. It is marked by focal disturbance of bone architecture caused by abnormally increased osteoblastic activity. It may involve a single bone (monostotic) or several bones (polyostotic), including the pelvis or vertebral bones. The alkaline phosphatase level is typically elevated, except in some early, limited, or monostotic forms. The disease may be asymptomatic or may cause focal pain. Involvement of the posterior pelvis or lumbar spine causes low back pain in some patients. Malignant transformation of Paget's lesion can occur, but this is uncommon. The lesions should be differentiated from those of hyperparathyroidism, fibrous dysplasia, myeloma, and metastatic tumors, particularly metastases from prostate cancer. The involved area shows significant uptake on radioisotope bone scan, but MRI findings can be surprisingly unremarkable.

• Treatment is needed only in symptomatic cases. Aspirin or nonsteroidal agents can reduce the pain. In active disease and when the pain is clearly related to the Paget's disease and not to other conditions (e.g., degenerative joint or degenerative disk disease), treatment with etidronate sodium (5 to 10 mg/kg/day orally for 6 months) can be considered. Alendronate, an amino-bisphosphonate, is taken as a single dose on arising in the morning and at least 30 to 45 minutes before breakfast (40 mg/day orally for 6 months). Pamidronate is infused over 4 hours for 3 consecutive days (30 to 90 mg/day intravenously). Systemic calcitonin (50 to 100 IU [0.25 to 0.5 mL] per day) is given subcutaneously or intramuscularly. The dose may be tapered to 50 IU twice a week. Calcitonin also may be given as a nasal spray. Continuous treatment with etidronate can result in side effects of osteomalacia with increased bone fractures and pain. Consequently, drug holiday periods of 3 to 6 months should be interspersed between the treatment courses.

Low Back Pain Due to Neoplastic Disease (pp. 880–881)

• Primary spinal cord tumors such as astrocytomas, and particularly spinal ependymomas, can cause low back pain. Extramedullary intraspinal tumors such as meningiomas or neurilemmomas, as well as primary tumors of the vertebral bones (whether benign or malignant), can also cause low back pain. The most common neoplastic diseases causing low back pain are the metastatic spinal or epidural cancers (multiple myeloma and malignant lymphomas included) (see Figs. 40–27 to 40–32 in the Textbook). One of the hallmarks of cancer pain is pain at rest, particularly nocturnal pain.
• Spinal cord compression because of metastatic cancer is found in about 5% to 10% of patients with bony metastases. The tumors that most commonly metastasize to the spine include cancers of the lung, prostate, breast, kidney, and colon; and malignant melanoma, myeloma, and lymphoma.
• Radiation is the palliative treatment of choice. In cases of cord compromise, in addition to the radiation therapy, high-dose dexamethasone is also often administered. In selected cases, surgical decompression or even corpectomy has been considered. Imaging studies, particularly MRI, are helpful for detection of spinal and epidural metastases, for determining the field of radiation therapy, and for post-treatment follow-up.
• Analgesic medications are often required, particularly for the acute pain. Proper bracing and spinal immobilization and support should be provided if they help to decrease the pain or if there is a suggestion of spinal instability. Ambulatory assistive devices such as a wheeled walker can reduce weight-bearing pain.

Ankylosing Spondylitis (pp. 881–883)

• Ankylosing spondylitis is a chronic inflammatory seronegative rheumatic spondyloarthropathy that affects skeletal and extraskeletal tissues. It mainly affects the spine and invariably involves the sacroiliac joints. Eighty percent to 90% of patients are HLA-B27-positive. The prevalence is about 1 per 1000 in the white population, and it is more common in males. The disease usually begins at age 20 to 35 years. Sacroiliitis is usually the first manifestation, presenting as unilateral or bilateral low back pain of insidious onset. Classically, significant morning stiffness and pain in the lower back are noted. These symptoms typically improve with activity during the day and return after rest or immobility. Many patients are awakened from sleep because of pain and stiffness of the lower back. Lumbar lordosis may be lost. Recurrent iritis, aortitis, and carditis are some of the peripheral manifestations of the disease.

- The diagnosis must be confirmed by radiography. The earliest radiographic findings are in the sacroiliac joints and include blurring of the margins of the lower two-thirds of these joints and widening of the joint space. With advance of sacroiliitis, increase in erosions and joint space destruction, and progression of sclerosis, total ankylosis and obliteration of the joint may finally occur. Early changes in the lumbar spine include squaring of the lumbar vertebral body and demineralization and spotty ligamentous calcification. In advanced cases with diffuse paraspinal ligamentous calcification, the classic picture of "bamboo spine" is produced.
- The prognosis is variable. Overall, women have less severe spinal disease but may have more peripheral joint involvement. The prognosis is less favorable in patients with refractory iliitis. Overall, most patients have mild disease and can lead full and productive lives.
- Conservative treatment is the basis of management of patients with ankylosing spondylitis. NSAIDs can help diminish the pain and stiffness. Surgical intervention (e.g., extension osteotomies for excessive thoracic and cervical kyphosis) only rarely becomes necessary.
- Evaluation should include periodic measurements (in centimeters) of height, chest expansion, and C7 to S1 spinal flexion. A back extension exercise program; deep-breathing exercises; posture training; range of motion of the proximal joints (shoulders and hips); range-of-motion exercises to the cervical spine (if possible); and stretching exercises for the pectorals, hamstrings, Achilles tendons, hip flexors, and low back are important and should be included in the overall management program. Every effort should be made to avoid a flexed posture because there is no cure for subsequent fusion in a flexed position. Certain assistive devices facilitate daily activities despite limited spine motion. These include prism glasses, reachers, and wide-angle rear view mirrors for the car. Activities that may unduly strain the spine (e.g., contact sports, motorcycle riding, and jumping) should be avoided because they could result in vertebral fractures.

Diffuse Idiopathic Skeletal Hyperostosis (DISH) (p. 883)

- Ankylosing hyperostosis is a fairly common nondeforming, ossifying disease that occurs in elderly and middle-aged patients, particularly men. Ossification occurs along the anterior and lateral spinal ligaments. The ossification may also involve peripheral muscular tenderness at insertions. Any level of the spine may be involved, but thoracic involvement is more common, followed by involvement of the lumbar region. The involvement may be unilateral. The condition may be asymptomatic or cause stiffness, pain, and some limitation of motion, but significant functional inability is rare. Management is conservative; nonsteroidal agents may also be helpful. Application of infrared heat and massage decrease the accompanying myalgias and stiffness.

Pyogenic Vertebral Spondylitis (pp. 883–885)

- This condition includes infectious discitis (intervertebral disk infection) and infectious vertebral osteomyelitis. Although these can occur postoperatively, the focus here is on childhood and adult pyogenic infectious spondylitis that occurs without a history of spinal surgery. The mechanism is from a contiguous infection or by hematogenous or lymphatic seeding from a remote site. Common sources of infection are pneumonia; urinary tract, cutaneous, and dental infections; and abdominal surgery. It is more common in patients with diabetes, malignancy, renal failure, alcoholism, and AIDS; in intravenous drug abusers; and in immunocompromised patients. The most common infectious agent is *Staphylococcus aureus.* Pyogenic vertebral spondylitis may become associated with spinal epidural abscess, which may cause compression of the spinal cord or cauda equina and create a surgical emergency.

• The clinical features are often different in children and adults. In children, the onset is often abrupt, with fever, malaise, back pain, and spine tenderness. In adults, the onset is more gradual; there is little or no fever and malaise is generally absent. Point tenderness is evident at the involved site, but in a small percentage of patients, back pain may not be evident, and it can take up to 3 months to reach a diagnosis. The erythrocyte sedimentation rate is usually elevated, but leukocytosis is more evident in acute cases.

Radiographic and Imaging Findings (p. 884)

• Radiographic abnormalities significantly lag behind the actual pathological changes that are taking place. The radiographic findings include narrowing of the intervertebral disk space in discitis, loss of definition and destruction of the cortical margins of the vertebral bodies facing the disk, bone loss and rarefaction, vertebral body collapse, and gibbus formation (see Fig. 40–35 in the Textbook).

• Myelography does not directly visualize epidural abscesses but demonstrates the associated mass effect on the thecal sac and neural structures. Myelography also carries the risk of introducing the infection to the spinal subarachnoid space and creating meningitis.

• CT may show the pathological alterations, including the epidural abscesses. CT can also demonstrate paravertebral soft tissue components of the infectious process. MRI is clearly superior to CT for evaluation of epidural abscesses, paraspinal masses, discitis, and osteomyelitis.

Treatment (pp. 884–885)

• The infection should be treated with antibiotics. In general, nonsurgical therapy is considered for patients without neurological deficits. Surgery for decompression and drainage of pus should be considered when pressure effects and neurological deficits develop. Childhood disk space infection often responds well to antibiotics and immobilization with application of a rigid orthosis for 6 to 12 weeks.

BACK PAIN IN CHILDREN (pp. 885–887)

• Low back pain in childhood is quite different from the low back pain in adults. Back pain in children is uncommon, and commonly, but not always, is the result of a serious underlying cause (Table 40–4).

Helpful Hints in the History (pp. 885–886)

• Nocturnal pain responding to aspirin or NSAIDs may suggest osteoid osteoma, and a higher than expected family history of spondylolysis or scoliosis may have

TABLE 40–4 Causes of Low Back Pain in Children

Etiological Factor	Comments
Trauma	
Strain	Ligamentous or muscle strain. Probably the most common cause of LBP in this group. Look for a history of fall, strenuous exercise, or other trauma. Localized tenderness and paraspinal spasm may be present
Disk herniation	Uncommon in children and often post-traumatic. LBP alone or with radicular symptoms in lower limbs
Infections	
Urinary tract infection	Back pain may be the primary complaint
Discitis	Most common at age 2–6 years (when disk space is still vascularized). Young children may refuse to walk. Back motion is limited. Low-grade fever and irritability may be present. May be associated with epidural abscess or vertebral osteomyelitis
Inflammatory	
Ankylosing spondylitis	Usually affects boys. Loss of back mobility; arthritis in hips or knees
Juvenile rheumatoid arthritis	Outlook typically better than in adults
Neoplastic	
Vertebral bones	
Benign	Osteoid osteoma, benign chondroblastoma, eosinophilic granuloma, aneurysmal bone cyst
Malignant	Ewing's sarcoma, osteogenic sarcoma, metastases
Spinal cord and roots	Astrocytoma, ependymoma, hemangioblastoma, teratomas, lipomas, neurilemomas, neurofibromas
Bony abnormalities	
Scheuermann's disease	Osteochondritis of upper and lower cartilaginous end-plate of several vertebrae, causing anterior wedging and kyphosis, "round back deformity," and back pain; often presents in adolescence
Spondylolisthesis	
Spondylolysis	Defect of pars interarticularis, probably due to stress fracture
Scoliosis	
Psychogenic	Reaction to stressful situations; affect may be inconsistent with symptoms; findings may be unexplainable. Can be risky diagnosis. Thorough workup may be needed to rule out organic disease.
Extraspinal	
Retrocecal appendicitis	
Pyelonephritis	
Hydronephrosis	
Psoas abscess	
Retroperitoneal mass	
Miscellaneous	
Tethered cord	
Cord AVM/dural AVF	
Diastematomyelia	

Abbreviations: AVF, arteriovenous fistula; AVM, arteriovenous malformation; LBP, low back pain.
Modified from Tunnessen WW Jr: Signs and Symptoms in Pediatrics, Ed 2. Philadelphia, JB Lippincott, 1988, pp. 467–470. By permission of the publisher.

diagnostic significance. A history of uveitis or iritis can suggest juvenile anky-losing spondylitis or juvenile rheumatoid arthritis. Improvement in morning stiffness (and uveitis) as the day progresses suggests ankylosing spondylitis, whereas stiffness that worsens as the day progresses suggests juvenile rheuma-toid arthritis. In a young child with back pain and a history of fractures, the pos-sibility of child abuse should be kept in mind.

Helpful Hints on Physical Examination (pp. 886–887)

• Many of the principles described for adults are applicable to children, but signs of spinal anomalies (e.g., skin lesions, café-au-lait spots, tufts of hair, dimples, or dermal cyst) should be particularly sought. Curvatures of the spine, a paraspinal mass, asymmetry, or spasm (including on flexion and extension) should be sought. Hamstring tightness is common in children with low back pain, including in spondylolysis, spondylolisthesis, discitis, and epidural abscess. Percussion may help differentiate spine pain from flank pain (often of renal origin).
• Back pain in children also can be related to lack of physical activity and decon-ditioning of truncal supportive muscles. The ratio of back extensor strength to back flexor strength is known to decrease with advancing age. In the clinical evaluation of children with back pain, muscle strength testing is important. The lack of ability in children age 5 or younger to perform a sit-up is not considered abnormal. Increased physical activity without proper development of strength in the back extensors as compared with flexors can be associated with back pain.

Lumbar Disk Disease (p. 887)

• About 1% of children presenting with low back pain have lumbar disk disease. Of these children, the vast majority are 10 years or older. Practically all patients have back pain, and 90% have radicular symptoms. Despite a trial of conserva-tive measures, more than 60% of patients need surgery. In 95% of the cases, the involved disk is at L4 to L5 and L5 to S1. A history of trauma is more com-monly elicited in adolescents with lumbar disk disease than in adults. Results of surgical therapy are encouraging, with a cure rate of about 90% to 95%. It is not uncommon for children who have undergone treatment for lumbar disk disease to have disk disease at a different level in the future.

Scheuermann's Disease (p. 887)

• Scheuermann's disease is another cause of low back pain in adolescents. It is more common in boys and is characterized by herniation of a disk through the end-plate into the vertebral body. Osteochondritis of the upper and lower verte-bral end-plates and trauma might play a role. Some patients have marfanoid fea-tures, and a familial tendency is present in some. The back pain typically responds to rest and immobilization through application of a proper spinal orthosis.

Spondylolysis and Spondylolisthesis (p. 887)

• In the pediatric age group, spondylolysis and spondylolisthesis are the most common causes of back pain associated with structural change. Older children and adolescents are more commonly affected than younger ones. In acute cases, a pars fracture may actually heal with immobilization for 10 to 12 weeks in a plaster body jacket. Restriction of activity and occasional bracing aid in resolution of the pain. In chronic cases, instructions in back care; abdominal muscle strengthening; and stretching of paraspinal muscles, hip flexors, hamstrings, and Achilles tendons are helpful.

Congenital Diseases (p. 887)

• With modern neuroimaging techniques, congenital spine and spinal cord problems and dysraphic anomalies are relatively easily detected in children with back pain. About 10% of patients have more than one spinal lesion, and imaging of the entire spine is therefore prudent.

Tumor (p. 887)

• Nocturnal pain, pain at rest, and pain on awakening are symptoms that may draw attention to tumors of the spinal column. Metastatic tumors of the spine are uncommon in children. The most common tumors of the spinal column in children include osteoid osteoma, osteoblastoma, histiocytosis X, and aneurysmal bone cyst.

CONSERVATIVE MANAGEMENT OF BACK PAIN: GENERAL CONSIDERATIONS (pp. 887–889)

Acute Low Back Pain Syndromes (pp. 887–889)

• Acute back pain is usually accompanied by anxiety and fear of possible debilitating causes. Conservative treatment is indicated for each case of acute back pain.
• A period of bed rest for 2 to 3 days can be helpful and does not result in excessive bone loss or debilitation. Prolonged bed rest is not recommended.

Chronic Low Back Pain Syndromes (p. 889)

• Back pain that has been present for more than 6 months is chronic and usually is accompanied by changes in the patient's lifestyle and behavior. The longer the pain has been present, the more resistive it becomes to therapeutic intervention. (See Chapter 42.)

PREVENTIVE MEASURES AND BACK SCHOOLS (pp. 889–890)

• Prevention of recurrence is of major importance in the management of low back pain syndromes. During the acute phase, the patient should be instructed in proper positioning techniques to decrease low back pain during dynamic or static posturing and to avoid reinjury. At this stage, pain is managed with the use of sedative physical therapeutic measures and analgesics. Meanwhile, the patient should be introduced to progressive isometric exercise programs to improve muscular support of the spine. Provision of a back education program (back school) very early in the patient's treatment program is helpful. Patients with low back pain should be instructed in basic body mechanics and the following measures:

1. If prolonged sitting is required for an occupation, one should get up every 20 minutes. In addition, to decrease strain on the low back during sitting, the patient can be instructed to perform pelvic tilt exercises, to sit with knees bent and one or both feet slightly elevated on a footrest, and to support the low back with a small cushion.
2. For driving a car, the seat should be brought close to the steering wheel so that the knees are slightly higher than the hips. In the presence of lumbar degenerative disk disease, getting out of the car frequently (e.g., every 20 to 30 minutes) to stretch is helpful.
3. Before coughing or sneezing, the stomach muscles should be tightened.
4. Begin a progressive low back isometric strengthening exercise program and perform stretching exercises to increase flexibility for performing daily activities.
5. Forward bending increases intradiscal pressure. Therefore, certain precautions (e.g., kneeling when trying to pick an object up from the floor or when making a bed) are advisable to decrease intradiscal pressure.
6. To decrease low back strain when getting into bed, one should sit on the edge of the bed, turn and roll slightly to one hip, bring the knees up with the feet hanging over the edge of the bed, and slowly recline, pushing up with the arms on the bed to support the body during this procedure. For getting out of bed, one needs to reverse this sequence.

• In summary, every effort should be made to prevent low back pain or to avoid its recurrence through education and instruction in proper body mechanics.

Acknowledgments. Supported in part by a research grant from the Donaldson Trust. The authors would like to thank LeAnn Stee and the Section of Scientific Publications for service, John Hagen for the illustrations, and Sandy Fitzgerald for secretarial assistance.

41

Original Chapter by Mehrsheed Sinaki, M.D., M.S.

Prevention and Treatment of Osteoporosis

• Osteoporosis consists of a heterogeneous group of syndromes in which there is reduced bone mass per unit volume in otherwise normal bone, resulting in fragile bone. The World Health Organization has defined osteoporosis as bone mineral density 2.5 standard deviations below the peak mean bone mass of young normal adults.

BONE FUNCTION AND STRUCTURE (p. 894)

• Bone serves as a mechanical support for musculoskeletal structures; as protection for vital organs; and as a metabolic source of ions, especially calcium and phosphate. To maintain its biomechanical competence, bone tissue undergoes continuous change and renewal so that older bone tissue is replaced by newly formed bone tissue. There are two types of bone cells: osteoclasts, which resorb the calcified matrix; and osteoblasts, which synthesize new bone matrix.

BONE REMODELING (pp. 894–895)

• Bone remodeling is a process that allows removal of old bone and replacement with new bone tissue.
• Bone remodeling has five phases: (1) activation—osteoclastic activity is recruited; (2) resorption—osteoclasts erode bone and form a cavity; (3) reversal—osteoblasts are recruited; (4) formation—osteoblasts replace the cavity with new bone; and (5) quiescence—bone tissue remains dormant until the next cycle starts. In osteoporosis there is a dysequilibrium between resorption and formation, favoring resorption that results in bone loss.
• The number of active remodeling units in trabecular bone is about three times higher than that in cortical bone. Consequently, more bone loss occurs at the trabecular areas when resorption is greater than formation. The vertebrae consist of 50% trabecular bone and 50% cortical bone, whereas the femoral neck consists of 30% trabecular bone and 70% cortical bone. When bone turnover increases, bone loss and osteoporosis occur in the vertebrae before the femoral neck.

PATHOGENESIS (p. 895)

• Peak adult bone mass is achieved between ages 30 and 35 years. Age-related bone loss is a universal phenomenon in humans. Circumstances that limit bone formation or increase bone loss increase the likelihood that osteoporosis will develop later in life.

• In the normal aging process, there is deficit between resorption and formation because osteoblastic activity is not equal to osteoclastic activity. The net result of the remodeling process is bone loss during each cycle of remodeling.

• Certain conditions, such as hyperparathyroidism or thyrotoxicosis, can increase the rate of bone remodeling. These conditions increase the rate of bone loss, which results in high-turnover osteoporosis. The secondary causes of osteoporosis are associated with an increased rate of activation of the remodeling cycle. Although environmental factors such as calcium intake, smoking, alcohol, physical exercise, and menopause are important factors in determining bone mineral density, genetic factors are the major determinant.

HORMONES AND PHYSIOLOGY OF BONE (pp. 895–896)

• The rate of bone remodeling can be increased by parathyroid hormone, thyroxine, growth hormone, and vitamin D $(1,25[OH]_2D_3)$; it can be decreased by calcitonin, estrogen, and glucocorticoids.

• The major hormone for calcium homeostasis is *parathyroid hormone* (PTH). The level of plasma calcium is the major moderator of the secretion of PTH. PTH regulates plasma calcium concentration in three ways: (1) In the presence of active vitamin D, it stimulates bone resorption; (2) it indirectly increases intestinal absorption of calcium and phosphate; and (3) it increases reabsorption of calcium ions in the renal distal tubal area. In general, PTH increases serum calcium and mostly tends to lower serum phosphate.

• *Calcitonin* is a hormone secreted by the parafollicular cells of the thyroid gland. The major stimulus of calcitonin is the serum level of calcium. Through inhibition of osteoclastic activity, calcitonin directly prohibits calcium and phosphate resorption, lowering the serum calcium level.

• The main regulators of vitamin D synthesis are the serum concentrations of $1,25(OH)_2D_3$ itself; calcium; phosphate; and PTH. PTH is the major inducer of the active form of vitamin D formation in the kidney. The active form of vitamin D stimulates osteoblastic activity and increases intestinal absorption of calcium and phosphate.

SEX STEROIDS (p. 896)

• The main endocrine function that occurs at menopause is loss of secretion of estrogen and progesterone from the ovaries. The circulating testosterone levels also decrease after menopause. Estrone is the major source of estrogen in postmenopausal women. Men do not have the equivalent of menopause, but in some elderly men, bone mass decreases along with decline in gonadal function.

OTHER FACTORS AFFECTING BONE MASS (p. 896)

• Several other factors can contribute to the reduction of gender-related steroids. In hyperprolactinemia, failure of the gonadal axis results in a significant loss of bone. Amenorrheic athletes who exercise excessively can have lower

circulating estradiol, progesterone, and prolactin levels. Their amenorrhea is associated with hypothalamic hypogonadism, which leads to excessive bone loss.
• Other factors such as race, genetics, nutrition, physical exercise, and lifestyle can also contribute to the rate of bone loss after ovariectomy or natural menopause.

EFFECT OF AGING (p. 896)

• Age plays a significant role in the rate of bone turnover. It has been clearly determined that bone turnover increases in women at menopause, but bone turnover does not increase significantly in men with aging.
• Plasma calcitonin levels are higher in men than in women. Calcitonin levels do not change with age. Thyroid hormone levels typically show no change or are slightly decreased with age. Growth hormone secretion is reduced in osteoporotic patients. Growth hormone and insulin-like growth factor I have several positive effects on calcium homeostasis.
• PTH level increases with age, perhaps because of mild hypocalcemia and decreased $1,25(OH)_2D_3$. This reduction in the active form of vitamin D can be caused by lower consumption of dietary vitamin D, lower exposure to sunlight, lower skin capacity for vitamin D conversion, reduced intestinal absorption, and reduced 1α-hydroxylase activity.
• Several studies have demonstrated that the level of physical activity decreases with aging. Optimal nutrition and physical activity are necessary to achieve the genetic potential for bone mass. Nutrition also can affect both bone matrix formation and bone mineralization. The recommended adequate calcium intake for ages 9 to 18 years is 1300 mg/day.

CLASSIFICATION OF OSTEOPOROSIS (pp. 896–897)

• Osteoporosis can be primary or secondary. Primary osteoporosis is also known as idiopathic osteoporosis because no specific etiologic mechanism is recognized. This type of osteoporosis is either postmenopausal (type I) or senile, or age related (type II). Another type of primary osteoporosis is the rare disorder of idiopathic juvenile osteoporosis, the cause of which is unknown. The most common causes of osteoporosis are listed in Table 41–1.

CLINICAL MANIFESTATIONS OF OSTEOPOROSIS
(pp. 897–898)

• Osteoporosis is typically a "silent disease" until fractures occur. The most common areas for osteoporotic fractures are the midthoracic and upper lumbar spine, hip (proximal femur), and distal forearm (Colles fracture). The highest incidence of fractures is in white females.
• The most concern is for hip fracture because the risk of death with osteoporotic hip fracture is 15% to 20%, despite all the developments in surgical and nonsurgical intervention. The management of an osteoporotic spine fracture requires immobilization of the involved vertebral bodies and analgesia. Fortunately, these fractures heal through becoming more condensed and do not require any specific treatment process, as is usually needed for the appendicular fractures. The duration of immobilization should be for only a limited time, sufficient to ensure

TABLE 41–1 Common Causes of Osteoporosis

Hereditary, congenital: osteogenesis imperfecta, neurologic disturbances (myotonia congenita, Werdnig-Hoffmann disease), gonadal dysgenesis

Acquired (primary and secondary)

    1. Generalized

        Idiopathic (premenopausal women and middle-aged or young men; juvenile osteoporosis)

        Postmenopausal (type I)

        Senile (type II)

        Secondary (type III):

            Nutrition: malnutrition, anorexia/bulimia, vitamin deficiency (C or D), vitamin overuse (D or A), calcium deficiency, high sodium intake, high caffeine intake, high protein intake, high phosphate intake, alcohol abuse

        Sedentary lifestyle, immobility, smoking

        Gastrointestinal diseases (liver disease, malabsorption syndromes, alactasia, subtotal gastrectomy) or small bowel resection

        Nephropathies

        Chronic obstructive pulmonary disease

        Malignancy (multiple myeloma, disseminated carcinoma)

        Drugs: phenytoin, barbiturates, cholestyramine, heparin

        Endocrine disorders: acromegaly, hyperthyroidism, Cushing's syndrome (iatrogenic or endogenous), hyperparathyroidism, diabetes mellitus (?), hypogonadism

    2. Localized: inflammatory arthritis, fractures and immobilization in cast, limb dystrophies, muscular paralysis

From Sinaki M: Rehabilitation in metabolic bone disease. In Sinaki M (ed): Basic Clinical Rehabilitation Medicine, ed 2. St Louis, Mosby, 1993, pp. 209–236. By permission of Mayo Foundation.

the primary fracture healing process. Prolonged immobilization is discouraged because it can contribute to osteoporosis.

FRACTURES AND MANAGEMENT (pp. 898–899)

Vertebral Fracture (p. 898)

• Vertebral fractures can create two types of pain: acute pain; and, later, chronic pain.

• *Acute pain* that occurs in the absence of a previous fracture is usually caused by compression fractures in the vertebrae. The compressed vertebrae might not be apparent on radiographs for up to 4 weeks after the injury. Compression fracture usually results in acute pain that later resolves (see Table 41–2 in the Textbook).

• Kyphotic postural change is the most physically disfiguring and psychologically damaging effect of osteoporosis. Recognition and improvement of decreased back extensor strength enhance the ability to maintain proper vertical alignment. Development of kyphotic posture not only can predispose to postural back pain, but also can increase the risk of falls.

• *Chronic pain* can be caused by the development of deformity caused by vertebral wedging, compression, and ligamentous strain. The intervertebral disks undergo the most dramatic age-related changes of all connective tissues.

TABLE 41–2 Management of Chronic Pain in Patients with Osteoporosis

Improve faulty posture, may need Posture Training Support (PTS)
Manage pain (ultrasound, massage, or transcutaneous electrical nerve stimulation [TENS])
If beyond correction, apply back support to decrease painful stretch of ligaments
Avoid physical activities that exert extreme vertical compression forces on vertebrae
Prescribe a patient-specific therapeutic exercise program
Start appropriate pharmacologic intervention

From Sinaki M: Rehabilitation in metabolic bone disease. In Sinaki M (ed): Basic Clinical Rehabilitation Medicine, ed 2. St Louis, Mosby, 1993, pp. 209–236. By permission of Mayo Foundation.

• Chronic back pain is related to postural changes caused by vertebral fractures. Chronic pain can also be caused by microfractures that are visible only on bone scanning and that occur continuously. Management of chronic osteoporosis-related pain is outlined in Table 41–2.

Hip Fracture (pp. 898–899)

• Hip fracture is an emergency situation. In typical cases, the extremity is rotated outward (externally rotated) and shortened. Radiographs are necessary to distinguish intracapsular from extracapsular hip fractures. The consensus is that surgery is the treatment of choice for femoral neck fracture and trochanteric hip fracture. However, in some unusual cases of impacted fracture, particularly in a patient who is severely debilitated and has impaired general health, conservative treatment might be advisable. Femoral neck fracture requires fixation, and the type of fixation varies among surgeons. Because of the high incidence of operative failures after internal fixation of these fractures, most orthopedists prefer performing arthroplasties.
• The trochanteric hip fracture creates lesser problems despite the fact that the fracture engages more bone than does the femoral neck fracture. The operative treatment of choice is internal fixation (see Fig. 41–4 in the Textbook). The postoperative course for all hip fracture is less eventful if physical therapeutic measures, such as use of gait aids with partial weight bearing on the operative side, are used postoperatively. Only in severely comminuted fractures or fractures in which the operative result has been unsatisfactory is the restriction of weight bearing to no weight bearing needed.

Sacral Insufficiency Fracture (p. 899)

• Other axial skeletal fractures, such as fractures of the sacral alae and pubic rami, can also occur. Fractures of the pubic rami can occur with minimal strain, and most patients can hardly recall having a severe strain. Healing typically occurs without invasive procedures. Weight bearing is limited, as dictated by the level of pain in the pelvic area. Fracture of the sacrum with minimal trauma also can occur, and the goal of management is to decrease weight-bearing pain with the use of proper assistive devices for ambulation.

DIAGNOSTIC STUDIES IN OSTEOPOROSIS (pp. 899–902)

• The diagnosis of osteoporosis requires a thorough history and physical examination, including family history of osteoporosis, type and location of muscu-

loskeletal pain, general dietary calcium intake, level of physical activity, and height and weight measurements.
• Several biochemical indices also are used in the differential diagnosis of metabolic bone disease or, in some instances, for therapeutic follow-up.
• Radiographic findings consist of increased lucency of the vertebral bodies with loss of horizontal trabeculae and increased prominence of the cortical end-plates and vertically oriented trabeculae, reduction in cortex thickness, and anterior wedging of vertebral bodies. Bone scan and magnetic resonance imaging can further define an area of bone loss (see Fig. 41–6 in the Textbook), if needed.
• Osteoporosis is typically not visible on conventional radiographs until at least 25% to 30% of bone mineral has been lost. Available methods in evaluating bone mass include photon absorptiometry (single or dual), finger x-ray spectrometry, ultrasound densitometry, qualitative computed tomography, and dual x-ray absorptiometry. The most commonly used technique is dual-energy absorptiometry. Dual-energy x-ray absorptiometry (DEXA) has high precision and is commonly used to measure the bone mineral density of the spine and hips (see Fig. 41–7 in the Textbook). More commonly measured is the bone mineral density of the femoral neck, because that of the spine can be erroneously high as a result of osteoarthritis of the spine.

TREATMENT (pp. 902–911)

• The World Health Organization has devised definitions for osteoporosis as follows: bone mineral density T-score greater than 1 to −1 SD, normal; T-score −1 to −2.5 SD, osteopenia; and T-score of −2.5 SD or more, osteoporosis. (SD = standard deviation below the peak, normal young adult mean.) These definitions facilitate decision making for therapeutic trials and are helpful for prescription of a proper exercise program (Table 41–3).

Exercise (pp. 902–903)

• Mechanical loading, when applied properly, can stimulate osteogenic activity. Individuals with normal bone mineral density can perform high-impact exercises such as aerobics, jogging, and skiing. For persons with osteoporosis, nonstraining exercises such as walking for 45 minutes three times a week or daily walking for 30 minutes are recommended. In-water exercises are recommended for patients who are unable to perform antigravity exercises because of pain or weakness. The nonstrenuous, low-resistance exercises can be advanced to antigravity and strengthening exercises as permitted by a patient's musculoskeletal status.
• Spinal extension exercises should be used along with exercises to reduce lumbar lordosis. Weakness in abdominal muscles adds to the problems of poor posture and protruded abdomen. To complement a posture training exercise program, isometric abdominal muscle-strengthening exercises should be included (see Figs. 41–9 and 41–10 in the Textbook).
• Certain exercises, especially spinal flexion exercises, should be avoided in patients with osteoporosis. The choice of physical activity is important and has to be individualized. Fitness programs such as swimming, fast walking, or short periods of stationary biking are not significantly osteogenic, but can fulfill the need for cardiovascular fitness without straining the osteoporotic frame. Knowledge of the bone mineral density is helpful before recommending a weight-training program.

TABLE 41-3 Suggested Rehabilitation Guidelines on the Basis of Bone Mineral Density T-Scores*

Reduction to −1 SD (normal)	−1 to −2.5 SD (osteopenia)†	−2.5 SD or more (osteoporosis)†
No treatment	Consultation for treatment	Pharmacologic intervention
Patient education, preventive measures	Patient education, preventive interventions	Pain management
Lifting techniques	Pain management	Range of motion, strengthening, coordination
Proper diet (calcium and vitamin D)	Back strengthening exercises	Mid-day rest, heat/cold, stroking massage if needed
Jogging (short distances)	Limit load lifting (≤10–20 pounds)	Back extensor strengthening
Weight training	Aerobic exercises, walking 30 min/day	Walking 30 min/day, Frenkel exercises
	Exercises: weight training three times a week	Aquatic exercises one or two times a week
	Postural exercises: Posture	Fall prevention program (see Table 41–3 in the Textbook)
	Training support combined with pelvic tilt and back extension	Postural exercises: Posture training support combined with pelvic tilt and back extension
Aerobics	Frenkel exercises, prevention of falls	Prevention of vertebral compression fractures (orthoses, as needed)
	T'ai chi, if desired	
Abdominal and back strengthening exercises‡	?Hormone replacement	Prevention of spinal strain (lifting ≤5–10 lb)
Postural exercises	?Other antiresorptive agents	Evaluation of balance, gait aid
		Safety and facilitation of self-care through modification of bathroom (grab bars), kitchen (counter adjustment), occupational therapy consultation
		Start strengthening program with 1–2 lb and increase as tolerated to 5 lb in each hand
		Hip protective measures

* T-score: Standard deviation below peak normal young adult bone mass.
† Osteopenia/osteoporosis as defined by the World Health Organization.
‡ See Figures 41–9 and 41–10 in the Textbook for proper exercise program and posture.

587

Posture-Training Program and the Osteoporotic Skeletal Frame (pp. 903–906)

• Any support that can improve posture and decrease pain-related paraspinal muscle co-contraction is desirable. With aging, reduced paraspinal muscle strength and forward tendency of head and trunk related to the effect of gravity can cause iliocostal friction syndrome and flank pain. Posture training programs that can decrease kyphosis can also subsequently reduce iliocostal friction syndrome. Posture training programs (e.g., the application of a weighted kypho-orthosis for half an hour twice a day or for 1 hour twice a day while trying to contract back extensors) can provide re-education for improvement of kyphotic posturing and reduction of the risk of falls (see Fig. 41–14 in the Textbook).

Orthoses and the Osteoporotic Spine (p. 906)

• Acute compression fracture usually results in severe pain and, if not managed well, can lead to prolonged immobility, chronic pain behavior, and subsequent psychological consequences. Acute pain needs to be actively managed with proper physical measures and modalities. Rigid thoracolumbar orthoses to promote extension of the spine are helpful (see Fig. 41–15 Textbook; see also Chapter 17). If thoracolumbar orthoses are not tolerated, a thoracic weighted kypho-orthosis or a combination of a kypho-orthosis and lower back support (elastic abdominal support) might suffice.

Pharmacological Interventions (pp. 906–911)

• Several agents can be used for treatment of osteoporosis. Estrogen, calcium, and vitamin D are the most commonly advocated pharmacological treatments for involutional osteoporosis. Antiresorptive agents include estrogens, androgens, calcitonin, and bisphosphonates. Osteoblast stimulator agents include fluoride and PTH. PTH is still an investigational supplement, and fluoride is not approved by the Food and Drug Administration at this time for the treatment of osteoporosis.

• Needless to say, cessation of tobacco and alcohol abuse is necessary. An adequate calcium intake is required to permit normal bone development and potentially to decrease bone loss.

• Estrogen acts directly on bone cells and is an antiresorptive agent that has been shown to decrease the rate of bone loss and fractures in postmenopausal women whether the menopause is natural or surgical. Estrogen is the most widely prescribed agent in the United States (except for calcium) for the treatment of established osteoporosis. Some clinicians use progestogen in patients with an intact uterus who are on estrogen. A recent study brought into question the safety of long-term use of estrogen and progestogen treatment.

• Calcitonin, an antiresorptive agent, acts directly on the osteoclasts. It is most effective in patients whose rate of bone turnover is high. Calcitonin is approved for therapy of established osteoporosis, but the long-term fracture-reducing efficacy of calcitonin has not been clearly demonstrated (Table 41–4).

• Bisphosphonates affect trabecular bone, especially the lumbar spine, where bone mineral density increases of 5% to 10% occur during the first 2 years of treatment. Alendronate sodium, an amino-bisphosphonate, has been shown to normalize the rate of bone turnover and increase bone mass. Risedronate is

TABLE 41–4 Commonly Used Agents in Osteoporosis

Agent	Common Dosage	Potential Side Effects
Calcium (type depends on patient's needs)	1000–1500 mg/day (Table 41–1)	
Vitamin D (multivitamin)	400–800 IU/day	
Estrogen		Headache, weight gain, change of mood or depression, increased blood pressure, gallbladder or liver disease, thrombophlebitis and increased blood clotting, increased serum triglycerides and blood glucose levels, abnormal vaginal bleeding, endometrial hyperplasia/cancer, breast cancer
Conjugated equine (Premarin)	0.625 mg (oral)/day	
Transdermal estradiol 17 (patch)	0.05–0.1 mg	
Progesterone (Provera), oral	2.5–5 mg (days 1–10 of cycle)	
Alendronate sodium (Fosamax)	5–10 mg/day	Esophageal irritation
Calcitonin	200 units nasal spray (Miacalcin) or 50 to 100 mg every-other-day injections	Nasal irritation/ulceration
Raloxifene (Evista)	60 mg/day (oral)	Leg cramps, hot flashes, deep vein thrombosis

another bisphosphonate that has been more recently introduced for the treatment of osteoporosis. Treatment with risedronate, 5 mg per day, was shown to significantly decrease the incidence of vertebral and nonvertebral fractures in postmenopausal osteoporosis.

• Anabolic steroids have an osteoblastic effect; however, because they have significant androgenic effects and induce liver function abnormalities, they are used only under the most extreme circumstances. Thiazide diuretics inhibit urinary excretion of calcium and can retard bone loss and reduce the rate of fractures in patients with osteoporosis.

• The estrogen-receptor mixed agonists/antagonists tamoxifen and raloxifene protect against bone loss in ovariectomized rats. They have an antiestrogenic effect on breast tissue. These agents also are known as selective estrogen-receptor modulators (SERMs). One of the side effects related to tamoxifen is uterine hyperplasia, but this is not a concern in treatment with raloxifene. Raloxifene decreases total cholesterol and serum low-density lipoprotein levels. Raloxifene is currently used only in the postmenopausal stage of osteoporosis (see Tables 41–8 and 41–9 in the Textbook).

• Treatment of osteoporosis in men includes the usual supplementation with calcium and vitamin D, limitation of alcohol use, and cessation of smoking. In cases of hypogonadism in men, endocrine consultation is necessary, and testosterone replacement therapy is a possibility.

• Management of steroid-induced osteoporosis requires calcium and vitamin D supplementation, use of antiresorptive agents such as alendronate sodium (10 mg/day orally), and implementation of a proper exercise program. If hyperparathyoidism or thyrotoxicosis is present, proper management should be implemented.

• A balanced diet is needed for maintenance of musculoskeletal health. Excessive dietary intake of sodium and phosphorus should be avoided. Studies of young women with malnutrition caused by anorexia nervosa have demonstrated poor muscle strength, significant loss of bone mass, irregularity of menstrual periods, and estrogen deficiency.

• Practical management of patients with osteoporosis requires not only pharmacological interventions, physical and rehabilitative measures, and good nutrition, but also consideration of the psychological consequences and reactions experienced by the patients. Public education can contribute to prevention, better understanding, and management of the consequences of osteoporosis.

42

Original Chapter by Donna Bloodworth, M.D., Octavio Calvillo, M.D., Ph.D.,
Kevin Smith, M.D., and Martin Grabois, M.D.

Chronic Pain Syndromes: Evaluation and Treatment

DEFINITION (p. 913)

• Perhaps the best way to define chronic pain is to compare and contrast it with acute pain (Table 42–1). Chronic pain syndrome is an abnormal condition in which pain is no longer a symptom of ongoing tissue injury, but one in which pain and pain behavior become the primary disease processes. In chronic pain syndrome, subjective and behavioral manifestations of pain persist beyond objective evidence of tissue injury. Some of the conditions that can cause chronic pain are listed in Table 42–2 in the Textbook.

• In chronic pain syndrome the original causes are often blurred by subsequent complications of multiple procedures, compensation factors, medication dependency, inactivity, and psychosocial behavior changes.

EPIDEMIOLOGY (pp. 913–914)

• One-third of all Americans are estimated to have a chronically painful condition (including headache, back pain, and degenerative joint disease), with 50% to 60% of these individuals partially or totally disabled by pain. This disability can be either transient or permanent.

ETIOLOGY (p. 914)

• Chronic pain can be caused by ongoing pathological processes (e.g., arthritis), chronic nervous system dysfunction (e.g., phantom limb pain), or a combination of both processes. The patient's perception of the pain is modified by psychological, social, and environmental factors to yield the presenting complaint. The evaluation of a chronic pain patient should focus on defining the pain sources as nociceptive, neuropathic, or neuropsychological, while recognizing potential modifiers of the complaints.

TABLE 42–1 Acute versus Chronic Pain

Acute	Chronic
Physicians trained in evaluation and diagnosis	Physician typically less interested and less trained
Short evaluation and treatment course	Long evaluation and treatment course
Pain is a biological symptom	Pain is a disease
Pain plus anxiety	Pain plus depression
Medications as needed	Nonnarcotic analgesics, antidepressants preferred
Little addiction concern	Polyaddiction concern
Diagnosis straightforward	Diagnosis complex
Cure likely	Cure usually not achieved

Adapted from Grabois M: Chronic pain. Evaluation and treatment. *In* Goodgold J (ed): Rehabilitation Medicine. St Louis, Mosby–Year Book, 1988.

Somatic Etiology (p. 914)

• For a somatic structure to be a source of pain, it must be innervated. Because nerve endings are stimulated by either mechanical or chemical irritation, any pathological process producing chronic stretching of connective tissues or inflammation of these innervated structures can lead to chronic somatic pain. This is usually manifested as aching, dull, or throbbing pain. Examples of this include rheumatoid arthritis, vertebral facet disease, and fibromyalgia.

Neuropathic Etiology (p. 914)

• Neuropathic pain results from alterations in nerve structure or function with or without associated deafferentiation. It is characteristically described as burning, shooting, or electrical in nature and is not associated with any ongoing nociceptive process. Trauma to or disease of the peripheral nerves can lead to chronic neuropathic pain. Spinal cord injury or dorsal root ganglion injury can lead to various deafferentiation pain syndromes, with pain being experienced in an area of sensory loss.
• Thalamic infarcts can cause "central pain," and postherpetic neuralgia can result from inflammatory injury with resultant deafferentiation of the dorsal root ganglia and dorsal horn. Metabolic derangement, as seen in diabetes, alcoholism, amyloidosis, and hypothyroidism, can lead to painful peripheral neuropathies.

Psychological Etiologies (p. 914)

• Psychogenic pain is often referred as a somatization disorder. The cause lies in an underlying emotional disturbance or stressor that often goes unrecognized by the patient. Although the pain can present in any area of the body, the most common forms are tension headaches, angina-like symptoms, colitis, non-specific vaginal pain, and myofascial pain involving the shoulder and upper and lower extremities.

CHRONIC PAIN MANAGEMENT (pp. 914–917)

• Because chronic pain syndrome is a complex problem with medical and psychosocial aspects, it requires a comprehensive and multidisciplinary approach to evaluation and treatment. In an attempt to maximize the treatment outcomes, pain programs have developed comprehensive and interdisciplinary approaches to evaluating and treating patients with chronic pain.

• There are several types of pain clinics. The International Association for the Study of Pain (IASP) has identified three such types, classifying pain clinics as modality-oriented, disease-oriented, or multidisciplinary.

• In a typical pain clinic, the clinical team regularly evaluates patients, sets goals, treats patients, and evaluates treatment outcomes. The physician leads the team, coordinates the program, and provides overall medical management. The psychosocial-vocational team, consisting of the psychologist, social worker, and vocational counselor, provides leadership in the evaluation and treatment of the behavioral changes that are a result of chronic pain, as well as appropriate vocational intervention. The therapy team typically consists of nurses, pharmacists, dieticians, physical therapists, and occupational therapists. They provide daily therapy to control medication levels, modulate the pain level, and increase patient activity.

• Opioids should be considered only after all other reasonable analgesic therapy has failed. Contraindications to chronic opioids use can include a history of substance abuse, severe character disorder, or chaotic home environment. A single practitioner should take primary responsibility for treatment. Fully informed consent should be obtained, as well as a written contract. Long-acting opioids are preferred for ease of administration. Fixed-schedule dosing is preferable for continuous or frequently recurring pain. "Rescue" doses can be used under clearly defined circumstances, but total (weekly/monthly) dose must be constant. Patients should initially be seen monthly for monitoring their improvement in function. Periodic assessment should specifically address degree of analgesia; adverse effects; functional status (e.g., physical, social, psychological); and indications of aberrant drug-related behaviors.

CLINICAL EVALUATION (pp. 917–918)

• It is important to obtain a complete history and physical examination (see Chapter 1) to assess the factors contributing to the patient's complaints and to assess the impact of the pain on the patient's functional capacity. Searching for a single cause to explain all of the patient's symptoms is typically futile. It can also be counterproductive, because it reinforces the patient's perception that "there's something seriously wrong with me and they just can't figure out what it is."

History (pp. 917–918)

• The history should focus on the time course, intensity, and location of the pain. The functional state of the patient before the onset of the problem should be established. Reactions to diagnostic and therapeutic interventions should be noted because they can be predictors of responses to future treatment. Have iatrogenic problems resulted from inappropriate or unnecessary procedures? Is there a past history of substance abuse or addictive behavior (a negative prognostic indicator)? What exacerbates and what relieves the pain? Is litigation a factor to be considered? All responses to prior and current medications should be noted.

Physical Examination (p. 918)

• A complete physical examination, focusing on the neurological and musculoskeletal systems, should be performed. The cranial nerves should be assessed, and exteroceptive sensations of pain, temperature, and touch documented. Anatomical patterns of pain and sensory loss often provide clues to the level of a lesion or to the lack of an organic basis for the complaint.

FUNCTIONAL EVALUATION (pp. 918–920)

• As with any patient requiring rehabilitation, an appropriate functional evaluation should be performed before, during, and after the completion of the program, and at follow-up evaluations. Objective, quantitative measurements give a baseline with which to evaluate the patient's progress and long-term outcome.
• Functional capacity evaluations (FCE) have existed in one form or another since the 1940s, although their use and application have changed over the decades.
• Tests of pain assessment, psychological distress, and self-perception of abilities and limitations describe the person's symptomatology but do not specifically assess the person's physical capacity for work. Researchers commonly use four test batteries for assessing personal functional status: the Roland disability questionnaire, the Oswestry Disability Questionnaire, the Million Visual Analog Scale, and the Waddell Disability Index.
• When evaluating an injured worker, the physician should establish the medical impairment and translate that impairment into functional limitation, including an estimate of work capacity (limited by appropriate restrictions). Physicians and patients have great difficulty estimating functional limitation and physical ability. Despite the scientific limitations of functional capacity evaluation testing, the literature supports obtaining an objective measure of the injured worker's physical abilities when indicated.
• An FCE may be indicated when: (1) the patient's rehab progress plateaus, (2) a difference exists between the patient's reported and observed function, (3) vocational planning calls for an accounting of the patient's physical abilities, or (4) case closure is indicated by judgment or statute. Third parties and allied health care personnel use FCEs as: (1) an objective independent medical evaluation, (2) a baseline of function for a work hardening or functional restoration program, and (3) a screening device for return to work.
• FCEs typically last 1 to 3 days, and usually require 2 to 6 hours per day to carry out. FCEs can be divided into four types: (1) simulation of the job requirements using trained observers, (2) simulation of the job requirements with no qualifications required for the observer, (3) generic evaluations of lifting and carrying abilities with a requirement for trained observers, or (4) generic evaluations of lifting and carrying abilities with no qualifications required for the observer.

• FCEs have scientific limitations in regard to standardization, validity, and reliability; but they do provide useful information about the injured worker's ability, as well as insight into effort and evoked symptomatology. Functional capacity testing does not predict return to work; but for the motivated patient who is returning to work or beginning a rehabilitation program, it can be a useful tool for scripting work restrictions or initial rehabilitation orders.

PSYCHOLOGICAL EVALUATION (pp. 920–921)

• The goal of the psychological evaluation is to determine the emotional, cognitive, behavioral, social, or vocational factors that are potentially affecting the patient's perception of the pain being experienced. Although it is true that patients with primary psychiatric disease can present with complaints of chronic pain that are largely psychogenic in nature, the use of the psychological evaluation solely for the purpose of determining whether pain is caused by an organic or psychogenic cause is problematic.

• There is a need to conceptualize chronic pain beyond the unidimensional construct of organic versus psychogenic, and to embrace a broader and more comprehensive scheme. Practitioners should be sensitive to the multifaceted aspects of chronic pain and not confuse the emotional consequences of pain with causation when no readily apparent medical explanation is available.

• The primary components of the initial psychological evaluation include the clinical interview(s) with the patient and family members, health questionnaires, pain inventories (e.g., McGill Pain Questionnaire and Multidimensional Pain Inventory), and measures of psychological and behavioral dysfunction (e.g., Minnesota Multiphasic Personality Inventory [MMPI], Symptoms Checklist-90, Beck Depression Inventory, and State-Trait Anxiety Inventory).

PAIN MEASUREMENT (p. 921)

• Measurement of induced acute pain is easier than measurement of chronic pain. A clear linear relationship between the quantity of noxious input and the intensity of pain experience is not readily apparent in chronic pain. In many cases all we have are the patient's words, his or her recollections of the experience, and the behavior exhibited when the pain is being experienced. For all these reasons, a pain scale should, at a minimum, include ease of administration and scoring, the potential for consistently accurate use by a variety of health care professionals, high inter-rater reliability, and validity.

• The three components of chronic pain measurement are: (1) the subjective, (2) the physiological, and (3) the behavioral. The subjective component of chronic pain management is reflected in rating scales, questionnaires, and diary cards. The visual analog scale (1 to 10) is the most commonly used rating scale.

• Questionnaires have gained wide acceptance, with the McGill Pain Questionnaire being the most popular. It evaluates three major classes of word descriptions (i.e., sensory, affective, and evaluative) that patients use to specify their subjective pain experience. It has a built-in intensity scale.

• Behavior measurement techniques use three categories of behavior: (1) somatic intervention, (2) impaired functional capacity, and (3) pain complaints.

• Clearly there is no current ideal method for evaluating and measuring chronic pain and the effectiveness of treatment techniques.

DIAGNOSTIC TESTING (pp. 921–922)

• Diagnostic testing should be undertaken with care in patients with chronic pain syndromes. The use of diagnostic testing should always be based on clinical findings or changes noted in the examination. If symptoms and findings have remained static since the last evaluation, the likelihood of finding a significant change in a repeated diagnostic test is low.

Laboratory Tests (pp. 921–922)

• Chronic pain usually does not produce distinct laboratory findings other than those that result from any underlying disease. Routine monitoring for drug effects is performed for patients taking anticonvulsants or other medications known to have adverse effects on specific organ systems. Urine or blood screening should be considered in any drug detoxification program.

Imaging Studies (p. 922)

• Diagnostic studies utilized in chronic pain patients are listed in Table 42–2.

TREATMENT GOALS (pp. 922–929)

• The cause of the chronic pain syndrome should be determined from a medical and psychosocial point of view and the location of "pain generator" should be noted.
• The goals of treatment in an interdisciplinary program center on moderating pain, increasing function, and decreasing health care utilization. These goals can be achieved by modifying pain medication and pain behavior, decreasing reliance on medical care utilization, and increasing activity through exercise.

TABLE 42–2 Diagnostic Studies Commonly Utilized in Chronic Pain Syndrome Patients

Imaging Study	Comment
Spinal plain films	Low specificity and predictive value
Computed tomogram (with myelography)	Demonstrates over 90% of herniated disks, but an have false-positives
Magnetic resonance imaging	Excellent soft tissue and disk images
Thermography	Can be used for confirmation of autonomic dysfunction in conditions such as reflex sympathetic dystrophy
Electromyography and nerve conduction studies	Objectively assess severity, location, and extent of nerve and muscular lesions
Bone scan	One of the few imaging techniques that detects physiological changes
Three-phase bone scan	Sensitive and specific for reflex sympathetic dystrophy

Behavioral Treatment (pp. 922–923)

• More recent developments in the theory and practice of pain management have led to the development of the cognitive-behavioral approach. The primary assumption from the cognitive-behavioral perspective is that the individual has learned maladaptive ways of thinking, feeling, and behaving. Cognitive-behavioral treatment (CBT) interventions are designed to change both the thoughts and behaviors of the individual to improve adjustment with chronic pain. Cognitive-behavioral interventions teach patients effective coping strategies, provide patients an opportunity to rehearse these new strategies, and work to prevent relapse following treatment.

• In the last several years, an effort has been made to identify specific cognitive-behavioral factors that can promote more successful patient outcome. One of the factors, a patient's "readiness to change," appears to have important utility for clinicians interested in identifying those patients who are most likely to benefit from cognitive-behavioral treatments for pain.

Medication Management Philosophy (pp. 923–924)

• Physicians have a long history of prescribing, and chronic pain patients have a long history of using inappropriate medications, and particularly opiate medications. Some physicians mistakenly believe that giving medication on an as-needed basis rather than on a scheduled dosage results in less addiction.

• Appropriate utilization of opioid medication can be a helpful strategy in some patients with chronic pain. When the goal of pharmacological management of a patient with chronic pain is to moderate or eliminate possible use of opiates, tranquilizers, and hypnotic medications, it usually requires detoxification in an organized treatment program. No new opiates, tranquilizers, or hypnotic drugs should be prescribed. Once the daily requirement for the patient is obtained over a few days, a "pain cocktail" approach is used on a time-contingent basis (see Table 42–10 in the Textbook).

• The pain cocktail typically consists of methadone or a similar preparation in a dose equivalent to the currently used opiate medication. It is mixed with a masking vehicle such as cherry syrup. The patient is fully informed in advance that the drug will gradually be withdrawn, but is not told the daily dose of the active ingredient. The cocktail is given at the dosage and on the time schedule the patient demonstrated in the daily requirement. Gradual reduction of the active ingredient with an equal increase in the masking vehicle is carried out over 3 to 6 weeks. Decrements are made slowly so as not to elicit withdrawal signs and symptoms. Eventually, the patient is receiving only the masking vehicle, and the cocktail is discontinued.

Pharmacological Management (pp. 924–925)

• Nonopioid analgesics can be subdivided into aspirin-like drugs (nonsteroidal anti-inflammatory drugs, [NSAIDs]) and acetaminophen. NSAIDs have analgesic, antipyretic, anti-inflammatory, and antithrombotic actions. These medications are well-absorbed, but demonstrate an analgesic ceiling. Gastropathy is the most common side effect and can be neutrophil or prostaglandin mediated. Renal complications include nephrotic syndrome and interstitial nephritis, which are reversible. Irreversible papillary necrosis can occur but is exceedingly rare.

NSAIDs should be used cautiously or avoided in patients with a past history of peptic ulcer disease or with decreased renal function.
• Acetaminophen's analgesic properties are equipotent with aspirin. Although it is antipyretic, it is not anti-inflammatory and does not affect platelet function. Doses exceeding 4 to 6 g/day can be hepatotoxic, and caution should be taken when using combination medications that contain this amount of acetaminophen.
• Opioid analgesics are generally not indicated for the treatment of nonmalignant chronic pain. Although efficacy without dependence has been reported for opioid treatment of somatic pain, opioid use for sympathetic pain and other chronic neuropathic pain disorders has been shown to have poor efficacy. For chronic somatic pain, opioids have improved efficacy, but dependence and tolerance remain a problem in some patients. Chronic malignant pain of somatic origin can be treated effectively with long-term opioid management.
• Tricyclic antidepressants have been shown in controlled trials to have analgesic effects independent of their antidepressant properties. They have also been shown in laboratory animals to enhance the effects of opioid analgesics with an efficacy 70 times that of aspirin. Amitriptyline is the best studied of the tricyclics, but its anticholinergic side effects (e.g., dry mouth, sedation, blurred vision, urinary retention, constipation, or delirium) can make this drug undesirable in some patients. Doses required to achieve analgesic effects are below those needed to relieve depression (usually in a range of 10 to 100 mg per day). It can be given at night to take advantage of its sedative properties to normalize sleep patterns and thus improve compliance. Caution should be taken in patients with hypertension or coronary artery disease because amitriptyline can cause a precipitous rise in blood pressure.
• Benzodiazepines are useful in relieving anxiety, but they have no intrinsic analgesic properties. Long-term use can lead to dependence and withdrawal effects including seizures, muscle cramps, and dysphoria. If given in combination with opioids they can potentiate respiratory depression, even in small doses.
• Steroids, in bolus doses, have been shown to be effective in the treatment of complex regional pain syndrome and can be helpful in cancer pain. Side effects with long-term use include Cushing's syndrome, weight gain, myopathy, psychosis, and gastrointestinal bleeding. Steroids should not be used in conjunction with NSAIDs. Abrupt withdrawal of steroids after long-term use can precipitate an Addisonian crisis with nausea, vomiting, hypotension, and hypoglycemia.
• The anticonvulsants carbamazepine, phenytoin, and valproic acid can also be effective in the treatment of neuropathic pain. Carbamazepine has been found to be useful in the treatment of trigeminal neuralgia, post-traumatic neuropathies, and phantom limb pain. Side effects that require routine monitoring with these medications include bone marrow suppression and hepatotoxicity.
• Clonidine, an α_2-adrenergic agonist, has been shown to enhance the effects of opioids and has independent analgesic properties when administered intrathecally. Potential side effects of clonidine include orthostatic hypotension and rebound hypertension upon withdrawal.

Pain Modulation (pp. 925–927)

• The complete eradication of chronic pain is rarely achieved, and the goal of most interventions is the modification of pain to a more tolerable level. A comprehensive pain management program utilizes an array of modalities to accom-

TABLE 42–3 Pharmacological and Nonpharmacological Pain Interventions

Pharmacological Interventions	Nonpharmacological Interventions
NSAIDs	Behavior modifiers
Antidepressants (TCAs)	Relaxation
Anticonvulsants	Biofeedback
Carbamazepine	Guided visual imagery
Phenytoin (Dilantin)	Music therapy
Invasive pain modulators	Distraction
Spinal opioids	Hypnosis
Peripheral nerve stimulators	Pain modulators
Dorsal column stimulators	TENS
Epidural and deep brain stimulators	Acupuncture
Invasive pain relievers	Conditioning exercises
Sympathetic nerve blocks	Stretching/flexibility
Epidural anesthetics/steroids	Myofascial release
Root sleeve injections	Spray and stretch
Trigger point injections	

Abbreviations: NSAIDs, nonsteroidal anti-inflammatory drugs; TCAs, tricyclic antidepressants; TENS, transcutaneous electrical nerve stimulation.

plish this goal. For the chronic pain population, the optimal techniques are those that can be used by the patient in the home setting, that are active rather than passive, and that can be used for the shortest time possible or gradually weaned. Table 42–3 lists commonly used pharmacological and nonpharmacological pain-modulating interventions.

Transcutaneous Electrical Nerve Stimulation (p. 926)
• TENS at rates of 50 to 100 Hz produces analgesia that is not reversible by naloxone. TENS can produce neuromodulation by three routes: (1) presynaptic inhibition of the spinal cord; (2) direct inhibition of an excited, abnormally firing nerve; or (3) restoration of afferent input.
• TENS is helpful in the treatment of many painful conditions. Proponents of TENS recommend its use early in a pain treatment program. The patients who respond best to TENS typically have neurogenic or musculoskeletal pain.
• TENS variables that can be adjusted by the patient include the stimulus amplitude, rate, pulse width, and location of the electrodes. Adverse reactions to TENS are infrequent; the most common is skin hypersensitivity. TENS should be avoided over the carotid sinus, in patients with demand-type pacemakers, and during pregnancy.

Heat and Cold (p. 926)
• The use of hot and cold modalities, particularly those that the patient can safely use at home, should be encouraged (see Chapter 21). The use of devices or treatments that require the help of other persons or professional settings (e.g., ultrasound or massage) are best reserved for acute pain syndromes or intermittently painful chronic conditions.

Biofeedback (p. 927)
• Relaxation training and biofeedback are behavioral treatment methods that have been successfully used to treat a variety of pain syndromes including myofascial and sympathetically maintained pain syndromes. Biofeedback utilizes instrumentation to provide feedback on a variety of physiological responses (e.g., hand temperature, muscle tension, and sweat gland activity). It is typically used to facilitate relaxation and enhance self-regulation.

Interventional Procedures (pp. 927–928)

• Interventional procedures are an important component of the therapeutic armamentarium for chronic pain management. Some of these techniques play an especially important role when used as diagnostic procedures. Interventional procedures can be powerful tools when used and interpreted intelligently in the context of a multidisciplinary approach to chronic pain. They can also help prevent the development of chronic pain syndromes. The most commonly employed interventional techniques are listed in Table 42–4.

Chemoneurolysis (p. 927)
• The injection of agents capable of interfering with neural conduction for prolonged periods is another common technique for pain control. Neurolytic agents include alcohol, phenol, ammonium sulfate, and chlorocresol. Chemoneurolysis can be done intrathecally and epidurally, as well at various plexuses or in some peripheral nerves.

TABLE 42–4 Commonly Utilized Interventional Treatments in Chronic Pain Syndrome

Treatment	Use/Comment
Nerve blocks	As diagnostic, prognostic, or therapeutic procedures
Diagnostic blocks	To ascertain source of pain, nerve pathway, or as tools for differential diagnosis
Prognostic blocks	Before neuroablative or neurolytic procedures to assess their possible effects
Therapeutic blocks	Can be performed with local anesthetics or with neurolytic agents
Trigger point injections	Treatment of myofascial pain
Facet or zygapophyseal blocks	Diagnostic or therapeutic
Epidural blocks	Useful especially when prolonged analgesia might be required for physical therapy, not for days but for weeks
Spinal blocks	Differential pain diagnosis
Neurolytic, epidural, and spinal techniques	Specific indications for the treatment of some intractable chronic pain syndromes
Sympathetic nerve blocks	Effective therapeutic tools in dealing with sympathetically maintained pain
Chemoneurolysis Cryoneurolysis/cryoanalgesia	Very effective in treatment of sympathetically maintained pain and cancer or noncancer chronic pain

• Sympathetic chemoneurolysis has a special indication in complex regional pain syndrome, either type I or II, with evidence of "sympathetically maintained pain." Somatic neurolytic techniques are used in the control of cancer and noncancer pain. Gasserian alcohol gangliolysis has been used extensively in trigeminal neuralgia, although this technique has been largely replaced by radiofrequency thermocoagulation of the Gasserian ganglion.

• Chemoneurolysis, even when meticulously performed, can be associated with serious complications such as neuritis. This can lead to increased pain, sexual dysfunction, or other serious side effects. Patients should be informed about such possibilities and informed consent must be obtained before any neurolytic procedure.

Cryolysis (pp. 927–928)

• Another technique commonly used in pain management is cryoanalgesia. This technique is based on the fact that freezing can induce a nerve lesion. Inducing cryogenic neural lesions, when done carefully, can be a powerful technique. Frustratingly, its effectiveness cannot be predicted; moreover, pain relief can last from 3 to 1000 days, with a mean of 60 to 90 days. Indications for cryolysis include facial pain, and cryolysis of the trigeminal nerve or its branches has been described in the literature. Thoracic pain such as acute post-thoracotomy pain or post-thoracotomy intercostal neuralgia can be treated by cryolysis. Spinal pain originating in the facets is often treated by cryolytic lesioning of the medial branch of the posterior primary ramus of symptomatic facets. Pelvic pain can be a particularly good indication for cryolysis, and it is often indicated in coccygodynia, or perineal pain from cancer of the rectum.

Radiofrequency Thermocoagulation (p. 928)

• Radiofrequency thermocoagulation (RFTC) has been used to ablate pain pathways in the trigeminal ganglion, sympathetic chain, spinal cord, dorsal root entry zone, dorsal root ganglion, and peripheral nerves.

• Because the neural lesion produced by RFTC is irreversible, it has to be considered an end-of-the-line procedure to be used only when other, more conservative modalities have failed. One complication that has been reported is the development of painful neuroma formation.

Steroid Injections (p. 928)

• Injection of steroids has been used widely for the treatment of chronic pain (see Chapter 24). Injections of steroids into the epidural space, onto peripheral nerves, and into joints have been done for many years with variable degrees of success. This variability of the success rate appears to depend on the condition being treated. The injection of steroids to treat pain caused by irritation of spinal segmental nerves secondary to intervertebral disk herniations has been used to avoid spinal surgery. A large number of patients experience significant relief of pain after epidural injection of steroids.

Lidocaine Challenge (p. 928)

Spinal Opiates (p. 928)

• Spinal opiates are used extensively for the management of chronic benign pain as well as for cancer pain. Opiates can be delivered epidurally or intrathecally. The delivery system can be fully implantable or use external pumps. The fully

implantable system is preferable for chronic use except when life expectancy is less than 6 months. Cancer pain can be treated efficaciously, thus providing adequate quality of life.
• Noncancer pain has been treated extensively with spinal opiates, and it has a special application in failed back syndrome and any type of orthopedic intractable pain. Even though neuropathic pain and complex regional pain syndrome are relatively insensitive to opiates, they can be managed successfully with spinal opiates.

Neuroaugmentation (Spinal Cord and Nerve Stimulation) (p. 928)
• Central and peripheral neuroaugmentation can be used in selected patients. Its mechanism of action is based on the notion that afferent input along low-threshold, large-diameter nerve fibers can exert a powerful inhibitory effect on nociceptive input conveyed along C fibers. This therapeutic modality is indicated when other, more conservative measures have failed.
• Failed back syndrome with radicular pain in either one or both extremities can be reasonably treated with spinal cord stimulation. Axial pain is not an indication for neuroaugmentation. Patients with complex regional pain syndrome of the upper or lower extremity are typically good candidates for spinal cord stimulation.

Increasing Activity Level (p. 929)

• Therapeutic exercises are intended to improve physical condition and functional capacities. They also indirectly provide pain relief and a better quality of life. Patients with chronic pain conditions tend to reduce or discontinue their activities because of fear of increased pain or harm. This can result in joint stiffness, decreased endurance, decreased muscle strength, muscle wasting, and even a general state of decompensation.
• Appropriate exercises that are specific for the pain area, and general conditioning exercises (e.g., bicycling, walking, and swimming) are usually indicated. The patient's baseline exercise level is determined by asking the patient to exercise to tolerance (i.e., until pain, weakness, or fatigue necessitates stopping) over a few days. Once the baseline has been established, the initial exercise goal is set within the patient's tolerance and then gradually increased, with new goals being set every few days. Rewards and reinforcement are given for accomplishing the established goals without demonstrating pain behavior.

Psychosocial Interventions (p. 929)

• Recent evidence suggests that the use of psychological modalities in conjunction with medical interventions and physical therapy increases the effectiveness of the chronic pain treatment program. Psychological treatments of chronic pain include psychoeducation, psychotherapy, biofeedback and relaxation training, and vocational counseling. Group psychotherapy has been used successfully to enhance the functioning of patients in a pain rehabilitation program. Individual and family therapy are other interventions often used with chronic pain patients to treat underlying psychosocial stresses.
• Several relaxation techniques can be used for chronic pain, the two most common being autogenic training and progressive muscle relaxation.

Vocational Rehabilitation (p. 929)

• Vocational counseling is an important component of the psychological approach to chronic pain. Each patient is evaluated to determine work history, educational background, vocational skills and abilities, and motivation to return to work. The vocational counselor can determine whether past work skills and current aptitudes can be transferred to alternative occupations if necessary. Vocational counseling is used to reduce functional impairment and disability, improve coping strategies, enhance effective use of pain medications, and decrease use of health care resources.

43

Original Chapter by Jeffrey M. Thompson, M.D.

The Diagnosis and Treatment of Muscle Pain Syndromes

• Muscles make up 40% of the mass of the human body. The forces muscles generate and the mechanical stresses they are subjected to are tremendous. It is not surprising, therefore, that many causes of muscle pain exist (Table 43–1). Those disorders with obvious pathological or laboratory findings are fairly easily defined and are well established as diagnostic entities. The muscle pain syndromes described in this chapter remain controversial largely because of the lack of such objective findings.

HISTORICAL REVIEW (pp. 934–937)

• The medical community has described muscle pain since the 1700s. See the Textbook for an in-depth review of the history of muscle pain syndromes.

PHYSIOLOGY OF MUSCLE PAIN (pp. 937–941)

• See the Textbook for an in depth discussion of the physiology of muscle pain.

MUSCLE PAIN SYNDROMES (pp. 941–954)

• Muscle pain syndromes are those entities that have muscle pain as a major component but do not have an established cause and therefore do not qualify as diseases.

Postexercise Muscle Soreness (p. 941)

• Postexercise soreness is most common following unaccustomed exercise using untrained muscles; it peaks 24 to 48 hours after the exercise. Serum muscle enzymes reach their peak at about the same time. Eccentric (lengthening) contractions provoke this pain much more efficiently than concentric (shortening) contractions. A few weeks of training can reduce or prevent this type of muscle soreness.
• The cause of postexercise muscle pain is not fully understood. With eccentric exercise the external forces acting on the muscle are greater than the forces generated by the muscle itself. These external forces are spread over a smaller percentage of motor units, leading to damage in the muscle fibers and

TABLE 43–1 Causes of Muscle Pain

Causes of Focal Muscle Pain	Causes of Generalized Muscle Pain

With Swelling or Induration
Neoplasm
Trauma (hematoma)
Ruptured tendon
Ruptured Baker's cyst
Thrombophlebitis
Infection
    Streptococcal myositis
    Gas gangrene
    Pyomyositis
    Trichinosis, hydatid cysts, sparganosis
    Painful leg weakness in children with
      influenza
Inflammation
    Localized nodular myositis
    Proliferative myositis
    Pseudomalignant myositis ossificans
    Eosinophilic faciitis
Sarcoidosis (nodular form)
Ischemia
    Muscle necrosis following relief of large
      artery occlusion
    Diabetes (infarction of thigh muscle)
    Embolism (marantic endocarditis)
    Azotemic hyperparathyroidism (muscle and
      skin necrosis)
Toxic and metabolic disorders
    Acute alcoholic myopathy
    Myoglobinuria in drug-induced coma
    Exertional muscle damage
      Normal persons (e.g., military recruits)
      Metabolic myopathies
    Motor unit hyperactivity states (stiff-man
      syndrome, tetanus, strychnine
      poisoning)
 	
No Swelling or Induration
Exertional myalgia
    Normal persons
    Vascular insufficiency (intermittent
      claudication)
    Metabolic myopathies
Acute brachial neuritis
Ischemic mononeuropathy
Parkinsonism
Resting leg pain of obscure cause
    Growing pains
    Restless legs
    Painful legs and moving toes
    Idiopathic leg pain
	With Muscle Weakness
	Inflammation (polymyositis,
	    dermatomyositis)
	Infection
	    Toxoplasmosis
	    Trichinosis
	    Toxic myopathy (influenza or other viral
	      infections, leptospirosis, gram-
	      negative infections, toxic shock
	      syndrome, Kawasaki's syndrome)
	    Poliomyelitis
	Toxic and metabolic disorders
	    Acute alcoholic myopathy
	    Hypophosphatemia
	    Potassium deficiency
	    Total parenteral nutrition (essential fatty
	      acid deficiency)
	    Necrotic myopathy stemming from
	      carcinoma
	    Hypothyroid myopathy
	    Drugs (ε-aminocaproic acid, clofibrate,
	      emetine)
	    Carnitine palmityltransferase deficiency
	Amyloidosis
	Bone pain and myopathy (osteomalacia,
	    hyperparathyroidism)
	Acute polyneuropathy (Guillain-Barré
	    syndrome, porphyria)
	
	Without Muscle Weakness
	Polymyalgia rheumatica
	Muscle pain-fasciculation syndrome
	Myalgia in infection or fever
	Myalgia in collagen-vascular disease
	Steroid withdrawal
	Hypothyroidism
	Primary fibromyalgia (fibrositis)
	Fabry disease
	Parkinsonism

Adapted from Layzer RB: Muscle pain, cramps, and fatigue. In Engel AG, Banker BQ (eds): Myology. New York, McGraw-Hill, 1986, pp. 1907–1922.

connective tissue. The release of nociceptor-sensitizing substances during repair of this damage may lead to the delayed muscle soreness. The pain probably is not caused by the mechanical muscle fiber damage directly because serum enzyme levels do not rise immediately. Because type I (oxidative) fibers are preferentially damaged, and because training can have a protective effect, disordered metabolism is probably a contributing component. The strengthening that occurs during the first few weeks of training is attributed to neural factors such as coordination of motor unit firing. This could explain how training of similar duration protects against postexercise muscle soreness.

• Treatment of postexercise muscle soreness is simple and effective. Rest and a more gradual approach to exercise cures most patients. Nonsteroidal anti-inflammatory drugs do not help, which eliminates prostaglandin from consideration as a sensitizing agent.

Overuse Syndromes (p. 941)

• The terms "overuse injury" and "repetitive strain injury" encompass a variety of musculoskeletal pain problems. Nerve entrapments, stress fractures, tendinitis and bursitis, and muscle pain have all been labeled overuse injuries. These are covered in more detail in Chapter 45 (occupational rehabilitation) and in Chapters 38 and 39 (upper and lower limb musculoskeletal disorders).

• Overuse pain arises from the repetitive use of a muscle, not from a single bout of exercise. These injuries are most common in athletes, musicians, and factory-line workers, where precise repetition of motor tasks is commonly a requirement for success.

• The cause of overuse muscle pain is thought to be microtrauma that outpaces the capacity of the muscle for repair. In laborers, continued use of fatigued muscles causes mechanical damage that is directly related to the heaviness of the work. Again, eccentric work seems to subject small numbers of muscle fibers to excessive loads.

• Many occupations, however, require precise manipulations, leading to excessive contraction of the proximal stabilizers that is unrelated to the heaviness of the task. The conflict of motor control between the postural stabilizers and the muscles needed for precise manipulation or movement leads to the fiber damage.

• The combination of mental stress and precise manipulations experienced by musicians can lead to occupational cramps believed to be of central origin (focal dystonia). These cramps occur more commonly early in the career of the artist, before the smooth, seemingly effortless motor patterns are established.

• Incoordination of movements and co-contraction of agonist-antagonists are often seen in the context of muscle pain. An example is the trapezius myalgia found in factory workers.

Myofascial Pain Syndromes (pp. 942–944)

• The myofascial pain syndromes owe their ever-widening acceptance (if not their existence) to the pioneering work of Travell and her later collaboration with Simons. In 1983, they combined their clinical experience in a detailed description of the multiple pain syndromes attributed to this disorder. In doing so, they further defined the major clinical components characteristic of myofascial pain, the most important being the trigger point, the "taut band," and the local "twitch" response.

The Trigger Point (p. 942)

• The trigger point got its name from its propensity to cause pain at a distant site. These points play a central role in the definition of myofascial pain syndromes and appear in predictable locations, usually in the midportion or belly of the affected muscle. Flat palpation of a relaxed muscle under passive stretch best locates these small (less than 1 cm^2), discrete, tender spots. Sustained pressure (10 seconds) or penetration by a needle usually causes referral of pain into the "zone of reference" typical of that muscle. There may or may not be a palpable nodule at the site. Often the trigger point is located within a taut band in a muscle with decreased range of motion. The significance of these trigger points is not clear. Some researchers believe they arise from localized areas of muscle trauma, but biopsy studies show mostly normal muscle.

The Taut Band (pp. 942–943)

• Trigger points are characteristically found within taut bands of muscle. The taut band is a shortened group of muscle fibers; it can be best palpated by sliding the skin and subcutaneous tissues perpendicularly across the fibers of the muscle. These bands are electrically silent and therefore not caused by "spasm." Localized contracture of a few muscle fibers is one proposed mechanism. Once the taut band is found, palpation along it will lead to the most tender: the trigger point. "Snapping palpation" of the band gives rise to another cardinal sign of myofascial pain, the local twitch response.

The Local Twitch Response (p. 943)

• When one "snaps" the taut band containing a trigger point, a transient contraction of the band's muscle fibers occurs. This sign is diagnostically important, as noted below, but its pathophysiological significance is unclear. The technique of snapping palpation requires significant skill, and its validity as a diagnostic sign has not been established.

Clinical and Research Criteria (p. 943)

• Simons' criteria for the clinical diagnosis of myofascial pain syndrome are listed in Table 43–2. Required features include regional pain, referred pain or disturbed sensation in a predicted location, a taut band, a tender point along the taut band, and restricted range of motion. One of three "minor criteria" must also be present: (1) pain complaint reproduced by pressure on the tender spot, (2) a local twitch response, or (3) relief of the pain by stretching or injecting. At the same time Simons listed research criteria for the identification of trigger points. To qualify, the point must be exquisitely tender, located in a taut band of a muscle with restricted range of motion, refer pain when pressed or needled, and exhibit a twitch response when needled.

Pathophysiology (pp. 943–944)

• The myofascial pain syndromes remain largely a clinical construct based more on case studies, anecdote, and clinical experience than on basic science. Travell and Simons combined facts of muscle physiology with some conjecture and arrived at the following sequence: acute muscle strain → tissue damage in a very localized area of muscle → tears in the sarcoplasmic reticulum → free calcium ions → sustained contraction → increased strain on vulnerable areas of muscle → free calcium ions, and so on. They further proposed that free calcium ions plus ATP leads to sustained contraction of fibers, causing a hypermetabolic state locally and local vasoconstriction (possibly via the sympathetic nervous system).

TABLE 43–2 Clinical Criteria for the Diagnosis of Myofascial Pain Syndrome Caused by Active Trigger Points

To make the clinical diagnosis of myofascial pain syndrome, the findings should include five major criteria and at least one of three minor criteria. The five *major criteria* are the following:

1. Regional pain complaint.
2. Pain complaint or altered sensation in the expected distribution of referred pain from a myofascial trigger point.
3. Taut band palpable in an accessible muscle.
4. Exquisite spot tenderness at one point along the length of the taut band.
5. Some degree of restricted range of motion, when measurable.

The three *minor criteria* are the following:

1. Reproduction of clinical pain complaint, or altered sensation, by pressure on the tender spot.
2. Elicitation of a local twitch response by transverse snapping palpation at the tender spot or by needle insertion into the tender spot in the taut band.
3. Pain alleviated by elongating (stretching) the muscle or by injecting the tender spot (trigger point).

Note: Additional symptoms such as weather sensitivity, sleep disturbance, and depression are often present but are not diagnostic because they may be attributable to chronic severe pain perpetuated by multiple mechanical and/or systemic perpetuating factors.
From Simons AG: Muscular pain syndromes. Adv Pain Res Ther 1990; 17:18.

Chronic Regional Myofascial Syndromes (p. 944)

• The single-muscle myofascial pain syndromes are usually acute and follow an episode of muscle overload. In some cases the pain persists and spreads to other, usually synergistic, muscles. This is referred to as a chronic regional myofascial syndrome. Many perpetuating factors encourage transformation to a more widespread muscle pain problem. Mechanical factors include postural stress, muscle imbalances, and skeletal asymmetries. Systemic perpetuating factors purportedly include anything jeopardizing the energy supply to muscle (e.g., anemia, endocrine imbalances, low thyroid function, and vitamin deficiencies).

Fibromyalgia (pp. 945–949)

The Search for a Definition (pp. 945–946)

• In 1990, the Multicenter Criteria Committee of the American College of Rheumatology (ACR 90) published its criteria for classification of fibromyalgia (Table 43–3). The emphasis was placed on the widespread nature of fibromyalgia, with the requirement of 11 of 18 tender points. Table 43–3 in the Textbook displays past criteria used to define fibromyalgia.

Prevalence and Epidemiology (p. 946)

• Fibromyalgia is common in the community, found in 2% to 4% of the general population. Eight percent of general medical patients meet previous definitions of fibromyalgia, as do about 15% to 20% of rheumatology clinic patients, making fibromyalgia the third most common diagnosis made by rheumatologists. Women make up 73% to 90% of those diagnosed with fibromyalgia, although this may represent a selection bias.

TABLE 43–3 The American College of Rheumatology 1990 Criteria for Classification of Fibromyalgia*

1. History of widespread pain
   Definition: Pain is considered widespread when all the following are present—pain in the left side of the body, pain in the right side of the body, pain above the waist, and pain below the waist. In addition, axial skeletal pain (cervical spine, anterior chest, thoracic spine, or low back) must be present. In this definition, shoulder and buttock pain is considered as pain for each involved side. "Low back" pain is considered lower segment pain.
2. Pain in 11 of 18 tender point sites on digital palpation
   Definition: On digital palpation, pain must be present in at least 11 of the following 18 tender point sites:
   Occiput—Bilateral, at the suboccipital muscle insertions
   Low cervical—Bilateral, at the anterior aspects of the intertransverse spaces at C5 to C7
   Trapezius—Bilateral, at the midpoint of the upper border
   Supraspinatus—Bilateral, at origins, above the scapular spine near the medial border
   Second rib—Bilateral, at the second costochondral junctions, just lateral to the junctions on upper surfaces
   Lateral epicondyle—Bilateral, 2 cm distal to the epicondyles
   Gluteal—Bilateral, in upper outer quadrants of buttocks in anterior fold of muscle
   Greater trochanter—Bilateral, posterior to the trochanteric prominence
   Knee—Bilateral, at the medial fat pad proximal to the joint line
   Digital palpation should be performed with an approximate force of 4 kg.
   For a tender point to be considered "positive," the subject must state that the palpation was painful. "Tender" is not to be considered "painful."

* For classification purposes, patients will be said to have fibromyalgia if both criteria are satisfied. Widespread pain must have been present for at least 3 months. The presence of a second clinical disorder does not exclude the diagnosis of fibromyalgia.
From Wolfe F, Smythe HA, Yunus MB, et al: The American College of Rheumatology 1990 criteria for the classification of fibromyalgia. Arthritis Rheum 1990; 33:160–172. Reprinted by permission of Wiley-Liss, Inc., a subsidiary of John Wiley & Sons.

Clinical Features (pp. 946–947)

WIDESPREAD PAIN AND TENDERNESS

• Widespread pain of 3 months' duration is required for the diagnosis of fibromyalgia; it is defined as pain both above and below the waist, on both the right and left sides of the body, along with axial pain (low back pain is considered below the waist). This may include more than 10% of the population, making the tender point count very important in the diagnosis of fibromyalgia. The sites in the ACR 90 criteria were chosen based on their utility in separating fibromyalgia patients from those with other painful conditions. It is implied that they are discrete points of tenderness.
• Three interpretations, singly or in combination, are possible regarding tender points: (1) they represent specific areas of pathological change; (2) they identify multiple regions of pain; or (3) they signify a generalized increase in tenderness. This has implications for the etiology of fibromyalgia.

SLEEP DISTURBANCE

• Almost all descriptions of fibromyalgia include poor sleep as a feature. At one time, and even recently, the alpha-delta sleep pattern was thought to be diagnostic, and possibly the cause of fibromyalgia. This alpha-delta sleep pattern, originally described by Hauri and Hawkins, correlates with subjective fatigue. The finding is very nonspecific and can be found in any chronically painful condition.

- Nonetheless, disturbed sleep is common in fibromyalgia, with reports of incidence ranging from 60% to 90%. Patients with myofascial pain have similar degrees of sleep disturbance, with the incidence of sleep disturbance correlating better with duration of pain than with diagnosis.

ASSOCIATED SYMPTOMS

- Multiple associated features commonly appear in reports of fibromyalgia. The most common are fatigue (75% to 100%), stiffness (75% to 90%), subjective swelling (30% to 100%), tension-type headache (45% to 75%), anxiety (40% to 70%), and irritable bowel syndrome (35% to 50%). Other common features include aggravation of symptoms by cold, humidity, change of weather, and physical activity. The prevalence of many of these features likely increases as the number of regions involved with pain increases and as the pain becomes more chronic.

PSYCHOLOGICAL ASPECTS

- Partly because of the high number of somatic complaints voiced by patients with fibromyalgia, many clinicians view the patients as psychologically disturbed. The majority of fibromyalgia patients do not have an active psychiatric disorder, but there is a greater prevalence of major depression and panic disorder. It may well be that the psychological aspects of fibromyalgia simply result from chronic pain and its effect on central pain modulation systems.
- Another view is that patients with a primary psychiatric disorder and symptoms of fibromyalgia represent one end of the spectrum of fibromyalgia disorders. In these patients the symptoms of fibromyalgia wax and wane with the psychiatric disorder and with psychosocial stressors. A particularly difficult differentiation is that between fibromyalgia and somatization disorder or somatoform pain disorder. Both of these require the presence of multiple symptoms or pain without causative organic pathological findings, or that the complaint or impairment be out of proportion to the physical findings. As muscle pain persists and becomes more widespread, the incidence of these psychiatric disorders increases.

Pathophysiology: Proposed Mechanisms (pp. 948–949)

- The pathophysiology of fibromyalgia remains a mystery. The few abnormalities found in various studies tend to be nonspecific and lend themselves to various interpretations. These have been combined liberally with conjecture to arrive at the leading theories of pathophysiology. The theories can be divided into three groups based on the location of the proposed mechanism: (1) primarily central, (2) a combination of central and peripheral, or (3) primarily peripheral.

Myofascial Pain Syndrome versus Fibromyalgia
(pp. 949–950)

- Although fibromyalgia and myofascial pain syndrome have many similarities, most investigators maintain that they are two distinct entities. In general, myofascial pain is thought to be a local or regional problem caused by acute muscle trauma, whereas fibromyalgia is a widespread pain problem affecting

more than just muscle and has systemic features. The presence of taut bands, referred pain, and twitch responses is often cited to differentiate myofascial pain.
• Myofascial pain and fibromyalgia might be labels for the two extremes of a single disorder. Under the right conditions, trigger points can develop in nearby muscles until widespread chronic pain involves multiple muscle sites associated with systemic features such as disturbed sleep, generalized fatigue, and anxiety, the characteristic features of fibromyalgia. At what point did the disorder change from myofascial pain to fibromyalgia? Is fibromyalgia myofascial pain plus chronic pain syndrome? Is myofascial pain simply localized fibromyalgia? These are questions yet to be answered.

Chronic Fatigue Syndrome (pp. 950–951)

• Chronic fatigue syndrome (CFS) has recently emerged as a popular diagnostic label for "a centuries-old disorder of fatigue and multiple somatic complaints."
• The 1987 Centers for Disease Control and Prevention (CDC) definition of CFS included fatigue of at least 6 months' duration in the absence of a known cause, and the presence of 8 of 11 symptoms that included sleep disturbance, muscle pain, postexertional fatigue, and migratory myalgias (Table 43–4). The large

---

TABLE 43–4 CDC Case Definition of Chronic Fatigue Syndrome (CFS)

A case of CFS must fulfill both major criteria as well as either eight symptom criteria or six symptom criteria plus two physical criteria.

Major Criteria
1. New onset of fatigue lasting 6 mo reducing activity to <50%
2. Other conditions producing fatigue must be ruled out

Minor Criteria

Symptom Criteria—beginning at or after onset of fatigue and persisting or recurring for at least 6 mo
1. Low-grade fever, temperature of 37.5 °C–38.6 °C (99.5 °F–101.5 °F) orally or chills
2. Sore throat
3. Painful cervical or axillary lymph nodes
4. Generalized muscle weakness
5. Muscle pain
6. Post-exertional fatigue lasting 24 hr
7. Headache
8. Migratory arthralgias
9. Neuropsychological complaints (e.g., photophobia, transient visual scotomata, forgetfulness, excessive irritability, confusion, difficulty thinking, inability to concentrate, or depression)
10. Sleep disturbance
11. Acute onset of symptoms over a few hours to a few days

Physical Criteria—documented by a physician twice, at least 1 mo apart
1. Low-grade fever, temperature of 37.6 °C–38.6 °C (99.7 °F–101.5 °F) orally or 37.8 °C–38.8 °C (100.0 °F–101.8 °F) rectally
2. Nonexudative pharyngitis
3. Palpable cervical or axillary lymph nodes up to 2 cm in diameter

Adapted from Klonoff DC: Chronic fatigue syndrome. Clin Infect Dis 1992; 15:812–823. Reprinted by permission of The University of Chicago.

number of symptoms required tended to select patients with psychiatric disorders. Because of this, the CDC criteria were modified to specifically exclude patients with psychoses and substance abuse.
• The cause of CFS is unknown. It most commonly begins suddenly after an infectious-like illness, but no link to any specific pathogen has been established. Initial findings in support of such a role for Epstein-Barr virus, Coxsackie B virus, and the human herpesvirus 6 have all been contradicted in more recent studies.
• There continues to be some discussion as to whether CFS is an organic or psychiatric illness. It is likely a combination of the two, with a link between organic and psychiatric factors similar to that found in chronic pain. In both, the symptoms and functional deficits are out of proportion to the identifiable pathological findings. In CFS, an underlying hyperresponsive immune system might provide the organic half of the link. Psychiatric disturbance (depression) could magnify this deranged immune response.
• The recommended treatment for CFS is very similar to that for fibromyalgia (see below). Recommendations include (1) exclusion of other conditions; (2) reassurance about the benign nature of the disorder; (3) use of antidepressants to treat both the depression and the sleep disorder, if present; (4) a graduated exercise program; (5) stress reduction; and (6) use of counseling and support groups.

Tension Myalgia (p. 951)

• The term tension myalgia covers patients who do not meet the strict criteria for fibromyalgia or myofascial pain (i.e., the majority). With the recent resurgence of interest in muscle pain disorders nationally, and the more widespread use of the terms fibromyalgia and myofascial pain (and the expansion of these terms to cover "localized fibromyalgia" and "generalized myofascial pain"), use of the diagnosis tension myalgia has declined. The concept of a continuum of muscle pain disorders remains, however, and tension myalgia remains a useful paradigm.
• The major utility of the term tension myalgia lies in patient education. Most patients have seen multiple health care providers without a specific diagnosis, resulting in the often less than subtle implication that it is "all in their head." They are concerned that something has been overlooked and that they may have cancer or some other debilitating disease. Receiving a definite diagnosis and an understandable explanation for their symptoms allays these fears and is the first step in successful treatment.
• "Myalgia" refers to the most characteristic symptom—local, regional, or widespread muscle pain, including pain at musculotendinous junctions and muscle attachments. "Tension" has two connotations. First, it suggests that a common finding (and possibly a causative factor) is muscle under tension, whether it is from "spasm," postural stress, overuse, or disordered motor sequencing. The presence or absence of "spasm" is not significant; rather, these patients misuse their muscles by habitually co-contracting them, by failing to fully relax them, by overusing them, by subjecting them to unrelenting postural stress, or by a combination of these.
• Second, the word tension suggests that psychological tension or stress may play a major role, especially in patients with more widespread pain. When the diagnosis is presented in this way, patients are more willingly accept the possi-

bility of psychological influences on their muscle pain disorder and are more likely to take the necessary steps to address them.

Diagnostic Approach to Muscle Pain Syndromes
(pp. 951–952)

• The approach to the diagnosis of muscle pain is fairly straightforward (Table 43–5). Despite a lengthy differential diagnosis (see Table 43–1), distinguishing these entities is seldom difficult in clinical practice. One difficulty can arise, however, if tension myalgia and another chronic disorder, such as rheumatoid arthritis, are present.

Treatment of Muscle Pain Syndromes (pp. 952–954)

• With the multiple theories of etiology for muscle pain syndromes come multiple, mostly unproven, methods of treatment. This section describes one approach to treatment, combining what little has been shown to be useful with what appears empirically to be useful (Fig. 43–1).
• The first step in treatment is establishing the diagnosis with the patient and spending the time to help the patient understand what the diagnosis is and is not (see Tension Myalgia, above).

Elimination of Contributing Factors (pp. 952–953)
• The next step in treatment is the elimination of contributing factors. A good diet is certainly important, including plenty of B vitamin sources. However, more common contributing factors include poor posture and poor body mechanics, which should be corrected to eliminate unnecessary muscle use
• Vocational and avocational muscle overuse is a common contributing factor and must be specifically pursued. It is important to specifically ask about hobbies, sports, daily tasks, and sleeping position. An ergonomic evaluation of the workplace is often valuable.
• The more chronic and widespread the muscle pain syndrome, the more likely that psychological stress plays a role. Instruction in stress management techniques can be useful, but if a major psychopathological disorder is suspected, formal psychiatric evaluation may be warranted. Often the more involved patients benefit from the cognitive-behavioral treatment approach used in comprehensive pain management centers (see Chapter 42).

TABLE 43–5 Suggested Laboratory Evaluation for Muscle Pain

Erythrocyte sedimentation rate
Serum creatine kinase
Complete blood count
Thyroid function tests

Also consider:
Electromyography
Rheumatoid factor
Antinuclear antibody
Muscle biopsy

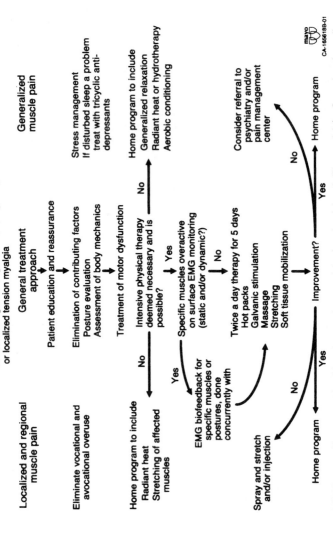

Establish diagnosis of generalized, regional, or localized tension myalgia

Localized and regional muscle pain

General treatment approach

Generalized muscle pain

Patient education and reassurance

Stress management
If disturbed sleep a problem treat with tricyclic anti-depressants

Eliminate vocational and avocational overuse

Elimination of contributing factors
Posture evaluation
Assessment of body mechanics
Treatment of motor dysfunction

Home program to include
Generalized relaxation
Radiant heat or hydrotherapy
Aerobic conditioning

Home program to include
Radiant heat
Stretching of affected muscles

Intensive physical therapy deemed necessary and is possible?

No → Home program

Yes

No ↓   Yes

EMG biofeedback for specific muscles or postures, done concurrently with

Specific muscles overactive on surface EMG monitoring (static and/or dynamic?)

No

Twice a day therapy for 5 days
Hot packs
Galvanic stimulation
Massage
Stretching
Soft tissue mobilization

Improvement?

Consider referral to psychiatry and/or pain management center

No

Yes → Home program

Spray and stretch and/or injection

No

Improvement?

Yes → Home program

FIGURE 43–1. Treatment algorithm for tension myalgia (myofascial pain/fibromyalgia). *Central column* lists approaches useful in both localized and generalized muscle pain problems. The approaches more specific to generalized muscle pain (fibromyalgia) are in the *right column*, and the approaches more specific for localized muscle pain (myofascial pain syndromes) are in the *left column*.

mayo
CA-1656188-01

- Poor sleep is another feature often found in the more chronic cases. If present, it often responds to low-dose tricyclic antidepressant medications (e.g., amitriptyline, 10 to 25 mg nightly). Trazodone, 25 to 75 mg nightly, appears to work equally well and is better tolerated. Even greater improvement may result from combination treatment with a selective serotonin reuptake inhibitor (SSRI) in the morning and a tricyclic at night to improve sleep (e.g., 20 mg of fluoxetine in the morning and 10 to 25 mg of amitriptyline in the evening).

Treatment of Motor Dysfunction (p. 953)
- The next major category of treatment addresses the problem of motor dysfunction. This often requires specific physical therapy. The goals of treatment are to decrease pain, restore normal range of motion, restore normal neuromuscular functioning, and improve fitness.
- Reducing pain will increase the patient's confidence in the treatment plan. The use of passive modalities should be limited to the early treatment phase to avoid patient dependence and the persistent notion that something must be done *to* them in order to get "fixed."
- A general stretching program with special emphasis on muscle groups found to be "tight" on examination is a basic part of treatment. The patient should learn to do this several times a day. Using heat before gentle prolonged stretching may improve its effectiveness and lessen its discomfort.
- The goal of neuromuscular re-education lies in restoring normal resting tone and fluid movement without co-contraction of agonists and antagonists. Surface EMG biofeedback over specific areas can be helpful, especially with the postural muscles, which often function subconsciously.
- Once pain has been reduced and motor dysfunction minimized, a very graduated aerobic fitness program can be instituted. The combination of biofeedback for relaxation and a moderate exercise program (e.g., stretching and aerobic walking) can help maintain significant improvement. It is important to stress a very gradual return to activity to avoid fatigue and increased muscle pain.

Local Treatments (pp. 953–954)
- Spray and stretch is the mainstay of myofascial pain syndrome treatment. The vapocoolant spray is used to reflexively relax the muscle to allow an adequate stretch. One maintains a sweeping pattern of spray in the direction of the muscle fibers as the muscle is passively stretched by the patient or the clinician's free hand. The prolonged stretch is the key element and is what provides pain relief through an as-yet-unknown mechanism.
- The second most commonly used treatment for localized muscle pain is injection. Dry needling appears to work as well as any other type, but most physicians use a local anesthetic for the sake of patient comfort. The addition of corticosteroids to the injection has many advocates but likely adds little but cost to the procedure. Proponents of injection focus on finding the primary trigger point, which, when treated successfully, leads to resolution of many of the secondary trigger points. Treating only the secondary points without finding the primary point is one reason for treatment failure.
- Even less well studied is the use of ischemic compression to treat trigger points. The theory is that sustained pressure over the pathological area induces increased blood flow on release of pressure, in turn reversing the assumed localized ischemia in the underlying muscle. The digitally applied pressure lasts for about 1 minute at gradually increasing pressure as tolerated up to 30 lb.

Medications (p. 954)

• Both amitriptyline and cyclobenzaprine have provided short-term relief in controlled studies of fibromyalgia patients as noted above in the discussion of contributing factors. Anti-inflammatory agents (including corticosteroids) and analgesics are generally not useful and should be avoided.

• The most important component of any treatment approach is the patient. The ultimate goal is to educate patients and provide them with the means to manage their own muscle pain disorder, eliminating dependence on (and overutilization of) health care providers.

44

Concepts in Sports Medicine

GENERAL CONCEPTS OF THE MUSCULOSKELETAL SYSTEM (pp. 957–958)

Muscle (pp. 957–958)

• Muscle injury can occur from direct macrotrauma, tissue invasion (via laceration), and repetitive microtrauma (overuse). During the healing process of a muscle injury—and after the inflammatory phase subsides and tissue healing, repair, and remodeling occur—concomitant changes take place in muscle function unless appropriate treatment is undertaken. Deficits in absolute strength, strength balance, flexibility, and proprioception can occur. If treatment is not initiated, these deficits are likely to predispose the patient to further injury at the same site or at a distal site in the kinetic chain. The kinetic chain, which is referred to often in this chapter, can be thought of as the linked system of muscles, joints, and body segments involved in a particular biomechanical movement or task.

Tendons (p. 958)

• Tendons connect muscle to bone. Their primary function is to transmit muscle force to the osseous skeleton, with minimal change in their inherent length. Tendons consist of densely packed collagen fibers, arranged in parallel with one another and oriented toward the tensile pull of the muscle. Tendons can be damaged if (1) a force is applied rapidly and obliquely through the tendon, (2) the tendon is under tension before the load is applied, (3) the musculotendinous group is stretched, (4) the attached muscle is maximally contracted, or (5) the tendinous structure itself is weak in comparison with the muscle.
• Tendon healing basically occurs in three phases. The first 48 to 72 hours of healing is known as the *inflammatory phase*. The second phase is reparative and entails collagen fibers laid down in a random, haphazard pattern. During the final phase of healing, the mechanical strength of the healing tendon increases with the maturation and remodeling of fiber architecture. The tensile strength of scar tissue is not optimum unless specific and gradually applied stressors are placed on the healing tissue.
• Chronic repetitive microtrauma to the tendon can lead to a condition of degenerative change and damage. This pathological condition has been called

617

tendinosis. Conditions in which tendinosis is common include plantar fasciitis, lateral epicondylitis, patellar tendinitis, and Achilles tendinitis. Tendinosis requires a complete analysis of kinetic chain function including flexibility, muscle balance, and proximal and distal mechanics and kinesiology, rather than mere control of inflammation.

Ligaments (p. 958)

• Ligaments consist of dense connective tissue and connect bone to bone. They have a mechanical stabilizing effect on joints. Ligaments contain proprioceptive afferents that provide feedback to the musculoskeletal system. Injuries to ligaments usually result from a large overload force. As with tendons, early motion is important to maximize tensile strength of a healing ligament.

Bursae (p. 958)

• Bursae are sacs formed by two layers of synovial tissue. The sacs usually contain a thin layer of synovial fluid. Bursae are located at sites of friction between tendon and bone. With overuse or repetitive trauma, bursae can be injured by friction or external pressure. They also can become inflamed through the degeneration and calcification of an overlying tendon (e.g., subacromial bursitis caused by calcific supraspinatus tendinitis). The response of bursae to injury usually consists of inflammation with resultant effusion and thickening of the bursal wall.

GENERAL CONCEPTS OF THE CARDIOVASCULAR SYSTEM (pp. 958–959)

• The importance of maintaining appropriate cardiovascular conditioning during sports participation and injury rehabilitation is well known. Complications of inactivity include cardiovascular and musculoskeletal deconditioning, bone loss, orthostatic hypotension, deep venous thrombosis, contracture, and pressure ulceration (see Chapter 32). In any musculoskeletal sports injury the principle of "relative rest" applies. This principle dictates that the injured body part should be "rested" and protected from further trauma or injury while the remaining muscle mass is used to provide appropriate stress to the cardiovascular system for maintaining optimal aerobic conditioning (see Chapter 32). In addition, strength training should continue in uninvolved body parts. "Crossover" training effects have been documented in the rested limb when the contralateral limb is exercised.

INJURY PREVENTION AND PRE-REHABILITATION (pp. 959–967)

• The term pre-rehabilitation, or *prehabilitation (prehab),* refers to rehabilitative exercises that are performed preoperatively to enhance the postoperative outcome. Theoretically, pre-rehabilitation can enhance the neuromuscular engram and hasten motor learning of the rehabilitative program after the surgical procedure. In addition, pre-rehabilitation can refer to exercises that are used to prevent injury or to prevent previously delineated biomechanical or kinetic chain deficits from contributing to musculoskeletal injury.

• The seven main components of a hypothetical protective exercise program include flexibility, strength training, aerobic training, analysis of kinetic chain function, proprioception, sport-specific and higher level skills training, and the incorporation of these elements into a practical training program.

Flexibility (pp. 959–962)

• Muscles that cross two joints can have an especially powerful impact on kinetic chain function. Tightness of these muscles can have more wide-ranging sequelae than that seen in muscles crossing only one joint. In the lower extremities, hamstring flexibility can be measured objectively by measuring the popliteal angle (Fig. 44–1).

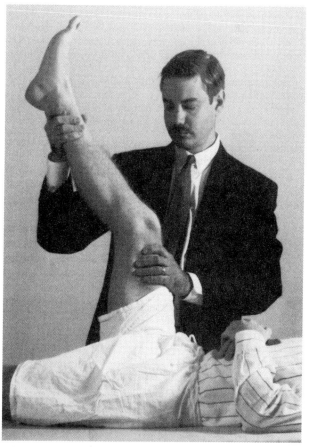

FIGURE 44–1. The popliteal angle is an objective measure of hamstring tightness. The angle is measured while the hip is flexed at 90 degrees.

• Quadriceps flexibility (specifically, the rectus femoris) can be measured with the Ely test, and the distance from the buttock to the heel (or the knee flexion angle) can be recorded to gauge improvement as the flexibility program progresses. Flexibility of the Achilles tendon can be gauged by measuring the degree of dorsiflexion that can be attained with the foot in a partially supinated position (see Fig. 44–3 in the Textbook). Iliotibial band tightness can be measured with the Ober test, although there is no reliable objective measurement for this maneuver.

• In the upper extremities, range of motion at the wrists and elbows can be measured goniometrically.

• Asymmetry might be the most important clinical aspect of flexibility, especially after an injury. One of the most important predictors of future injury is a history of past injury, and any flexibility deficit and asymmetry can increase the risk of musculoskeletal injury or reinjury. Even without previous injury, stretching can help physiologically to prevent injury in many ways.

• Proper stretching technique is crucial because both the positioning of the body during the stretch and the duration of hold are important in maximizing the result of the stretch. For example, a common mistake in the gastrocnemius-soleus stretch occurs when the patient externally rotates the rear foot (see Fig. 44–5 in the Textbook). This takes the vector of stretch off the main bulk of the Achilles tendon.

• The optimal duration for a stretch is still a matter of controversy, but the evidence favors holding the stretch for 15 to 30 seconds and repeating it three to five times. Ideally, the stretch should be performed before and after the competition or exercise period. If stretching is going to be done only once, it should be *after* the exercise session. After a session of exercise, increased deep muscle blood flow can increase tissue temperature and facilitate stretching.

• There are also age-specific and sport-specific stretching concerns. For example, specific muscle tightness during adolescence can have an impact on growth-related musculoskeletal problems such as Osgood-Schlatter disease. More concentrated stretching on two-joint muscles (e.g., the hamstrings, hip flexors, and rectus femoris) is important during this stage. Older adults have specific flexibility concerns with respect to posture and biomechanics. Hamstring and hip flexor flexibility are particularly important as a person ages. Stretching the muscles that are used in specific sports should also be considered. The hip adductors and shoulder rotators, for example, are especially important in tennis; the hamstrings in running (especially sprints); and the hip flexors and hip adductors in soccer.

• Finally, one of the most effective means of stretching a chronically tight muscle is to strengthen the antagonist muscle. As an example, tight gastrocsoleus muscles can often be passively stretched by strengthening the anterior tibialis, and tight hamstrings can be passively stretched by strengthening the quadriceps group.

Protective Strength Training (p. 962)

• The role of strength training in preventing injury depends primarily on two mechanisms. First, a stronger muscle is able to absorb more tensile loading and force before breakdown occurs either in the muscle itself or at the musculotendinous junction. Second, it is important clinically to address any relative muscle weakness, asymmetry, or imbalance.

Aerobic Training (pp. 962–963)

• Aerobic exercise can be a key component of a preventive musculoskeletal exercise program. Aerobic exercise should be an essential component of training to prevent early musculoskeletal fatigue because this might help prevent injury. Increased capillary density also helps combat the relative ischemia of a tight muscle group, perhaps contributing to earlier washout of lactic acid. Strength training can negate some of the beneficial effects of increased capillary density, and a regular aerobic component can help balance this seemingly counterproductive effect.

• With respect to sport-specific upper extremity training for exercises or sports that primarily use the arms (e.g., swimming and kayaking), the onset of lactate accumulation occurs earlier during arm exercise than during leg exercise.

ATP-Phosphocreatinine Energy System. The ATP-phosphocreatinine system provides for explosive power and is extremely short-lived (5 to 10 seconds). Training in this system helps to improve speed and quickness. Traditionally, this system has been thought to be enhanced through plyometric-type activities that stress muscle power. Lower-weight, higher-repetition weight training that emphasizes speed and explosiveness of movement is thought to enhance this energy system. Rather than plyometric activities, one-repetition maximal resistance training sessions might also help to neuromuscularly train the development and availability of maximal motor unit activity.

Anaerobic Energy System. Intermediate-duration (60 to 90 seconds) power comes from the anaerobic energy system (glycolysis). Training of this type enables high-speed, high-intensity activity to be sustained over short periods. Exercises that enhance this energy system include 220- and 440-yard sprints; stair runs; and interval training on a bicycle, running, or with in-line skates.

Aerobic Energy System. Aerobic training enables sustained intervals of higher intensity exercise and quicker recovery between exercise sessions. It also allows more frequent periods of high-intensity exercise.

Kinetic Chain Function (pp. 963–964)

• The importance of analyzing kinetic chain mechanics cannot be overstated. Attending only to the local area of pain and treating this area exclusively can contribute to perpetuation of symptoms. For example, lateral epicondylitis (tennis elbow) is manifested as tenderness to palpation at the lateral epicondyle and forearm extensor muscle mass. This area can be iced and anti-inflammatory medication can be given, but if the biomechanical deficits of suboptimal wrist or shoulder strength, flexibility, or mechanics are not addressed, and if potential problems with sports equipment (e.g., high tension of the strings in a graphite racquet) are not considered, the problem will continue.

• With respect to overuse and macrotraumatic musculoskeletal injuries, a therapeutic intervention must occur to make the person "different" before he or she returns to the sport or activity that originally caused the problem. The injured tissue must be modified to deal more effectively with the loads and mechanics of the sport or activity and be reintegrated into the functional kinetic chain through a logical progression of sport-specific exercises.

• There are many ways of incorporating kinetic chain exercises that occur in a proprioceptively enriched environment and that can be specific for integration

of various upper extremity and lower extremity biomechanical movements. Various functional upper extremity and lower extremity exercises include the use of multiple joints and muscle co-contraction. These exercises are sport- and life-specific and use muscle groups in a coordinated fashion rather than in an isolated one.
• Isolated stretches can help to heal and to modify tissue at the site of injury, but true functional stretch can occur only when the tissue is incorporated into the loads it will be experiencing in the kinetic chain.

Proprioception (pp. 964–966)

• Proprioception can be thought of as a complex neuromuscular process that allows the body to maintain proper stability and orientation whether moving or standing still. Injury to a joint can cause direct or indirect alterations in the innervation of mechanoreceptors. As a consequence, messages to and from these joint receptors are disrupted, and deafferentation (disruption of input information) leads to insufficient or uncoordinated activation of muscle groups. One of the most important predictors of future injury is a history of previous injury.
• After an injury, "pain free" does not mean "cured" and, unless the proprioceptive deficit has been addressed, complete rehabilitation has not been accomplished. To improve dynamic joint stability, the proprioceptive system must in some way be challenged. Balance training (e.g., single-leg stance exercises) and closed kinetic chain exercises are effective ways to challenge the dynamic and reflexive aspects of proprioception in the lower extremities. Functional testing (e.g., figure-8 cuts, vertical jumps, or single leg hops) and sport-specific testing (e.g., timed, backward running for a defensive back in football) are ways to ensure that the proprioceptive neuromuscular system has been sufficiently retrained for safe participation in sports.

Sport-Specific Higher Level Skills (pp. 966–967)

• Before a person returns to a sport after an injury, or before initial participation in a sport, sport- and position-specific skills are necessary to ensure that the skills related to a sport are performed with the greatest facility and dexterity. These exercises include higher-order gait and coordination exercises, plyometrics, and sport-specific drills. In addition to sports specificity, position specificity is important. The job description for a lineman on a football team is different from that for a wide receiver, and each of these jobs requires a specific exercise program.
• The key purpose of sport-specific practice is to solidify and to hardwire the neuromuscular engrams required for the execution of sport movements. Integral to this principle is the concept that "only perfect practice makes perfect."

Incorporation of Components into a Practical Training Program (p. 967)

• Education is essential and can be incorporated on three levels. The person should receive information from the sports medicine team (e.g., physician, physical therapist, athletic trainer, coach, and others as applicable). At local and regional levels, high school and college sports programs can have considerable impact by implementing the above prehabilitation or injury protection elements into their programs.

EXTRINSIC CONTRIBUTORS TO INJURY AND SUBOPTIMAL SPORTS PERFORMANCE (pp. 967–968)

• The major factors that contribute to injury can be grouped into extrinsic and intrinsic factors. Extrinsic factors consist primarily of elements external to a person, whereas intrinsic factors are related to a person's anatomical and biomechanical characteristics.
• Extrinsic factors that can contribute to injury or suboptimal sports performance are listed in Table 44–1.

Conditioning and Preparation (p. 967)

• It is important to analyze an athlete's training history (e.g., the types of terrain on a runner's running route, the volume of training, and the intensity of training). The *terrible too's*—"too much, too soon, too fast, and too hard"—contribute to many overuse injuries. It is also important to ensure that sport-specific conditioning and sport preparation have taken place, as outlined above in the section on sport-specific practice.

Climate, Fluids, and Hydration (p. 967)

• The importance of adequate hydration and fluid replacement should be stressed for persons competing in endurance events. Because water constitutes most of the fluid that is lost in events lasting less than 90 minutes, water replacement is the best mode of restoring fluid status. The athlete should drink at least 16 oz of fluid approximately 2 hours before starting physical activity, and 20 to 40 oz per hour of a cool, noncarbonated beverage during exercise. Drink 16 oz of fluid for each pound of weight lost during physical activity. Carbohydrate supplementation can be helpful during exercise that lasts longer than 90 minutes. Athletes who use creatine supplementation should pay special attention to adequate hydration because creatine draws water inside muscle cells and can lead to a relative extracellular volume depletion.

Kinesiology of the Sport (p. 967)

• Each sport places unique kinesiological and biomechanical stresses on the components of the kinetic chain that are involved in performing the sport. If training focuses on optimizing the mechanics of the sport, injuries might be prevented. A video camera recording can often help delineate the suboptimal components of the kinetic chain and provide feedback for technique correction.

TABLE 44–1 Contributors to Injury: Extrinsic Factors

Training errors—conditioning and preparation	Epidemiology
Climate, fluids, and hydration	Equipment
Kinesiology of the sport	Playing field

Epidemiology (p. 968)

• Certain sports have an inherent risk and predispose to injury of specific parts of the body, and each sport has certain risk factors that pretraining can help minimize. It is important to identify injuries that are specific for a sport or activity and to maximize the kinetic chain function related to the particular part of the body at risk.

Equipment (p. 968)

• Equipment can play a significant role in injury. For example, tennis racquets strung at an excessively high tension can contribute to the development of lateral epicondylitis.

Playing Field (p. 968)

• The playing field should be considered an extrinsic contributor to injury. Various artificial turf surfaces can alter foot and lower limb torque, and certain injuries (e.g., "turf toe" in football) seem to be more prevalent on artificial surfaces. The composition of the playing surface should be considered in relation to the particular sport training and game requirements. For example, cross-country runners should not be trained exclusively on concrete surfaces.

INTRINSIC CONTRIBUTORS TO INJURY AND SUBOPTIMAL SPORTS PERFORMANCE (p. 968)

• The intrinsic contributors to injury are listed in Table 44–2. Malalignments and anatomical variations (e.g., excessive forefoot pronation, cavus foot, varus/valgus malalignment, excessive tibial torsion, excessive leg-length discrepancy [more than 2 cm], and excessive femoral anteversion) can contribute to numerous biomechanical problems that can cause injury. Orthotic interventions such as supports to preserve the longitudinal arch of the foot can help to optimize foot biomechanics and to improve the distribution of force throughout the lower extremity. In addition, adequate shock absorption can help reduce the incidence of overuse injury in such sports as running.

• Ensuring symmetrical and sport-specific flexibility is important, as is maintaining balanced muscle group strength. Signs of incomplete or improper rehabilitation from a previous injury (e.g., strength asymmetries or deficits, flexibility asymmetries, or a poor aerobic base) should be addressed.

• Lack of appropriate neuromuscular skills for a particular sport or position within a sport can contribute to an increased risk of injury. For example, there have been many instances of players injured after a change in position. If an

TABLE 44–2 Contributors to Injury: Intrinsic Factors

Malalignment/Anatomical variation	Muscle imbalance
Leg-length discrepancy	Decreased neuromuscular skills
Poor flexibility	Kinetic chain dysfunction
Muscle weakness	

athlete returns to competition after an injury and before sport-specific skills are gained, the risk of reinjury is also increased.

• Gait, stance, and the biomechanics of a particular sport movement should be examined for possible dysfunction of the kinetic chain. It is important to look at static and dynamic alignment as well as at function.

• Principles of sports psychology are important in injury prevention because they can help a person to focus his or her concentration. They also provide techniques for relaxation and stress management. Neuromuscular engrams and motor learning can be facilitated through the use of such techniques as imagery.

GENERAL PRINCIPLES OF MUSCULOSKELETAL REHABILITATION (pp. 969–977)

Assessment of Injury (p. 969)

• Most musculoskeletal injuries can be divided into two broad categories: (1) acute; and (2) subacute, or chronic. Acute injuries are often related to macrotrauma and a breach of integrity of the musculoskeletal system (e.g., bone fracture or ligamentous disruption). The range of severity is broad. The evaluator must be capable of recognizing the signs and symptoms of a neurological problem. It is important to know the indications for and use of spinal stabilization and transport techniques to prevent spinal cord injury. Some sports injuries and conditions benefit from early surgical intervention to maximize function, to enable early return to activity, and to prevent reinjury. Early identification of these conditions is crucial.

• Subacute or chronic injury can usually be thought of as repetitive damage to or overuse of the musculoskeletal system. Treatment of these injuries typically involves the principle of relative rest, in which the injured body part is protected from further trauma and then gradually rehabilitated to normal function. During the treatment, aerobic fitness is maintained by using other, noninjured parts of the body. Essential to the successful treatment of chronic injury is an understanding of the factors that put the injured tissue at risk and contributed to musculoskeletal stress.

Treatment (p. 969)

• The basic principles of rehabilitation after musculoskeletal injury include pain reduction by means of various modalities (e.g., ice, superficial and deep heat, and interferential current) and through appropriately prescribed medications; restoration of range of motion and flexibility; therapeutic strengthening; and maximization of sport specific agility, coordination, and proprioception before return to sports. Another basic principle is the use of relative rest to maintain aerobic conditioning and cardiovascular fitness.

Relative Rest (p. 969)

• The principle of relative rest means that the injured part of the body is rested and protected from further trauma or injury while the remaining muscle mass is used to provide appropriate stress to the cardiovascular system for maintaining optimal aerobic conditioning.

• Relative rest of an injured part of the body is achieved with splinting, bracing, taping, or specialized adaptive equipment that permits performance of aerobic exercise. Exercise of the contralateral limb can be continued by use of devices such as resistance bicycles that provide for both upper extremity and lower extremity movement for bi- and tri-limb work. Wet-vest running (i.e., running in deep water with a buoyancy vest to keep the head above water) is also an effective method of non-weight-bearing training. Similar benefits with minimal weight-bearing stress can be achieved by walking in water that is only waist deep.

Pain Relief and Inflammation Control (pp. 969–970)

• The initial goals of the treatment of a sports injury should be to limit as much as possible the extent of the initial injury, to aid healing, and to provide for early institution of rehabilitation measures. The mainstay of early treatment (i.e., 24 to 48 hours after the injury) follows the principles of PRICE, as listed in Table 44–3.

• Ice is efficacious for decreasing pain and swelling by producing local vasoconstriction. Ice packs can safely be applied for 20 minutes of every hour. For focal injuries, ice massage is easy to apply and it can be particularly time effective. Compression around the injured area also helps to limit swelling and enhances comfort and earlier range of motion. If compression initially is instituted with elastic wraps (e.g., Ace bandages), rewrapping should be performed every 4 hours to ensure appropriate compression. Compression and cold can be applied simultaneously with an intermittent pneumatic compression pump. The injured extremity should be raised to a level higher than the heart to facilitate venous return.

• Superficial ice (acute and chronic) and heat (subacute and chronic) modalities are likely to continue to be the mainstays of pain relief because of the low risk of complications, the ease of application, and the therapeutic efficacy. Ultrasound treatment, short-wave diathermy, interferential current, and transcutaneous electric nerve stimulation can also be used safely with the usual precautions and with appropriate prescription (see Chapters 21 and 22).

Overuse Injury (pp. 970–971)

• Early treatment of an overuse injury is different from that of an acute injury. The activity that contributed to the microtrauma must be avoided or at least greatly modified. Patients must be educated about appropriate biomechanical and kinesiological principles of the sport-related movement. Ice can be an effective method of pain control, but heat might be especially beneficial. Heat causes blood vessel dilation, provides pain relief, and can help decrease muscle

TABLE 44–3 PRICE Principles

P:	protection
R:	relative rest
I:	ice
C:	compression
E:	elevation

tightness. General and muscle-specific relaxation and stretching techniques can help diminish muscle tightness and enhance whole body relaxation. Massage techniques, appropriately used, can be a beneficial adjunct, and cross-fiber or friction massage can be used to help mobilize contracted scar tissue. Myofascial interventions such as strain/counterstrain can also be useful tools in an attempt to reset chronically altered muscle proprioceptors.

• Biofeedback is effective for re-educating the patient regarding the kinesthetic sensation of achieving and maintaining relaxation in a particular muscle. This can be helpful in cases of painful muscle splinting that are refractory to other treatment. Biofeedback can also enhance activation of a specifically inhibited muscle group. Electrical stimulation can help athletes regain kinesthetic awareness of a particular muscle group, and biofeedback can verify voluntary activation and be effective in learning to enhance selective muscle use. This is particularly efficacious in entities such as patellofemoral pain, in which an afferent nociceptive stimulus causes neuromuscular inhibition or asynchronous firing of the oblique portion of the vastus medialis.

• Whether NSAIDs have any direct effect on the rehabilitative course is unclear. If used initially and for a short time, these drugs can assist in starting the rehabilitation process by decreasing the level of pain. However, in the early stages of macrotrauma with significant bleeding, NSAIDs may increase bleeding by decreasing platelet aggregation. Long-term use of NSAIDs is not advisable for either able-bodied or physically challenged athletes.

Range of Motion, Flexibility, and Muscle Balance (pp. 971–972)

• Restoring joint range of motion, establishing symmetric flexibility, and regaining strength often can be facilitated concurrently in the rehabilitation program. Depending on the injury, range of motion might need to be protected, passive, or limited in the initial stages, but should progress to full range as tolerated. To achieve full range of motion, gentle terminal stretching might be necessary, especially after treatment with superficial heat or ultrasound. During the healing process, specific stresses must be applied to the tissue by range of motion and stretching to promote linear alignment of collagen. Without stress, collagen fibers tend to be arranged in a chaotic fashion.

• Stretching in combination with a strengthening program that emphasizes muscle balance is essential in athletic rehabilitation. Dominance of an agonist over a weakened or nonfunctioning antagonist group can produce contracture and joint dysfunction. Dominance of one muscle group can result from strength imbalances (e.g., greater development of anterior shoulder muscle groups than of posterior shoulder muscle groups). This unbalanced system creates a potential for overuse and stress at the weak link (i.e., the point of imbalance). The entire kinetic chain mechanics must be assessed in relation to the particular task or movement of a sport.

Strength Training (p. 972)

• Strength training can begin in some fashion early in rehabilitation, with progression as tissue healing and joint range of motion permit. The more efficient use of muscle provided by strengthening exercises has a positive effect on early return of function and performance. The various types of strength training include isometric, isotonic, isokinetic, resistance band, variable resistance, plyometric, and kinetic chain exercise (see Chapter 19).

Isometric (p. 972)

• Isometric, or equal length, exercise is essentially a static muscular contraction. It entails exerting a maximal force against a relatively immovable object, with no appreciable change in muscle length. Isometric training is not a functional type of exercise. It does, however, protect the joint from undue stress, and it creates less inflammatory response in the joint than does isotonic exercise. Isometric exercise can prepare the muscle for functional kinetic chain strengthening at a later stage.

• The most important role of isometric contractions might be in body stabilization. Proper training of stabilization is essential to ensure that we can use muscles effectively in an isolated fashion and that we do not put other elements of the kinetic chain at risk because of an excessive or unbalanced load.

Isotonic (pp. 972–973)

• Isotonic, or equal tension, exercise ideally consists of constant muscle contraction with constantly applied tension. Isotonic exercise is dynamic and occurs when the muscle contraction itself is used to move a joint that ultimately moves a load through a range of motion. Isotonic strength depends on the contractile force and mechanics of movement about a joint. The muscle is not contracting at constant capacity or a specific percentage thereof throughout the entire range of motion. For this reason, the term *isotonic* technically is not accurate, because equal tension is not exerted throughout the joint range of motion. Isotonic exercise can further be divided into concentric and eccentric components. Concentric contractions require the loading of the muscle while it is shortening, whereas eccentric contractions load the muscle while it is lengthening.

Isokinetic (pp. 973–974)

• Isokinetic, or equal speed, exercise allows maximal force production through full range of motion (e.g., Cybex machines, Ronkonkoma, NY). Isokinetic exercise consists of exercising at a predetermined constant velocity of joint motion. This type of exercise provides objective information about peak muscle torque, power, and endurance at reproducible velocities.

• This type of exercise for strength training purposes is nonfunctional because only one joint and one muscle system are used at maximal contraction. Isokinetic exercise does not simulate the way we use our muscles either during a sport or in activities of daily living.

• Although objective data are obtained, athletes still must regain agility, coordination, and sport-specific skills before returning to competition. There is also no direct correlation between machine scores and athlete performance.

Resistance Band (p. 974)

• Resistance-band exercise usually involves the use of a progressive resistance band (e.g., Theraband) that provides gradually increasing resistance when stretched. The band can be used in multiple planes of motion. It can also be used to simulate functional and sport-specific activities. With this type of resistance, it must be remembered that the most resistance occurs at the extreme of joint range of motion. At low levels of resistance, this might not be a problem, but with higher loads and healing tissue, care must be taken to ensure optimal technique to prevent excessive shear or compressive force across a joint.

Variable Resistance (p. 974)

• Variable resistance training means that the resistance is altered through the use of cams or pulleys in an attempt to match the force-producing capability of the muscle throughout the full range of motion (e.g., Nautilus machines). This training is an isolated and nonfunctional exercise and does not stimulate associated proximal and distal components of the kinetic chain. Velocity and acceleration are variables in this type of exercise training, which is more useful for isolated strengthening than for sport-specific training.

Plyometric Exercise and Power Training (pp. 974–975)

• Plyometric exercises emphasize speed and power. They consist of concentric muscle contractions after a previous stretch of the same muscle groups. Plyometric exercises contain both eccentric and concentric components and load both the elastic and the contractile elements of a muscle. Examples of higher-level plyometrics include jumping rapidly onto and off different-sized boxes and jumping back and forth over a low object.

Kinetic Chain Exercise (pp. 975–977)

Closed and Open Kinetic Chain Exercises (pp. 975–976)
• Closed kinetic chain exercises involve predictable coordinated muscle contractions with motion at multiple joints and a limb whose segment meets fixed or constrained resistance (e.g., leg press or squat). In the upper extremities, a push-up can be considered a closed chain exercise. In general, closed chain exercises are more function-based and sport-specific for the lower extremities. For example, squats involve co-contraction of the quadriceps, hamstrings, and gastrocnemius-soleus muscle groups in a functional manner similar to that used in many sports and general daily living activities (e.g., getting up from a chair). Closed kinetic chain exercise should be the predominant type of exercise for the lower extremities in sports medicine and in rehabilitation of the lower extremities in general. However, there are still many appropriate indications for use of open kinetic chain exercise.
• Open kinetic chain exercises such as knee extensions tend to isolate a particular muscle group (in the case of knee extensions, the quadriceps) and involve motion distal to the axis of the joint. For the upper extremities, open kinetic chain exercises are essential before return to sports because these exercises are similar to the limb movements used in most sports (e.g., the throwing motion).

AGILITY, PROPRIOCEPTION, AND SPORT-SPECIFIC SKILLS (pp. 977–978)

• Athletes should work to regain optimal agility and coordination either after strength has been maximized or in tandem with strength training. In many injuries, a muscle, tendon, or ligament and a joint are "detuned," and the proprioceptive feedback that the muscle or joint capsule normally provides is disrupted. Examples of exercises that help regain this function include wobble board exercises, which help maximize balance and refine coordinating movements of lower extremity muscles, especially at the ankle. Knee proprioception can be better maximized with both standing and supine exercises involving a pediatric ball (Swiss ball) and knee-specific movements. If lower extremity ambulation has been hindered by the injury, therapy should focus on higher-order gait activities (including carioca or crossover walking) and balance activities specific to the athlete's sport.

• Evidence strongly supports specificity in training. Exercise gains are specific to the type and pattern of movement addressed by training, the velocity of training, and the range of motion and angle at which training occurs. Thorough knowledge of an athlete's sport and kinesiological demand is essential in designing an appropriate rehabilitation program for return to sports. The ultimate goal is for an athlete to be at maximal strength and agility to maximize performance and to prevent recurrence of injury.

YOUTH SPORTS MEDICINE CONSIDERATIONS
(pp. 978–979)

• Resistance training in young athletes must be used judiciously before closure of the growth plates occurs. These areas of growth are relatively weak in comparison with the surrounding ligamentous and fibrous supports, and if this "weak link" is injured, bony deformity and unequal growth can result. Proper technique prevents these problems by not overloading any bone or muscle and joint complex. In this regard, prepubescent weight lifters should be encouraged to emphasize lower weight and higher repetitions, with impeccable technique, instead of trying to see how much weight they can lift. During periods of rapid growth, strength training should be decreased and flexibility exercises should be emphasized.

• Children and adolescents are entering organized sports at earlier ages, resulting in increased musculoskeletal injuries and a change in distribution of injuries among young athletes. Skeletally immature athletes have growth centers that are susceptible to repetitive microtrauma or more acute injuries. Gross injuries include compression epiphysis and traction epiphysis (apophysis) injuries. Most commonly, comparison radiographs of the uninjured side are obtained to judge asymmetries. Avulsion injuries can occur when tensile forces through the muscle-tendon units or ligaments cause separation of the vulnerable cartilaginous zone between the apophysis and bone. The ischial apophysis and the anterior superior iliac spine (ASIS) apophysis are common areas where avulsions can occur; if there is significant displacement of the ischial avulsion, surgical fixation may be indicated. Pediatric articular surface injuries can also occur as an osteochrondritis of the knee or osteochrondritis of the talar dome.

• The preparticipation examination for school sports is an excellent opportunity for physicians to help affect injury prevention and to assess at-risk areas in young athletes. Musculoskeletal and cardiovascular concerns are two areas in which intervention and identification of problems can contribute to reducing morbidity and, possibly, mortality.

UNIQUE CONSIDERATIONS FOR PHYSICALLY CHALLENGED ATHLETES (pp. 979–980)

• It is estimated that 2 to 3 million athletes with physical and mental disabilities participate in organized athletic activities in the United States. The groups that make up the Committee on Sports for the Disabled, a standing committee of the United States Olympic Committee, are excellent resources with respect to sports for physically challenged persons and participation requirements. These groups include the American Athletic Association for the Deaf, the Dwarf Athletic Association of America, Disabled Sports USA (DS/USA), the National Wheelchair Athletic Association, the Special Olympics, the United States Association of Blind Athletes, and the United States Cerebral Palsy Athletic Association.

• Individuals who treat and advise physically challenged athletes should understand how the adaptive equipment required for the sport can affect injury risk. New aerodynamic body positions in wheelchair racing can increase the risk of pressure ulcers, and if the splashguards on high-performance wheelchairs are not adjusted properly, they can cause skin breakdown. With respect to downhill snow skiing, monoskiers can risk skin breakdown if seating positions create too much ischial shear. Amputees can require special residual limb protectors or warmers (or both) if tissue blood flow is compromised. Athletes with cerebral palsy, multiple sclerosis, or spasticity require special containment provided by straps to enable more isolated limb movement, especially during resistance training. Wheelchair road racers benefit greatly from the use of gloves and from wearing friction-reducing material on the biceps and triceps regions of the arms and on the chest wall region of the axilla.

• Another external factor is the environment, which can pose risk of thermal injury to physically challenged athletes. The main group of athletes who need to use extra caution during temperature extremes are those with spinal cord injuries, especially with lesions above the T8 level. In these persons autoregulation is impaired, and the body temperature tends to equalize with that of the ambient environmental temperature. Athletes with ischemia or vascular dysfunction and those who are insensate are also at risk in a cold environment, and frequent skin checks are necessary to ensure that skin damage is not occurring.

SPORTS PSYCHOLOGY (pp. 980–981)

• The sports counselor or sports psychologist has recently had a larger presence as a member of the treatment team. Sports medicine professionals should be aware that the response of an athlete to injury can differ from that of other patients, and early identification and treatment of concurrent psychological issues by appropriate professionals often facilitate rehabilitation and maintenance of health. Many studies suggest that severe depression, tension, and anger are common among seriously injured athletes. Many techniques have been advocated to provide psychological assistance and to facilitate rehabilitation, including visualization, relaxation, goal-setting, prioritization, and elimination of negative thoughts.

• Reinstilling self-confidence is another key aspect of the rehabilitation process. Even though the physiological damage might not be severe, athletes who perceive an injury as serious are likely to experience more intense depression and to have a slower recovery than those who do not perceive an injury as serious. Athletes should believe that they will be able to resume competitive sports, take command of their rehabilitation, and commit time and effort to the sometimes long and arduous rehabilitation process.

• Strategies for performance enhancement and stress management are ways in which sports psychology professionals can help to improve focus in competition and to maximize physical execution. Visualization and imagery also can be used in training to enhance neuromuscular engrams, to assist in rehabilitation, and to control pain.

• For optimal rehabilitation, athletes need the services of a multidisciplinary team that functions in an interdisciplinary manner. Each contributor plays an important role in helping an injured athlete to resume sports activities and to return to other activities of daily living.

45

Original Chapter by John A. Schuchmann, M.D.

Occupational Rehabilitation

- The cost of workplace injuries in 1996 was estimated to be $121 billion.
- Industrial injuries are costly because the industry loses productivity and sales and the worker loses wages. Health care costs, as well as costs for retraining and replacing workers, add to the loss.
- A team effort is often required to ensure the successful outcome of returning the injured worker to work.

COMMON MEDICAL PROBLEMS SEEN IN A REHABILITATIVE INDUSTRIAL PRACTICE (pp. 985–986)

Low Back Pain (pp. 985–986)

- Low back pain is second only to upper respiratory illnesses as the most common cause of time missed from work. Chronic low back pain has a major economic and personal impact because it is the leading cause of disability for individuals between the ages of 19 and 45 years.
- Low back pain is most prevalent in heavy industry. The low back injury rate has been found to be about 3 to 5 per 1000 employees per year in light industries, as compared to 200 per 1000 employees per year in heavy industries.
- Despite advances in automation, humans are still required by many industries to perform considerable manual material handling. Stresses on the spine vary depending on the lifting techniques utilized as well as on the load handled. Improper handling of work materials, overuse with muscular fatigue, and repetitive vibratory stresses can precipitate back injuries.
- Only 1% to 2% of patients with low back pain usually require surgical treatment. Overall, about 90% of patients with low back pain improve with minimal or no medical intervention. A small percentage of cases, however, become chronic, leading to long-term disability associated with increased medical expenses and compensation costs. Recurrence of low back pain is also quite common, with a recurrence rate of approximately 70%. (See Chapter 40 for additional information about low back pain.)

Cumulative Trauma Disorders (p. 986)

- Cumulative trauma disorders, also referred to as repetitive motion disorders, repetition strain injuries, or occupational overuse injuries, have recently gained more attention throughout industry and in the health care sector. In the United States, such disorders accounted for 40% to 50% of all workers' compensation claims. More recent statistics point to a slow and progressive decrease in the number of cases of cumulative trauma disorders reported as industries aggressively institute preventive ergonomic and early intervention programs.

• A variety of tissues can be affected by cumulative trauma disorders, including muscles, tendons, bursae, ligaments, peripheral nerves, bones, cartilage, and intervertebral disks. Many clinical problems fall under the category of cumulative trauma disorder, including muscle strains, tendinitis, bursitis, ligamentous injuries, compression neuropathies, fractures, cartilage damage, and disk disease.

• The common etiological feature of these disorders is that repetitive trauma occurs faster than the tissue's ability to heal itself. Cumulative trauma disorders usually develop slowly and gradually over many weeks, months, or years. A number of activities and related equipment have been implicated as etiological and aggravating factors for the development of cumulative trauma disorders; some of these are listed in Table 45–1.

• In the workplace, upper extremity cumulative trauma disorders far outnumber lower extremity disorders. Some of the more common disorders seen in clinical practice are listed in Table 45–2.

• Chronic muscle soreness in a worker might be an early warning sign of the development of a cumulative trauma disorder. The prolonged persistence of symptoms can indicate that tissues are not able to adapt to the stress. Continuing the activity could lead to tissue damage and the development of a cumulative trauma disorder.

PREVENTION (pp. 986–991)

Back Injury (pp. 986–990)

X-Ray Screening (p. 987)

• There is no definite correlation between an abnormality seen on a lumbar x-ray and the chance of an individual's sustaining an on-the-job back injury. With the advent of computed tomography (CT) and magnetic resonance imaging (MRI), it has been found that disk abnormalities, including disk bulges and herniations, occur in 30% to 50% or more of asymptomatic individuals. The use of pre-employment or preplacement spine radiographic studies is in disrepute, and some consider the practice a violation of the Americans With Disabilities Act.

Education: The Back School Approach (pp. 987–988)

• Most individuals learn how to lift by trial and error. Proper lifting, however, is something that must be taught. Today, many industries realize that an investment in a "back school" for employees can help decrease on-the-job back injuries. An effective back school program incorporates individual or small group instruction along with actual practice and skill development. Items actually lifted and manipulated at work are used for training, and the worker is coached and reinforced in proper lifting and handling techniques.

• The recommended lifting technique generally requires the worker to be positioned directly in front of and as close to the load as is feasible. The worker is taught to squat while keeping the shoulders back and the low back in a neutral

TABLE 45–1 Sampling of Etiological or Aggravating Factors and Activities in Cumulative Trauma Disorders

Activities

Forceful grasping
Highly repetitive work
Activities causing rapid or extreme joint movements
Overhead work
Maintaining static work positions for prolonged times

Occupations

Assembly line worker
Carpenter
Butcher
Typist/data entry worker
Cashier
Driver
Factory worker performing repetitive activity
Food preparer
Postal worker
Musician
Electrician
Professional athlete

Tools and Equipment

Repetitive assembly lines, on which worker performs at "machine pace"
Undampened pneumatic tools
Hammers
Screwdrivers
Pliers
Scissors
Knives
Keyboards
Musical instruments
Use of gloves

TABLE 45–2 Common Cumulative Trauma Disorders Related to Work Activities

Tendinitis and tenosynovitis at wrist and in forearm
Epicondylitis
Rotator cuff tendinitis and shoulder bursitis
Myofascial syndromes
Hand-arm vibration syndrome
Median nerve-carpal tunnel syndrome, nerve trauma in palm
Ulnar nerve compression in elbow, hand, or wrist
Thoracic outlet syndrome

position, with the lumbar lordosis maintained. Footing should be secure, and the lift should be performed in a slow and controlled fashion.

Evaluation and Enhancement of Strength, Flexibility, and Fitness (pp. 988–989)

• It has been hypothesized that a fit worker is less likely to be injured on the job. Many facilities perform screening with job-specific testing that measures the ability to safely perform specific job tasks. Some industries, especially those that require much physical work, are now realizing the importance of emphasizing physical fitness in their work force. The military has for many years realized the necessity of soldiers' maintaining physical fitness and combat readiness. Other professions, such as police and firefighters, have also emphasized fitness in their workers. Workforce fitness programs have resulted in lower injury rates and worker's compensation costs.

• Other interventions, such as flexibility programs, have been used to try to improve performance on the job and to decrease injuries. Some industries have established their own fully staffed fitness centers. Smaller industries typically find it more feasible and cost effective to encourage the use of existing community fitness facilities and programs.

Ergonomic Assessment and Intervention (pp. 989–990)

• Injuries often occur because a worker is mismatched with a job, such as when a physically deconditioned worker is placed in a job that is very strenuous and demanding.

• Jobs should be analyzed ergonomically to determine the amount and frequency of lifting required. Postures utilized by workers on the job should be noted. Other factors to be considered include the following: (1) What are the sizes and the shapes of the objects lifted? (2) Can the worker get a firm grasp on the object? (3) Is twisting required along with the lifting? (4) What speed of lifting is required to keep up with the expected productivity? (5) Does awkward placement of bins (or other equipment) require the worker to flex the spine into a position that creates a higher back injury risk?

• Proper lifting and materials-handling techniques are impossible to utilize in some circumstances. In these cases, an assessment should be performed to ascertain whether the load can be subdivided into lighter loads, whether a mechanical lifting device can be used, whether loads can be positioned to allow lifting without concomitant spine rotation, or whether help from another individual can produce a safer lift.

• Low back pain is also common in sedentary workers such as secretaries and drivers. Properly fitted and supportive seating is essential to minimize stress on the back. Chairs can be properly fitted and adjusted to meet the specific needs of the workers who will occupy them for 8 or more hours per day.

• Job descriptions that actually quantify the amount and frequency of lifting, pushing, pulling, climbing, stooping, and squatting are helpful when trying to make a successful fit between a prospective worker and a specific job.

Lumbar Support Orthoses (p. 990)

• Lumbar support orthoses are widely marketed to industry as aids to help decrease the incidence of low back injuries. There might be some value in using back supports to prevent initial back injuries, but their across-the-board use for all workers in manual industries has not yet been shown to decrease overall injuries, injury severity, or overall cost per injury.

Preplacement Screening: ADA Approach (p. 990)
- The Americans With Disabilities Act (ADA) (Public Law 101-336) became effective on July 26, 1992. Under this act, an employer can require an employee to undergo *job-specific* preplacement testing only after a job offer has been made to the prospective employee. This preplacement examination can test the ability to safely perform the *usual tasks* of the specific job. The goal of testing is to ensure that the employee is physically and emotionally capable of performing the job safely so that the worker or co-workers will not be endangered. If the employee is unable to successfully perform the testing because of some functional limitation, the employer is obliged to determine whether job accommodations could reasonably be implemented that would allow the successful performance of the required job tasks. Preplacement examinations cannot be performed randomly.

EVALUATION OF THE INJURED WORKER (pp. 991–994)

The Detailed History (pp. 991–992)

- It is very important for the examining physiatrist to obtain a complete history from the worker. A description of the overall job tasks and requirements is helpful, as is a detailed history of what happened at the time of the accident. Incurring an injury on the job is often an emotionally charged event for both the employee and employer. The attitude and response that the injured worker perceives at the time of injury are vitally important. The injured worker should be treated with kindness and compassion. When handled properly, the initial response can help develop a cooperative relationship between the worker and the employer. When handled poorly, the initial response can distance the employee from the employer and result in a chronic adversarial relationship. Part of history taking is to learn the worker's perception of how he or she has been treated.
- The physiatrist is often asked by the worker's compensation carrier to respond to a number of questions to help determine whether a work-related problem really did occur. The history should be sufficiently detailed to be able to answer these commonly asked questions:

1. Do the history and physical findings clearly support a work-related illness or injury?
2. Is there consistency between the history of the illness or injury and the clinical findings and diagnosis?
3. Was there sufficient job-related exposure to provide a clear cause-and-effect relationship between the work activities and the clinical presentation?
4. Are any other pre-existing problems or causative factors present that could have led to the development of this clinical problem?

- In more chronic worker's compensation cases, it is important to extend the history to include additional information (Table 45–3).
- The worker's perception of and satisfaction with his or her job can strongly influence the course of the initial injury as well as the ultimate recovery and return to work.

TABLE 45–3 Important Areas to Assess with Chronic Injuries

1. Ask the worker to describe the initial medical examination and treatment. What did the worker understand the diagnosis to be? What was the response to initial treatment? Did the worker attempt to return to work? If so, what happened?
2. If improvement did not occur, what other testing, treatments, and physicians have been involved? Has surgery been performed? If so, how many operations, and how effective were they in providing relief?
3. Has the worker been involved in rehabilitative efforts such as active physical therapy, work conditioning, or work hardening?
4. Does the worker have a job to return to? What is the worker's current relationship with the employer? Does the employer seem willing to accept the worker back on the job?
5. How is the worker currently spending a typical day? How much time does the worker spend in bed every day? In front of the television? Does the worker get out of the house regularly? Does the worker participate in hobbies and recreation?
6. Does the worker participate in any regular exercise? This includes specific exercises to correct the condition as well as general exercises to improve overall aerobic fitness. What is the worker's estimate of his or her own level of physical fitness?

- It is also important to assess the individual's current lifestyle and plans for the future. Some workers focus on keeping productive, taking the necessary steps to return to work and maintaining favorable relationships with their employers. Others, however, blame the employer for all their problems and take a passive or even a passive-aggressive role in returning to any meaningful productivity. Litigation that is pending is also important because it often slows down recovery and limits response to treatment.

Concurrent Medical or Psychological Illnesses (p. 992)

- The evaluation should include an assessment of the worker's overall health. Pre-existing health problems are occasionally present that could have contributed to the accident or injury or that can affect the recovery process.
- The patient should be evaluated for the abuse of drugs, alcohol, and tobacco. Accidents and injuries can occur from working under the influence of these substances. Prescription medication overuse should also be considered. Tobacco use should also be addressed because a number of studies have shown a correlation between tobacco use and back pain, disk degeneration, and slower healing.

Physical Examination (pp. 992–993)

- A meticulous physical examination is essential for optimal management of injured workers. A general assessment of the worker's health, as well as a thorough assessment of the musculoskeletal system, should be performed. How much pain behavior is present during this portion of the examination? Is the individual able to walk on toes and heels, to squat, and to forward flex and touch the toes?
- The amount of spine mobility and flexibility should be assessed, including forward flexion, extension, lateral bending, and rotation. Do any specific move-

ments aggravate the symptoms? Leg-length inequalities or spinal deformities should be noted. Palpation is helpful to evaluate for areas of local tenderness (e.g., trigger points or local areas of injury) or widespread tenderness.

• For shoulder girdle problems, the shoulder region should be observed from all sides. Is there any scapular winging with either forward flexion or abduction of the upper extremities, with or without resistance? Is pain produced at any point in the arc of motion? Are the shoulders symmetrical? Is any atrophy present? (For additional information, see Chapter 38.)

• Range of motion of the spine and joints in the affected area should be measured (see Chapter 1). Limitation of motion should be noted, as well as pain produced with movement.

• A systematic evaluation of spinal and extremity strength is useful to identify areas of weakness. Muscle atrophy, either focal or generalized, should be noted. True organic weakness results in a smooth "giving way" during muscle testing. Muscle giving way in a ratchety pattern often suggests a possible "functional" nonorganic component to the symptoms. The examiner should also avoid mistakenly ascribing true weakness to a patient who actually has only pain inhibition of function.

• Measurement of handgrip strength can be helpful during the evaluation. A handheld dynamometer can be utilized to assess grip strength in various positions. These measurements can be useful in assessing the amount of weakness present, as well as in following progress during treatment.

• Sensation should also be addressed to assess whether deficits follow specific peripheral nerve, nerve root, or neuropathic patterns. Sensory deficits that incorporate the whole leg or the whole arm often suggest the presence of a nonphysiological, functional sensory deficit. Vibratory sensation measured with a tuning fork can be used to help determine the validity of otherwise questionable sensory findings. A right-to-left difference in vibratory sensation in a midline bone strongly suggests a functional, nonorganic deficit.

• Muscle stretch reflexes need to be evaluated to assess integrity of the reflex arc. Straight-leg-raising can be measured in both the sitting and supine positions to assess for consistency. Special tests (e.g., Tinel's sign, Phalen's wrist flexion test, Spurling's test, Finkelstein's test, Patrick's test, and tests for thoracic outlet syndrome) can provide helpful information at times.

• The examiner needs to continually analyze the findings as the examination progresses. Injured workers can occasionally demonstrate "symptom magnification," with inconsistencies in findings being common in these examinations. Tests such as those described by Waddell and co-workers (Table 45–4) can help to differentiate nonorganic from organically mediated physical findings. Pain behavior and inconsistencies are important to recognize to ensure that the patient is not medically overevaluated or subjected to potentially risky tests or treatments. Identifying functional issues also allows for the institution of appropriate psychologically and behaviorally based intervention.

• When indicated, appropriate testing (e.g., radiography, CT, MRI, radionuclide scintigraphy, laboratory testing, or electrodiagnostic testing) can also be useful in confirming the diagnosis.

Diagnosis (pp. 993–994)

• After the evaluation is completed, a working diagnosis should be formulated and explained to the worker in clear and understandable terms. It is important

TABLE 45–4 Nonorganic Findings in the Low Back Evaluation: Waddell's Signs

1. Tenderness of the skin to light pinch over a widespread area
2. Deep tenderness in a nonanatomical distribution
3. Reproduction of back pain with axial loading by pressing down on the worker's head while he or she is standing
4. Reproduction of back pain when the shoulders and pelvis are rotated together as a unit
5. Inconsistencies between straight-leg testing done when the worker is otherwise distracted versus that done when worker is aware of the test being performed
6. "Giving way" weakness in a widespread and nonanatomical pattern
7. Inconsistent and nonanatomical sensory deficits
8. Overreaction (e.g., disproportionate verbalization, facial expression, muscle tension and tremor, collapsing, or sweating) during the examination

Adapted from Waddell G, McCulloch JA, Kummel E, et al: Nonorganic physical signs in low-back pain. Spine 1980; 5:117–125.

to try to avoid emotionally charged words such as "ruptured" disk or "degenerative" arthritis, which might frighten the worker. The overall prognosis and treatment plan should be clearly provided to the worker. Approximate time frames for treatment and return to work should be provided to the patient. These time frames are also helpful for the employer and insurer.

TREATMENT (pp. 994–999)

Early Intervention (p. 994)

• Early treatment of the injured worker can occur in a number of settings, including (1) an on-site clinic at work, (2) the company physician's office, (3) an occupational medicine clinic, (4) a minor emergency clinic, or (5) the emergency department of a hospital. The goals of early intervention are accurate diagnosis and appropriate treatment to facilitate the worker's return to work as soon as possible, in a manner consistent with safety and quality medical care. The worker needs to be seen promptly after the injury and followed up closely with scheduled, short-interval follow-up appointments.
• Pain is the major symptom of most acute injuries and is usually reflective of some degree of tissue damage. The early treatment of an acute injury focuses on control of pain and tissue damage. Rest should be limited in duration for most musculoskeletal injuries, with 2 days of bed rest often being preferable to 7 days of bed rest for back injuries. Specific rest of an injured part for other injuries can be provided with appropriate casts, splints, or braces. Prolonged bed rest or immobilization can perpetuate disability by causing deconditioning. Appropriate analgesics can help control pain, as can physical modalities such as heat, cold, transcutaneous electrical nerve stimulation (TENS), massage, and gentle stretching.
• During the early intervention phase, it is often possible and desirable to provide treatment while the worker is still performing light duty or a modified job. As long as the medical outcome will not be compromised and no further tissue damage will occur, it is usually best to facilitate early return to work.
• As acute symptoms subside, use of medications and physical modalities should decrease. The worker should be instructed in specific flexibility and

strengthening exercises that will improve conditioning and lessen the chance of recurrence. Identification of pre-existing deconditioning gives the physician an opportunity to recondition the worker more extensively and to return a worker to the workplace in better condition than before the injury. Before returning the worker to work it is helpful to fully understand the worker's job. Ergonomic modifications or worker training in proper biomechanics could be helpful in avoiding recurrence of the injury.

• Any identified problems with drug or alcohol overuse should be addressed, with referral to appropriate treatment programs. Cessation of smoking should also be encouraged.

Chronic Treatment (pp. 994–995)

• About 10% of workers still have pain complaints and physical disability that prevent return to work after the completion of acute and subacute care programs. These workers might be candidates for more highly structured treatment programs such as work conditioning, work hardening, vocational rehabilitation, or chronic pain therapy.

• It is well recognized that the longer workers are off the job, the more difficult it becomes to return them to work. There is about a 50% chance of return to work when a worker is off for 6 months, with the rate dropping to 25% when the worker is off for 1 year.

• When cases enter the chronic stage, the initial injury is often resolved but the worker is left with chronic weakness, deconditioning, loss of flexibility, and poor endurance. In addition to being physically deconditioned, the worker is often psychologically deconditioned. It is common for such workers to let other positive health habits deteriorate, and they often increase the use of tobacco, alcohol, and medications. Prolonged absence from work can also be reinforced by a number of factors (see Table 45–7 in the Textbook). Such an individual can be a candidate for a more intense program of work conditioning, work hardening, chronic pain treatment, or structured vocational rehabilitation.

Work Conditioning: A Sports Medicine Approach (p. 995)

• Work conditioning is a program of progressive structured reconditioning to prepare the worker for return to the job. These programs are often provided by physical and occupational therapists in coordination with the primary physician, the employer, and the injured worker.

• The treatment focus for work conditioning shifts away from passive modalities and medications and toward more active rehabilitation and physical restoration. This stage of care is often best presented to the worker as a "sports medicine" model of treatment. The worker might be considered an "occupational athlete" because many workers perform vigorous repetitive physical activities on a daily basis. The goal is to return them to their game, which is their job.

• Understanding the physical requirements of a specific job should start with an analysis of the job description.

• Communicating with the worker's employer during job site visits can help overcome obstacles to returning the employee to the job. Employers can also be educated about the value of light duty programs and about how they can help return workers to productivity earlier while helping to minimize injury-related compensation costs.

• Work conditioning often begins on a three- to five-times-a-week schedule. When the worker is sufficiently conditioned to meet the requirements of light duty, the worker is usually returned to a light duty job. Arrangements are made to continue the conditioning until the worker has maximally improved or has met the requirements for returning to the original job.
• Work conditioning treatment usually lasts 3 to 6 weeks. The outcome is that the vast majority of workers return to their jobs at the completion of the program.

Work Hardening (pp. 995–998)
• Workers who have been off work for long periods, such as 3 months or more, might need a more comprehensive program than can be provided by work conditioning. Work hardening programs focus on physical conditioning but also address psychological issues and vocational issues that often interfere with return to the job.
• Success is facilitated if the work hardening team has a complete understanding of the worker's job and work conditions. Work hardening usually incorporates general as well as job-related physical conditioning.
• Work hardening programs also incorporate job specific work simulation activities. If the worker is required to lift boxes, for example, the program includes lifting boxes.
• The program also tries to simulate actual work conditions. The worker is often required to clock in and out daily. To minimize the worker's perception of illness and sickness, the program is often housed in a warehouse or other work-like setting rather than in a medical clinic or hospital. The treatment duration is usually 5 half-days or whole days per week for up to 6 weeks.
• The goal is to progressively increase exercise tolerance and work activities until they simulate a typical day on the job. Education is an important part of the program.
• Psychological counseling can help the worker overcome fears and anxieties about returning to work.
• The cost of these programs is relatively high, but well-organized programs often have favorable success rates. Individuals selected for these programs should be motivated to return to work, should have jobs available, and should be free of overwhelming psychological or secondary gain issues that can undermine successful return to work.

Vocational Rehabilitation (p. 998)
• If at all possible, it is preferable to assist the injured worker to return to work with the previous employer in some capacity. Close communication between the worker, the employer, and the rehabilitation team can help achieve this goal and help to avoid misunderstandings that can inhibit the employer's willingness to accept the worker back on the job. The case manager can play a vital role in promoting this communication and facilitating return to the job.
• For a number of potential reasons, some workers do not have the option of returning to their former jobs. With no available job to return to, a more comprehensive vocational rehabilitation approach can be needed.
• The process starts with a thorough assessment of the individual. It is helpful to survey areas of interest and aptitude to help ascertain the appropriate vocational possibilities. Psychological testing can be helpful to determine aptitude for specific vocations, as well as for various levels of vocational or educational training. Physical evaluation is helpful to determine the individual's work capac-

ity and whether this level can be enhanced with physical reconditioning programs such as work conditioning.

• The vocational counselor should be familiar with job options in the geographic area and able to assist the individual with formulating a reasonable plan for vocational rehabilitation. In many instances the resources of the state vocational rehabilitation services can be called on to assist with the vocational rehabilitation effort.

• A successful vocational rehabilitation plan usually requires consideration of specific job adaptations or modifications to enable success in the work force. The prospective worker with a physical impairment (e.g., a previous brain or spinal cord injury) might need ergonomic adaptations.

• Job coaching and education are important for the individual who has been out of the work force for some time.

• Vocational rehabilitation is a team effort. The vocational counselor usually coordinates the effort, with assistance provided as needed by physicians, psychologists, neuropsychologists, physical and occupational therapists, ergonomists, industrial engineers, employers, and educational facilities.

Chronic Pain Treatment (pp. 998–999)

• Some individuals with work-related injuries develop chronic pain. The chronic pain might be related to the original injury, or it can be an aftermath of the treatment efforts. In otherwise psychologically well-adjusted individuals, chronic pain can sometimes be treated effectively using the traditional medical model of care. Treatment modalities such as physical therapy, epidural blocks, TENS, or even implanted stimulators or pumps can be helpful and allow increased activity and productivity.

• Many other individuals have chronic pain but no specific medical condition that can be readily treated or cured. This is often referred to as chronic pain syndrome. Psychological factors can be present. There is often overuse of medications, alcohol and tobacco, and medical and surgical services. Secondary gain issues are often prominent. Such patients often live sedentary and even dependent lifestyles. Return to work is not the initial priority with these individuals. Initial pain management efforts typically revolve around medication detoxification, psychological counseling, and progressive reconditioning. Such patients might be best treated in an interdisciplinary program that focuses on the behavioral treatment of chronic pain syndrome. If the chronic pain program proves successful, patients might later qualify for one of the programs more strictly focused on preparation for returning to the work force, such as work conditioning or vocational rehabilitation. (For more information on chronic pain and chronic pain syndrome, see Chapter 42.)

WRAPPING IT UP: RETURN-TO-WORK ISSUES
(pp. 999–1000)

Case Management (p. 999)

• Case management can play a useful role in assisting the worker and the treatment team during the treatment process. Case managers can be employed by the rehabilitation facility, the employer, the insurance carrier, or even by the physician. They can communicate with the health care team, the insurer, the employer, and the worker to ensure that smooth, unhindered communications take place.

Functional Capacity Evaluation (pp. 999–1000)

• After completion of medical treatment, the physician is often required to make a determination about whether the worker is capable of returning to the full-duty job or if specific limitations in performance remain. This is often a difficult determination because most medical offices are not set up in a way that enables testing of the worker's abilities. A more rigorous approach is to assess the worker with a functional capacity evaluation.

• Functional capacity evaluations are typically performed by physical or occupational therapists. The therapist methodically tests the worker with actual or simulated job tasks to determine the worker's capabilities for performing the required job tasks. Routine performance measures, specific to the worker's job and including physical skills, strength, flexibility, and endurance should be assessed. The worker's effort is often determined using the Borg Rating of Perceived Exertion Scale (see Table 45–9 in the Textbook).

• A comprehensive report is prepared for the referring physician and is extremely useful when communicating with the employer about job abilities and limitations. The work capacity evaluation helps ensure that the worker-job fit is appropriate and reduces the risk of reinjury.

Impairment Evaluation (p. 1000)

• After treatment is completed, and the patient's progress has plateaued and is not expected to change further, it is concluded that the maximum medical improvement has been achieved. In accordance with worker's compensation program rules in many states, an impairment evaluation must be performed when the worker reaches this plateau. (See Chapter 6 for more information on impairment rating.)

Litigation Resolution (p. 1000)

• After completion of treatment, it is important to document any residual impairment. Specific limitation of motion, sensory deficit, or muscle weakness is important to note in case the worker becomes involved in litigation about the injuries. Thorough documentation of the initial encounter and any pre-existing injuries and disorders is important, as is documentation of diagnostic procedures and their results, working diagnoses, treatments rendered, response to treatment, and patient compliance and participation in the treatment program.

OPPORTUNITIES FOR THE FUTURE (p. 1000)

• Physical medicine and rehabilitation has for many years been active in the development of various programs for injury prevention. In the future, physical medicine and rehabilitation should expect to play a major role in enhancing worker fitness, preventing injuries, enhancing job safety, and restoring workers to full function in an expedient and cost-effective manner.

Internet Resource Guide (pp. 1002–1004)

• When dealing with injured workers, it is essential to practice in accordance with the appropriate worker's compensation rules and regulations for the jurisdiction. Please refer to Appendix A in the Textbook for a list of Internet sites helpful in obtaining basic information and updates for various worker's compensation programs.

Accreditation Issues (p. 1005)

• The Rehabilitation Accreditation Commission (CARF) helps ensure the quality of various occupational rehabilitation programs by surveying and accrediting programs that meet appropriate standards. CARF recognizes and accredits several different types of work-specific occupational rehabilitation programs. Appropriate standards exist for each type of program accredited, with these standards developed by experts in the respective fields with feedback provided from facilities that use these standards (see Appendix B in the Textbook).

46

Original Chapter by James C. Agre, M.D., Ph.D.,
and Dennis J. Matthews, M.D.

Rehabilitation Concepts in Motor Neuron Diseases

CLASSIFICATION OF MOTOR NEURON DISEASES
(pp. 1006–1014)

Motor Neuron Diseases Can Be Classified in a Number of Ways (Table 46–1)

Upper Motor Neuron Disorders (pp. 1006–1007)

Primary Lateral Sclerosis (p. 1006)
• Primary lateral sclerosis (PLS) is a rare, nonfamilial, slowly progressive corticobulbar and corticospinal tract disease of unknown cause.

Clinical Features. The onset of spasticity is usually noted in the lower limbs, although occasionally spasticity is first noted in the upper limbs or the bulbar musculature. As the disorder progresses, spasticity affects all limbs and the bulbar musculature. Urinary incontinence can occur, but usually not until late in the course. Survival is usually two to three decades or longer. Spastic dysphagia can be life threatening in these patients. On physical examination, no signs of lower motor neuron dysfunction, such as muscle atrophy or fasciculations, are found. Electromyographic (EMG) examination of these patients does not reveal signs of denervation. These findings differentiate this disorder from classic amyotrophic lateral sclerosis (ALS).

Pathology. The pathogenesis of PLS is unknown. Pathological findings include a reduced number or absence of Betz's cells in the primary motor cortex or precentral gyri accompanied by degeneration of the corticospinal pathways while other structures are spared.
• (Please see the Textbook for a discussion of rare diseases in this category such as tropical spastic paraparesis, Lathyrism, and epidemic spastic paraparesis.)

Familial (Hereditary) Spastic Paraplegia (p. 1007)
• Familial spastic paraplegia can be transmitted as an autosomal dominant trait, occasionally as an autosomal recessive trait, and very rarely as an X-linked

TABLE 46–1 The Motor Neuron Diseases

Upper motor neuron disorders
    Primary lateral sclerosis
    Tropical spastic paraparesis
    Lathyrism
    Epidemic spastic paraparesis
    Familial (hereditary) spastic paraplegia
Combined upper and lower motor neuron disorders
    Amyotrophic lateral sclerosis (ALS)
    Familial ALS
    Western Pacific ALS–parkinsonism dementia complex
    Groote Eylandt motor neuron disease
    Postencephalitic (encephalitis lethargica) ALS
    Juvenile inclusion body ALS
Lower motor neuron disorders
    Spinal (bulbospinal muscular) atrophies
    Monoclonal gammopathy and motor neuron disease
    Cancer and motor neuron disease
    Poliomyelitis and post-polio syndrome

Modified from Hudson AJ: The motor neuron diseases and related disorders. In Joynt RJ (ed): Clinical Neurology, vol 4. Philadelphia, JB Lippincott, 1991, pp. 1–35.

recessive disease. The disorder can appear at any age, but usually occurs in childhood or early adult life. The onset of familial spastic paraplegia is accompanied by complaints of stiffness and unsteadiness of the legs and gradually results in a spastic paraplegia. Muscular atrophy has been reported, but often in only one or two members of a large pedigree. The pathogenesis of familial spastic paraplegia is unknown. The pathological findings in this disease, reflecting its genetic transmission, are diverse.

Combined Upper and Lower Motor Neuron Disorders
(pp. 1007–1008)

Classic Amyotrophic Lateral Sclerosis (pp. 1007–1008)
• Amyotrophic lateral sclerosis is the benchmark of the motor neuron disorders. ALS encompasses two conditions, progressive bulbar palsy and progressive muscular atrophy, which differ only in their site of onset. Progressive bulbar palsy initially affects the bulbar motor neurons, whereas progressive muscular atrophy initially affects the spinal motor neurons. These two diseases tend to overlap the longer the patient survives.

Epidemiology. The classic form of ALS is so named because it is the most prevalent motor neuron disease and because it was one of the first to be recognized. The incidence of this disease is approximately 1.6 to 2.4 cases per 100,000 population, but incidence varies with age. The average age at the time of diagnosis is 62 years. The average survival from time of diagnosis is approximately 2.5 years but varies with age. Survival is reported to be somewhat shorter for patients over the age of 50 years. The male-female ratio varies from 1.2:1 to 1.6:1.

Clinical Features. Most patients with classic ALS complain of weakness. During the initial examination lower motor neuron signs of atrophy, weakness, and fasciculations are commonly noted. In addition to these signs, muscle stretch reflexes can be depressed in regions where there is primarily lower motor neuron involvement or where atrophy is so advanced that upper motor neuron signs cannot be demonstrated. Otherwise, it is common to find brisk muscle stretch reflexes in areas of muscle atrophy. Occasionally, patients present with only mild spasticity, suggesting a purely upper motor neuron disorder. The most notable of these cases are patients who present initially with spastic dysarthria or facies (or both) with no detectable lower motor neuron signs. Muscle cramping is a common complaint.
• The most striking feature of ALS is the focal, often asymmetrical onset of weakness, which then spreads from the initial site to adjacent areas of the body. Spasticity can be very disabling and can produce significant deformities of the hand. Spasticity and clonus can make ambulation difficult. Except for constipation caused by poor nutritional intake or inactivity, the bowel and bladder are spared in this disease. Sensation is generally spared, although subtle symptoms and signs of sensory involvement, complaints of paresthesias, and decreased vibratory sense occur in up to 25% of patients. A small percentage of individuals with classic ALS also show signs of dementia (about 3.5%) or parkinsonism (about 1.5%).

Pathology. The pathogenesis of classic ALS is unknown. Characteristic pathological findings in classic ALS include degeneration or complete loss of motor neurons in the brainstem and spinal cord areas corresponding to the muscle atrophy and degeneration of the large pyramidal neurons in the primary motor cortex and of the pyramidal tracts. Onuf's nucleus (controlling the striated muscles of the pelvic floor and the bowel and bladder sphincters) is preserved.

Familial Amyotrophic Lateral Sclerosis (p. 1008)
• Familial ALS is clinically identical to classic ALS except for a somewhat younger average age at onset (46 years). A bimodal distribution of survival is found in these patients, with peaks of survival at 2 years and 12 years from the time of initial diagnosis. The pattern of inheritance is reported to be autosomal dominant, but a recessively inherited form of chronic juvenile ALS has been reported.

Clinical Features. The clinical features of familial ALS are similar to those of classic ALS.

Lower Motor Neuron Disorders (pp. 1008–1014)

Infantile Forms of Spinal or Bulbospinal Muscular Atrophies (1009–1010)
ACUTE INFANTILE SPINAL MUSCULAR ATROPHY (WERDNIG-HOFFMAN DISEASE, TYPE I SPINAL MUSCULAR ATROPHY, ACUTE PROXIMAL HEREDITARY MOTOR NEUROPATHY)
• The chronic form of acute infantile spinal muscular atrophy was first described by Werdnig and by Hoffmann. It is an autosomal recessive disorder with an estimated incidence ranging from 1 in 15,000 to 1 in 25,000 live births. The disease is already manifest in one-third of affected children by the time of birth through decreased fetal movements or congenital arthrogryposis. The diagnosis is usually made by the age of 3 months and certainly by the age of 6 months. The average survival from time of diagnosis is 6 to 9 months; survival does not exceed 3 years.

Clinical Features. The clinical picture is dominated by severe hypotonia and weakness. There are resultant delays in motor milestones. At birth the baby is usually floppy (hypotonic), with generalized weakness and absence of reflexes. Feeding difficulty and poor breathing are soon apparent. Progressive muscle weakness, atrophy of the trunk and limbs, hypotonia, and feeding difficulties are the primary clinical features. The infants characteristically lie motionless with the lower limbs abducted in the frog-leg position. The face often lacks expression with an open mouth because of facial muscle weakness. Intercostal muscle paralysis is evident, and fasciculations are present. Fasciculations of the tongue are almost pathognomonic for the disease. The cause of death is typically respiratory failure.

CHRONIC INFANTILE SPINAL MUSCULAR ATROPHY (CHRONIC WERDNIG-HOFFMAN DISEASE, TYPE II SPINAL MUSCULAR ATROPHY, CHRONIC PROXIMAL HEREDITARY MOTOR NEUROPATHY)

• The chronic form of Werdnig-Hoffmann disease is much more slowly progressive than the acute form of this disease. This actually was the form of the disease initially described by Werdnig and Hoffmann. Clinical signs indicative of this disease are usually present by age 3 years but occasionally are seen by 3 months of age. This disease has variable progression, and the median age at death is about 12 years, with some individuals surviving into the third decade. This disease is autosomal recessive, and the gene for chronic spinal muscular atrophy has been found on chromosome 5q.

Clinical Features. Weakness and atrophy are predominantly proximal, with the lower limbs being more involved initially than the upper limbs. Muscle stretch reflexes are reduced or absent. Sensation is normal. Owing to the gradually progressive weakness, scoliosis, thoracic deformities, and equinus deformities of the feet usually develop as the disease progresses.

Juvenile and Adult Forms of Spinal or Bulbospinal Muscular Atrophies (pp. 1009–1010)
JUVENILE AND ADULT PROXIMAL SPINAL MUSCULAR ATROPHY (KUGELBERG-WELANDER DISEASE, TYPE III SPINAL MUSCULAR ATROPHY, RECESSIVE PROXIMAL HEREDITARY MOTOR NEUROPATHY; TYPE IV SPINAL MUSCULAR ATROPHY, [JUVENILE] DOMINANT PROXIMAL HEREDITARY MOTOR NEUROPATHY; TYPE V SPINAL MUSCULAR ATROPHY, [ADULT] DOMINANT PROXIMAL HEREDITARY MOTOR NEUROPATHY)

• The juvenile and adult forms of spinal muscular atrophy (Kugelberg-Welander disease) are characterized by slowly progressive weakness and atrophy of the proximal limb and girdle musculature. The disorder is genetically transmitted, usually as an autosomal recessive trait (type III proximal hereditary motor neuropathy), but an autosomal dominant inheritance (type IV juvenile and type V adult proximal hereditary motor neuropathy) is also possible. The clinical onset of the disease can occur anytime between childhood and the seventh decade of life, but is usually between the ages of 2 and 17 years. The duration is also quite variable, ranging from 2 to more than 40 years. It occurs predominantly in males.

Clinical Features. Both the juvenile and the adult forms of proximal spinal muscular atrophy begin with symmetrical atrophy and weakness of the pelvic girdle and proximal lower limbs. This is followed by involvement of the shoulder girdles and upper arms. The leg and forearm musculature are affected later. Fasciculations are noted in about half of the cases. Dysphagia and dysarthria can occur late in the disease and are usually mild.

• (See the Textbook for a description of Bulbar Disease of Childhood [Fazio-Londe Disease and Brown-Vialetto-van Laere Syndrome].)

DISTAL SPINAL MSUCULAR ATROPHY (DISTAL HEREDITARY MOTOR NEUROPATHY)

• Distal spinal muscular atrophy is also known as the spinal form of Charcot-Marie-Tooth disease and distal hereditary motor neuropathy. There are a number of different forms of distal spinal muscular atrophy with different inheritance patterns: (1) autosomal recessive juvenile mild (onset between 2 and 10 years of age) and juvenile severe (onset between 4 months and 20 years), and (2) autosomal dominant in the juvenile (onset between 2 and 20 years) and in the adult (onset between 20 and 40 years). The majority of the cases reported, however, are sporadic, and a recessive inheritance is suspected. Life expectancy is normal except in some severe juvenile cases. Weakness and atrophy are most often initially noted distally in the legs, especially in the anterior tibial and peroneal muscles. Usually the upper limbs are spared, but they are rarely predominantly affected.

Adult Forms of Bulbar and Bulbospinal Muscular Atrophies (p. 1010)
SCAPULOPERONEAL (FACISOSCAPULAOPERONEAL) MUSCULAR ATROPHY

• Scapuloperoneal muscular atrophy has an autosomal dominant inheritance. The atrophy typically begins between 30 and 50 years of age. The disease progresses slowly. Patients do not become incapacitated until at least 10 to 20 years after its onset and have a normal life expectancy. Weakness and atrophy begin in the muscles of the legs, but the intrinsic muscles of the feet are spared. Several years later the shoulder girdle musculature, and later the musculature of the thigh, pelvic girdle, upper arm, neck, and face, are affected. At this stage the disorder appears similar to facioscapuloperoneal muscular dystrophy, but in the latter disorder the shoulder girdle musculature is affected first.

• (See the Textbook for descriptions of Chronic Bulbospinal Muscular Atrophy of Late Onset, Monomelic [Segmental] Spinal Muscular Atrophy and Monoclonal Gammopathy and Motor Neuron Disease.)

Cancer and Motor Neuron Disease (p. 1011)

• The possibility of motor neuron disease occurring as an effect of cancer is difficult to evaluate at the present time because of the many other explanations for neurological signs (e.g., metastases to the nervous system and meninges, and cachexia). However, there are reports of individuals who had apparent motor neuron disease related to cancer or lymphoma.

Acute Poliomyelitis (pp. 1011–1013)

• Acute poliomyelitis occurs as a result of a generalized viral infection that has an affinity for motor neurons. The virus is a single-stranded RNA enterovirus (picornavirus) and is comprised of three antigenically distinguishable viruses. Acute poliomyelitis is presently very rare in the United States. It can occur in severely immunocompromised persons or in persons who did not receive the vaccination and were exposed to someone who recently received the oral vaccine, which has the live, attenuated virus. Although there is a worldwide attempt to eradicate poliomyelitis, acute poliomyelitis still occurs in developing nations with poor health care delivery systems.

• The virus usually enters the body via the oral route. It replicates in the lymphoid tissues of the pharynx and the intestine. It then spreads to the regional lymphoid tissues and a viremia can follow, leading to a nonspecific illness. Viremia is the most accepted mechanism for direct nervous system exposure to the virus.

- The poliovirus is an extremely infectious agent, but only a fraction of those infected have symptoms. The disease progresses to central nervous system involvement and paresis or paralysis in 1% to 2% of cases, whereas in 90% to 95% of cases the infection is inapparent, and in 4% to 8% of cases only a nonspecific illness is noted.

Clinical Features. The incubation period is from 1 to 2 weeks. The onset is usually accompanied by malaise, muscle aches, and low-grade fever lasting from 1 to 3 days. These findings may cease and no further symptoms might occur. Alternatively, a symptom-free period can be followed by recurrence of systemic symptoms.

- The potentially paralytic illness is characterized by fever, generalized headache, and neck and back stiffness. The illness may regress or may proceed, with paralysis appearing by the second to fifth day after onset. Muscle soreness and a sensation of tightness are present, as well as shooting pains and hyperesthesia. Sensory loss is rare. The weakness appears and evolves over hours to a few days. Autonomic dysfunction with cardiac arrhythmia, hypertension, hyperhidrosis, urinary retention, and constipation can occur. Changes in mental status ranging from anxiety to stupor can occur and are attributed to reticular formation or hypothalamic involvement.

- Death is usually the result of bulbar or respiratory involvement. Survivors commonly gradually recover muscle function in muscles not completely paralyzed, and some ultimately have minimal or no residua. Improvements begin in the first weeks, but can continue for several years after the acute illness. The mechanisms of recovery include both resolution of dysfunction of partially damaged motor neurons and reinnervation of denervated muscle fibers by surviving motor units.

Post-Polio Syndrome *(pp. 1013–1014)*

- A number of reports document the complaints registered by poliomyelitis survivors several decades after the acute poliomyelitis illness. In particular, new musculoskeletal and neuromuscular symptoms are reported by these patients. Table 46–2 lists the most common new health and activities of daily living (ADL) problems of post-polio patients, whether they were seen in a post-polio clinic or had responded to a national survey. The most prevalent new health-related complaints were fatigue, muscle or joint pain, and weakness. The most prevalent new ADL complaints were difficulties with walking and stair climbing. Fatigue was described by many (43% in one survey) as though they were "hitting the wall." Of this group, 68% reported that this phenomenon occurred on a daily basis. Most commonly, this "wall" was experienced in the mid- to late afternoon. Fortunately, for almost all patients it could be ameliorated or aborted by increasing rest time, napping, or reducing the overall level of activity during the day.

- The typical post-polio patient seen in a post-polio clinic had the acute poliomyelitis illness in childhood (average age at onset between 5 and 10 years), had gradually improving function over a period of 5 to 8 years after the acute illness, remained clinically stable for 25 to 30 years, and then noted the onset of new health or ADL problems about 5 to 8 years before seeking evaluation in a post-polio clinic.

TABLE 46–2 New Health Problems and New Problems in Activities of Daily Living in Post-Polio Patients in Three Studies

Symptom	Percent of Patients Affected, by Study		
	Halstead and Rossi (n = 539)	Halstead and Rossi (n = 132)	Agre et al (n = 79)
New health problems			
Fatigue	87	89	86
Muscle pain	80	71	86
Joint pain	79	71	77
Weakness			
Previously affected muscles	87	69	80
Previously unaffected muscles	77	50	53
Cold intolerance	—	29	56
Atrophy	—	28	39
New ADL problems			
Walking	85	64	—
Stair climbing	83	61	67
Dressing	62	17	16

- It can be estimated that approximately one-fourth to one-third of persons who had acute poliomyelitis in the past may be experiencing post-polio syndrome at the present time. This proportion may well increase as these persons age.
- Post-polio syndrome is essentially a diagnosis by exclusion. A good definition of post-polio syndrome has been given by Halstead and Rossi and is based on five criteria:

1. A confirmed history of paralytic polio
2. Partial to fairly complete neurologic and functional recovery
3. A period of neurologic and functional stability of at least 15 years' duration
4. The onset of two or more of the following health problems since achieving a period of stability: unaccustomed fatigue, muscle and/or joint pain, new weakness in muscles previously affected and/or unaffected, functional loss, cold intolerance, new atrophy
5. No other medical diagnosis to explain these health problems

- Among the suggested causes are premature aging of motor neurons damaged by the poliovirus, premature aging of the motor neurons because of the increased metabolic demand, loss of muscle fibers within the surviving motor units, death of motor neurons because of the normal aging process, disuse weakness, overuse weakness, or weight gain.

EVALUATION OF THE PATIENT WITH MOTOR NEURON DISEASE HISTORY (pp. 1914–1915)

- The major complaints of the patients and their parents (in the case of children) should be noted. The pattern of weakness can be helpful in determining the spe-

cific motor neuron disease. It can be difficult at times to distinguish between some of the motor neuron disorders, muscular dystrophies, and neuropathies. A careful history is essential in this regard. In general, patients with neuropathic disorders usually give a history of distal rather than proximal weakness, often accompanied by sensory abnormalities (which are rare in the motor neuron disorders).
• A careful family history is also important because a number of the motor neuron disorders are genetically transmitted.

Physical Examination (p. 1014)

• Visual inspection usually reveals areas of significant muscular atrophy, muscular hypertrophy (which can be found in some of the muscular dystrophies), and fasciculations. Visual inspection for atrophy assists in determining whether the disease involvement is greater in the proximal or the distal limb musculature. Palpation of the limbs can reveal the muscle tenderness that is found in inflammatory myopathies, but which is rare in motor neuron diseases other than acute poliomyelitis.
• The sensory examination detects any sensory loss, which is very rare in motor neuron diseases but common in the neuropathic disorders. Muscle stretch reflexes can be increased in the upper motor neuron disorders or in the combined upper and lower motor neuron disorders, but such reflexes are reduced or absent in the lower motor neuron disorders. In the combined upper and lower motor neuron disorders, the muscle stretch reflexes can be increased or decreased, depending on the associated muscular weakness and atrophy. Manual muscle testing demonstrates the level of residual muscle function and shows the distribution of the weakness (e.g., proximal, distal, or asymmetrical).
• Assessment of range of motion allows for the detection of contractures. It is important to determine passive range of motion in these patients because muscle weakness can significantly limit active range of motion.
• A thorough functional assessment of the patient allows the rehabilitation team to determine the patient's present level of functional abilities including the patient's abilities to be mobile in bed, to transfer, to ambulate with or without assistive devices or be mobile in a wheelchair, and to perform all of the usual ADL.

Laboratory Evaluation (pp. 1014–1015)
• In the evaluation of a patient suspected of having a motor neuron disease, it is important to carefully investigate laboratory studies to rule out other potentially remediable causes of motor neuron disorder.

Electrodiagnosis. Nerve conduction studies can confirm the presence or absence of peripheral neuropathy (see Chapters 10 and 11). The EMG can be of assistance in differentiating neuropathy and myopathy and in determining loss of motor neurons, the amount of denervation, and the presence of collateral reinnervation.

Muscle Biopsy. The muscle biopsy can help determine whether the disorder is an inflammatory myopathy because most inflammatory myopathies are amenable to treatment.

Other Laboratory Evaluations. Depending on the clinical presentation of the patient, the clinical laboratory investigation can consist of a number of other evaluations, including serum protein electrophoresis (looking for evidence of monoclonal gammopathy or paraproteinemia); antiacetylcholine receptor antibodies (looking for evidence of myasthenia gravis); various antiviral antibody titers (e.g., HLTV-1 and human immunodeficiency virus [HIV]); serum hexosaminidase A determination (looking for GM_2 gangliosidosis) of anti-GM_1 and GD_{1a} ganglioside IgM antibodies (which may be elevated in ALS and motor neuropathy); endocrine tests (looking for such disorders as diabetes mellitus or thyrotoxicosis); metabolic and blood cell studies (looking for amyotrophic choreic acanthocytosis); serum creatine kinase (usually normal in the motor neuron diseases but often elevated in myopathies); and heavy metal analysis of the urine (looking for such problems as lead and mercury intoxication). The spinal fluid evaluation of patients with motor neuron diseases is usually normal; any elevation of the spinal fluid protein above 80 mg/dL should lead the clinician to suspect another disorder.

GENERAL PRINCIPLES OF REHABILITATION MANAGEMENT (pp. 1015–1018)

• Specific treatment for the pathophysiological processes in motor neuron disease is lacking at the present time. The best approach currently is prevention, with vaccination for the viral diseases, education to prevent toxic exposures, and genetic counseling for the hereditary diseases. Overall management should be divided into prospective care and expectant care. The rehabilitation team should assist the patient in maximizing function and independence for as long as is possible.

• *Prospective care* takes in all the usual measures provided to all people regardless of their health status and includes such things as vaccinations and health screening tests. *Expectant care* includes anticipation of complications that might be expected during the course of the patient's motor neuron disease. Aggressive measures can be taken to prevent or minimize these complications and maximize the patient's function and independence for as long as possible. The expected complications include pain, muscle tightness, deformities of bones and joints, weakness, impaired ventilation, and impaired functional abilities.

Muscle Tightness (pp. 1015–1016)

• Soft tissue contractures can occur at all stages in motor neuron disease. Muscles that span two joints are often the first to become tight, usually with the joint in the flexed position (contracture) (Table 46–3). Depending on the condition of the patient, physical treatment includes passive, active-assistive, and active stretching, usually after the application of superficial heat. A heated pool allows heat treatment and exercise to be combined. Appropriate positioning also facilitates prolonged stretching and prevents deformity. Bracing to aid in the prevention of contractures requires careful assessment of kinesiological factors. When preventing or correcting shortening of a muscle that spans two joints, the physiatrist must be certain that the muscles are stretched at both joints that they cross.

Spasticity (p. 1016)

• In some motor neuron diseases, considerable spasticity can occur. This is treated in the same way as spasticity in other conditions (see Chapter 29).

TABLE 46–3 Movements Commonly Affected by Tightness in Soft Tissue

Neck flexion	Hip flexion
Shoulder adduction	Hip internal rotation
Elbow flexion	Knee flexion
Forearm pronation	Ankle plantar flexion
Finger adduction	Foot inversion
Finger extension	

From Pease WS, Johnson EW: Rehabilitation management of diseases of the motor unit. In Kottke FJ, Lehmann JF (eds): Krusen's Handbook of Physical Medicine and Rehabilitation, ed 4. Philadelphia, WB Saunders, 1990, pp. 754–764.

Deformity (p. 1016)

• Malalignment of body segments leads to contracture and deformity. Care must be taken in the prospective treatment of patients with motor neuron disease to prevent or minimize the development of contracture or deformity. Appropriate stretching, bracing, and positioning can help prevent contractures.

Management of Scoliosis (pp. 1016–1017)

• Abnormal spinal curvature occurs with increasing age and with advancing disability in neuromuscular disorders. Most children with motor neuron disease develop a collapsing, paralytic type of scoliosis. Initially, paraspinal muscular weakness is usually symmetrical, and if the child is still ambulatory, the development of scoliosis is uncommon. Once the weakness progresses sufficiently to prevent ambulation, scoliosis develops rapidly. Preventing scoliosis or limiting its effect is important because scoliosis alters sitting tolerance, leading to skin and pressure relief problems and a decrease in pulmonary function.
• The initial approach to scoliosis management is to prescribe the most appropriate wheelchair for the individual child (see Chapter 18).
• An erect spine is necessary for proper sitting balance. A variety of orthoses have been developed to manage the scoliosis curve from 20 to 40 degrees. Children tolerate the sitting support orthosis or the thoracolumbar orthosis well until the curve reaches more than 40 degrees. Once the curve is more than 40 degrees, a relatively rapid progression continues that generally cannot be managed orthotically.
• Surgical stabilization of the spine has been advocated in a number of neuromuscular disorders. Various segmental instrumental and fusion techniques have been described. Postoperative complications are primarily pulmonary. It is believed that the earlier the spine is stabilized, the less likely are the secondary pulmonary and cardiac complications (see Chapters 32 and 33).

Weakness (p. 1017)

• Proximal weakness interferes with such activities as gait, transfers, and gross motor movements, whereas distal weakness interferes with more fine motor skills. Treatment of weakness, however, might include strengthening exercises, if prescribed judiciously and followed carefully. Although not well studied, it appears that vigorous, fatiguing progressive resistive exercise is contraindicated in most motor neuron diseases because such exercise can lead to overuse weakness. Low-intensity, nonfatiguing exercise, however, may be quite beneficial for maintenance or improvement in muscle strength (as has recently been demonstrated in several studies on post-polio patients) and for enhancing cardiorespiratory fitness.

Respiratory Assistance (p. 1017)

• When motor weakness or deformity sufficiently limits the patient's ability to ventilate, mechanical ventilatory assistive devices are needed to allow for adequate ventilation. Early signs and symptoms of hypoxia include difficulty with sleeping, night-time dyspnea, nightmares, and somnolence during the day. As these signs appear, appropriately prescribed ventilatory aids (e.g., a cuirass or plastic wrap) enhance gas exchange in the recumbent position. In the later stages of motor neuron disease, oral positive pressure ventilation, a pneumobelt, or cuirass ventilators can be used throughout the day, energized by the wheelchair battery. Although noninvasive management is preferable, tracheostomy may be useful if the patient has severe scoliosis or if control of aspiration is a major problem (see Chapter 33).

Functional Ability (pp. 1017–1018)

• The primary goals of the rehabilitation team in treating a patient with motor neuron disease are to assist the patient in the maintenance of function, independence, and quality of life for as long as possible. Appropriate preventive and therapeutic interventions for the treatment of pain, soft tissue tightness, deformity, scoliosis management, motor weakness, and respiratory dysfunction can minimize complications and maximize the patient's ability to function. Functional training for locomotion, dressing, eating, and other ADL are practiced as developmentally appropriate (see Chapter 25).

TREATMENT OF THE PATIENT WITH MOTOR NEURON DISEASE (pp. 1018–1020)

Treatment of Post-Polio Syndrome (pp. 1018–1019)

• Fatigue is a very common complaint of post-polio patients. Many patients describe this phenomenon as "hitting the wall." The origin of this complaint is unknown but may be central in nature in at least some patients. Regardless of the cause, however, it has been reported that most post-polio patients have found that fatigue could be significantly reduced by increasing rest time, napping, or reducing the overall level of activity during the day. Table 46–4 lists some of the more common interventions and recommendations made for post-polio patients as a result of their clinical evaluation. The use of new or modified aids (e.g., corsets, lumbar rolls, neck pillows, wheelchair positioners, canes, and crutches); energy conservation techniques; or the use of new orthotic devices enhances the patient's ability to function and minimizes overuse problems. Psy-

TABLE 46–4 Common Clinical Interventions and Recommendations Made to Post-Polio Patients

Intervention	Percentage of Patients Given the Recommendation, by Study	
	Halstead and Rossi (n = 132)	Agre et al (n = 79)
New or modified aids*	87	—
Energy conservation techniques	64	73
Change in exercise program	64	—
Change in orthoses	52	34
Weight loss	52	27
New/modified wheelchair	26	—
Gentle exercise program		
Aerobic exercise	—	23
Stretching exercises	—	46
Strengthening exercises	—	43

*Durable products used to improve posture, diminish pain, and enhance comfort. These include corsets, lumbar rolls, neck pillows, wheelchair positioners, canes, and crutches.

chological counseling or participation in a post-polio support group to learn new coping skills is also recommended for many patients.

• Up to 78% of patients seen in follow-up after a treatment program report improvement in their symptoms. Improvements include decreased muscle and joint pain, decreased level of fatigue, improved gait pattern (with the use of an orthosis or cane), and improved coping abilities. Patients who do not report improvement are typically less compliant with the recommendations made.

• Early reports of exercise in post-polio patients yielded conflicting results. Some studies showed that muscle-strengthening exercises were beneficial, whereas other reports indicated that vigorous exercise or activity was detrimental. It appears that a key difference between these studies was the intensity of the exercise program. It appears most probable that the exercise regimens in the studies reporting deleterious effects were too vigorous for the patients and subsequently led to overuse problems. Current studies have shown that judicious exercise can improve muscle strength, cardiorespiratory fitness, and the efficiency of ambulation. These benefits occur when the patient's exercise program avoids excessive fatigue, muscle pain, and joint pain.

• It is important to protect the weakened muscles and affected joints of post-polio patients from overuse during exercise. At the same time, the patient needs to exercise those body areas that can tolerate exercise so that function is not reduced as a result of disuse. At present, it appears that muscles with antigravity or greater strength on manual muscle testing can tolerate strengthening exercises. Swimming and aquatic exercise may be one of the best types of exercise in these persons because the buoyancy of the water reduces the effect of gravity on the patient's joints and limbs, protecting them from overuse.

Treatment of Amyotrophic Lateral Sclerosis (pp. 1019–1020)

• The progression of ALS is quite variable. It may be rapidly progressive or slowly progressive, with some patients surviving up to 15 to 20 years after the initial diagnosis is made. Most patients with ALS go through three phases.

• In the first phase, the patient is independent. This phase can be separated into three distinct stages. In the first stage, the patient is ambulatory, independent in ADL, and has mild weakness or clumsiness. Treatment at this time includes encouraging the patient to perform range-of-motion exercises and strengthening exercises of the unaffected musculature to compensate for the weakened muscles. Strenuous exercise, however, is discouraged because it might lead to increased fatigue and disability. Psychological support is very important at all stages. In the second stage the patient is still ambulatory but has moderate selective weakness and slightly decreased independence in the performance of ADL (e.g., difficulty with climbing stairs, raising arms overhead, or buttoning clothing). Treatment at this stage includes substituting Velcro closures for buttons, encouraging the use of ankle-foot orthoses, prescribing wrist-and-thumb splints, and encouraging selective strengthening for unaffected muscles and stretching exercises to avoid contractures. Patients are advised to avoid overuse and fatigue. In the third stage, the patient is still ambulatory but becomes easily fatigued with long-distance ambulation. There is severe selective weakness in the ankles, wrists, and hands, with a moderate decrease in independence in ADL. Treatment in this stage is designed to keep the patient independent for as long as possible. Deep breathing exercises should be added in this stage and the patient should receive an appropriate wheelchair or motorized scooter for longer-distance mobility.

• In the second phase, the patient is partially independent. This phase can be divided into stages 4 and 5 of the overall course of ALS. In the fourth stage, the patient is no longer ambulatory and is confined to a wheelchair. The patient has severe weakness in the lower limbs, with or without spasticity. The patient has moderate upper limb weakness but is able to perform many ADL independently or with partial assistance. The patient may have shoulder pain caused by weakness about the shoulder girdle musculature and may have edema of the hand. Treatment at this time includes supporting the shoulder and using heat and massage for shoulder pain. Antiedema preventive measures should be utilized. Passive range-of-motion exercises and stretching should be performed to prevent contracture. The patient should be encouraged to perform isometric exercises of the few remaining uninvolved muscles. In the fifth stage, the patient's strength continues to decline. The patient has severe lower limb weakness and moderate to severe upper limb weakness. The patient progressively needs more and more assistance with all ADL. The patient needs assistance in transferring into and out of the wheelchair. Pressure ulceration may also occur as a result of immobility and pressure. Treatment at this stage includes continuing with range-of-motion and stretching exercises to avoid contracture formation. The patient's family should be encouraged to learn proper transfer and positioning principles. Modifications of the home environment are needed to aid the patient's mobility and independence. Use of a water mattress may be helpful in preventing pressure ulcer formation.

• In the third phase, the patient is totally dependent. The patient is essentially bedridden and is completely dependent in all ADL. Treatment includes continuance of range-of-motion and stretching exercises to prevent the formation of contractures. For dysphagia, a soft diet might be helpful; otherwise the patient may need tube feeding. For accumulation of saliva, the use of suction, medications, or surgery to decrease salivary flow may be helpful. For dysarthria, the use of palatal lifts or electronic speech amplification may be helpful. For breathing difficulty, the airway needs to be carefully monitored and cleared as needed. Tracheostomy or respirator use may be required. During this phase, the physical ability of the family to care for the patient at home needs to be considered.

SUMMARY (p. 1020)

• The overall aim in the treatment of a patient with a motor neuron disease is to prolong functional abilities, independence, and quality of life for as long as possible.

47

Original Chapter by Lois Buschbacher, M.D.

Rehabilitation of Patients with Peripheral Neuropathies

- Peripheral neuropathies can be localized or generalized, proximal or distal. They can be due to a variety of causes including compression, toxic exposure, metabolic derangements, neoplasm, infection, inflammation, amyloidosis, autoimmune phenomena, or hereditary causes. Peripheral neuropathies can involve the axon, the myelin sheath, or both.

NERVE ANATOMY AND PHYSIOLOGY (pp. 1024–1028)

- Each peripheral nerve is surrounded by an outer connective tissue sheath, called the epineurium, which protects the nerve from compression. Inside the epineurium the nerve fibers are arranged in bundles, or fascicles, which are surrounded by a perineurium. The perineurium is the primary strengthening connective tissue of the nerve and also acts as a diffusion barrier. Nerve fibers can intermingle and cross from one fascicle to another along the course of the nerve. Each individual nerve fiber is surrounded by a membrane called the endoneurium.
- Axons are the long cellular processes of both motor and sensory nerves. To increase the speed of nerve conduction, all axons are surrounded by an insulating layer of myelin (see Chapter 10). Some axons share myelin with other axons and are poorly insulated. These axons are commonly called "unmyelinated fibers" and are reserved for functions that do not require rapid transmission through the body. Other axons are surrounded by individual sheaths of the Schwann cells. These axons are more effectively insulated and transmit impulses much more rapidly. These axons, which carry information that must be rapidly disseminated, are commonly called "myelinated fibers."
- The fibers that must transmit impulses rapidly are, in general, larger in diameter, because larger fibers have less electrical resistance. There is a wide array of fibers of varying diameters and degrees of myelination. Larger fibers tend to be myelinated. Table 47–1 is a common classification scheme for all nerve fibers. Table 47–3 in the Textbook is an alternative classification system for sensory fibers only. Both classification schemes are in widespread use.

TABLE 47-1 Nerve Fiber Types in Mammalian Nerve

Fiber Type	Function	Fiber Diameter (μm)	Conduction Velocity (m/sec)	Spike Duration (ms)	Absolute Refractory Period (ms)
A					
α	Proprioception; somatic motor	12–20	70–120	0.4–0.5	0.4–1.4
β	Touch, pressure	5–12	30–70		
γ	Motor to muscle spindles	3–6	15–30		
δ	Pain, temperature, touch	2–5	12–30		
B	Preganglionic autonomic	<3	3–15	1.2	1.2
C					
Dorsal root	Pain, reflex responses	0.4–1.2	0.5–2.5	2	2
Sympathetic	Postganglionic sympathetics	0.3–1.3	0.7–2.3	2	2

From Ganong WF: Review of Medical Physiology, ed 13. East Norwalk, CT, Appleton & Lange, 1987.

TYPES OF NEUROPATHY (p. 1028)

• Peripheral neuropathies are divided into two major categories, demyelination and axonopathy, depending on whether they primarily affect the axon or the myelin sheath. The interruption of the myelin sheath causes a slowing in nerve conduction. This slowing can be localized, as in a focal neuropathy like carpal tunnel syndrome; or generalized, as in Guillain-Barré syndrome (GBS). GBS and Dejerine-Sottas syndrome are examples of diseases that predominantly cause demyelination.

• *Axonopathy* can be caused by toxic or metabolic derangements, trauma, compression, traction, or transection. If the damage is severe enough to block nerve conduction, nerve conduction studies show a decrease in amplitude of the resulting motor unit action potential (MUAP) (see Chapter 10).

CLASSIFICATION SYSTEMS (pp. 1028–1030)

• Localized nerve injuries can be classified by degree of severity. There are two main classification schemes: the Seddon system and the Sunderland system (Table 47–2). The Sunderland system is an expansion on Seddon's divisions.

Seddon's Classification (pp. 1028–1029)

• Seddon proposed categorizing localized nerve injury into three divisions: (1) neurapraxia, (2) axonotmesis, and (3) neurotmesis.

ETIOLOGY OF NEUROPATHY (pp. 1030–1035)

• There is a wide array of neuropathic disorders, which are usually categorized by etiology. These etiologies include hereditary (Table 47–3), toxic (Table 47–4), those associated with diseases and inflammatory processes (Table 47–5), idiopathic (Table 47–6), entrapment (Table 47–7), nutritional (Table 47–8), and those secondary to infectious processes (Table 47–9).

• The most common causes of diffuse peripheral neuropathy seen in the developed world are diabetes and alcoholism. Worldwide, however, the primary cause is leprosy. In up to one-third of cases a specific cause for peripheral neuropathy cannot be identified.

• A diagnostic algorithm is presented in Figure 47–1.

TABLE 47-2   The Seddon and Sunderland Classification Systems

Seddon	Sunderland	Description
Neurapraxia	First-degree injury	Focal conduction block; axons remain intact
Axonotmesis	Second-degree injury	Axonal damage and Wallerian degeneration; intact supporting structures
Neurotmesis	Third-degree injury	Interruption of axon and endoneurium
	Fourth-degree injury	Interruption of perineurium and endoneurium
	Fifth-degree injury	All supporting structures and axon damaged

TABLE 47–3   Hereditary Peripheral Neuropathies

Charcot-Marie-Tooth disease (hereditary motorsensory
   neuropathy [HMSN] types I and II)
Dejerine-Sottas disease (HMSN type III)
Refsum's disease (HMSN type IV)
Neuropathies associated with
   Spinocerebellar degeneration (HMSN type V)
   Optic atrophy (HMSN type VI)
   Retinitis pigmentosa (HMSN type VII)
Friedreich's ataxia
Pressure-sensitive hereditary neuropathy
Acute intermittent porphyria
Familial amyloid neuropathy
Fabry's disease
Hereditary sensory neuropathy
Giant axonal neuropathies
Lipoprotein neuropathies
Roussy-Lévy syndrome
Riley-Day syndrome
Pelizaeus-Merzbacher disease
Metachromatic leukodystrophy
Krabbe's leukodystrophy
Tangier disease

TABLE 47–4   Toxic Peripheral Neuropathies

Drugs	*Heavy Metals*
Amiodarone	Antimony
Chloramphenicol	Arsenic
Corticosteroids	Gold
Dapsone	Lead
Diphenylhydantoin	Mercury
Disulfiram	Thallium
Halogenated hydroxyquinolones	*Organic Compounds*
Heroin	Acrylamide
Hydralazine	Carbon disulfide
Isoniazid	Dichlorophenoxyacetic acid
Lysergide (LSD)	Ethyl alcohol
Misonidazole	Ethylene oxide
Nitrofurantoin	Methyl butyl ketone
Pyridoxine	Triorthocresyl phosphate
Sodium cyanate	
Tetanus toxoid	
Thalidomide	

TABLE 47–5   Diseases Associated with Peripheral Neuropathy

Alcoholism
Amyloidosis
Benign monoclonal gammopathy (IgG, IgA, IgM)
Chronic liver disease
Chronic obstructive pulmonary disease
Cryoglobulinemia
Diabetes mellitus
    Distal symmetrical neuropathy
    Autonomic neuropathy
    Proximal asymmetrical painful motor neuropathy
    Cranial mononeuropathies
Giant cell arteritis
Gout
Hypothyroidism
Necrotizing angiopathy
Neuropathies in malignant diseases
    Lymphomas—focal and systemic
    Multiple myeloma
    Bronchogenic carcinoma
    Tumors of the ovary, testes, penis, stomach, or oral cavity
    Meningeal carcinomatosis
    Oat cell carcinoma
    Osteosclerotic myeloma
    Vasculitis/connective tissue disease

Evaluation of the Patient with Peripheral Neuropathy
(pp. 1031–1035)

History (p. 1031)
• The physician must take a careful history to assess the patient with peripheral neuropathy. An in-depth family and social history is useful, particularly if there have been familial occurrences or toxic exposures.

Physical Examination (pp. 1031–1032)
SENSORY EXAMINATION
• All sensory modalities should be tested, including pinprick, light touch, proprioception, vibration, graphesthesia, and temperature. If sensory deficits are detected, the extent and pattern of the loss should be determined.

TABLE 47–6   Idiopathic Neuropathies

Brachial neuritis (Parsonage-Turner syndrome)
Chronic inflammatory polyradiculopathy
Chronic relapsing polyneuropathy
Fisher syndrome
Acute inflammatory demyelinating polyradiculoneuropathy (Guillain-Barré syndrome)
Steroid-responsive polyneuropathy
Multifocal motor neuropathy

TABLE 47–7   Common Peripheral Nerve Injury and Entrapment Syndromes

Nerve	Entrapment
Radial nerve	At the radial groove of the humerus (Saturday night palsy)
	Posterior interosseous nerve syndrome
Ulnar nerve	At the olecranon groove
	Tardy ulnar palsy
	Cubital tunnel syndrome
	Injury at the wrist (can be at the canal of Guyon)
Median nerve	At the supracondylar ligament of Struthers (at elbow)
	Pronator teres syndrome
	Carpal tunnel syndrome
	Anterior interosseous syndrome
Sciatic nerve	Injection palsy—injury to lateral division
	Injury to medial division
Femoral nerve	Above or below the inguinal ligament
Peroneal nerve	At head of fibula
Tibial nerve	Tarsal tunnel syndrome

MOTOR EXAMINATION
• Muscle strength should be graded by the make-and-break system and with functional tests of multiple muscles and muscle groups (see Chapter 1).

Reflex Testing (p. 1032)
• In peripheral neuropathy the muscle stretch reflexes are usually depressed, especially distally. Superficial skin reflexes can be elicited by stroking the skin rather than striking a tendon. Abnormal superficial reflexes are usually signs of upper motor neuron disorders and are typically not present in peripheral neuropathy. Their presence can help differentiate a central from a peripheral condition.

TABLE 47–8   Nutritional Neuropathies

Beriberi or pellagra—thiamine (vitamin B_1) deficiency
Riboflavin (vitamin B_2) deficiency
Pyridoxine (vitamin B_6) deficiency
Pernicious anemia (vitamin B_{12} deficiency)
Protein or calorie deficiency in children

TABLE 47–9   Infectious Causes of Peripheral Neuropathy

Cytomegalovirus in human immunodeficiency virus (HIV) infection
Diphtheria
Herpes zoster
Leprosy
Rabies

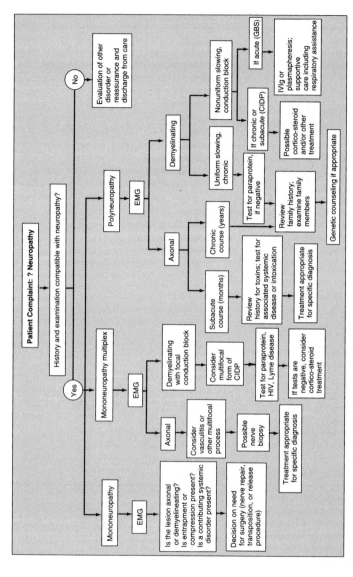

FIGURE 47–1. Diagnostic algorithm for neuropathies.

Electrodiagnostic Examination in Peripheral Neuropathy (pp. 1032–1035)

NERVE CONDUCTION STUDIES

• Nerve conduction studies (NCS) are the most helpful part of the electrodiagnostic examination for peripheral nerve disorders (Table 47–10). The conduction velocity is typically moderately to severely slowed, and the distal latency is prolonged, whereas the amplitude of the evoked responses is relatively preserved in severe demyelination. If conduction block is present in some fibers of a nerve, the amplitude of the evoked response is reduced because of temporal dispersion (see Chapters 10, 11, and 12).

• In diseases where axonal degeneration predominates, the conduction velocity generally remains normal or only slightly decreased. If the larger (faster) nerve fibers are predominantly involved, there can be more significant slowing. More typical of axonopathy, however, is a reduction in amplitude of the evoked responses. This is caused by the fact that as some of the fibers die, they no longer contribute to the amplitude of these responses. This is especially true when recording directly from nerves. When recording from the muscles, the remaining axons can continue to innervate a constant number of muscle fibers (through reinnervation) and the evoked muscle response can be maintained well into the disease process. Temporal dispersion is usually minimal until well into the disease process.

• Many peripheral neuropathies involve a component of both axonal degeneration and demyelination, and the resultant findings on nerve conduction studies suggest a mixed picture: there is slowed conduction and temporal dispersion, as well as decreased amplitude of the recorded responses (see Chapters 10, 11, and 12).

ELECTROMYOGRAPHY

• This part of the examination is useful in determining the extent of muscle denervation and in localizing nerve lesions. It can also aid in determining the time course of the neuropathy because it helps in analyzing the process of reinnervation. It is less useful in evaluating purely demyelinating lesions because the muscle fibers retain their innervation in these disorders (see Chapter 11).

• In mild peripheral neuropathy the EMG findings are generally minimal. In mildly affected muscles the changes include increased polyphasicity of the MUAPs. In more severe neuropathies there is muscle membrane instability. As reinnervation progresses, polyphasic motor units of prolonged duration and high amplitude are seen. Demyelination typically causes little abnormal muscle membrane irritability, and fibrillation potentials and positive sharp waves are only occasionally seen (see Chapters 10, 11, and 12).

COMMON COMPLICATIONS OF PERIPHERAL NEUROPATHY (pp. 1035–1036)

• Muscle weakness, sensory loss, and autonomic problems occur commonly in patients with peripheral neuropathies. Muscle weakness can lead to joint contractures and muscle shortening. Sensory loss can result in more frequent and severe injuries to insensate areas. Autonomic problems can affect many functions including heart rate, blood pressure, and sweating; and can cause gastroparesis, neurogenic bladder, and impotence. Patients with peripheral neuropathy often complain of pain.

TABLE 47–10 Typical Electrodiagnostic Findings in the General Categories of Neuropathy*

Type	Motor Nerve Conduction Velocities	Amplitude of CMAP	Amplitude of Sensory Action Potential	EMG Findings
Hereditary	↓	NL/↓	↓	Usually denervation potentials
Toxic	NL/↓	NL/↓	NL/↓	Usually denervation potentials
Associated with disease	↓	↓	↓	Usually denervation potentials
Idiopathic	↓	↓	↓	Variable
Entrapment	↓	NL/↓	NL/↓	Variable; usually NL
Infectious	NL/slight ↓	Slight ↓	↓	Denervation potentials
Nutritional	↓	Slight ↓	↓	Denervation potentials

*Exceptions are common.
Abbreviations: CMAP, compound motor action potential; EMG, electromyography; NL, within normal limits.

Muscle Weakness (p. 1035)

• Joint contractures and muscle shortening are associated with muscle weakness. They can be prevented with daily range-of-motion (ROM) and muscle-stretching exercises. Depending on the degree of weakness, this exercise can be passive, active-assistive, or active. When in bed or at rest, proper positioning is essential, as is splinting (if needed).

Sensory Loss (p. 1035)

• When protective sensation is compromised, patients should carefully examine the anesthetic or dysesthetic areas daily. Because they are the most distal body part, the feet are most commonly affected by loss of sensation in neuropathy. Repetitive joint trauma can lead to the development of neuroarthropathic (Charcot's) joints. In either case, the prescription of extra-depth or custom-molded shoes might be indicated. A shoe insert helps to prevent foot trauma and ulcers.

Autonomic Dysfunction (p. 1035)

• Autonomic problems are seen in a variety of peripheral neuropathies, but are perhaps most commonly associated with diabetes mellitus and Guillain-Barré syndrome. Cardiovascular symptoms can include orthostatic intolerance or cardiac arrhythmias. Genitourinary symptoms include a flaccid bladder and male impotence. Gastrointestinal symptoms can include vomiting, dysphagia, diarrhea, and constipation. Sweating abnormalities are seen with autonomic involvement as well.

Pain (pp. 1035–1036)

• Pain is a common problem in peripheral neuropathy, and it can be difficult to treat. Analgesics are often ineffective. The first line of treatment for neuropathic pain includes tricyclic antidepressants. The side effects of these drugs include orthostatic hypotension and worsening of urinary retention. The second line of treatment can include carbamazepine or gabapentin. Topical capsaicin can also be beneficial in some patients and transcutaneous electrical nerve stimulation (TENS) can be added as well. Often a multiple drug regimen is needed to control pain; care should be taken to avoid drug interactions.

REHABILITATION MANAGEMENT OF THE MORE COMMON PERIPHERAL NEUROPATHIES (pp. 1036–1042)

Diabetic Neuropathies (pp. 1036–1038)

• These are subdivided into whether they are symmetrical or asymmetrical (see Figs. 47–12 to 47–14 in the Textbook). In the symmetrical group are polyneuropathies, including: (1) a primarily sensory peripheral neuropathy, the most common of the diabetic neuropathies; (2) autonomic peripheral neuropathy, which is often seen in conjunction with the sensory form; (3) acute painful neuropathy; (4) subclinical neuropathy; and (5) proximal lower extremity motor neuropathy, also known by the less descriptive term *diabetic amyotrophy*.
• The asymmetrical neuropathies include: (1) neuropathy of individual nerves (mononeuropathy), (2) some painful neuropathies, (3) truncal neuropathy or

radiculopathy, and (4) entrapment neuropathies. Some cases of proximal lower extremity motor neuropathy are also asymmetrical.
• Every neuropathy in a patient with diabetes should be separately evaluated and not automatically diagnosed as a diabetic neuropathy. Hyperglycemia in a newly diagnosed or poorly controlled diabetic can also cause a reduction in nerve conduction velocity. This is usually reversible. Diabetes predisposes the patient to other neuropathies, especially focal neuropathies such as carpal tunnel syndrome. Both insulin-dependent and non-insulin-dependent diabetes mellitus can cause neuropathies.

Symmetrical Peripheral Neuropathy in Diabetes. The initial symptoms of diabetic symmetrical polyneuropathy are usually sensory. They include burning, itching, and a "pins-and-needles" sensation. On physical examination the greatest abnormalities are in light touch and vibration, with preservation of conscious proprioception until late in the course. Patients complain of muscle cramping or tightness, especially at night. They also present with hypoesthesia or analgesia that may go unnoticed because of its gradual onset. The symptoms begin in the toes and progress proximally over the course of months to years. The longest nerves are affected first. Eventually the fingers and hands become involved, giving the typical stocking-and-glove distribution.
• Weakness is generally seen later in the course of diabetic complications. It starts distally and progresses proximally. A foot slap is a common result of this. Patients with diabetic polyneuropathy can also have an ataxic gait. This is due to abnormal proprioceptive sensation, which typically is involved only in the late stages of neuropathy.
• If the diabetic patient with peripheral sensory impairment does not care for his or her affected areas meticulously, repeated trauma can result in skin ulceration, Charcot's joint, or even amputation.

Autonomic Peripheral Neuropathy. Autonomic symptoms are often seen together with sensory loss. They can involve the cardiovascular, genitourinary, gastrointestinal, cutaneous, and thermoregulatory systems. The primary cardiovascular abnormalities are orthostatic hypotension, cardiac arrhythmias, and impaired heart rate control. The cause of the orthostatic hypotension is most likely an impaired vasoconstriction reflex.
• Gastrointestinal dysautonomia can manifest as esophageal dysmotility, gastroparesis, bowel incontinence, and constipation or diarrhea.
• Common genitourinary abnormalities are neurogenic bladder and erectile dysfunction. Diabetic impotence is common in the male and is usually irreversible. The early signs of neurogenic bladder include decreased urinary frequency, followed by difficulties with initiating micturition. The bladder eventually becomes flaccid and urinary retention with overflow voiding occurs as the neuropathy worsens.
• When the cutaneous system is also affected there can be impaired distal sweating. This often results in compensatory sweating of the trunk and face.

Acute Painful Neuropathy. Acute painful diabetic neuropathy occurs rarely, and is characterized by severe pain in the distal lower extremities, described as a burning dysesthesia. It is often associated with depression, insomnia, and weight loss. Examination reveals only a mild sensory loss, if any. It is often referred to inappropriately as diabetic "neuritis."

Lower Extremity Proximal Motor Neuropathy. This disease entity has been called "diabetic amyotrophy" and was initially described as being a unilateral

proximal leg weakness. The term is now also used to describe bilateral proximal leg weakness. Electrodiagnostic studies have shown that the dysfunction is in the proximal peripheral nerve (lumbosacral polyradiculopathy, plexus lesion, femoral neuropathy, or obturator nerve lesion).
• The onset of this neuropathy can be acute or subacute. The disorder is characterized by weakness of the quadriceps, iliopsoas, or thigh adductors, individually or in combination. The gluteal muscles, hamstrings, and gastrocnemius can also be weak. Pain is often a prominent component of this problem and is worse at night. The pain is described as severe, deep, and aching. Sensation is usually intact, but this disorder can coexist with a sensory neuropathy. Recovery occurs over a 12- to 24-month period, and the prognosis for significant improvement is generally good.

Mononeuropathy. Mononeuropathy, an asymmetrical form of diabetic peripheral neuropathy, can affect the cranial or peripheral nerves. The third cranial nerve is most commonly affected, although the abducens, trochlear, and facial nerves can be involved as well. The pupil is usually spared in oculomotor palsy. Multiple asymmetrical nerve involvements, referred to as mononeuropathy multiplex, can occur. In these cases, other causes of mononeuropathy multiplex have to be ruled out.

Truncal Neuropathy or Radiculopathy. Truncal neuropathy or radiculopathy occurs most often in diabetic patients older than 50 years. Onset can be acute or gradual. The distribution is usually unilateral, involving primarily T3 through T12. The condition can be painful and includes a differential diagnosis of myocardial infarction, an intraspinal pathological process, abdominal disease, or malignancy.

Entrapment Neuropathy. Persons with diabetes have long been thought to be at increased risk for entrapment neuropathies. Some studies have found no clearcut relationship between the mononeuropathies and duration of diabetes, diabetic control, or the presence of other diabetic complications. Nevertheless, evidence seems to support the common belief that diabetes does indeed predispose to focal pressure neuropathies.

Electrodiagnostic Findings in Diabetic Neuropathy (pp. 1037–1038)
• In symmetrical peripheral sensory neuropathy, nerve conduction studies often show a mixed picture of an axonal and segmental demyelinating process. Increased temporal dispersion of the sensory potential is one of the earliest signs of diabetic peripheral neuropathy. The longest nerves are usually the first affected. They are slower distally than proximally. Sensory nerve amplitude is decreased and motor conduction velocity is slowed. Single-fiber EMG studies indicate that the primary dysfunction is due to demyelination. Moderate slowing occurs proximally and distally as determined by F-wave and other studies.
• Early needle examination reveals reduction in the number of MUAPs and only subtle changes of increased polyphasicity of the MUAP. There are few if any fibrillation potentials, and the MUAP is close to normal in configuration, amplitude, and duration. Later the needle EMG changes can be pronounced.
• Lower extremity proximal motor neuropathy, thoracolumbar neuropathy, and acute painful diabetic neuropathy all have similar electrodiagnostic findings. Nerve conduction studies are usually within normal limits unless there is concomitant peripheral sensory neuropathy. Mononeuropathies are found most commonly in the peroneal nerve, with findings of slowed conduction in the segment

of the nerve traversing the fibular head. Other commonly affected nerves include the median and ulnar. Up to one-half of patients with diabetes have findings consistent with subclinical carpal tunnel syndrome.

Management of Diabetic Peripheral Neuropathy (p. 1038)

Medical Management. Although this has not been proven to prevent diabetic complications, there is evidence that better diabetic control lowers the incidence and severity of neuropathy.

Sensory Changes. Sensory loss is the most common symptom of diabetic peripheral neuropathy. Because decreased protective sensation is often compounded by vascular insufficiency and dry skin (caused by autonomic impairment), skin breakdown can occur. Careful daily inspection of the affected areas is necessary. Proper footwear, with appropriate in-shoe orthoses, is imperative. When indicated, a podiatrist should be involved in the patient's care. If such preventive measures are not undertaken, ulceration and neuroarthropathy are common. Poor healing of ulcers can lead to gangrene and ultimately to amputation.

Pain. Neuropathic pain in diabetic patients is often a difficult and frustrating problem. Usually, the pain of diabetic neuropathy decreases spontaneously over time, and patients should be encouraged to remain active to avoid the complications of inactivity.

Autonomic Dysfunction. Autonomic neuropathy is a common complication of diabetes, and treatment should be directed to the specific system affected. Gastroparesis is typically treated with metoclopramide. Diarrhea or constipation can be treated with a proper diet. The initial treatment of postural hypotension is to teach the patient to change position slowly and consider sleeping with the head of the bed elevated. Compression stockings and an abdominal binder can improve venous return and decrease symptoms. When these fail, use of a mineralocorticoid such as fludrocortisone might benefit the patient.

- Postvoiding residual measurements often help in guiding management. In cases of mild to moderate impairment of bladder emptying, the patient should be encouraged to empty the bladder every 2 to 3 hours while awake. As severity increases, an intermittent catheterization program can be necessary to assure adequate drainage. Use of a parasympathomimetic agent can also be helpful (see Chapter 27).
- Impotence is a common problem in diabetes. Treatment choices include counseling, medication, suction erection devices, and penile implants (see Chapter 30).
- Sudomotor dysfunction can leave the skin dry and subject to cracking and fissuring. Regular skin care and lubrication are necessary (see Chapter 56).

Alcoholic Neuropathy (pp. 1038–1039)

- The neuropathy of alcohol abuse appears to be, at least in part, related to malnutrition (especially the B vitamins). The ensuing neuropathy is a mixed motor and sensory disorder, with the symptoms first occurring in the lower extremities. Paresthesias are often present.
- The affected patients have decreased sensation (especially of proprioception), distal muscle weakness and wasting, and depressed distal reflexes. As the disorder worsens, these changes appear more proximally in the lower extremities and begin to occur in the upper extremities.

- Electrophysiological studies show decreased sensory action potential amplitudes. There is minimal slowing of motor conduction velocity, and distal latencies are minimally prolonged. Needle examination typically shows positive sharp waves and fibrillation potentials in the distal muscles, with polyphasic units of increased amplitude (see Chapter 12).

Management of Alcoholic Neuropathy (p. 1039)
- The primary treatment is to stop the use of alcohol. Vitamins (especially B vitamins) and magnesium should be supplemented and a good diet instituted. Unlike diabetic polyneuropathy, alcoholic neuropathy has a good prognosis if treated promptly, or at least while it is not too advanced. The complications of alcoholic neuropathy are treated similarly to those of diabetes described above.

Acute Inflammatory Demyelinating Polyradiculoneuropathy (pp. 1039–1040)
- Diagnostic criteria for Guillain-Barré syndrome (GBS) typically includes areflexia and progressive weakness in all extremities. The etiology is usually unknown, but the condition often follows a viral or bacterial infection, immunization, or surgery. Strong supporting features include a progression of the symptoms over a 4-week period, relative symmetry, mild sensory symptoms, cranial nerve involvement, recovery beginning 2 to 4 weeks after progression ceases, autonomic dysfunction, elevated concentration of protein in the CSF, and typical electrodiagnostic features. On physical examination there is symmetrical limb weakness, and bilateral facial weakness in one-third of the patients. The muscle stretch reflexes are absent and there is minimal change in sensation. If the respiratory muscles are involved, the vital capacity may be significantly diminished. The vital capacity should be carefully monitored because the patient might require ventilatory support. Autonomic function is often affected (71%) and can precipitate abnormalities in heart rate, heart rhythm, and blood pressure. Patients who require ventilatory support generally have a longer period of recovery. The insult to the nerve appears to be primarily of a demyelinating type, but in more severe cases there can also be prominent axonal loss.

Electrodiagnostic Findings in Guillain-Barré Syndrome (p. 1039)
- Because the earliest involvement of GBS is at the nerve root level, the earliest electrodiagnostic abnormalities are prolongation or absence of the late responses (F wave and H reflex). Later there can be a slowing of motor nerve conduction, but this is a less consistent finding. Temporal dispersion of the evoked responses, as well as significantly prolonged distal latencies, can also be noted. If serial studies are performed, the electrodiagnostic findings commonly lag behind the clinical course, both during worsening and during recovery of function. Patients with weakness typically show a reduction in the number of motor units firing on maximal effort.
- The best prognostic indicator is the needle EMG. EMG signs of denervation indicate that the patient has axonopathy rather than just demyelination, and will have a slower recovery with poorer outcome.

Management of Guillain-Barré Syndrome (pp. 1039–1040)
- Patients with acute GBS should be hospitalized for observation. It is particularly important to serially monitor the pulmonary and cardiovascular systems. If the vital capacity is rapidly declining or if there is cardiovascular dysautono-

mia, the patient should be monitored in an ICU. DVT prophylaxis should be instituted for immobile patients.

• Large randomized trials have shown the usefulness of plasmapheresis in treating GBS. The duration of mechanical ventilation can be halved with such treatment, and overall recovery time is significantly decreased. Contraindications to plasma exchange include recent myocardial infarction, angina, sepsis, or cardiovascular dysautonomia.

• Patients should be warned about having surgery after recovery from GBS because surgery can cause a recurrence, even years later. The recurrence is often worse than the original GBS episode. The exact part of the surgical experience that causes the recurrence is unknown.

Rehabilitation Methods. In the early stages of GBS the patient can have quadriplegia. During this time, prevention of contractures by ROM exercise, positioning, and the use of static splints is important. Careful positioning should also be done to prevent peripheral nerve compression and pressure ulcer formation. Meticulous pulmonary care is indicated to prevent atelectasis and pneumonia.

• The rehabilitation program is gradually advanced in intensity as the patient improves. Because the patient with GBS is susceptible to overwork weakness, the strengthening program should initially be nonfatiguing. When muscles regain greater than antigravity strength, they can generally be stressed with more aggressive strengthening exercises. If the exercises are advanced too quickly, however, there can be a regression of strength. This should alert the clinician to reduce the activity level.

• During recovery, GBS patients often benefit from the use of orthoses and assistive devices. It is more common for GBS patients to develop tightness of two-joint muscles than joint capsule contractures. Stretching of these muscles will alleviate this problem, and should include the hamstrings, tensor fascia lata, and gastrocnemius.

• Gait retraining typically begins with the use of the tilt table because it helps prevent deterioration in orthostatic tolerance. This can also be started in bed by having the patient sit upright for extended periods, as tolerated. There is a cardiovascular and autonomic adaptation as the patient is gradually elevated to the upright position. Patients are next allowed to stand in a standing table, which improves their muscular endurance and permits them to work on other tasks. Eventually the patient is advanced to the parallel bars, with the close assistance of the therapist. Next, the patient can be advanced to ambulation with assistive devices. Eventually, the patient is advanced to ambulation without assistive devices. Lower extremity orthoses are used as indicated throughout the course of treatment (see Chapter 16).

• In addition to progressive ambulation training, patients develop upper extremity strength and endurance through a combination of functional and weight-lifting exercises. The goal is to achieve independent self-care, using assistive devices as needed. Most patients tolerate such a rehabilitation program and go on to an essentially complete recovery. The 5% to 10% who do not recover completely benefit from the long-term use of assistive devices and rehabilitation strategies.

Uremic Neuropathy (p. 1040)

• Chronic renal insufficiency is associated with a sensorimotor peripheral neuropathy, which causes a diffuse slowing of both motor and sensory conduction.

Symptoms of peripheral weakness and decreased sensation are often most severe in the lower extremities, despite an approximately equal slowing of conduction in both the upper and lower extremities. The amplitude of the sensory nerve action potential and the H reflex latency are the most sensitive indicators of uremic neuropathy. Improvements in the electrodiagnostic findings are noted with dialysis and more significantly with kidney transplantation. Needle examination typically shows signs indicative of denervation in the weak muscles, with MUAPs decreased in number and increased in amplitude (see Chapters 11 and 12).

Charcot-Marie-Tooth Disease (Hereditary Motor Sensory Neuropathy, Types I and II) (pp. 1040–1041)

• Charcot-Marie-Tooth (CMT) disease includes a group of hereditary symmetrical distal polyneuropathies. It is one of the most commonly inherited neurological diseases, with an estimated prevalence of 125,000 persons in the United States. The most common type is hereditary motor sensory neuropathy type I. It is usually inherited in an autosomal dominant fashion. CMT type II is also common.

• CMT is usually detected in the first or second decade of life, although foot deformities can be noted even during infancy. The initial symptoms include progressive distal lower extremity weakness and then atrophy. Pes cavus deformity is common, and is exaggerated (if not caused) by the distal motor dysfunction. The most severely affected muscles are the intrinsic foot muscles and peroneal muscles. Distal sensory deficits are often present. Physical examination typically reveals peripheral weakness. The ankle muscle stretch reflexes are often absent and other reflexes can be hypoactive. Gait abnormalities are common and include drop foot, foot slap, and steppage gait. As the disease progresses, the distal upper extremities can become involved, with atrophy and decreased strength and dexterity (see Fig. 47–15 in the Textbook). Nerves can be palpably enlarged.

• In HMSN-I there is a segmental demyelination with secondary Schwann cell proliferation. The Schwann cells form "onion bulbs"—concentric arrays around the demyelinated nerve—that account for the peripheral nerve enlargement. HMSN-II is sometimes known as the "axonal" form of CMT. It is marked by axonal loss with subsequent Wallerian degeneration.

• CMT disease has variable penetrance. A carrier might have only mild foot deformities, whereas members of the same family exhibit significant difficulties with ambulation, hand dexterity, and even diaphragmatic involvement.

• The symptoms of CMT-I and CMT-II are remarkably similar, although they tend to be milder in type II. In both conditions the symptoms generally progress slowly, with only gradual deterioration in function and a normal life span. Despite distal weakness, these patients typically remain ambulatory throughout their lives.

• Electrophysiological studies are helpful in diagnosing CMT and in distinguishing type I from type II. In HMSN-I, motor nerve conduction velocities are significantly reduced (to about one-half of normal). As the disease progresses, the muscle action potential amplitude decreases. Sensory nerve action potential amplitudes are also significantly decreased. In HMSN-II the conduction velocity is normal or near normal, whereas both the motor and sensory action potential amplitudes are diminished. In both types, needle EMG examination can show signs indicative of denervation in the affected muscles.

Management of Charcot-Marie-Tooth Disease (p. 1041)
• Treatment of CMT is aimed primarily at maintenance of function because currently there is no known way to alter the progression of the disease. Ankle-foot orthoses may be indicated if there is significant leg weakness or ankle instability or for protection if sensory symptoms are a significant issue. Careful selection of shoes is important. Custom-molded shoes might be necessary in some cases.
• The patient with CMT is at risk for decreased ROM and contractures, especially loss of ankle dorsiflexion. The patient should be taught appropriate ROM and stretching exercises. Careful daily inspection of hypoesthetic areas should be encouraged.

Mononeuritis Multiplex (p. 1041)

• Mononeuritis multiplex is characterized by sensory and motor neuropathies that occur asymmetrically and asynchronously. It is most commonly due to multiple nerve infarctions. It is commonly seen in vasculitic conditions and it is also associated with diabetes mellitus and multiple nerve compressions. Diagnosis is critical if mononeuropathy multiplex is due to a vasculitis because treatment with steroids can arrest or limit the condition. Failure to recognize and treat vasculitis can have fatal consequences.
• Electrodiagnostic studies show multiple nerve lesions. The rehabilitation management depends on the sites involved and generally includes positioning, bracing (static and functional), and a strengthening program. Precautions for insensate areas should be instituted if appropriate.

Idiopathic Brachial Neuritis (Parsonage-Turner Syndrome) (pp. 1041–1042)

• Idiopathic brachial neuropathy, or brachial neuritis, is a peripheral neuropathy that most commonly affects the radial, long thoracic, phrenic, suprascapular, or spinal accessory nerves. Men are affected twice as often as women. In approximately one-third of the cases the shoulders are affected bilaterally. This condition classically begins with a sharp pain in one shoulder followed by an aching sensation. Approximately 1 week later the patient notes weakness in the affected muscles. Atrophy typically develops later. The motor nerves are usually more affected than the sensory nerves. If sensory nerves are affected, the most likely to have deficits are the axillary, radial, or cutaneous nerves of the upper extremity.
• Latencies from Erb's point to the affected muscles can be slightly prolonged with decreased amplitude and temporal dispersion. Needle EMG examination reveals signs of denervation in the affected muscles as well as polyphasic motor unit potentials and a reduced interference pattern.
• Prognosis is generally good, but recovery can take a few years in more severe cases. Rehabilitation management includes maintaining shoulder ROM and preventing contractures so that the limb is functional when recovery eventually occurs. Orthotic prescription is often appropriate.

Ischemic Monomelic Neuropathy (p. 1042)

• Ischemic monomelic neuropathy results from infarction of all the nerves of a distal extremity. It can be caused by spontaneous or iatrogenic arterial occlusion or embolization, such as during surgical procedures. The patient complains of a deep burning pain that persists even after arterial flow has been restored. Symptoms are predominantly caused by a distal sensory loss in all nerve distributions. In more severe cases there is weakness as well, although the motor involvement is not usually as severe. Symptoms can persist for months. Electrodiagnostic evaluation reveals sensory and motor axonal loss distally. Treatment is supportive with gait aids and orthoses as indicated.

48

Rehabilitation Concerns in Myopathies

• Myopathies are a group of muscle diseases whose most common primary symptom is proximal limb muscle weakness. There are a variety of myopathies, and they differ in etiology, course, specific muscle involvement, and associated problems (Table 48–1).

DYSTROPHIES (pp. 1045–1059)

• Muscular dystrophies can be either hereditary or congenital disorders of muscle (Table 48–2).

Duchenne Muscular Dystrophy (pp. 1045–1055)

• DMD has an incidence of 1 in 3500 live male births with a prevalence approximating 3 per 100,000 live males. Approximately one-third of DMD cases are thought to occur secondary to a spontaneous mutation. The absence or severe abnormality of the protein dystrophin is the cause of DMD.
• DMD typically becomes clinically evident at approximately 3 to 5 years of age. Early difficulties noted are clumsiness, poor walking, and frequent falls. Symmetric weakness begins in the pelvic and then the shoulder girdle muscles, and finally progresses to the respiratory and distal limb muscles. Muscle pain, especially in the calves, can occur. Death is usually caused by respiratory insufficiency and generally occurs at approximately 20 years of age unless ventilatory assistance is given.
• DMD is seen rarely in females. Because this is an X-linked recessive disorder, it can occur in a girl with Turner's syndrome. Female carriers can also have varying degrees of mild muscle weakness and elevation of muscle enzymes.
• Physical findings at the time of DMD diagnosis often include calf pseudohypertrophy. This finding is believed to represent fatty and fibrotic replacement of muscle. Another common sign is difficulty rising from the floor and demonstration of Gower's sign, where the boy stabilizes his legs with his arms and pushes his arms up the front of his thighs to stand up. Pelvic girdle weakness is generally present earlier than shoulder girdle weakness. Gait is commonly wide-based, and the child will progress to walking on tiptoe with tight Achilles tendons. Muscle stretch reflexes can be decreased or absent.

TABLE 48–1   Types of Myopathies

Dystrophies	Endocrine myopathies
Duchenne muscular dystrophy	Hyperthyroidism
Becker's muscular dystrophy	Hypothyroid myopathy
Facioscapulohumeral dystrophy	Hyperparathyroidism
Limb-girdle dystrophy	Corticosteroid myopathy
Myotonic dystrophy	Inflammatory myopathies
Emery-Dreifuss muscular dystrophy	Polymyositis
Congenital myopathies	Dermatomyositis
Central core myopathy	Sarcoidosis
Nemaline myopathy	Infectious myopathies
Myotubular (centronuclear) myopathy	Trichinosis
Congenital fiber disproportion	Cysticercosis
Metabolic myopathies	HIV/AIDS
Muscle phosphorylase deficiency (McArdle's disease, type	Toxic myopathies
V glycogenosis)	Alcoholic myopathy
Phosphofructokinase (type VII) deficiency	Medications
Acid maltase deficiency (type II glycogenosis; infantile	
[Pompe's disease])	
Debranching enzyme deficiency	

Abbreviations: HIV, human immunodeficiency virus; AIDS, acquired immunodeficiency syndrome.

- Intelligence is affected by DMD, although the exact cause of this is unknown. Twenty-five percent of boys with DMD have intelligence quotients (IQs) lower than 75, which is not a progressive loss. Cardiac involvement can lead to arrhythmias and tachycardia. Upper gastrointestinal tract dysfunction and gastric hypomotility can also be present.
- Patients with DMD and other myopathies have been reported as having malignant hyperthermia (MH) as an adverse response to general anesthesia. This is manifest by tachycardia, cardiac arrhythmia, tachypnea, unstable blood pressure, cyanosis, fever, and possibly convulsions. Immediate treatment improves the outcome.
- The most useful laboratory finding in DMD is an elevated creatine kinase (CK), which can be 300 to 400 times normal. This decreases with age as muscle mass declines with disease progression. The electrocardiogram (ECG) is abnormal in two-thirds of patients, usually demonstrating a tall right precordial R wave with deep Q waves in the limb and left precordial leads.
- Needle electromyography (EMG) and nerve conduction studies (NCSs) are a useful part of the evaluation (also see Chapters 10, 11, and 12). Sensory NCSs are normal. Motor NCSs have normal latencies, conduction velocities, and F-wave latencies, but the amplitude of the compound muscle action potential (CMAP) typically decreases as the disease progresses. The EMG shows an increase in insertional activity early in the disease, which can decrease later as fibrotic tissue replaces muscle. Motor units in DMD show the classic short-duration, low-amplitude polyphasicity (often called "myopathic") accompanied by satellite potentials.
- Muscle biopsy shows increased fibrosis with circular fibers.

TABLE 48–2   Muscular Dystrophies

Type	Genetic	Signs at Presentation	Age at Presentation	Associated Findings
Duchenne muscular dystrophy	XLR	Poor walking Frequent falls Gower's maneuver Pseudohypertrophy of calves	3–5 yr	Cardiac disease Restrictive lung disease Scoliosis Decreased IQ
Becker's muscular dystrophy	XLR	Decrease in walking Pseudohypertrophy of calves	10–15 yr— varies	Cardiac disease
Facioscapulohumeral dystrophy	AD	Facial weakness Shoulder weakness	Teenage— varies	Dry sclera Facial droop
Limb-girdle dystrophy	AR	Hip weakness	Teenage–20s	Cardiac disease Pulmonary disease
Myotonic dystrophy	AD	Myotonia (cramping or stiffness) Long face Distal extremity weakness	Late teenage– 20s	Cataracts Cardic conduction defects Endocrine abnormalities
Emery-Dreifuss muscular dystrophy	XLR	Early contractures Cardiac conduction defect	Childhood	Denial Cardiac disease

Abbreviations: IQ, Intelligence quotient; CK, creatine kinase; ECG, electrocardiogram; CRDs, complete repetitive discharges; LDH, lactic dehydrogenase; XLR, X-linked recessive; AD, autosomal dominant; AR, autosomal recessive.

- The DMD gene is a large genetic locus including over 2.5 million base pairs of a human X chromosome. Once the mutation is identified in a family member, the specific genetic lesion present in that family can be searched for in DNA prenatal diagnosis. For deletion-positive patients, DNA screening of carriers and intrauterine diagnosis are recommended. For those families without a known

Chromosome	Disease Course	Laboratory Studies	Electrodiagnosis	Biopsy
Xp21	Severe, progressive	Early: very high CK ECG abnormal	Positive sharp waves, fibrillations, CRDs, small-amplitude polyphasics	Fibrosis, circular fibers, basophilic fibers, abnormal or no dystrophin
Xp21	Slowly progressive —varies	Increased CK ECG abnormal	Positive sharp waves, fibrillations, CRDs small-amplitude polyphasics, paraspinal	Abnormal quality or quantity of dystrophin
	Varies	Normal or mildly increased CK	CRDs early, may be normal. Positive sharp waves, fibrillations, small-amplitude polyphasics	Tiny fibers "moth-eaten" fibers
	Varies	Increased LDH Increased CK	CRDs Small-amplitude polyphasics,	Varied fiber size, increased internal nuclei Fiber splitting, "moth-eaten" whorled fibers
Chromosome 19	Varies	Increased CK	Myotonic discharges (wax and wane) Small-amplitude polyphasics	Internal nuclei, type I fiber atrophy
Xq28	Slowly progressive	CK normal to increased	Small- and large-amplitude polyphasics	Type I predominance and atrophy

deletion, genetic linkage analysis studies and muscle biopsy of a potential carrier or male fetus are available, as well as chorionic villus DNA analysis.
• The clinical course in DMD includes progressive respiratory and limb muscle weakness, contractures, and reduction of physical function. Ambulation ceases at approximately 10 years of age, ranging from 7 to 13 years. Ambulation past 14 years should lead to consideration of other diagnoses.

• Scoliosis is present in approximately 75% of patients. Surgery for scoliosis is generally considered when the curve is greater than 35 degrees. Forced vital capacity (FVC) is generally improved or stable after surgery for scoliosis, particularly when the FVC is greater than 1.5 L at the time of surgery. Bracing of the spine is typically not indicated in DMD because surgical treatment is much preferable.
• There is a correlation between development of pneumonia and an FVC of approximately 1 L or less. Patients who are weaker tend to die from respiratory failure and pneumonia, whereas patients who are stronger have preserved respiratory function and might eventually die from cardiac failure.

Treatment (pp. 1048–1050)
• There is currently no cure for DMD, although intensive research is under way.

VENTILATION
• Maximizing ventilatory assistance in patients with DMD is critical. Approximately 90% of these patients die secondary to chronic respiratory insufficiency.
• Respiratory assistance is typically initiated when vital capacity (VC) decreases to approximately 20% of predicted normal and symptoms of hypercapnia begin. VC generally maximizes at approximately age 10 years in children with DMD. In the ensuing years, the VC decreases, generally to 30% to 50% of predicted by the mid-teenage years. Some caregivers then recommend the use of mouth intermittent positive pressure breathing (MIPPB) with the use of an intermittent positive pressure–breathing (IPPB) device.
• Glossopharyngeal breathing (GPB), or frog breathing, can be a useful tool for DMD patients. GPB can decrease the time of ventilatory assistance. Additionally, GPB is a useful backup for any mechanical failure of ventilatory assistance. GPB can be used to take deep breaths, shout, and increase the effect of coughing. Intact oropharyngeal muscles are necessary for GPB.
• Respiratory assistance is usually considered when the VC falls to approximately 10% of the predicted normal, or when a patient begins to have symptoms of nocturnal hypoventilation. Symptoms of hypercarbia include irritability, daytime somnolence, morning headaches, nausea, restless sleep, palpitations, dysphoria, and decrease in daytime vigor. The workup of a patient with falling VC typically consists of continuous overnight capnography (measurement of partial pressure of carbon dioxide [PCO_2]). Arterial blood gases can also be done and oxygen saturation using pulse oximetry can be monitored. With a night PCO_2 of 55 mm Hg, the patient can have daytime symptoms, even if blood gases during the day are normal. If the PCO_2 levels are increased during the day, there is commonly severe nocturnal hypoventilation, with the PCO_2 as high as 80 to 95 mm Hg. Treatment is initiated with the use of noninvasive negative or positive pressure ventilators.
• Commonly used types of negative pressure ventilation include the iron lung, Porta-Lung (Lifecare, Lafayette, Colo.), chest cuirass, negative pressure wrap, and rocking beds. All except the cuirass ventilator require the patient to be supine. Negative pressure pumps drive these systems.
• There are several forms of positive pressure ventilation (PPV) available. Noninvasive intermittent PPV (NIPPV, bipap) can be done with mouth or nasal access. Alternatively, the more commonly used PPV is the invasive method using a tracheostomy. NIPPV methods include the exsufflation belt or pneumobelt,

which has an elastic inflatable bladder within an abdominal corset. This mechanism is effective only in the seated position, and ineffective in patients with severe scoliosis.

• Bipap is PPV noninvasively delivered with an oral or nasal interface. For oral PPV a mouth seal (Puritan-Bennett, Boulder, Colo.) is often used to keep the mouthpiece in place and prevent excessive leakage. Both the PPV system devices and the negative pressure devices are generally initiated with nighttime use (see Chapter 33).

• Invasive PPV is done with a tracheostomy and positive pressure ventilator. Tracheostomy is deemed mandatory when oral pharyngeal muscle strength is inadequate to control secretions or speech, when patients are unreliable or uncooperative, when severe intrinsic lung disease is present, when there are seizures, or when there are severe orthopedic facial problems. Tracheostomy intermittent positive pressure ventilation (IPPV) is the most common method of respiratory support offered to DMD patients requiring ventilatory assistance. There are a number of potential problems associated with tracheostomy ventilation: airway colonization, increased risk of respiratory tract infection, tracheal necrosis, tracheoesophageal fistula, tracheostenosis, laryngeal complications, swallowing problems, food aspiration, cardiac arrhythmias, chronic granulation tissue formation, painful tracheostomy tube change, mucous plug, and death either from sudden respiratory arrest secondary to mucous plug or from accidental disconnection of the ventilator.

• Patients with DMD have a progressive decrease in VC, even with ventilatory assistance. They can anticipate an increased use of assisted ventilation each year. The treatment is not giving oxygen; it is the mechanical work of ventilation. With assisted ventilation, survival is increased by approximately 6 years. Ventilatory assistance in DMD is controversial.

• Because of the inherently personal nature of the decision, information about ventilation and its consequences should be made available to patients and families early in the disease course. This will enable them to make an informed decision based on their own assessment, as opposed to their physician's assessment, of the quality of life.

• Other aspects of pulmonary care include vaccination against influenza beginning at age 6 months and against *Haemophilus influenzae* and pneumococcus beginning at age 2 years. During upper respiratory infections, antibiotics, chest physical therapy, postural drainage, and assisted cough with suction should be used. Supplemental oxygen might be necessary during these times. Careful monitoring of any spinal orthoses must be made to ensure that they do not impair respiratory muscle function.

Contractures *(pp. 1050–1051)*

• Contractures are a severe problem in DMD. Mild heel cord, ITB, and hip flexion contractures are typically present by age 6 years. Significant contractures are rare before age 9 years. Night-time use of bilateral ankle-foot orthoses (AFOs), along with a regular stretching routine, has been shown to delay development of contractures of the Achilles tendon. Boys who regularly wear AFOs and stretch their legs walk independently for a longer time, and children who do not stretch or use splints lose the ability to ambulate much earlier. Standing is described as an excellent stretching activity. Stretching of the tensor fascia latae (TFL) is crucial. Good positioning includes lying prone to promote extension of the hip and knees.

Mobility (p. 1051)

• Many attempts have been made to maximize ambulation time for boys with DMD. AFOs or ischial weight-bearing plastic knee-ankle-foot orthoses (KAFOs) are often used to maximize gait. The KAFOs are commonly used with locked knees. Surgical intervention for contracture release has also been used to maximize and prolong ambulation. The commonly involved areas for surgical tendon release are the hip flexors, TFL and ITB, hamstrings, and Achilles tendons. The progression of weakness in DMD typically involves the hip girdle muscles first, with contracture of these muscles and of the Achilles tendon. As contractures progress, patients often end up in a position of hip flexion and abduction, with heel varus angulation and equinus of the foot. A compensatory increase in lumbar lordosis occurs to balance the weight line with respect to the center of gravity. Tendon releases are sometimes performed in an attempt to stop this cycle of contractures, worsening posture, and decreasing stability.

Scoliosis (pp. 1051–1052)

• Scoliosis is an almost inevitable progressive problem in DMD. Onset of scoliosis is seen in 50% of DMD patients between the ages of 12 and 15 years. The progression of scoliosis causes problems in several areas, including skin ulceration, back pain, decreased sitting balance, possible limitations on cardiopulmonary reserve, cosmetic difficulties, wheelchair seating problems, and limitations of the variety of assisted ventilation techniques that can be used.

• Scoliosis progresses in patients without any spinal intervention until the time of death.

• Bracing is not effective in the prevention of scoliosis or its progression. Some bracing can be used to facilitate wheelchair seating. For correcting the scoliosis, spinal fusion has been found to be effective. The most common procedure currently is the use of Luque rods with double sublaminar wires, unit rod fixation, and placement of bone grafts. The timing for surgery is based on the balance between scoliosis progression, remaining FVC, and spine growth.

• The trend recently has been to operate on scoliosis earlier in an attempt to minimize the residual scoliosis left after surgical intervention, maximize seating and standing position postoperatively, and minimize respiratory complications. There is controversy over the impact of scoliosis surgery on future VC progression, with no hard evidence of stabilization or deterioration of VC. There is a known minimal decrease in FVC when the thoracic region is fused following fixation of the ribs.

• Problems with spinal fusion include anesthesia risks, blood loss, respiratory problems, and potential neurological injury. There is significant blood loss during these procedures, averaging between 3400 and 3700 mL. Many centers are using a "cell saver" to treat and reinfuse the patient's own red blood cells during the procedure.

• Mobilization should begin as quickly as possible postoperatively. Children are generally able to move about initially on the second day postoperatively. They begin in physical therapy for mobility and strengthening exercises immediately. A plastic body jacket is commonly used for sitting in a wheelchair approximately 1 week postoperatively and for several months afterward.

Other Complications (p. 1052)
• Other complications in DMD include osteoporosis secondary to disuse, and with it, the risk of pathological fractures. Fractures should be treated with minimal immobilization to encourage continued ambulation and mobility.
• Obesity also becomes a common problem once patients become nonambulatory. The change in calorie expenditure from walking to wheelchair mobility is the major contributing factor. Weight management for obesity consists of a low-calorie, well-balanced diet, taking care to monitor calorie intake and output. Weight loss can become a problem in later stages, likely because of hypercatabolic protein metabolism, and is most commonly reported in those aged 17 to 21 years.

Loss of Strength (pp. 1052–1053)
• Muscle strength declines with age with a predictable pattern. There is a fairly steady decrease of strength with symmetrical weakness that is most severe proximally and in the extensor muscles. Muscle strength, motor ability, and performance are closely correlated. Neck flexor weakness is the earliest reported, often in the preschool years. Ankle dorsiflexors are weaker than plantarflexors, ankle everters are weaker than inverters, hip abductors are weaker than adductors, and hip and knee extensors are weaker than flexors. The strength levels of knee extensors and hip abductors are key in maintaining ambulation, along with the degree of contractures and the problem of maintaining balance. Treatment is directed at maintaining range of motion, strength, and the use of earlier involved muscles.

Exercise (p. 1053)
• The effect of exercise on muscle in DMD—both its beneficial effects and possible detrimental side effects—has long been the subject of research and a source of controversy. A major concern in trying to prevent a decrease in muscle function in DMD is that of overwork weakness, which includes a prolonged decrease in both absolute strength and endurance of a muscle. Overwork weakness is reversible if noted early and corrected by rest.
• In supervised resistive exercise programs there is no negative effect on muscle in DMD. Objective increases in muscle strength are found, but these diminish as the disease advances. The overall gain in strength noted in DMD is the strength increase from the exercise program offset by the progression of disease and loss of strength. Exercise programs should be carried out early in the course of DMD when more relatively healthy muscle fibers are present.

Muscle and Gene Research (pp. 1053–1054)
• Current areas of DMD research include myoblast implantation and gene transfer. Myoblast transfers have been attempted in patients with DMD, but without success to date. Researchers are attempting gene transfers in animals by transplanting portions of a dystrophin copy DNA (cDNA) into skeletal muscle fibers.

Hand Function (p. 1054)
• Hand function is critical in DMD because the hands are useful not only for activities of daily living (ADL), but also for assistance in mobility as the disease progresses.

- ADL problems in older patients with DMD typically manifest as a limited ability to pick up heavy objects, whereas fine motor ability is relatively preserved. Functional deterioration of the arms begins around age 10, with the deterioration plateauing approximately 2.2 years later.
- Older children with DMD exhibit some common physical abnormalities in the wrist and hand that can contribute to decreased upper limb function. These abnormalities include extrinsic and intrinsic digital muscle shortness, swan neck and boutonniere deformities, and hyperextension of the interphalangeal joints, as well as wrist flexion and ulnar deviation contractures. Decreased wrist extensor strength occurs by age 8 years. The goals of therapy are to maintain optimal range of motion of the wrist, prevent wrist ulnar deviation contractures, and maintain wrist extensors strength. Therapy includes stretching exercises and positioning of the wrist and fingers. Splint use is necessary in some cases. Balanced forearm orthoses (BFOs) can be used to compensate for proximal strength deficits when distal function remains intact. Minimal elbow flexion contractures of up to 15 degrees can actually be of benefit in initiating flexion and certainly are not a detriment to ADL function.

Psychosocial Management (pp. 1054–1055)

- Psychosocial management is crucial in the care of a DMD patient and his family. It is important for physicians to anticipate medical changes and deterioration and to prepare the family for them. Boys in the early stages of DMD often have a great deal of anxiety, along with fear of falling. Later there is a tendency toward social withdrawal, frustration, and anxiety secondary to a fear of dying. Counseling services should be available for the children and families throughout the lifetime of the boys, and beyond that for the parents. Proper school placement can be extremely helpful in this regard.

Becker's Muscular Dystrophy (p. 1055)

- Becker's muscular dystrophy (BMD) is a milder variant of DMD and is caused by a mutation of the same gene as that in DMD. It is a slowly progressive X-linked recessive disorder and has an incidence of approximately 1 in 50,000 live male births. The onset of weakness generally manifests between 10 and 15 years of age. Motor milestones are met, but the pattern of weakness follows that in DMD, although to a much milder degree and with a better prognosis. Pseudohypertrophy of the calves is commonly seen. The presentation of BMD is much more variable than DMD, with variable age of onset, progression, distribution, and severity of muscle involvement. Associated findings in BMD include cardiac disease, which can be noted at an early age or during adulthood.
- An elevated CK is noted in BMD, but it is usually lower than in boys with DMD. Needle EMG can show primarily symmetrical changes in the proximal limb muscles, including positive waves, fibrillations, and CRDs. Motor unit potentials (MUPs) generally are small, polyphasic, and have early recruitment. Muscle biopsy shows an abnormal quantity and quality of dystrophin, but not as severe as in DMD.
- The clinical course of BMD is similar to that of DMD, although it is milder, with later onset, and is more variable. Proximal weakness leads to difficulties in walking, climbing stairs, and rising from the floor. Contractures can develop late in the disease. Myocardial disease usually (but not always) presents in later years. Survival is generally into middle adulthood.

• Because the course of BMD is milder than that of DMD, the treatment is less aggressive. Medications are not used except in those persons with the most severe form of the disease. AFOs for ambulation and a wheelchair for mobility can become necessary as the disease progresses. Stretching to prevent contractures is important, and surgical treatment of severe contractures can be helpful when they interfere with gait or posture. Patients with BMD can gain significant increases in muscle strength, endurance, and work capacity with a weight-training program.

Facioscapulohumeral Dystrophy (pp. 1055–1057)

• Facioscapulohumeral dystrophy (FSH) is an autosomal dominant myopathy with complete penetrance but variable expressivity. There can be a spectrum of mild to severe cases within the same family. There is typically a normal life span. The incidence is approximately 3 to 10 cases per million. When FSH is first noted in infancy, its course is more severe. A common presentation is facial weakness at approximately 15 years of age, with facial and proximal weakness progressing very slowly.

• The weakness is generally present in the face, shoulder girdle, and anterior portion of the leg. Facial weakness causes an inability to whistle, drink through a straw, and blow up a balloon. During sleep, the eyes can remain open. Proximal upper limb muscles are weak. The hip musculature gradually weakens and drop foot can eventually occur. This progression usually occurs over decades. The face is characteristically smooth and unlined. There is loss of contour of the mouth with a horizontal appearance of the lower lip and a pouting expression of the lips. Neck muscles are often weak.

• There are no echocardiographic abnormalities in FSH. Nerve deafness is associated with the infantile onset of FSH.

• In FSH the CK is elevated two to four times normal in 50% of the patients. The needle EMG can be normal early on but will eventually show myopathic motor units, with fibrillations and repetitive discharges occasionally seen. The biopsy in FSH usually shows an increased variability in the size of fibers, with small fibers called tiny fibers.

• Treatment is focused on assistance in ADL with hand or foot orthoses (see Chapters 15 and 16). There is a lack of consensus regarding statistically significant improvement in muscle strength following exercise. Studies show, however, that a carefully supervised strength-training program with a gradual increase in activity does not cause damage to the muscle or increase weakness.

• Some patients with FSH gradually develop scapular instability secondary to weakness of the scapular stabilizing muscles. Because of this, they cannot flex or abduct the arm. In assessing the potential effectiveness of scapular surgical fixation to the thorax, a preoperative assessment can include manually holding the scapula stable bilaterally while the patient attempts to raise the arm above the head. If the patient can do so, it predicts that the stabilizing operation would be helpful.

• FSH patients can have weak eye closure and drying of the sclera. Artificial tears can control this problem; but if artificial tears prove ineffective, plastic surgery should be considered. Plastic surgery can also help with difficulties in eating, drinking, and cosmetic appearance because of facial weakness in FSH.

Limb-Girdle Dystrophy (p. 1057)

• Limb-girdle dystrophy (LGD) is a group of disorders producing weakness about the hips and shoulders. It can be either autosomal recessive or dominant. LGD is a less well-defined myopathy, which actually represents a heterogeneous spectrum of diseases. The weakness most commonly begins in the second or third decade. Facial muscles are generally spared. Associated findings can include cardiopulmonary difficulties, although cardiac conduction defects are rare. Intellect is normal.

• Laboratory findings show an increase in CK and lactic dehydrogenase. The increase is generally mild, but can be up to 10 times normal. Needle EMG shows small-amplitude polyphasic MUPs of short duration and, rarely, CRDs. Muscle biopsy shows variation in fiber size with increased internal nuclei, fiber splitting, and "moth-eaten," whorled fibers.

• The clinical course is varied but classically is described as beginning with hip weakness (flexors and extensors), quickly followed by shoulder weakness. There also can be weakness of both neck flexors and extensors.

• Ventilatory assistance, including intermittent positive or negative pressure ventilation, can be helpful in the treatment of LGD. A monitored strength training program has been shown to have no adverse effects and, in some cases, shows an increase in strength, at least for the short term.

Myotonic Dystrophy (pp. 1057–1059)

• Myotonic muscular dystrophy (MMD) is an autosomal dominant disease with a prevalence of 3 to 5 per 100,000. In MMD there is progressive muscle weakness (generally worse distally) and atrophy with characteristic involvement of facial, jaw, anterior neck, and distal limb muscles; and myotonia. *Myotonia* is defined as a delayed relaxation of muscle contraction. The onset of weakness is generally gradual in late teenage years or early adulthood. Distal muscle weakness is generally symmetrical and slowly progressive. A long face and slightly nasal voice are often noted early in the course. Patients with MMD can complain of muscle stiffness or cramps, but weakness of the feet and hands is usually their first complaint. The myotonic phenomenon can be elicited by striking the abductor pollicis brevis with a reflex hammer, which causes the thumb to move across the palm.

• MMD is described as a multisystem disease because of the many associated findings. Cataracts are noted in over 90% of patients. Smooth muscle abnormalities are present and can cause dilation of the esophagus. There is an increase in gallbladder problems. Weakness in the bowel musculature can cause significant problems with constipation.

• Cardiac abnormalities in MMD include cardiomyopathy and conduction defects. Cardiac conduction disturbances are present in one-half to two-thirds of patients. Arrhythmias and mitral valve prolapse are increased in MMD. Because an abnormal exercise response of the left ventricle has been reported in MMD patients, any exercise program should be closely prescribed and monitored.

• Males with MMD have degeneration of testicular tubular cells with low sperm formation and low testosterone levels. In females, variable abnormalities are present including amenorrhea and menstrual irregularities. Infertility is common in MMD patients of both sexes. Increased denial of abnormalities has been noted in patients with MMD, along with common mild mental retardation.

• Infants born to mothers having MMD can have a much more severe form of MMD; this form, which is present at birth, is called congenital myotonic dystrophy. In this group there is mental retardation as well as respiratory difficulties and motor delay. In congenital MMD there is hypotonia and facial paralysis with the upper lip having an inverted V appearance.

• MMD patients have an increased pulmonary risk associated with general anesthesia and with use of barbiturates and other medications that depress respiratory drive.

• Evaluation of MMD patients typically shows facial weakness as described above, as well as weakness of the hands and feet. Percussion myotonia is present, and a slow handshake release can be the first indication of MMD. Needle EMG shows myotonic discharges that wax and wane in amplitude and frequency. The sound is often described as similar to a dive bomber or motorcycle. There can also be brief, small polyphasic potentials (see Chapters 10, 11, and 12). CK is generally increased. Muscle biopsy shows internal nuclei and atrophy of type I fibers.

• Treatment for patients with MMD includes orthoses for distal weakness, including AFOs or wrist-hand orthoses. When myotonia is a severe functional problem, medications can be tried to stabilize the muscle membranes. Quinine and procainamide have been used, although they can depress cardiac conduction. Phenytoin (Dilantin), calcium channel blockers, and carbamazepine (Tegretol) can also be used. Because weakness is generally a more severe problem than myotonia, the success of these medications is variable and many patients choose not to use them.

Emery-Dreifuss Muscular Dystrophy (p. 1059)

• Emery-Dreifuss muscular dystrophy (EDMD) is an X-linked recessive dystrophy with a classic triad of findings. These include: (1) early contractures, particularly of the elbows, Achilles tendon, and posterior cervical muscles; (2) cardiac conduction defects; and (3) a slowly progressive weakness and atrophy in a humeroperoneal distribution. The incidence is estimated to be 1 in 100,000 but is not well defined. This disorder is believed to be a slowly progressive myopathy, but the disease spectrum includes patients whose disease is much more severe. Survival is generally into middle age. Cardiomyopathy can present with heart block, commonly in the late teens or the early 20s, and all adult patients with EDMD have this disorder. The severity of the cardiac disease is much greater than the myopathy. The early onset of contractures before the onset of any significant weakness is unique to this disease.

CONGENITAL MYOPATHIES (pp. 1059–1062)

• The congenital myopathies are a group of nonprogressive or slowly progressive myopathies presenting with hypotonia or weakness in the neonatal period. These babies commonly have decreased spontaneous movement and delayed motor milestone achievement. Physical anomalies such as high palate, pectus excavatum, elongated face, and scoliosis can be present as an indication of long-standing weakness (see Table 48–3 in the Textbook).

Central Core Myopathy (p. 1060)

• Central core myopathy (CCM) is an autosomal dominant myopathy with the gene involved located on the long arm of chromosome 19. The child with CCM is floppy at or shortly after birth, with common congenital hip dislocation. The milestones are delayed, although weakness never becomes a severe problem. The child is commonly clumsy, slender, and short. The diffuse weakness typically includes the face and neck, as well as the extremities. Reflexes are normal or decreased. Skeletal deformities, including lordosis, kyphoscoliosis, and clubfeet, can be present. There is relative sparing of the bulbar muscles. Significant muscle atrophy is not seen.

• The CK level is usually normal. Needle EMG shows small-amplitude, short-duration, polyphasic MUPs. Single-fiber EMG shows abnormalities because of an increased number of fibers innervated per anterior horn cell. Biopsy shows a type I fiber predominance with central cores (i.e., an unstained central area running through the center of the fibers) present in type I and some type II fibers. Electron microscopy shows an absence of mitochondria in the central core. The disease course is very mild and the life span is normal. The weakness is generally so mild that no specific treatment is usually needed.

Nemaline Myopathy (p. 1060)

• Nemaline myopathy (NM) is a congenital myopathy that is distinguished by small, rodlike particles on muscle biopsy. The gene is located on the long arm of chromosome 1. There is an autosomal dominant pattern of inheritance with reduced penetrance and variable expressivity.

• In NM, hypotonia with diffuse mild weakness of the extremities and facial muscles with common dysmorphic appearance is noted. Facial muscle weakness often results in poor suck and swallow. Clubfeet and kyphoscoliosis are present. A more severe form of NM can arise that involves the respiratory muscles to a greater degree. This can actually cause death in young adulthood from respiratory failure. Cardiomyopathy is also present in severely affected patients. The disease, however, is believed to be slowly progressive in the large majority of patients.

• A nasal voice is observed in all children with NM. During preschool, two-thirds of the children are susceptible to respiratory infections; some require hospitalizations.

• CK is normal to mildly elevated and needle EMG shows a nonspecific myopathic pattern. The muscle biopsy reveals type I fiber predominance (up to 90%) as well as selective type I fiber atrophy and nemaline rods.

• Treatment includes appropriate bracing for weakness and limb function, surgery for severe skeletal anomalies, and close follow-up and treatment of cardiomyopathy. Respiratory care must be diligent, particularly during times of pulmonary infection. Therapy for improving strength, ADL, range of motion, and endurance is useful, and work simplification is important. Wheelchairs are required for some patients.

Myotubular (Centronuclear) Myopathy (pp. 1060–1062)

• Myotubular (centronuclear) myopathy (MTM) is a congenital myopathy with two distinct forms. The first form is autosomal recessive and has delayed motor milestones and hypotonia, with weakness beginning early in life. There is also ptosis, ophthalmoplegia, slowly progressive weakness, generalized facial weak-

ness, and equinovarus. Seizures can be present. This form is variable in severity. Patients survive into adulthood with minimal motor deficits.
• The second form of MTM is an X-linked recessive disorder that leads to early respiratory failure. There is severe weakness of the face, poor suck and swallow, and weak neck muscles, but ptosis is not severe. The X-linked form has an 80% fatality rate in the first year. Ventilatory support can decrease the early deaths.
• In both forms of MTM, CK is normal or slightly elevated. Needle EMG can show low-amplitude polyphasic MUPs as well as fibrillations, positive sharp waves, and CRDs. Myotonic discharges can also be present. The muscle biopsy shows a type 1 fiber predominance, with increased central nuclei with increased staining of the fiber with oxidative enzymes, and a pale area centrally with adenosine triphosphatase reactions. An electroencephalogram (EEG) typically shows paroxysmal abnormalities in the patient with the autosomal form.
• Treatment is variable depending on the type of MTM. Antiseizure medication is important for patients with the autosomal recessive form. Ventilatory assistance is important for survival in patients with the X-linked type of MTM. Therapy and bracing can be helpful, depending on the extent of weakness and deficits.

Congenital Fiber Disproportion (p. 1062)

• In congenital fiber type disproportion (CFTD), no classic structural abnormalities are noted, but there is abnormalities in the size of muscle fibers and fiber type predominance. Children with CFTD present with floppiness at birth, with weakness most severe in the first 2 years. The weakness subsequently improves or stabilizes. There are delayed motor milestones. Congenital hip dislocation is common, as are other skeletal abnormalities. The patients are short and commonly have low weight as well. Cognitive function is intact. The proximal muscles are more involved than the distal. Reflexes can be decreased or absent. Respiratory infections and complications are common in the first 2 years of life. CK is normal or mildly elevated and needle EMG is myopathic.
• Treatment emphasizes respiratory care, particularly in the first 2 years of life. Subsequent therapy and bracing are used depending on individual patient status. Range of motion and stretching exercises are advisable early in the disease course because of the potential for contractures.
• Over time the children demonstrate a decrease in muscle bulk and an onset of foot deformities and scoliosis. Patients often require some assistance with ADL, ranging from requiring help with heavy lifting to complete dependence.

METABOLIC MYOPATHIES (pp. 1062–1064)

• There are a variety of myopathies that are secondary to metabolic abnormalities. Ten glycogen storage diseases have been well described, with four demonstrating significant muscle involvement: types II, III, V, and VII (see Table 48–4 in the Textbook).
• The glycogen storage diseases present in one of two ways: (1) progressive muscle weakness, as in acid maltase deficiency and debranching enzyme deficiency; or (2) exertional cramps and myalgias, as in muscle phosphorylase deficiency (McArdle's disease).

Muscle Phosphorylase Deficiency (Type V Glycogenosis, McArdle's Disease) (pp. 1062–1064)

• Muscle phosphorylase deficiency (McArdle's disease) presents in a heterogeneous manner. Without this enzyme a person cannot use glycogen as an energy source. In McArdle's disease there is exercise intolerance, easy fatigability, and stiffness of the exercised muscles. Patients have symptoms brought on by bursts of exercise. There also can be episodes of myoglobinuria and cramping after exercise. This cramping can proceed to the hallmark of full contracture with electrical silence.

• McArdle's disease is generally inherited in an autosomal recessive manner, although some persons have an autosomal dominant form. This disease is more common in males than females. Most patients can be diagnosed from their leukocytes, avoiding the need for muscle biopsy. There are no other organs primarily involved in McArdle's disease, but renal involvement can occur secondary to myoglobinuria.

• Physical findings vary with age, but are typically normal between episodes. Proximal muscle weakness might develop late in the disease. Reflexes are normal. CK is elevated at rest in more than 90% of patients, and needle EMG commonly shows fibrillations and positive waves, as well as polyphasic MUPs. Repetitive nerve stimulation at 20 Hz can show a marked decremental response.

• Muscle biopsy typically shows excessive glycogen in vacuoles in the subsarcolemmal region, with variability of fiber size. A biochemical test for phosphorylase shows no activity or up to 10% of normal activity.

• McArdle's disease is usually first noticed late in the first decade when the child complains of fatigue and is unable to keep up with peers. In early adolescence there is typically mild aching of the legs that increases in severity. During the teenage years, painful cramps after exercise are noted that can last for hours. In later years there can be permanent proximal muscle weakness. Renal failure secondary to myoglobinuria can occur.

• Treatment for patients with McArdle's disease is through use of the second wind phenomenon (i.e., taking a brief rest after the onset of myalgia, with resumption of exercise at a lower level) and careful timing of exercise and rest. A graduated exercise program with aerobic activity is helpful. Some patients benefit from a high-fructose diet.

Phosphofructokinase Deficiency (p. 1064)

• Phosphofructokinase deficiency glycogenosis (type VII, PFKD) is an autosomal recessive disease with symptoms closely resembling McArdle's disease. The episodic exercise-induced symptoms are similar to those of McArdle's disease except that they are commonly associated with nausea and vomiting. Gout may be a complication of PFKD. There can be episodes of hemolysis and jaundice. CK, needle EMG, muscle biopsy, and glycogen accumulation are much like those in McArdle's disease. The diagnosis of PFKD can be made by direct measurement of muscle phosphofructokinase activity. Three gene mutations have been identified in Ashkenazi Jews. A molecular diagnosis is now possible to screen for the known allele mutations, which account for 95% of patients. No treatment has been described, but the gradual exercise with intermittent rest, as in McArdle's disease, can be utilized.

Acid Maltase Deficiency (p. 1064)

• Acid maltase deficiency (type II glycogenosis, AMD) is an autosomal recessive disease that can occur in three different forms. In the first or infantile form (Pompe's disease), children have severe hypotonia that develops shortly after birth. These children die in the first 2 years from cardiac or respiratory failure. Abnormal glycogen deposition results in an enlarged tongue, heart, and liver. The second or childhood-onset type produces proximal limb and trunk weakness with motor milestone delay. The liver and tongue can be enlarged. There is respiratory muscle involvement, and death occurs approximately by age 20 years. In the third or adult variety of AMD, there is a slow progression of proximal weakness beginning in the third or fourth decade. Bulbar musculature is spared, as are the heart and liver. Respiratory failure is seen in one-third of the adults, with the diaphragm selectively involved. Pulmonary hypertension can also be present.

• The CK is elevated in AMD and needle EMG shows increased insertional activity with fibrillations and positive sharp waves, as well as CRDs. There are brief myopathic MUPs and myotonic discharges. The ECG is abnormal in the infantile form of AMD. Prenatal diagnosis is available by fetal cell culturing, which shows absence of enzyme activity. Muscle biopsy shows abundant vacuoles with high glycogen content, affecting type I more than type II fibers. Treatment with specific diet or medications has not been found to be effective.

Debranching Enzyme Deficiency (p. 1064)

• Debranching enzyme deficiency (type III glycogenosis, DED) is an autosomal recessive glycogen storage disease. Glycogen with short-branched outer chains accumulates in muscle and liver tissues. Infants are hypotonic with proximal weakness noted. Hepatomegaly is present, and there can be episodes of hypoglycemia. Symptoms tend to improve around puberty, with myopathy appearing in adulthood and progressing as proximal muscle weakness.

• CK is elevated in DED. EMG can show fibrillations, CRDs, and brief small polyphasic MUPs. Biopsy shows subsarcolemmal periodic acid–Schiff positive vacuoles, particularly in type II fibers. Biochemical muscle assay reveals an absence of the debranching enzyme. Prenatal diagnosis with enzymatic marker methods is difficult and cannot distinguish carriers from affected patients. Treatment is with small, frequent meals to avoid hypoglycemia. Cardiac status is also carefully monitored because heart disease can be present.

ENDOCRINE MYOPATHIES (pp. 1065–1066)

• Proximal muscle weakness can be seen, with abnormalities of thyroid and parathyroid function as well as secondary to endogenous or exogenous steroids (see Table 48–5 in the Textbook).

Hyperthyroidism (p. 1065)

• Hyperthyroid or thyrotoxic myopathy is present in a large percentage of patients with thyrotoxicosis. The myopathy is more common in men with thyrotoxicosis than in women. Proximal weakness develops, most commonly about the shoulders. Extraocular muscles can be tethered, causing exophthalmic ophthalmoplegia. Reflexes are normal or hyperactive. CK can be normal, with muscle biopsy demonstrating nonspecific abnormalities. The EMG shows brief, small-amplitude MUPs with early recruitment. Successful treatment of the thyroid disease cures the muscle disease.

• Thyrotoxic patients have been reported to have episodes of periodic paralysis. In exercise tests of 2 to 5 minutes with serial measurements of compound MUP amplitude, an initial amplitude increase is noted immediately post-exercise with a subsequent decrease. When a patient is treated and becomes euthyroid, the above pattern remains but is less dramatic.

Hypothyroid Myopathy (p. 1065)

• Hypothyroid myopathy produces proximal muscle weakness, occasionally associated with muscle cramps. There is a slowed relaxation of muscle stretch reflexes. CK can be elevated and needle EMG shows increased insertional activity and repetitive discharges. Successful treatment of the thyroid disease causes subsequent improvement of muscle symptoms.

Parathyroid Disease (p. 1065)

• In *hypoparathyroidism*, tetany is a neuromuscular complication secondary to chronic hypocalcemia. *Hyperparathyroidism* can lead to proximal muscle weakness, which is more severe in the pelvic girdle than in the shoulder region. Reflexes are normal to increased. There may be fatigue and muscle aching, along with atrophy. Bulbar findings are also noted. The severity of the disease is not correlated with calcium or phosphate levels. On needle EMG there are brief small-amplitude MUPs and early recruitment, with no spontaneous activity. NCSs can show reduced amplitude of the compound MUP with normal conduction velocities. Muscle biopsy shows changes indicative of denervation with type II atrophy. Treatment is of the underlying hyperparathyroidism.

Corticosteroid Myopathy (pp. 1065–1066)

• Myopathy can be caused by excessive corticosteroids. Weakness can occur in Cushing's syndrome as well as with corticosteroid treatment. The weakness generally begins in the hip and proximal lower limb muscles, later affecting the proximal upper limb muscles and, in severe cases, the distal limb muscles. Weakness gradually begins from a few weeks to several years after the onset of corticosteroid administration.

• Severe myopathies have recently been reported related to the use of high-dose intravenous corticosteroids in patients with asthma who required mechanical ventilation and neuromuscular blocking agents (pancuronium bromide and vecuronium). The neuromuscular blocking agents appeared to facilitate a steroid myopathy with an increase in severity.

• The CK is normal in steroid myopathy. Needle EMG shows no spontaneous activity, but can reveal small polyphasic potentials that are recruited early. The myopathy improves within days or weeks after a decrease or discontinuation of the steroid.

INFLAMMATORY MYOPATHIES (pp. 1066–1069)

Polymyositis and Dermatomyositis (pp. 1066–1068)

• Polymyositis (PM) and dermatomyositis (DM) are generally described together as variants of the same disease, but there is evidence that their etiologies are different. PM and DM are acquired myopathies, each with an acute or subacute course (see Table 48–4 in the Textbook). Pain and muscle aches are sometimes present but certainly are not diagnostic. DM has a bimodal distribution, being more common in childhood and in middle age (the 40s and 50s). PM or DM can be associated with neoplasms, vasculitis, or collagen-vascular diseases. Neoplasms are more commonly associated with dermatomyositis, except in children. Childhood dermatomyositis is more commonly associated with collagen-vascular disease. DM is distinguished from PM by a violet rash over the upper and lower eyelids and cheeks with periorbital edema. An erythematous rash can also be present in any exposed part of the body. Calcinosis can occur, particularly in children.

• Associated findings can include vasculitis, especially in children; this can affect the gastrointestinal tract and myocardium. Initial symptoms generally are nonspecific systemic complaints of malaise, fever, anorexia, and weight loss. Raynaud's phenomenon is present in approximately 20% of patients. Dysphagia is common and can necessitate tube feeding. Neoplasms involving the breast, lung, ovary, or stomach are the classic diseases associated with the adult form of PM or DM. Other collagen-vascular diseases are commonly present.

• Physical examination shows proximal weakness involving first the hips, then the shoulders, and also the anterior neck muscles. As the disease progresses, it involves the distal limb muscles. In children the rash is almost invariably seen.

• Reflexes are normal until depressed late in the course of the disease. Mild muscle atrophy can be noted.

• CK is elevated in 90% of patients. The myoglobin and erythrocyte sedimentation rate can also be increased. The needle EMG shows fibrillations, positive sharp waves, CRDs, and small, brief-duration polyphasic MUPs with early recruitment. Ten percent of patients have a normal EMG study. Muscle biopsy shows necrosis, phagocytosis, inflammatory cells, and degeneration, along with regeneration.

• The clinical course is variable and more severe in DM than in PM. Unfavorable prognostic factors include an underlying malignancy, previous diagnosis of collagen-vascular disease, advanced age, and a delay in corticosteroid treatment. Some patients have a complete recovery after one episode, whereas others can have a remitting and relapsing course, with some weakness between severe episodes. A third type is a chronic form of DM or PM. In this last form pulmonary function can ultimately be compromised and the patient can die from respiratory failure.

• Improved treatment of DM and PM is currently an area of active research. The one point of agreement is that steroids must be instituted as early as possible for maximal effectiveness. Prednisone is generally begun at 60 to 80 mg/day or 1 to 2 mg/kg/day in children. If steroids are ineffective, other immunosuppressants (e.g., methotrexate, cyclophosphamide, azathioprine, and chlorambucil) are generally used. Cyclosporine has been shown to be effective in some patients resistant to steroid treatment. High-dose immunoglobulin monthly for 3 months can increase muscle strength and decrease neuromuscular symptoms.

Low-dose total body irradiation (150 rads) has been used in cases not responding to medications.

Sarcoidosis (pp. 1068–1069)

• Sarcoidosis is a multisystem granulomatous disorder that commonly involves pulmonary, skin, and eye tissues. Muscle involvement in sarcoidosis is present in at least 50% to 80% of patients, but is most commonly asymptomatic. Symptomatic muscle presentation is often one of chronic, slowly progressive proximal weakness, along with atrophy. There can also be acute myositis with myalgias and weakness. Postmenopausal women are more commonly affected. CK is generally normal to mildly elevated, and needle EMG shows myopathic changes. Muscle biopsy shows noncaseating granulomas. There is generally bilateral hilar lymphadenopathy on chest radiography. MRI shows abnormalities suggestive of a nodular type of muscular sarcoidosis. Treatment with steroids or adrenocorticotropic hormone (ACTH) is generally effective.

INFECTIOUS MYOPATHIES (p. 1069)

• Documented parasitic infections of the muscle are uncommon outside of tropical areas. Subclinical infection can be more common, however. *Trichinella* larvae can get into human muscle after infected pork is eaten. Fever can be present with muscle pain and stiffness, along with periorbital edema. The masseter muscle is commonly involved, causing painful chewing. *Trichinella* preferentially invade the extraocular muscles. Muscle biopsy shows a parasite and commonly a hypersensitivity reaction. Treatment is with prednisone and thiabendazole.
• Viral infections of muscles may be very common. In influenza B virus infections, acute calf muscle pain is often present. Echovirus, influenza A virus, herpesvirus, coxsackievirus, and adenovirus 21 have all been associated with muscle pain. Muscle biopsies show necrosis; or, if less severe, vacuolar degeneration.
• The *human immunodeficiency virus* (*HIV*), along with its treatment, can cause muscle disease (see Chapter 60). There are two separate myopathies noted in the HIV-positive population. Patients with AZT myopathy have early prominent proximal weakness and myalgia. They fulfill the criteria for *acquired immunodeficiency syndrome* (*AIDS*) and have generally taken AZT for more than 9 months. Muscle biopsy shows ragged red fibers. Withdrawal of AZT results in reversal of the myopathy. Restarting AZT at a lower dose after recovery can prevent recurrence. CK is generally markedly elevated.
• The other form of myopathy is noted in HIV patients who are not taking AZT. This type of inflammatory myopathy occurs early in the infection. There is a relatively painless, severe proximal weakness with elevated CK. Biopsy shows inflammation and nemaline rod bodies. The weakness is generally improved with use of steroids or plasmapheresis. In both of these disorders, needle EMG shows spontaneous activity and short-duration MUPs.

TOXIC MYOPATHY (p. 1069)

• The most common toxic myopathy is *alcoholic myopathy*. There is an acute type and a chronic type. Acute alcoholic myopathy occurs after a bout of excessive drinking, with an acute attack of muscle pain, weakness, and muscle swelling. There can be myoglobinuria and subsequent renal failure. It can resolve completely or residual weakness might be present. In chronic alcoholic myopathy there is generally leg weakness, with the shoulders involved somewhat less commonly. Vincristine and chloroquine have also been implicated in toxic myopathies. Treatment for toxic myopathies is removal of the toxin, which allows for partial or complete improvement.

49

Original Chapter by Corwin Boake, Ph.D., Gerard E. Francisco, M.D.,
Cindy B. Ivanhoe, M.D., and Sunil Kothari, M.D.

Brain Injury Rehabilitation

• Traumatic brain injury (TBI) is the most common form of brain injury. Less commonly, brain injury may be caused by anoxia and certain types of strokes, infections, and brain tumors. Despite different etiologies, many patients with brain injury have a similar clinical course, one that starts with a global impairment of brain function, progresses through a period of functional recovery, and terminates in a stable level of functioning without further deterioration.

TERMINOLOGY OF BRAIN INJURY (pp. 1073–1074)

Traumatic Brain Injury. The term *traumatic brain injury* (TBI) is endorsed as the general term for all injuries to the brain caused by external force. although several older terms, chiefly *head injury* (or *head trauma*), are still used to refer to TBI, such terms can be misleading.

Nontraumatic Brain Injuries. The terminology of nontraumatic brain injuries indicates a specific etiology and pathology, and is therefore readily understood. *Anoxic brain injury* refers to injuries caused by decreased oxygen supply to the brain, and is equivalent to *hypoxic brain injury* and *hypoxic encephalopathy.* Major causes of anoxic brain injury are cardiac arrest, respiratory arrest, and carbon monoxide poisoning.

PATHOPHYSIOLOGY OF BRAIN INJURY (pp. 1074–1075)

Traumatic Brain Injury (pp. 1074–1075)

• The pathophysiology of TBI differs between closed or open head injury, on the one hand; and penetrating head injury on the other. The large number of mechanisms that cause traumatic brain damage can be categorized into primary and secondary mechanisms. *Primary* mechanisms occur at the moment of impact; *secondary* mechanisms are triggered by primary mechanisms and, in turn, cause additional brain damage.

Closed or Open Head Injury (pp. 1074–1075)

- In closed or open head injury, the brain can be damaged by contact between the head and another object, and/or by acceleration or deceleration of the brain within the skull. In a fall, for example, the brain rapidly decelerates when the head hits the ground, and in an assault the brain rapidly accelerates when the weapon hits the head. Motor vehicle crashes typically involve both acceleration and deceleration.
- Most of the primary mechanisms of brain damage are caused by acceleration-deceleration. Primary brain damage produced by acceleration-deceleration include diffuse axonal injury, multiple petechial hemorrhages, contusions, and cranial nerve injury. *Diffuse axonal injury* refers to the widespread stretching of axons caused by rotation of the brain around its axis. The distribution of axonal damage is consistent with the centripetal model of closed head injury, which postulates that the force exerted by rotation of the brain is greatest at the brain's surface and weaker in deeper brain structures. The model correctly predicts that neuroimaging abnormalities in milder TBI tend to be located near the cortex, but in more severe TBI are located in deep as well as surface brain regions. In severe TBI, axonal damage tends to be greater in longer fiber tracts (e.g., corpus callosum). Regardless of the point of contact of the head against an external object, contusions are most commonly situated in the inferior frontal and anterior temporal lobes, where the adjacent skull surfaces are irregular.
- Secondary mechanisms of traumatic brain damage include intracranial hemorrhage (e.g., epidural, subdural, and intracerebral hematomas), brain swelling (e.g., vasogenic or cytogenic edema), excitotoxicity, oxidant injury, and hypoxia because of decreased cerebral perfusion pressure. Both primary and secondary brain damage can lead to increased intracranial pressure (ICP), which in turn can potentiate the mechanisms of secondary brain damage in a positive feedback loop. Brain shift and herniation can be produced by mass effect from brain swelling or intracranial hemorrhage. Hydrocephalus is a treatable cause of secondary brain damage that can occur remotely postinjury.
- *Excitotoxicity* refers to neuronal damage caused by above-normal release of excitatory neurotransmitters by injured neurons. Excitotoxic brain damage can be reduced by moderate hypothermia.

Gunshot Wounds of the Brain (p. 1075)

- In gunshot wounds, most brain damage is located along the track of the bullet and in-driven bone fragments. A major rehabilitation implication is that gunshot wounds of the brain generally cause syndromes of focal brain damage (e.g., hemiplegia, hemianopsia), with relatively spared functioning of brain regions located away from the missile track.

Anoxic Brain Injury (p. 1075)

- The mechanism of brain damage in anoxic brain injury is ischemia caused by hypoxemia or decreased cerebral perfusion. Although anoxic brain injury typically causes diffuse neuronal death and injury, there is selective vulnerability of neurons in parts of the hippocampus, cerebellum, and basal ganglia; and in arterial boundary zones (i.e., watershed areas) of the cerebrum. Neurons in parts of the hippocampus appear to be the most vulnerable, which correlates with the high frequency of amnesia following anoxic brain injury.

EPIDEMIOLOGY OF TRAUMATIC BRAIN INJURY
(pp. 1075–1077)

• TBI is one of the most common neurological disorders resulting in death and disability, and the annual incidence of hospitalized TBI is approximately 200 per 100,000 persons. Approximately 80% of new hospitalized TBI cases are mild and have a survival rate of nearly 100%. The true incidence of mild TBI could be double the estimate based on hospital admissions because many mild TBI patients fail to seek medical attention or are discharged home from the emergency department. The remaining 20% of new hospitalized TBI cases can be divided evenly between moderate and severe TBI. Severe TBI has a survival rate of approximately 40%, as compared with 90% to 95% for moderate TBI.
• The risk of TBI is highly predictable from demographic factors. Males are at higher risk in all age groups. The peak risk is during young adulthood and particularly between 18 and 25 years of age.
• The single largest indirect cause of TBI is probably alcohol abuse. The single largest external cause of TBI is motor vehicle crashes, followed in frequency by auto-pedestrian accidents, falls, and assaults (including gunshot).

ASSESSMENT TECHNIQUES AND PROGNOSIS
(pp. 1077–1081)

Measuring Severity of Brain Injury: Glasgow Coma Scale
(pp. 1077–1079)

• **Glasgow Coma Scale.** Lacking a direct way to measure severity of brain injury, most centers use the Glasgow Coma Scale (GCS) to measure brain injury severity, particularly during the early stages of recovery. Although the GCS was initially designed for TBI, it is also used with anoxic brain injury and other nontraumatic brain injuries that cause impairment of consciousness. The GCS, shown in Table 49–1, consists of rating the patient's best motor and speech responses and the weakest stimulus needed to elicit eye opening. Ratings of these three responses are summed to yield a GCS score that ranges from a minimum of 3 to a maximum of 15. Lower GCS scores indicate lower levels of consciousness and therefore imply greater severity of brain injury. Conversely, higher GCS scores indicate levels of consciousness that are closer to normal, implying less severe brain injury. It has been repeatedly demonstrated that the depth and duration of unconsciousness, as measured by the GCS score, is the single best predictor of outcome from TBI. A modification of the GCS is available for children.
• The lowest postresuscitation GCS score, obtained at any time following resuscitation, is the preferred index of severity. The major advantage of using the lowest postresuscitation GCS score is that it can reflect later deterioration that would not be reflected by a GCS score obtained at the scene or immediately upon hospital arrival.

Classifying Severity of TBI (pp. 1079–1080)

• It is now accepted that the severity of TBI should be graded into the three categories (i.e., mild, moderate, and severe) based on the patient's GCS score (Table 49–2).

TABLE 49–1   Glasgow Coma Scale

Patient's Response	Score
Eye opening	
Eyes open spontaneously	4
Eyes open when spoken to	3
Eyes open to painful stimulation	2
Eyes do not open	1
Motor	
Follows commands	6
Makes localizing movement to pain	5
Makes withdrawal movements to pain	4
Flexor (decorticate) posturing to pain	3
Extensor (decerebrate) posturing to pain	2
No motor response to pain	1
Verbal	
Oriented to place and date	5
Converses but is disoriented	4
Utters inappropriate words, not conversing	3
Makes incomprehensible nonverbal sounds	2
Not vocalizing	1

Instructions: Rate best response in the verbal and motor categories and the stimulus needed to elicit eye opening. Sum the three ratings to obtain the score.

- *Severe TBI,* defined by a lowest GCS score of 8 or less, implies that the patient was in coma. *Coma* is defined as the state in which the patient does not open the eyes and does not demonstrate evidence of cognition, such as following commands or communicating. Severe TBI accounts for the large majority of inpatients in acute brain injury rehabilitation units. In terms of prognosis, the large majority of severe TBI survivors have permanent neurological and neuropsychological impairments that result in functional disabilities.
- *Moderate TBI,* which corresponds to a lowest GCS score in the range of 9 to 12, implies that the patient's level of consciousness is combative or lethargic. At a GCS score of 9 to 12, it is possible for the patient to follow commands, but not to answer questions appropriately. Moderate TBI accounts for a minority of inpatients in acute TBI rehabilitation. With respect to prognosis, the major-

TABLE 49–2   Classifying Severity of Traumatic Brain Injury (TBI) Based on the Glasgow Coma Scale (GCS)

Mild TBI—GCS score of 13–15 at lowest point after resuscitation and no TBI-related abnormalities on neurologic examination
- *Uncomplicated mild TBI*—normal CT scan of the brain
- *Complicated mild TBI*—CT scan of the brain reveals brain trauma

Moderate TBI—GCS score of 9–12 at lowest point after resuscitation

Severe TBI—GCS score of 3–8 at lowest point after resuscitation

ity of patients with moderate TBI and without complicating extracranial injuries are able to resume their preinjury activities despite mild, permanent cognitive deficits in an undetermined proportion of this population.

• *Mild TBI,* defined by a lowest GCS score of 13 or greater, indicates that the patient might be confused or disoriented, but is awake (or wakes when spoken to), follows commands, and speaks coherently. The commonly used term *concussion* is equivalent to mild TBI. The diagnosis of mild TBI can be made despite a GCS score of 15 if there is neuroimaging evidence of brain trauma or if the injury caused altered mental status such as loss of consciousness, a period of confusion or disorientation, or amnesia for the injury itself. On the basis of studies showing that neuroimaging findings are the single best prognostic indicator for mild TBI, it is recommended that patients in the GCS 13 to 15 range be categorized according to whether computed tomography (CT) scanning of the head reveals any brain trauma. Specifically, it is recommended that mild TBI patients with evidence of brain trauma on CT scanning should be classified as *complicated mild TBI* or *high-risk mild TBI.* Conversely, TBI patients without evidence of brain trauma on CT scanning should be classified as *uncomplicated mild TBI* or *low-risk mild TBI.* Although mild TBI is not by itself an indication for inpatient rehabilitation, mild TBI often co-occurs with spinal cord injury and musculoskeletal injuries that do receive inpatient rehabilitation. The long-term prognosis of mild TBI is controversial, as discussed later in this chapter; however, it has been demonstrated that the outcome of a single uncomplicated mild TBI to a child or young adult generally is return to preinjury activities without detectable cognitive impairments. Moreover, the time needed for neurological recovery from mild TBI in such cases is at most 3 months, and probably less than 1 month in most cases.

Neuroimaging of Brain Injury (p. 1080)

• In TBI, CT is the technique of choice during the acute-care stage because of its sensitivity to the presence of blood, facial or skull fractures, and most other intracranial injuries requiring emergency treatment. CT scans of the head can be obtained quickly and are not contraindicated by the presence of metallic material in the body or in life support equipment. Relationships between early results of CT brain scanning and later gross outcome (i.e., conscious survival versus deceased or vegetative) are well understood. Normal CT findings point to the best prognosis, and CT findings of acute subdural hematoma, intracerebral hemorrhage, and massive bilateral hemispheric swelling point to a worse prognosis.

• MRI of the brain is generally more sensitive than CT to traumatic brain lesions because of its greater resolution. MRI is selectively more sensitive than CT to nonhemorrhagic shear injuries and to contusions in certain areas, such as the inferior frontal region and brainstem, which are located near bony surfaces that produce artifacts in CT scanning. Disadvantages of MRI are the relatively long time needed for scanning, inaccessibility of the patient during this time, and its contraindication by metallic materials in the patient's body or medical equipment.

Neurophysiologic Studies (pp. 1080–1081)

• Whereas CT and MRI provide structural information, electroencephalography (EEG) and other electrophysiologic assessment tools, such as evoked potentials,

give information about neurophysiologic functions. EEG is more commonly used in seizure assessment. Focal slowing, a common EEG abnormality, can persist for a long time without clinical seizures.
• In the acute setting, EEG is a powerful predictor of survival from traumatic brain injury. As a predictor of functional outcome, however, the role of conventional EEG and quantitative EEG is still being delineated.
• Somatosensory evoked potentials (SEP) have also been shown to predict long-term outcome of severe brain injury.

Neuropsychological Testing (p. 1081)

• Neuropsychological tests are the major tools used to evaluate cognitive functions in brain-injured patients.

Summary of Acute Prognostic Indicators (p. 1081)

• Table 49–3 presents the major prognostic indicators for TBI available upon admission to acute rehabilitation. The best predictors of outcome from TBI are the GCS score and other indicators of overall severity of brain injury.

Measures of Outcome from Brain Injury (p. 1081)

• Because brain injury can affect different aspects of a person's life, measurement of the outcome of brain injury needs to be multidimensional. However, to

TABLE 49–3   Prognosis of Traumatic Brain Injury at Rehabilitation Admission

Predictor	Description
Glasgow Coma Scale (GCS)	Strongest predictor of survival and functional outcome from traumatic brain injury; basis for grading severity as mild, moderate, or severe
Duration of unconsciousness	Interval from injury to following commands. Alternative to GCS as an injury severity indicator
Age	School-age children and young adults (<45 years) achieve better outcomes than infants or older adults (>45 years).
Post-traumatic amnesia (PTA) duration	PTA duration may be a stronger predictor than GCS score in survivors of moderate-severe TBI. Predictive value of PTA in mild TBI is not established.
Pupillary light reflex	One or both nonreactive pupils predict a worse outcome because of association with brain swelling and/or herniation.
Neuroimaging findings	CT scanning is a strong predictor of outcome from mild TBI. In severe TBI, worse prognosis is predicted by midline shift, herniation, or cisterns compressed by swelling.
Multiple trauma	Musculoskeletal or internal injuries predict worse outcomes.

avoid the need for multiple outcome measures, brain-injury researchers have favored rating scales that reduce different outcomes to a single rating of global outcome. The Glasgow Outcome Scale (GOS), shown in Table 49–4, is the most commonly used measure of outcome in brain injury research. (See Table 49–8 in the textbook for a comparison of the major outcome measures used in brain injury rehabilitation.)

CONTINUUM OF BRAIN INJURY REHABILITATION SERVICES (pp. 1081–1093)

• Rehabilitation of the brain-injured patient is typically divided into acute rehabilitation and postacute rehabilitation.

Acute Brain Injury Rehabilitation (pp. 1081–1085)

• Rehabilitation of the brain-injured patient should begin during critical care. At this stage the rehabilitation physician can intervene to prevent complications that could magnify later disability. For example, the unconscious patient without contraindications should undergo passive range of motion twice daily in order to prevent contractures and other joint abnormalities, and should be positioned to prevent pressure ulcers, edema, and contractures. Additional interventions can be recommended for spasticity, nutrition, and incontinence. Although definitive orthopedic management of fractures in TBI patients can often be delayed, early surgical treatment of orthopedic injuries can minimize later disability.
• The initial rehabilitation evaluation can determine whether the patient is appropriate for acute rehabilitation (e.g., in either a general rehabilitation unit or a specialized brain injury unit); for a subacute program; or for treatment in a postacute program. Transfer to an acute rehabilitation program should be done at the point when the patient is medically stable and when the ongoing medical care will not substantially interfere with progress in rehabilitation.
• Indications for admission to a specialized brain injury rehabilitation unit, instead of to a general rehabilitation unit, include: (1) unconsciousness or

TABLE 49–4   Glasgow Outcome Scale

Category	Definition
Good recovery	Able to resume all preinjury activities despite mild deficits. Psychosocial factors may prevent return to work.
Moderate disability	Able to care for self for at least 24 hours and to travel by public transportation. May work at a noncompetitive level.
Severe disability	Needs on-site assistance during each 24-hour period. May require full-time supervision even if independent in self-care.
Persistent vegetative state	Spontaneous eye-opening without evidence of consciousness (e.g., following commands, speaking words, communicating by gesture).
Death	

inconsistent evidence of consciousness; (2) agitation requiring environmental modifications; (3) risk of complications (e.g., spasticity) requiring specialized management; and (4) severe cognitive impairment requiring modifications of therapy and nursing procedures.

Stages of Neurobehavioral Recovery from Brain Injury
(pp. 1085–1093)

• Compared with other neurological disorders treated in rehabilitation, brain injury has an unusually long course of recovery. For example, TBI patients generally make more functional progress during inpatient rehabilitation than do patients in other diagnostic groups. The Levels of Cognitive Functioning scale, shown in Table 49–10 in the Textbook, describes the sequence of neurobehavioral recovery from TBI and provides a rationale for cognitive rehabilitation at each recovery stage.

Coma and Unconsciousness (pp. 1085–1086)
• The natural history of recovery from severe brain injury begins with coma, a state in which the patient shows no evidence of cognition and does not open his or her eyes, even to painful stimulation. In brain injury caused by trauma, coma and unconsciousness are caused by the disruption of input to surface brain structures from deeper structures that subserve arousal and wakefulness. This disruption can, in turn, be produced by disconnection of ascending fiber pathways because of diffuse axonal injury, or by compression of brainstem or diencephalic structures because of mass effect from supratentorial lesions. In surviving patients, there is a fairly consistent sequence of recovery of function from coma that begins with eye opening and sleep-wake cycles, and then progresses to following commands and, finally, to speaking. This recovery sequence is consistent with the centripetal model of TBI, which predicts that functions subserved by deeper brain structures, such as sleep-wake cycles, should recover earlier than functions subserved by surface brain structures, such as memory. Cognition is usually first demonstrated by the patient's ability to communicate, such as following commands or gesturing.

• In previous studies of severe TBI, 10% to 15% of survivors were still unconscious at the time of discharge from acute care. Most patients who remain unconscious after 1 month have regained sleep-wake cycles, and therefore spontaneously open their eyes part of the time. They typically also exhibit pupillary reactivity and oculocephalic reflexes, primitive behaviors such as chewing and roving eye movements, and vegetative functions such as spontaneous respiration, all of which reflect preserved brainstem and hypothalamic functions. Although there is general agreement on diagnostic criteria for coma, diagnostic inaccuracies and confusion attend attempts to distinguish vegetative from minimally conscious or minimally responsive states. The term *persistent vegetative state* (PVS) has been used to describe a state in which a previously comatose patient has recovered sleep-wake cycle and progressed to a state of wakefulness without awareness. Patients in PVS have no reproducible, purposeful, or voluntary behavioral response to stimuli, and no evidence of language comprehension or expression. PVS is a diagnosis rather than a prognosis. A related condition, *permanent vegetative state,* signifies irreversibility and is therefore a prognosis.

Rehabilitation of Patients with Impaired Consciousness (pp. 1086–1088)

• Patients who remain unconscious upon discharge from acute care present difficult assessment and treatment problems, and should be admitted to a brain injury rehabilitation program. In the absence of treatments with proven efficacy to facilitate recovery of consciousness, the goals of rehabilitation of unconscious TBI patients are (1) to remove obstacles to recovery, thereby allowing patients who have the potential to regain consciousness to do so; (2) to treat medical complications that can increase disability in those patients who do recover; and (3) to provide education, counseling, and support to family members.

• Rehabilitation of unconscious patients remains controversial. In particular, the efficacy of *sensory stimulation* (also termed *coma stimulation*), in which patients are presented with directed stimulation in multiple modalities, has not been supported by clinical trials.

• Pharmacological treatment remains the most promising intervention to directly increase arousal and facilitate recovery of consciousness of these patients. See Table 49–13 in the Textbook for a summary of some medications used for neurostimulation.

• Potentially sedating medications that are often given to unconscious patients are listed in Table 49–5.

Post-Traumatic Amnesia and Agitation (pp. 1089–1091)

• Following recovery of consciousness, patients with brain injury typically pass through a period of confusion and disorientation termed *post-traumatic amnesia* (PTA). PTA is defined as the period during which the patient's ability to learn new information is minimal or nonexistent. For example, early in PTA, patients might not be aware of being in a hospital and may instead state that they are at home or at work. This false recall of fictitious events, termed *confabulation,* is an organic rather than a functional symptom. Toward the end of PTA, patients become less confabulatory but still fail to recall specific episodes (e.g., visitors received the previous day). After emerging from PTA, patients have a permanent memory gap for events that occurred during the period of PTA. They usually also have a memory gap for events that occurred a short period before the moment of injury (termed *retrograde amnesia*) (Fig. 49–1).

• Different measures are available to assess whether a patient is in PTA or is recovering out of PTA. The most widely used measure is orientation to place and time, but this can be less suitable in rehabilitation units where patients are given frequent "reality orientation" drills. A standard technique for assessing PTA is the Galveston Orientation and Amnesia Test (GOAT), a brief structured interview that quantifies orientation and recall of recent events. The GOAT score can range from 0 to 100, with a score greater than 75 defined as normal. The end of PTA can be defined as the date after which the GOAT score is consistently greater than 75.

• Duration of PTA is an indicator of the severity of brain injury and should be used to supplement the GCS score, duration of unconsciousness, and neuroimaging findings.

• During PTA many patients exhibit a neurobehavioral syndrome, termed *agitation,* which includes cognitive confusion, extreme emotional lability, motor overactivity, and physical or verbal aggression. The agitated patient is typically unable to sustain attention and effort long enough to perform simple tasks, such as dressing, and can overreact to frustration by crying or shouting. The patient

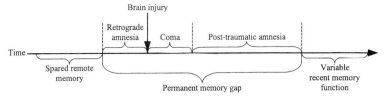

FIGURE 49–1. Recovery of Memory after Brain Injury. Timeline showing the stages of cognitive recovery that apply to most survivors of severe brain injury. Mild and moderate TBI will demonstrate the same stages as depicted, except for coma. Some survivors do not recover from unconsciousness or from posttraumatic amnesia (PTA). The majority of patients emerge from PTA and have a permanent memory gap for experiences that occurred during unconsciousness, PTA, and a shorter preinjury period (retrograde amnesia).

can be easily frustrated and irritated, and show grossly inappropriate behavior toward staff or family members.

Rehabilitation of the Agitated Patient (pp. 1091–1092)
• Although agitation is commonly observed in brain injury, it should be a diagnosis of exclusion. Concurrent medical or neurological problems can cause or aggravate delirium and agitated behavior. Metabolic derangement, hyperthyroidism, infection and sepsis, hypoglycemia, hypoxemia, medications (e.g., anticholinergics), and drug withdrawal (e.g., baclofen, sedatives, and hypnotics) are some medical causes of delirium and agitation. Among the neurological complications that might present as delirium or agitation are seizures, hydrocephalus, intracranial mass lesions (e.g., hematoma and hygroma), and migraine. Pain, especially in a patient who is confused and unable to communicate, is a com-

TABLE 49–5 Alternatives of Commonly Used Sedating Medications

	Sedating Medications	Less Sedating Alternatives
Antiepileptics	Phenytoin	Carbamazepine
	Phenobarbital	Valproic acid
		Gabapentin
Drugs for excesses of behavior (e.g., agitation, episodic dyscontrol)	Haloperidol and other neuroleptics	Risperidone
		Carbamazepine
	Lorazepam	Valproic acid
	Diazepam	Buspirone
Antidepressants	Tricyclic antidepressants	Selective serotonin reuptake inhibitors
		Venlafaxine
Antispasticity medications	Baclofen (oral)	Botulinum toxin
	Diazepam	Baclofen (intrathecal)
Gastrointestinal drugs	Cimetidine	Antacids
	iMetoclopramide	Erythromycin

monly overlooked cause of agitation. It is reasonable to perform various tests in the evaluation of the confused and agitated patient (Table 49–6).

• Treatment of agitation involves medications, behavioral strategies, and environmental management. If needed, restraints should be applied to the minimal degree necessary (e.g., padded hand mittens and soft lap belts for wheelchair safety). Traditional behavioral modification techniques, such as using rewards for desired behaviors, are not considered effective for agitation because the patient is generally confused and amnestic. Nonpharmacological efforts are directed toward environmental management and restructuring of therapies (Table 49–7). The goal of environmental management is to lower the level of stimulation and cognitive complexity in the patient's immediate surroundings.

• No guideline exists in the use of medications for agitation. Sedation should be used only when environmental strategies have failed and in emergency situations. Drugs such as carbamazepine, tricyclic antidepressants (TCAs), trazodone, amantadine, and β-blockers are preferred over haloperidol and benzodiazepines (Table 49–8). In situations where agitation is uncontrollable and has progressed to violent behavior, intramuscular lorazepam (Ativan), 1 to 2 mg, might be required. This is recommended only for emergency situations when there is immediate danger to the patient or others, and the physician should also be aware of a paradoxical increase in agitation, which can occur with the use of lorazepam.

Rehabilitation During and After Post-Traumatic Amnesia (pp. 1092–1093)

• The rehabilitation program during PTA should be modified for the patient's severe memory impairments. The rehabilitation unit should have a system (e.g., colored wristbands) for identifying how closely each patient needs to be supervised. Patients who are at high risk of eloping or of harming themselves or others might need a locked area or direct supervision by nursing staff. To reorient patients to their environment, the place and date and a daily schedule should be posted in patient rooms, and orientation information can be repeated through the day. The team should avoid overstimulating the patient with a demanding therapy schedule, unrealistic therapeutic expectations, and unpleasant emotional interactions with family or staff. Patients who are capable of walking can require close supervision because of safety concerns and might be safer using a

TABLE 49–6 Suggested Tests for the Evaluation of the Confused and Agitated Patient

Serum electrolytes
Blood urea nitrogen (BUN), serum creatinine
Glucose, calcium, magnesium, and liver enzymes
Thyroid function
CBC with differential
Urinalysis
Serum B-12 and folate levels
Drug and alcohol screen
Brain CT or MRI
EEG
Plain radiograph (to evaluate for occult fractures or heterotopic ossification causing pain)

TABLE 49–7 Environmental Management of Agitation

1. **Reduce the level of stimulation in the environment**
   - Avoid overstimulation by decreasing background noise (e.g., radio, television) and visual distraction in the patient's room and in therapy areas. Monitor room temperature for comfort.
   - Room should be in an area with low traffic but where the patient can be easily monitored.
   - Limit visitors. Orient visitors regarding strategies.
   - During therapies, eliminate or reduce activities that appear to cause annoyance, frustration, and overstimulation.
   - Avoid excessive touching and handling.
   - Provide frequent breaks during therapy sessions.
   - Staff needs to maintain calm demeanor. Keep voice volume and pitch low.
2. **Reduce the patient's confusion**
   - Provide consistent staffing.
   - Avoid moving rooms.
   - Allow one person to speak at a time.
   - Communicate clearly and concisely (i.e., one idea at a time).
   - Keep a consistent schedule for therapies and activities.
   - Reorient to place, time, and purpose through the day.
3. **Protect the patient from harming self or others**
   - Keep the patient in a locked unit or use an alarm system to prevent elopement.
   - Consider using a floor bed with padded walls (e.g., Craig bed).
   - Use stable wheelchair with appropriate safety straps.
   - Avoid use of physical restraints (e.g., Posey) that may heighten agitation.
   - Consider the option of a 1:2 or 1:1 sitter for close supervision.
   - Staff responsible for close supervision can wear a bracelet.
4. **Tolerate restlessness as much as possible**
   - Review with staff specific therapy and environmental strategies to be used for each patient and "crisis intervention" techniques.
   - Allow patient to thrash about in floor bed.
   - Allow ambulatory patient to pace around the unit, with supervision.
   - Allow confused patient to be verbally inappropriate.

TABLE 49–8 Some Drugs Used to Treat Post-Traumatic Agitation

Class	Drug
β-blockers	Propranolol
Antiepileptics	Carbamazepine
	Valproic acid
Dopamine agonist	Methylphenidate
	Amantadine
	Bromocriptine
Tricyclic antidepressants	Amitriptyline
	Nortriptyline
Benzodiazepine	Lorazepam
Others	Buspirone
	Risperidone

wheelchair when not in therapies. As the patient's safety awareness and endurance increase toward the end of PTA, the team can clear the patient for walking, toileting, and other activities at a reduced level of supervision.

Postacute Brain Injury Rehabilitation (p. 1093)

• Postacute rehabilitation includes interventions designed to help patients reenter the community. Most postacute interventions are based on training patients to use compensatory strategies to overcome their permanent deficits (e.g., memory notebooks), or altering the environment so that the patient is more functional despite these deficits (e.g., following a routine schedule). The rehabilitation physician should be familiar with local postacute programs in order to make appropriate referrals and monitor progress (see Table 49–17 in the Textbook).

MEDICAL COMPLICATIONS OF BRAIN INJURY
(pp. 1093–1105)

• In recent years there has been a trend toward shorter stays in acute care and, therefore, toward earlier admission to rehabilitation. Medical examination of brain-injured patients is typically made difficult because of inability to communicate or cooperate with procedures. For these reasons, a thorough evaluation by the rehabilitation physician is needed once the patient has been admitted to the rehabilitation unit.

Spasticity (pp. 1093–1095)

• Cerebral origin spasticity characteristically presents with greater extensor tone in the lower extremities and a lesser tendency to "spasms" than with spinal cord injury.
• Although spasticity can be beneficial, decreasing the risk of thrombophlebitis and in some cases aiding in function, it can also create impressive deformity, pain, and other medical complications. Spasticity that interferes with functional goals warrants treatment. Potential complications of spasticity (e.g., heterotopic ossification, pressure ulcers, and respiratory infections) should be considered.
• The evaluation of the patient with spasticity should include not only the usual neurological examination, but also consideration of such factors as gait, balance, synergy patterns, speed of movement, distribution of tone, modified Ashworth scores (Table 49–9), goniometric evaluation, and functional assessment.
• In the past, a pyramid approach to spasticity treatment was advocated. This began with prevention of nociceptive stimuli and education and progressed to therapy (e.g., ROM, stretching, casting, orthoses, and modalities), and then to more invasive options such as motor point blocks. A "complementary approach," wherein various treatment strategies are employed concurrently based on therapeutic goals, is currently favored.
• Antispasticity drugs such as diazepam and oral baclofen can impair cognition. Dantrolene sodium has been considered the oral medication of choice in the TBI population because it acts peripherally, at the muscle. It can also be sedating, however, and can lead to generalized weakness. Liver enzymes also need to be monitored when using dantrolene sodium. Tizanidine, which is an α-2 agonist

TABLE 49–9 Modified Ashworth Scale

0	= No increase in muscle tone
1	= Slight increase in tone, minimal resistance end of range
1+	= Slight increase in tone with minimal resistance throughout less than half the remainder range
2	= More marked increase in muscle tone through most of the range; affected part easily moved
3	= Considerable increase in tone, passive movement difficult
4	= Part fixed

Source: Bohannon RW, Smith MB: Interrater reliability of a modified Ashworth scale of muscle spasticity. Phys Ther 1987; 76:206–207.

like clonidine, has demonstrated effects in the multiple sclerosis and spinal cord injury populations.

• Serial casting refers to the practice of applying and removing casts to a limb as joint range of motion increases. Modalities such as heating and cooling can also be helpful for improving range in the short term, and can be used in conjunction with casting to allow for greater stretch. In rare instances, tone is too great to allow for casting because of potential skin breakdown and behavioral issues. In these cases, injections of botulinum toxin and/or phenol should be considered to decrease the spasticity and thereby decrease this risk.

• The role of positioning techniques in spasticity management is often underappreciated. Appropriate positioning should maximize muscle relaxation as well as improve alignment, symmetry, and function. Positioning can also be used to decrease the primitive reflexes that can recur in patients after brain injury. For example, lying supine can increase the tonic labyrinthine supine reflex (TLSR), thereby increasing extensor tone. One of the acceptable goals of rehabilitation can be providing equipment prescriptions to allow for optimal positioning. The antispasticity ball splint for the spastic hand is commonly used. Abduction of the thumb from the palm and spread of the digits can decrease flexor tone in the hand. Like casting, splinting techniques can also be used both to decrease tone and to stretch soft tissues. These techniques can also be combined. For instance, the inhibitory footplate fabricated into lower extremity casts improves support and alignment of the forefoot. These concepts can be incorporated into orthoses as well.

• Other treatment options include injections such as neurolytic procedures and chemodenervation with botulinum toxin. Phenol, alcohol, or anesthetic agents are injected to impair conduction of impulses. Chemical neurolysis refers to destruction of a portion of nerve with alcohol or phenol.

• Botulinum toxin A is also effective in the treatment of spasticity, although it is not FDA approved for this indication. It binds irreversibly at the neuromuscular junction, blocking contraction of muscle. Side effects are rare but include atrophy, pain, and infection. Unlike motor point blocks, there are no immediate restrictions on activity following injection. To minimize the potential for antibody production to the medication, it is recommended that injections not be repeated more often than every 3 months and that the total toxin dose be limited to 400 units per session. However, these stipulations are evolving as more experience is gained with the medication and different strains become available for future use.

• The FDA approved intrathecal baclofen therapy (ITB) for the treatment of cerebral origin spasticity in 1996. It effectively reduces spasticity across the greatest number of joints and often produces a dramatic change in tone. Administration of baclofen directly into the intrathecal space allows effective cerebrospinal fluid concentrations with plasma concentrations 100 times less than with oral administration. The systemic side effects are decreased or absent and the clinical response is greater when used intrathecally. Effects of this treatment are greatest on the lower limbs because the concentration of baclofen is four times greater in the lumbar region than in the cervical region. Changes in upper extremity spasticity are also seen, but this is not considered a primary indication for this treatment at this time.

• Other surgical procedures available for spasticity management include tendon lengthenings and transfers. Whereas surgeries can weaken spastic muscles, residual spasticity can lead to recurrent deformity. More clinicians now recognize the inherent value in combining spasticity-reducing techniques. Adequate spasticity management with ITB therapy can decrease the need for surgical intervention. Rhizotomies are generally not performed on adult patients, and their performance on children varies regionally. This is a permanently destructive procedure. Anterior rhizotomies provide denervation of the muscle whereas posterior rhizotomies interrupt IA and IB afferents from muscle spindles.

Post-Traumatic Epilepsy (pp. 1095–1096)

• It is estimated that approximately 5% of all persons who are hospitalized for TBI will develop *late seizures,* defined as those that occur a week or more after the injury. However, the presence of certain risk factors can increase the probability of developing late seizures or post-traumatic epilepsy (PTE). In particular, penetrating injuries seem to significantly increase one's risk.

• In the past, patients were placed on long-term seizure prophylaxis acutely; however, recent studies have shown that using phenytoin beyond the first week following a brain injury does not prevent the development of late PTE. In addition, the neurobehavioral side effects of phenytoin and other sedating anticonvulsants, such as phenobarbital, can be detrimental to the patient with already slowed thinking and memory loss.

• Seizure prophylaxis in patients with nonpenetrating injuries who have not demonstrated any seizure activity is no longer indicated. If a patient has a penetrating injury, or if he or she had seizures during the first week (early seizures), then the decision on prophylactic medication needs to be based on the individual clinical situation.

• If late seizures develop, then the patient has PTE and the issue becomes treatment rather than prophylaxis. In these cases, carbamazepine appears to be the drug of choice.

• Valproic acid (Depakote, Depakene), although initially sedating, can be useful as well because it can have fewer cognitive and behavioral side effects than carbamazepine. Gabapentin (Neurontin), another new antiepileptic medication, may prove to be helpful for patients with PTE. It is approved as adjunctive therapy, does not have significant cognitive side effects, and does not require monitoring of blood levels. Newer antiepileptics, whose benefits for PTE are unknown, include lamotrigine (Lamictal) and topiramate (Topamax).

Post-Traumatic Hydrocephalus (pp. 1096–1097)

• Hydrocephalus is a well-recognized complication of traumatic brain injury, and depending on the study, ranges in incidence from 9% to 72%. The fundamental abnormality in hydrocephalus is an imbalance in the production and absorption of cerebrospinal fluid (CSF). Overall, impaired absorption accounts for most cases of hydrocephalus.

• Traditionally, hydrocephalus is categorized as either communicating or noncommunicating. In the former, there is a free flow of CSF in the various portions of the ventricular system, the cisterns, and subarachnoid spaces. However, CSF flow from the cisterns to the arachnoid villi is blocked or CSF absorption by the villi is impaired. The latter occurs with inflammation or subarachnoid hemorrhage. Other commonly used terms to categorize hydrocephalus include obstructive hydrocephalus, which describes the pathomechanism, normal pressure hydrocephalus (NPH), and hydrocephalus ex vacuo. NPH is defined as a clinical triad of gait disturbance, mental deterioration, and urinary incontinence associated with ventricular enlargement and normal CSF pressure. Despite radiographic evidence of ventricular enlargement, hydrocephalus ex vacuo is not "true" hydrocephalus. Instead, it represents changes resulting from brain atrophy.

• Timely diagnosis and treatment are important during rehabilitation because failure to do so may hamper recovery and minimize the chances of benefiting from therapies. Diagnosis in individuals with severe brain injuries is difficult because the classic triad of NPH is already present as a direct result of brain trauma. The clinician often has to rely on atypical or more subtle symptoms (e.g., functional decline, failure to progress, seizures, emotional problems, abnormal posturing, or increased spasticity) and confirm the suspicion through CT.

• If suspicion for the development of PTH is high, serial monthly CT scans for comparison can help make the diagnosis. In situations where the radiographic findings are equivocal, determining which patients might benefit from shunting is usually based on a constellation of findings. A lumbar puncture for craniospinal-axis pressure can be considered. Shunting is usually successful if the pressure is elevated above 180 mm H_2O or if the ventricles have progressively increased in size. The patient will also likely benefit from shunt placement if there is a clinical picture of normal pressure hydrocephalus.

• CSF diversion, such as ventriculoperitoneal shunting, is the definitive treatment of hydrocephalus. Alternative methods of shunting include ventriculoatrial, ventriculojugular, and lumboperitoneal. Complications may arise from mechanical failure of the shunt, functional failure resulting from an inadequate flow rate of a working shunt, and infection.

Cranial Nerve Damage (pp. 1097–1098)

• Cranial nerve damage is a common consequence of brain injury. The resulting impairments, such as compromise of sensation (e.g., sight, hearing, smell, or taste) and swallowing, can lead to further impairment of function in an already confused patient.

• Studies have shown that cranial nerve VII is injured most commonly (9% of patients), followed by cranial nerve III (6% of patients); least commonly injured were cranial nerves IX and XI. The true incidence of cranial nerve damage related to traumatic brain injury cannot be determined, however, because many studies and common clinical practice tend to ignore testing certain cranial nerves such as I (olfactory).

- Cranial nerve I can be damaged directly as it goes through the cribiform plate by a frontal blow or via contrecoup injury. Impaired olfaction, or dysosmia, can be complete (anosmia) or partial (hyposmia). Dysosmia commonly results in taste alterations and can cause patients to have strange or new food preferences. Patients with an impaired sense of smell might require cueing for hygiene, cooking, storage of food, and use of perfumes.

- Damage to cranial nerve II results in optic neuropathy that presents as visual loss of varying degrees. Injury to the motor system of the eye (i.e., cranial nerves III, IV, and VI) can occur at several levels, both centrally and peripherally. Secondary insults can occur after impact, as with temporal herniation because of edema (uncal herniation with cranial nerve III injury). The resulting strabismus can be caused by cranial nerve injury, but some gaze deviations in the early stages after brain injury might not be because of cranial nerve injury. Objective testing to determine ocular alignment can be simply performed by noting symmetrical placement of the corneal reflection of a pen light in each of the cardinal eye positions (Hirschberg reflex). Convergence and accommodation testing should be performed carefully. Side effects of drugs, most commonly phenytoin and phenobarbitol, can also impair these reflexes. Diplopia occurring at near-vision only can be the result of an impaired vergence system.

- Early neuro-ophthalmologic or neuro-optometric evaluation can be valuable in diagnosing subtle abnormalities, recommending corrective measures for visual abnormalities, and preventing secondary complications such as exposure keratitis of the cornea. In the authors' center, a weekly "Low Vision Rounds" run by a neuro-optometrist serves this purpose. The use of corrective prisms, when a patient's alignment is several diopters off, is helpful for the patient who can utilize them.

- Injury to the facial nerve most commonly occurs within its passage through the temporal bone. The most deleterious effect is inadequate lid closure, and the patient may be susceptible to exposure keratitis of the cornea. If cranial nerve V has also been injured, resulting in the loss of corneal sensation, the problem is compounded. It is imperative that the eye be protected by the use of lubricants and by taping the lid closed with eye pads. Alternatively, occlusive transparent film, which covers the ocular area and creates a "wet chamber," has been utilized to keep the cornea lubricated with some success. Lid tarsorrhaphy might be necessary to prevent further damage, especially in a low-level patient.

- Evaluation of cranial nerve VIII (vestibulo-cochlear nerve) usually occurs during the acute neurosurgical phase. Direct examination can reveal Battle's sign, mastoid fracture, otorrhea, bleeding from the ear, hemotympanum, and lacerations of the tympanic membrane. Hemorrhage from the ear and lacerations of the tympanic membrane might indicate a longitudinal fracture of the temporal bone. As the patient stabilizes, audiometry and the tuning fork test can be utilized. Brainstem auditory evoked potentials can provide further information about the integrity of the auditory system. If hearing loss is significant, hearing aids of the CROS (Contralateral Routing of Signal) type, which transfer sound to the intact ear, can help the patient compensate.

- Vestibular disturbances can result in dizziness, impaired balance, ataxia, and nystagmus. The Barany test, a provocative test using head rotation, is useful in evaluating nystagmus. Patients will commonly compensate by tilting their heads to decrease the nystagmus. In patients complaining of dizziness, it is reasonable to implicate vestibular etiology; however, other possible etiologies need to be ruled out (Table 49–10).

• Common medications used for vestibular problems (e.g., meclizine or dimen-hydrinate) are antihistamines and can cause sedation in patients with brain injuries. Vestibular therapy employing habituation is preferred. The patient uses provocative exercises, which increase the symptoms, to decrease the sensitivity of the vestibular response.

• The lower cranial nerves are only occasionally affected by brain injuries. They are more often damaged by direct trauma.

Post-Traumatic Hyperthermia (p. 1098)

• Hyperthermia is a common occurrence during recovery from trauma. It is tempting to attribute fever in an individual with brain injury to central dysfunction, especially if the results of the initial workup do not suggest an infectious or inflammatory process. However, post-traumatic hyperthermia of central origin is relatively uncommon, occurring in just 4% in one series. A thorough evaluation is usually needed to investigate other, more common etiologies. (See Fig. 49–10 in the Textbook for a suggested algorithm for the workup of hyperthermia in an individual with brain injury.)

• When an extensive fever workup fails to identify an etiology, the clinician is led to label the condition "fever of unknown etiology" or attribute the fever to central origin. Central fever usually results in a modest temperature elevation. In some cases, however, it can present as temperature lability. The goal of treatment is to prevent further complications because elevation of body temperature is associated with increased metabolic demands, exacerbation of neuronal excitotoxicity, and disruption of the blood-brain barrier. Management includes the use of cooling blankets and antipyretics, such as aspirin, acetaminophen, and nonsteroidal anti-inflammatory drugs. Other medications that have been used include dopaminergics (e.g., bromocriptine or amantadine), dantrolene sodium, chlorpromazine, clonidine, and propranolol.

Sleep Disorders (pp. 1098–1099)

• Although disturbance of sleep is a common observation in brain injury survivors, its exact incidence is not well known. One study reports an incidence of 73% and 52% in inpatient and outpatient settings, respectively. Sleep disorders following brain injury can be classified as either insufficient or excessive sleep.

TABLE 49–10 Some Common Causes of Dizziness in TBI

Brainstem involvement	Perilymphatic fistula
Posterior circulation insufficiency	Labyrinthine concussion
Vestibular impairment (cranial nerve VIII involvement)	Meniere's syndrome
	Cervical vertigo
Ocular abnormalities	Migraine
Orthostatic hypotension	Medications
Benign paroxysmal positional vertigo	

Insufficient sleep can be further categorized as a problem with either initiation or maintenance, or both. Excessive daytime sleepiness might be caused by poor night-time sleep, narcolepsy, or sleep apnea, among others. Too much or too little sleep can impair an individual's arousal, cognition, behavior, and ability to participate in therapies.

• Various neurochemicals have been implicated in the sleep-wake cycle. Disruption of these chemicals following a brain injury might theoretically form the basis for post-traumatic sleep disturbance; however, other causes need to be identified in order to render the appropriate treatment. Causative or aggravating conditions include medications, pain, hypoxia, sleep apnea, stress, prior sleep history, poor environmental conditions, excessive caffeine intake, and nicotine use.

• Once other correctable etiologies have been identified, appropriate measures need to be instituted. Nonpharmacological strategies include environmental management (e.g., low noise and light, comfortable room temperature), discontinuation or change in administration time of alerting medications, and the avoidance of caffeine and nicotine. Table 49–22 in the Textbook lists some commonly used hypnotics.

Pulmonary Complications (pp. 1099–1101)

• Pulmonary complications associated with brain injuries can directly result from the trauma itself (e.g., pneumothorax), subsequent instrumentation (e.g., intubation), or associated neurological deficits. Even when promptly managed, these problems prolong the need for acute intensive management, prevent early mobilization, and hinder full participation in rehabilitation.

• Acute pulmonary complications resulting from trauma include pneumothorax, hemothorax, atelectasis, bacterial and chemical pneumonia, prolonged mechanical ventilation, and neurogenic pulmonary edema (NPE). In addition to complicating medical recovery, these conditions also increase the risk of secondary hypoxic injury. Neurogenic pulmonary edema, associated with isolated brain injury or hemorrhage, is probably related to adult respiratory distress syndrome (ARDS). Increased intracranial pressure, heightened sympathetic activity, and alteration in pulmonary capillary permeability are implicated in its causation. Clinical findings suggestive of NPE include dyspnea, hypoxia, decreased pulmonary vascular compliance, and appearance of "fluffy" infiltrates on chest radiographs. It is usually a self-limiting complication treated with supportive measures. Sympatholytic and inotropic agents might also play a role in treatment.

• Pneumonia is a common complication of TBI. Up to 80% of patients with TBI develop early onset pneumonia during the first 7 days postinjury. Early pneumonia is usually nosocomial. Intubated TBI patients are at particular risk because of instrumentation, mechanical ventilation, and compromise of the immune system. Common organisms include *Staphylococcus aureus, Haemophilus influenzae,* and *Pseudomonas aeruginosa.* Important risk factors include intubation at the scene of the injury, GCS score less than 5, evidence of aspiration, and swallowing dysfunction.

• In the rehabilitation setting, aspiration is a significant concern because it is a potential cause of pneumonia. Individuals with TBI are at risk of aspiration of stomach contents because of disruption of the normal cough reflex, decreased level of consciousness, decreased oropharyngeal sensation, and reduction in lower esophageal sphincter tone. Early tracheostomy plus percutaneous endoscopic gastrostomy has been shown to decrease the risk of clinically significant aspiration. It is important for the clinician to recognize that the presence of an inflated tracheostomy tube is not an absolute protection against aspiration. Bypassing the oral route through a gastrostomy or jejunostomy tube also does not guarantee protection from aspiration. In fact, the presence of a feeding tube can decrease the lower esophageal sphincter tone. Moreover, there appears to be no significant difference in the occurrence of aspiration pneumonia in individuals with intragastric or transpyloric feeding tubes.

• In most brain injury rehabilitation units, newly admitted patients are assessed for swallowing function by a speech pathologist. The appropriate fluid and diet consistency is then prescribed. This procedure is performed regardless of diet recommendations from the transferring hospital because patients' swallowing abilities can change rapidly in the course of recovery. Bedside evaluation of oral motor strength and coordination, management of secretions, ability to swallow different fluid and diet consistencies, and estimation of laryngeal elevation can be helpful in identifying those at risk for aspiration. The authors have not found the "gag reflex" helpful for this purpose. The presence of a right middle or lower lobe infiltrate on the chest radiographs should raise the suspicion of aspiration pneumonia. Because some individuals are "silent aspirators" (i.e., have actual tracheal penetration or aspiration of food in the absence of clinical symptoms such as coughing or choking), modified barium swallow or videofluoroscopic study are important diagnostic adjuncts.

• Early in recovery, an artificial airway is often necessary to prevent hypoxia and improve pulmonary toilet. As recovery progresses, the need for the artificial airway lessens; once this stage is reached, the clinician should consider decannulation (removal of the tracheostomy tube). Timely decannulation may prevent many complications, and is typically considered when the patient does not require oxygen support, is able to effectively manage secretions, and is at a low risk for aspiration.

• Decannulation is commonly accomplished by first weaning down the tube size; then plugging the tracheostomy tube over a continuous 24-hour period; and, finally, by removal. In the authors' center, the tube is downsized to a cuffless variety before plugging in order to prevent accidental suffocation. Tracheostomy tube plugging is begun for about 2 hours. If the patient is able to tolerate this (i.e., able to maintain good oxygenation as gauged by symptoms and pulse oximetry) and able to handle his or her secretions, plugging is advanced by 2- to 6-hour intervals daily, depending on patient tolerance. This continues until the tube is plugged continuously for 24 hours. The tube is then removed.

Gastrointestinal and Nutritional Complications
(pp. 1101–1103)

Early Nutrition (pp. 1101–1102)
• It is estimated that resting energy expenditure in patients with severe TBI increases by an average of 40%. Hyperglycemia with increased rates of glucose turnover and resistance to insulin are found in those with TBI, even in the absence of physical trauma. Most trauma centers now take into account the nutritional needs of acutely injured patients by quickly initiating enteral tube feedings. Patients who have suffered severe visceral trauma can require supplementation by hyperalimentation. Although total enteral nutrition (TEN) is pre-

ferred over total parenteral nutrition (TPN), TPN should be promptly given while increasing TEN to a goal of 2 to 2.5 g protein/kg/day and 25 to 35 nonprotein kcal/kg/day. Despite aggressive efforts at early nutritional support, it can take up to 3 weeks to achieve a positive nitrogen balance, even if positive caloric balance has been reached. Many TBI patients still need aggressive nutritional management upon admission to rehabilitation. The physiatrist and dietitian should also pay attention to fiber, vitamins, minerals, and isotonicity of enteral feedings, in addition to calories and protein. Weekly weights, as well as monthly measurements of serum prealbumin, are appropriate ways to monitor nutritional status during the rehabilitation phase.

Dysphagia (p. 1102)
• The incidence of dysphagia in patients with TBI at the time of transfer to rehabilitation is about 27%. Videofluoroscopy typically shows that the majority of patients have a delay or absence of swallowing responses; about half show reduced tongue control; about a third have reduced pharyngeal transit; and some will also have reduced laryngeal closure, elevation, or spasms. Acutely, thin liquids are to be avoided because they are typically the most difficult to handle from a swallowing perspective and, as a result, can lead to aspiration pneumonia.
• Patients with swallowing difficulties often have concomitant cognitive impairments. They typically need to be reminded and monitored to employ compensatory strategies. Their diets need to be changed in a sequential fashion (i.e., from pureed, to ground, to chopped, to soft, to regular) as their use of compensatory mechanisms increases and/or their swallowing improves. During this time the patient is at high risk for developing aspiration pneumonia.
• Patients who fail to progress cognitively, are unable to follow commands, have significant swallowing difficulties, and are documented to aspirate or are at high risk for aspiration need to be fed via an enteral tube. If enteral feeding will be necessary for longer than 3 to 4 weeks, a gastrostomy or jejunostomy tube is preferable to a nasogastric tube. The tube can be placed through an open surgical procedure or using an endoscopic technique. Prolonged use of a nasogastric tube may lead to nasal ulceration, nasopharyngeal irritation, sinus infection, and discomfort. Nasogastric tubes can also aggravate agitation and cause the patient to pull out the tube. When this happens, frequent tube reinsertions might have to be done, increasing the risk for nasopharyngeal trauma.

Other Gastrointestinal Complications (pp. 1102–1103)
• Stress gastritis can occur acutely in patients with TBI. Almost all patients are still on ulcer prophylaxis at the time of admission to rehabilitation. The clinician should discontinue the medication, when feasible, to minimize adverse drug effects and drug-drug interactions, simplify the drug regimen, and save unnecessary expense.
• Nausea and vomiting are commonly encountered gastrointestinal complications of TBI. Although these appear to be relatively minor symptoms, they can increase the risk of aspiration pneumonia, interrupt therapies, and cause distress to the patient and family. The etiologies of nausea and vomiting in TBI are multifactorial (Table 49–11).
• Small bowel feeding through a jejunostomy is a treatment option. Jejunostomy was thought to decrease the risk of aspiration because it bypasses the pylorus. A recent study, however, failed to demonstrate this purported advantage

TABLE 49–11 Some Causes of Nausea and Vomiting in TBI

Intracranial
    Increased intracranial pressure
    Space-occupying lesion
    Hydrocephalus
Ophthalmologic
    Ocular muscle imbalance
Vestibular
Respiratory
    Associated with excessive gagging and coughing
Gastrointestinal
    Gastritis and ulcer
    Impaired LES (lower esophageal sphincter) tone
    Impaired gastric emptying
    Constipation
    Pancreatitis
    Hepatitis
Infection
Iatrogenic
    Medications that cause gastric irritation
    Medications that directly induce nausea and vomiting
    Medication overdose
Migraine
Psychogenic

of a jejunostomy over a gastrostomy tube. Jejunostomy can give rise to problems with nutrition and medication administration because the absorptive capacity of the small bowel is less than that of the stomach. Jejunostomy also requires continuous feedings, and is not ideal during rehabilitation because it limits mobility and therapies. Unless the patient is suffering from severe reflux and aspiration, gastrostomy is the preferred route.

• There can be advantages to having both a jejunostomy and gastrostomy concurrently in those with impaired gastric emptying. The jejunostomy can be used for feeding and the gastrostomy for medication administration and decompression to prevent aspiration. If reflux remains a concern, the head of the bed needs to be elevated and the patient should be tried on various formulas or smaller feedings.

• The "blue dye test" can help identify individuals with tracheostomies who aspirate oral secretions. This is performed on patients who have a good reflexive swallow and are able to tolerate tracheostomy cuff deflation. On the morning of the test, 4 drops of blue dye are placed orally and the tracheostomy cuff is deflated. More dye may be added at least every 4 hours. The night before the test, blue dye in the tube feedings is discontinued. The presence of blue dye in tracheal secretions is indicative of aspiration or tracheo-esophageal fistula.

• Prokinetic agents can be used to facilitate gastric emptying. The use of metoclopramide (Reglan) should be avoided. This drug is like the phenothiazines; although it can help initially with reflux by increasing gastric emptying in a small percentage of patients, it is not particularly useful in the long term. More-over, it is known to cause significant cognitive difficulties for patients, especially for those regaining consciousness. Cisapride (Propulsid) is a more attractive alternative because, unlike metoclopramide, it does not cause central dopamin-ergic blockade and extrapyramidal effects are rare. In the event that cisapride cannot be used, erythromycin might be a useful alternative to improve gastric emptying.

Incontinence (p. 1103)
• Fecal incontinence following brain injury is fairly common, especially in patients with significant cognitive impairments. Following brain injury, patients can have an uninhibited neurogenic bowel and be unaware of the need to defe-cate in a timely and appropriate manner. Constipation or diarrhea can also be significant problems. The development of a daily bowel-training program is appropriate regardless of the patient's cognitive status. This can be accomplished through the use of high-fiber enteral feedings or oral supplementation of fiber and the use of a glycerin rectal suppository daily or every other day. Use of digital stimulation should be avoided because it can be misinterpreted by patients who have cognitive difficulties.
• Diarrhea can be the result of impaction, osmolar overload from tube feeding, or *Clostridium difficile* colitis. Both osmolar overload and impaction can be pre-vented by the use of high-protein isotonic feedings that provide essential vita-mins and minerals (e.g., Jevity or Enrich).

Gastrointestinal Bleeding (p. 1103)
• As with most polytrauma patients, the patient with a brain injury has an increased risk of gastrointestinal bleeding secondary to stress ulceration during the acute care phase. It is not unusual for patients to be placed on prophylaxis with H_2 antagonists such as cimetidine or ranitidine. Because cognitive and behavioral disturbances have been noted in patients on H_2 antagonists, these medications should be withdrawn once the risk of gastrointestinal bleeding has passed.

Thrombophlebitis (pp. 1103–1104)

• Deep venous thrombosis (DVT) is estimated to occur in up to half of cases following major head trauma. Important risk factors for DVT following brain injury include immobility, muscle weakness, associated bone fracture, direct vascular trauma, and venous catheterization. Typical clinical signs, such as calf pain and leg swelling, are not present in all cases. This is a concern because of the potential for pulmonary embolism (PE), which is the initial clinical presen-tation in up to 80%. Early detection is important to avoid morbidities and poten-tial fatal consequences (the incidence of fatal PE is estimated at 1%). Impedance plethysmography (IPG), Doppler ultrasound, D-dimer assay, I-fibrinogen scan-ning, and radionuclide and contrast venography are commonly used methods of DVT detection. Their sensitivities and specificities vary greatly, especially in the absence of clinical findings.
• Commonly used prophylactic measures include intermittent pneumatic compression, graded compression elastic stockings, and anticoagulants (e.g., low-dose unfractionated and low-molecular-weight heparin, warfarin, and aspirin). The treatment of PE or DVT proximal to the calf includes anticoagu-

lation. Following initiation of treatment with unfractionated heparin, warfarin is initiated once an activated partial thromboplastin time 1.5 times the control is reached. An initial dose of 5 mg of warfarin is recommended in order to avoid adverse effects such as excessive anticoagulation and the development of a potential hypercoagulable state. The treatment goal with warfarin is an International Normalized Ratio (INR) between 2 and 3. In those at high risk for bleeding complications, inferior vena cava (IVC) filter placement (Greenfield Filter or Modified Bird's Nest Filter) should be considered. The use of anticoagulants following TBI with associated intracranial hemorrhage is controversial. It should also be used with caution in agitated or confused patients at significant risk for falls. Currently, there are no guidelines as to the optimal time of initiation of anticoagulation following trauma with associated intracranial bleeding.

Genitourinary Complications (p. 1104)

• Neurogenic bladder following TBI is rare; if it does exist, it is usually because of uninhibited detrusor hyperreflexia causing the patient to void small amounts frequently with complete bladder emptying. Patients can usually be adequately managed with an external collection device, such as a condom catheter in males or a diaper in females. These measures should be continued until patients are aware of their surroundings and have sufficient memory to benefit from being offered a commode or bedpan on a regular basis. Patients can also have detrusor hyporeflexia as a result of bladder overdistension that occurs with iatrogenic or traumatic outlet obstruction. These patients usually require prolonged intermittent catheterization (ICP) or an indwelling Foley catheter until this problem has resolved, which may take weeks to months. It is the rare, primarily brainstem-injured patient with detrusor sphincter dyssynergia who needs intermittent catheterization or prolonged Foley drainage and complete urologic studies.

Musculoskeletal Complications (p. 1104)

Heterotopic Ossification (p. 1104)
• Heterotopic ossification (HO) is the formation of mature lamellar bone in soft tissue and periarticular areas. The reported incidence of HO ranges from 11% to 76%, reflecting differences in study populations and detection methods. However, only 10% to 20% of cases have clinically significant HO.
• Significant risk factors in TBI include prolonged coma (longer than 1 month), immobilization, and limb spasticity. Ectopic bone following TBI usually forms around major joints including elbows, shoulders, hips, and knees. HO often causes limitation of joint range of motion, joint deformity, and pain. It can also cause peripheral nerve compression, vascular compression, and lymphedema. Diagnostic findings include transient depression in serum calcium in the early stages and elevated serum alkaline phosphatase, which reflects osteoblastic activity. Increased alkaline phosphatase is not specific for HO because concurrent fractures or hepatic abnormalities can have a similar effect. Triple-phase bone scan demonstrates abnormalities sooner than plain radiographs.
• Prophylaxis with etidronate disodium is controversial. By the time physiatrists receive these patients, typically a few weeks postinjury, HO might have started

to develop, and prophylactic therapy becomes moot. In the presence of clinical findings suggestive of HO (e.g., loss of range of motion and joint or limb pain), efforts should be concentrated on early detection and treatment of HO.
• Surgical excision is the definitive treatment of HO. In general, surgery should be considered after several months from the time of diagnosis to allow the HO to "mature" and therefore lessen the chances of excessive blood loss during the procedure.

Sexual and Reproductive Functioning (pp. 1104–1105)

• In addition to physical impairments that might hinder sexual functioning and satisfaction, personality changes, impulsiveness and inappropriateness, and changes in libido can all contribute to the problem in patients with TBI. Patients with frontal lobe lesions reported a higher level of sexual functioning and satisfaction than those without a similar lesion. But patients with frontal lobe lesions are also more likely to display disinhibition and inappropriate sexual behavior, which can pose difficulties not only for patients, but also for their interactions with families, the hospital staff, and the public at large. At the other extreme, some TBI patients appear to lose interest in sex. This can also be true of their partners, who may be affected by a change in their roles from partner to caregiver. Obviously, this has the potential to disrupt relationships because many couples draw upon sex as an expression of love and intimacy.
• Medical treatment (e.g., drugs for erectile dysfunction or penile prostheses) are available, but contributing factors to loss of sexual drive, such as depression and medications, should be addressed first.
• It is not uncommon for menstruation to cease after a TBI. In many cases, it can take up to 1 year for normal menses to return. In the event that resumption of menses is delayed, or if there are significant changes in menstrual characteristics (e.g., metromenorrhagia), it is reasonable to refer the patient to an obstetrician for further gynecologic, and possibly endocrinologic, evaluation. For sexually active patients and their partners, counseling regarding birth control may also be carried out. It should be noted, however, that the use of oral contraceptives is a concern for those at risk for venous thrombosis.
• In some cases, pregnancy during TBI has affected therapeutic decisions during and after rehabilitation. Certain medications used to treat TBI complications have teratogenic potential, some documented (e.g., phenytoin) and others unknown (e.g., botulinum toxin for spasticity). For patients desiring to resume parenting after recovery, parenting activities (e.g., diaper changes or breast-feeding) can be incorporated into the various physical and occupational therapies. (See Chapter 30 for further information on sexuality.)

REHABILITATION OF PATIENTS WITH PEDIATRIC BRAIN INJURY (p. 1105)

• Pediatric brain injury differs in several important ways from brain injury in the adult. Pathologically, TBI in infants and children produces a higher incidence of diffuse cerebral swelling and a lower incidence of intracranial hemorrhage than seen in adults. Special assessment techniques, such as pediatric coma scales and the Children's Orientation and Amnesia Test (COAT), are needed to evaluate the level of consciousness and duration of PTA in infants and children. Severe childhood TBI appears to have a better prognosis for recovery of consciousness and mobility. One unique feature of pediatric brain injury is that certain injuries suffered at younger ages can lead to functional outcomes worse than those arising from the same injuries suffered in adulthood (e.g., severe TBI during infancy producing mental retardation). This vulnerability has been attributed to disruption of the normal development process, leading to a slower rate of skill acquisition.

• A second unique component of pediatric brain injury rehabilitation is the need for long-term follow-up of the child's progress in school because the child with brain injury is presented with increasing challenges at higher grades.

MANAGEMENT OF MILD TRAUMATIC BRAIN INJURY
(pp. 1105–1106)

• Diagnostic criteria for mild TBI are presented above in Table 49–2. The American Congress of Rehabilitation Medicine defines mild TBI as a traumatic disruption of brain functioning manifested by at least one of the following: (1) loss of consciousness; (2) loss of memory for events occurring pre- or post-injury; (3) alteration in mental status at the time of injury; (4) physical symptoms attributable to brain injury (e.g., tinnitus, visual changes, memory disturbances, fatigue, and anosmia); and (5) post-traumatic cognitive impairment.

• A rational strategy for managing mild TBI is based on chronicity, objective evidence of brain injury, and presence of extracranial injuries. During the acute stage following mild TBI, patients should receive a CT scan of the head because the presence or absence of a traumatic brain lesion on CT scanning is the most reliable indicator of prognosis. In a healthy pediatric patient or young adult with mild TBI and without disability from associated injuries, the absence of brain trauma on CT scanning (i.e., uncomplicated mild TBI) should cause activity restrictions for a few days or weeks. However, when brain trauma is present on CT scanning (i.e., complicated mild TBI), the resumption of preinjury activities might be delayed beyond this time and, in a minority of patients, some preinjury activities cannot be resumed.

• Techniques in the management of acute mild TBI are education and activity restrictions. Complaints of headache and dizziness are common for several months postinjury and should be investigated. The patient and family should be forewarned about cognitive and behavioral changes and about circumstances that might worsen them (e.g., inadequate sleep, substance abuse, and stress). The likelihood of a rapid return to preinjury activities should be emphasized to the patient and family. Brief neuropsychological testing might be useful in identifying cognitive deficits during this stage. If injury-related cognitive deficits are present, the patient should be encouraged to temporarily limit activities and to resume them gradually. For example, a patient with memory deficits might be encouraged to delay returning to work until cleared to do so. Return to work can begin on a part-time or light-duty basis, possibly for only a few days before resuming full duty. In some cases it might be necessary to resume work duties through one or more intermediate steps.

• Although isolated mild TBI is not usually seen in rehabilitation settings, it commonly co-occurs with orthopedic or spinal cord injuries that do require rehabilitation. In the case of mild TBI patients who are undergoing rehabilitation for other injuries, the strategy of recommending activity restrictions might be impossible to implement. Instead, it might be necessary to modify the rehabilitation program in order to avoid or circumvent problems related to TBI (e.g., minimize sedating antispasticity or analgesic medications, direct teaching toward family members, or extend the length of stay).

• Management of mild TBI in the chronic stage remains controversial. The label of postconcussional syndrome has traditionally been applied to multiple post-injury complaints of dizziness, headache, emotional instability, and cognitive difficulty. In recent years, it has been established that the incidence of secondary gain and somatoform disorders in causing chronic postconcussional complaints is greater than previously recognized. Useful techniques in determining the validity of symptom complaints include specialized neuropsychological tests (e.g., forced choice recognition testing). MRI of the brain detects traumatic lesions in a minority of mild TBI patients whose brain CT findings are normal, but the prognostic value of MRI findings in uncomplicated mild TBI patients is undetermined.

POST-TRAUMATIC HEADACHE (p. 1106)

• Headache is a common complaint of patients after trauma to the head or neck. It must be emphasized that post-traumatic headache (PTH) is not a diagnosis: it is merely a symptom that can have various etiologies (Table 49–12). Treatment of post-traumatic headache is directed to correcting the underlying etiology. Treatment often includes both pharmacological agents (see Table 49–25 in the Textbook), and other treatment strategies such as biofeedback and relaxation training.

SPORTS-RELATED TRAUMATIC BRAIN INJURY
(pp. 1106–1107)

• Increased awareness of TBI resulting from sports and recreation parallels the continued popularity of sports and growing attention from the media. It is esti-

TABLE 49–12 Some Causes of Post-Traumatic Headache

Intracranial
Injury to pain-sensitive structures (venous sinuses, dura in the base of the brain, blood vessels, cranial nerves)

Extracranial
Neuroma
Injury to skin, muscle, arteries
Injury to periosteum
Sinusitis
Temporomandibular joint dysfunction
Cranial nerve abnormalities (e.g., ophthalmoplegia)
Myofascial pain

Others
Adverse effect of medications and other substances (e.g., caffeine)
Co-morbid medical conditions (e.g., uncontrolled hypertension)
Seizures
Poor sleep
Psychological factors

mated that up to 87% of boxers have either clinical or radiologic evidence of TBI. Indeed, the cognitive impairment in boxers has a special designation: *dementia pugilistica.* Nevertheless, boxing's popularity is unabated, despite the fact that the American Medical Association is on record favoring a ban of the sport. Approximately 250,000 concussions have been attributed to football injuries per year. Practically every contact sport—basketball, soccer, and wrestling included—has the potential for TBI. The same is true for some recreational activities such as snow- and jet-skiing.

• The American Academy of Neurology recently published a report of its Quality Standards Subcommittee on practice parameters for the management of concussion in sports. The common symptoms of concussion were categorized as either early, occurring minutes to hours after the event; or late, occurring days to weeks afterward. Among the early symptoms are headache, dizziness or vertigo, lack of awareness of surroundings, and nausea or vomiting. Late symptoms include persistent low-grade headache, lightheadedness, poor attention and concentration, memory dysfunction, easy fatigability, irritability and low frustration tolerance, intolerance of bright lights or difficulty focusing vision, intolerance of loud noises, anxiety, depressed mood, and sleep disturbance. Based on a review of the literature, a grading scale and treatment recommendations were established.

ETHICAL ISSUES (pp. 1107–1108)

• Brain injury raises many profound and difficult ethical issues. Although some of these ethical issues can be addressed only at a collective level (e.g., how society allocates resources for people with brain injuries), others arise in the daily practice of rehabilitation professionals.

• One of the most commonly encountered problems in brain injury rehabilitation is the assessment of competency. Determining a patient's competence to make decisions is crucial because, as clinicians, we have an obligation to honor the wishes of competent adult patients. At the same time, we are committed to preventing the harm that can result from decisions made by an incompetent patient. The practical question of whether or not to accede to a patient's wishes depends on our assessment of their competence to make decisions. Unfortunately, evidence suggests that clinicians working with people with brain injuries tend to neglect issues of competence and consent.

• To begin with, the clinician should recognize that competence is domain specific. That is, patients can be determined to be competent to make certain decisions (e.g., regarding medical treatment) but not others (e.g., regarding financial management). In addition, recent commentators have emphasized evaluating the process by which a decision is made. That is, the focus is on how a decision is made, not what is decided.

• The assessment of this process involves the direct examination of the abilities central to decision-making capacity. These include the abilities to *choose,* to *understand* relevant information, to *appreciate* its significance for one's own situation, and to *reason* logically with that information.

• If a person is found to be incompetent to make treatment decisions, substitute or *surrogate* decision makers must be identified. Clinicians should be guided by the relevant laws in their states to determine who the surrogate may be and what sort of limits (if any) apply to their decision-making authority.

• One of the most difficult questions a family member or clinician is called upon to make is that of withholding or withdrawing life-sustaining treatments.

This issue has dominated bioethics for the last two decades, and many of the most prominent cases have involved people with severe brain injuries. Most often, the family of a severely injured patient makes the request to withhold or withdraw treatment. The patient is usually in a vegetative state; however, the number of similar requests for minimally conscious patients appears to be rising.

• Although controversy continues, a bioethical and legal consensus is beginning to coalesce around certain fundamental principles. The primary obligation of the clinician in these situations is to ascertain what the patient's prior beliefs and preferences were. This information is most often obtained from the patient's family. A recent U.S. Supreme Court decision has confirmed that decisions regarding withholding or withdrawing life-sustaining treatments from incompetent patients can be guided by their previously expressed wishes.

• Clearly, there is no societal consensus on how to proceed when a patient's previous wishes are not known. In these situations, clinicians should seek the guidance of hospital ethics committees as well as legal counsel. In addition, physicians who are uncomfortable with the decisions reached can consider transferring the care of the patient to another physician. Finally, it should be emphasized that hasty decisions are rarely necessary. Especially if a patient is in a vegetative state, little harm is done in taking time to address all considerations.

• A less dramatic but far more common ethical issue confronting physicians involves the decision to initiate psychoactive medications or physical restraints. Some of the considerations that should guide the use of psychoactive agents were discussed in the section on the management of agitation. These same principles (e.g., obtaining consent, ensuring that the intervention is in the patient's best interest, exhausting less restrictive alternatives) apply when choosing to physically restrain a patient.

• It is also important to recognize the disadvantages of physical restraints. Evidence is accumulating that restraints are not particularly effective (e.g., in preventing falls). Moreover, the restraints themselves pose a physical risk to the patient, including reported cases of death. Because of the ethical issues involved, many institutions are adopting a minimal-restraint or restraint-free policy.

CHAPTER

50

Original Chapter by Elliot J. Roth, M.D., and Richard L. Harvey, M.D.

Rehabilitation of Stroke Syndromes

- The ultimate goal of the stroke rehabilitation program is long-term, safe, independent, energy-efficient, pleasurable, and high-quality functioning in the community. Achieving this goal requires addressing a variety of medical, functional, and psychosocial issues.
1. Prevention, recognition, management, and minimizing the impact of preexisting medical conditions, ongoing general health functions, and secondary medical complications
2. Training for maximal functional independence
3. Facilitating optimal psychosocial adaptation and coping by both the patient and family
4. Promoting community reintegration; resumption of prior life roles; and the return to home, family, recreational, and vocational activities
5. Enhancing quality of life

DEFINITIONS (pp. 1118–1119)

Stroke or Cerebrovascular Accident? (p. 1118)

- The term *stroke* connotes the sudden and surprising nature of symptomatic cerebrovascular disease and is preferred over the more scientific sounding phrase *cerebrovascular accident* (or CVA). We define stroke as a nontraumatic brain injury caused by occlusion or rupture of cerebral blood vessels that results in sudden neurological deficit. This definition excludes nonvascular conditions that can present with stroke-like symptoms (e.g., seizure, syncope, traumatic brain injury, and brain tumor).

Pathophysiological Classification of Stroke (p. 1118)

- Stroke is a neurological syndrome caused by vascular etiologies. Intracranial hemorrhage accounts for 15% of all strokes and can be further divided into intracerebral (10%) and subarachnoid (5%) hemorrhage. Subarachnoid hemorrhages typically result from aneurysmal rupture of a cerebral artery. Rupture of weakened vessels within brain parenchyma as a result of hypertension, arteriovenous malformation, or tumor results in intracerebral hemorrhage.

727

• Some 85% of strokes are caused by ischemic brain injury resulting from large-vessel (40%) or small-vessel (20%) thrombosis; cerebral embolism (20%); and other less common causes (5%), such as cerebral vasculitis or cerebral hypo-perfusion. Vessel occlusion from thrombosis occurs most commonly in the presence of atherosclerotic cerebrovascular disease. Vascular changes found in small, deep, penetrating arteries as associated with chronic hypertension can lead to small-vessel thrombosis. Cerebral emboli are usually of cardiac origin and are often a result of chronic ischemic cardiovascular disease with secondary ventricular wall hypokinesis or atrial arrhythmia.

Temporal Classification of Stroke (pp. 1118–1119)

• A transient ischemic attack (TIA) is an event in which neurological symptoms develop and disappear over several minutes and completely resolve within 24 hours. TIAs are most commonly associated with atherosclerotic carotid artery disease and they should provoke an urgent diagnostic evaluation.
• A transient neurological event that lasts longer than 24 hours is called a reversible ischemic neurological deficit (RIND). Such events are clinically rare and their etiology is unknown. It is likely that RINDs result from small infarctions (lacunes) of the deep subcortical gray and white matter.
• Embolic strokes generally have a quick onset and fully develop in a matter of minutes, whereas hemorrhagic strokes often evolve over 1 to 2 hours. Thrombotic strokes can have a rapid or a prolonged interval of onset, lasting many hours. *Stroke in evolution* denotes an unstable ischemic event characterized by the progressive development of more severe neurological impairment, and it is often associated with active occlusive thrombosis of a major cerebral artery. Once a stable neurological status is reached, clinicians refer to the event as a *completed stroke.*

EPIDEMIOLOGY (pp. 1119–1120)

Stroke Mortality in the United States (pp. 1119–1120)

• Stroke is the third leading cause of death in the United States. A reduction in annual stroke mortality has taken place within the United States in the last century. In particular, a sharp decline in the annual stroke deaths began in the 1970s and continued into the 1980s. The improved detection and treatment of hypertension is directly responsible for the steep decline in stroke mortality.
• Beginning in the 1980s the steep decline in mortality began to flatten, coincident with improved diagnostic sensitivity of cranial CT and MRI. Improved stroke detection may explain the decline and more recent increase in stroke incidence.

Stroke Survival (p. 1120)

• The prevalence of stroke survivors has doubled over the past 25 years. The major contributor to the increased proportion of stroke survivors is reduced mortality as a result of better management of medical co-morbidity and complications. Better detection and management of coronary artery disease, prevention of aspiration pneumonia by identification and treatment of dysphagia, prevention of pulmonary embolism using prophylactic measures, and reduction of general disability and immobility by active rehabilitation care has improved long-term survival after stroke.

STROKE RISK FACTORS (pp. 1120–1122)

Hypertension (pp. 1120–1121)

• Evidence supports public health efforts aimed at reducing the prevalence of poorly controlled blood pressure, thereby reducing the risk of stroke and heart disease. Improved public education, detection, and treatment of hypertension will have a positive impact on the further decline of stroke incidence and mortality. Hypertension is defined as a systolic pressure greater than 165 mm Hg or a diastolic pressure greater than 95 mm Hg. Hypertension increases the relative risk of stroke by a factor of 6. Among stroke survivors, 67% have chronic hypertension.

• Reduction of diastolic blood pressure is associated with a reduction in stroke risk in both hypertensive and normotensive subjects.

• Isolated systolic hypertension is more common among individuals older than 60 years and is an independent risk factor for stroke and cardiovascular disease.

Risk Factors Modifiable by Lifestyle Changes (p. 1121)

• Smoking is independently associated with an increased risk of atherothrombotic and hemorrhagic stroke. Cessation of smoking reverses risk to that of non-smokers within 5 years after quitting.

• The influence of hypercholesterolemia in the development of coronary artery disease and atherosclerosis indicates at least an indirect risk factor for stroke. Reduced dietary intake of cholesterol and saturated fatty acids has been recommended for adults with total cholesterol levels greater than 200 mg/dL or low-density lipoprotein (LDL) cholesterol levels greater than 160 mg/dL. If dietary measures are ineffective, cholesterol-reducing medications are recommended.

• Obesity at least indirectly increases stroke risk. Weight loss has a positive influence on blood pressure and diabetic control and likely has a risk-reducing effect on stroke and cardiovascular disease.

• Heart disease increases stroke risk by two to six times normal. Control of hypertension, cessation of smoking, and reduction of serum cholesterol can reduce the development of heart disease as well as prevent stroke. Prevention of heart disease through lifestyle changes has a positive influence on stroke prevention. However, in the presence of established conditions such as atrial fibrillation or left ventricular failure, the use of medical means to reduce stroke risk can become important.

Risk Factors Modifiable by Medical Means (pp. 1121–1122)

• Transient ischemic attacks are associated with carotid artery disease and are an important sign of stroke risk. Medical or surgical treatment for carotid artery disease in patients experiencing TIA can considerably reduce stroke incidence and mortality. The presence of an asymptomatic carotid bruit is an indication of atherosclerotic disease, and is a predictor of myocardial infarction and cardiovascular death as well as stroke.

• Diabetes mellitus increases the relative risk of ischemic stroke to three to six times. This risk can be partly attributed to the higher prevalence of hypertension and heart disease among those with diabetes, but even after controlling for these factors, diabetes independently doubles stroke risk. Two factors that increase blood viscosity, hematocrit and serum fibrinogen, have also been implicated as risk factors for stroke.

Nonmodifiable Risk Factors (p. 1122)

• Risk factors for stroke that are not modifiable include age, sex, race, and previous stroke.

STROKE PREVENTION (pp. 1122–1124)

• Public awareness of modifiable risk factors for stroke, medical management of risk factors, and the active promotion of lifestyle changes have the potential to decrease stroke.

Antiplatelet Therapy (pp. 1122–1123)

Primary Prevention (p. 1122)
• Currently, the *routine* use of antiplatelets for stroke and cardiovascular disease prophylaxis is not recommended. Decisions to use aspirin for primary prevention should be based on the patient's age, risk for stroke or MI, and risk for bleeding.

Secondary Prevention (pp. 1122–1123)
• Antiplatelet agents reduce the risk of nonfatal stroke by 31%. Subgroups of hypertensive and diabetic subjects also benefited from treatment.
• Aspirin is the most commonly prescribed antiplatelet agent for secondary stroke and cardiovascular disease prevention. By irreversibly inhibiting cyclo-oxygenase-dependent platelet aggregation, aspirin achieves a significant antiplatelet effect. Trials have supported the use of doses between 30 and 1500 mg/day. The principal advantage that aspirin has over other antiplatelet agents is its low cost and over-the-counter availability.
• Clopidogrel and ticlopidine are newer agents that prevent platelet aggregation for the life of the cell by directly inhibiting adenosine diphosphate (ADP)-induced platelet aggregation. They both lack antipyretic, anti-inflammatory, and analgesic effects, and they do not affect the integrity of the gastric mucosa. Although both medications are effective antiplatelet agents and prevent secondary stroke, the use of ticlopidine is limited by the important side effects of rash and diarrhea and reversible neutropenia. Clopidogrel lacks these side effects, making it a good choice for secondary stroke prevention in patients who cannot tolerate the gastric effects of aspirin.

Anticoagulation and Antiplatelet Therapy in Atrial Fibrillation (pp. 1123–1124)

• Individuals with nonvalvular atrial fibrillation have five times the relative risk for cardioembolic stroke, and those with rheumatic heart disease have a 17-fold increase. Clinical trials have supported the use of aspirin to prevent primary cardioembolic stroke in nonvalvular atrial fibrillation. Use of warfarin anticoagu-

lation for primary stroke prevention in nonvalvular atrial fibrillation also reduces relative stroke risk.
• Warfarin is more effective than aspirin for stroke prevention in atrial fibrillation. Care must be taken when considering anticoagulation in patients older than 75 years because the risk of intracranial hemorrhage is higher in elderly persons.
• Individuals with rheumatic valvular disease and atrial fibrillation benefit from anticoagulation with warfarin for stroke prevention.

Surgical Management of Carotid Artery Disease (p. 1124)

• Recent evidence supports the use of carotid endarterectomy in combination with aspirin as the treatment of choice for both symptomatic and asymptomatic high-grade carotid artery disease. Antiplatelet therapy after carotid surgery remains critical for successful overall outcome.

STROKE PATHOPHYSIOLOGY (pp. 1124–1126)

Ischemic Stroke (pp. 1124–1125)

• The unifying pathophysiology is cerebral ischemia from compromise of cerebral blood flow.

Thrombosis (p. 1124)

• Infarction from cerebral thrombosis is strongly associated with atherosclerotic cerebrovascular disease. Atherosclerotic plaque formation occurs commonly at major vascular branching sites, including the common carotid and vertebrobasilar arteries.
• It is unclear whether symptoms of TIA are caused by transient thrombotic occlusion of major cerebral arteries or by microemboli that break away from a thrombus. Symptoms of transient monocular blindness, or amaurosis fugax, are likely due to microemboli from the internal carotid artery to a branch of the ophthalmic artery.
• A large arterial thrombus can occlude a major extracranial artery, producing a low-flow state that causes ischemic injury to neural tissue supplied by the most distal arterial branches. The volume of damage that results from such hemodynamic compromise is dependent on the length of time the vessel is occluded, the rate of flow through the occluded site, and the effectiveness of the collateral circulation.
• Ischemic injury from a cerebrovascular thrombus results in simultaneous distal branch occlusions from microemboli and compromise of blood flow proximally.

Embolism (pp. 1124–1125)

• Many embolic strokes have a cardiac origin. Thrombus formation within the cardiac chambers is generally caused by structural or mechanical changes within the heart. Atrial fibrillation is a significant risk factor for embolic stroke as a result of poor atrial motility and outflow, with stasis of blood and atrial thrombus formation. Atrial fibrillation is often caused by rheumatic valvular disease or coronary artery disease, but can be idiopathic. Mural thrombus within the left ventricle after MI, in the presence of cardiomyopathy or after cardiac surgery, is the other major cause of embolic stroke. Mechanical heart valves cause cerebral emboli if anticoagulation is insufficient. Infectious endocarditis can lead to septic emboli.

• Paradoxical embolism is a rare cause of embolic stroke that occurs in the presence of a deep vein thrombosis (DVT) and an atrial or ventricular septal defect. On modern echocardiography, a patent foramen ovale is a common finding, indicating that paradoxical embolism might be more common than previously thought.

• Cerebral emboli cause single or multiple branch occlusions resulting in sudden focal neurological impairment. These branch occlusions significantly compromise flow distally, inducing ischemic injury to neural tissue, glia, and vascular endothelium. Reperfusion of the occluded vessel can occur in response to endogenous fibrinolysis, but because ischemic damage to the vascular bed is often significant, the capillaries become incompetent and secondary cerebral hemorrhage ensues.

• In contrast to thrombotic stroke, microemboli probably do not precede cardioembolic strokes because TIAs are uncommon. Commonly no cardiac thrombus can be found after the event, and the only clue to an embolic cause is the sudden neurological deficit without previous or progressive symptoms.

Lacunes (p. 1125)

• Lacunar infarcts are small, circumscribed lesions located in subcortical regions of the basal ganglia, internal capsule, pons, and cerebellum. The area corresponds to the vascular territory supplied by one of the deep perforating branches from the circle of Willis or major cerebral arteries. Lacunar strokes are pathologically associated with microvascular changes that often develop in the presence of chronic hypertension and diabetes mellitus.

Hemorrhagic Stroke (pp. 1125–1126)

Intracerebral Hemorrhage (p. 1125)

• The deep perforating cerebral arteries are also the site of rupture preceding intracerebral hemorrhage (ICH). However, unlike lacunar strokes, ICH does not obey the anatomical distribution of a vessel but dissects through tissue planes. Such damage can be significant, resulting in increased intracranial pressure, disruption of multiple neural tracts, ventricular compression, and cerebral herniation. Acute mortality is high, but those who survive ICH often experience rapid neurological recovery during the first 2 or 3 months after the hemorrhage.

• Nearly one-half of all ICHs occur within the putamen and the cerebral white matter. Sudden hemorrhage into brain parenchyma is related to both acute elevations in blood pressure and chronic hypertension. Microvascular changes associated with hypertensive hemorrhages include lipohyalinosis and Charcot-Bouchard aneurysms. The latter are not true aneurysms of the vessel wall but are pockets of extravasated blood or "pseudoaneurysms," a sign of previous microscopic ruptures within the vascular wall.

• Cerebral amyloid angiopathy is gaining recognition as an important cause of ICH in the elderly.

• Other notable causes of ICH include the use of anticoagulants, intracranial tumor, and vasculitis.

Subarachnoid Hemorrhage (pp. 1125–1126)

- Bleeding that occurs within the dural space around the brain and fills the basal cisterns is most commonly caused by rupture of a saccular aneurysm or an arteriovenous malformation. Saccular aneurysms develop from a congenital defect in an arterial wall followed by degeneration of the adventitia, which causes ballooning or outpouching of the vessel. Saccular aneurysms often rupture during the fifth or sixth decade of life. When a rupture occurs, the extravasation of blood into the subarachnoid space is irritating to the dura and results in a severe headache often described as the "worst in my life." A sudden drop in cerebral perfusion pressure often results in acute loss of consciousness. Focal neurological changes or coma can ensue. Approximately one-third of patients with aneurysmal hemorrhage die immediately. Patients who present with coma, stupor, or severe hemiplegia have the worst prognosis for survival. The risk of rebleeding from an unoperated aneurysm is as high as 30% within the first month and declines thereafter. The risk for long-term rebleeding remains 3% per year.
- Saccular aneurysms are most often found in the anterior region of the circle of Willis, but they can also be found at the junction of almost any branch site within the cerebral circulation. Early surgical management using clipping techniques is as safe as late surgery, and it significantly reduces risk of rebleeding.
- Arteriovenous malformations present with hemorrhage, often in the second or third decade. Vascular malformations are also important causes of ICH and intraventricular hemorrhage. An AVM is a congenital tangled web of tissue that contains multiple arteriovenous fistulas. They can be located anywhere in the CNS and may grow quite large, usually without disruption of function. The patient often presents with seizure, migraine, or hemorrhage.
- The incidence of lifetime hemorrhage with AVM is 40% to 50%, with a rebleeding rate of 4% per year and a mortality rate of 1% per year. Treatment options include neuroradiological embolization, surgical resection, and radiotherapy.

Hydrocephalus (p. 1126)

- Acute and chronic hydrocephalus can complicate both SAH and intraventricular hemorrhage. Blood coagulum within the ventricular system can block the foramen of Sylvius or the fourth ventricle, causing acute obstructive hydrocephalus over minutes to hours after hemorrhage and leading to lethargy, coma, or death. Placement of an external ventricular drain can be lifesaving. If the obstruction does not resolve, a ventriculoperitoneal shunt is placed for long-term decompression.
- Normal pressure hydrocephalus is very common after SAH. The cause is a disruption of CSF resorption caused by fibrosis of the arachnoid granulations from subarachnoid blood. The classical symptoms of dementia, incontinence, and gait disorder are clues to the presence of hydrocephalus. The physiatrist should also have a high level of suspicion when a patient with recent hemorrhage is not making expected functional gains.

STROKE-RELATED IMPAIRMENTS (pp. 1126–1128)

- Disability in stroke is a result of CNS injury by which physical, cognitive, and psychological functioning become impaired.

Motor Control and Strength (p. 1126)

Anatomy (p. 1126)
• The primary motor area is located along the cortex of the precentral gyrus anterior to the central sulcus, and extends from the paracentral lobule within the longitudinal fissure to the frontal operculum within the Sylvian fissure. The classic "motor homunculus" is useful for visualizing the topography of motor control.

Recovery (p. 1126)
• Weakness and poor control of voluntary movement are present initially, associated with reduced resting muscle tone. As voluntary movement returns, nonfunctional mass flexion and extension of the limbs are first noted. Synergy patterns, or mass contraction of multiple muscle groups, are seen. Later, movement patterns can be independent of synergy.

Motor Coordination and Balance (pp. 1126–1127)

• Trunk control and stability, coordination of movement patterns, and balance all involve complex extrapyramidal systems that are commonly disrupted by stroke. Extrapyramidal disorders are often amenable to therapeutic exercise.

Anatomy (p. 1127)
• Anterior to the precentral gyrus within the frontal lobe is the premotor area, which is important in motor planning. Fiber tracts descend via the anterior limb of the internal capsule to the basal ganglia and the cerebellum, with input from the vestibular, visual, and somatosensory systems. Injury to the efferent or afferent systems can cause poor static and dynamic balance as well as movement disorders.

Spasticity (p. 1127)

• Spasticity can cause reduced flexibility, functional mobility, and poor posture as well as joint pain, contracture, and difficulty with positioning. Spasticity develops shortly after completed stroke, and is initially manifested as an increased phasic response to tendon tap and a slight catch with passive ranging. Later, ranging can become difficult and the patient might show tonic positioning in flexion or extension. Often, as voluntary motor activity returns, a reduction in tone and reflex response is noted, but if recovery is incomplete, spasticity usually remains.

Sensation (p. 1127)

• Loss of sensation after stroke can have a significant effect on joint and skin protection, balance, coordination, and motor control.

Anatomy (p. 1127)
• Pain and temperature sensation are relayed centrally by fibers that enter the spinothalamic tract from the contralateral dorsal root ganglion and ascend to the thalamus.
• Although injury to the sensory pathways typically causes hypoesthesia or reduced sensation, patients with lesions in the thalamus or spinothalamic tract

occasionally experience severe pain that can interfere with functional recovery. Treatment options include tricyclic antidepressants, anticonvulsants, and physical modalities.

Language and Communication (pp. 1127–1128)

• Aphasia is an impairment of language. Typical lesions that cause aphasia affect comprehension and the use of symbolic material for the purpose of communication and meaning. Testing of language should include an examination of oral expression, verbal comprehension, naming, reading, writing, and repeating. A simple and commonly used classification system for aphasia is listed in Table 50–1.

• Although language is considered a function of the left or dominant hemisphere, some elements of communication such as *prosody* have nondominant hemisphere control. Prosody is the rhythmic pattern and vocal intonation of speech that adds emphasis and emotional content to language. There is evidence that prosody might have similar anatomical topography as verbal language in the nondominant hemisphere.

Anatomy (pp. 1127–1128)

• Patients with Broca-type aphasia have lesions near the frontal operculum, anterior to the precentral gyrus. This location is named *Broca's area*. Broca-type aphasia is a primary language deficit with mildly compromised comprehension as well as impaired oral expression. The topographical location for the Wernicke type of aphasia is *Wernicke's area*, which is found in the posterior superior portion of the first temporal gyrus. Lesions near but not involving Broca's or Wernicke's area are associated with transcortical motor and sensory aphasias, respectively.

• Aprosody has been associated with lesions of the frontal operculum of the nondominant hemisphere. Patients who have aprosody speak at an even tempo with flat intonation; however, they are able to hear and comprehend the emotional content of language. In contrast, patients with a lesion in the temporoparietal region have an affective agnosia in that they are unable to recognize the emotional prosody of spoken language.

TABLE 50–1 Clinical Characteristics of the Common Aphasic Syndromes

Aphasia	Fluency	Expression	Comprehension	Repetition	Naming
Broca's	Impaired	Impaired	Mildly impaired	Impaired	Impaired
Wernicke's	Normal	Impaired	Impaired	Impaired	Impaired
Global	Impaired	Impaired	Impaired	Impaired	Impaired
Transcortical motor	Impaired	Moderately impaired	Minimally impaired	Normal	Impaired
Transcortical sensory	Normal	Minimally impaired	Moderately impaired	Normal	Impaired
Transcortical mixed	Impaired	Impaired	Impaired	Normal	Impaired
Conduction	Normal	Impaired in repetition	Normal	Impaired	Mildly impaired
Anomia	Normal	Normal	Normal	Normal	Impaired

• Conduction aphasia, with severely impaired repetition of language, is associated with a lesion of the arcuate fasciculus, which is a bundle of fibers that passes from the temporal to the frontal lobe. Disorders of reading (alexia) and writing (agraphia) are associated with disconnection of the primary language area from the primary visual cortices, which correlates to lesions in the angular gyrus at the junction of the occipital and temporoparietal lobes.

Apraxia (p. 1128)

• Disorders of skilled movement in the absence of motor, sensory, or cognitive impairment are called *apraxia*. Patients with apraxia often have difficulty performing simple functional activities. It is often difficult to test for apraxia in the presence of a language deficit because the examiner must be assured that the patient understands the command. Apraxia is most commonly seen in left hemisphere strokes and affects the left nonhemiplegic limb.
• Patients with right parietal strokes often have significant difficulty in dressing, despite adequate strength and flexibility. This has been called "dressing apraxia," but it is not a true apraxia because it is not a disorder of skilled motor function. It is actually a disorder of spatial perception that impairs the patient's ability to find the sleeves and neck of a shirt. Similarly, patients with "constructional apraxia" have difficulty copying a figure because of visuospatial deficits consistent with right parietal stroke.

Neglect Syndrome (p. 1128)

• Hemispatial neglect has been described as a failure to report, respond, or orient to novel or meaningful stimuli presented to the side opposite a brain lesion. It is important to exclude visual, somatosensory, or motor impairments. Hemispatial neglect significantly contributes to disability after stroke because it has a negative impact on sitting balance, visual perception, wheelchair mobility, safety awareness, skin and joint protection, and fall risk. Patients with neglect have difficulty completing hygiene and self-care on the affected side, fail to eat food items in the neglected visual space, and commonly run into objects and walls. Neglect is a disorder of visual and spatial attention and is associated with temporoparietal strokes and lesions of the frontal eye fields, cingulate gyrus, thalamus, and reticular formation.

Dysphagia (p. 1128)

• Dysphagia is common after stroke. Risk for aspiration pneumonia is strongly associated with a delayed initiation of pharyngeal swallow and reduced pharyngeal transit times commonly seen on video-fluoroscopic swallow evaluation. Other neurological factors that influence risk for aspiration after stroke include reduced labial and lingual mobility and sensation, unilateral neglect, pooling of pharyngeal residue within the vallecula and pyriform sinuses, and cricopharyngeal dysmotility. Laryngeal elevation during swallow normally declines with age and can have a negative influence on aspiration risk after stroke.

Uninhibited Bladder and Bowel (p. 1128)

• Bladder and bowel incontinence are common consequences of stroke. Because the pontine micturition center is typically preserved, reflex voiding usually shows normal synchronous internal sphincter relaxation with detrusor contraction. Postvoid residual volumes are generally low in the absence of bladder outlet obstruction. Incontinence is caused by a lack of voluntary inhibition to void and results in urgency. Immobility, unilateral neglect, and communication deficits often impair a patient's ability to ask for assistance or use equipment. Diabetic stroke survivors might also have a hypotonic bladder from neuropathy. Bowel incontinence results from uninhibited reflex rectal emptying by the same mechanism as the uninhibited bladder.

NEUROANATOMICAL BASIS FOR CLINICAL STROKE SYNDROMES (pp. 1128–1131)

Middle Cerebral Artery Syndromes (p. 1129)

• These are very commonly seen in the inpatient rehabilitation setting. The anatomical distribution includes a large proportion of cerebral cortex, and ischemia imparts significant impairment and disability. The MCA is vulnerable to cardioembolic and thrombotic disease.

MCA Stroke (p. 1129)

Main Stem. The impairments following occlusion of the MCA main stem (M1 segment) are listed in Table 50–2. The hemiplegia in a main-stem stroke affects the upper and lower limbs and lower portions of the face equally. This results primarily from ischemia within the lenticulostriate circulation to the posterior limb of the internal capsule. Sensory deficit is not as severe because only the inferior portion of the primary sensory cortex is supplied by the MCA. Complete hemianopia, dysphagia, and uninhibited voiding are commonly found.

Upper Division. MCA upper division strokes are listed in Table 50–3. Hemiplegia and language comprehension deficits are usually not as severe as in

---

TABLE 50–2 Middle Cerebral Artery Stroke: Main Stem

Contralateral hemiplegia
Contralateral hemianesthesia
Contralateral hemianopia
Head/eye turning toward lesion
Dysphagia
Uninhibited neurogenic bladder
Dominant hemisphere:
   Global aphasia
   Apraxia
Nondominant hemisphere:
   Aprosody and affective agnosia
   Visuospatial deficit
   Neglect syndrome

TABLE 50–3 Middle Cerebral Artery Stroke: Upper Division

Contralateral hemiplegia*	Dominant hemisphere:
Contralateral hemianesthesia	Broca's (motor) aphasia
Contralateral hemianopia	Apraxia
Head/eye turning toward lesion	Nondominant hemisphere:
Dysphagia	Aprosody
Uninhibited neurogenic bladder	Visual-spatial deficit
	Neglect syndrome

*Leg relatively more spared than hand and face.

main-stem infarction. Ischemia is limited to the inferolateral portion of the primary motor cortex. Thus motor strength and control are better in the lower limb than in the hand and face. A classic Broca-type aphasia is typical in a dominant hemisphere stroke, and aprosodia is found in nondominant hemisphere stroke.

Lower Division. Branch obstruction of the MCA lower division is less common and is usually caused by an embolic event. Patients can have significant functional disability from impaired language and vision and poor awareness of deficits. Table 50–4 lists the impairments associated with lower division strokes.

Anterior Cerebral Artery Syndromes (p. 1130)

Anatomy (p. 1130)
• The anterior cerebral artery (ACA) supplies the interhemispheric cortical surface of the frontal and parietal lobes.

ACA Stroke (p. 1130)
• The disorders resulting from an ACA infarction are listed in Table 50–5. The hemiplegia in ACA strokes shows weakness of the shoulder and foot with relative sparing of the forearm, hand, and face. Unilateral footdrop can be a long-term impairment. Upper limb apraxia to verbal commands can also result from an infarction of the anterior corpus callosum.
• Occlusion involving the anterior communicating artery and the recurrent artery of Heubner can extend the infarction through the anterior limb of the internal capsule, causing complete hemiplegia. The proximity of such a stroke to Broca's area can also result in a transcortical motor aphasia.

TABLE 50–4 Middle Cerebral Artery Stroke: Lower Division

Contralateral hemianopia
Dominant hemisphere:
    Wernicke's aphasia
Nondominant hemisphere:
    Affective agnosia

TABLE 50–5 Anterior Cerebral Artery Stroke

Contralateral hemiplegia*	Grasp reflex—groping
Contralateral hemianesthesia	Disconnection apraxia
Head/eye turning toward lesion	Akinetic mutism (abulia)

*Hand relatively more spared than arm and leg.

Posterior Cerebral Artery Syndromes (p. 1130)

Anatomy (p. 1130)
• The vertebral arteries pass through the transverse foramina of the cervical vertebra and intracranially via the foramen magnum. At the junction of the medulla and pons, the vertebral arteries unite to form the basilar artery, which divides into the posterior cerebral arteries (PCAs). The thalamus is supplied by perforating arteries called the *thalamoperforans* and *thalamogeniculates.*

PCA Stroke (p. 1130)
• The syndrome of PCA infarction is listed in Table 50–6. Infarcts can cause hemisensory deficits including hypoesthesia; dysesthesia; and hyperesthesia, or pain. Visual disturbances result from injury to the lateral geniculate, temporal, and occipital visual radiations and the calcarine cortex of the occipital lobe. Damage to visual association areas can cause altered color discrimination. A disorder of reading without impaired writing associated with a right visual field deficit results from an infarction of the left occipital cortex and posterior corpus callosum. Impaired memory can result from infarction of the temporal lobe and the hippocampal gyri.

Vertebrobasilar Syndromes (pp. 1130–1131)

Anatomy (p. 1130)
• The major arterial branches supplying the brainstem and cerebellum are the posterior inferior cerebellar artery (PICA), the anterior inferior cerebellar artery (AICA), and the superior cerebellar artery (SCA). The PICA wraps dorsally around the medulla. The AICA circles around the pons. Both supply the inferior lobe of the cerebellum. The superior lobe of the cerebellum receives its blood supply from the SCA at the level of the midbrain. Perforating arteries supply the brainstem.

Brainstem Stroke Syndromes (pp. 1130–1131)
• The bulbar nuclei form afferent and efferent cranial nerves that innervate the ipsilateral side of the body, whereas the ascending and descending bulbar and spinal tracts innervate contralaterally. Unilateral strokes often cause loss of cranial nerve function ipsilaterally and sensorimotor dysfunction contralaterally.

TABLE 50–6 Posterior Cerebral Artery Stroke

Hemisensory deficit	Dyschromatopsia
Visual impairment	Alexia without agraphia
Visual agnosia	Memory deficits
Prosopagnosia	

TABLE 50–7 Brainstem Syndromes and Their Anatomical Correlates

Syndrome	Location	Structural Injury	Characteristics
Weber's	Medial basal midbrain	Third cranial nerve	Ipsilateral third nerve palsy
		Corticospinal tract	Contralateral hemiplegia
Benedikt's	Tegmentum of midbrain	Third cranial nerve	Ipsilateral third nerve palsy
		Spinothalamic tract	Contralateral loss of pain and temperature sensation
		Medial lemniscus	Contralateral loss of joint position
		Superior cerebellar peduncle	Contralateral ataxia
		Red nucleus	Contralateral chorea
Locked-in	Bilateral basal pons	Corticospinal tract	Bilateral hemiplegia
		Corticobulbar tract	Bilateral cranial nerve palsy (upward gaze spared)
Millard-Gubler	Lateral pons	Sixth cranial nerve	Ipsilateral sixth nerve palsy
		Seventh cranial nerve	Ipsilateral facial weakness
		Corticospinal tract	Contralateral hemiplegia
Wallenberg's	Lateral medulla	Spinocerebellar tract	Ipsilateral hemiataxia
		Fifth cranial nerve	Ipsilateral loss of facial pain and temperature sensation
		Spinothalamic tract	Contralateral loss of body pain and temperature sensation
		Vestibular nuclei	Nystagmus
		Sympathetic tract	Ipsilateral Horner's syndrome
		Nucleus ambiguus	Dysphagia and dysphonia

The common brainstem syndromes are listed in Table 50–7, along with their anatomical correlates.

• The *Wallenberg* or lateral medullary syndrome is characterized by ipsilateral limb ataxia, loss of pain and temperature sensation on the ipsilateral face and contrateral body, ipsilateral Horner's syndrome, dysphagia, dysphonia, and nystagmus. Vertebral artery thrombosis near the PICA branch is the usual cause. The prognosis for functional improvement is excellent.

• The *locked-in* syndrome is a severe pontine stroke causing quadriplegia, oral motor and laryngeal weakness, and disruption of conjugate eye movements. Patients usually have voluntary vertical eye movements that they can use for communication.

• Cerebellar strokes are common and can cause hydrocephalus if cerebellar edema obstructs the fourth ventricle. PICA and AICA strokes are generally caused by thrombosis of the vertebrobasilar system. SCA strokes are more commonly cardioembolic.

Lacunar Strokes (p. 1131)

• Lacunar strokes are located within the cerebral white matter, basal ganglia, thalamus, and pons, and result from occlusion of perforating arteries. The most common syndromes are listed in Table 50–8.

TABLE 50–8 Lacunar Syndromes and Their Anatomical Correlates

Syndrome	Anatomical Sites
Pure motor stroke	Posterior limb internal capsule
	Basis pontis
	Pyramids
Pure sensory stroke	Thalamus
	Thalamocortical projections
Sensory-motor stroke	Junction of internal capsule and thalamus
Dysarthria-clumsy hand	Anterior limb internal capsule
	Pons
Ataxic hemiparesis	Corona radiata
	Internal capsule
	Pons
	Cerebellum
Hemiballismus	Head of caudate
	Thalamus
	Subthalamic nucleus

ACUTE STROKE MANAGEMENT (pp. 1131–1135)

Saving the Ischemic Penumbra (pp. 1131–1132)

• Acutely, surviving but inactive neural cells are located at the rim of the ischemic injury, where collateral circulation provides minimal tissue perfusion. Improved blood flow to this *ischemic penumbra* can theoretically restore normal neurological function. Recent acute stroke management protocols have focused on vascular reperfusion of the ischemic zone. From the standpoint of public education regarding stroke, the National Stroke Association has emphasized that to reduce neural impairment, acute stroke management should be implemented within the first 6 hours of the event.

The First 6 Hours (pp. 1132–1133)

• Current research has focused mainly on four pharmacological treatments: thrombolytic agents, heparin, calcium channel blockers, and neuroprotective medications.

• IV administration of rt-PA increases plasmin generation, resulting in significant thrombolytic activity. The FDA has approved rt-PA for the treatment of acute ischemic stroke. It is clear that rt-PA can reduce unfavorable outcome in selected patients who present to the emergency department (ED) within the first 3 hours after acute stroke onset.

• Heparin is commonly administered IV to arrest stroke progression or to prevent its recurrence, but there is little support for its efficacy, and clear guidelines for its use are lacking. Evidence supports the use of antiplatelet agents for the management of acute *thrombotic* stroke, regardless of thrombolytic treatment. The use of heparin followed by warfarin is warranted to prevent recurrent *cardioembolic* stroke. Many clinicians advocate delaying initiation of anticoagulation by a minimum of 48 hours to avoid hemorrhage of the ischemic infarct. Low-dose subcutaneous heparin is safe to administer early.

• Calcium channel–blocking agents are effective in preventing death from vasospastic complications of SAH and are recommended for 21 days after hemorrhage.

• The *N*-methyl-D-aspartate (NMDA) receptor antagonists have shown the potential to delay neuronal injury. Several studies testing the NMDA antagonists have been discontinued because of safety concerns or lack of benefit. One solution may be to combine neuroprotective agents with thrombolytic therapy.

Emergency Department Evaluation and Treatment (p. 1133)

• Based on the need for rapid diagnosis, the NINDS has recommended that a physician assessment, laboratory testing, and CT with its interpretation be completed within 45 minutes of arrival in the ED with acute stroke symptoms. The goal of the initial evaluation is to establish medical stability, develop a differential diagnosis, and initiate the management protocol if indicated.

• Laboratory tests performed in the ED include electrolytes, blood urea nitrogen, creatinine, glucose, total cholesterol levels, complete blood cell count with platelets, prothrombin time, partial thromboplastin time, erythrocyte sedimentation rate, and urinalysis.

• Cranial CT identifies whether the stroke is ischemic or hemorrhagic. In cases of ischemic infarct the CT findings are often negative for the first 24 to 48 hours after symptom onset. Early signs of a cortical infarct include loss of definition at the gray-white junction and effacement of the sulci. During the first 48 hours the image begins to show a hypodense area. Lacunar strokes appear as small punctate hypodensities. Strokes in the brainstem and cerebellum are more difficult to visualize using cranial CT because the thick bone of the skull base creates image artifacts.

• ICH has a hyperdense appearance on CT and can be distinguished from infarction. Hemorrhage confined to the basal ganglia or thalamus is likely a result of hypertensive ICH. Saccular aneurysm and AVM should be considered if intraventricular or subarachnoid blood is seen.

• The decision to use thrombolytic agents is not based only on the absence of hemorrhage. Patients with recent bleeding or surgery, a history of ICH, hematological abnormalities, or uncontrolled hypertension should not be given rt-PA.

Acute Medical Management (pp. 1133–1134)

• Initial medical care requires careful and frequent monitoring to manage complications that compromise cerebral tissue perfusion. Airway protection is critical. Cerebral edema and hydrocephalus may develop rapidly, requiring hyperventilation or placement of an external ventriculostomy device to relieve intracranial pressure. Surgical decompression of the posterior fossa can be lifesaving.

• Blood pressure is often acutely elevated and often falls over the following week. Higher mean arterial pressure (MAP) is needed to maintain cerebral perfusion pressure. Acute hypertension after stroke should be treated only if it is symptomatic, if there is evidence of end-organ injury, or if the diastolic pressure rises above 120 mm Hg. When treated, blood pressure should be lowered gently, and it is best to allow the systolic pressure to remain above 150 mm Hg

and the diastolic pressure above 90 mm Hg. Calcium channel blockers can cause reduced perfusion. Better choices are mixed β- and α-antagonists, such as labetolol; or α-2-receptor antagonists, like clonidine.
• Hyperglycemia occurs in both diabetic and nondiabetic patients during stroke. Frequent monitoring and control of serum glucose levels during acute stroke have been recommended.

Further Diagnostic Evaluation (pp. 1134–1135)

• Additional laboratory tests can be ordered as indicated. In young patients with stroke it is important to consider hereditary diseases that increase the risk for hypercoagulability. Serum hemoglobin electrophoresis can detect sickle cell disease or trait. Plasma levels of protein C, protein S, or antithrombin III can be tested. Elevated ESR prompts an evaluation for vasculitis, anticardiolipin antibody, or lupus anticoagulant.
• MRI is useful to determine the extent of brain injury and identify structural abnormalities. MRI is more sensitive than CT in demonstrating the changes of stroke in the first 48 hours, for lacunar strokes after the first 24 hours, and for imaging the posterior fossa. Diffusion-weighted MRI detects early ischemic changes and can be performed rapidly.
• Cranial CT remains the test of choice for examination of ICH in the acute setting. With subacute or chronic hemorrhagic stroke, MRI is better.
• MR angiography is indicated as a screening test for extracranial and intracranial disease
• Transthoracic echocardiography (TTE) after suspected cerebral embolism is standard practice. However, the detection of thrombi within the left atrium and the atrial appendage is unreliable. Transesophageal echocardiography (TEE) provides a tenfold improvement in left atrial thrombus detection. Atrial septal defects are also well visualized with TEE.
• Arterial duplex scanning is a useful screening tool for carotid atherosclerosis. A negative carotid duplex scan excludes the need for carotid endarterectomy but does not rule out intracranial atherosclerosis.
• Transcranial Doppler imaging can measure flow characteristics of the intracranial vessels and is most useful when measurements of CBF are needed, such as in vasospasm after SAH.
• Conventional contrast-enhanced cerebral angiography is the most accurate method of detecting and anatomically defining extracranial or intracranial cerebrovascular disease. It is the method of choice for detecting and defining the anatomy of cerebral aneurysms and AVMs. It is invasive and not without complications.

NATURAL SPONTANEOUS NEUROLOGICAL RECOVERY (pp. 1135–1136)

• Reduction in the extent of neurological impairment results from spontaneous recovery, treatments that limit the extent of the stroke, or from other interventions.
• Also seen is the improved ability to perform daily functions, within the limitations of impairments. The ability to perform these tasks can improve through adaptation and training. There is some controversy over the extent to which rehabilitation interventions might promote *remediation* of primary deficits. Rehabili-

tation activities are thought to exert their greatest effectiveness in providing compensatory training to reduce disability.

• Alternative compensatory functional strategies play a major role in the performance of functional tasks when neurological recovery is minimal or absent.

• The degree and time course of recovery of neurological functioning is variable. Generally, deficits decline in frequency one-third to one-half. Most improvements in physical functioning occur within the first 3 to 6 months. Many variables determine outcome.

Recovery of Motor Function (pp. 1135–1136)

• For many, the pattern of spontaneous recovery of motor function follows a sequence in which lower extremity function recovers earliest and most completely, followed by upper extremity and hand function. Return of tone precedes return of voluntary movement, proximal control precedes distal control, and synergy patterns precede isolated volitional motor functions. This sequence of recovery can stop at any stage.

Recovery of Language and Perceptual Functions (p. 1136)

• Recovery from aphasia usually occurs at a slower rate and over a more prolonged time course than does motor recovery. Most aphasia recovery occurs in the first 3 to 6 months; however, global aphasia can show the greatest improvement during the latter half of the first year. The amount and pattern of recovery are usually related to the initial severity of the aphasia and the specific type. Patients with nonfluent aphasia generally have a less favorable prognosis than those with fluent aphasia, although both can improve. Comprehension usually returns earlier and to a greater extent than expression.

Proposed Mechanisms of Recovery of Neurological Function (p. 1136)

• Resolution of local harmful factors usually accounts for early spontaneous improvement. These processes include resolution of local edema, resorption of local toxins, improved local circulation, and recovery of partially damaged neurons.

• Neuroplasticity can take place early or late after brain damage. Plasticity refers to the ability of the nervous system to modify its structural and functional organization. The two most plausible forms of plasticity are sprouting of new synaptic connections and unmasking of latent functional pathways. Other mechanisms include assumption of function by redundant pathways, reversibility from diaschisis, denervation supersensitivity, and regenerative proximal sprouting of transected neuronal axons.

MEDICAL CO-MORBIDITIES AND COMPLICATIONS (pp. 1136–1138)

• Medical problems can be categorized as (1) pre-existing illnesses that necessitate ongoing care, (2) general health functions affected by the stroke, (3) secondary poststroke complications, and (4) acute poststroke exacerbations of pre-existing chronic diseases.

• Medical complications can limit the patient's ability to participate in a therapeutic exercise program, inhibit functional skill performance, and reduce the likelihood of achieving favorable outcomes from rehabilitation. The rehabilitation interventions also might adversely affect the medical condition. Medical complications can occur during the rehabilitation program that demand diagnostic evaluation, prompt recognition, and appropriate medical management.
• Table 50–10 in the Textbook lists some common diagnoses that accompany stroke.

Select Complications (pp. 1137–1138)

• *Physiological deconditioning* accompanies acute medical illness and prolonged bed rest. Deconditioning can contribute to fatigue, endurance limitations, poor exercise tolerance, orthostatic hypotension, lack of motivation, and depression. Preventive techniques include early mobilization, participation in rehabilitation, and a schedule that balances rest and activity.
• The incidence of *venous thromboembolism* is between 40% and 50% for deep vein thrombosis and 10% for pulmonary embolism. Some form of prophylaxis for venous thromboembolism should be instituted. In patients in whom hemorrhagic stroke has been ruled out, low-dose heparin or low-molecular-weight heparin compounds are effective.
• *Pneumonia* occurs in about one-third of patients with stroke. The incidence is higher in patients who have subarachnoid hemorrhage. Dysphagia can cause aspiration. It is important to evaluate swallow function. Other factors that might predispose to pneumonia include abnormal central breathing patterns, general debility causing impaired immune response, and hemiparetic weakness of ventilatory muscles causing weakened cough.
• *Cardiac abnormalities* can be causal, consequential, or coincidental in stroke, with rates of association of 75% for hypertension, 32% to 62% for coronary artery disease, 40% to 70% for various arrhythmias, and 12% to 18% for congestive heart failure. Because the presence of heart disease can adversely affect functional outcome, it may be necessary to screen stroke patients prior to initiating exercise, to closely monitor stroke patients during rehabilitation, or modify therapy.
• *Central poststroke pain* is estimated to occur in about 2% of patients. It can be a limiting factor in functional recovery and often is refractory to treatment. Interventions include treatment of other conditions; positioning; psychological techniques; antiepileptic and/or antidepressant medications; and, rarely, surgical intervention.
• *Preventing recurrent stroke* is a key component because patients are at substantial risk for another stroke. Measures are directed toward risk factors. Surgical treatment of cerebral aneurysms after subarachnoid hemorrhage can be effective in reducing recurrences in most patients. Education is one of the major preventive interventions.
• *Bowel and bladder incontinence* is seen in one-third to two-thirds of stroke survivors during the early period and in about one-fifth to one-fourth after 6 months. Continued incontinence is often predictive of limited functional outcome. Urinary incontinence can result from urinary tract infection, neurogenic bladder, cognitive or sensory dysfunction, or mobility deficits. Planned toileting programs are often effective. Bowel problems following stroke might be due to immobility and inactivity, inadequate fluid or nutritional intake,

psychological depression, neurogenic bowel, lack of transfer ability, cognitive deficit, or reduced consciousness.

- *Shoulder pain, contracture, and other musculoskeletal disorders,* resulting from glenohumeral subluxation, impingement syndromes, rotator cuff tears, frozen shoulder, brachial plexus injuries, complex regional pain syndromes, bursitis, or tendinitis, occur in about 70% to 80% of hemiplegic patients. Shoulder problems occur with greater frequency during the spasticity phase of recovery than during flaccidity. Treatment includes the use of wheelchair arm troughs and lap trays, shoulder slings, physical modalities, medications, and ROM exercises.

- *Falls* occur with striking frequency in stroke survivors. Prevention approaches emphasize balance training, cognitive training, safety training, ensuring supervision during mobility activities, eliminating environmental hazards, and use of assistive devices.

PRINCIPLES OF STROKE REHABILITATION
(pp. 1138–1140)

- Common features of stroke rehabilitation programs are shown in Table 50–11 in the Textbook.

Holistic Care (pp. 1138–1139)

- The effects of stroke are broad, and the course of stroke and the outcomes of care following stroke depend on a number of factors. Social, vocational, and economic factors often play an important a role in determining rehabilitation participation and outcome, as do physical and emotional issues.

Team Management (p. 1139)

- Interdisciplinary team care allows specialists from different backgrounds to treat the patient simultaneously and collaboratively with the goal of enhancing function.

Goal-Directed Treatment (p. 1139)

- An early *and recurring* step is establishing realistic, practical, and feasible goals that are mutually agreed upon by the patient, family, and professionals.

Focus on Learning and Adaptation (p. 1139)

- Principles of learning theory suggest that patients reacquire old skills or develop means to compensate for new impairments in a logical, coherent manner. Supervised practice is a necessary component. Ideally, rehabilitation programs train patients in skills that are meaningful to them. Concrete phrasing is used, and attempts are made to ensure that instructions are understood. Tasks should be tailored to meet the patient's level of skill. Another component is frequent and timely support, education, reassurance, direct physical assistance, and feedback on progress.

Therapy Environments (p. 1139)

• Patients can benefit greatly from practice in therapy environments that closely reflect natural home or community settings. Some programs use mock kitchens, apartments, community shops, and other similar facilities to allow patient practice.

Timing of Therapy (p. 1140)

• Therapy schedules should be individualized. Endurance, medical stability, mood, motivation, and other considerations affect the degree and duration of physical and cognitive activity that an individual patient can tolerate.

Attention to Psychosocial Issues (p. 1140)

• Disability can give rise to a variety of reactions in patients including sadness, grief, anxiety, depression, despair, anger, frustration, and confusion. Addressing these issues is critical. Dealing with the emotional issues at times forms the major focus of the care activities. Addressing these issues facilitates improved participation in the program. Reactions are often dependent on *prestroke* coping styles, levels of frustration tolerance, and ability and mechanisms used to deal with adversity.
• Families might experience a variety of emotions including grief, sadness, depression, anxiety, and guilt. Families often serve as caregivers; they might experience the care as burdensome, and might feel guilt over their feelings. The complexity of these emotional reactions underscores the importance of ongoing counseling, support, and care for the family caregivers.

Emphasis on Community Issues (p. 1140)

• Rehabilitation includes planning for ways to meet the patient's needs in the home environment, educating family members on care techniques in the home, encouraging the practice of skills by patients and family members, providing instruction in medication administration and exercise technique, explaining potential medical complications and their warning signs, recruiting community resources and introducing these resources to the patient, and training community members in functional care skills and equipment use.

REHABILITATION ASSESSMENT AND INTERVENTIONS DURING THE ACUTE PHASE
(pp. 1140–1141)

• Many problems are related to the immobility and deconditioning imposed by prolonged bed rest. Early poststroke rehabilitation is both preventive and therapeutic (Table 50–9).
• The patient should undergo an evaluation to determine the optimal type, level, setting, and timing of the program. In addition to the nature, pattern, and severity of physical impairments, some of the key components of the assessment include health status, endurance level, and medical stability; functional capabilities and disabilities in the areas of mobility, self-care, and instrumental

TABLE 50–9 Rehabilitation Activities during the Acute Poststroke Phase

Evaluate and manage medical problems
Monitor and adjust medications
Maintain hydration and nutrition
Facilitate rest and sleep
Venous thromboembolism prophylaxis (physical or pharmacological measures)
Proper bed and chair positioning
Frequent turns and position changes
Range-of-motion exercises
Deep breathing and cough exercises
Frequent skin inspections
Swallowing evaluation
Safety measures
Removal of indwelling catheter, if possible, with planned, timed toileting program
Bowel evacuation regimen
Sitting in chair
Supervised bedside exercises
Self-performance of activities of daily living
Mobilization exercises
Standing and gait training as able
Educational programs on stroke, recovery, and personal care
Communication evaluation and training
Psychological support to the patient
Family education and support
Evaluation of social supports and available resources
Evaluation for formal continued rehabilitation
Transition to rehabilitation

ADL; mood and coping ability; community resources and family supports; social situation and vocational/educational status; and cognitive, communicative, perceptual, and behavioral functioning.

LEVELS OF POSTACUTE STROKE CARE (pp. 1141–1142)

• Factors that are useful in determining the ideal setting of care for a patient at a particular point in time include the patient's cognitive ability, motivation level, prior and present levels of functioning, medical stability, level of available social resources, medical and nursing needs, and likelihood of achieving significant functional gains during rehabilitation.

Acute Inpatient Rehabilitation (p. 1141)

• Acute inpatient stroke rehabilitation refers to the traditional interdisciplinary hospital-based coordinated program of medical, nursing, and therapy services. Care in this setting is directed by a physician and carried out by a team. This level of care is most appropriate for patients who need and can tolerate 3 or more hours of therapy a day, and who need both around-the-clock nursing care and at least daily physician supervision. Patients must have a reasonable likelihood of achieving significant functional gains.

Subacute Inpatient Rehabilitation (pp. 1141–1142)

• Subacute inpatient rehabilitation is appropriate for stroke survivors who need comprehensive and coordinated therapy services for functional training in an institutional setting, but in a less intensive program than is used at the acute level of rehabilitation. Patients in this level of care usually receive between 1 and 3 hours of therapy per day.

• Subacute inpatient rehabilitation is usually conducted in a skilled nursing facility and occasionally in the hospital setting. In this level of care, patients receive 24-hour-a-day nursing care, but physician visits typically average only one to three times per week.

Day Rehabilitation (p. 1142)

• Day rehabilitation is a comprehensive and coordinated program of therapy that takes place in an outpatient setting. The rehabilitation is directed by a physician and facilitated by a team with regularly scheduled team conferences. Therapy services typically are provided between 3 and 8 hours a day. Relative medical stability is necessary.

Outpatient Therapy (p. 1142)

• Many patients need traditional outpatient therapy. These services do not entail the coordination, comprehensiveness, and team conferences that characterize day rehabilitation. These services include single-modality training (e.g., physical therapy, occupational therapy, speech-language pathology services, or psychological support) for patients with focal deficits and for whom specific functional training might be useful.

Home Therapy (p. 1142)

• Therapy in the home allows the patient and family to learn specific functional tasks in the setting in which those skills will be used most often. A potential disadvantage is the limitation in available resources.

THERAPEUTIC INTERVENTIONS DURING REHABILITATION (pp. 1142–1146)

• The therapeutic interventions include skills training, demonstration, providing opportunity for practice, offering feedback, therapeutic exercises, physical modalities, adaptive devices, education, and supportive counseling. Medications and surgical techniques also can be used.

Sensorimotor and Functional Training (pp. 1142–1143)

• Traditional therapeutic exercise programs consist of positioning, ROM exercises, and progressive resistive exercises. Endurance training also can be implemented.

- Training in the performance of self-care tasks, mobility skills, and advanced or instrumental ADL form the central focus of most programs. The patient is encouraged to make use of residual abilities to develop new ways of achieving old goals and to perform routine tasks.
- Several neuromuscular facilitation exercise approaches have been developed. Proprioceptive neuromuscular facilitation relies on several mechanisms such as quick stretch and spiral diagonal movement patterns of the extremities. Brunnstrom movement therapy encourages and facilitates the use of synergy patterns as a means of developing voluntary control. Cutaneous sensory stimulation provides facilitatory or inhibitory inputs into the system. In Bobath neurodevelopmental treatment approach, inhibition of abnormal tone, synergies, and postures are combined with facilitation of normal automatic motor responses to develop skilled movements. The motor relearning program emphasizes functional training for specific tasks such as standing and walking, and carryover of those tasks. Many therapists combine elements of various procedures.

New Approaches for Sensorimotor and Functional Training (p. 1143)

- Partial weight-bearing treadmill training (PWBTT) is an emerging method of improving quality of gait in hemiparetic patients. It consists of combining partial body weight support, by using a body harness suspended from the ceiling, with enforced stepping, by using a motor-driven treadmill.
- There is a renewed interest in behavioral approaches to motor control enhancement, including kinesthetic and positional biofeedback. Electromyographic biofeedback technology makes the patient consciously aware of his or her own muscle activity. Although some favorable results have been noted, these findings have not been substantiated on a consistent basis.
- A potentially favorable effect of therapeutic exercise maneuvers that involve the hemiparetic extremity is to prevent or overcome "learned nonuse." This concept suggests that attempts to use the affected limb should be reinforced. It could even be beneficial to inhibit or immobilize the function of the unaffected limb to encourage or "force" the use of the hemiplegic extremity. Reported successful work with animals, and more recently in humans, supports the usefulness of this "forced-use" approach, now known as "constraint-induced movement therapy."
- Functional electrical stimulation of muscles that lack voluntary control could help facilitate their movement or compensate for their lack of voluntary movement.
- An emerging body of literature demonstrates that sensory stimulation and acupuncture may have a beneficial effect on motor control following stroke.

Spasticity Management (p. 1143)

- Spasticity can interfere with functional performance, cause muscle and joint contracture and pain, and result in skin breakdown.
- Treatment begins with good general medical care designed to prevent and treat infections or other secondary problems and is supplemented by ROM exercises, positioning, and splinting. The use of oral medications is usually attempted but is often unsuccessful. Injections of neurolytic agents such as phenol have been used with variable success. The selective local intramuscular injection of extremely low doses of botulinum toxin A has been found to be effective.

Speech, Language, and Visuospatial Perceptual Disorders
(pp. 1143–1144)

• Many procedures have been developed to manage various aspects of speech and language disorders. One goal of therapy is to improve the patient's ability to speak, understand, read, and write. Another goal is to assist patients to develop strategies that compensate for or circumvent problems.

• Treatment of aphasia focuses on the most effective means by which the patient can communicate.

• For dysarthria, exercise modalities include sensory stimulation procedures, exercises designed to strengthen oromotor speech muscles, respiratory training procedures, and retraining of articulatory patterns and sequences of gestures. Alternative forms of communication and augmentative devices can be used.

• Visual-spatial perceptual deficits are troublesome problems. Treatment methods include the use of prism glasses, increasing awareness of deficits with cues, using computer-assisted training, and providing compensatory strategies.

Swallowing Training (p. 1144)

• Impaired swallowing places the patient at risk for aspiration and pneumonia, malnutrition, and dehydration. Compensatory treatments include changing posture and positioning for swallowing, learning new swallowing maneuvers, and changing food amounts and textures.

Psychosocial Considerations (pp. 1144–1145)

• One of the major factors influencing both the degree of participation in a therapy program and the outcome achieved is patient motivation. Examples of techniques used to enhance or direct motivation include: explanation, positive reinforcement, behavioral modification, and coaxing. Counseling interventions have proved to be effective in improving family functioning and patient adjustment.

• Depression occurs in one-third to two-thirds of survivors. Most patients experience a combination of organic and reactive causes of mood disorders. Treatment consists of psychotherapy, psychosocial support, milieu therapy, and medications. Antidepressant medications can improve not only mood, but also functional performance. Anxiety and fear are common.

• Sexual dysfunction has been reported in 40% to 70% of stroke survivors. Its cause is largely psychological rather than organic. Issues related to self-esteem, affection, and relationships should be emphasized, as should specific practical suggestions on positioning, timing, and techniques.

• Lack of social support is a major problem. Recruiting available resources and supports, securing appropriate entitlements, and advocating on behalf of the patient are major tasks for the team.

• Problematic psychosocial functioning is related to physical function or motor skill performance.

• Recreational activities often have the effect of improving affect, focusing therapy of meaningful activities and desirable goals, and facilitating a smooth transition to the community.

• The presence of other patients with similar disabilities on the rehabilitation unit can assist the patient in several ways. First, it can help to reduce the fear and anxiety often associated with the new onset of physically disabling or disfiguring conditions. Second, patients often can counsel and support each other in ways that professionals cannot. Finally, patients often not only gain insight into their disability, but also garner specific suggestions for functional skill performance or about adaptive equipment from other patients who have already been through the experience.

Specialized Equipment (p. 1145)

• Adaptive equipment and durable medical equipment assist the patients to become more independent and to facilitate functional skill performance. It is important to consider the patient's functional level, level of adaptation to the disability, architecture of the living environment, and instruction in the use of all devices and equipment.

• A wheelchair can greatly enhance quality of life by improving positioning and mobility. Generally, a wheelchair for a hemiplegic patient has a lowered base to allow the nonhemiparetic lower extremity to touch the floor and to allow the patient to use that limb in wheelchair propulsion. There is usually also a one-arm drive mechanism to enable the patient to use the nonhemiplegic upper limb for wheelchair propulsion.

• Upper extremity resting hand splints are usually used to prevent deformity and to maintain the wrist in a functional, slightly extended position. Orthoses are used to an optimal gait pattern.

• The various types of commonly used specialized equipment for stroke survivors are noted in Chapter 25.

Caregiver Training (pp. 1145–1146)

• One of the most important interventions is the training of families and other caregivers in specific care techniques to prevent complications, perform physical functions, and encourage the patient. Family education has been found to contribute to the long-term maintenance of rehabilitation gains.

TRANSITION TO THE COMMUNITY, FOLLOW-UP, AND AFTERCARE (p. 1146)

• Realizing the goal of optimal long-term quality of life is accomplished through an interdisciplinary approach that includes helping the patient achieve maximal independent functioning in daily activities and training personal caregivers in specific skills.

• Major efforts for discharge are directed toward securing community resources (e.g., attendant care, home nursing visits, outpatient or home therapy, and community transportation and recreational programs). Teaching patients about stroke, medications, fluid intake, diet, exercises, catheter care, feeding tube use, tracheostomy management, signs and symptoms of common complications such as infections, and specific functional task performance greatly facilitates a smooth transition to home.

• Specific functional issues that are relevant around the time of transition to the community are the "higher level" community skills that are related to the postdischarge lifestyle. Important examples include sexual functioning, driving ability, grocery shopping, housekeeping, laundry management, safety considerations, socialization outside of the home, vocational pursuits, recreational activities, and others. The emphasis on education, mobilization, activity, independence, coping, family involvement, and especially quality of life should be incorporated into the patient's lifestyle.

REHABILITATION OUTCOMES (pp. 1146–1147)

Functional and Social Outcomes (pp. 1146–1147)

• Physical performance, functional abilities, and quality of life are considerably better after rehabilitation and during long-term care than immediately after the stroke. Most studies show that a substantial proportion of stroke survivors achieve independence in their ability to complete mobility and self-care skills. Social and vocational outcomes are not as favorable as functional independence figures.

Predictors of Outcome (p. 1147)

• Several factors influence the outcome of an individual who is involved in a stroke rehabilitation program. The strongest and most consistent predictor of discharge functional ability is admission functional ability.
• Specific reported predictors are listed in Table 50–16 in the Textbook. Caution is needed in using the predictors for clinical purposes. Identification of some of these factors can help to better direct patient management activities.

EVIDENCE FOR EFFECTIVENESS OF STROKE REHABILITATION (pp. 1147–1150)

• Much of the early effectiveness research consisted of observational descriptions of patient outcomes achieved after participation in rehabilitation programs, but more recent investigations have reported empirical results derived from prospectively conducted controlled clinical trials; the application of epidemiological principles to clinical research; the development and use of meta-analysis techniques; and, most recently, the publication of the U.S. Agency for Health Care Policy and Research (AHCPR) *Post-Stroke Rehabilitation Clinical Practice Guidelines.*

Common Themes of the Effectiveness Studies
(pp. 1149–1150)

• In addition to early initiation of rehabilitation treatment, several other common characteristics of the intervention programs appear to have been important in the achievement of favorable outcomes. These include focused personal care and mobility training; a comprehensive approach to care by a team of professionals, with coordination of treatment interventions; patient and family education; active participation by family; staff education; and care that is systematic, standardized, uniform, and consistent. Despite limitations in the amount and quality of the research on the effectiveness of stroke rehabilitation, and despite several persisting questions on the effectiveness of the interventions that make up the programs, there is growing evidence that stroke rehabilitation programs improve the outcome of individuals who are disabled by stroke.

U.S. AGENCY FOR HEALTH CARE POLICY AND RESEARCH POSTSTROKE REHABILITATION CLINICAL PRACTICE GUIDELINES (pp. 1150–1151)

- The guidelines focus on five major points:

1. Thorough and consistent assessment of status at each stage of the recovery process to help guide treatment and to monitor progress.
2. Early implementation of rehabilitation interventions during acute care to promote recovery and prevent complications.
3. Selection of the type of rehabilitation program and services best suited to meet the patient's needs.
4. Establishment of realistic rehabilitation goals and provision of treatment in accordance with a carefully developed rehabilitation management plan.
5. Combined follow-up and treatment during transition to a community residence.

- Emphasis was also placed on the importance of active patient and family involvement.
- The AHCPR relied on evidence derived not only from an exhaustive literature review, but also from the development of consensus opinions by an expert panel.
- According to the AHCPR Clinical Practice Guidelines, several factors are critical to the appropriate implementation of a rehabilitation program. First, there is a fundamental recommendation to use an interdisciplinary team approach. Thorough, consistent, and fully documented patient assessment is key at several points, including at the time of screening for rehabilitation, at rehabilitation admission, throughout the course of rehabilitation, at discharge, and during long-term follow-up.
- Patient and family involvement in the rehabilitation process enhance the likelihood of achieving favorable outcomes. Principles derived from learning theory should be applied to ensure that appropriate training is occurring.
- Stroke rehabilitation should begin as soon as the diagnosis is established, life-threatening problems are brought under control, and activity is deemed medically feasible. Specific measures should be taken to prevent recurrent stroke, to prevent secondary medical complications, and to address ongoing functional health issues. The patient should be mobilized and encouraged to resume self-care activities.
- During the acute phase after stroke, the patient should be screened for whether or not there is a need for rehabilitation, and if so, screened for the level, type, and setting. Criteria for admission to specific levels or types of settings are not uniformly applied. However, the AHCPR guidelines attempt to provide threshold criteria for determining the need for rehabilitation, including medical stability, the presence of functional deficits, the ability to learn, enough physical endurance to allow the patient to sit up for at least 1 hour, and the ability to participate actively in the rehabilitation program. Within the group of patients who meet those criteria and who are candidates for rehabilitation, one criterion for admission to a comprehensive interdisciplinary program is the presence of at least two types of disability that would require at least two disciplines of professionals to assist in management.
- One important aspect of management is the performance of a thorough and accurate assessment. This assessment is used to establish the goals of the

rehabilitation program. The assessment is also used to drive the development of the management plan that is implemented to promote the attainment of those goals. Another reason for the assessment is to provide a baseline for comparing functional progress. Ongoing monitoring of progress allows the team to adjust the plan and the specific interventions. The interventions in the treatment program should be designed and implemented to *match* and meet the patient's needs.

• A list of potentially useful modalities is available in the AHCPR guidelines and in other references.

• Discharge planning should be performed during the rehabilitation program and should include family teaching and securing community resources.

• It is important to monitor progress and status after discharge. Specific attention should be paid to important long-term issues as the availability of community supports, safety and fall prevention, health promotion, sexuality issues, leisure and recreational activities, driving, and return to work.

SPECIAL PATIENT CONSIDERATIONS (pp. 1151–1152)

Pediatric Stroke (p. 1151)

• Stroke is unusual in children, with an estimated incidence of 2.5 per 100,000 children per year. The presentation in neonates and children often is different from that in older individuals; seizures, fever, and delayed achievement of developmental milestones are not uncommon. Causes of stroke include hereditary conditions, congenital heart disease, metabolic disorders, coagulopathy, drugs, and intracerebral vascular anomalies. The prognosis after stroke in children is generally thought to be better than in adults. Some residual deficit is present in the majority of children. Rehabilitation emphasizes functional restoration and compensation, psychosocial support, and the attainment of normal developmental abilities.

Stroke in Young Adults (p. 1151)

• Hemorrhagic strokes account for about one-third of all strokes in young adults. Common causes of cerebral infarctions include atherosclerosis, cardiogenic embolism, cerebral vasculitis, and coagulopathy. The approach to the diagnostic workup of the younger stroke patient is aggressive, and often calls for pro-

---

TABLE 50–10 Rehabilitation and Long-Term Issues in Young Stroke Survivors

1. Employment
2. Sexuality
3. Child care, parenting
4. Instrumental activities of daily living—homemaking, meal preparation, shopping
5. Psychological aspects of life-role changes
6. Spouse vs. personal caregiver role
7. Financial management
8. Driving
9. Relationship changes
10. Leisure planning, hobbies, socializing

cedures such as cerebral angiography, coagulation tests, collagen vascular disease evaluation, and cardiac workup.

• Young adults tend to present with unique rehabilitation needs and long-term issues. Table 50–10 lists many of the specialized problems and needs that are more prevalent and prominent among younger adults compared to older individuals.

Ethical Considerations (p. 1152)

• An issue that commonly arises in the treatment of patients with stroke (and other conditions treated in rehabilitation units and centers) is whether and to what degree autonomy in decision making can be undertaken safely and reliably by the patients.

• Other problems arise when an individual insists on living independently when it is unsafe to do so, or when patients or their families insist on continued hospitalization or rehabilitation program participation when there is little or no clinical indication to do so. Many of these decisions involve the determination of the patient's competency and establishment of guardianship.

51

Original Chapter by Mary L. Dombovy, M.D., and Barbara A. Pippin, M.D.

Rehabilitation Concerns in Degenerative Movement Disorders of the Central Nervous System

• The general category of movement disorders includes a number of central nervous system (CNS) neurodegenerative diseases such as Parkinson's disease and other brainstem-basal ganglia degenerations, the hereditary ataxias, and the dystonias (Table 51–1). Parkinson's disease is by far the most common, affecting 1% of the population aged 65 years and over. Many of the symptoms and signs of Parkinson's disease can be seen in other neurodegenerative disorders, as well as in anoxic encephalopathy, multiple lacunar infarcts, drug effects, and the normal aging process (Table 51–2).

PARKINSON'S DISEASE (pp. 1164–1174)

Pathophysiology, Clinical Presentation, and Differential Diagnosis (pp. 1164–1168)

• The primary biochemical defect in Parkinson's disease is the loss of striatal dopamine resulting from the degeneration of dopamine-producing cells in the substantia nigra. There is an associated hyperactivity of cholinergic neurons in the caudate nuclei contributing to the symptoms.

• Although Parkinson's disease can present with an array of clinical symptoms and signs (Table 51–3), the cardinal features of the disease are: (1) resting or postural tremor, (2) bradykinesia, (3) rigidity, and (4) postural instability. In the early stages of Parkinson's disease, rigidity (often described as "stiffness" or "achiness" by patients) can be mistaken as a symptom of arthritis. Masked facies and bradykinesia can lead to the most common early misdiagnosis, that of depression. The onset and progression of the disease are slow and insidious. The disease can begin either with tremor or with bradykinesia and rigidity as the initial presentation. Symptoms and signs typically begin in one extremity or one side but eventually spread to involve the other limbs and trunk. Lack of arm swing when walking and changes in handwriting (micrographia) are early signs.

• Although tremor can become disabling, it usually does not impair function as much as bradykinesia and rigidity, which eventually lead to problems in all areas of mobility and activities of daily living (ADL). When ambulating, patients have

TABLE 51–1 Selected Central Nervous System Movement Disorders

Idiopathic	*Secondary*
Parkinson's disease	Birth injury
Progressive supranuclear palsy (Steele-Richardson-Olszewski syndrome)	Chorea gravidarum
	Neuroleptic medications
Multiple system atrophy (Shy-Drager syndrome)	Head injury
Corticobasal degeneration	Cerebral infarct/hemorrhage
Most dystonias	Anoxia
Blepharospasm	Carbon monoxide poisoning
Meige's disease	Manganese poisoning
Gilles de la Tourette's syndrome	Mercury poisoning
	Basal ganglia tumor
Genetic	Liver disease
Huntington's disease	Oral contraceptives
Wilson's disease	Hyperthyroidism and hypothyroidism
Some dystonias	
Inherited ataxias	Hypoparathyroidism
Numerous metabolic defects	Alcohol
Ataxia telangiectasia	Sydenham's chorea
Olivopontocerebellar degeneration	von Economo's encephalitis
Friedreich's ataxia (and others)	
Familial nonprogressive chorea	
Essential tremor	
Hallervorden-Spatz disease	

difficulty in changing direction or moving around objects and can "freeze." Patients with Parkinson's disease have great difficulty in carrying out two simultaneous but unrelated motor acts, such as talking while walking.

• Impairment of speech is one of the most frustrating disabilities for patients with Parkinson's disease. Speech becomes rapid, monotonous, and of low volume (hypokinetic dysarthria).

• Because the basal ganglia play an important role in motor planning and programming, Parkinson's disease patients display various degrees of difficulty with initiating activity such as walking, reaching for objects, or changing course when walking.

• As Parkinson's disease progresses, autonomic symptoms, dysphagia, and postural instability become bothersome. Dementia is often a late feature and ultimately appears in about one-third of the patients. Depression can affect as many as 50% of the patients. Dementia and depression can be difficult to diagnose in the presence of psychomotor retardation (i.e., a slowness in producing the motor response). Hallucinations, insomnia, nausea, lack of appetite, weight loss, and dystonia are often encountered as side effects of dopaminergic medications. Insomnia is also seen as the result of nocturnal bradykinesia.

• Typically there is a gradual increase over time in all of the manifestations of Parkinson's disease. Before the advent of levodopa therapy, 25% of patients with symptom duration of less than 5 years were severely disabled, and 75% of survivors with symptom duration of 10 to 15 years were totally disabled. Patients having rigidity as the predominant initial symptom tend to experience disability

TABLE 51–2 Differential Diagnosis of Parkinsonism

Idiopathic Parkinson's disease*,†
Progressive supranuclear palsy*
Multiple system atrophy*
Oliropontocerebellar atrophy*
Striatonigral degeneration
Wilson's disease†
Westphal variant of Huntington's disease†
Corticobasal degeneration
Hallervorden-Spatz disease
Alzheimer's disease (late stages)
Parkinson-ALS-dementia complex
Postencephalitis
Drug-induced*† (neuroleptics,*† metaclopramide,*† reserpine†)
Toxin-induced*† (MPTP,† manganese,† carbon monoxide,*† carbon disulfide,† cyanide†)
Metabolic*,† (anoxia,* hypothyroidism,*† hypoparathyroidism*†)
Multi-infarcts*†
Subdural hematoma*†
Multiple head injuries (boxer's dementia†)
Basal ganglia tumor*†
Normal-pressure hydrocephalus*†

*Most common considerations.
†Important to consider and rule out.
Abbreviations: ALS, amyotrophic lateral sclerosis; MPTP, 1-methyl-4-phenyl-1,2,3,6-tetrahydropyridine.

TABLE 51–3 Clinical Features of Parkinson's Disease

Symptoms and Signs	*Common Presenting Complaints*
Rigidity	Stiffness, aching muscular pain, slowed
Bradykinesia (slowness of movement)	movements
Resting/postural tremor	Trouble getting out of a chair
Hypokinesia (small-amplitude movement)	Trouble rolling over in bed
Loss of postural reflexes	Falling, tripping over objects on floor
Loss of preparatory and associated movements	Tremor, "shaking"
("en bloc" movements, decreased arm swing,	Depression
decreased blinking)	Memory loss
Akathisia (inability to sit still, relieved by	Stooped posture
walking about)	Rapid or whispering speech
Dementia	Change in handwriting
Autonomic dysfunction (orthostatic hypotension,	Slowness in activities, dressing, grooming
slowed gastrointestinal motility, urinary	Trouble walking
retention, impotence)	Slow to respond to questions and requests
Hypokinetic dysarthria	Drooling; trouble controlling saliva
Festinating gait	
Masked facies (stare with decreased blinking)	
Dystonia	
Flexed posture	
Dysphagia	
Sudden "freezing" of motor activity	

TABLE 51–4 Common Side Effects of Medications Used in Parkinson's Disease

Carbidopa-levodopa compounds	Nausea, hypotension, arrhythmias, hallucinations, nightmares, hypomania, paranoid psychosis, delirium, insomnia, dystonia, dyskinesias
Deprenyl (selegiline)	Cardiac toxicity, hallucinations; potentiates side effects of levodopa
Amantadine	Hallucinations, insomnia, nervousness, edema, livedo reticularis, headache
Dopaminergic agonists	Hallucinations, vivid dreams, psychosis, paranoia
Anticholinergics	Impaired memory, confusion, urinary retention, blurred vision, dry mouth, constipation, orthostatic hypotension

earlier than those with tremor as the presenting feature. The introduction of levodopa, deprenyl (selegiline), and novel medication management strategies has prolonged independence and has allowed for continued employment in many cases.

• Early Parkinson's disease can be difficult to distinguish from other subcortical degenerations. The hallmarks of Parkinson's disease are a definite response to levodopa treatment and the absence of symptoms and signs such as early vertical eye movement abnormalities (progressive supranuclear palsy), early autonomic failure (Shy-Drager syndrome), hyperreflexia, Babinski's signs, ataxia, and peripheral neuropathy (multisystem degeneration).

• A number of medications are utilized in the management of Parkinson's disease (Table 51–4). Levodopa combined with carbidopa remains the cornerstone of pharmacological therapy for Parkinson's disease, although controversy exists as to when treatment with levodopa should begin. More than half of the patients with Parkinson's disease who receive treatment with conventional levodopa preparations later develop response complications, including a shortened response duration. Some treating physicians delay levodopa therapy until symptoms significantly interfere with function, or they begin treatment with a direct dopamine receptor agonist such as pergolide or bromocriptine.

• Monoamine oxidase B inhibitors such as selegiline may exert a mild dopaminergic effect and may inhibit generation of oxygen radicals. Some treating physicians begin treatment of early Parkinson's disease with selegiline because of its therapeutic effects and the potential that it might slow disease progression. Selegiline also can be used to smooth out levodopa-related fluctuations later in the disease.

• With sustained-release levodopa combination preparations, the potential for symptom fluctuation is reduced. An additional advantage of sustained-release preparations is the reduction of the profound alterations in levodopa plasma concentrations that are thought to contribute to some of the later problems with dyskinesia and other dose-response fluctuations. Although the manufacturer indicates that twice-daily dosing is adequate with Sinemet CR, most patients achieve a smoother response dosing three times a day and eventually four times a day. The use of catechol O-methyltransferase (COMT) inhibitors has been shown to prolong the biologic half-life of levodopa. COMT inhibitors increase the bioavailability of levodopa and smooth the fluctuations of plasma levels of levodopa.

- Variable gastric emptying is often a feature of advanced Parkinson's disease and can lead to an apparent lack of response to oral medication. Jejunal infusion has also been used in instances in which motor fluctuations and wearing-off effects are prominent, even if gastric retention is not a problem. Enteral tubes are a consideration when dysphagia has progressed to the point of inadequate nutrition or there is a high risk of aspiration. Improvement in gastric emptying can also be achieved by administering a large glass of water with oral levodopa or carbidopa.
- Direct dopamine agonists (DAs) such as bromocriptine and pergolide have emerged as a significant therapeutic addition to levodopa. These compounds directly stimulate dopamine receptors independent of levodopa. The potential neurotoxic effects of levodopa are avoided. DAs also scavenge oxygen radicals, suppress lipid peroxidation, and decrease dopamine release and turnover, all of which are neuroprotective. DA monotherapy has been shown to be effective for a majority of patients at 1 year, but was effective only for a small percentage (2% to 17%) at 5 years. A number of studies have shown that the combination of DA and levodopa is more effective than levodopa alone in preserving motor activity and minimizing dyskinesia at 5-year follow-up. Some investigators suggest the use of DA monotherapy early, with addition of levodopa only when DA can no longer satisfactorily control the symptoms. The use of DA monotherapy and its timing is clearly still controversial.
- Amantadine, which has both pre- and postsynaptic dopaminergic effects, is also used both as early treatment and later as an adjunct. Anticholinergics (e.g., trihexyphenidyl [Artane] and benztropine [Cogentin]) are helpful when tremor is the predominant problem, but become less well tolerated as Parkinson's disease progresses. This is because of such side effects as sedation, impaired memory, and urinary retention. The use of anticholinergics to treat Parkinson's disease has decreased over the past 5 years.
- A reasonable approach to initial treatment of Parkinson's disease would be to: (1) introduce selegiline (Deprenyl) at the time of early diagnosis; (2) begin a low dose of a dopamine agonist, either with or without a long-acting levodopa preparation, when symptomatic treatment becomes functionally indicated; and (3) titrate levodopa dosages as symptom control warrants, using the lowest dose required for adequate function. This approach is particularly reasonable for younger and middle-aged patients with Parkinson's disease. It should be noted that there appears to be declining enthusiasm for the use of deprenyl. Multiple drug approaches can produce significant side effects in the elderly and can lead to decreased compliance with the medication program. Many treating physicians prefer to initiate the treatment of older patients with immediate release Sinemet and to titrate the dose depending on the patient's tolerance and the therapeutic response. The management of dose-response fluctuations, dyskinesia, and the "on/off" phenomenon is complex and can be frustrating.
- The potential side effects of these medications are numerous, and it is important to be aware of them in the rehabilitation setting (see Table 51–4).

The Rationale for Rehabilitation (pp. 1168–1170)

- Many experts in the treatment of Parkinson's disease recommend rehabilitation to prevent complications and to either maintain or assist with function.
- In general, evidence suggests Parkinson's disease patients benefit from an exercise program that focuses on improving range-of-motion (ROM),

endurance, balance, and gait. Parkinson's disease patients report that the provision of equipment and instruction in adaptive techniques provided by OT in the home was helpful to them.

• There is some evidence that rehabilitation leads to an improvement in ADL and motor function (i.e., bradykinesia and rigidity) but no improvement in tremor, timed finger tapping, mentation, or mood. Unfortunately, there is also evidence that patients do not continue the exercise program at home, causing a return to baseline. Continued exercise might be needed to maintain function, but permanently incorporating such a program into a patient's lifestyle without continuation of an organized program appears unlikely.

• Exercise tends to produce improvements in gait, tremor, motor coordination, and grip strength in Parkinson's disease patients in an exercise program, regardless of whether the program is formal rehab or karate training. Such a program could be more easily continued in a group format at a community gymnasium or other facility in a more cost-effective fashion, with the additional benefit of increasing socialization.

• Although speech and swallowing disorders are commonly a source of disability in Parkinson's disease, speech therapy is likely underutilized. Families often complain that speech is improved as long as the patient is receiving therapy, but as soon as the therapy ends, speech reverts to the previous pattern.

• Another speech disorder common in Parkinson's disease is palilalia. Palilalia is characterized by the repetition of a word or phrase with increasing rapidity and decreasing distinctiveness, and eventually becoming inaudible. The use of a pacing board has been noted to be helpful in decreasing palilalia.

Exercise and Muscle Physiology (p. 1170)

• In prescribing exercise programs for patients with Parkinson's disease, the ability of the patient to tolerate the exercise must be taken into account. Lowered mechanical efficiency in leg muscles has been demonstrated in Parkinson's disease patients, resulting in these patients performing twice the work of normal controls. Physical inactivity and deconditioning in subjects with Parkinson's disease might be as important a factor as an altered metabolic state of muscle. It has also been shown that levodopa therapy reduces the externally measured work of walking in subjects with varying stages of Parkinson's disease.

Psychological and Social Aspects (p. 1170)

• Psychological and cognitive impairments and their resultant impacts on disability are often overlooked. Most patients with Parkinson's disease perform less well on a wide range of cognitive tests than age- and education-matched controls. It appears that dementia in Parkinson's disease has both a cortical and a subcortical origin. Pathological changes similar to those found in Alzheimer's disease are commonly found in patients with Parkinson's disease. The changes do not always correlate with the presence of dementia.

• Adaptation to change in daily routine or environment can be difficult and result in undue anxiety. It is as if the same rigidity, bradykinesia, and difficulties with planning and adapting to change that affect the motor system in Parkinson's disease also affect the mind and thought processes. Patients with Parkinson's disease develop a sensitivity to drugs that affect the CNS, and often develop delirium when they are used.

- Sleep disturbances are common, and difficulty falling asleep can occur early in the disease. Sleep problems can be accentuated by the vivid dreams and hallucinations that can occur as a side effect of dopaminergic medications. Fatigue and an increased tendency to daytime napping also contribute to what eventually can become a totally reversed sleep-wake cycle.
- Depression is common in Parkinson's disease. It might be related to a deficit in serotonergic neurotransmission or to the diminution of cortical levels of norepinephrine and dopamine. Depression is difficult to treat in patients with declining mental function because of the anticholinergic side effects of the tricyclic antidepressants. A serotonergic agent might be the logical first choice in these patients. If that is ineffective, a tricyclic with low anticholinergic side effects (e.g., desipramine or nortriptyline) can be tried.
- Social dysfunction is also quite common, with the most common problem being lack of socialization because of anxiety related to bodily symptoms. Patients with akinesia rigidity tend to experience more emotional stress than those with tremor-predominant Parkinson's disease. Group counseling activities involving both patients and caregivers were found in one study to be helpful in reducing stress in 74% of patients.
- Maintaining the ability to drive is also important to independence. When motor or cognitive function becomes impaired such that driving could be affected, the physician should suggest a detailed assessment, which can include retaking the driver's test.

Specific Therapy Approaches (pp. 1171–1174)

Gait, Station, and Posture (pp. 1171–1172)

- The typical patient with moderate Parkinson's disease assumes a flexed posture, has difficulty initiating gait, and ambulates with short shuffling steps at an increasing rate. The base of support is usually narrow. Once walking begins, the patient has great difficulty changing direction, stepping over or moving around objects, or stopping (the festinating gait). Before beginning ambulation, the patient with Parkinson's disease does not make the normal preparatory movements of the trunk and extremities. During gait, associated movements (e.g., arm swing, trunk rotation, and pelvic motion) are reduced or absent. Postural reactions are impaired so that the patient with Parkinson's disease is unable to correct for mild perturbations in the center of gravity (e.g., being brushed by another person or taking a slight misstep). Sudden "freezing" can also occur and can precipitate a fall. (See Table 51–5.)
- Useful approaches to these problems include exercises emphasizing trunk extension and lateral and rotational trunk mobility, weight shifting and balance training, and instruction in falling safely and getting up off the floor. Widening the stance provides a better base of support. Conscious strategies to initiate gait and maintain a cadence are often quite helpful and include mental rehearsal and counting or singing, either aloud or to oneself; and marching to the rhythm. Exaggeration of arm swing and leg excursion is also helpful.
- Balance activities can be made a part of other functional activities such as washing, grooming, and household activities. A rolling walker typically works better than a standard walker because patients who are at a stage where a walker is needed usually cannot incorporate lifting a walker into their gait pattern. Care should be taken to set the walker at a higher height than usual so as not to further promote flexion. Inability to stop once started can be a problem with rolling walkers, and supervision is often required.

TABLE 51–5 Example of Rehabilitation Approach in Parkinson's Disease

Functional Problem	Underlying Impairments	Goals	Interventions
Slow and hesitant gait, problem reversing or changing direction, short steps	Bradykinesia, hypokinesia, loss of associated movements, loss of range of motion (ROM) in lower extremities	Decrease hesitancy; increase stride length; improve arm swing; allow for movement around obstacles	Mental rehearsal; marching to metronome and other external cues; exaggerate steps and arm swing; lower extremity ROM exercise and stretching
Kyphosis, reduced respiratory capacity	Rigidity, hip and knee flexion contractures, thoracic rigidity	Improve posture; improve respiration	Trunk extension exercises; breathing exercises; hip flexor and hamstring stretch
Rapid monotone speech with poor intelligibility	Hypokinesia, motor control disintegration	Improve intelligibility	Control breathing; pace rate; exaggerate enunciation
Falling	Rigidity, truncal and extremity contractures, loss of postural reflexes	Improve balance; decrease falls; improve safety	Stretching and ROM exercise of trunk, upper and lower extremities; balance training; instruction in falling and getting up from floor

• A visit to the patient's home by a physical or occupational therapist can result in environmental safety measures such as the removal of throw rugs; rearrangement of furniture; and installation of railings, grab bars, and other adaptive equipment. They can also help develop patient-specific home management strategies.

• In the newly diagnosed patient, there is an opportunity to prevent loss of motion and the development of flexed posture. Vigorous exercise that improves coordination and balance and promotes general fitness is helpful. Walking, bicycling, dancing, low-impact aerobics, and other group exercise programs not only improve function but also provide the opportunity for socialization.

Tremor, Bradykinesia, Hypokinesia, and Rigidity (p. 1172)

• Although tremor does not usually cause the same degree of functional impairment as other aspects of Parkinson's disease, it can become a factor if it is severe. The tremor is typically a resting-postural tremor that often ceases (or at least does not become worse) during movement. Anticholinergic medications can be helpful if tolerated. Because the tremor becomes worse with anxiety or stress, relaxation techniques are often helpful. Distal weights have not been proven to be of benefit in improving function.

• Bradykinesia, hypokinesia, and rigidity affecting the flexor muscles more than the extensors underlie the disability caused by Parkinson's disease. ROM exercises and stretching on a daily basis are important in preserving flexibility.

Initiation of movement, larger excursions during movement, and coordination should be addressed as a part of functional activities. There is increasing evidence that exercise is most effective when it is task-specific. Task-specific exercise might be especially important for the patient with Parkinson's disease in light of the impairments in motor planning and programming that are characteristic of the disease. Helpful strategies and techniques include measures such as rocking to and fro in the chair before arising, and other preparatory motions to provide momentum. A raised chair and toilet seat and arm rests also make arising easier.

• Rigidity can also result in musculoskeletal pain, which often responds to heat, massage, stretching, and ROM exercise.

Speech and Swallowing (pp. 1172–1173)
• Speech disturbances in patients with Parkinson's disease include initial hesitancy, low volume, rapid rate, monotone voice, poor articulation, hesitations or inappropriate periods of silence, stuttering, palilalia, and trailing off of the voice with an increasing rate. All of these combined are referred to as "hypokinetic dysarthria." The initial deficit is a failure to control respiration for the purpose of speech. Following this is gradual breakdown in the complex sensorimotor integration of speech production complicated by stiffness of facial and pharyngeal muscles.

• Speech typically improves somewhat with levodopa treatment. Speech therapy interventions consist of exercises emphasizing breath and rate control, improved (often exaggerated) articulation, and increased volume.

• Dysphagia tends to occur later in the disease and results in drooling, poor nutrition, and inability to take oral medications, and can lead to aspiration pneumonia. Common abnormalities include food-pocketing and a delayed swallowing reflex. Aspiration pneumonia is a major cause of morbidity and mortality in Parkinson's disease. Therapeutic interventions include positioning of the neck in flexion, smaller amounts of food, thickened liquids, avoidance of foods with mixed consistencies (e.g., vegetable soup), and a double swallow (see Chapter 26). The caregiver should be instructed in the Heimlich maneuver. In later stages, placement of a gastrostomy tube and tracheostomy might be considered. Consultation with a dietitian is helpful to ensure adequate nutrition. A decrease in protein intake can be necessary to promote adequate levodopa absorption. Patients with frequent and severe dyskinetic reactions can require large amounts of calories.

• A videofluoroscopic swallowing study is helpful in determining the cause of the swallowing difficulties and helps direct the treatment approach. The swallowing study is also able to assess the severity of the problem and the potential for and actual occurrence of aspiration (see Chapter 26).

Autonomic Dysfunction (p. 1173)
• Orthostatic hypotension becomes a problem in later stages of the disease. Arising slowly and pausing in the sitting position before standing, elevating the head of the bed, and using pressure garments are helpful conservative approaches. Mineralocorticoids can also be helpful.

• Slowed gastric and intestinal motility lead to early satiety, vomiting, poor absorption of medications, and constipation. Useful strategies include frequent small meals, increased fiber intake, bulking agents, stool softeners, suppositories, and timed voiding. Metoclopramide facilitates gastric emptying but should

generally be avoided because of its tendency to cause parkinsonian side effects.
• Urinary incontinence, difficulty voiding, retention, and infections can also occur. Recurrent urinary infections often indicate neurogenic bladder dysfunction, although other causes such as prostatic hypertrophy are common in this age group. An appropriate investigation typically includes postvoid residual; cystoscopy; assessment of renal function; and, in some cases, cystometrogram-sphincter electromyography (CMG-EMG). The results of this workup can guide the practical and pharmacological interventions. An indwelling catheter should be used only as a last resort and if it will facilitate the care of a severely disabled patient (see Chapter 27). Impotence can also occur as a result of autonomic dysfunction or psychological factors.
• "Sympathetic pain" and complex regional pain syndrome can be seen in Parkinson's disease. The pain is often alleviated by levodopa. If it is not, the use of a tricyclic antidepressant is often helpful and can also decrease tremor. In later stages, the anticholinergic effects on cognition are less well tolerated. The effectiveness of the serotonergic antidepressants in alleviating neurogenic pain is unclear.

Cardiopulmonary Function (p. 1173)
• Flexed posture leads to kyphosis, which reduces lung capacity. Rigidity can result in a "restrictive" pulmonary disease pattern, further complicating respiratory function. Endurance often decreases secondary to a sedentary lifestyle. A focus on breathing exercises, proper posture, and trunk extension early in Parkinson's disease is helpful in preventing these musculoskeletal complications, which contribute to the high incidence of pulmonary dysfunction. Cardiopulmonary conditioning should also be a component of the early treatment program (see Chapters 32 and 33). Later in the course, breathing and extension exercise should be continued, with the addition of coughing, incentive spirometry, and respiratory therapy techniques as needed. Instruction in energy conservation techniques and pacing can preserve the ability to continue in a productive role.

Cognition and Depression (p. 1173)
• Management of declining cognitive function becomes a major issue in many cases. Although Parkinson's disease has its peak incidence in the sixth decade, the disease begins in some patients in the 40s or 50s. As noted above, patients with Parkinson's disease can have deficiencies in cognitive function very early in the disease that might not be apparent on a social level but which can cause problems at work. Full neuropsychological assessment is prudent in such cases. In other cases more limited testing to assess for safety to continue independent living or driving is adequate. Making the family aware of safety issues and providing both the family and the patient with compensatory cognitive techniques are essential.

ADL and Adaptive Equipment (pp. 1173–1174)
• A thorough functional assessment is key to the development of an integrated program for the patient with Parkinson's disease. Instruction in compensatory techniques and the use of various devices can allow the patient to remain functional for a prolonged period. A home visit not only helps in assessing the need for home modification but also allows the therapist to see how the patient functions in the home. Numerous assistive devices are available (see Chapter 25).

The Home Program and Follow-up (p. 1174)

• Patients with Parkinson's disease require a regular and ongoing exercise program to maintain or, in some cases, improve function. A specific exercise format does not appear to be as critical as covering the following areas: (1) relaxation and breathing; (2) posture principles; (3) active, active-assistive, and passive ROM exercises and stretching; (4) balance and gait activities; (5) coordination; (6) general conditioning; and (7) specific functional activities, including speech, ADL, and other tasks.

PARKINSON-LIKE SYNDROMES (pp. 1174–1175)

• The approach to other degenerative disorders with features similar to Parkinson's disease (e.g., progressive supranuclear palsy and multiple system atrophy) is similar to that used with Parkinson's disease. Many of these diseases have a more rapidly debilitating course that needs to be considered when developing the rehabilitation plan.

Huntington's Disease (p. 1174)

• Huntington's disease is an autosomal dominant disorder caused by a genetic mutation on chromosome 4. The mutation is ubiquitous, although the striatum manifests the most severe neuropathological damage. Huntington's disease usually presents with chorea, dementia, and behavioral and mood disorders. In a small percentage of patients, hypokinesia and rigidity are the presenting features. This is referred to as the Westphal variant and tends to have its onset at an earlier age. It is now possible to identify patients while they are still asymptomatic with the use of genetic testing. In addition to chorea and neuropsychological changes, dysarthria, dysphagia, and gait abnormalities can also occur.

• Rehabilitation efforts are functional and patient care and caregiver oriented. Chorea does not respond to PT, although dopaminergic-blocking agents can be helpful. Chorea can consume a large amount of energy and calories, making nutrition a prime concern. Many communities have active support groups for patients and families affected by Huntington's disease.

Hereditary Ataxias (pp. 1174–1175)

• The hereditary ataxias include a wide range of disorders. Some of these present with intermittent ataxia, and some have ataxia that is progressive and combined with other neurological features such as upper motor neuron signs (e.g., olivopontocerebellar atrophy) and peripheral nerve signs (e.g., absent ankle reflexes in Friedreich's ataxia). Ataxia can result from disorders of the cerebellum or its connections, the brainstem, the vestibular system, the dorsal columns and spinocerebellar tracts of the spinal cord, the dorsal root ganglia, or the peripheral nerves. Some of these disorders also have associated systemic involvement (e.g., cardiomyopathy and diabetes mellitus in Friedreich's ataxia), which also have an impact on the rehabilitation program.

• Ataxia and ataxic (intention) tremor cannot be treated with medication in the same way that the symptoms of Parkinson's disease are diminished by levodopa. The mainstay of treatment is the provision of physical and occupational therapy directed at maintaining function for as long as possible. Gait training and instruction in the use of assistive devices to prevent falls and enhance mobility are useful. Distal weights can dampen the intention tremor. Speech therapy can be helpful in improving articulation dysphagia. Specific coordination exercises are rarely useful or practical in progressive disorders, at least as compared to their utility in static causes of ataxia (i.e., head injury or stroke). Social services and psychological support are especially important, as they are for all progressive disorders.

Dystonia (p. 1175)

• Dystonia is a syndrome characterized by sustained muscle contractions resulting in abnormal movements or sustained postures. These movements and postures are the result of sustained co-contraction of both the agonist and the antagonist. Dystonia can be focal, multifocal, segmental, or generalized. Dystonic syndromes can be primary (idiopathic) or associated with or caused by another disorder (e.g., Parkinson's disease, anoxia, head injury, Wilson's disease, and inherited metabolic defects).

• Most focal dystonias respond to injections of botulinum toxin. Anticholinergics, levodopa, baclofen (Lioresal), carbamazepine, and clonazepam have all been used with some success in selected patients with more generalized forms. Thalamotomy is reserved for severe cases of generalized dystonia that have not responded to intensive pharmacological trials.

• Physical therapy techniques (e.g., massage and slow stretching) and modalities such as ultrasound and biofeedback are sometimes helpful in the focal or regional dystonias. Patients with generalized dystonia often benefit from gait and mobility training and instruction in the use of assistive devices.

52

Original Chapter by Ronald S. Taylor, M.D.

Rehabilitation of Persons with Multiple Sclerosis

• Multiple sclerosis (MS) is an inflammatory disease of the central nervous system (CNS) characterized by areas of demyelination. It is the third most common cause of disabling illness in individuals between the ages of 15 and 50 years. The exact cause remains uncertain. Evidence supports that MS is an illness of viral exposure during puberty that affects individuals with a genetically determined defect in their immune system. Functional and cognitive impairments develop in the majority of patients, with common involvement of gait, coordination, bladder, and sexual function.

EPIDEMIOLOGY (p. 1177)

• Studies from Olmstead County, Minnesota, indicate an incidence of 171 per 100,000, with females accounting for approximately 70% of cases. The average age at onset is 32.4 years for females, 34.3 years for males.
• Human lymphocyte antigen (HLA) linkages to MS have been noted, but vary with different populations. There appears to be increased incidence of MS in families, but no true Mendelian pattern of inheritance has been detected. In twin studies, concordance rates are 26% for monozygotic twins and 2.3% for dizygotic twins.

DIAGNOSTIC STUDIES (pp. 1177–1178)

Cerebrospinal Fluid Examination (pp. 1177–1178)

• No cerebrospinal fluid (CSF) abnormalities are specific for MS. CSF protein is elevated in approximately one-fourth of patients during exacerbations. Sixty to 75% of patients with MS have increased levels of CSF protein. The oligoclonal nature of IgG in the CSF of patients with MS was recognized more than two decades ago.

Magnetic Resonance Imaging (p. 1178)

• Magnetic resonance imaging (MRI) has been used as an adjunct in the diagnosis of MS since 1991, with positive findings seen in up to 95% of definite cases. Typical findings are multiple white matter lesions appearing as bright areas on T2-weighted (proton-density) sequences. Lesions are often seen in the brainstem, periventricular region, and cerebellum, with lesions in the corpus callosum being relatively specific for MS. Many other conditions can give similar changes on MRI. These conditions include aging, vasculitis, trauma, HIV infection, and irradiation. A commonly used criterion for diagnosis on MRI is four lesions greater than 3 mm in size (three lesions, if one is periventricular in location). One study has shown 100% specificity for MS when periventricular or infratentorial lesions greater than 6 mm are detected.

• The use of gadolinium adds to the utility of MRI. This tracer crosses the disturbed blood-brain barrier seen in MS exacerbations and allows the identification of acute inflammatory lesions and reactivated chronic plaques.

• Sixty-five percent of patients with positive MRI findings go on to develop clinically definite MS within 5 years, whereas only 3% of those with negative studies are subsequently diagnosed as having the disease. It is also to be noted that in patients with MS, the lesions detected on 75% of MRI studies do not correlate with the patient's neurological status.

Evoked Potential Recordings (p. 1178)

• Evoked potentials are useful in the diagnosis of MS because of altered conduction time in the CNS myelinated pathways. Visual-evoked potentials (VEP) are abnormal in 75% of patients with definite MS, and in 15% to 60% of patients with possible MS. Subclinical abnormalities are detected in 20% to 30% of cases.

• Brainstem auditory-evoked potentials (BAEP) are also useful, with abnormalities seen in 67% of persons with definite MS, 41% of those with probable MS, and 30% of subjects with possible MS. Subclinical abnormalities are detected in 21% to 55% of studies. Similar values are noted for somatosensory-evoked potentials (SSEPs), with higher rates of abnormality found in the lower extremities than in the upper extremities. Combining all three potentials can be helpful when the diagnosis is questionable.

PATHOPHYSIOLOGY (pp. 1178–1179)

• Postmortem studies reveal areas of demyelination, with relative preservation of axons. These areas are called plaques and are found only in the CNS. They have a predilection for the optic nerve; the perivenous areas; and the periventricular white matter of the cerebrum, brainstem, and spinal cord.

• The earliest abnormality typically detected on MRI is a localized breakdown in the blood-brain barrier. Such breakdown is seen as an area of enhancement on gadolinium-enhanced MRI and can precede the onset of neurological deficits. The area of abnormality increases in size over an average of 6 weeks and eventually decreases to the size of the original enhancing lesion. The lesions disappear completely in up to 20% of cases. The decrease in size of the lesions is thought to be caused by resolution of brain edema.

• Demyelination is the hallmark of MS, but it remains unknown whether it precedes or follows the changes in the blood-brain barrier discussed above. Signs of remyelination have been noted, but remyelination appears to take place predominantly in the early part of the illness. Recent studies imply that axonal transection exists in patients with MS.

IMMUNOREGULATION (pp. 1179–1180)

• Recent clinical data indicate that MS could be an autoimmune disease triggered by an infectious agent. Abnormalities of T lymphocytes have been documented in MS patients since the early 1970s. IgG has been shown to be increased in the CSF of patients with MS. Various studies have implicated measles, rubella, or even "nonsense antibody" as the trigger. Further theories postulate that these cells may have "escaped" more normal regulation and are synthesizing antibodies on their own.

• Recent studies of acute MS lesions have detected antibody against myelin-oligodendrocyte glycoprotein, a minor protein component of myelin. This is the first solid evidence of the presence of autoantibodies against myelin in patients with MS.

SIGNS AND SYMPTOMS (p. 1180)

• The initial signs and symptoms of MS are quite variable (Tables 52–1 and 52–2). Fifty percent of patients have symptoms related to one site or system at onset. Optic neuritis is present at the onset in up to 48% of patients, and 40% present with weakness. Weakness is often accompanied by an increase in muscle stretch reflexes and is one of the more common symptoms found in patients with MS. The distribution of the weakness is most commonly in both lower extremities, with the next most common pattern being one leg, or one leg and the ipsilateral arm. Weakness confined to one or both upper extremities is unusual.

• Paresthesias can be present at any stage of the disease and often are described as painful. True radicular pain is unusual, and other causes should be sought when this occurs. Cerebellar signs increase during the course of the disease and often lead to marked disability.

• The general course of the illness in MS is variable but generally falls into a benign category (with one or two episodes followed by long periods of remission), a relapsing and remitting course, a relapsing-progressive course, or a chronic progressive course.

DIAGNOSIS AND COURSE (p. 1181)

• Because of the pleomorphic aspects of MS, the diagnosis depends on a skilled clinician's recognition of signs of demyelination. Visual, gait, and sensory disturbances are the most common presentations at the onset of the disease.

TABLE 52–1 Symptoms Present at Onset of Illness in Definite MS

Symptom	% of Patients
Weakness	40
Paresthesia	30
Gait difficulty	25
Optic neuritis	20
Diplopia	15
Ataxia	10
Disturbed nutrition	10
Vertigo	5

TABLE 52–2 Signs and Symptoms Present during the Course of MS

Sign/Symptom	% of Patients
Paresthesia	100
Weakness	100
Abnormal reflexes	80
Cerebellar signs	80
Spasticity	75
Fatigue	75
Decreased alternating movements	70
Heat intolerance	60
Nystagmus	50
Cognitive impairment	40
Erectile impotence	40
Lhermitte's sign	40
Pain	30
Depression	30
Muscle wasting	20
Dementia	10
Facial weakness	3
Unilateral hearing loss	3
Epilepsy	2
Visual failure	1
Trigeminal neuralgia	1

Diagnostic criteria for MS are listed in Table 52–3. In up to 91% of patients, MS begins with a relapsing and remitting course, with a majority of the exacerbations occurring in the first 5 to 10 years of the illness. In many patients the disorder becomes stable or progresses only slowly after this point. Chronic progressive MS is more likely to occur in patients with disease onset after age 40 years. In many cases the disease is characterized by a long latent period, with minimal symptoms of progression. It is not clear whether the disease is active during these periods. Factors associated with an increase in MS exacerbations are listed in Table 52–6 in the Textbook.

• The course of MS is extremely variable, ranging from death within 5 years in 5% of affected people, to many cases that are manifested by only one episode. In some cases MS can be diagnosed only postmortem. A decrease in life expectancy by $9^{1}/_{2}$ years in men and 14 years in women has been reported, but this is skewed by the rapid downhill course of a small percentage of patients. In the remainder of the MS population, life expectancy is not significantly affected. Severe disability is noted in 10% of patients within 5 years, in 25% of patients within 10 years, and in 50% of patients within 18 years. Approximately 20% of patients have no disability after 15 years of having MS. Annual relapse rates in MS vary in different studies, ranging from 0.1 exacerbations per year to 1.5. Factors associated with poor prognosis in MS include: progressive course at onset; male sex; age at onset greater than 40 years; cerebellar involvement at onset; and multiple system involvement at onset.

TABLE 52–3 Diagnostic Criteria

Possible MS

History of relapsing and possibly remitting signs without prior neurogenic symptomatology
Only one site of involvement in CNS determined by clinical, laboratory, or imaging studies
No other diagnostic explanation

Probable MS

Two documented attacks with clinical, laboratory, or imaging evidence of at least one lesion
One documented attack with clinical, laboratory, or imaging evidence of two separate lesions

Definite MS

Two attacks, separated by at least 1 month, with clinical, laboratory, or imaging evidence of at
  least two lesions

SOME FEATURES (pp. 1181–1182)

Cranial Nerve Involvement (p. 1181)

• Optic neuritis is more common early in the illness. It is usually associated with pain in the eye or forehead that can occasionally be severe. The visual field defect is typically a central scotoma. Bilateral simultaneous optic neuritis is not unusual, and is especially common in patients of Japanese descent. The visual-evoked potential after optic neuritis never returns to normal even if normal vision returns.
• Trigeminal neuralgia is present in 1% of patients. It can be bilateral and often is the presenting symptom. Facial palsy can be seen. Facial myokymia, manifested by rapidly firing muscular contractions of the facial muscles, is not unusual. Vertigo is common and can be severe and associated with vomiting. This might be the only initial symptom in patients with MS, but it is almost always transient.

Epilepsy (p. 1181)

• Epilepsy occurs in 1% to 2% of patients with MS, making it perhaps no more common than in the general population. Tonic seizures are the most common seizures seen in MS. They generally involve one arm or leg, and last for a few seconds. They can occur many times during the day.

Pain (pp. 1181–1182)

• Pain occurs in up to 50% of patients with MS. It is chronic in 90% of cases and manifests as dysesthetic extremity pain, chronic back pain, or painful leg cramps. The dysesthetic pain is the most common and also the most difficult to treat. Acute pain most commonly takes the form of trigeminal neuralgia or transient dysesthetic extremity pain.

DIFFERENTIAL DIAGNOSIS (p. 1182)

• The differential diagnosis in MS encompasses many entities. Care should be taken in diagnosing MS in the absence of eye findings, during a clinical remission, or in the presence of localized or atypical clinical features.

TREATMENT (pp. 1182–1186)

• Because of its variable presentations, the treatment of MS should be individualized for each patient. Treatments can be divided into symptomatic therapies and those that are designed to affect the natural course of the disease or to alter the length and severity of individual exacerbations. A sample of drug treatments is listed in Table 52–4. It is important to recognize and convey to the individual with MS that relapse rates decrease as the disease progresses, with the vast majority of relapses occurring in the first 5 to 10 years after the onset of initial symptoms.

• Treatment results in MS should be based on both objective findings and the subjective complaints of each patient. Objective findings do not always correlate with the clinical presentation. Many measurement devices have been proposed to monitor treatment efficacy. The most commonly used is the Kurtzke Disability Status Scale in either its original or expanded forms (Table 52–5; see also Fig. 52–9 in the Textbook).

Treatment Designed to Alter the Course of the Disease (pp. 1182–1185)

Steroids (pp. 1182–1183)

• The role of steroids in decreasing the length and severity of MS exacerbations has been documented in many articles. The mechanism of action is unknown but might relate to a decrease in CNS edema or to an effect on the immune system. Oral prednisone, in a dose of 60 to 100 mg tapered over 1 to 3 weeks, is commonly used for the treatment of a documented exacerbation of MS. If the exacerbation does not respond or is severe, intravenous doses of 500 to 1000 mg of methylprednisolone given daily for 3 to 7 days are recommended.

• The use of steroids in the treatment of chronic progressive MS has not been shown to be effective. Drug management for this entity remains controversial and unsatisfactory, although recent studies with interferon-beta-1B might change this situation. Cyclophosphamide, with or without ACTH, has been shown to be beneficial by some investigators.

Immunosuppressive Agents (p. 1183)

• Other attempts at immunosuppression in chronic MS have included the use of azathioprine and, more recently, cyclosporin A. Cyclosporin A has been shown to delay the time to becoming in need of a wheelchair in patients with chronic progressive MS, but nephrotoxicity has limited its usefulness. Plasmapheresis has also been used in addition to these medications, with mixed results.

Disease-Modifying Treatment: Interferon and Copaxone (pp. 1183–1184)

• Three disease-modifying immunosuppressive therapy treatments are currently in widespread clinical use: two interferons and glatirimer acetate (Copaxone). Each of these has been shown to be safe, to decrease the number of exacerbations by one-third, and possibly to slow the progression in chronic MS.

• Interferons as a class impede viral replication, slow cell proliferation, and alter immune responses. Studies with interferon-beta have demonstrated a one-third decrease in incidence of exacerbations in patients with relapsing-remitting MS and a 50% decrease in severe exacerbations. A decreased accumulation of plaque has been measured on MRI in 60% of patients taking this medicine.

TABLE 52-4 Sample Drug Treatments for MS

Medication	Dosage	Effects
Medications for Use in Exacerbations		
Prednisone	80–100 mg daily with taper over 7–21 days	Decreases length and severity of exacerbation
ACTH	40 units b.i.d. × 7 days	
Solumedrol	1000 mg IV over 2–4 hr, daily × 7 days, followed by 7–21 days of taper oral steroids	
Disease-Altering Medications		
Interferons		
INF-*β*-1B	8 million units SQ, QD	
INF-*β*-1A	30 micrograms 1M qw	
Copolymer-1	25 mg SQ qd	Decreases number of exacerbations
Medications for Chronic MS		
Cyclophosphamide with or without ACTH	By protocol	Slows progression in chronic MS
Azathioprine	By protocol	Slows progression in chronic MS
Cyclosporin A	By protocol	Slows progression in chronic MS

Table continued on following page

TABLE 52-4 Sample Drug Treatments for MS—cont'd

Medication	Dosage	Effects
Medications for Fatigue		
Amantadine	200–300 mL/day	Decreases fatigue
Pemoline		Liver toxicity
Medications for Spasticity		
Baclofen	20–120 mg/day	Decreases spasticity
Dantrolene	75–250 mg/day	Decreases spasticity
Tizanidine	4–16 mg/day	Decreases spasticity
Valium	5–40 mg/day	Decreases spasticity
Medications for Paroxysmal Symptoms		
Carbamazepine	200 mg b.i.d. or TIW	Decreases pain and parynchemal spasms
Gabapentin	300–2400 mg/day	Decreases pain and spasticity
Phenytoin	200–400 mg 1 day	Decreases pain and parynchemal spasms
Medications for Ataxia		
Clonazepan	1–6 mg/day	Decreases ataxia
Isoniazid	900 mg/day	Decreases ataxia

TABLE 52–5 Neurological Assessment: Kurtzke Disability Status Scale (DSS)

0 Normal neurological examination (all grade 0 in functional systems*)

1 No disability and minimal signs such as Babinski sign or vibratory decrease

2 Minimal disability (e.g., slight weakness or mild gait, sensory, or visuomotor disturbance)

3 Moderate disability though fully ambulatory (e.g., monoparesis, moderate ataxia, or combinations of lesser dysfunctions)

4 Relatively severe disability though fully ambulatory and able to be self-sufficient and up and about for some 12 hours a day

5 Disability severe enough to preclude ability to work a full day without special provisions. Maximal motor function: walking unaided no more than several blocks

6 Assistance (e.g., canes, crutches, or braces) required for walking

7 Restricted to wheelchair but able to wheel self and enter and leave chair alone

8 Restricted to bed but with effective use of arms

9 Totally helpless bedridden patients

10 Death due to multiple sclerosis

*Excludes cerebral function grade 1.
From Hart RG, Sherman DO: The diagnosis of MS. JAMA 1982; 247:498–503.

• The two FDA-approved types of interferon for MS are interferon-beta-1A (Avonex) and interferon-beta-1B (Betaseron). The major side effects include flu-like symptoms in approximately 60% of patients, which can usually be successfully treated with either anti-inflammatory medication or low-dose prednisone. Injection site reactions are also very common with interferon-beta, but rarely proceed to develop skin necrosis. Emphasizing proper injection technique can usually control such reactions.

• In a 2-year study of relapsing-remitting MS, glatirimer was found to decrease exacerbations by 29%. It also showed a significant slowing of cumulative disability. Other studies, however, have demonstrated a lack of response in patients with chronic progressive MS. Major side effects include flu-like symptoms and occasional injection site reactions. These problems are generally well tolerated. A transient flushing associated with chest tightness and dyspnea lasting for 30 seconds to 30 minutes is experienced by 15% of patients. This typically resolves spontaneously.

• A recent study in Europe of 700 patients with secondary progressive MS utilized 8 million units of interferon-beta subcutaneously every other day. The study was discontinued early because of the excellent response of treated patients when compared with those given placebo.

4-Aminopyridine (4-AP) (pp. 1184–1185)

• In one study, 70 patients with relapsing-remitting MS were treated with intravenous and oral 4-AP and placebo. Subjective improvement (defined as improvement in activities of daily living capabilities) was noted in 29% of the patients taking the medication but in only 1.6% of those taking placebo. Unfortunately, the clinical use of 4-AP has been delayed because of significant side effects, primarily seizures.

Treatment Designed to Ameliorate the Course of the Disease (pp. 1185–1186)

• The overall goal of rehabilitation in MS is to maximize function, regardless of whether the impairment is stable or worsening. Individuals with MS commonly present with problems in gait, sexuality, driving, shopping, cleaning house, urinary function, and socioeconomic stability. All of these factors lend themselves to intervention by the rehabilitation team.

Ameliorating Weakness (p. 1185)

• Because weakness is often a significant problem in MS, it is important that general conditioning be maintained as long as possible. This has to be done in a way that does not increase fatigue or body temperature. Because elevated body temperature can worsen MS symptoms, it is important that these patients have air conditioning in their homes and cars, especially if they live in southern climates. They might even consider moving to a more temperate zone to alleviate these problems. An individualized exercise program should be adapted to any ongoing changes in the patient's disease process. The use of air resistance stationary bikes (air movement minimizes temperature fluctuation), cool therapeutic pools, or upper extremity ergometers has proved beneficial in maintaining general aerobic conditioning. Such aerobic exercise has a significant impact not only on aerobic capacity but also in decreasing depression, anger, and fatigue.

• If patients wish to do additional exercises, a lightweight progressive resistance exercise program can be performed as tolerated. The use of weights, although often beneficial, is often not feasible, especially if the patient's primary disability relates to ataxia rather than weakness. Maintaining function of the musculoskeletal system is certainly helpful in minimizing the disability associated with MS. Not to be overlooked, however, is the significant psychological benefit and increase in overall self-esteem garnered from participating in a "can do" program.

Ameliorating Fatigue (p. 1185)

• The actual source of the fatigue is not well understood, but might represent a combination of weakness, spasticity, ataxia, depression, and heat. Patients with characteristic afternoon fatigue might benefit from Pemoline, 18.75 to 75 mg/day as needed. Patients on this medicine must be watched closely for liver toxicity. Amantadine (Symmetrel) in doses of 200 to 300 mg/day has also been documented to be useful.

Improving Mobility (p. 1185)

• Up to 60% of patients with MS have a need for some assistance with mobility. Maintaining mobility and functional independence is a constant challenge to the rehabilitation team, mainly because of the ever-changing clinical picture. Appropriate assistive devices should be prescribed to increase safety and decrease energy expenditure. Careful attention should be paid to psychological changes triggered by the need for these devices and the resultant implication that the disease is progressing. Patients should be informed that, on average, individuals with MS are still ambulating 27 years after diagnosis. Proper prescription and instruction in the use of wheelchairs often prolongs and increases the patient's functional independence. Motorized three-wheeled scooters are often preferred by the patient with MS because of the perception of greater societal acceptance. Care should be taken to ensure that the patient does not lose remaining functional ambulation by becoming overly dependent on these aids (see Chapter 18). Such aids should initially be used for long distances and difficult tasks, with patients continuing to ambulate on their own when doing less stressful activity.

Rehabilitation in Activities of Daily Living (pp. 1185–1186)

• Activities of daily living are often affected in patients with MS. Problems with balance, mobility, ataxia, spasticity, and weakness commonly lead to difficulty with hygiene, dressing, toileting, and communication. These problems are often amenable to the efforts of a rehabilitation team trained to deal with the unique and variable patterns of MS. Visits by an occupational therapist to a patient's home or office to recommend ergonomic considerations often lead to a marked increase in the patient's quality of life (see Chapter 25).

Assistance with Vocational and Avocational Activities (p. 1186)

• MS affects people in the prime of their lives, often after they have made and developed career choices. One-third of patients with MS are able to continue on their regular career path without modification, whereas another third can continue working with the help of the rehabilitation team and vocational counseling. The average patient suffers a 40% decrease in total lifetime earning capacity. Employers should be given information on the specific needs of the MS workers, including the elimination of architectural barriers and the role of fatigue in the patient's illness.

OTHER PROBLEMS TO BE ADDRESSED IN TREATING MS (pp. 1186–1188)

Cognitive and Psychiatric Aspects (p. 1186)

• Cognitive and psychiatric changes contribute substantially to the patient's level of disability. Memory appears to be the most affected function, with conceptual and abstract reasoning diminished to a lesser extent. One study reported mild intellectual deficits in 41% of people with MS, moderate deficits in 14%, and severe deficits in 6.5%. Although the severity tends to increase with duration, significant mental impairment can exist even in the presence of otherwise mild MS. MRI studies have demonstrated that patients with more severe cognitive impairments typically have more extensive brain lesions.

• Several authors characterize the dementia of MS as being of a subcortical type, marked by impaired manipulation of acquired knowledge, slowness of cognitive process, apathy, and lack of initiative. These cognitive problems are very important to identify because patients with such deficits are also less likely to be employed and more likely to engage in fewer social and avocational activities, to have increased sexual difficulties, and to exhibit more psychopathology.

• Psychiatric changes in MS have been described since the time of Charcot, with euphoria noted in 63% of patients in an early study by Cottrell and Wilson. An increase in the incidence of depression has recently been noted to correlate with the degree of neurological impairment but not with functional disability. One study of 108 patients with MS found depression that was mild in 17%, moderate in 7%, and severe in 4%. It remains to be clarified whether these psychiatric changes are an organic result of the MS or are a reaction to the illness. This could be of clinical significance because some patients with MS respond to very low doses of antidepressants and are thought to exhibit depression as a result of plaques in areas of the brain controlling emotions.

Neurogenic Bladder (pp. 1186–1187)

• Bladder dysfunction is a common complaint in MS patients. Early changes include either an increase or decrease in detrusor, bladder neck, or external sphincter control. Later stages of the disease are marked by bladder hyperreflexia and dyssynergia. The evaluation for these problems should include laboratory assessment of general renal function, with several determinations of post-voiding residuals. Cystometric evaluation with associated electromyographic monitoring of the pelvic floor musculature (see also Chapter 27) is helpful in categorizing bladder dysfunction. The constantly changing nature of the neuro-logical and urological deficit in the patient with MS should be recognized before treatment is begun.

• Management of mild neurogenic bladder symptoms should begin with regu-lation of fluid intake. If postvoid residuals exceed 100 mL, consideration should be given to a program of intermittent catheterization. Oxybutynin can be used for its anticholinergic and direct smooth muscle relaxant effects on the bladder. Detrusor tone can be increased with the use of bethanechol. Alpha-adrenergic drugs such as ephedrine can be used to increase bladder tone. Alpha-adrenergic-blocking agents (e.g., prazosin or phenoxybenzamine) can decrease bladder neck tone. Baclofen can decrease external sphincter dyssynergia. Antibiotics are often used prophylactically in conjunction with intermittent catheterization, but should be avoided when an indwelling catheter is utilized.

Neurogenic Bowel (p. 1187)

• Stool incontinence or constipation is often a disconcerting problem for the individual with MS. A bowel program that includes a high-fiber diet, a bulk former, a stool softener, and adequate fluid intake should be developed early in the course of the disease before significant difficulties develop. The use of lax-atives and enemas should be discouraged. It constipation becomes a problem, glycerin or Dulcolax suppositories, taken 45 minutes after the day's major meal, can be useful in maintaining bowel function (see also Chapter 28).

Spasticity (p. 1187)

• Spasticity is a common problem in the management of the patient with MS. Severe spasticity can be totally disabling. Management should always begin with instructing the patient and family in a program of stretching the affected muscles and joint range of motion. Attempts should be made to identify and correct sources of nociceptive input to the CNS because they can worsen spasticity. Such irritating stimuli can include urinary tract infections, skin ulcers, constipation, and deep venous thrombosis.

• If spasticity remains a problem, the carefully monitored use of medications should be instituted. Baclofen is the initial drug of choice when spasticity is of spinal origin, but it is less useful in spasticity of supraspinal origin. Baclofen treatment should begin at 10 to 20 mg/day in divided doses, with titration up to a dose of 80 to 100 mg/day if necessary. Care should be taken that the patient does not abruptly discontinue the medicine because seizures can result. Tizanidine (Zanaflex) is another helpful drug, but its usefulness is often limited by sedation. Benzodiazepines such as diazepam can be added if spasticity persists. They work at the spinal level but must be used cautiously as they can enhance previously existing fatigue, weakness, depression, and sedation. In refractory cases, dantrolene can also be utilized. Its mechanism of action is peripheral (i.e., it prevents myofibrillar contraction). Hepatotoxicity can occur, with the greatest incidence in women over 35 years of age.

• Recent trials have utilized localized botulinum toxin injection for treatment of intractable spasticity. In refractory cases, phenol nerve blocks can be attempted. The long-term nature of phenol blocks, as well as the possible side effect of painful paresthesias, can limit their usefulness. If spasticity remains a problem, the use of intrathecal baclofen, neurectomy, rhizotomy, tenotomy, or myelotomy might be required. For further information about spasticity treatment, see Chapter 29.

Ataxia and Tremor (pp. 1187–1188)

• Ataxia and tremor are especially vexing symptoms in the person with MS because they are often nonresponsive to rehabilitative or drug treatment. If exacerbated by weakness, appropriate strengthening can be beneficial. Repetitive coordinative exercises, such as those recommended by Frankel, are rarely useful owing to the progressive nature of the illness. In patients with extremity ataxia that interferes with dressing or feeding, appropriate proximal splinting can be beneficial. Drug therapy is of limited usefulness.

Sexual Function (p. 1188)

• In the early stages of MS there can be varied types of sexual dysfunction, most of which are usually transient. As the illness progresses, these symptoms typically become more common. In one study 91% of men and 72% of women reported changes in their sexual life. Disturbances in erection were noted in 62% of males. Failure to achieve orgasm (33%), loss of libido (27%), and spasticity (12%) were the most common complaints in women. Treatment involves identifying the problem as early as possible and providing appropriate counseling. Sildenafil (Viagra) is often helpful in this population for erectile dysfunction.

Pregnancy (p. 1188)

• The effects of MS on pregnancy are very important but remain controversial. In a recent study of 254 pregnant women with MS, no excess pregnancy-related complications were found. In the year prior to becoming pregnant, the patients averaged 0.7 MS relapses. This number dropped to 0.5 relapses during the first trimester of pregnancy, 0.6 during the second trimester, and 0.2 during the third trimester. The relapse rate increased to 1.2 per year during the first 3 months postpartum, however, leading to an overall relapse rate unchanged for the year dated from the onset of pregnancy to the first 3 months postpartum. Epidural anesthesia and breast-feeding had no effect on the results.

Charlatanism (p. 1188)

• The chronic and variable nature of MS, coupled with the lack of a cure, makes the individual with this illness especially susceptible to medical quackery.

Numerous miracle treatments have been proposed for MS, and they are often nothing more than a hoax. The physician must be sensitive to the desire of the MS patient to "try anything" and counter these claims with education and the utilization of the full line of available rehabilitation resources.

INPATIENT REHABILITATION (pp. 1188–1189)

• Patients with MS are often underserved in inpatient rehabilitation. This is despite the fact that rehabilitation, especially on an inpatient basis, can enhance the quality of a patient's life, improve functional status, and reduce overall health care costs. In patients with significantly diminished functional capacities, an admission to an inpatient rehabilitation unit can often provide the skills necessary to avoid placement in a long-term care facility.

53

Original Chapter by Lynne M. Stempien, M.D., and Deborah
Gaebler-Spira, M.D.

Rehabilitation of Children and Adults with Cerebral Palsy

• Cerebral palsy (CP) is a disorder of muscle tone and posture caused by a non-progressive injury to the immature brain. In most definitions, the neurological insult must occur by age 2 years. Neurological maturation can result in some early improvement, causing overestimation of children with permanent neuromotor dysfunction. Diagnosis of CP may not become clear until the child has difficulty reaching developmental milestones.

EPIDEMIOLOGY (pp. 1191–1192)

• Cerebral palsy is one of the most common disabilities affecting children. The prevalence rate is 5.2 per 1000 live births at 1 year of age, but resolution is reported in up to half of these children by 7 years of age.

• CP prevalence in full-term infants has remained relatively constant. Improved neonatal survival has decreased the risk of CP for neonates weighing more than 2500 g. In recent decades there has been a trend toward higher survival rates for smaller and premature infants with medical complications. Despite improved neonatal outcomes in general, the survival of these low-birth-weight (less than 2500 g) and very low-birth-weight (less than 1500 g) infants with higher CP risk has kept the prevalence of CP in childhood relatively constant.

• Gestational age less than 32 weeks is one of the most powerful predictors of CP. Maternal factors that increase CP risk include mental retardation, seizure disorder, hyperthyroidism, two or more prior fetal deaths, and a sibling with motor deficits. Long menstrual cycles and low socioeconomic class are also associated with increased CP risk. Intrauterine factors including fetal growth retardation, twin gestation, congenital malformations, third-trimester bleeding, increased urine protein excretion, fetal bradycardia, chorionitis, low placental weight, and abnormal fetal presentation are risk factors for CP. During labor and delivery, premature placenta separation poses an increased CP risk. In the early postnatal period, newborn encephalopathy increases risk of CP.

• Evidence is mounting that CP is most often the result of brain injury in utero. Peripartum difficulties are increasingly being regarded as the sequelae of an in vivo neurological insult and not necessarily as the cause of a neurological insult.

ETIOLOGY (p. 1192)

• The brain injury that leads to CP can occur in the prenatal, perinatal, or post-natal period. Currently, most common causes are related to premature births. The combination of fragile brain vasculature and the physical stresses of prematurity predispose these children to compromise of cerebral blood flow. Blood vessels are particularly vulnerable in the watershed zone next to the lateral ventricles. Bleeding in this area is often arterial in origin and can occur in differing degrees: cerebral intraventricular hemorrhage isolated to germinal matrix (grade 1), intraventricular hemorrhage with normal ventricular size (grade 2), intraventricular hemorrhage with ventricular dilatation (grade 3), or intraventricular hemorrhage with parenchymal hemorrhage (grade 4).

• Very low-birth-weight infants also have an increased incidence of periventricular hemorrhagic infarction. With healing of this bleeding, symmetrical necrosis of white matter adjacent to the lateral ventricles (periventricular leukomalacia) can develop. Periventricular leukomalacia is one of the strongest predictors of CP in the premature neonate.

• Fortunately, the large majority of children who are born prematurely do not develop CP, although they can have neuromotor and developmental abnormalities during early life. Even the most sophisticated pediatric developmental assessment tools are not sufficiently sensitive to detect deficits that will persist until after 1 year of age. Consequently, it is common for families to suspect motor problems long before the diagnosis of CP is given.

• In term births that result in CP, the cause of brain injury is often elusive. Most known perinatal injuries that cause CP are because of severe anoxic or ischemic brain injury. This can occur with mechanical difficulties of the placenta, umbilical cord, or the actual delivery itself. Intrapartum asphyxia must be severe to be the cause of CP. Unfortunately, injuries of this type tend to be more global and are more likely to cause a severe disability. Anoxia, ischemia, infection, or trauma can all cause injury in the postnatal period that results in a CP-type picture.

CLASSIFICATION (pp. 1192–1194)

• Cerebral palsy is generally characterized by the muscle tone abnormality and the body parts involved (Table 53–1). Spastic CP is the most common form, affecting approximately three-fourths of all patients with CP. This spasticity can occur in a velocity-dependent or velocity-independent manner. Resistance to passive movement may result in rigidity.

• Dyskinetic disorders with involuntary movements are less common. Dyskinetic disorders cause postural instability and sometimes involve fluctuations in tone. These patients often begin with hypotonia and develop the discrete involuntary movements over the first few years of life. Athetoid disorders are caused by damage to the basal ganglia, most commonly by hyperbilirubinemia or severe anoxia. The involuntary, slow writhing movements of athetosis involve large muscle groups. Small muscle involuntary movements such as chorea can also be seen. Rarely, ballistic, rotary, and flailing movements have been described. Ataxic disorders that mimic cerebellar dysfunction with wide-based gait and dysmetria are very rare in CP. The hypotonic form of CP is also uncommon. Some patients are classified as "mixed-type" CP if they have a combination of tone abnormalities.

• The distribution of affected limbs is used to name the type of CP. *Diplegia* refers to spastic paresis with predominant lower limb involvement, and is the most common form. *Quadriplegia,* involving abnormalities of both upper and lower extremities, is another common form. Rarely, a child has obvious abnormalities of both legs and one arm, and is referred to as having *triplegia.* Patients with arm and ipsilateral leg involvement are labeled as having *hemiplegia.* For unclear reasons, right hemiplegia is twice as common as left hemiplegia.

• Diplegia, or leg-dominated symptoms, is most common in low-birth-weight, premature patients. Quadriplegia is more common in those with normal birth weight. It should be noted, however, that most children with CP are "total body–involved." Close examination of motor control in the more normal-appearing limbs, trunk, and oral-motor musculature often reveals some abnormalities.

CLINICAL EFFECTS (pp. 1194–1197)

• The most pronounced symptoms in CP are disorders of neuromuscular control. Problems in infancy that suggest CP include irritability, lethargy, a weak suck, poor head control, high-pitched cry, oral hypersensitivity, asymmetrical movements, or unusual posturing. Motor delay can also be suggested by persistent abnormal motor activities such as rolling for mobility, combat crawling, "W-sitting," "bunny hopping," or adopting a hand preference before the first birthday (see Figs. 53–5 and 53–6 in the Textbook).

• Abnormalities of muscle tone are often accompanied by muscle weakness. Identifiable movements such as "scissoring," "guarding" of the upper extremities, and extensor posturing may result from imbalances in muscle tone and strength. Scissoring is the simultaneous adduction, knee hyperextension, and plantar flexion of the lower limbs (Fig. 53–1). Upper limb flexion synergy patterns include flexion at the fingers, wrists, and elbows with shoulder abduction. As this upper extremity pattern becomes stronger, the child may produce a low, mid, or high guard position. Some patterns of movement can be recognized as

TABLE 53–1 Classification of Cerebral Palsy Types

By Tone Abnormalities	By Body Parts Involved
Spastic	Diplegia
Dyskinetic	Quadriplegia
Athetoid	Triplegia
Choreiform	Hemiplegia
Ballistic	
Ataxic	
Hypotonic	
"Mixed"	

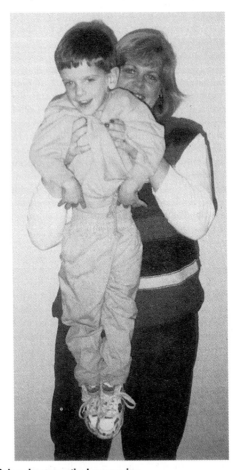

FIGURE 53–1. Scissoring on vertical suspension.

components of persistent primitive reflexes, such as the asymmetric tonic neck reflex (ATNR) (Fig. 53–2), symmetric tonic neck reflex (STNR), or tonic labyrinthine reflex (TLR).

• These movement patterns can be seen as the child attempts voluntary movement, triggered by passive positioning, in response to sensory stimuli, or as an "overflow" of uninvolved limbs. A primary difficulty in CP is this inability to separate out individual movements. The activation of remote muscle groups is one of the major impediments to more normal movement. Abnormalities of muscle tone and weakness often co-exist. Thus measuring muscle strength is problematic in CP patients because tone abnormalities may mask the patient's ability to generate force.

• Difficulty with head and trunk control interferes dramatically with balance. The development of appropriate, adequately implemented equilibrium and right-

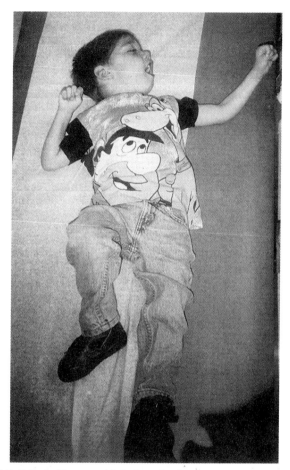

FIGURE 53–2. Patient with asymmetric tonic neck reflex.

ing reactions is delayed or sometimes absent. Abnormal coordination causes difficulty with executing movements. Even children with minimal involvement can exhibit apraxia when attempting high-level motor activities.

• Children with CP are often sensitive to normally innocuous stimuli because of a disordered kinesthetic sense. The abnormal sensory experience of disordered motor control can contribute to disordered sensory perception, which further interferes with the child's ability to perform high-level motor activities. Impaired two-point discrimination has been found in the upper extremities of children with all types of CP. Children with hemiparetic CP have also been found almost universally to have impaired stereognosis, with impaired proprioception in about half of patients tested.

• Contracture and deformity may result from disordered muscle tone, control, and balance. Contracture, or passive shortening that can limit joint and soft tissue movement, often affects the adductor, hamstring, and plantar flexor muscles of the lower limbs and the flexors of the upper extremities. This reflects the presence of spasticity, scissoring, or upper extremity flexion patterns that are present in most children with CP. Spasticity interferes with muscle lengthening in a growing child and can cause a biomechanical disadvantage that impairs strength and function.

• Bony deformity can occur because abnormal muscle forces are acting on a growing skeleton. The typical increase in hip flexion, adduction, and internal rotation of the femur often directs the femoral head in an upward posterolateral direction out of the acetabulum. This causes the hip to be more prone to subluxation (see Fig. 53–14 in the Textbook). Spinal deformities are not quite as common but have severe consequences. Asymmetrical muscle pull and immobility can contribute to significant spinal deformities including kyphosis and scoliosis. These spinal deformities can significantly affect comfort, tone, sitting and standing alignment, and balance. Spondylolisthesis and spondylolysis are not increased in CP.

• Bony abnormalities of the feet are common. The most common is deformity of the hindfoot with exaggerated heel valgus or varus. Hyperpronation occurs often, along with calcaneovalgus or cavus. A rocker-bottom foot is occasionally seen.

• Motor control for effective speech may be inadequate and can interfere with communication skills. Language production and processing problems can occur, and correlate with cognitive impairments. Difficulty controlling oral secretions can cause significant drooling.

ASSOCIATED MEDICAL AND FUNCTIONAL PROBLEMS (pp. 1197–1198)

• Esotropia, or exotropia, often requires strabismus surgery. Visual field deficits are less common but occur most often in hemiplegic patients. Visual acuity is affected more in quadriplegics than diplegics.

• A large number of children with CP have oromotor dysfunction, leading to eating and speaking problems. Incomplete lip closure, low suction pressure, and delay between suction and propulsion cause inadequate bolus preparation. In more involved children, this can interfere with the pharyngeal swallowing mechanism. Abnormalities in strength, tone, and coordination can be severe enough to cause difficulty protecting the airway. Testing of swallowing function with videofluoroscopy is helpful in determining which food textures are safe. Motor impairment can interfere with accessing food or communicating hunger. Feeding difficulties can contribute to substantial malnutrition. Malnutrition correlates with significantly reduced linear growth.

• Asymmetry of linear growth, particularly in the limbs, can result from motor and tone imbalances. Severely motor-impaired limbs can have decreased length and girth at maturity. Interestingly, there is a tendency for hemiplegic children with impaired sensation to have inadequate limb growth.

• Gastrointestinal symptoms are common in children with CP. Gastroesophageal reflux can cause episodic emesis. Reflux can interfere with ingestion and absorption of nutrients, thus compromising adequate nutrition and growth. Constipation, exacerbated by immobility and abnormal diet, can usually be managed with medications. Fecal incontinence appears to be related to abnormalities in neuromotor control (see Chapter 28).

- Incontinence is the most commonly reported urinary symptom. Increased incontinence has been attributed to decreased mobility, communication, and cognitive skills. Urodynamics in patients with urinary dysfunctional revealed that upper motor neuron injury is most common, but lower motor neuron disorders and vesicoureteral reflux have also been described.
- The prevalence of mental retardation in CP patients is estimated at 30%. The risk increases with the severity of motor disability. Learning disabilities and mental retardation are more common in premature children. Up to 50% of normal-birth-weight children with CP may have some degree of cognitive impairment.
- Seizure disorders occur in up to a third of children with CP. Epilepsy is more common in severely motor-affected children and those with mental retardation, reflecting the greater extent of brain injury in these cases. Hearing disabilities are rare in CP and are most commonly associated with congenital nervous system infections.

FUNCTIONAL PROGNOSIS (pp. 1198–1199)

- Children who are able to sit independently by age 2 years often become independent walkers, with or without equipment. The persistence of primitive reflexes (e.g., ATNR, STNR, tonic labyrinthine, Moro's, positive supporting reflex, or extensor posturing) is a poor prognostic indicator for independent ambulation. Most children who become ambulators have fewer than three primitive reflexes present at 18 months. Independent ambulation is typically achieved by age 2 years, and perhaps up to age 7 years. Seventy-five percent of children with spastic CP eventually ambulate, as do about 85% with diplegia and 70% with quadriplegia. Most children with hemiplegic or ataxic CP ambulate independently, the majority by age 3 years. Unfortunately, those with hypotonic CP rarely walk.
- Abnormal neuromotor control leads to a decrease in independence and mobility. One of the hallmarks of CP is motor delay despite normal development in other areas. The increased muscle tone during movement and standing greatly increases the energy expended for motor activity. Children typically have an inefficient gait, with much shorter step length, decreased range of motion at the hip and knee, more energy expenditure, and decreased velocity as compared with their peers.
- Inefficiencies of muscle control contribute to decreased endurance. Endurance correlates with the overall motor capabilities of the individual. Contractures and bone or joint deformities can greatly limit a child's function. Impairment in coordination may become more apparent with challenging motor activities.

EFFECTS OF AGING (p. 1199)

- Life expectancy for all but the most severely involved children is close to that of the unaffected population.
- Painful sequelae of childhood deformities occur and may become problematic for the adult. Positioning equipment, anti-inflammatory medication, bursal injections, mobilization by physical therapy, and spasticity treatment can improve

activity tolerance and decrease pain. Dislocated hips and the chronic effects of asymmetric posture create uncomfortable sitting. Adults with athetoid CP are susceptible to cervical spondylosis from excess movement.
• Adults with CP often require repetition of a surgical intervention performed during childhood. Careful planning is needed, and rehabilitation is usually undertaken to address the deconditioning that ensues after postoperative immobilization.
• Communication, activities of daily living (ADL), and mobility are ranked as higher-priority goals than ambulation in adults with CP. In the past, vocational rates among adults with CP were only 30% to 50%. The Americans With Disabilities Act, however, holds promise with respect to employment, housing, and accessibility to the community.

THERAPEUTIC MANAGEMENT (pp. 1199–1202)

• The therapeutic management of the child with CP emphasizes a functional, aim-, or goal-oriented approach. The two major goals of rehabilitation are to decrease complications of CP and to enhance the acquisition of new skills. Emphasizing parent and caregiver education, decreasing skeletal deformity, and improving mobility are important. In general, children should not be considered only in terms of deficits. The evaluation begins with an assessment of the strengths and deficits of the child and family.
• From the first evaluation, the family and child should be encouraged to become active participants in the process of setting priorities and goals. The physician should provide an accurate description of therapies and interventions available to the child and family.

Early Intervention (pp. 1199–1200)

• Current thinking emphasizes early identification of the infant with developmental delay so that intervention can be instituted as soon as possible. There is a discrete group of children who initially appear to have manifestations of CP but appear to normalize with age. The quality and quantity of verbal interactions with parents, maternal sensitivity, and the existence of a social support network are associated with a child's development.

Therapy Approaches (pp. 1200–1202)

• There are a number of schools of therapy that have influenced therapy for CP children (Table 53–3). Therapy services rarely rely on any one approach and are generally tailored to meet the child and family's goals. Crothers encouraged participation of severely involved children and stressed active movement and stimulation activities to prevent contractures. Phelps used conventional techniques from poliomyelitis treatment regimens. He emphasized inhibiting abnormal movement. Deaver emphasized functional ability rather than patterns of movement; this method is also known for its extensive use of bracing. Fay postulated that motor developmental levels of the brain were comparable to the evolutionary process. This highly controversial concept is expressed by the aphorism "ontogeny recapitulates phylogeny." Doman integrated patterning into therapy. Patterning has been subjected to critical review by the pediatric community and is not recommended.

• The neurodevelopmental treatment (NDT) approach, developed by the Bobaths, has been recommended for infants who display signs of CP. The main goals of NDT are to normalize tone, to inhibit abnormal primitive reflex patterns, and to facilitate automatic reactions and subsequent normal movement. Therapists emphasize "key points of control" throughout the body, theoretically providing kinesthetically normal feedback. The Bobaths emphasized family involvement. For the older child, the Bobaths shift emphasis to ADL skills. Rood developed a sensorimotor approach to activate movement and postural responses at an automatic level while following a developmental sequence similar to Bobath's.

• Children with CP can participate in integrated school therapy programs with physical therapists, occupational therapists, and speech therapists acting as consultants. The current trend in schools is to include disabled children as much as possible in the regular classroom. Mainstreaming has a positive psychological benefit to the child and increases academic expectations of the disabled student.

• In the past, CP children were advised to not participate in sports: that has changed. There is no evidence that strengthening adversely affects muscle tone. There is also no evidence to preclude children from vigorous activities (e.g., downhill skiing) that once were thought to increase orthopedic deformity. Therapeutic benefits of swimming and horseback riding for children with motor disabilities have been established. Whereas sports can improve endurance and strength, they also promote interpersonal growth and improve self-esteem.

• Most studies of the effectiveness of PT and other treatment are inconclusive. Investigators have found that the children most likely to improve in motor abilities were those children with higher intelligence quotients (IQs) and lesser involvement of the neuromuscular system.

Equipment Concerns (p. 1202)

• Assistive devices play an important role in household and community ambulation. Independent mobility increases exploration of the environment and improves self-esteem. A reverse walker can assist with upright posture better than the traditional forward walker. A wheelchair for community mobility becomes practical once a child has outgrown commercially available strollers. When standardized equipment does not meet the postural support needs of the severely involved child, adaptive seating is essential. Not only does a specialized seating system preserve a child's capacity to interact in a conventional posture but it can also improve pulmonary function (see Chapter 33). Typically, the child who is adequately seated has better feeding, digestion, and vocal production.

• The early introduction of technology to improve communication, either written or oral, is warranted. Adaptive specialists provide access to computers, environmental control units, and various adaptive equipment (see Chapter 25). The child with CP is often assisted in mobility and ADL tasks by the use of splints or orthoses. The decision to brace and the type of orthosis is dictated by the child's age, functional level, motor control, type of deformity, and compliance. Splinting is a common conservative method of managing a spastic but flexible deformity. Low-temperature tone-reducing ankle-foot orthoses

TABLE 53–3 Similarities and Differences between Neuromotor Therapy Approaches to Cerebral Palsy (CP)

	Neurodevelopmental Treatment (Bobaths)	Sensorimotor Approach to Treatment (Rood)
Central nervous system model	Hierarchical	Hierarchical
Goals of treatment	1. To normalize tone 2. To inhibit primitive reflexes 3. To facilitate automatic reactions and normal movement patterns	1. To activate postural responses (stability) 2. To activate movement (mobility) once stability is achieved
Primary sensory systems utilized to effect a motor response	1. Kinesthetic 2. Proprioceptive 3. Tactile	1. Tactile 2. Proprioceptive 3. Kinesthetic
Emphasis of treatment activities	1. Positioning and handling to normalize sensory input 2. Facilitation of active movement	1. Sensory stimulation to activate motor response (tapping, brushing, icing)
Intended clinical population	Children with CP Adults postcerebrovascular accident (CVA)	Children with neuromotor disorders such as CP Adults post-CVA
Emphasis on treating infants	Yes	No
Emphasis on family involement during treatment	Yes Handling and positioning for activities of daily living	No
Empirical support	Few studies Conflicting results	Very few studies Conflicting results

From Harris SR, Atwater SW, Crowe TK: Accepted and controversial neuromotor therapies for infants at high risk for cerebral palsy. J Perinatol 1988; 8:3–13.

(TRAFOs) have tone-reducing aspects incorporated into their construction. TRAFOs have been useful in some children but are not universally recommended. High temperature total contact orthoses can decrease energy expenditure when used in conjunction with therapy, surgery, and other treatment. Compression garments theoretically increase proprioceptive input to the neuromuscular system and improve motor function.

Sensory Integration Approach (Ayres)	Vojta Approach	Patterning Therapy (Doman-Delacato)
Hierarchical	Hierarchical	Hierarchical
1. To improve efficiency of neural processing 2. To better organize adaptive responses	1. To prevent CP in infants at risk 2. To improve motoric behavior in infants with fixed CP	1. To achieve independent mobility 2. To improve motor coordination 3. To prevent or improve communication disorders 4. To enhance intelligence
1. Vestibular 2. Tactile 3. Kinesthetic	1. Proprioceptive 2. Kinesthetic 3. Tactile	All sensory systems are utilized
1. Therapist guides, but child controls sensory input to get adaptive purposeful response	1. Trigger reflex locomotive zones to encourage movement patterns (e.g., reflex crawl)	Sensory and reflex stimulation, passive movement patterns, encouragement of independent movements
Children with learning disabilities Children with autism	Young infants at risk for CP Young infants with fixed CP	Children with neonatal or acquired brain damage
No	Yes	No
No	Yes	Yes
Supportive role encouraged	Family administers treatment at home daily	Family and friends administer treatment several times daily
Many studies Conflicting results with school-age children Positive results for tactile and vestibular input with infants	Few studies Conflicting results	Few studies Conflicting results

MEDICAL AND SURGICAL MANAGEMENT
(pp. 1202–1207)

Medications (p. 1202)

• Studies have demonstrated clinically useful reduction in spasticity following the initiation of medication (see Table 53–5 in the Textbook). Commonly used antispasticity drugs include Baclofen (Lioresal), Zanaflex (Tizanadine), and Dantrolene (Dantrium). Side effects may preclude long-term use. Other commonly used drugs are oxybutynin (Ditropan), to improve bladder control; and scopolamine to reduce drooling. Pain medications are often needed.

TABLE 53–4 Common Orthopedic Surgeries in Cerebral Palsy

Surgical Procedure	Purpose
Hip flexor lengthening	Increase extension ROM
Usually iliopsoas	Decrease muscle imbalance—risk of hip subluxation
Sometimes proximal rectus femoris	Improve alignment stance, gait
Rarely sartorius	
Hip adductor lengthening	Increase hip abduction
Usually proximal—origin	Decrease scissoring
Adductor longus, gracilis	Decrease abnormal muscle imbalance—risk of hip
Sometimes adductor brevis	subluxation
	Increase base of support
	Improve hygiene, positioning
Hamstring lengthening	Increase knee extension
Medial/lateral hamstrings	Improve standing alignment
Almost always distal	Decrease crouch posture
	Increase stance-phase stability in gait, improved alignment
	Increase step length → increased terminal swing phase and heel-strike ability
	Increase positioning options
Achilles tendon lengthening	Increase dorsiflexion ROM
Five different types: Baker, percutaneous, sliding, fractional	Increase full-foot contact for standing and gait
lengthening, vulpius	Increase ability for heel-strike in gait
	Allow for bracing

Abbreviations: ROM, range of motion; AFO, ankle-foot orthosis: TAL, tendoachilles lengthening.
From Feathergill B: Personal communications, 1993.

Orthopedic Intervention (pp. 1202–1204)

• Children with CP should have regular orthopedic consultations to evaluate musculoskeletal deformities. Physiatrists work in conjunction with orthopedists and therapists to address musculoskeletal issues that arise (Table 53–4).

Surgery for Sitting (p. 1204)

• Sitting is a realistic functional goal for every child. A level pelvis and a reasonably straight spine are necessary to sit. The loss of motion associated with hip dislocation can alter seating (see Chapter 18). Excessive pelvic obliquity

Positioning Considerations	Treatment
Avoid prolonged sitting Prone wedge preferred Standing frame with foot control (casts/AFOs) Prone at night (with or without body splint) Abduction at night, usually prone With/without night splint Abduction wedge on prone wedge/wheelchair	Maintain length of hip flexor muscles Strengthen hip flexors (need for stairs, gait) Strengthen hip extensors Maintain length of hip adductors (knees flexed and extended) Strengthen hip adductors and abductors
Avoid prolonged sitting Prone wedge preferred (consider soft knee splints) Standing frame with foot control Prone at night with soft knee splints or night splints	Maintain length of hamstrings (avoid knee hyperextension) Strengthen hamstrings and quadriceps (proximal and distal), especially terminal knee extension Monitor for overactive quadriceps, increase in extensor tone → knee hyperextension
Initially no dorsiflexion beyond neutral Standing with neutral dorsiflexion only Temporary splint/cast initially to maintain ROM—begin early supportive weightbearing Sitting OK, if TALs only and other muscles not tight If prone wedge—feet off edge with AFO/cast/splint AFO approximately 6 mo (surgeon discretion) AFO/cast/splint at night	Maintain length of plantar flexors Strengthen plantar flexors and dorsiflexors Avoid overstretching—could lead to crouch posture (Special attention when considering hinged AFOs) (Repeat procedures common—especially if done at early age)

reduces the sitting surface area and causes excessive pressure on the bony prominences of the pelvis.
• The management of the hip is complex. Early detection of hip subluxation is possible with radiographs as subluxation may not be detectable on physical examination. If the hip is subluxed, the surgeon may lengthen the iliopsoas and adductor muscles to reduce overpowering muscle forces. This brief procedure allows easier dressing, diapering, cleaning, and positioning by improving femoral head coverage under the acetabulum. If the hip progresses to dislocation, a more extensive procedure involving reconstruction of the femur and acetabulum may be necessary. A combination of muscle lengthenings, varus derotational osteotomy of the femur, and augmentation procedures of the acetabulum are done in some cases. Postoperative immobilization may be necessary for as long as 6 to 8 weeks. Rehabilitation plays an important role following cast

removal. Complications of these procedures include femoral fractures, heterotopic ossification, and peripheral neuropathy. Hip fusion, artificial joint replacement, and resection of the femoral head can afford relief of pain in the refractory patient.

• Hamstrings act as hip extensors but also tilt the pelvis posteriorly. Sacral sitting with constant sliding out of a wheelchair can be partially corrected by a hamstring release. Distal hamstring lengthening is the more common surgery, but a proximal lengthening can also be considered.

• Scoliosis or kyphosis can be progressive. Early treatment usually involves a molded thoracic lumbar orthosis. The orthosis improves trunk support and may slow the rate of progression. Total contact support can be incorporated into a contoured seating system. If a curve progresses beyond 40 degrees, fusion is considered to avoid compromise of the respiratory system. If the deformity is rigid and extends over a long segment, staged procedures are performed.

Surgery for Standing (p. 1204)

• Supported standing and transfers are possible when the ankle can be held in the neutral position and the knee has less than 20 degrees of flexion contracture. The surgical procedures used to improve alignment for standing and transfers are hamstring lengthenings and Achilles tendon lengthenings. Hip flexion contractures greater than 20 degrees can also hinder standing and may need surgical intervention.

Surgery for Ambulation (pp. 1204–1207)

• Surgery to improve ambulation remains problematic. Difficulty in predicting outcome for the ambulator has led to caution in recommending orthopedic surgery. Adductor myotomies in combination with hamstring lengthenings can create a better base of support and a more upright posture. Recently, rectus femoris transfers and lengthenings have decreased the problem of stiff-knee gait following hamstring release. A braceable foot or a foot that allows for foot-flat or heel-strike is desirable for stance.

• Gait analysis provides objective information that enhances orthopedic decision making and analysis of outcome following surgery (see Chapter 5). Energy expenditure is an important consideration for continued community ambulation because energy expenditure for some children with spastic CP is as high as 350% of normal.

Other Surgeries (p. 1207)

• Selective posterior rhizotomy (SPR) and intrathecal baclofen pumps hold promise in reducing spasticity. Reduction in tone, as recorded by the modified Ashworth scale, is achieved in both procedures (see Chapter 29). Gait analysis studies after SPR have consistently shown improved range of motion at the knee and hip, resulting in an increased stride length. However, neurosurgical procedures such as stereotactic ablation of thalamic nuclei and chronic electrical stimulation of the cerebellum or posterior columns have thus far been unsuccessful in reducing spasticity in CP.

Other Interventions (p. 1207)

• Motor point blocks and botulism injections are used in management of spasticity. Functional electrical stimulation and biofeedback can be helpful for training specific muscles. The use of low-voltage, high-frequency electrical stimulation increases blood flow and improves muscle growth and strength.

54

Original Chapter by Ross M. Hays, M.D., and Teresa L. Massagli, M.D.

Rehabilitation Concepts in Myelomeningocele

HISTORICAL BACKGROUND (p. 1213)

• Tulpius coined the term *spina bifida* in 1652. In the 1860s, both Lamarck and Darwin commented that environmental influences may be involved in myelomeningocele. Effective neonatal surgical back closure occurred in the 1940s. Invention of the one-way shunt valve in 1952 effectively reversed survival curves from 10% survival in 1956 to 10% mortality in 1985.

DEFINITIONS (pp. 1213–1214)

• *Myelomeningocele* (MMC) is the failure of fusion of the neural folds during the neurulation phase of embryologic development. Defects of bone, meninges, and spinal cord may result in a neurogenic bowel and bladder, lower extremity paralysis, and sensory loss.

• *Meningocele* describes a hernia of the meningeal membranes with little or no dysgenesis of the underlying nervous system. Most meningoceles contain all the neural elements, are skin-covered, and produce little paralysis.

• *Lipomeningomyeloceles, lipomeningoceles,* and *lipomyeloceles* are lipomas that occur within the neural canal. They most commonly accompany some degree of meningocele formation and interfere with neural function by increasing pressure on the lower spinal cord.

• *Diastematomyelia* is a splitting of the lower spinal cord in association with mesodermal elements, bone or cartilage spurs, and fibrous bands. It may occur alone or in association with meningomyelocele.

• *Myelocystocele* describes a cystic defect that communicates with the central canal of the spinal cord. Myelocystoceles vary in size and may be either dorsal or ventral. They produce neurological symptoms by exerting pressure on the spinal cord during growth.

• *Spina bifida* denotes a bony defect resulting from failure of mesodermal closure around the neural canal. Meningomyelocele and meningocele are examples of *spina bifida aperta. Spina bifida occulta* is a defect of the posterior bony elements without involvement of the underlying meningeal or neural elements. Spina bifida occulta is not uncommon and is usually asymptomatic.

EPIDEMIOLOGY (pp. 1214–1215)

Incidence (p. 1214)

• Geographical and racial variations in the incidence of MMC have been reported. From 1970 to 1989, the incidence of neural tube defects in the United States dropped from 1.3 to 0.6 per 1000 live births. This decreased incidence may be attributable to improved prenatal diagnostic testing, increased termination of affected pregnancies, and environmental factors. About two-thirds of neural tube defects are MMC cases, translating into about 2000 affected infants born each year in the United States.

Etiology (pp. 1214–1215)

• Myelomeningocele occurs as a result of incomplete closure of the neural tube during fetal development. Closure typically occurs 26 to 30 days after fertilization. Determining the cause and implementing prevention strategies is difficult because malformation occurs soon after conception, often before women are aware they are pregnant.
• **Genetics.** Open neural tube defects have occurred in multiple births and in infants with chromosomal disorders, but most occur as isolated defects. There is a slight sex preference with a female to male ratio of 1.3:1. Low sacral lesions are more common among males, whereas thoracic lesions are more common among females. Recurrence rate is related to the incidence of neural tube defects in the region. A frequency of 1% has been reported in children of maternal sisters and when one of the parents has a neural tube defect. Consanguinity between parents also increases risk.
• Neural tube defects are multifactorial in origin. The increased incidence of MMC in families, certain ethnic groups, and in cases of parental consanguinity suggests that there is a strong genetic component. The interaction of predisposed individuals to certain environmental triggers may cause neural tube malformation.
• **Environmental Factors.** Nutrition, drugs, and heat have been proposed as environmental factors. For instance, the use of valproic acid during pregnancy is associated with a 2.5% to 6.3% prevalence of MMC. An increased incidence of MMC has been noted among people of low socioeconomic status and among children conceived in spring months.
• Heat exposure has long been suspected of being a teratogen in humans. Strong associations between maternal heat exposure during early pregnancy and neural tube defects have been reported. Taking hot tubs, hot baths, or a febrile illness during the first trimester have been associated with twice the risk of fetal neural tube defects. The amount of heat exposure necessary for teratogenicity is unknown, as is the mechanism of action in preventing neural tube closure.
• Folic acid supplementation is an important preventive measure against MMC. The U.S. Public Health Service recommended that all women who are capable of becoming pregnant consume 0.4 mg of folic acid daily to reduce their risk of neural tube defects. Women who have had an affected child should consider peri-

conceptional consumption of 4 mg of folate per day. The mechanism of action of folate in preventing MMC is unknown.

MANAGEMENT (pp. 1215–1226)

Early Management (pp. 1215–1217)

Prenatal Management (p. 1215)

• Prenatal screening can identify the majority of cases of MMC. This information can be used to plan for termination of pregnancy or to enhance perinatal management. Prenatal diagnosis begins with measurement of maternal serum alpha-fetoprotein (AFP) at 16 to 18 weeks after conception.

• High-resolution US can reveal the presence of MMC by 14 to 16 weeks of gestation. Because of advances in US technology, scanning alone may be sufficient to diagnose a neural tube defect. The diagnosis should be confirmed by amniocentesis to measure the amount of AFP in amniotic fluid. Although elevated levels of AFP are seen in a number of conditions, isoenzymes of acetylcholinesterase are seen only in open neural tube defects and are independent of the length of gestation.

• Prenatal detection of MMC is even important for families who would not choose to terminate the pregnancy because it enhances perinatal management. Families have time to learn about the diagnosis and prepare for a safe delivery. High-resolution US can accurately predict functional motor outcome. Infants with neural tube defects should be delivered in the medical center where surgical closure will occur. It has also been suggested that infants with MMC be delivered by cesarean section to avoid injury to the sac and contents. Prenatal diagnosis allows physicians to plan for elective cesarean section prior to labor, when the fetus has achieved pulmonary maturation.

Neonatal Management (pp. 1215–1217)

Back Defect. The first priority of medical treatment is management of the open neural tube defect (Fig. 54–1). There are three goals managing the back defect: (1) reduce the risk of infection, (2) preserve existing neurological function, and (3) decrease the deformity if severe kyphoscoliosis is present. Most centers advocate closure within the first hours after delivery. The risk of central nervous system (CNS) infection in lesions closed before 48 hours averages 7%; the infection risk for later closure rises to an average of 37%. The back defect must be carefully protected to prevent contamination or further damage because of trauma or desiccation. The lesion and CSF are cultured and the infant is treated with antibiotics at dosages sufficient to treat meningitis. Back closure is performed in three stages: (1) the neural plaque is returned to the canal and a watertight closure of dura and arachnoid is constructed; (2) the reformulated neural tube is then protected by myofascial closure; and (3) the skin is then closed with a tension closure.

• Back repair may produce alterations in CSF fluid dynamics by closing the open conduit at the caudal end of the central canal. In some cases, fluid pressures spontaneously readjust after closure. In others, hydrocephalus becomes rapidly apparent. Kyphectomy to treat severe kyphoscoliosis in the newborn is difficult and often complicated by poor bone growth, high blood loss, and intraoperative mortality. Minimal osteotomy repair is a compromise that provides less immediate correction but is better tolerated by the infant.

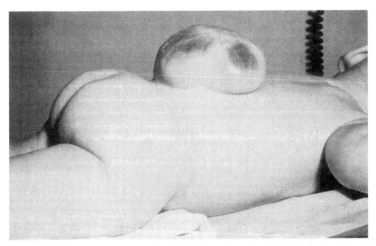

FIGURE 54–1. Typical appearance of a child with myelomeningocele lesion prior to surgical closure.

Hydrocephalus. Ninety percent of children with myelomeningocele will develop clinically significant hydrocephalus. Some children have true aqueductal stenosis, and others have communicating hydrocephalus that worsens after back closure. Nearly all children with MMC have displacement of the cerebellum caudally with elongation and kinking of the fourth ventricle and medulla. These combined defects are known as the Arnold-Chiari II malformation. Recently, the term *constrictive hydrocephalus* has been used to describe the relationship between Arnold-Chiari II malformation and the restricted flow of CSF that causes hydrocephalus in the majority of children with MMC.

• Hydrocephalus is often present at birth or discovered prenatally on US. It usually does not progress immediately and may show no evidence of additional ventricular enlargement until 3 to 7 days of age. The onset of hydrocephalus in some patients does not require treatment for months or even years. Progressive hydrocephalus in the newborn manifests as increasing head size; older children with delayed-onset hydrocephalus develop signs and symptoms of increased intracranial pressure (e.g., vomiting, headache, somnolence, or irritability). Insidious onset of hydrocephalus may appear as lethargy, personality alterations, or subtle changes in intellectual performance.

• Ventriculoperitoneal (VP) shunting is the treatment of choice for hydrocephalus. Surgical advances can be credited with better outcomes as well as a decreased likelihood of shunt failure.

Early Bladder Management. The neurogenic bladder in the newborn can be evaluated by physical examination. Babies with large, distended bladders on abdominal examination are likely to have sphincter dyssynergia. A nonpalpable bladder and constant dribbling suggest weak or nonexistent sphincter tone. Abdominal US can detect the presence of a distended, poorly emptying bladder; hydronephrosis; or renal agenesis. US should be repeated after back closure to rule out urinary tract obstruction resulting from damage to the spinal cord.

• Postvoid residual urine volumes should be checked by US. A postvoid residual of 20 mL or greater in the newborn period indicates clinically significant urinary retention and requires intermittent catheterization, treatment with phenoxybenzamine, or both. Blood urea nitrogen (BUN) and creatinine levels must be monitored and routine urine cultures obtained during the first month of life. The first voiding cystourethrogram may be safely deferred until 6 months of age if all other tests suggest that bladder emptying is reasonable.

Assessment of Neurological Level. The motor level is important in predicting ambulation and intellectual potential, but it does not correlate well with the level of vertebral abnormality on radiographs, the anatomical site of the skin lesion, or the level of abnormality on sensory examination. The best method of motor examination is careful inspection for muscle bulk, stimulation with postural challenges, and gentle opposition of major muscle groups to elicit voluntary activity. The presence of considerable muscle bulk without any observed voluntary movement may indicate temporary spinal cord shock after delivery or back closure. In 37% of MMC newborns, motor strength improves within a week after delivery. Joint movement, especially hip and knee flexion in response to painful stimuli, may result from reflex-mediated activity below the level of the lesion rather than true voluntary control.

Therapy. Experienced therapists can assist with positioning and handling of the newborn and provide anticipatory guidance for the parents. Contractures of the hips and knees benefit from a range-of-motion exercise program implemented by the family. Babies with higher-level lesions may require custom-fabricated seating and support devices that protect the surgical site and assist with trunk and head control.

Family Counseling. The need for parents to be completely and accurately informed about all aspects of their infant's care, medical needs, and future potential cannot be overemphasized. A successful approach is to have one physician and one nurse act as the primary support for each family and child. Good communication among primary care physician, nurses, specialists, and the parents is the best assurance of achieving the desired medical outcome.

Long-Term Management (pp. 1217–1226)

The Central Nervous System (pp. 1217–1218)
Shunts. Approximately 90% of children with MMC need a VP shunt placed to manage hydrocephalus. The two most common late complications associated with shunts are obstructions and infections. Of these, infections have the greater morbidity. The overall risk of shunt infection is 12% per child. The most common infections are caused by *Staphylococcus epidermidis* and are associated with the surgical insertion of the shunt. Each shunt placement or revision carries a 5% risk for infection. Delayed infections with culture-proven *S. epidermidis* likely represent indolent, late postoperative infections.
• Children with hydrocephalus and shunts are at greater risk for epidemic meningitis caused by β-hemolytic streptococcus, meningococcus, pneumococcus, and *Hemophilus influenzae*. The other common source of infection is erosion of the VP shunt into intra-abdominal organs and resulting contamination with gram-negative organisms.

- Infections in the shunt downstream from the CNS are the least serious and the most easily treated. Low-grade ventriculitis is often associated with shunt obstruction; shunt infection with ventriculomeningitis carries the most severe morbidity. The relationship between shunt infection, CNS infection, and intellectual functioning in children with MMC is controversial. Several studies suggest that a reduction in cognitive function is associated with the frequency and severity of infections.
- Fifty percent of children with VP shunts experience obstruction and need shunt revision in the first year of life. Among children whose shunts obstruct during the first year, 31% need shunt replacement in the second year, and 12% per year thereafter. In children who do not need shunt revision during the first year of life, the risk of obstruction is only 8% per year.

Complications of Arnold-Chiari II Malformation. Nearly all children with MMC have Arnold-Chiari II malformation of the hindbrain; the majority are asymptomatic. The term *central ventilatory dysfunction* (CVD) describes the 7% to 30% of children who have severe manifestations with Arnold-Chiari II. Severe manifestations of CVD include upper airway obstruction because of vocal cord abductor paralysis (30%), vocal cord abductor paralysis with other cranial nerve involvement (17%), and central apnea (22%). The mechanism of action probably involves traction on upper cervical nerves because of downward displacement of the medulla, brainstem compression with the abnormally located hindbrain, and increased intracranial pressure resulting from hydrocephalus.
- The mainstays of treatment are management of increased intracranial pressure, treatment of CNS infection, and vigorous airway management. Placement or revision of CSF shunts to reduce intracranial pressure may provide improvement. Close attention to the airway obstruction and apnea is essential.
- CVD is not associated with the lesion level, severity of hydrocephalus, or the presence of CNS bleeding and infection. Children with CVD who survive because of aggressive ventilatory support often experience remission of symptoms by 30 months of age. At the present time, CVD is the most common cause of death in children with MMC.

Hydromyelia. Hydromyelia is analogous to dilation of the ventricles in hydrocephalus and occurs in 50% to 80% of children with MMC. The most common symptoms are rapidly progressive scoliosis, weakness of the upper extremities, spasticity, and ascending motor strength changes in the lower extremities. Hydromyelia is best demonstrated by magnetic resonance imaging (MRI) of the brain and spinal cord. When symptoms warrant treatment, decompressing subclinical hydrocephalus may be effective. In more aggressive cases, decompressive laminectomy, plugging of the obex, and direct shunting may be required.

Tethered Cord Syndrome. Tethered cord syndrome refers to progressive neurological deficits resulting from traction of the conus medullaris and the cauda equina. It has been reported in 11% to 15% of children after myelomeningocele repair. The diagnosis is based on progressive symptoms, not the radiographic finding of a low-lying conus. Routine MRI studies have demonstrated that 80% to 90% of MMC patients have an abnormally low conus medullaris, most of whom never develop clinical symptoms.
- The most common symptom of tethered cord is change in motor strength (62%), followed by recent onset of spasticity (56%) and changes in mobility (43%). Back pain is reported in 37%. Some 25% of patients report a recent

change in bowel and bladder function or recent onset of scoliosis. Because the diagnosis of tethered cord syndrome is clinical rather than radiographic, and because symptoms are superimposed on existing pathological conditions, a high level of suspicion is required to diagnose the syndrome.

Urological System (pp. 1218–1219)

Patterns of Involvement. The type of neurogenic bladder in MMC does not correlate with the lesion level. More than 80% have partial or complete denervation of the bladder with poor compliance and poor contractility, producing high residual volumes. In 86%, the internal sphincter is incompetent, causing incontinence when intravesical pressure exceeds urethral resistance. The external sphincter is usually at least partially functional, and in about one-third of patients detrusor-sphincter dyssynergia causes abnormally high intraluminal pressures. Bladder function may change with time or because of tethered cord syndrome. Most changes occur in the first year after birth. For these reasons, early assessment of bladder and kidney function, followed by reassessment at least annually, is necessary.

Preventing Renal Involvement. Management of neurogenic bladder focuses on prevention of urinary tract damage and achievement of continence. Urodynamic examination of intravesical and bladder neck pressures is routine in newborns with MMC. About 75% of infants have normal upper tracts, whereas the rest have hydronephrosis because of such problems as vesicoureteral reflux (VUR), detrusor-sphincter dyssynergia, an enlarged bladder, or a structural abnormality. Infants with normal upper tracts and satisfactory bladder emptying are monitored twice a year by renal US during early childhood. If the bladder does not empty efficiently and there is no outlet resistance or reflux, parents can be taught the Credé maneuver to improve emptying. If detrusor-sphincter dyssynergia is present, there is a significant risk for development of hydronephrosis, and such infants are managed with anticholinergic medications and clean intermittent catheterization.

• If the child has VUR, prophylactic antibiotics are prescribed because VUR of infected urine can cause upper tract damage or even renal failure. Risk factors for upper tract damage and VUR include detrusor-sphincter dyssynergia, decreased bladder compliance, and elevated leak pressures. VUR is seen when detrusor pressure exceeds $40\,cm\,H_2O$ before leakage of urine occurs. If the child develops persistent febrile urinary tract infections or if hydronephrosis does not improve, antireflux surgery is indicated. Surgical options include vesicostomy, reimplantation of ureters, or bladder augmentation. Outcomes from urinary diversion into an ileal conduit have been disappointing and many patients have subsequently had reversal of the diversion.

• Asymptomatic bacteriuria is prevalent in children with MMC. Urine culture screening is indicated for those with VUR or when signs or symptoms of urinary tract infection occur. Prophylactic antibiotics have not been found to reduce the occurrence of clinical urinary tract infection.

Continence. Less than 10% of children with MMC have normal urinary control. Knowledge of bladder capacity and sphincter function is vital when considering options for management. For boys with reflex emptying, external collection devices may be feasible if they do not have VUR or large residual urine volumes.

Condom catheters require careful attention to skin integrity when sensation is impaired.
- There are no effective external collection devices for girls. Girls and boys with incomplete emptying rely on clean intermittent catheterization and, sometimes, medications. Only about one-fourth of children can become continent with clean intermittent catheterization alone. Commonly used medications include anticholinergics to inhibit contractions and α-adrenergics to increase outlet resistance. Compliance may be a problem for complicated regimens in this population. Some children need to empty their bladders very frequently, often at intervals of less than every 4 hours. The entire daily bladder management can require more than 1.5 hours per day.
- Surgery may be considered for children who fail to become continent using medications and clean intermittent catheterization. The options depend on bladder size, sphincter competence, and the ability to perform clean intermittent catheterization. Bladder augmentation may be necessary for the child with a small or noncompliant bladder and can be done in conjunction with an artificial sphincter if the outlet resistance is low. Ileum, sigmoid colon, and stomach have all been used for augmentation. An artificial urethral sphincter may be created for those with low outlet resistance. About half of patients need to use clean intermittent catheterization after sphincter implantation. Overall success for long-term continence is over 60%. If the patient has difficulty performing clean intermittent catheterization, continent diversion is another option. The appendix can be used as a conduit to the bladder to create an abdominal stoma, which is easier for the patient to access.

Development and Bladder Management. Independent toileting is delayed more than any other self-care task, even in those with normal intelligence. Children with MMC may not achieve independent bladder and bowel function control until 10 to 15 years of age. Factors affecting this delay include the level of paralysis, intelligence, visual-spatial imperceptions, kyphoscoliosis, obesity, degree of parental support, degree of sensation, sphincter control, and bladder capacity.
- Parents need to help children accept responsibility for these tasks once the child is physically and mentally capable. Children can learn to catheterize themselves using clean technique as early as age 5 years. Unfortunately, as many as 30% of teenagers with MMC still need assistance from a caregiver for bladder management.

Allergy to Latex. Children with MMC have recently been found to have high incidence of allergy to latex products. This IgE-mediated allergic response can manifest as contact dermatitis, allergic rhinitis, asthma, angioedema, or intra-operative anaphylaxis. Patients may encounter latex in such products as rubber balloons, rubber gloves, condoms, or ostomy bags. Patients with MMC who require surgery should be protected by a latex-free environment, regardless of latex reactivity. Many clinics advocate nonlatex catheters for all MMC children.

Neurogenic Bowel (pp. 1219–1220)
Description of Patterns. About 20% of children with MMC have normal bowel control. Bowel continence may be compromised by inconsistent parental expectations, impaired rectal sensation, impaired sphincter function, or altered colonic motility. Children with MMC may experience relative intestinal stasis because

of loss of sacral parasympathetic input. It is not known whether the gastrocolic reflex is intact in patients with neurogenic bowel. If the external sphincter is partially or wholly denervated, incontinence results when the pressure in the rectum is high enough to produce reflex relaxation of the internal sphincter. In patients with MMC above L3, the internal sphincter tonic pressure is low, possibly because of loss of sympathetic input. Rectal sensation is also related to lesion level and is usually absent in those with lesions above L3 and more likely present, though often abnormal, with lower lesions. It is important to know whether the child has any voluntary control over the external anal sphincter, but the anocutaneous reflex has not been shown to correlate with internal sphincter tone. Although sphincter status can be determined with anorectal manometry, it is not clear whether this alters the management. However, the presence of either a bulbocavernosus or anocutaneous reflex is associated with a greater likelihood of achieving continence.

Management Strategies. Children with MMC need efficient, regular, and predictable emptying of soft stool. The goal is to empty the rectum before it becomes full enough to stimulate reflex relaxation of the internal sphincter. If the child lacks rectal sensation, the emptying should be done according to a regular schedule. It is not known if the gastrocolic reflex is present with MMC. Thus there may no reason to perform bowel regiments after meals. Classic bowel programs utilize stool softeners or bulking agents, but families often prefer dietary measures. Suppositories, digital anorectal stimulation, manual removal of stool, dolusate or glycerine mini-enemas, saline enemas, and use of biofeedback if the child has adequate rectal sensation are potentially useful. Surgical diversion may be helpful in children who suffer from intractable bowel incontinence.

Social Implications. It is important for parents to establish an effective program of bowel continence at an early developmental stage. Children are subject to severe peer criticism if "accidents" occur in preschool or kindergarten. The child also needs to be encouraged to assume increasing responsibility for performing the bowel program. Clinicians can facilitate this learning experience for the child by keeping the program simple and as short as possible.
• In one study, up to 86% of teenagers needed assistance from a caregiver for their bowel program. As with bladder management, the reasons for this are not entirely clear. Children who are fearful of bowel accidents will try to avoid incontinence by staying constipated, but this strategy inevitably results in impaired bowel emptying. Parents perceive urinary and fecal incontinence as more stressful than impaired motor function in their children with MMC.

Musculoskeletal Complications *(pp. 1220–1223)*
Motor Innervation. It is important to appreciate that the level of neurological lesion often does not match the radiographic vertebral level. Of the vertebral defects, 1% are cervical, 1% are upper thoracic, 6% are lower thoracic and upper lumbar, 27% are midlumbar, 42% are lumbosacral, and 21% are sacral. Another 2% have large lesions encompassing the entire lumbosacral spine, 92% have lesions at or below L2, and essentially half have defects at or below L5 or S1. Only 4% present with lower sacral level paralysis with intact lower extremity strength and some degree of bowel and bladder dysfunction.
• The majority of patients exhibit a variety of motor abnormalities, including incomplete flaccid paraplegia, spasticity, mixed paraplegia and spasticity, asym-

metry of involvement, intact regions of voluntary control below the other segments of paralysis, and combinations of these impairments within the individual. Only one-third of children actually demonstrate flaccid paralysis. The level of neurological impairment influences the types of musculoskeletal deformities and complications. However, children with MMC often do not present in straightforward manner from a neurological standpoint.

Hips. The majority of patients have some hip deformity that interferes with ambulation, seating, or bracing. Only those with functional deficits or pain need treatment. Muscle imbalance at the hip accounts for most of the hip flexion deformity. A small number of patients develop hip flexion contractures from spasticity in the iliopsoas, rectus femoris, or sartorius. Hip flexion contracture of 20 degrees or more will increase the anterior pelvic tilt, create excessive lumbar lordosis, and interfere with ambulation. Patients with high level lesions may require soft tissue releases and anterior capsulotomy to improve seating and comfort. Patients with lower levels lesions who are over 10 or 11 years of age may require a subtrochanteric extension osteotomy to preserve ambulation. This approach is less successful in younger ambulatory patients, for whom continued growth is likely to result in bone remodeling. Younger patients may respond to hip flexor releases using free tendon grafting using the tensor fasciae latae.
• Hip flexion-abduction-external rotation deformity is seen in patients with higher lesion levels and may necessitate radical hip releases for seating. Iliotibial band and tensor fasciae latae strength may be asymmetrical and lead to hip abduction contracture and pelvic obliquity. Hip adduction contracture is the deformity that is most often associated with secondary hip dislocation. The goal in treating this deformity is to release the adductors to regain 45 to 60 degrees of passive abduction.
• Fifty percent of children with myelomeningocele have subluxed or dislocated hips at some time. Hip dislocation at birth occurs with lesions that are very high (thoracic level) or very low (sacral level). Some 50% to 70% of hip dislocations are associated with the muscle imbalance of mid-lumbar-level lesions. When hip dislocation occurs in later childhood or adolescence it may signal new-onset, late neurological changes (e.g., hydromyelia or tethered cord).
• Reducing dislocated hips in the active, ambulatory child may decrease dependence on assistive devices and reduce energy expenditure. Reducing dislocations that are bilateral and very high is often contraindicated. Nonambulatory children with high lesion levels commonly need only soft tissue releases. The most common complication of hip surgery is hip flexion contracture that interferes with mobility in later life. Repeat procedures are associated with greater hip stiffness and greater disability.

Knees. The most common knee deformity is a flexion contracture. Knee flexion contracture may be caused by congenital joint stiffness because of decreased intrauterine movement, from spasticity in the knee flexors, or from progressive crouched posture with ambulation. The incidence of knee flexion contractures is related to neurological level and the child's age. About 70% of patients with lesions at L3 or higher develop knee flexion contractures by 8 years of age. Only 25% of patients with lesions at L4 or L5 have contractures by age 12 years. Most patients with sacral lesions do not suffer knee flexion contractures. Knee extension contractures and valgus and varus deformities occur rarely and are seen most often with higher level lesions.

Feet. Foot deformities occur in 85% of children and are the most common orthopedic abnormality in MMC. Both muscular imbalance and spasticity contribute to deformities. Impaired sensation and autonomic dysfunction with vasomotor instability contribute to skin injury and poor wound healing. The goals of treatment are braceable plantar-grade feet and balanced muscle control around the ankle joint.

• Equinovarus results from retained tibialis posterior and tibialis anterior function in the child with a midlumbar neurological deficit (see Fig. 54–3 in the Textbook). The first line of treatment is casting to reduce the deformity, but surgery to produce a stable ankle joint is usually inevitable. A hindfoot valgus deformity with residual forefoot adduction is a common complication. Rigid fusions such as triple arthrodesis are associated with development of neuropathic joints. Children with tibialis posterior paresis are at risk for congenital rocker-bottom deformity. Surgical correction is designed to balance the hindfoot and forefoot musculature. Spasticity of foot muscles is more commonly associated with calcaneus deformities than with equinus deformities.

• Flexible, flail feet may drift into pure equinus deformity, which can be treated with a neutrally positioned ankle-foot orthosis. Plantar flexion contracture of greater than 20 degrees is unlikely to improve with stretching and may require serial casting or soft tissue releases. Pes cavus requires little treatment until adolescence, when weight bearing may lead to skin ulceration. When necessary, metatarsal osteotomies and orthoses can successfully redistribute forces around the foot. Hindfoot valgus can be treated with orthoses until it exceeds 7 degrees. Deformity beyond this amount typically requires surgery.

Spine. Spinal deformity in MMC usually occurs in one of three forms: (1) scoliosis with lordosis, (2) kyphosis, or (3) rigid congenital malformation. The level of spinal lesion direct correlates with the incidence of scoliosis. All patients with thoracic lesions develop a scoliosis of 45 degrees or more. Scoliosis occurs in only 60% of patients with L4 lesions, and less than half of them will need surgical correction. Scoliosis in high-level paraplegia occurs in early childhood and is progressive. Scoliosis as a result of hydromyelia or syrinx may improve after treatment of the hydromyelia if the curve has not progressed beyond 50 degrees. Scoliosis that presents in later childhood may be the first sign of secondary CNS complications (e.g., lipoma, dermoid tumors, or tethered cord).

• Kyphosis in MMC is almost always progressive, and conservative management is rarely effective. Curves of 100 degrees or more are commonly seen by age 3 years. The apex may be at any point from the lower thoracic vertebrae to the lumbosacral joint. The kyphosis that presents at birth is associated with vertebral malformations. The rigid apex is commonly in the high- to midlumbar region, and there is a compensatory lordosis above it. Rarely, children present with partial aplasia of the lumbar spine, which also results in kyphosis. The goals of treatment in kyphosis are to maintain abdominal height, to relieve pressure on the diaphragm, and to prevent pressure ulcers. If kyphosis approaches 180 degrees, treatment becomes extremely difficult. Children with large vertebral column malformations may require anterior and posterior fusion in infancy. Those who do not undergo early correction may develop additional, progressive curves with growth.

• In all three forms of scoliosis, the timing of surgical correction is critical. Spinal fusion performed too early will further limit vertebral growth and waiting may lead to progressive curves that are more difficult to treat.

Fractures. Fractures occur in approximately 20% of children with MMC, and the femur is the most commonly broken bone. In ambulatory patients, fractures often accompany falls. In nonambulatory children, fractures may occur with minor trauma to osteopenic extremities. In the insensate lower extremity, fractures may escape detection initially. Fractures tend to heal quickly in children with MMC. The bone forms exuberant calluses and rarely needs rigid fixation. Soon after a cast or surgery, patients are relatively more osteopenic and are at greatest risk for new fractures.

Mobility *(pp. 1223–1224)*
Lesion Level. Using motor level to predict ambulation is difficult because the classic neurosegmental levels and motor correlates are probably more variable than originally thought. There is a wide range of mobility among patients with similar patterns of segmental innervation. In a large recent study, iliopsoas strength was a robust predictor of independent ambulation. Grade 4 to 5 iliopsoas strength was most often associated with community ambulation; grade 0 to 3 iliopsoas strength was always associated with wheelchair use. The ability to walk without assistive devices was strongly associated with grade 4 to 5 gluteal and tibialis anterior strength. Patients with a combination of strong hip flexors and weak gluteus medius muscles were most likely to experience deterioration in muscle strength regardless of age. Other factors are involved in mobility including cognitive ability, musculoskeletal complications, surgery, motivation, obesity, and age.

Orthoses. Orthotic devices may be used to prevent deformity, to provide support or augment mobility, to maintain correction of deformities after casting or surgery, and to support normal joint alignment and mechanics. Orthoses may be effective in controlling muscular weakness that interferes with normal gait. Their ability to alter the progression of spontaneous deformity is not well established in this population.
• In addition to the many variations of knee and ankle-foot orthoses, three unique and extensive bracing systems are used to facilitate function for children with MMC. The parapodium provides structural support from the midthorax to the floor. It is often jointed at the hip and knee to accommodate both standing and sitting positions. This allows the child to maintain an upright, weight-bearing position and to ambulate with a swing-through gait regardless of the level of paralysis. The swivel walker is a modification of the parapodium that has a dual footplate system which translates trunk rotation into forward movement. The reciprocating gait orthosis (RGO) joins two hip-knee-ankle-foot orthoses (HKAFOs) with an elaborate cable system to link hip flexion with hip extension on the contralateral side. All three of these systems have the advantage of simulating upright ambulation, but none approaches the energy efficiency of normal walking. Children using HKAFOs with a swing-through gait have greater gait velocity than children using the RGO and a reciprocating gait pattern, but they walk with higher energy consumption (see Chapter 15).

Functional Mobility. With appropriate support, surgery, extensive bracing, and therapy, many children with MMC with high-level lesions become community ambulators. Standing and walking may have great value in the minds of individual children and their parents and should be supported for these reasons. Efficient, functional mobility, however, is often better achieved by providing these children with a wheelchair.

• An upright stance may improve urinary tract and bowel function because of gravity. Improved cardiopulmonary fitness is provided as an argument for aggressive ambulation with assistive devices, but abundant research suggests that energy expenditure for patients with disabilities is usually constant because of decreased velocity and endurance. Often, more opportunities for aerobic fitness are available to wheelchair racers than to people depending on braces and crutches for ambulation.

• The most commonly cited argument for weight bearing is the development of osteopenia and the increased risk of fractures in nonambulatory patients. It is true that these patients are more osteopenic than ambulatory children, but the risk of fracture is more closely associated with surgery and immobilization than with lack of weight bearing. Ambulatory children with MMC have a higher frequency of orthopedic procedures and therefore more risk of fractures. Weight bearing is encouraged to counteract the risk of lower extremity contractures and deformity, but the association has never been clearly defined. It has been suggested that keeping children upright and weight bearing will prevent the development of obesity, but a recent study comparing the users of standing frames and wheelchairs found the opposite to be true. Maintaining an upright posture does not reduce the risk of decubitus formation; it only changes the pattern of skin breakdown. Wheelchair users have more gluteal lesions and ambulators have more foot involvement.

Skin Breakdown (pp. 1224–1225)

Morbidity and Cost. The overall incidence of skin breakdown with MMC is typically about 43%. The prevalence of skin breakdown tends to increase annually from infancy to age 10 years, then plateau at 20% and 25% of patients.

Common Sites. Skin breakdown occurs most commonly as a result of unrelieved pressure over anesthetic areas. Lacerations, burns, dermatitis, and even cold injury in anesthetic areas can also cause serious skin breakdown. In patients with MMC, higher rates of skin breakdown are seen in those who have mental retardation, large head size, kyphoscoliosis, or chronic soiling. Bony prominences and orthopedic deformities cause skin ulceration from pressure or shear forces. Nonambulatory patients have common ulceration in the perineum, whereas the highest frequency of lower extremity breakdown occurs in ambulatory patients with lower lumbar motor levels.

Prevention. All patients with MMC should receive periodic examinations for and preventive guidance against skin breakdown. The child must learn that meticulous hygiene and daily inspection of insensate skin are important. Whenever a child receives a new spinal or lower extremity orthosis, a sequential wearing schedule should be used to monitor for sites of excessive pressure. Ambulatory patients should be cautioned against walking barefoot, especially outdoors or on hot pavement. Patients who use wheelchairs need adjustment of seating to prevent pelvic obliquity or pressure over bony prominences. There is no preferred wheelchair cushion for patients with MMC, but gel cushions should not be left outdoors in cold climates because they may become cold enough to induce freeze burns.

Treatment. The medical management of skin breakdown is similar to that for other diagnoses. Attention to relief of pressure or shear forces, hygiene, debridement, and nutrition is important. Deep wounds may require surgical closure.

Primary closure or skin rotation is preferable to myocutaneous flaps for first procedures (see Chapter 31).

Obesity (p. 1225)
• Dieting studies document that, on average, children with MMC ingest 25% fewer calories than their peers, and yet 27% to 90% are reported to be obese. Daily energy expenditure is inversely related to the level of the lesion (i.e., higher-level lesions result in lower energy expenditure). Once a child with MMC becomes obese, the reduced energy expenditure makes weight loss even more difficult. Dietary management should begin in infancy with anticipatory guidance and nutritional education. Weight reduction is extremely difficult, requiring professional assistance to maintain adequate protein and vitamin intake while severely restricting calories.

Psychological and Social Issues (pp. 1225–1226)
Intellectual and Personal Development. Many children with MMC perform in the lower ranges of intelligence tests. IQ scores have been correlated with level of lesion (i.e., higher-level lesions are associated with lower scores, lower lesions with better performance). IQ scores are adversely affected by the presence of CNS infection and shunt malformation. The combination of cognitive impairment and significant physical disabilities makes training in self-care both challenging and difficult.
• Children with MMC typically view themselves as less competent in academic, athletic, and social domains than their unaffected peers. Peer acceptance is highly valued by children with MMC, but they feel less supported by classmates than nondisabled children do. Clearly, interventions to foster independence and to increase self-perception are necessary.

Family. The family is irreversibly changed by the presence of a disabled child, and the child is affected by the family's response. Most social science research now agrees that the family's response to the disabled child probably plays a greater role in emotional development than the disability itself.

MYELOMENINGOCELE IN ADULTS (pp. 1226–1227)
Description of a New Disease (pp. 1226–1227)
• The combination of improved surgical practices, new antibiotics, and the willingness of health care professionals to manage patients with MMC using a team approach has made long-term survival possible. With aging, periodic screening for change in neurological status, development of joint disease, deterioration of renal function, or development of pressure ulcers is essential.

Skin Breakdown. Pressure ulcers are a major cause of morbidity in adolescents and adults with MMC. In one series of young adults aged 19 to 27 years, 85% had had skin breakdown requiring hospitalization and 70% had continuing problems with skin ulcers. About half had only occasional breakdown, but one-fourth had nearly continuous problems. Skin breakdown over the feet can be extremely difficult to heal and can cause loss of ambulation because of need for pressure relief or surgical amputation.

Musculoskeletal Complications and Joint Disease. Joint pain and degeneration can cause adults to become more dependent on a wheelchair for mobility. Those with sensory levels at L3 or L4 are particularly likely to lose the ability to be community ambulators in young adulthood. Upper extremity joints such as the shoulder and elbow may become painful from overuse. Lower extremity joints may become Charcot joints in the second and third decade as a result of an orthopedic deformity, abnormal dynamic forces, and impaired sensation. Clinicians should give careful consideration to joint protection for young children with MMC. Scoliosis does not appear to progress beyond adolescence.

Late Neurological Changes. Neurological deterioration in adults with MMC can occur as a result of shunt obstruction, syringomyelia, or tethering of the spinal cord. Most children with MMC and hydrocephalus do not seem to outgrow the need for a shunt as adults. Hydromyelia causing upper extremity pain, paresthesias, and weakness has been reported as a late development in adults. Tethering of the spinal cord and herniated disks have occurred in adults, often in association with pregnancy. Symptoms from tethered cord can be exacerbated by forward bending, childbirth, and trauma.

Renal and Urological Problems. Renal failure is one of the most serious complications facing adults with MMC. In one study of 61 adults at age 25 years, 31% had renal damage and 15% were being treated for hypertension. Whereas the primary causes are most often reflux and recurrent infection, other contributing factors include hypertension, shunt nephritis, amyloidosis, and calculi. Regular urological follow-up is important to monitor renal function, treat infections, and identify complications such as calculi formation or renal failure. Patients with MMC appear to be good candidates for dialysis, and renal transplantation has also been used successfully.

Fertility. Adolescents with MMC have similar expectations regarding marriage and reproduction as do adolescents without MMC, but they have considerably less experience with dating and knowledge of sexual functioning, family planning, and birth control. Girls, but not boys, with MMC have been observed to physically mature earlier than peers and same-sex family members without MMC. They also tend to reach menarche sooner than the national mean.
• Women report various degrees of genital sensation, whereas many men report the ability for erection and ejaculation, but none of these correlates with level of motor function. Most adults with MMC are reported to have satisfactory sexual function. Primary testicular failure with low serum testosterone and elevated follicle-stimulating and luteinizing hormones may be common, but men with MMC have been reported to father children. Women with MMC have successfully conceived and carried to term without major complications, although urinary tract infections have been commonly reported.

Affective Disorders (p. 1227)

• Adolescents with MMC often have low self-esteem and frequent doubts concerning their health, physical condition, and sexual functioning. Delayed social responsibility is prominent, as is a paucity of friends. Social isolation is a common problem. Adults with MMC are reported to have a range of adjustments from well adapted to poorly motivated, apathetic, and dependent personalities. Although psychosocial problems are common, suicide has not been reported in higher-than-expected frequency.

Vocational Issues (p. 1227)

• Most adults with MMC are reported to have completed high school and about half continued in postsecondary education. About 25% of adults with MMC report employment, mainly in routine, nonmanual work. They had average working hours, but received below-average pay. Most enjoyed their jobs and were well accepted by peers at work, but job retention was poor. Adolescents with MMC appear to have unrealistic ideas about training and skill requirements compared with their peers.

Independent Living (p. 1227)

• Various rates of living away from parents have been reported in different cultures, ranging from over 60% in the United States to 15% in Great Britain. In one study, one-third of adults with MMC were fully independent, employed, financially independent, homeowners, and free of psychological problems. The other two-thirds required Social Security income and various levels of support from family and friends. Many have limited abilities to do cooking, shopping, or use public transportation. Factors associated with independence include sensory level below L3, no ventriculoperitoneal shunt, IQ of 80 or greater, no epilepsy, community ambulation skills, no pressure sores, and freedom from incontinence pads.

• Planning for postsecondary education, vocation, and independent living should begin in early adolescence. Schools must include transition services in the Individualized Education Program (I.E.P.) to help move the child beyond school to vocational training, employment, adult services, independent living, and community participation.

55

Original Chapter by Frederick S. Frost, M.D.

Spinal Cord Injury Medicine

• The benefits of SCI programs utilizing a system approach (e.g., coordination of emergency rescue, acute, rehabilitation, follow-up, and vocational services) have been documented. Patients admitted immediately after injury to such coordinated centers demonstrate better outcomes including fewer medical complications, increased efficiency of rehabilitation gains, higher percentages of discharges to private residences, and reduced length of acute hospitalization and hospital charges. Improvements in the acute treatment of SCI now allow even the most severely injured individuals to survive, placing a greater emphasis on the goal of improving quality of life. The rate of rehospitalization for medical complications actually declines as years pass after injury, suggesting that adaptation to injury occurs on both a physiological and a psychological level.

EPIDEMIOLOGY (pp. 1231–1232)

• The differential diagnosis of spinal cord diseases resulting in paralysis is noted in Table 55–1. Persons with cancer metastatic to the spinal cord, and those with degenerative spinal diseases, outnumber patients with traumatic SCI. This heterogeneous group of patients is often overlooked in the provision of medical and rehabilitation services, usually because of advanced age or co-morbid medical conditions. Most of the concepts of care related to traumatic SCI are pertinent and applicable to nontraumatic myelopathies.

• Traumatic SCI is an uncommon condition. Not including persons who die at the scene of the accident, approximately 10,000 persons sustain SCI in the United States each year. Estimates of incidence in industrialized nations are similar, typically between 20 and 40 new cases per 1 million in population each year. Prevalence studies estimate that 200,000 persons with SCI are living in the United States. The majority of injuries occur in young people, and the cumulative loss of years of potential employment, productivity, and good health creates a huge financial burden that, in many cases, must be absorbed by the social welfare and public health care systems.

• SCI primarily affects young men. There has been no variation in the 4:1 male to female ratio of injury over the last two decades, although the average age at injury (currently 31.5 years) has slowly risen. The proportion of those older than 60 years at injury has doubled (4.7% versus 9.7%) over the last 20 years. Both of these trends are consistent with the increase in median age of the general

TABLE 55-1 Differential Diagnosis of Spinal Cord Injury

Traumatic (e.g., Fractures, Dislocations, Contusions)
Cervical (C1–C8)
Thoracic (T1–T12)
Lumbar (L1–L5)
Sacral
Multiple

Nontraumatic
Motor Neuron Diseases
   Amyotrophic lateral sclerosis
   Spinal muscular atrophy
   Other motor neuron diseases
Spondylotic Myelopathies
   Spondylolysis, spondylolisthesis
   Spinal stenosis
   Disk herniation, ruptures
   Atlantoaxial instability
Infectious and Inflammatory Diseases
   Multiple sclerosis
   Epidural abscesses
   Transverse myelitis
   Poliomyelitis, postpoliomyelitis
   Osteomyelitis
   Arachnoiditis
   Human immunodeficiency virus infection
   Chronic inflammatory demyelinating polyradiculoneuropathy
   Acute inflammatory demyelinating polyradiculoneuropathy
Neoplastic Diseases
   1. Intradural intramedullary
      Primary: ependymoma, astrocytoma
      Metastatic: lung, breast, lymphoma, colorectal, head/neck, renal
   2. Intradural extramedullary
      Primary: meningioma, neurofibroma, nerve sheath schwannoma, embryonal tumors
      Metastatic: leukemia/lymphoma, adenocarcinoma, untreated primary CNS tumors
   3. Extradural
      Primary: myeloma, neuroblastoma, osteosarcoma, Ewing's sarcoma
      Metastatic: breast, lung, prostate, thyroid, kidney, lymphoma, gastrointestinal
Vascular Disorders
   Ischemic myelopathy
   Arteriovenous malformations
Toxic/Metabolic Conditions
   Radiation-induced myelopathy
   Subacute combined degeneration
Congenital/Developmental Disorders
   Spina bifida
   Developmental syringomyelia
   Myelodysplasia

population. More than half (63.4%) of SCI patients were employed or in school at the time of their injury, and 53.7% were unmarried.

• Motor vehicle collisions (36.6%) have remained the most common cause of injury since 1991, followed by acts of violence (27.9%), falls (21.4%), and sports injuries (6.5%). After age 45 years, falls supplant motor vehicle collisions as the most common cause of injury. As might be expected, women incur fewer injuries in sporting activities than men. In the African-American and Hispanic populations, acts of violence, not motor vehicle collisions, account for the majority of injuries.

• Many of these injuries are preventable. Estimates of the rate of alcohol intoxication among those sustaining SCI range between 17% and 49%. The majority of injuries occur on Saturday and Sunday, and the peak incidence occurs in the month of July.

ANATOMY, TERMINOLOGY, AND CLASSIFICATION OF INJURY (pp. 1232–1235)

• The classification of injuries is based on knowledge of the anatomy and function of the spinal cord and segmental nerves (Fig. 55–1). The spinal cord extends from the foramen magnum to the lower border of the first lumbar vertebra, where it reaches a conical termination, the conus medullaris. The first cervical nerve, which usually lacks dorsal root fibers, has no corresponding dermatome. It exits the vertebral canal between the atlas and the occiput. The first seven cervical nerves exit the foramina above the vertebrae of their same number. The eighth cervical nerve emerges between C7 and T1. All the spinal nerves below this level exit the vertebral canal from the foramina beneath the vertebrae of the same number.

• The spinal cord is supplied by branches of the vertebral arteries and by anterior and posterior radicular arteries that arise from segmental vessels.

• Each vertebral artery gives rise to a posterior and an anterior spinal artery, but the anterior spinal arteries unite to form a single anterior midline vessel at the level of the medulla. The anterior spinal artery supplies the anterior two-thirds of the spinal cord, and is dependent on anastomotic branches from the anterior radicular arteries as it descends below the cervical spinal cord. In the thoracic region, the anterior spinal artery can be narrow and irregular, which places the spinal cord at risk should segmental vessels be occluded. The paired posterior spinal arteries supply the posterior third of the spinal cord, receiving blood from the posterior radicular arteries. They form a discontinuous plexus of vessels on the posterior surface of the spinal cord medial to the dorsal roots.

• Radicular arteries vary considerably in number, and are most commonly located along the left side in the thoracic and lumbar regions. A large-caliber anterior radicular artery, the artery of Adamkiewicz, usually enters with a left lower thoracic or upper lumbar spinal root. This region of the spinal cord, along with the upper thoracic levels (which receive weak supply from the intercostal arteries), is particularly vulnerable to vascular compromise.

• A useful SCI examination in the emergency setting requires the participation of an alert and cooperative patient but is often limited by concomitant brain injury, therapeutic sedation, or the influence of drug or alcohol intoxication. The initial examination is important in establishing an initial level of injury and for detecting secondary injuries to the cord during the first few days of hospitalization. For prognostic purposes, however, an examination at 72 hours

STANDARD NEUROLOGICAL CLASSIFICATION OF SPINAL CORD INJURY

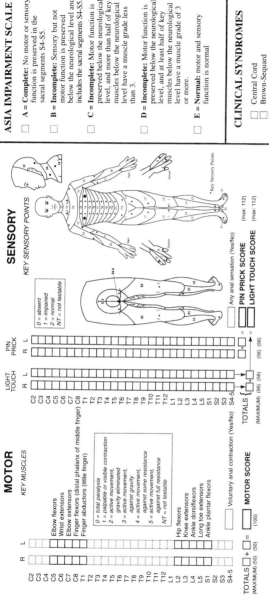

FIGURE 55-1. Standard neurological classification of spinal cord injury. (From American Spinal Injury Association: International Standards for Neurological and Functional Classification of Spinal Cord Injury. Atlanta, American Spinal Injury Association, 1996.)

is more reliable. Evaluations of residual muscle and sensory function are the central elements of the examination. Examination of muscle stretch reflexes, including the bulbocavernosus reflex, is useful in assessing lesions of the lower motor neurons. In many instances, however, *spinal shock* can be encountered, in which upper motor neuron sensory and motor loss is associated with areflexia below the level of injury. Spinal shock is a poorly defined phenomenon. If lower motor neuron injury is not present, reflex activity typically returns over the course of weeks or months. The presence of spinal shock is of marginal prognostic significance because a reliable examination and prognostic evaluation can be carried out when spinal shock is present.

- The American Spinal Injury Association (ASIA) Impairment Scale (see Fig. 55–1) describes the degree of motor and sensory preservation below the level of injury and allows for description of the residual function of the injured spinal cord. Injuries are rated along a spectrum ranging from complete (grade A) to full motor and sensory preservation (grade E). Other clinical syndromes describe lesions that affect specific areas of the spinal cord. *Tetraplegia* results from an injury to the spinal cord within the cervical canal, with neurological deficits observed in the upper extremities, trunk, lower extremities, and visceral functions. In *paraplegia,* arm and hand function is normal, but deficits in neural control of the trunk, lower extremities, and visceral functions are brought about by SCI in the thoracic, lumbar, or sacral segments.

- *Central cord syndrome,* the most common of these clinical syndromes, is often associated with neck hyperextension injuries in older individuals with spondylosis. This is an incomplete injury, characterized by weakness that is more severe in the arms than in the legs. Pathological findings of necrosis in the central spinal cord have been attributed to the sparse vascular supply in this area and to injury mechanics that place the greatest pressures on the center of the cord. The pattern of neurological deficit has traditionally been explained by the claim that the corticospinal tract is somatotopically organized, with fibers supplying upper extremity function lying medially, closer to the area of injury. However, there is limited evidence to support such organization.

- *Brown-Séquard syndrome* is seen in association with a cord hemisection. Lesions of this type are characterized by ipsilateral muscle weakness and proprioception deficits. On the contralateral side, there is loss of pinprick and thermal sensation. A clean hemisection injury is rare, and patients often exhibit lesions that mix characteristics of Brown-Séquard and central cord syndromes.

- The *anterior cord syndrome* results from a lesion involving the anterior spinal artery or from direct trauma to the anterior two-thirds of the spinal cord. This can occur with retropulsion of disk or bone fragments and is sometimes associated with flexion injury of the cervical spine. Anterior cord syndrome allows relative preservation of proprioception and light touch and deep-pressure sensation, but pain sensation and motor function are diminished below the level of injury.

- The terms *conus medullaris syndrome* and *cauda equina syndrome* are often confused and misapplied in the description of lesions at the caudal region. A lesion of the conus medullaris is characterized by devastating deficits in bowel and bladder function, a symmetrical sensory deficit in the saddle distribution, and relatively minor deficits in lower extremity function. The deficits associated with cauda equina syndrome are asymmetrical and areflexic. The muscles affected exhibit atrophy and atonia. Patients with symmetrical weakness in lower extremity muscles across multiple myotomes are likely to have sustained a traumatic myelopathy above the level of the conus.

- The *neurological level of injury* (see Fig. 55–1) is defined as the most caudal neurological segment that retains normal sensory and motor function on both sides of the body. Often the neurological level of injury is different from the skeletal level of injury, and the segments where normal function is found often differ by side of body and in terms of sensory versus motor testing. Up to four different segments can identify the neurological level (i.e., R-sensory, L-sensory, R-motor, and L-motor). In these instances, the assignment of a single neurological level might be misleading, and the injury is best described by detailing the four segments. Dermatomes and myotomes are assessed at 28 key sensory points and 10 key muscles on each side. Muscles are graded from 0 (total paralysis) to 5 (provides full resistance). The motor level (the lowest normal motor segment) is defined by the lowest key muscle that has a grade of 3 or better, provided that all the key muscles represented by segments above that level are judged to be normal (grade 5). Light touch and pinprick are used to determine the Sensory Index Score. The Motor Index Score is determined by adding the manual muscle test scores of the 10 key muscles on each side, with a maximum of 100 points.
- A careful rectal examination is required to determine whether the injury is complete or incomplete. A complete lesion is defined as the absence of sensory or motor function in the lowest sacral segment. The use of this definition, proposed by Waters and colleagues, identifies a distinct subpopulation of injured persons who rarely change to incomplete status. If deep anal sensation or sensation at the anal mucocutaneous junction is reliably demonstrated, or if there is voluntary control of the external anal sphincter, the lesion is incomplete.

NEUROLOGICAL PROGNOSIS AND FUNCTIONAL OUTCOMES (pp. 1235–1237)

- Virtually all patients who survive traumatic SCI experience some neurological recovery. For some patients this recovery results in an improved level of function. Recovery can be monitored by clinical examination and electrodiagnostic studies. Recovery of neurological function in the segments near the zone of injury, or "root recovery," is distinguished from global improvements in spinal cord function that result in changes of injury grades within the ASIA Impairment Scale.
- A number of studies have shown that in the interval between 1 month and 1 year postinjury, the rate of motor recovery rapidly declines in the first 6 months, although gains in strength can be seen as late as 2 years after injury. Patients with incomplete injuries recover faster in the zone of injury than those with complete injuries, but their degree of recovery is not necessarily greater. Nearly all muscles with grade 1/5 or 2/5 strength 1 month after injury recover up to 3/5 (antigravity) strength by 1 year. Muscles with 0/5 strength that are located at the first neurological level below the most caudal segment having motor function typically recover antigravity strength in about one-third of cases. If the 0/5 muscle is two segments below the most caudal level exhibiting motor function, functional recovery is extremely rare.
- Longitudinal studies utilizing the ASIA Impairment Scale and its predecessor, the Frankel classification, have generated considerable data to describe the potential for recovery caudal to the zone of injury. Patients with complete injuries (grade A) have a poor prognosis for improvement, with estimates of

changes in grade after such an injury ranging between 0% and 9%. Although late conversion of ASIA impairment grade A cases certainly can occur, retrospective analysis of these relatively rare cases has, in many instances, shown that concurrent conditions (e.g., concurrent brain injury or sedation) might have prevented an accurate initial examination.

• Preservation of pinprick sensation conveys a greater potential for ambulation recovery than preservation of light touch sensation, presumably because of the proximity of the spinothalamic and corticospinal tracts. Persons with sparing of motor function below the zone of injury, including those with central cord syndrome and Brown-Séquard syndrome, have the best prognosis for recovery. The majority of persons with central cord syndrome ultimately attain functional use of their hands and control of bladder and bowel function. Recovery of ambulation in these patients correlates with a younger age at injury. Patients with Brown-Séquard-type injuries have the best outlook; over 90% reach ambulatory status at 6 months postinjury.

Functional Outcomes (pp. 1236–1237)

• The functional abilities of persons with SCI should be assessed in the areas of mobility, locomotion, feeding, dressing, grooming, bathing, and toileting (Table 55–2). Many persons can master tasks that would not be predicted from the level of lesion alone. Performance is influenced by such variables as age, body habitus, general health, concurrent injuries, spinal instrumentation, intelligence, and motivation. A careful assessment of the patient's personal needs and social support is necessary to correctly identify the functional tasks that will be the most relevant after discharge from the rehabilitation setting. Insistence on independent functioning at all costs is often counterproductive. The most productive disabled individuals develop strategies to make the most of help that is available from family, friends, hired assistants, and co-workers.

THE REHABILITATION PROCESS (pp. 1237–1238)

• It is impossible to measure the magnitude of personal loss experienced by a person with tetraplegia. Readjustment and adaptation can be a slow process, a critical point to consider when planning for the provision of rehabilitation services. Although physical restrictions might be overcome fairly rapidly by environmental modifications and assistive equipment, the loss of freedom and change in body image cannot be reconciled so quickly.

• The initial therapy process focuses on joint protection and maintenance of range of motion (ROM). Proper positioning in bed is critical, and ROM exercises are carried out one to three times a day depending on the degree of muscle tone present in the extremities. In tetraplegic persons, particular care is taken to guard against shortening of shoulder adductor muscles, which would limit shoulder abduction. The wrists and ankles often need protective splints to preserve ROM.

• In the face of such a devastating medical condition, patients, family, and staff members often place an inappropriate urgency on starting strengthening exercise and aggressive conditioning programs. This can be particularly harmful in tetraplegic persons with borderline pulmonary reserve. Many of these patients are in a catabolic state, using all of their energy just to breathe and clear their lungs of secretions. There is nothing to be gained at this point by insisting

TABLE 55–2 Expectations for Function by Motor Level of Injury

Motor Level of Injury	Activities of Daily Living	Mobility and Locomotion
C1–C4	Feeding possible with balanced forearm orthoses Computer access by tongue, breath, voice controls Weight shifts with power tilt and recline chair Mouth stick use	Operate power chair with tongue, chin, or breath controller
C5	Drink from cup, feed with static splints and setup Oral/facial hygiene, writing, typing with equipment Dressing upper body possible Side-to-side weight shifts	Propel chair with hand rim projections short distances on smooth surfaces Power chair with hand controller
C6	Feed, dress upper body with setup Dressing lower body possible Forward weight shifts	Bed mobility with equipment Level surface transfers with assistance Propel chair indoors with coated hand rims
C7	Independent feeding, dressing, bathing with adaptive equipment, built-up utensils	Independent bed mobility Independent level surface transfers Wheelchair use outdoors (power chair for school or work)
C8	Independent in feeding, dressing, bathing Bowel and bladder care with setup	Propel chair, including curbs/wheelies Wheelchair-to-car transfers
T1	Independent in feeding, dressing, bathing Independent in bowel and bladder care	Transfer from floor to wheelchair
T2–L1	Independent in all self-care	Stand with braces for exercise Independent in transfers and wheelchair mobility
L2	Independent in all self-care	Potential for swing-to gait with long leg braces indoors Use of forearm crutches
L3	Independent in all self-care	Potential for community ambulation
L4–S1	Independent in all self-care	Potential for ambulation with short leg braces Potential for ambulation without assistive devices

that the patient sit in a chair for extended periods or engage in resistive exercises.

• Patients and families benefit from meeting with members of the rehabilitation team early in the hospital course. Education regarding the rehabilitation process often helps reduce feelings of ignorance and helplessness. There is no single best way to counsel patients and families regarding prognosis. These discussions must take into account the patient's premorbid personality, maturity, and status in life. Clinicians worried about creating false hope are as likely to create false pessimism. An overview of the rehabilitation process must not ignore the obvious; most persons with SCI are young, and 80% are male. Many were injured by violent acts or have a history of risk-taking behavior. Their disability occurs at a time when they are only beginning to develop an adult identity.

SPECIAL COMPONENTS OF THE REHABILITATION PROCESS (pp. 1238–1245)

• Traditional therapeutic exercise, functional training, and aerobic conditioning are augmented by the use of adaptive equipment and orthotic devices, tendon transfer surgery, and functional electrical stimulation. These modalities facilitate community reintegration by enhancing community reintegration and vocational rehabilitation.

Assistive Devices (p. 1239)

• The ability of the person with SCI to manipulate the environment might depend on the proper prescription of assistive devices and adaptive equipment (Table 55–3). Occupational therapists specialize in the instruction of patients in the use of devices that circumvent deficits in upper extremity function (see Chapter 25). Although some assistive devices may cost only a few dollars, items such as wheelchairs, adapted vehicles, and environmental control devices are expensive. These products should be prescribed by a person knowledgeable in the field. A higher level of technology does not guarantee a higher level of function. As devices become more complicated, breakdowns become more common, and the crucial fit at the user-device interface becomes more tenuous.

• The best SCI rehabilitation programs make available a variety of sample assistive devices (e.g., wheelchairs, computers, and adapted vehicles) that allow the patient to evaluate each item before a prescription is made. A wheelchair that is appropriate for a young SCI patient at 8 weeks postinjury, for example, might be quite inappropriate at 12 weeks because balance, strength, weight distribution, and even neurological status continue to change.

• The goals of wheelchair prescription are to enhance mobility and locomotion; maximize pulmonary function; and prevent postural deformities, pain, and pressure ulcers (see Chapters 18 and 31). The treatment team helps the patient establish priorities for wheelchair use, anticipating the variety of situations and environments that the patient will encounter. Compromises must be made with any prescription. The fastest and lightest wheelchair might be too unstable. The best cushion might restrict transfers to and from the chair, or it might require considerable maintenance.

• Persons with lower level tetraplegia, despite being able to self-propel a wheelchair, are often appropriate for powered mobility. The energy saved from

TABLE 55-3 Interventions and Supplies

International Classification System by Motor Level	C2	C3	C4	C5	C6	C7	C8	T1	T2–T5	T6–L1	L2	L3	L4	L5	S1	S2–S4
Self-Care/Orthoses																
Mouth stick	S	S														
Balanced forearm orthosis			S													
Drop-arm commode				U	S							S	S			
Bath bench				U	U	U	U	U	U	S	S	S	S		S	
Utensil cuffs/adaptation				U	U	U	S				S	S		S		
Skin mirror				S	U	U	U	U	U	U	S	S				
Reacher/long-handled sponge					U	S	S	U	U	S						
Resting hand splints	S	S	S	S	S	S	S									
Long opponens splint	U	U	U	U	S	U	S									
Short opponens splint					U	U	S	S								
Suppository inserter					S	S	S	S								
Rope ladder/leg lifter			S	U	U	U	S	S	S							
Rolling shower chair	S	S	S	S	S	S										
Electric leg bag opener	U	U	U	S	S	S	U									
Adapted leg bag clamp							U	S	S							
Mobility/Functional Restoration																
Tongue touch controller	S	S	S													
Sip-and-puff/chin switch	S	S	S													
Adapted personal computer	U	U	U	U	U	S	S	S								
Power recline wheelchair	U	U	U	U	S	S	S	S								

Table continued on following page

TABLE 55-3 Interventions and Supplies—cont'd

International Classification System by Motor Level	C2	C3	C4	C5	C6	C7	C8	T1	T2-T5	T6-L1	L2	L3	L4	L5	S1	S2-S4
Power wheelchair	U	U	U	U	U	S	S	S	S							
Lightweight manual chair			U	U	U	U	U	U	U	U	S	S	S			
Wheelchair ramp	U	U	U	U	U	U	U	U	U	U	U	U	U			
Wheelchair cushion	U	U	U	U	U	U	U	U	S							
Transfer board	U	U	U	U	S	S	S	S	S							
Transfer lift device	U	U	U	U	U	S										
Auto hand controls						U	U	U	U	U	U	U	U			
Van with lift	U	U	U	U	S	S	S	S	S	S						
Adapted van driving system											U	U	U	U		
Leg braces									S	S	U	U	U	U	S	
Tendon Transfer and Neuroprostheses																
Phrenic nerve pacemaker	S	S	S													
Hand grasp neuroprosthesis				S	S											
Elbow extension transfer				S	S											
Tenodesis grip transfer					S	S										
One-stage pinch transfer					S	S										
Two-stage finger transfer					S	S										
Intrinsic transfers					S	S										
Bladder neuroprosthesis	S	S	S	S	S	S	S	S	S	S						
Medical Devices																
Primary and backup ventilator	U	U	S													
Aerosol nebulizer	U	U	S													

Portable suction machine	U	S								
Abdominal binder	U	U	U	U	U	U				
Elastic stockings	U	U	U	U	S	S	S	S	S	
Ankle-foot boots	U	U	U	U	U	S	S	S	S	
Blood pressure cuff and stethoscope	U	U	U	U	U	U	U			
Electric hospital bed	U	U	U	U	S	S	S	S		
Special mattress	S	S	S	S	S	S	S	S		
Urinary catheter supplies	U	U	U	U	U	U	U	U	S	S
Suppositories/gloves	U	U	U	U	U	U	U	U	U	U
Incontinence pads	U	U	U	U	U	U	S	S	S	S
Grab bars		S	S	S	S	S	S	S	S	S
Arm ergometer		S	S	S	S	S	S			

Key: U Usually required
  S Sometimes required
  Rarely required

pushing the chair can be used for wheelchair transfers, weight shifts, and vocational activities, reducing the long-term wear and tear on joints and soft tissues. For those who need advanced technology and customized seating systems, rehabilitation engineers can help patients navigate through the enormous array of commercial components that are available.

• Computers play an ever-increasing role in SCI rehabilitation. Modifications of workstations in the rehabilitation hospital computer laboratory can allow the patient to improve arm strength and hand function while learning computer skills. Keyboards and peripheral devices can be adapted in a fashion that requires the patient to use specific muscle groups in isolation. Many disabled persons find unique opportunities to socialize, network, and gather information over the Internet.

Upper Extremity Functional Intervention (pp. 1239–1242)

• Techniques used to augment upper limb function range from simple splinting and positioning to complex neuroprosthetic interventions. In the intensive care setting, attention to basic joint positioning sets the stage for later work on strengthening and dexterity. For persons with tetraplegia through the C7 level, proper hand position is maintained by resting splints, which allow tightening of the flexor tendons. Many families and patients desire a cosmetic, "flat hand" position, and education regarding the use of tenodesis for hand function needs to be undertaken. Preventing elbow flexor shortening can spell the difference between independent and assisted wheelchair transfers. Maintenance of pronation range is also critical, allowing patients to work with palms down in tabletop activities. As spinal and medical stability is achieved, work on strengthening innervated muscles can begin. For anxious patients with only a few functioning muscles, there is a high risk of muscle overwork and soft tissue strain. Most patients with SCI report shoulder, neck, and arm pain early on, and these symptoms should be carefully monitored by the physician.

• Patients can learn to compensate for impaired muscles by substitution movements, utilizing gravity and momentum and creating multiarticular closed kinetic chains. These substitution movements can be used to improve respiratory function, to assist with weight shifting and transfer skills, and to facilitate proper hand positioning and dexterity.

• Upper limb orthoses are commonly prescribed for persons with injury levels between C4 and C8. Balanced forearm orthoses and mobile arm supports augment weak deltoid and biceps muscles. These devices employ a counterweight/fulcrum mechanism to support the distal forearm, allowing the patient with a C4 or C5 injury to position the hand for tabletop activities (see Chapters 15 and 25). The devices can be used for strengthening, training, and as functional assist devices.

• Persons with a C5 injury can position their hands but need long opponens orthoses to provide wrist stability. This static splint can be fabricated to include utensil slots and penholders.

• Functional abilities improve significantly with functional wrist extensor muscle strength that is present at the C6 level. Active wrist extension results in tenodesis of the hand. This passive movement is characterized by the opposition of thumb and index finger, with flexion of the fingers occurring as the wrist extends against static finger flexor tendons. With wrist control at the C6 level, patients can use short opponens orthoses or utensil cuffs to feed themselves. A

simple tenodesis orthosis can be fabricated by the occupational therapist for the purposes of training and evaluation.
• Patients with injury levels C7 and C8 need few orthotic interventions. The addition of finger extension and wrist flexion can augment grasp strength. Short opponens splints and utensil cuffs are often utilized. Pencil and utensil use can often be accomplished by weaving the device through the fingers, provided that sufficient tightness of the finger flexors is present. For those with C8 finger flexors, utensils with built-up handles can improve grip stability.

Upper Extremity Tendon Transfers (pp. 1242–1243)

• Tendon transfers and upper limb reconstructive surgery have recently gained more acceptance as a means of restoring elbow extension, wrist extension, and rudimentary hand function. These procedures are considered 1-year postinjury, keeping in mind that upper limb muscle recovery can occur over the course of 2 years or more. This period allows patients to assess their upper extremity capabilities and compensatory strategies in their home and vocational environment. Patients with remote tetraplegia can also be considered, but outcomes are often less predictable. Although the surgery itself is typically brief, splinting and prolonged immobilization of the arms might make the patient totally dependent for 3 to 6 weeks, and preoperative functional abilities can be temporarily lost. This can result in a major disruption in the patient's personal and vocational life, and requirements for caregiver assistance are commonly altered.
• Restoring elbow extension in persons with C5 level injuries by posterior deltoid to triceps muscle transfer enables overhead and forward reaching and enhances performance of grooming, hygiene, and tabletop activities. Brachioradialis transfers to the wrist extensors produce a weak tenodesis grip and allow patients to manipulate light objects without an orthosis. For those with C6 and C7 level injuries, there are many surgical options that can restore key-pinch and palmar grasp function (Table 55–4).

Lower Extremity Functional Interventions (pp. 1243–1244)

• Walking is a goal of every person with newly acquired paralysis. Persons who ambulate at the community level after SCI usually have retained at least 4/5 strength in both hip flexors and in at least one quadriceps muscle. It is possible for almost every patient to achieve some type of vertical posture through the use of orthoses, standing frames, or standing wheelchairs. The psychological benefit of standing can be high. It is uncommon for patients with thoracic level paraplegia to use long leg braces for ambulation outside of the house. Rejection rates for long leg braces can be as high as 75%. The energy expenditure of ambulation with long leg braces can be increased as much as 12 times per unit distance.
• Ambulation outcomes are optimized when attention is given during the acute phase of injury to maintenance of hip extension and ankle dorsiflexion ROM through exercises and splinting. Factors that contribute to loss of joint ROM (e.g., heterotopic ossification, spasticity, and pain) should receive aggressive treatment. Patients with leg weakness might need excessive lumbar lordosis to balance in the standing position, but this degree of spinal range of motion can be absent in those with lumbosacral spinal fusions. These persons also place unusual and excessive forces across sites of spinal fractures during standing

TABLE 55–4 Surgery to Enhance Upper Extremity Function in Tetraplegia: International Classification

	Available Muscles Grade 4–5/5	Transfers and Reconstruction—Examples
Motor Groups		
0	None below elbow	Posterior deltoid to triceps (Moberg, 1975, 1975)
		Biceps to triceps (Zancolli, 1979)
1	Brachioradialis (BR)	BR to ECRB (Freehafer, 1967)
		Flexor pollicus longus (FPL) tenodesis (McDowell, 1986)
2	ECRL	BR to ECRB/L
		BR or FPL (Waters, 1985)
3	ECRB	ECRL to flexor digitorum profundus (FDP) (Lamb, 1972)
4	Pronator Teres (PT)	BR to FDP + PT opponensplasty (Freehafer, 1984)
		Two-stage House procedure (1985)
5	FCRB	As above
6	Finger extensors	As above, without finger extensor transfer
7	Thumb extensors	As above, without thumb extension transfer
8	Partial finger flexors	FDS lasso for intrinsic balance (House, 1985)
9	Lacks intrinsics only	Two-stage Zancolli procedure (1979)
Sensory Groups		
0	Ocular sensibility; two-point discrimination >10 mm in the thumb	
Cu	Cutaneous sensibility; two-point discrimination <10 mm in the thumb	

Abbreviations: ECRL, extensor carpi radialis longus; ECRB, extensor carpi radialis brevis; FCRB, flexor carpi radialis brevis; EDC, extensor digitorum communis; EPL, extensor pollicis longus; FDS, flexor digitorum sublimis.

activities, raising the risk of instrumentation and fusion failure in the first few months after injury.

• There is a strong correlation between the physiological determinants of gait and the ASIA lower extremity motor score. Lower extremity motor score at 1 month is predictive of further motor recovery and the achievement of community ambulation status at 1 year. The majority of patients with lower extremity motor score greater than 10 at 1 month achieve community ambulation status at 1 year. The lower extremity motor score of incomplete tetraplegic patients might be the same as that for persons with incomplete paraplegia, but upper extremity deficits limit the use of assistive devices.

• Lower extremity bracing (see Chapter 16) can help compensate for deficits in muscle strength, but energy costs associated with extensive bracing usually prohibit community-level ambulation. Traditional knee-ankle-foot orthoses (KAFOs), or long leg braces, include an upper and lower thigh band, drop locks, and a double-action ankle joint. Custom-molded thermoplastic calf and shank sleeves are now commonly used in place of leather bands and extended metal uprights. Extension of the brace to include hip and trunk bands is possible for persons who lack hip control, but this does not enhance function. The lighter Scott-Craig KAFO design allows easier donning and doffing and more efficient ambulation. The lower calf and thigh bands of the standard KAFO are eliminated. In addition, this brace includes a hinged anterior tibial band, with snap locks, a bail knee lock, a proximal thigh band, and a reinforced footplate. The tibial band generates a force close to the knee for added stability, analogous to a patellar tendon-bearing prosthesis. It is not likely that patients will continue to use their braces after training unless they can ambulate nonstop more than 300 yards and use their braces all day.

• Community ambulation is promoted through the use of a reciprocal gait pattern, a pattern that is virtually impossible using bilateral long leg braces. Reciprocating orthoses have been developed that transform a passive rigid orthosis into an active, articulating orthosis by simulating hip flexion (see Chapter 16). These devices allow the lower limb to advance when body weight is shifted from side to side as a reciprocating cable is incorporated into articulated hip joints. These orthoses are expensive to fabricate and require considerable formal therapy training for safe use. There is no evidence that these braces offer a better long-term acceptance rate than standard KAFOs. Children with SCI might be better candidates for these interventions than adults, owing to differences in body habitus and energy levels.

• At present the clinical applications of lower extremity functional neuromuscular stimulation systems are limited, and decades of research have failed to achieve results that are superior to standard orthotic management. The cost of fitting such systems and their rehabilitation is high, and the distances that can be traveled are short. Electrical stimulation reverses the natural recruitment order of muscle fibers, resulting in severe and accelerated fatigue compared with that induced by normal muscle contraction. Fatigue of electrically stimulated muscles is an important limiting factor in lower extremity applications. Patients with intact or partial sensation can also find the stimulation painful or uncomfortable. It has been estimated that less than 11% of SCI persons are appropriate for these systems.

Driver Rehabilitation (pp. 1244–1245)

• Driver rehabilitation is a critical component of successful community reintegration. The driver rehabilitation program evaluates driving ability and training needs, assists with state licensing issues, recommends passenger vehicles and modifications, and offers counseling regarding utilization of community transit services. A prescription for van modifications should not be dispensed until the driver has been tested using the specific adapted driving equipment being considered.

Vocational Rehabilitation (p. 1245)

• Return to work after injury is recognized as one of the indicators of recovery. Estimates of employment rates after injury range from 13% to 48%. Those with paraplegia have higher re-employment rates than those with tetraplegia. Persons with incomplete injuries and those who incur SCI at a younger age are more likely to become employed. A lower employment rate occurs with low preinjury education levels, minority race, and poor preinjury vocational experience. Several disincentives, chiefly the risk of losing disability income and public-funded medical insurance, make a return to work an unattractive proposition for many. Despite the Americans With Disabilities Act, persons with disabilities are often subjected to discrimination and prejudice in the employment setting.

MEDICAL CONDITIONS (pp. 1245–1257)

• Most patients at the time of SCI also suffer associated trauma to other organ systems. The most common concurrent injuries are fractures (29%), loss of consciousness (28%), and pneumothorax and hemothorax (17%). There is an average 15-day acute care hospital length of stay, followed by an average of 44 days in the rehabilitation hospital. Persons with tetraplegia and those with complete injuries need longer hospitalizations. The costs of hospitalization account for over 80% of the total injury costs during the first year postinjury.

• Medical illnesses prompting readmission are common in the first years postinjury, with a slight decline in frequency as years pass. Risk factors for readmission include younger age, nursing home residence, fewer trips outside the home, more complete injuries, and a lower educational level. Urinary tract infections are the most common admitting diagnosis, although admissions for pressure ulcers account for more hospital days and generate greater human and financial costs.

• Changes in survival and injury demographics have resulted in an increased interest in the problems faced by elderly persons with SCI and persons who have survived their injury for many decades. Older persons with new-onset SCI have a different course than their younger counterparts, one that is characterized by a slower pace of rehabilitation and longer hospitalizations. Most elderly patients with adequate cognitive abilities benefit from rehabilitation services after injury, although goals are typically less ambitious.

• Renal diseases accounted for the majority of deaths after SCI in previous decades secondary to the presence of unresolved, recurrent infectious. The causes of death after SCI now approach those seen in the general population, although many cause-specific mortality rates remain above normal. Although pulmonary causes are now the most common cause of death, the ratio of actual to expected deaths is highest for septicemia. Clinicians should be aware of the high risk for suicide in SCI patients. A large epidemiological study showed that unintentional injuries and suicides are the leading cause of death in persons with paraplegia as well as in all SCI patients less than 55 years old. Statistics regarding cause of death differ for injury subgroups, including age and level and grade of injury. For ventilator-dependent quadriplegia, the overall 1-year survival rate is approximately 25% and the 15-year survival rate is 17%.

Psychological Issues (p. 1246)

• Traumatic SCI has been described as one of the most devastating calamities in life. Counseling services should be made available to all patients with SCI. It is unfortunate that some of the most pressing psychological and social needs of the patient are met by resources that are often diminished by financial cutbacks. The psychologist can be helpful to other team members as well, recommending approaches to the patient and helping to clarify patients' behavior in terms of adaptation to injury.

• The assumption that most persons with SCI are clinically depressed is incorrect. Several studies have shown that the overall incidence of depressive illness on the SCI rehabilitation unit is only moderate. Many persons need several years to adapt psychologically to SCI. Poor adaptation and depression often lead to medical complications, which can cause more adaptation and depression problems.

- Alcohol and substance abuse can be involved as a cause of the injury itself and can continue after discharge from rehabilitation. Up to 50% of persons develop problems with substance abuse after SCI. Substance abuse treatment should be initiated during the initial rehabilitation period and continued after discharge as needed. Substance abuse often leads to covert self-destructive behavior and can be disruptive to the family as well.
- Cognitive deficits are common in persons with SCI and can interfere with the rehabilitation process. Closed head injury occurs in up to 57% of SCI persons. Cognitive deficits are often multifactorial and can relate to substance abuse, learning disabilities, and other medical conditions. The team should be aware of these deficits and how they affect the person's ability to cooperate and participate in therapy. Neuropsychological evaluation gives insight into the person's behavior (see Chapter 4).
- The most pressing need for counseling support in this population arises after hospital discharge. For disabled persons with suboptimal support systems, the cumulative effect of years of isolation, inactivity, or neglect can have a profound effect on health and quality of life. The aging or death of a patient's caregiver can bring about devastating life changes. Disability is often associated with poverty. Physical and sexual abuse of disabled persons is common.

Respiratory System (pp. 1247–1249)

- The leading cause of death in persons with SCI is pneumonia, and diseases of the respiratory system are the underlying cause of death in over 20% of this population. The clinical manifestations of pulmonary disease in this population are numerous and include ventilatory failure, pulmonary edema, pneumonia, atelectasis, restrictive lung disease, pneumothorax, hemothorax, lung contusion, and the need for tracheostomy. Persons with high cervical SCI or concomitant chest injuries and those injured later in life are at particular risk. The pulmonary complications seen during the acute phase of injury are the most debilitating and the most difficult and expensive to treat. Up to 50% of acutely injured persons develop pulmonary complications during the first month postinjury, most commonly those with injuries from the C1 to C4 levels.
- The muscles involved in normal pulmonary ventilation include the diaphragm, the intercostal muscles, the accessory neck muscles, and the abdominal muscles. Following SCI, the nature and magnitude of the changes in ventilatory function and cough depend on the level of neurological injury. Injuries between T7 and T12 impair abdominal muscle function, reducing forceful expiration and cough. In higher-level thoracic and cervical injuries, intercostal muscle function is diminished or absent, affecting both inspiratory and expiratory function. In the first weeks after injury, flaccid intercostal muscle paralysis can result in paradoxical collapse of the rib cage during inspiration, further reducing ventilatory efficiency. As spasticity develops after a few weeks, this paradoxical movement is reduced and function improves. Because the diaphragm is supplied by C3, C4, and C5, it is common for persons injured above the C4 level to need ventilator support. For those with high-level injuries, accessory muscles of respiration in the neck can sustain acutely injured patients long enough to survive until emergency treatment arrives. These muscles can generate tidal volumes of several hundred cubic centimeters. They are particularly effective during the chronic phase of injury, but are effective only during waking hours and are easily fatigued. Accessory muscles can also help produce the small active

expiratory volumes seen in tetraplegic patients during the acute phase of injury. Tetraplegic patients usually have a reduction in all measures of pulmonary function with the exception of residual volume. Residual volume is increased because of lack of active expiratory effort.

- The chief pulmonary concerns during the acute phase of care are ventilation, oxygenation, secretion management, atelectasis, and segmental collapse. For acutely injured tetraplegic patients, initial energy requirements and tissue oxygen consumption are low. If no associated chest injuries are present, pulmonary status can remain stable for the first few days after injury. Persons with neurological injuries between C1 and T12 have a 67% incidence of significant pulmonary complications, most commonly atelectasis. Ventilatory failure and aspiration occurs earliest (mean 4.5 days), followed by atelectasis (mean 17.7 days) and pneumonia (mean 24.5 days). This late decline coincides with the onset of mucous hypersecretion and muscle fatigue. Although the sputum quickly becomes colonized with bacteria in the intensive care setting, relatively few white cells are noted. This hypersecretory state is likely neurological in nature and has been attributed to unopposed vagal nerve stimulation of the airway submucosal glands. A tracheostomy tube is commonly inserted to facilitate airway suctioning and secretion clearance. Cough assistance maneuvers produce a modest increase in expiratory flow. Insufflation-exsufflation machines can be used with or without tracheostomy tubes and have been shown to facilitate air stacking and achieve expiratory flow rates nearer to the 6 to 7 liters per second necessary for an effective cough. Drying of secretions increases the risk of mucous plugging. Patients must be kept well hydrated, but overzealous hydration (e.g., in an attempt to normalize typical low blood pressures) can result in pulmonary edema.

- The problem of secretion management, combined with diminished ventilation of the lower lung segments, places these patients at high risk for pneumonia and segmental collapse. Over 36% of tetraplegic patients experience atelectasis with lung volume loss, and 31% develop pneumonia (most commonly in the left lower lobe). Curved-tip suction catheters can assist in suctioning the left mainstem bronchus, which is commonly missed with standard suctioning techniques. Treatment with frequent bronchoscopic suctioning, combined with larger ventilator tidal volumes (15 mL/kg of ideal body weight) can be helpful. In many cases segmental collapse follows a protracted and relapsing course. Prone Trendelenburg positioning promotes postural drainage of the left lower lobe, but unfortunately the hospital staff may resist this positioning because of difficulty in viewing the patient's face.

- Body positioning is also important to facilitate ventilation. In contrast to other pulmonary conditions, patients with tetraplegia exhibit higher vital capacities when positioned flat in bed. The mechanisms underlying this phenomena is likely relate to improved diaphragm function as the abdominal contents splint the lower rib cage. The reduction in vital capacity seen when these patients are seated upright can be counteracted to some extent by placement of an elastic abdominal binder. For obese persons and those already on positive pressure ventilation, these positioning effects are less significant, but their importance increases during periods of weaning.

- Intubation and ventilation are usually undertaken based on objective measures of pulmonary function. Patients with new cervical injuries commonly experience a reduction in vital capacity of 24% to 31% of the predicted value. Blood gases in these patients exhibit hypoxemia and normal $PaCO_2$, and the ventilation-perfusion mismatch is usually attributed to microatelectasis. Signs of impending ventilatory failure include: (1) a climbing respiratory rate and arterial CO_2 concentration in conjunction with a dropping tidal volume, (2) a drop in vital capacity to a level less than 15 mL/kg ideal body weight, (3) a drop in maximal inspiratory pressure to less than 20 cm H_2O, and (4) a neurological level of C3 or higher. Pulmonary function can improve steadily over the acute course, even without concurrent neurological recovery. By 3 months, most tetraplegic patients can be expected to attain 60% of predicted vital capacity. Ventilator weaning has been demonstrated in 80% of C4 SCI patients and in 57% of C3 SCI patients. Considerable patience is required because weaning protocols used for emphysema and heart failure patients are not applicable in this situation. Most authors argue for timed, progressive ventilator-free breathing, as opposed to synchronized intermittent mandatory ventilation (SIMV) weaning. The benefits of pressure support are yet to be clearly defined in this population, although intermittent positive pressure ventilation techniques have been shown to enhance noninvasive treatment of ventilatory failure via nasal or mouth masks. These promising noninvasive approaches decrease the need for tracheostomy ventilation but are not yet widely used. Measurements of arterial CO_2 must accompany pulse oximetry measurements during the weaning process because they provide an early and more sensitive indicator of respiratory muscle fatigue.

• There are several special considerations in the management of tracheostomy care in this population. Decannulation can usually be carried out in the weeks after injury as the need for suctioning and positive pressure treatments is reduced. Early on, a cuffed tracheostomy tube is usually needed that provides a good airway seal and anchors against heavy ventilation tubing. When pressure support is not needed, cuff deflation or a switch to cuffless cannulas can be considered. Cuffless tubes allow air to pass the vocal cords for phonation. For persons on ventilators, delivered volumes are increased to compensate for the air that passes cephalad through the vocal cords during the inflation phase.

• A variety of special tracheostomy tubes are available that promote vocalization. Fenestrated tubes and one-way-valve devices work well, but they can become clogged by secretions and require frequent manipulation of the sensitive tracheostomy site. Fenestrated tubes can irritate the posterior airway and promote formation of granulation tissue. Progression to a cuffless tube and progressive downsizing of the tube give the patient a sense of accomplishment during a time when functional gains are typically slow in coming. Tracheostomy tube changes should be carried out by an experienced individual. Patients who are not able to move air around a deflated cuff need special attention. The tracheal rings can be weakened by chronic inflammation, and excessive granulation tissue might be present. The tracheostomy tube might be serving as a splint for a damaged airway, and removal can result in airway collapse under the negative pressure of a deep breath. The removal of the tracheostomy tube is warranted when the patient demonstrates an effective cough. With proper noninvasive support, decannulation can be carried out when peak cough flows are greater than 160 L/min.

• Patients with injuries above the segments innervating the phrenic nerve are candidates for phrenic nerve pacemaker implantation. Although this technology is expensive and requires a lifelong tracheostomy, it has been shown to be a safe and reliable method for long-term ventilatory support. Benefits include reducing the need for heavy ventilator equipment, a reduction in sinus symptoms through better humidification of the upper airway, and improved taste sensation.

• In the chronic phase of SCI, pulmonary issues remain at the forefront. Breathlessness and wheezing are common complaints, and bronchial hyperreactivity has been described. Development of kyphoscoliosis can result in a reduction in lung compliance and vital capacity. Pregnancy and gastrointestinal dysmotility with gaseous distention of the viscera can interfere with diaphragmatic function. Night-time oxygen desaturation is often noted in patients with chronic tetraplegia, presumably because of the reduced use of accessory muscles during sleep. Resistive inspiratory muscle training can be useful in reducing respiratory complaints and complications. Smoking cessation and vaccination programs are important components of long-term care.

Changes in Body Composition and in Metabolic and Endocrine Function (p. 1249)

• Striking changes in body composition and physiological processes occur after acute SCI. Soon after injury, body weight declines. There is a decrease in total body water, fat, and protein. Loss of protein results in increased urea nitrogen excretion. Both extracellular and intracellular water are decreased, but the preferential loss of intracellular water leads to the relative expansion of extracellular fluid stores. Muscle tissue loss leads to decreased exchangeable potassium and increased exchangeable sodium, further exacerbating the expansion of extracellular fluid. Hyperosmolar hyponatremia (Na less than 130 mmol/L) is also seen, especially in acute tetraplegia. Most patients are asymptomatic, but serious complications can result if the condition is ignored. Disorders in sodium regulation can occur as a result of excessive fluid resuscitation or impaired cortisol response. Anemia is common after acute SCI. This anemia is normochromic normocytic, with low levels of iron and transferrin. Erythropoietin levels are usually normal.

• A number of abnormalities in endocrine function accompany acute injury. At rest, serum measures and steady-state excretion of corticosteroids in the urine are similar to those of resting, healthy subjects. In the stimulated state, such as after surgery, the expected increases in these measurements are absent in persons with SCI, probably because of loss of integrated neuroendocrine function.

• Changes in energy expenditure occur in the acute phase of paralysis. Acute SCI patients require up to 54% fewer calories than would be predicted by their weight. The higher the level of injury, the greater the reduction in basal energy expenditure. The inability of tetraplegic and high paraplegic patients to control their body temperature (poikilothermia) is most striking in the period immediately after injury. Close monitoring of ambient and body temperature is required in the acute phase after injury. These patients retain the ability to mount a febrile response to infectious conditions. Patients without leukocytosis should be evaluated for venous thromboembolism and heterotopic ossification as a source of their fever. As a patient progresses into the rehabilitation hospital and into the chronic phase of injury, sensitivity to ambient temperature remains, although the striking dysregulation seen in the intensive care unit typically resolves.

• Other body changes are most marked in the chronic phase of injury. Glucose intolerance is a common finding. The insulin resistance is due in part to abnormal muscle utilization, decreased lean body mass, and increased fat body mass. Muscle fiber types can change during the chronic phase, with a gradual increase in the percentage of type II fibers, a factor that exacerbates insulin resistance. Anemia in chronic SCI persons is common, ranging in incidence from 30% to 56%, with blood indices indicating an anemia of chronic disease. Chronic SCI patients continue to demonstrate lower rates of energy expenditure than predicted.

Calcium Metabolism and Osteoporosis (pp. 1249–1250)

• Any form of immobilization alters calcium metabolism, but the structural and physiological changes associated with SCI predispose these patients to a variety of complications. These include hypercalcemia, bone fractures, nephrolithiasis, and renal failure. As early as 10 days postinjury, hypercalciuria develops, reaching a peak between 1 and 6 months postinjury. There is an initial suppression of parathyroid hormone (PTH) that reaches its nadir at 3 months and returns to the normal range at 6 months. Pathological studies demonstrate an increased number of osteoclasts in bone, reaching a peak at 16 weeks postinjury, with diminished bone formation and mineralization. Hypercalcemia is seen in some patients. Risk factors for hypercalcemia include childhood or adolescent SCI, male sex, complete injuries, tetraplegia, dehydration, and prolonged immobilization. Treatment of hypercalcemia in adults is similar to that used in children, including use of IV fluids, loop diuretics, pamidronate, and calcitonin. Limitation of dietary calcium and vitamin D intake is not recommended.

• The degree of lower extremity bone loss after injury has been correlated with the occurrence of fractures. Bone loss is most severe in regions having neurological deficits. A study of the bone density found that 50% of the acutely injured patients and 90% of those with chronic SCI had proximal tibial densities below the fracture threshold. The weight-bearing vertebral column is generally spared these severe effects, and spinal bone density can even improve as time passes after injury, especially in females. Patients with significant osteopenia of the spinal column should be investigated to determine whether secondary causes of osteoporosis are present.

• A number of interventions have been studied in the hope of preventing and treating disorders of calcium metabolism in these subjects. Physical activity, including wheelchair use, frame-assisted standing, and tilt table, might improve calcium balance in the acute phase, but no effect on bone density has been demonstrated. Functional electrical stimulation cycle ergometry can provide modest reductions in the rate of bone loss, sustained only during the period of application. Patients with chronic SCI can benefit from correction of nutritional deficiencies. Patients often restrict dietary calcium because of fear of renal lithiasis. Many individuals with chronic SCI are prone to secondary hyperparathyroidism and further bone loss, remediable by vitamin D and calcium supplementation.

• Antiresorptive therapies, including calcitonin and third-generation bisphosphonates, offer treatment alternatives. The utility of these agents has been demonstrated in other diseases featuring rapid bone turnover. Estrogen therapy should be considered for women with SCI, with the same caveats as with ablebodied women.

Cardiovascular Conditions (pp. 1250–1251)

• The alterations in cardiovascular physiology and risk factors for coronary heart disease after SCI merit special attention. Cardiac arrhythmias and orthostatic hypotension are common problems, especially during the acute phase of treatment. Over the long term, patients are predisposed to the development of accelerated and premature coronary artery disease. Cardiovascular diseases account for 46% of all deaths in SCI persons more than 30 years postinjury, and the prevalence of asymptomatic coronary disease in persons with tetraplegia can be as high as 70%.

- The vagus nerve exits the central nervous system (CNS) at the brainstem and is spared in SCI. Injuries to the spinal cord above the upper thoracic levels block the compensatory sympathetic impulses that exit toward the sympathetic cervical ganglia, resulting in impaired vasoconstrictor tone and reduced cardiac contractility and heart rate. Bradycardia is seen in all patients with complete tetraplegia and in up to 71% of patients with Frankel class C or D tetraplegia. Severe sinus slowing can necessitate treatment with temporary transvenous pacemakers, atropine, or sympathomimetic drugs. The response to atropine can be blunted in this group. Bradycardia peaks around injury day 4 and resolves over the next 2 weeks in most instances. Bradycardia can be exacerbated by hypoxia and by activation of vagovagal reflexes during tracheal suctioning. Hyperoxygenation before suctioning can help remedy this problem. Atrioventricular block, ventricular tachycardia, supraventricular tachyarrhythmias, and cardiac arrest have also been described in cervical and high thoracic level injuries. Decreased heart rate and cardiac index can be treated with dopamine and dobutamine; however, pulmonary and systemic vascular resistance, as well as central venous pressures, are typically not as responsive to treatment.

- As the SCI patient enters the rehabilitation phase of care, orthostatic hypotension can occur, resulting in lightheadedness, dizziness, nausea, loss of consciousness, and seizures. This condition is most prominent in persons with higher injury levels. Plasma adrenaline and noradrenaline levels respond to changes in body position significantly less than in noninjured control subjects. Symptom relief can often be obtained through the use of recliner wheelchairs with elevating leg rests, elastic compression stockings, and abdominal binders. In some instances, short-term (i.e., 1- to 2-month) treatment with salt, ephedrine, or fluorinated steroids is helpful. Tilt table treatments are sometimes employed, but the patient's tolerance of such sessions has little bearing on the ability to achieve wheelchair sitting without symptomatic hypotension.

- Although symptomatic orthostatic hypotension usually resolves soon after injury, persons with high injury levels can retain low blood pressure readings on a lifelong basis. Healthy, asymptomatic patients sometimes present with blood pressures that are virtually inaudible. Other long-term issues relate to the alteration in cardiovascular risk factors, including reduced cardiac output, glucose intolerance, an unfavorable lipid profile, a decrease in lean body mass, and reduced physical conditioning. Because of interruption of cardiac nociceptive afferent fibers, tetraplegic patients with coronary artery disease often do not experience angina, necessitating a higher index of suspicion when the clinician is faced with intermittent or exercise-induced symptoms. Angina must remain in the differential diagnosis of left shoulder and arm pain. Reduced serum HDL cholesterol is seen in both tetraplegic and paraplegic patients, possibly related to hyperinsulinemia and increased hepatic triglyceride production.

- Indications for lipid-lowering drugs are the same as for the general population. Bile acid–binding resins are usually avoided in this group, however, because of the side effects of constipation, gas, and interference with absorption of nutrients. Exercise in persons with SCI, both with arm ergometry and electrically stimulated programs, can bring about increased HDL cholesterol levels, reversal of ventricular atrophy, and a reduction in the risk for developing cardiovascular disease. For SCI persons at risk, exercise tolerance tests can be performed via arm ergometry, or thallium stress testing can be used (see Chapter 32).

Venous Thromboembolism (pp. 1251–1253)

- The potentially devastating consequences of venous thrombosis make prevention, diagnosis, and appropriate treatment very important in SCI patients. Autopsy studies of deaths in acute SCI patients report the incidence of death from pulmonary embolism (PE) to be as high as 37%. PE is the third leading cause of death in all SCI patients in the first year postinjury. The risk of DVT during the months immediately following injury is also high. Studies of the incidence of DVT vary widely. Studies employing modern diagnostic techniques (e.g., Doppler ultrasound [US], fibrinogen scanning, venography) place the risk of DVT between 40% and 100%. Risk prior to 72 hours post-SCI appears to be low, but over 80% of DVTs will occur within the first 2 weeks. The risk of DVT is maximal between days 7 and 10. PE is estimated to occur in approximately 5% of acute SCI patients. Venous stasis in the flaccid lower extremities plays the principal role in clot development. Another factor could be the transient hypercoagulable state that has been described. In immobilized patients without paralysis, thromboses are rare, suggesting that impaired autonomic input to the venous system might also play a role.
- The risk profiles for venous thrombosis differ when considering DVT and PE. Those with complete injuries are at higher risk for DVT than those with incomplete lesions. Patients with paraplegic injuries are at higher risk than tetraplegic patients for DVT, whereas an increased risk of PE is associated with tetraplegia, less spasticity, and greater body mass. The incidence of DVT is similar for SCI persons in all age groups, where the incidence of PE peaks in ages 61 to 75 years. Both DVT and PE occur with higher frequency in males with SCI.
- Physical examination is especially unreliable in the diagnosis of DVT in SCI patients. Because of impaired vasomotor tone in the legs, changes in volume and appearance are seen daily, and serial leg measurements are of little value. The clinician is armed only with a strong index of suspicion and a willingness to employ more sensitive diagnostic tests, either as routine surveillance or as an adjunct to frequent leg examinations. Signs of DVT include unilateral edema, an increase in collateral vein markings, low-grade fever of unknown etiology, and changes in pain or leg sensation patterns in persons with incomplete SCI.
- Duplex US with manual compression has become widely used as a convenient, sensitive, and specific noninvasive method of DVT diagnosis in symptomatic patients. Duplex US is limited, however, in that there is poor visualization of the venous system proximal to the femoral veins, poor sensitivity for calf vein thrombosis, and difficulties with imaging in the presence of heterotopic ossification. If vena cava thrombosis is suspected, spiral computed tomography (CT) and magnetic resonance imaging (MRI) are particularly useful, with sensitivities and specificities in the 80% to 90% range.
- Ventilation-perfusion lung scans are regarded as definitive only when normal or high probability readings are obtained. Scans read as low or intermediate

probability are best followed by another study, such as US of the legs or pulmonary angiography. Contrast venography is still the gold standard for diagnosis of DVT, although it is underutilized because of inconvenience, patient discomfort, and the risks of allergic reactions and phlebitis. A number of d-dimer assays are now commercially available. A low d-dimer concentration has a high negative predictive value for thromboembolism, but significant methodological problems with the test limit the usefulness of published estimates of d-dimer diagnostic accuracy. D-dimer levels are elevated by a variety of co-morbid conditions (e.g., infections and surgery), and these elevations can persist for months after acute SCI. In addition, the specificity of d-dimer in DVT diagnosis is low in asymptomatic patients, so its use as a surveillance test is limited.

• The Consortium for Spinal Cord Medicine published practice guidelines for the prevention of thromboembolism. Both mechanical and pharmacological methods of prevention were analyzed, and prophylaxis regimens were stratified based on estimates of relative patient risks.

• A number of mechanical treatments have proved effective in reducing the incidence of DVT, including ROM exercises, rotation beds, gradient elastic stockings, lower extremity electrical stimulation, external pneumatic leg compression, and the venous foot pump. External pneumatic compression devices are widely available and have been applied successfully in the SCI population. If their use is instituted later than 72 hours postinjury, testing to exclude the presence of leg thrombi should be undertaken.

• Vena cava filter insertion is often considered in patients with complete motor paralysis caused by lesions in the high cervical cord, patients with poor cardiac reserve, and in patients for whom bedside clinical assessment for DVT might be obscured by obesity or dark skin color. Vena cava filters are also employed in the setting of failed prophylaxis, in those with contraindications for pharmacological prophylaxis (e.g., bleeding risks in the CNS, lungs, or GI tract), and for the treatment of thrombus in the vena cava. Filter use can be complicated by caval perforation or thrombosis and by filter migration or dislodgment during cough assistance maneuvers.

• Considerable progress has been made in the development of pharmacological strategies to prevent thrombosis. Evidence supporting the use of subcutaneous low-dose unfractionated heparin (5000 units, two or three times a day) comes chiefly from small, retrospective studies. Higher doses of subcutaneous unfractionated heparin (10,000 to 15,000 units, twice daily) are more effective, but bleeding complications are significant, and monitoring of aPTT levels is cumbersome. Prophylaxis with oral warfarin carries the same need for frequent blood tests. In SCI patients, the presence of vitamin K deficiency and the potential for interactions with the multiplicity of drugs makes monitoring of warfarin prophylactic therapy even more problematic.

• New low-molecular-weight heparins have shown promise for use in prophylaxis when used alone or in combination with mechanical modalities. Like standard heparin, low-molecular-weight heparins bind to antithrombin III, potentiating inhibitory actions against activated factor Xa and thrombin. The low-molecular-weight heparins, however, are unable to bind thrombin directly, do not reduce platelet activity, and do not change vascular permeability. These factors can allow for equivalent anticoagulant effects with reduced bleeding risks. These preparations also exhibit better subcutaneous absorption, longer half-life, and smoother anticoagulant response. They require only once or twice daily dosing. Initial experience with low-molecular-weight heparins in SCI patients has demonstrated both an improved safety profile and superior thrombosis prevention when compared with earlier modes of treatment. There is little scientific data dealing with the duration of prophylaxis. For some patients, thrombosis development might only be delayed for the period during which preventive measures are employed.

• When the diagnosis of proximal DVT or PE is confirmed, either low-molecular-weight heparin or unfractionated IV heparin should be administered. Therapies and mobilization are usually withheld for 4 to 7 days after diagnosis. Treatment of calf vein thrombosis has been more controversial. As an alternative to anticoagulation, some clinicians choose to follow calf thromboses with serial noninvasive tests to monitor for proximal extension. This approach is often impractical, however, and there is mounting evidence that the long-term complications of calf DVT can be as problematic as proximal DVT. In light of this, most of the patients with calf DVT in this high-risk group are best treated with full anticoagulation for at least 3 months.

• The FDA recently approved one of the low-molecular-weight heparins (enoxaparin) for an indication in the treatment of DVT. Enoxaparin is administered subcutaneously, on a weight-based dose, once or twice a day. When compared to IV unfractionated heparin, these drugs present a lower risk of thrombocytopenia and osteopenia. Because of their favorable dose-response characteristics, monitoring is unnecessary in most patients. Warfarin remains the drug of choice for long-term treatment, and is begun on the first day of anticoagulant therapy in most settings. Careful monitoring of the International Normalized Ratio (INR) is essential in the SCI patient. Dietary changes, drug interactions, and co-morbidities interfere with dosing and response to the drug. The INR of 2.5 provides good protection against further thrombosis and is associated with no more bleeding complications than an INR of 2.0. Warfarin therapy should be administered for a minimum of 3 to 6 months in hopes of reducing the recurrence rate and the risk of chronic post-thrombotic syndrome, with chronic lower extremity edema and skin ulceration.

• There are few studies that examine the long-term risk of venous thromboembolism, but there is a much lower rate of occurrence than in the acute phase of SCI. Persons with long-standing SCI who are readmitted to the hospital for medical or surgical illnesses are at similar risk for thrombosis development as other immobilized, hospitalized patients. Reinstitution of prophylactic measures should be considered in this setting.

Autonomic Dysreflexia (pp. 1253–1254)

• Autonomic dysreflexia is an acute syndrome of massive sympathetic discharge that is triggered by a noxious stimulus. It occurs in persons with spinal cord lesions above the level of the sympathetic splanchnic outflow, which usually couples with the spinal cord at T6. It is characterized by severe paroxysmal hypertension, pounding headache, sweating, nasal congestion, facial flushing, piloerection, and reflex bradycardia. The incidence has been reported to range from 48% to 83% of tetraplegic and high paraplegic patients. Most persons do not experience signs and symptoms in the first 2 months postinjury. Autonomic dysreflexia occasionally is seen in persons with injury levels as low as T10. It can be seen in association with both incomplete and complete injuries. All patients with injuries above the midthoracic spinal cord levels will exhibit *autonomic dysregulation,* with very low baseline blood pressures and orthostatic hypotension.

• *Autonomic dysreflexia* is episodic in nature, and extremely high blood pressure is the sentinel sign. The most common cause by far is bladder distention. Other causes include bowel impaction, pressure sores, ingrown toenails, tight clothing, tight shoes and leg bag straps, urinary tract infections, and uterine contractions in pregnant women. Invasive procedures such as bladder catheterization, rectal stimulation, cystometrography, and extracorporeal shock wave lithotripsy are known to precipitate this response.

• This condition is generated by spinal cord and splanchnic reflex mechanisms that remain operative despite the SCI. The triggering events noted above produce afferent impulses that are transmitted to the dorsal column and spinothalamic tracts. As these tracts ascend, they synapse with sympathetic neurons in the intermediolateral columns and generate a generalized sympathetic reflex response. Normally, descending supraspinal inhibitory signals modulate these autonomic reflexes, but because of the spinal lesion above the sympathetic outflow, inhibitory impulses cannot effectively descend in the sympathetic chain to block the autonomic response. The result is peripheral and splanchnic vasoconstriction and the development of acute hypertension. Sweating and piloerection also occur as a result of the mass sympathetic discharge. Baseline serum catecholamine levels are low after SCI, raising the suspicion that a denervation hypersensitivity to adrenergic stimulation contributes to this condition.

• With the increase in blood pressure, the aortic arch and carotid sinus receptors are stimulated, which can result in reflex bradycardia and vasodilation above the level of the lesion. The vasodilation is manifested as facial flushing, sweating, and nasal congestion (see Fig. 55–5 in the Textbook). Signs and symptoms can vary slightly between patients (e.g., some patients exhibit tachycardia, not bradycardia), but the bedside diagnosis of this condition is rarely ambiguous. A diagnostic challenge might exist in elderly patients or in pregnant women. Some elderly patients with recent motor incomplete injuries will exhibit the essential systolic hypertension that afflicted them prior to their injury. In pregnant women, hypertension can be due to preeclampsia. In both of these situations, hypertension is asymptomatic and nonepisodic.

• Complications that develop from autonomic dysreflexia are usually secondary to severe hypertension. The elevated blood pressure can result in life-threatening complications including confusion, visual disturbance, loss of consciousness, encephalopathy, intracerebral hemorrhage, seizures, electrocardiographic changes, atrial fibrillation, acute myocardial failure, and pulmonary edema. In pregnant women with SCI, intracerebral hemorrhage and death during labor also have been reported.

• Treatment of an acute episode generally focuses on identifying and eliminating the cause. The first action taken is to place the patient in an upright sitting position with, if possible, the legs dangling over the bedside. This maneuver makes use of the natural orthostatic hypotensive response in SCI patients and can lower the blood pressure and reduce headache symptoms. Tight clothing and constrictive devices should be removed. The blood pressure and pulse are frequently monitored. A quick survey of the possible instigating causes should be done, beginning with the urinary system. This step might require bladder catheterization; irrigating an existing indwelling catheter; changing a catheter; or utilizing lidocaine anesthetic jelly.

• If these steps do not result in a reduction in blood pressure, rectal impaction should be suspected. Pharmacological management should be considered at this point because stool removal digitally can exacerbate the episode. Opinion varies regarding the level of blood pressure that warrants pharmacological treatment. The treating physician should be aware that the baseline systolic blood pressure after a tetraplegic or high paraplegic injury falls in the 90 to 100 mm Hg range. Systolic pressures in the 150 mm Hg range typically represent significant hypertension. Rapid-onset, short-duration antihypertensive medications that can be used include nitrates, nifedipine, prazosin, hydralazine, mecamylamine, and IV diazoxide. If 2% nitroglycerin ointment is used, 1 inch can be applied to the skin above the level of SCI and wiped off as the blood pressure is lowered. Nifedipine has been used safely in autonomic dysreflexia, but its use has declined as a result of multiple reports of hypotensive complications in patients with essential hypertension. Once the blood pressure is lowered, examination for fecal impaction and for other inciting causes can be done. Headaches can persist for hours after the hypertension is treated; they usually respond to acetaminophen. Oral medications and regional, spinal, and epidural anesthesia have been used as pretreatment for episodes that are anticipated in association with surgical or diagnostic procedures.

• Although most episodes of autonomic dysreflexia are easily remedied, the patient who experiences recurrent episodes presents a therapeutic challenge. The triggering mechanism is often obscure or not easily remedied (e.g., pressure ulcer, bowel distention, or fractures). In these situations, a suppressive therapeutic agent is usually needed. Ganglionic blocking agents (e.g., guanethidine, mecamylamine, and phenoxybenzamine) have been used in this setting, but these drugs are difficult to obtain and are questionable in efficacy. Newer α-adrenergic receptor blockers (e.g., terazosin) are reasonable options.

• Prevention of recurrent episodes includes proper bladder and bowel management and skin care. Also vital is patient and family education regarding the prevention, causes, presentation, and treatment of autonomic dysreflexia. At discharge from rehabilitation, patients at risk for autonomic dysreflexia should be prescribed appropriate antihypertensive medications to use in an emergency setting.

Pressure Ulcers (pp. 1254–1255)

• The importance of preventing pressure ulcers in the SCI patient cannot be overemphasized. Their impact in terms of morbidity, diminished quality of life, and monetary expense can only be estimated.

• Some 33% of SCI patients have had at least one pressure ulcer, and 14% have had a stage 3 or 4 ulcer. In the acute phase of injury, most pressure sores occur on the sacrum. After 2 years postinjury, the ischium is the most common site of involvement, followed by the sacrum, trochanter, and heel. Pressure ulcers are preventable.

• Pressure ulcers will not heal unless the pressure is removed. An hour of sitting on an ischial ulcer can cause damage that might require weeks of bed rest to reverse. Special beds and cushions by themselves neither prevent nor heal pressure sores. The patient or caregiver must carry out regular weight-shifting and pressure relief maneuvers. Extensive counseling should be started early and continued in the years following injury. Most patients cannot appreciate the disastrous implications until a serious pressure ulcer develops.

• Treatment of a pressure ulcer can require weeks or months of restricted activity, increased caregiver support, and time lost from work or school. The prevention of pressure ulcers usually involves many factors such as genetic/physical predisposition, environmental and social resources, good health maintenance habits, and good luck. To say that pressure ulcers are preventable is not to say that they are easily prevented. Ulcers will heal if the basic elements of care are followed, medical status is optimized, pressure is removed, the ulcer is cleaned, and a moist environment for re-epithelialization is provided (see Chapter 31).

• Surgical consultation is usually needed if the ulcer has eroded to underlying bone or bursa. It is possible to treat these ulcers without surgery, but draining sinuses and large scars are commonly encountered that can predispose to chronic tissue breakdown. Surgical treatment can provide the individual with well-padded, durable, weight-bearing areas. On the other hand, each pressure ulcer operation "steals" tissue from an adjoining area of the body to fill the defect. For ulcers on the seated surface of the body, there are only a limited number of procedures that can be performed, short of lower limb amputation. Each surgical option that is used represents an option that is no longer available should a recurrence develop.

• Surgery does not cure the problem of pressure ulcers. Repair and healing of ulcers has to be accompanied by a graduated program of remobilization and rehabilitation, a thorough review of remediable environmental precipitants, and education in the rehabilitation setting to teach methods to prevent recurrence.

Urological Issues: Implementing a Bladder Management Program (pp. 1255–1256)

• There are many reasonable options for bladder management after SCI. It is best when the SCI center staff selects a small number of applicable management options and teaches them well, rather than confuse patients and caregivers with an eclectic mix of techniques.

• The medical priorities of urological management in this population are simple: regular voiding with low bladder residual urine, low baseline bladder pressures, and continence. Intermittent catheterization comes to the mind of many clinicians when confronted with a person with SCI. A successful intermittent catheterization program involves much more than a timed catheterization schedule. It requires the active participation of the patient to monitor and adjust oral fluid intake, and constant adjustments of the intermittent catheterization schedule in response to a variety of variables. Intermittent catheterization is usually inappropriate in the ICU setting when dietary intake and urinary output are inconsistent. In the hospital setting, urinary bacterial colonization occurs in just 3 or 4 days. In the acute setting it is better to have a low-pressure colonized urine (with indwelling catheter) than a distended bladder with high-pressure colonized urine. Avoidance of mechanical detrusor damage from bladder overdistention in the ICU is extremely important.

• Some patients, particularly those with incomplete injuries, regain normal voiding function. Those with more severe deficits who retain hand function can be expected to maintain a long-term catheter-free state with intermittent self-catheterization. Another group of SCI patients, mainly men who can use condom catheters, can potentially maintain a catheter-free state by triggering regular reflex bladder emptying. Intermittent catheterization can be used for these groups, either as a definitive program or as a means to achieve continent or reflex voiding.

- Education should begin in the hospital, with nurses teaching proper catheterization technique that is then carried out every 4 to 6 hours. Catheterization volume in the 400 to 500 mL range is the goal. Care must be taken to avoid both overdistention and excessive voluntary fluid restriction and low urine output. Catheterization volumes are often large at night because renal plasma flow increases in the supine position. Wide variability in catheterization volumes is expected early on. When large volumes occur, the patient is typically discouraged. The staff should offer reassurance.
- Some patients begin to pass urine between catheterizations. If the long-term goal is to remain on intermittent catheterization, continence can be promoted by the use of anticholinergic medication. This helps avoid the inconvenience of an incontinence pad or condom catheter. After discharge, "clean technique" rather than sterile catheterization is tolerated in most situations. Specialized catheters with self-contained urinary collection bags are convenient, but funding for them is often limited. If the goal is reflex or continent voiding, a neurourology evaluation is important. In these patients, intermittent catheterization is continued until adequate bladder emptying and low baseline bladder pressures are demonstrated by cystometrography. There is no magic number that designates a safe postvoid residual urine. Volumes in the 100-mL range are reasonable, but higher residual volumes might be tolerated if the patient empties the bladder at shorter (e.g., 2- to 3-hour) intervals. High pressure or overflow voiding secondary to high outflow resistance (detrusor-sphincter dyssynergia) must be avoided. A variety of methods are available to promote complete bladder emptying with reasonable bladder pressures.
- There is no external collecting device useful for women, and some men are unable to wear a condom catheter. A few highly motivated persons who lack hand function can reliably engage caregivers to perform intermittent catheterization. Other patients, despite a variety of sophisticated interventions, cannot maintain proper detrusor pressures. Indwelling catheters are a convenient and reasonable alternative for these individuals. Although there are many known complications associated with their use, they can be used successfully with proper self-care and regular medical follow-up. Suprapubic catheters can be used and have many advantages, although the risk of bladder stones is similar to that seen with urethral catheters. Suprapubic catheters do not restrict sexual function, are easily replaced, reduce the incidence of urethral erosions, and avoid catheter contact with other structures that are potentially infected (e.g., urethra, prostate, and seminal vesicles). All SCI persons with indwelling catheters benefit from anticholinergic medication (to block the bladder reflexes from "fighting" the foreign object) and from regular follow-up with cystoscopy. Persons with indwelling catheters are at slightly higher risk for bladder neoplasms and at high risk for stone development. Cystoscopy is the best means of surveillance for these conditions. Calcium bladder sludge, not free floating stones, is the most common cause of catheter blockage. Bladder sediment is rarely detected by US or plain radiography.
- Asymptomatic bacteriuria is generally not treated in persons who use catheters. Even persons on intermittent catheterization commonly develop urinary colonization. Antibiotics are generally reserved for persons symptomatic with fever and leukocytosis and for those demonstrating catheter blockage, increased spasticity, or very foul urine. Overuse of antibiotics is common in SCI persons.

• Several new surgical options are available. Continent diversion and bladder augmentation procedures have been studied in this population, and promising results have been seen, especially in the treatment of females with neurogenic bladder dysfunction. It is important that these operations be performed by a team of clinicians who have sufficient experience in their implementation in persons with SCI.

Gastrointestinal Complications and Practical Management (pp. 1256–1257)

• Gastrointestinal disorders rank seventh as a cause of death in persons with SCI. Dysfunction of this system has a profound impact on medical morbidity, maintenance of body image, need for caregiver support, and hospital discharge destination. More than one-third of surveyed persons with paraplegia ranked the loss of bowel and bladder control as the most significant functional loss associated with their respective injury—more important than the paralysis of their legs. Difficulties in maintaining bowel continence can have an impact on virtually every aspect of life, interfering with fulfillment of interpersonal, sexual, and employment roles (see Chapter 28).

• Studies of GI complaints have traditionally focused on the acute postinjury period when ileus, fecal impaction, and upper GI bleeding are most prominent. More recent investigations have assessed the importance of GI problems over the long term, finding that delayed bowel emptying, hemorrhoids, and lower GI tract bleeding are common problems.

• In the intensive care unit, swallowing and nutritional problems are common. Dysphagia affects nearly 20% of tetraplegic patients, brought about by excessive neck extension in halo devices, soft tissue swelling after anterior neck surgery, poor coordination with ventilator cycling, tracheostomy pain, and concomitant head or cranial nerve injuries. In most cases dysphagia is caused by pharyngeal stage problems. Videofluoroscopy can be employed as a diagnostic aid in this setting. In all persons with cervical spine injury, special attention must be given to ensure that esophageal perforation has not occurred at the time of initial trauma. Treatment includes careful supervision of feeding, use of compensatory positioning, and training in supraglottic swallowing and Mendelsohn maneuvers. The prognosis for return of normal swallowing is good in this population.

• Even with supplemental tube feeding, nutritional support can be inadequate. Poor tolerance of tube feeding and ileus commonly limit replacement of the huge protein losses associated with injury. Appetite is often poor early on but improves with the establishment of a good bowel routine, correction of dehydration, and resumption of activity. Most patients are constipated at the time of discharge from the intensive care unit. In some instances, only liquid stool passes around a fecal impaction, giving the false impression of diarrhea. Diarrhea can occur in this setting, especially when *Clostridium difficile* and other pathogens colonize the bowel as a complication of liberal antibiotic use. A plain radiograph of the abdomen can be very helpful in patients with constipation. Typically, solid stool is seen in the cecum, which is an abnormal finding. Constipation is best relieved through digital and chemical rectal evacuation, avoiding the use of strong oral cathartics that invariably further distend a poorly motile GI tract.

• Although upper GI problems are commonly seen in this population (e.g., slow stomach emptying, gallstones, and superior mesenteric artery syndrome), bowel emptying is the major concern for most patients. In the acute setting, accurate records of stool output are critical to the development of a bowel routine. In persons with complete SCI, the primary deficits are the lack of sphincter control and reduced bowel motility associated with diminished physical activity.

• Persons with injuries in the lumbar cord or conus can lack the rectal reflex actions that normally expel stool. These patients are best managed with a program of digital stool removal, usually carried out daily. Often mobility and self-care skills are mastered long before the bowel routine is stabilized—a problem with reduced length of acute hospital stay. Those with SCI in the cervical and thoracic regions who lack sphincter function can use suppositories or enemas. These chemical methods save time and provide an extended period of continence between bowel routines. Daily suppository use is usually not recommended because it may result in overstimulation of the rectum and leads to mucous incontinence. Strong oral cathartic medications are avoided; their time of onset is unpredictable and their use precludes the development of a normal column of stool in the colon, increasing the risk of incontinence. Stool consistecny is regulated by the use of medium-grade dietary fiber.

NEUROLOGICAL ISSUES AFTER INJURY (pp. 1257–1260)

Pain Syndromes (pp. 1257–1259)

• Most SCI persons experience problems with pain. The pain associated with trauma to bone and soft tissue structures usually disappears within weeks of injury, but subsequent chronic pain problems are estimated to affect between 48% and 94% of this population. For some of these patients, pain problems become disabling. *Nociceptive pain,* generated by noxious stimuli in normally innervated body parts, can often be effectively managed by standard therapeutic modalities, injections, NSAIDs, and remediation of the pathological process that precipitates the pain stimulus. *Neurogenic pain,* associated with injury to nerve roots, cauda equina, and the spinal cord, however, constitutes one of the most enigmatic clinical syndromes faced by patients, clinicians, and researchers.

• Some special causes of nociceptive pain after SCI warrant mention. Nociceptive pain sensation can vary in quality and localization can be inaccurate, but symptoms usually follow a reproducible pattern. Visceral pain (possibly transmitted through sensory fibers in the vagus nerve, pleura, peritoneum, and diaphragm) is often perceptible even in higher level injuries, and can indicate pelvic or abdominal pathology. Shoulder dysfunction, compression mononeuropathies, degenerative joint disease, trauma, and late spinal deformity and spasticity can precipitate pain complaints.

• Neurogenic pain can be further described as radicular, segmental, or deafferentation central pain (DCP). Pain near the level of the cord lesion can be nociceptive, radicular, or segmental. *Radicular pain,* caused by nerve root damage or arachnoiditis, can be unilateral or bilateral. It is confined to predictable areas near the root dermatomes. Nerve root blocks offer pain relief for many of these patients. *Segmental pain* is bilateral in many instances and has also been described as "border zone pain," associated with hyperalgesia and hypersensitivity in two or three dermatomes adjacent to the level of SCI. Pain with cauda equina syndrome is a well-recognized variant of segmental pain, often described as a burning or tingling in the buttocks, anus, genitals, and feet. A constricting band can be felt around the trunk in persons with thoracic injuries. Another form of segmental pain, "burning hands syndrome" (or "stingers"), is experienced in many persons with incomplete tetraplegia or minor cord contusions. This is often difficult to distinguish from complex regional pain syndrome.

• *Deafferentation central pain* is characterized by vague, nondermatomal symptoms originating caudal to the cord lesion that lacks reliable nociceptive precipitants. This type of pain is common and extremely difficult to treat. Symptoms can be worsened by a variety of events (e.g., changes in body position, bladder infections, or pressure ulcers) but are neither precipitated by them or relieved when these secondary conditions are remediated. The terms dysesthesias and phantom pain are often used in this setting, but are less specific than DCP. This pain is variably described, but once it starts, it is continuous. It can begin weeks or months after SCI. It is likely that the pain impulses are generated in segments of the spinal cord just above the lesion, although a complex interaction involving supraspinal deafferentation changes in the thalamus and cortical sensory areas has also been postulated. Persons who develop neurogenic pain in the chronic phase of injury should be evaluated for syringomyelia.

• There is no single intervention, invasive or noninvasive, that is reliably effective in the treatment of segmental and deafferentation central pain. Judicious treatment of these conditions involves recognition of this fact and an appreciation of the complex physical and psychosocial factors that influence the impact that pain exerts on a patient's life. Despite the frustrating nature of the problem, patients must be reassured that, in the vast majority of instances, the usual pattern is for pain to become more tolerable or manageable.

• Medications are considered if symptoms restrict activity or sleep. Tricyclic antidepressants (e.g., amitriptyline and doxepin) have been used for decades in this setting. These drugs act by diminishing the presynaptic uptake of serotonin and norepinephrine. Newer antidepressants (e.g., fluoxetine, sertraline, and venalafaxine) have not been well studied in this population. Anticonvulsants (e.g., carbamazepine, clonazepam, phenytoin, and gabapentin) have also been prescribed, often in combination with antidepressant medication. Opiate analgesics are sometimes prescribed.

• Although some pain specialists have advocated more liberal use of opiate drugs in chronic pain conditions, these recommendations are difficult to put into daily practice. Patients with DCP typically experience their symptoms with or without opiate medication. Constipation can become a significant side effect of these medications.

• Over the years persons with spinal cord pain syndromes have been subjected to a large variety of ablative and invasive procedures. Spinal subarachnoid anesthesia has been used for diagnostic purposes and has temporarily reduced pain symptoms in the majority of subjects. Intrathecal baclofen, morphine, and clonidine have also been studied. Transcutaneous nerve stimulation is best employed in the setting of nociceptive, radicular, or segmental pain. Dorsal column electrical stimulation has also been attempted. In addition, ablative surgical and injection procedures have been carried out at virtually every level of the neuraxis, with marginal benefit.

Progressive Post-Traumatic Cystic Myelopathy (Syringomyelia) (p. 1259)

• Syringomyelia is a recognized cause of progressive myelopathy. Syringomyelia is idiopathic in some cases, but usually it is associated with developmental anomalies of the foramen magnum, spinal cord tumors, or as a late complication of spinal cord trauma. Post-traumatic syringomyelia has been termed progressive post-traumatic cystic myelopathy (PPCM). The classic clinical signs of PPCM include a dissociated loss of pain and temperature sensation, usually in the distal upper extremities. The most common initial symptom of PPCM is pain. PPCM has been noted as early as 2 months postinjury and as late as 23 years. Estimates of the incidence of PPCM range from 0.3% to 8%. Spinal cord cysts and myelomalacia are commonly seen on MRI after traumatic injury. This condition is probably more common in persons with paraplegia. The pathological processes that generate cystic spinal cord changes are not well understood.

• Symptoms of post-traumatic syringomyelia commonly consist of segmental or radicular pain, late motor and sensory loss, increased spasticity, and hyperhydrosis. Horner's syndrome and respiratory insufficiency can be seen with cysts that extend into the brainstem. Symptoms can also be positional. Radiological diagnosis is now much improved with the use of T1-weighted high-resolution MRI. Gadolinium images are helpful in differentiating between syrinx and myelomalacia in post-traumatic cases. Electrodiagnosis, including central motor conduction times and motor-evoked potentials, can also be a sensitive diagnostic modality.

• The treatment of PPCM has long been controversial. Asymptomatic cysts and those smaller than 1 cm are not considered for surgical treatment and are followed with serial clinical examinations and follow-up MRI. Surgery is considered if one or more signs or symptoms are encountered in the presence of larger cysts. Surgical treatment usually consists of a midline myelotomy, with placement of a shunt tube to continuously drain the cyst into the subarachnoid space. Desired surgical outcomes include resolution of clinical symptoms and persisting collapse of the cyst cavity. Treatment outcomes vary considerably among investigators. Studies that report long-term postoperative results are less favorable than those that reporting shorter postoperative results.

Spasticity (pp. 1259–1260)

• The evaluation and treatment of spasticity in persons with SCI are comparable to that done in persons with other types of upper motor neuron neurological diseases. The evolution of uncontrolled muscle stretch reflexes is common during the period of initial inpatient rehabilitation and is a source of great interest to and misunderstanding among patients and families. The acknowledgment that this new movement is expected and is of little prognostic significance can be difficult. Spasticity is usually not painful. In some cases, however, spasticity can be so powerful as to make wheelchair use and transfers dangerous. Spasticity is not a problem that is separate from SCI; it is inseparable from the problem of muscle weakness and is part and parcel of upper motor neuron disease. Functional restrictions often arise, less from poorly functional spastic muscles than from the interference that spastic limbs present to positioning and the functional movements of normally innervated muscles.

• Spastic hypertonia does not always require treatment. Many SCI patients use extensor muscle tone to assist with standing, transfers, and ambulation. Spasticity preserves muscle mass and might lessen the incidence of venous thrombosis. Treatment is indicated only if the spasticity interferes with the performance of self-care, gait, wheelchair positioning, and transfer activities, disrupts sleep, or causes excessive pain or joint deformity. Spasticity also contributes to the development of pressure ulcers. An unexplained worsening of spasticity can signal the development of a secondary condition such as spinal instability or syringomyelia. Virtually any noxious stimulus (e.g., pressure ulcers, urinary tract infections, urolithiasis, or constipation) can worsen muscle spasms. Evaluation for such contributing factors is the first element in the comprehensive management of this condition.

- A daily routine of prolonged muscle stretching is the foundation for management of spasticity. The reduction in hypertonia that follows can last for several hours. Spasticity is probably most severe in persons with motor incomplete spinal cord lesions. Early after injury, flexor tone usually predominates, but this can change to an extensor pattern as time passes. In some instances, the problem is focal. Flexor spasticity at the elbow, for example, might respond to local treatment with muscle or nerve blocks, serial splinting, or orthopedic surgery intervention. If the problem with abnormal tone is generalized, medications are considered. Four medications—baclofen, diazepam, dantrolene, and tizanidine—are indicated for use in SCI. Symptom relief can be modest with these drugs; clinicians must be familiar with their mechanisms of action and their significant side effects (see Chapter 29).

- Baclofen, diazepam, and tizanidine act on the CNS. Baseline liver function tests are useful before initiating treatment with these antispasticity medications. Baclofen is often used as a first-line agent. The maximum recommended dosage is 80 mg/day, but many clinicians exceed this dose. Abrupt discontinuation of the drug can result in seizures, and SCI persons with renal insufficiency require dose adjustment.

- Diazepam is a safe and effective drug. Tolerance to its cognitive effects develops rapidly, and the antispasticity effects can persist indefinitely. Adult dosages of 10 to 40 mg/day are typically used. Its use is contraindicated in persons with a history of alcohol, drug, or medication abuse. A paradoxical response is occasionally seen with diazepam, resulting in insomnia, hostility, or anxiety. Dosage increases in diazepam should be undertaken carefully.

- Tizanidine treatment starts with 4 mg taken at bedtime. Its dose can be increased in very small increments to obtain the desired effects, an advantage over treatment with clonidine. Most patients will require 12 to 36 mg/day in three or four divided doses. Problems with low blood pressure are expected with α-2 agonist drugs but are uncommon in the SCI population. The concurrent use of tizanidine and clonidine is not recommended.

- Dantrolene acts peripherally at the neuromuscular junction. It is initiated at a dose of 25 mg, which can be increased slowly to a maximum of 400 mg/day in divided doses. This agent weakens innervated and noninnervated muscles in a nonselective fashion. Rarely, serious hepatotoxicity can occur. This risk is higher in females, persons older than 35 years, persons on estrogen therapy, and those taking high doses of the drug.

- Clonidine, both in oral and in transdermal forms, has been used as a spasticity agent in SCI patients. Its use can be limited by the side effects of constipation, hypotension, and lethargy. Gabapentin has also been studied. Doses above 400 mg three times a day are usually needed to produce a clinical response. A number of other drugs have been suggested, including cannabis.

- Intrathecal baclofen, delivered through an implanted programmable pump and catheter system, has been used for more than a decade for spasticity in persons with SCI (see Fig. 55–6 in the Textbook). The magnitude of spasticity relief is remarkable in comparison with that achieved with oral medication, but this invasive treatment is not appropriate for all patients. Regular pump refills are needed on a lifelong basis and must be carried out by experienced nursing staff. In some instances, tachyphylaxis is encountered, and intrathecal morphine is temporarily substituted. It is also quite useful in persons who are chronically bed-confined. In these patients, severe spasticity often prevents proper positioning and hygiene of the perineal area. Other surgical options exist for the treatment of spasticity (see Chapter 29).

ORTHOPEDIC AND MUSCULOSKELETAL ISSUES
(pp. 1260–1264)

Spinal Fractures (pp. 1260–1261)

• Although most persons with spinal fractures do not sustain SCI, most persons with SCI have spinal fractures. There are as many types of spine fractures as there are mechanisms of injury, and the study of spinal fractures occurring in conjunction with myelopathy has been limited by the lack of a widely accepted system to describe the bone trauma.

• Initial orthopedic trauma care attempts to identify and immobilize fractures to lessen the risk of further neurological injury. The degree of spinal instability is then assessed, with consideration of the severity and stability of the neurological deficit. Even patients who have undergone spinal instrumentation and spinal immobilization with an orthosis can still have a high degree of spinal instability.

• The goals of spinal treatment are to realign the spine, promote proper healing, prevent late deformity, and protect damaged neural tissue. Great controversy exists regarding the indications for spinal surgery and the timing of its application. It is of extreme importance that these patients be treated by an experienced spine traumatology team. There are dozens of compelling reasons to treat the spine surgically, but there is sparse evidence in human studies that surgery promotes neurological recovery over and above that expected on the basis of spontaneous improvement, either at the root or at the spinal cord level. Surgery is sometimes advocated as a means of providing early patient mobilization, but for patients with severe neurological injuries at the cervical or high thoracic level, this benefit is questionable. With expert nursing and therapy care, little time is lost when the spinal immobilization period is used to enhance healing of associated injuries, nutrition, pulmonary status, and strength in preparation for the added stress imposed by sitting.

Spinal Orthoses (p. 1261)

• Proper management of spinal orthoses is an important part of the acute rehabilitation process (see Chapter 17). The rehabilitation team works closely with the spinal surgeon and orthotist to ensure that braces are applied and maintained properly and that consistent directions for wear are given. Achievement of some therapy goals might have to be delayed until the spine has healed and the brace has been removed.

• The halo orthosis is an effective means of reducing spinal motion, both for conservative and for postoperative management. This device provides superior restriction of cervical motion at most levels, although this restriction is not complete. When properly applied it is remarkably well tolerated and needs little adjustment. Extra caution should be used when considering halo placement for persons with delirium, acute psychosis, or schizophrenia, and for patients with severe skull osteoporosis (e.g., elderly rheumatoid patients). Swallowing difficulties and choking sensations can occur when the halo ring locks the neck in excessive extension. Most patients report occasional creaking and popping noises associated with the halo superstructure. Adjustment is usually not necessary unless there is obvious motion in the halo frame. Halo pin sites are cleaned daily.

Heterotopic Ossification (pp. 1261–1263)

• Heterotopic ossification is a poorly understood medical condition characterized by the development of para-articular ossification, usually on the flexor surfaces of larger joints. It occurs in persons with neurological diseases, usually within the region of their motor deficits. It also is seen in persons who have sustained burns and in persons who have undergone total hip arthroplasty. The factors that connect these three disparate groups of patients and predispose to the development of heterotopic bone are unknown. This process of true ossification (i.e., trabecular bone formation) is distinct from ectopic calcification, or mineralization of soft tissue structures, which is noted in a variety of medical and traumatic conditions. Its incidence in persons with SCI has been reported to range from 16% to 53%. In the majority of SCI patients, ectopic bone is an incidental finding on plain radiographs and without clinical or functional significance. Of those developing heterotopic ossification, only 18% to 37% have disabling ROM limitations, and less than 5% develop ankylosis of the affected joint.

• The onset of heterotopic ossification is generally within 6 months after injury, with the most common occurrence between 1 and 4 months. It has been reported to occur as early as 20 days postinjury. The initial presentation of heterotopic ossification rarely occurs more than 1 year after injury. The most commonly involved areas, in decreasing order, are the hips, knees, shoulders, and elbows. Involvement of the axial skeleton and smaller joints in the extremities is very rare. In comparison to heterotopic ossification found in traumatic brain injury and hip replacement patients, there appear to be specific patterns of formation in SCI patients. About the hip, heterotopic ossification is most commonly located anteriorly and generally forms between the anterior superior iliac spine and the lesser trochanter. At the knee, involvement of the medial aspect is most commonly noted.

• The presence or absence of spasticity has not been shown to be associated with the development of heterotopic ossification. Although the presence of a pressure ulcer near a proximal joint increases the risk of developing heterotopic ossification, other conditions, including severe spasticity and aggressive ROM exercise, have not been demonstrated to be risk factors.

• Ectopic bone is extra-articular, often leaving the joint capsule intact. It forms in the connective tissue between the muscle planes and not within the muscle itself. The bone can be contiguous with the skeleton but generally does not involve the periosteum. Mature heterotopic ossification has histological features similar to those of a fracture callus.

- The initial clinical features of heterotopic ossification are nonspecific. The most common presentation is a warm, swollen, erythematous extremity. It can be confused with acute deep venous thrombosis. Swelling in the extremity is usually localized, and within several days a more circumscribed, firm mass can be noted within the area of edema. Early symptoms can include pain and restriction of joint motion. During the initial presentation, the differential diagnosis includes cellulitis, septic arthritis, bone tumor, Baker's cyst, and venous thrombosis.
- Plain radiographs are of limited use in the early diagnosis of this condition. The first evidence of calcification might not appear for weeks after the clinical presentation. An elevated serum alkaline phosphatase level can assist in differentiating early heterotopic ossification from other conditions, but serum levels are often abnormal secondary to other causes (e.g., spinal fracture or concomitant long bone injuries). Serial alkaline phosphatase levels are better used in following the progression of bone deposition rather than in the initial diagnosis. The triple-phase bone scan, performed using radiolabeled diphosphates, is very helpful for early detection of heterotopic ossification. The first two phases, dynamic blood flow study and static scan for blood pool, are the most sensitive for early detection (see Fig. 55–8 in the Textbook). Ultrasonography is essential in differentiating this process from thrombosis and is also helpful in the diagnosis of heterotopic bone.
- When the diagnosis is confirmed, initial treatment involves passive ROM exercises to maintain joint mobility. There is no evidence in human studies that this approach increases the ultimate amount of bone formation. Misguided discontinuation of passive ROM exercise can result in decreased motion in the affected joint and possibly in ankylosis. Disodium etidronate is effective in limiting the extent of heterotopic ossification when this treatment is started early in the course. It appears to be much less effective when used later in the disease course, regardless of dosage or duration of treatment. Larger doses of disodium etidronate have recently been employed in hopes of producing greater reduction in bone formation. Other medications, most notably indomethacin and warfarin, have been studied in the treatment of this condition. In some instances these drugs are combined with radiation therapy to the affected joint.
- The complications of heterotopic ossification can include peripheral nerve entrapment, the development of pressure ulcers, an increased risk of DVT, and extra-articular joint ankylosis. In these situations, surgical resection of the bone can be considered. Surgical resection of the bone would seem to be a simple solution to the problem, but complication rates approach 80%, even in experienced hands. There is conflicting opinion regarding the timing of surgery and the modes of perioperative care. Conventional surgical approaches have included a delay of 12 to 18 months between diagnosis and surgery, ostensibly to allow the bone mass to mature before resection. Problems arise when conventional tests for bone maturity (e.g., bone scan, radiography, and alkaline phosphatase levels) fail to correctly identify those with mature bone. Nuclear medicine scans can show activity for many months after the initial diagnosis, and the patient can have progressive loss of joint mobility during this waiting period. Recent reports of early resection of heterotopic bone in combination with drug and radiation treatment appear promising. The surgical procedure is often more complicated than anticipated. The surgeon often encounters a "nest" of bone that is perforated by tortuous blood vessels and nerves, and no distinct

tissue planes are apparent. Total resection is not undertaken. The goal of free ROM is obtained with a limited wedge resection to reduce postoperative "dead space." A hematoma develops in the dead space soon after surgery. A fever can be present, and the operate limb is often warm and swollen. The question of perioperative DVT is always a consideration in this setting, where anticoagulation can certainly aggravate the healing process. The majority of patients exhibit recurrence of bone after surgery. With proper care, joint ROM can be preserved despite this recurrence. Many surgeons begin drug treatment with disodium etidronate and use radiation in the perioperative setting. Careful positioning and turning in bed is necessary to protect the operated limb from excessive stretching and to prevent trauma to the swollen operative site.

Limb Fractures (p. 1263)

• In the acute setting, limb fractures are the most common traumatic condition associated with SCI. Despite striking changes in bone metabolism during this phase, long bone and spinal fractures heal well with standard orthopedic care, including internal and external fixation. The presence of longstanding myelopathy markedly raises the risk of leg fractures. Fractures that occur in the chronic phase of injury present a number of unique treatment challenges. These fractures are often discovered after a minor or incidental trauma. In some instances the patient cannot identify the precipitating event. Most of these fractures occur just above or just below the knee. The patient presents with malaise, clinical signs of fever, and swelling and redness of the affected limb. Venous thrombosis and cellulitis are always included in the differential diagnosis.

• In the chronic phase of injury, upper extremity fractures (and leg fractures in ambulatory patients) are treated with the same techniques that are used in nondisabled populations. The treating physician confronts a unique set of circumstances when faced with leg fractures in persons who are nonambulatory. These fractures are radiographically striking, and osteopenia is severe. The temptation to instrument the fracture is great; however, severe muscle and soft tissue atrophy is present, the patients often lack sensation in the area, and they might not be able to properly splint the area because of spasticity. Patients often benefit from a short (2- to 3-day) period of bed rest when fever is present. After this, quick mobilization is undertaken with fracture stabilization provided by soft splint materials. In the nonambulatory patient, a limited degree of limb shortening and angulation of the fracture site is tolerated, but avoidance of rotational deformities is a priority. Hard cast materials can produce pressure ulcers. If the patient is careful with limb positioning and wheelchair transfers, hard cast immobilization is not necessary.

• Persons with fractures of the leg are usually advised to elevate the limb while in the wheelchair. This practice is risky because elevation of the leg changes wheelchair positioning, shifting weight over the seated surface and placing the patient at high risk for seated pressure ulcers. If tissue edema is an issue, frequent recumbent rest periods out of the wheelchair are a better option. Although conservative care is used if possible in the chronic phase, subtrochanteric and proximal femur fractures rarely heal properly without internal fixation.

Contractures and Overuse Syndromes (p. 1264)

• Pain and restrictions in joint ROM are an important problem in both the acute and the chronic setting. The intensity of ROM exercises needed to prevent joint deformity varies among patients, but education regarding the consequences of range restrictions (e.g., pressure sores, pain, and mobility restrictions) is important for every patient. Joint ROM restrictions result from muscle shortening, spasticity, capsular adhesions, trauma, and joint ankylosis. In the acute phase, splints at the wrists and ankles and proper positioning of the shoulders and elbows are important. Nonambulatory patients who can lie in the prone position greatly reduce their risk of pressure ulcers and hip and knee flexion contractures. Achieving the prone position should be a goal for every SCI patient in the acute setting as soon as spinal and pulmonary stability permit. Regional injection of neurolytic agents or botulinum toxin can be used in selected instances if spasticity restricts joint mobility and pharmacological management has not been satisfactory. Muscle release surgery requires special expertise and postoperative care.

• Patients with lower extremity motor deficits place an inordinate amount of weight-bearing stress on the upper extremities, either for wheelchair propulsion, transfers, or crutch walking. In the weight-bearing upper extremity, there is an increased prevalence of shoulder impingement, tears of the rotator cuff, carpal instability, and carpal tunnel syndrome. These conditions probably arise from muscle imbalance, repetitive loading, and postural abnormalities. Shoulder pain is reported in more than one-half of surveyed patients with SCI. Patients with upper extremity dysfunction can be treated with standard musculoskeletal modalities, including NSAIDs and injection, and a review of their mobility techniques is of utmost importance. The emphasis of treatment must be on joint conservation. A power wheelchair is sometimes the best means of preserving shoulder function into the later years for those with the potential to perform independent wheelchair transfers. Persons with progressive signs of nerve entrapment, shoulder impingement, and rotator cuff pathology are candidates for standard surgical decompression or repair.

PEDIATRIC SPINAL CORD INJURY (pp. 1264–1267)

• Across the United States, 5% of SCIs occur in children and adolescents under the age of 15 years. Just as in the adult population, motor vehicle collisions are the most common cause of injury (38% to 64%). Young children are at special risk for sustaining automobile-inflicted injuries as pedestrians. Sporting activities, acts of violence, and falls are other common causes of traumatic paralysis. Sporting injuries, mostly from diving, account for 23% of injuries in this group and are seen more commonly in older children and adolescents. Injuries from violence have increased over the past two decades. Even the youngest children are not spared; 15% of children under age 8 years are injured by violent acts.

• Other injury mechanisms are rare but unique to this group. Neonatal SCIs are seen in approximately 1 in 60,000 births. Rotational injuries from forceps trauma result in high cervical injuries. Cervicothoracic injuries can occur with breech deliveries, and thoracic lesions can arise as a result of perinatal umbilical artery trauma or paradoxical air embolism through transitional cardiovascular shunts. In older children, injury can be associated with atlantoaxial instability (e.g., in Down's syndrome); juvenile rheumatoid arthritis; and in the setting of skeletal dysplasias, such as Morquio's syndrome or metatopic dwarfism.

• In contrast to SCI adult patients, girls and boys are equally represented in the youngest injury cohorts. In addition, the mechanisms and epidemiology of spinal injury differ between children and adults. Nearly 70% of spinal injuries in children result in paraplegia, probably because of the high incidence (64%) of motor vehicle trauma in this group. Lap belt injuries, commonly seen in children weighing less than 40 lb, are brought about by flexion-distraction trauma over a restraint situated above the pelvic brim. Neurological lesions in this setting are variable. Deficits can be seen as high as the midthoracic spinal cord, implicating vascular trauma. In the cervical spine, very high lesions (C1 to C3), which are rare in adults, are overrepresented in this group, accounting for 10% of injuries. This is most likely because of the proportionately large head and weak neck muscles in small children. In the emergency setting, these anatomical differences necessitate the use of pediatric spine immobilization boards with cranial openings to allow an anatomical alignment during transport and initial treatment.

- In the immature spine, excessive elasticity, shallow, horizontal facet joints, and fragile vertebral end-plates contribute to the high incidence of SCI in the setting of normal spinal radiographs. The incidence of SCI without radiographic abnormality is 63% in children under the age of 10 years. Despite the normal radiographic appearance, these children are more likely to develop a complete neurological injury and to have a poor neurological prognosis. In up to 25% of children with SCI there is a delay, lasting hours to days, between the traumatic episode and the appearance of neurological deficits. Newer MRI techniques are extremely helpful in this setting, detailing soft tissue injury in 65% of children with SCI without radiographic abnormalities.

- Even the youngest children should be given a role in decision making. Children injured at birth present altogether different problems for the treatment team than those injured in adolescence. Clinicians must be prepared to spend extra time with family members, providing anticipatory guidance and support. Centers that treat adults with SCI might not be able to meet the unique medical and psychological needs of this heterogeneous group.

- In many respects, the medical management of children with SCI parallels that of adults. Although venous thromboembolism is diagnosed less often in children, the disastrous potential of clots that go undetected has led to the recommendation that all children should receive thromboprophylaxis, with aggressive physical and pharmacological measures. The goals of acute pulmonary management are the same in children as in adults: to maintain appropriate oxygenation and reduce the effects of atelectasis and pneumonia. Alveolar ventilation requirements, however, are higher in children because of a higher metabolic rate. The compliance of the immature rib cage is also increased, necessitating bilateral pacing in infants by means of phrenic nerve electrostimulation.

- Methods of neurogenic bowel management in children are analogous to those used in adults. For children with intact sacral reflexes, a regular schedule of rectal emptying promoted by chemical or digital stimulation of the anorectum should be established. Children with lumbar and sacral injuries might lack sacral reflexes and need daily digital removal of stool. Considerable latitude should be given to younger children, who typically approach the problems of bowel continence at their own pace. Older children and adolescents are prone to bowel emptying difficulties secondary to irregular dietary habits.

- The presence of nonspecific GI complaints in an adolescent with SCI can indicate the presence of hypercalcemia. This usually appears within the first 3 months postinjury and affects 10% to 23% of persons with SCI; it is most common in young males. Clinical manifestations can include nausea, abdominal pain, vomiting, poor appetite, polydipsia, and mental status changes. The increase in bone turnover characteristic of growing children, combined with the increased bone resorption seen in acute SCI, might be responsible for the high incidence of hypercalcemia in this population. In most instances, IV hydration, combined with administration of furosemide, facilitates renal excretion of calcium and symptom relief within 3 to 4 days. If this treatment is not successful, the use of calcitonin should be considered. Etidronate disodium is not used in growing children because of the potential for development of a rachitic syndrome. Close follow-up is needed after treatment because prolonged hypercalcemia is associated with the development of urinary tract lithiasis and renal failure.

• Proper urological management of the pediatric patient also minimizes the risk of renal complications by reducing risk factors such as cystitis, pyelonephritis, vesicoureteral reflux, and trauma from long-term catheter use. Children should undergo routine urodynamic evaluations, renal US, and voiding cystourethrography to assess the function and coordination of the bladder and sphincter. The goals of treatment are the same as in adults—establishment of a plan that maintains low detrusor pressures and allows complete bladder emptying. For children under the age of 4, continence is not a primary concern, and diapers can be used if detrusor pressures are low and reflux is not present. Intermittent catheterization can be started at any age, even in infants, if recurrent infections or vesicoureteral reflux are noted. Bladder volumes range from 30 mL in neonates to over 350 mL in preadolescents. An attempt to wean children from diapers should begin at an age-appropriate time, usually around 4 years. Parents are trained to perform clean intermittent catheterization, and continence is facilitated by pharmacological treatment with such agents as oxybutinin, imipramine, terazosin, propantheline, desmopressin, and pseudoephedrine. Self-catheterization can be introduced as early as age 5 years, but many children, especially boys, might not be developmentally ready until age 8 or 9 years.

• Intermittent catheterization programs are not successful in many children. Poor hand function, high-pressure, low-capacity bladders unresponsive to drug treatment, unacceptable drug side effects, inability to restrict fluid intake, and inconvenience are common reasons for abandoning intermittent catheterization. In older boys, condom catheters can be used, but they are only appropriate after a thoughtful and detailed analysis of baseline voiding function because sphincterotomy is rarely performed in this setting. Indwelling urethral or suprapubic catheters allow the child considerable autonomy and convenience in the school setting, advantages that must be weighed against the increased risks of lower urinary tract trauma and calculus formation.

• Even the best intermittent catheterization programs do not eliminate the risk of instrumentation trauma and infection. Counseling should emphasize the minimal use of antibiotics. The indications for prophylactic and acute antibiotic treatment are the same for children as they are for adults. Surgical reconstruction of the lower urinary tract, including construction of bowel loop diversions, continent catheterizable stomas, and bladder augmentation procedures, remains a reasonable option for children with recurrent symptomatic infections and evidence of upper urinary tract deterioration despite best efforts at conservative management.

• Planning for any surgery should involve consideration of latex allergy and the risk of anaphylaxis when exposed to latex products in the operating suite.

Up to 18% of children with SCI demonstrate positive skin testing for latex, precipitated by early and repeated contact with the allergenic proteins present in catheters and latex gloves. Life-threatening anaphylactic reactions can be the presenting sign of latex allergy in up to 30% of latex-sensitive children. Contact dermatitis and urticaria, wheezing, and angioedema are other presenting factors.

• Notwithstanding the considerable attention given to medical concerns, the central focus of injured children and their parents relates to disability, and walking is their primary goal. The medical, orthopedic, and musculoskeletal benefits of achieving standing and walking are regularly misrepresented and overstated. Studies demonstrating that upright activities change the natural history of this condition are lacking. Standing facilitates childhood recreational, educational, vocational, and leisure activities.

• Success in achieving ambulation depends on a number of factors, chiefly neurological level of injury, motivation, body size, and musculoskeletal integrity. For patients with residual arm function, castor carts can be used at 9 to 12 months to allow exploration of their environment. At 18 to 24 months, a wheelchair can be prescribed as a primary means of mobility for tetraplegic children, and as a concurrent mobility device for those who are learning to walk with assistive devices. As in adults, children with lesions at L3 and below and those with International Classification D injuries have a favorable prognosis for long-term community ambulation. They can sometimes achieve surprising levels of mobility despite higher neurological lesions. The use of standing frames and parapodia can be initiated at 10 to 12 months of age, even in individuals with quadriplegia. These devices allow children free use of their hands and, given flat terrain, good head control, and joint flexibility, they can be used for rudimentary ambulation using a swivel-rocking motion. Cosmetic issues and reduced stability as the child grows taller usually restrict the use of these devices beyond the third grade. For children with thoracic and lumbar injuries, progression to orthoses that promote gait can begin at 12 to 18 months.

• The muscle requirements for gait and orthosis prescription in this population are similar to those in adults. Children with good pelvis control and hip flexor strength are candidates for KAFO bracing. The hyperlordotic posture required for KAFO use places excessive stress on a recently fractured spine and can exacerbate the spinal deformities commonly seen in these patients. Because of this, children should begin standing only after sufficient spinal healing and stability are attained, and those with higher injuries are best served with KAFOs or reciprocating gait orthoses (RGOs). RGOs are expensive, heavy, and require considerable maintenance. Although RGOs are designed to promote a reciprocal gait, many children use them with crutches and a swing-to pattern. Children fitted with RGOs are likely to use them only for household ambulation. Newer RGOs with hydraulic assist components have been developed and might offer greater potential for community ambulation. Functional electrical stimulation to promote standing and gait has also been studied in children. These systems have demonstrated a good safety profile and show potential for providing a higher level of mobility for those with thoracic injuries.

• Special attention should be given to orthosis prescription and fabrication in the pediatric setting. Particular vigilance for the development of pressure ulcers is required. Many braces allow for adjustment as the child grows, but repair, replacement, and training costs are not avoidable. Children who do not, for whatever reason, make use of their preliminary, simple orthoses will not use more complex and advanced systems. Social goals, motivation, body habitus, and physical capabilities undergo major changes as the child reaches adolescence. In many instances, progressive musculoskeletal complications tip the balance toward use of a wheelchair for locomotion.

• Acquired deformities at the hip are common after pediatric SCI. Hip instability is found in 78% of spastic hips and 89% of flaccid hips, and occurs with increased frequency in children injured before age 5. Over the course of time, hip flexion contractures and subluxation occur as a result of muscle imbalance, poor socket development, and trauma. In those with paraplegia, it is unclear whether this represents the cause or the result of reduced ambulation as the child grows. As in adults, the hip is especially difficult to target with conservative treatment. The muscles and nerves responsible are not easily isolated or stretched. It is best to place the emphasis of care on prevention. Once the joint demonstrates ankylosis or frank dislocation, attempts at surgical repair are complicated and rarely successful.

• Family members should be well versed in stretching techniques, and prone sleeping is encouraged. Spasticity management with baclofen and clonidine can be initiated. In children under the age of 6 years, diazepam might be the best choice owing to difficulties with dosing of the other drugs and the constipation associated with clonidine. Although the radiographic appearance and examination findings of hip dislocation are striking, this condition is often irrelevant from a functional standpoint. Children with hip dislocation can continue to use long leg braces, and the sitting position is rarely compromised. Advanced hip flexion deformities, however, might bring about more functional restrictions. For young people who are community ambulators, frequent examination allows the clinician to discover abnormalities in hip ROM at their earliest stage, when surgical soft tissue releases can best be utilized.

• Frequent examination is even more critical in the management of late spinal deformity. As periods of rapid growth occur, spinal deformity can advance, sometimes over just a few months. Scoliosis is ubiquitous in children with spinal injuries that occur before skeletal maturity. Up to 67% will need surgery to prevent further loss of thoracoabdominal capacity, cardiopulmonary reserve, and musculoskeletal integrity. The concepts applied to treatment of scoliosis in the able-bodied child have little pertinence for this population. Noting a prevalence of 91% to 100%, Betz has advocated the use of prophylactic spinal bracing in all children before any curve develops, along with prescription of an appropriate wheelchair and encouragement of ambulation. Lightweight plastic spinal orthoses are used, and refitted frequently as the child grows. The goal is to reduce or forestall the progression of spinal deformity until at least age 10 years, when the child has developed sufficient adult trunk height. At this time, corrective surgery for curves measuring more than 40 degrees are best considered.

• The life satisfaction of adults who had SCI as children is inversely associated with medical complications, but issues of education, socialization and recreation, and employment are also of extreme importance. Rehabilitation services focus on family attitudes and resources, with the acknowledgment that the child's adaptation strategies will change as new challenges are faced. Psychological support is important in helping the patient and family deal with the issues of independence, social development, and self-esteem. Education of parents regarding community recreation resources, peer support groups, camp opportunities, and financial resources is as important as education regarding medical issues.

THERAPEUTIC AND REGENERATIVE THERAPIES
(pp. 1267–1271)

- Because of the numerous mechanisms of trauma and the variety of neurological manifestations of SCI, the prospect for discovery of a single, effective drug treatment for paralysis remains remote. Nevertheless, enthusiasm for cure research has risen in the past three decades, based on the exciting possibility that a combination of pharmacological, bioengineering, genetic, surgical, and rehabilitative strategies can be used to reduce or reverse neurological deficits.

- Of all the venues of research, the most exciting has been the study of treatments that might salvage or preserve residual function during the period of secondary injury to the spinal cord. The study of high-dose methylprednisolone in acute cord injury arose out of numerous encouraging animal studies. These reports noted that a single bolus of this drug given after injury significantly improved spinal cord blood flow, prevented decreases in extracellular calcium, and reduced total lesion volume.

- The mechanisms of neurological improvement in the months after injury are not well understood. Initial recovery in the zone of injury, related to reversal of conduction block, occurs within 6 weeks of injury. Strength change after this period is attributed to peripheral nerve sprouting and muscle hypertrophy, but there is limited evidence to support these concepts. In animal models, nascent axons are seen traversing necrotic central spinal cord cavities, raising the possibility that recovery in the months following injury is a result of CNS regeneration and plasticity. See the Textbook for further discussion of spinal cord injury research.

56

Original Chapter by Karen L. Andrews, M.D., Thom W. Rooke, M.D., and Phala A. Helm, M.D.

Vascular Disease: Evaluation and Management

ARTERIAL DISEASE (pp. 1283–1292)

Epidemiology (p. 1283)

- Peripheral arterial disease is a relatively common manifestation of systemic atherosclerosis; it affects 5% of persons 50 years of age and 20% of persons older than 70 years. The most common presentation of arterial occlusive disease is intermittent claudication. Epidemiologic studies have demonstrated that limb-threatening ischemia develops in as few as 2% to 5% of patients with intermittent claudication monitored for up to 10 years. There is an overall reduction of 10 years in life expectancy among patients with peripheral vascular disease, with mortality primarily caused by coronary artery disease and diabetes mellitus with its associated complications.

Etiology (pp. 1283–1284)

- There are many causes of arterial occlusive disease, the most common of which is atherosclerosis obliterans (ASO). Other disease processes include thromboangiitis obliterans (Buerger's disease); vasospastic disorders (Raynaud's phenomenon, livedo reticularis, and acrocyanosis); thrombosis; embolism; dissection; vasculitis; and fibromuscular dysplasia.

Atherosclerosis (pp. 1283–1284)

- Atherosclerosis in its advanced form is a systemic disorder involving the coronary, cerebral, pulmonary, renal, and peripheral vessels. Atheroscerotic plaques tend to develop at branch points, bifurcations, zones of rapid tapering, and areas where arteries follow a tortuous course. In patients with diabetes, ASO occurs with equal frequency in both femoral and tibial arteries, whereas in nondiabetics the most common sites of severe disease are the abdominal aorta and iliac and femoral arteries.
- Potentially reversible factors that increase the risk of atherosclerosis include smoking, hyperlipidemia, hypertension, diabetes, and obesity. Cigarette smoking

is by far the most common risk factor, competing with juvenile diabetes mellitus and certain rare congenital hyperlipidemias as the most serious. Smoking acts synergistically with other risk factors such as hypertension or hypercholesterolemia to enhance progression of atherosclerotic lesions.

Thromboangiitis Obliterans (Buerger's Disease) (p. 1284)
• Thromboangiitis obliterans (Buerger's disease) is a disease involving thrombosis and inflammation of small peripheral arteries and veins. Lesions are usually located distal to the knee or elbow. Most theories implicate some component of cigarette smoking that predisposes the arterial wall to inflammation, possibly through the formation of immune complexes.

Vasospasm (p. 1284)
• Raynaud's phenomenon most commonly involves the hands but can also affect the feet. With exposure to cold or emotional stress, spasm of the small arteries and arterioles results in ischemia (pallor or cyanosis), pain, and subsequent vasodilatation with hyperemia. Raynaud's phenomenon can be idiopathic or occur as a manifestation of a potentially serious underlying systemic disease.

Other Causes of Arterial Occlusive Disease (p. 1284)
• Thrombosis, embolism, and arterial dissection are discussed in the following sections on acute and chronic arterial occlusion.

Clinical Evaluation (pp. 1284–1285)

Acute Arterial Occlusion (p. 1284)
• The clinical presentation in acute arterial occlusion includes sudden onset of toe, foot, and leg pain associated with absence of pulse and coolness and discoloration of the skin in a patchy irregular configuration. The findings are commonly described as the "6 Ps"—pulselessness, pain, polar (cold), pallor, paresthesia, and paralysis. The major causes of acute arterial occlusion are embolism, thrombosis, trauma, and dissection. The most common cause of acute arterial embolism is cardiac (e.g., atrial fibrillation; recent myocardial infarction; cardiomyopathy; native or prosthetic heart valve replacement; and, rarely, atrial myxoma). If previous symptoms of claudication are present in a patient with no cardiac dysfunction, the diagnosis of thrombosis is most likely.

Chronic Arterial Occlusion (pp. 1284–1285)
• Chronic arterial occlusive disease can usually be diagnosed from the history and physical examination. The most common symptom is intermittent claudication. Lower extremity claudication is reproduced with a consistent level of exercise from one occasion to the next, and completely resolves within minutes after the exercise has been discontinued.
• The site of claudication is a rough indicator for the level of occlusion. For example, patients with occlusion at or above the ankle can present with claudication in the arch of the foot. Elevation pallor is determined by raising the leg to a 90-degree angle; if pallor develops within 60 seconds, the patient has mild occlusive disease; within 30 seconds, moderate disease; and within 15 seconds, severe disease. When the legs are returned to a dependent position, the venous filling time (i.e., the time it takes for the small veins of the feet to distend with

blood) can be determined. Normal venous filling time is classically described as 20 seconds, but this value is altered with associated congestive heart failure, venous insufficiency, pulmonary hypertension, or tricuspid regurgitation.

• As the disease process advances, resting blood flow rates are affected, and ischemia at rest and impaired skin metabolism result. Clinical findings of ischemia can include trophic changes, dependent rubor, paresthesias, cutaneous ulceration, and gangrene.

Vascular Testing (pp. 1285–1287)

Noninvasive Studies (pp. 1285–1287)

• If ischemia is noted on clinical examination, noninvasive studies can delineate the degree and level of ischemia and the potential for healing (Table 56–1). They can also provide a baseline for future comparison. When patients present with symptoms that occur during exercise, some form of exercise evaluation should be performed.

SEGMENTAL PRESSURE

• Measurement of supine resting ankle pressure is the most common noninvasive study performed on patients with suspected vascular disease. The arterial systolic blood pressure in a given limb segment is determined by inflating a cuff around that segment and slowly deflating the cuff until pedal arterial blood flow is detected with continuous-wave Doppler or by feeling for the return of pulses. (A stethoscope is not sensitive enough to reliably assess the return of blood flow.) Variations in systemic pressure between individuals are corrected by expressing the absolute ankle pressure as a ratio relative to the brachial pressure (ankle/brachial index, ABI). The ABI is interpreted as follows: 0.9 or greater, normal; 0.8 to 0.9, mild; 0.5 to 0.8, moderate; and 0.5 or less, severe. In patients with mild symptoms of claudication, the ABI might be normal at rest but reduced after exercise.

• Segmental limb pressure measurements extend the application of ankle pressure measurements and provide a more precise determination of the anatomy of the occlusive process. Continuous-wave Doppler is still used to assess posterior tibial or dorsalis pedis blood flow, but this time the occlusion cuffs are placed

TABLE 56–1 Noninvasive Vascular Studies Used to Diagnose Arterial Disease

Vascular Disease	Anatomic	Hemodynamic/ Functional	Disadvantages
Arterial	Continuous wave Doppler	Continuous wave Doppler	Operator dependent
			Limited ability to quantify disease severity
	Pulse volume recording		Poor reproducibility
	Segmental pressure	Segmental pressure	
	Ankle/brachial index		Cannot be interpreted if vessels noncompressible
	TcPO$_2$ (amputation level)	TcPO$_2$	Limited availability
"Small vessel" (arteriolar)		TcPO$_2$	Limited availability

at high-thigh, above-knee, below-knee, and ankle locations. Limb pressure equal to or less than the brachial artery pressure indicates significant aortoiliac or proximal femoral arterial occlusive disease. A gradient of more than 20 mm Hg between any adjacent segments is an abnormal finding.

CONTINUOUS WAVE DOPPLER

- A normal flow waveform in peripheral arteries is characterized by a triphasic Doppler signal during each cardiac cycle. Biphasic signals are observed in the absence of disease in distal arteries or when the peripheral resistance is low. Distal to a stenosis, the waveform becomes monophasic, characterized by a blunted peak velocity and the absence of a reverse component.

PLETHYSMOGRAPHY

- Plethysmography can be used to measure mean blood flow by recording the rate of increase in limb volume after sudden interruption of venous outflow.
- Digital plethysmography can be performed with either strain-gauge or photoelectric instrumentation. This test is useful for the evaluation of patients with noncompressible ankle or leg arteries because it is unusual for digital arteries to be affected by this process. A toe/brachial index greater than 0.60 is normal. If the absolute pressure is 30 mm Hg or less, healing is unlikely to occur.

TRANSCUTANEOUS OXYGEN TENSION

- Transcutaneous oxygen tension ($TcPO_2$) is an objective indicator of ischemia of the skin in a patient with peripheral occlusive arterial disease. $TcPO_2$ measurements are relatively simple and reproducible. In a standard study of the lower extremities, two electrodes are placed on the dorsum of each foot. With the patient supine, $TcPO_2$ values are recorded and the regional perfusion indices ($TcPO_2$ foot/$TcPO_2$ chest) are calculated. The feet are then elevated to 30 degrees for 3 minutes, and the $TcPO_2$ measurements are repeated. If the $TcPO_2$ value is 20 torr or less, healing is not likely to occur, whereas $TcPO_2$ values of more than 40 torr are associated with healing.

DUPLEX ULTRASONOGRAPHY

- Duplex ultrasonography combines a pulsed Doppler with real-time B mode scanning. Duplex scanning combines exact anatomic localization of disease with physiologic blood flow studies to define the hemodynamic significance of the lesion. The expense of this equipment limits its utilization as a general screening tool (see the section on venous studies later in this chapter).

MAGNETIC RESONANCE ANGIOGRAPHY

- Magnetic resonance imaging can yield images of sufficient quality that peripheral vascular disease might also be diagnosed and visualized by noninvasive means.

Invasive Studies (p. 1287)

ARTERIOGRAPHY

- Although physiologic testing is excellent for screening and follow-up, arteriography remains the most accurate procedure for evaluation of arterial anatomy. If surgery is anticipated, arteriography is usually needed to determine the length of arterial occlusion, level of distal reconstruction, and patency of the plantar arch.

Testing for Associated Diseases (pp. 1287–1288)

• When evaluating the patient with atherosclerotic occlusive disease, especially if surgical intervention is planned, it is important that the clinical evaluation define and quantify any associated cardiovascular, renal, and pulmonary problems.

Exercise Thallium-201 Scintigraphy (p. 1288)

• Exercise thallium-201 scintigraphy (or related tests using provocative agents such as adenosine or dipyridamole and uptake agents such as sestamibi) are useful for screening patients with peripheral vascular disease for coronary artery disease because they are minimally invasive and can assess the extent of myocardium at risk. Exercise (or dobutamine, dipyridamole, or other agents) cause coronary vasodilation. During exercise (or drug administration in the case of patients who are unable to exercise), the difference in perfusion between myocardium supplied by normal coronary arteries and that supplied by stenotic, nondistensible vessels is accentuated. Thallium-201 is promptly absorbed by areas of normal perfusion and serves as a marker for viable myocardium. When the patient is rescanned 3 hours later, uptake of thallium-201 is delayed in areas of potentially ischemic myocardium. No uptake is noted in areas of infarcted tissue. Patients with a history of more severe cardiac disease and thallium-201 redistribution involving two or more vessels are at increased risk for postoperative cardiac complications, and further cardiac evaluation such as cardiac catheterization should be considered.

Treatment (pp. 1288–1292)

Acute Arterial Occlusion (pp. 1288–1289)

THROMBOSIS

• Acute thrombosis is generally best managed with an initial course of heparin therapy followed by arteriography to define the lesion and the status of the inflow and outflow vessels. Lytic therapy or urgent surgical revascularization might be required. Early intervention can prevent neuromuscular injury; enhance limb salvage; and avoid myonecrosis, myoglobinuria, and associated renal failure. In less severe cases where immediate revascularization is unnecessary, elective revascularization at a later date might be required to alleviate symptoms of chronic ischemia.

EMBOLIC ISCHEMIA

• Heparin should be given as soon as the diagnosis of acute arterial embolus is suspected. When results of sensory and motor examination are normal, the limb generally shows rapid improvement with anticoagulation. Early recognition and correction of an offending proximal lesion or cardiac abnormality are important.

• Advanced ischemia is characterized by absent motor and sensory function, muscle tenderness and rigidity, limb pallor (without elevation), and prolongation of the venous filling time to more than 1 minute. With marked motor deficit, muscle rigidity, or anesthesia on clinical examination, early amputation must be considered. Revascularization of such an ischemic limb can result in a mortality rate of 50% to 75% because of the effects of metabolic products on the renal and pulmonary systems (reperfusion syndrome).

DISSECTION

- Treatment of aortic dissection depends on location. If the dissection is located in the ascending aorta (Stanford type A), management includes control of arterial systolic blood pressure and emergency surgical repair. If the dissection occurs in the descending thoracic or abdominal aorta (Stanford type B), medical management of pain and arterial blood pressure is usually the treatment of choice. Surgical repair is generally reserved for patients who have significant vascular occlusion, persistent pain, progression of the dissection, or aneurysm formation.

Chronic Arterial Occlusion (p. 1289)

- The ultimate goal is to develop effective therapy that prevents progression of the disease process and possibly promotes regression of existing lesions. It is important that the correct diagnosis and cause of the underlying disease process be identified before proceeding with treatment. Controllable risk factors, as discussed previously, should be addressed appropriately.

PATIENT AND FAMILY EDUCATION

- It is important to discuss in detail, with the patient and family, the diffuse and progressive nature of atherosclerosis, the importance of controlling risk factors, and measures to protect the ischemic limb.

PROTECTION FROM TRAUMA

- Thermal injury is prevented by avoiding excess heat (e.g., heating pad or hot water). Warm outer footwear is recommended in the winter to protect against cold. Vascular boots made of cotton fleece and bandage material are good for keeping an ischemic limb warm, but are not designed to protect ischemic or neuropathic feet during ambulation. Chemicals, corn remedies, and antiseptics should be avoided to prevent chemical trauma. Mechanical trauma can be caused by poorly fitting footwear.

FOOTWEAR

- The use of rocker-sole shoes, which lessen the work of the gastrocnemius soleus muscle groups during ambulation, increases walking distance and can be a useful addition to the nonsurgical management of calf claudication. Ankle-foot orthoses to eliminate ankle motion can also help increase walking distance.

Exercise (pp. 1289–1290)

- Exercise increases the demand for blood to the lower extremities. In a normal arterial system, demand is primarily met by arterial vasodilatation. With atherosclerosis, the capability of the arterial system to supply peak blood flow is progressively reduced. At rest, maximal blood flow goes to the skin; during exercise, most of the increase in blood flow is shunted to the active muscle beds. Several studies have shown the beneficial effects of physical training in patients with intermittent claudication. Improved peripheral utilization of oxygen, walking technique, and glycolytic and oxidative metabolic capacity have been suggested as reasons for the improvement with training. Biochemical evidence suggests that the activity of glycolytic and mitochondrial enzymes in calf muscle tissue is positively correlated with walking distance in patients with claudication who receive physical training. Walking programs must be individualized; however, the usual prescription has a goal of 30 to 60 minutes, 3 to 5 days per week at a pace of 2 miles per hour, as allowed by cardiac precautions. The patient should rest after symptoms of claudication develop. Improvement will be gradual over a period of 3 to 6 months.

Risk Factor Modification (pp. 1290–1291)
• Peripheral artery disease and coronary artery disease are both manifestations of atherosclerotic disease and have similar risk factors: age, gender (estrogen status), family history, tobacco abuse, hypercholesterolemia, hypertension, diabetes mellitus, and physical inactivity. Patients should be counseled to modify these risk factors. In addition, if premature atherosclerosis is detected, the patient's first-degree relatives should be screened for heritable risk factors such as homocysteine and possibly familial lipoproteinemia.

Medication (p. 1291)
• **Vasodilators.** Although vasodilator drugs have been shown to increase blood flow to the limbs and various organs in animal experiments and in humans with vasospastic disorders, their use in peripheral obstructive vascular disease remains questionable. An ideal vasodilator for use in peripheral vascular disease would increase blood flow only in areas of deficient blood supply. In some circumstances, vasodilation in areas without diseased vessels can actually steal flow from the affected area. β-adrenergic blockade can cause peripheral vasoconstriction, and therefore, β-adrenergic blockers should be avoided in patients with arterial occlusive disease.
• **Anticoagulants and Antiplatelet Agents.** Platelet aggregation can exacerbate arterial occlusive disease by causing mechanical occlusion of small arteries or by releasing serotonin and stimulating local vasospasm. There is no evidence that fibrinolytic agents, anticoagulants, or antiplatelet agents are directly effective in the treatment of intermittent claudication.
• **Hemorrhelogic Agents.** Pentoxifylline (Trental) increases red cell deformability, decreases plasma viscosity, and diminishes platelet aggregation by decreasing fibrinogen concentration. It also increases resting and hyperemic extremity blood flow, presumably through its rheologic effects. Reports in the literature about the degree of clinical improvement in patients taking pentoxifylline for the treatment of intermittent claudication have been variable. Because pentoxifylline is a methylxanthine derivative, this drug should not be used in persons intolerant of this class of compounds (e.g., caffeine and theophylline).
• **Antioxidant Agents.** Oxidation of low-density lipoprotein cholesterol tends to promote atherosclerotic disease development. There might be a role for treatment of patients with peripheral arterial occlusive disease with antioxidant medications (e.g., vitamins E and C); however, final recommendations await a large-scale study of the effects of antioxidants in patients with peripheral arterial disease.

Revascularization (pp. 1291–1292)
Angioplasty. Percutaneous transluminal angioplasty is an established treatment for claudication in patients with arterial occlusive disease. Angioplasty is indicated for focal stenosis or short segmental occlusions in which the adjacent vessels are relatively free of disease. Angioplasty is associated with a low incidence of morbidity, and 5-year patency rates of 80% to 90% have been reported for iliac lesions, as opposed to 60% to 70% for superficial femoral artery lesions.

Surgery. Vascular reconstruction is indicated in patients with incapacitating claudication, rest pain, gangrene, and tissue loss, especially when the ankle/brachial index is less than 0.4 or the forefoot $TcPO_2$ is less than 30 mm Hg.

Aortoiliac Occlusive Disease. The standard operation for aortoiliac disease is an aortobifemoral bypass. In selected patients with unilateral disease, limited operations such as femoral-femoral (fem-fem) bypass or iliofemoral bypass can be considered. Contralateral disease progression or atherosclerotic occlusive disease of the donor iliac artery in the fem-fem bypass can result in steal, from which ischemia develops in the previously asymptomatic donor leg.

Infrainguinal Occlusive Disease. Patients with superficial femoral or proximal popliteal occlusion in whom the arteries distal to the popliteal area are patent might be candidates for a femoral-popliteal bypass. When a femoral-popliteal bypass is not possible, a more distal bypass to the posterior tibial, anterior tibial, or peroneal arteries can be considered. The patency and limb salvage rates for inframalleolar revascularization are comparable to those obtained with femoral popliteal or femoral tibial bypasses. The dorsalis pedis bypass is beneficial for patients with diabetes whose occlusive disease commonly involves the tibial and peroneal vessels and spares the inframalleolar circulation.

Other Measures (p. 1292)

Sympathectomy. Limbs with inoperable arterial disease, ischemic cutaneous ulceration, pain at rest, or pregangrenous changes can be considered for sympathetic denervation. The primary effect of sympathectomy seems to be enhancing pain relief rather than augmenting blood flow to the ischemic limb. A diabetic neuropathy can commonly cause autosympathectomy. It is imperative to document the presence of sympathetic nerve function with neuroautonomic testing or a temporary sympathetic block before proceeding with surgical sympathectomy.

Intermittent Venous Occlusion/Pneumatic EndDiastolic Leg Compression. Skin blood flow, as reflected by $TcPO_2$, can be augmented acutely in ischemic limbs by intermittent venous occlusion with an externally applied inflatable cuff. The mechanism proposed to explain the increased flow is analogous to the pumping action of the calf muscle during walking. A cuff is strapped to the leg and connected to a compressor that rapidly inflates the cuff with air, delivering a short pulse of 80 to 100 mm Hg every 20 seconds. Other devices, which apply intermittent circumferential pneumatic compression to the foot or lower limb during cardiac diastole, show promise as adjunct measures to augment limb perfusion.

Amputation. With advances in limb salvage procedures, it is important to review carefully the risk-to-benefit and cost-to-benefit ratios with the patient before each intervention. Although in the later stage of disease each patient has a choice between amputation or delay, the choices often are a relatively pain free, comfortable prosthesis or salvage of a painful, ulcerated, or gangrenous foot. Most patients choose a shorter procedure enabling them to spend as much as possible of their remaining lives in comfort.

VENOUS DISEASE (pp. 1292–1296)

Epidemiology (pp. 1292–1296)

• More than 250,000 new cases of DVT occur each year, resulting in approximately 500,000 patients presenting for the treatment of venous stasis ulcers.

Etiology and Pathogenesis (pp. 1293–1294)

Venous Thromboembolism (p. 1293)

• Thrombi commonly arise from clots that form in the cusps of venous valves and propagate into the major venous channel. Many small venous thrombi fortunately undergo rapid thrombolytic dissolution. For large thrombi, organization begins after 3 to 4 days. Recanalization can require a period of several months or more. Usually, but not always, venous valves are destroyed or lose their normal function as a fibrotic process thickens the venous wall and cusp. Superficial venous thrombosis alone is not thought to have any serious morbidity unless a saphenous vein thrombus propagates and involves the common femoral vein.

• Risk factors associated with the development of acute DVT include prior history of DVT, immobilization, postoperative state, age (older than 40 years), cardiac disease, limb trauma, post-thrombotic state or coagulation abnormalities, hormonal therapy, pregnancy and postpartum state, obesity, and advanced neoplasm. A complete medical workup should be done for any patient with an unexplained deep or superficial venous thrombosis to rule out cancer, inflammatory bowel disease, blood dyscrasias, or intrinsic clotting disease.

Chronic Venous Insufficiency (pp. 1293–1294)

• Many factors can result in the development of venous insufficiency including heredity, local trauma, thrombosis, and intrinsic defects in the veins or valves themselves. The venous system of the lower extremity is divided into three groups: (1) the superficial veins (great and small saphenous veins and their tributaries) (Fig. 56–1); (2) the perforating (communicating) veins, which connect the superficial venous system with the deep venous system; and (3) the deep veins, which are supported externally by a strong fascial layer and the surrounding musculature.

• Venous flow is based on a force that pushes the blood proximally (e.g., gravity or the calf muscle), an adequate outflow, and the presence of competent valves limiting reflux. Any disruption of these components results in chronic venous hypertension. Venous insufficiency develops only when the valves in the perforator or deep veins are incompetent. Ultimately, venous hypertension is the result of valve damage and retrograde venous blood flow to the superficial veins. Retrograde flow can occur with (1) faulty communication and superficial venous valves; (2) damage to the deep vein valves; (3) deep vein occlusion; and (4) muscle dysfunction and pump failure from fibrosis, neuropathies, and inflammatory disease.

• Chronic venous insufficiency is usually the result of congenital or acquired valvular incompetence and, less commonly, obstruction of the veins. Post-thrombotic syndrome (venous occlusion and/or valve destruction after thrombosis) develops in 67% to 80% of patients after DVT.

• The true mechanism by which venous hypertension leads to induration and fibrosis of the skin (lipodermosclerosis) and ulceration remains unclear. It is apparent, however, that venous hypertension sets the stage for adverse conditions that eventually lead to skin damage and impaired healing.

History and Clinical Findings (p. 1294)

Venous Thromboembolism (p. 1294)

• Relevant history includes the patient's symptoms or presence of potential risk factors. Clinical findings associated with DVT include pain, tenderness, unilat-

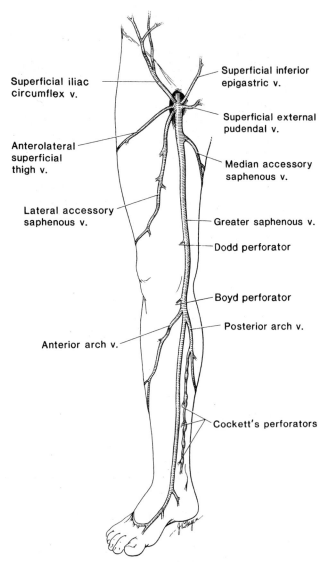

FIGURE 56–1. Normal anatomy of the greater saphenous vein and its tributaries. (Courtesy of Mayo Foundation.)

eral ankle or calf edema, palpable induration or cord, and pain produced by extreme dorsiflexion of the foot. Unfortunately, most clinical signs and symptoms attributed to DVT have a poor predictive value for determining the presence or absence of DVT. It is therefore essential to perform objective testing (e.g., ultrasound duplex scanning) when DVT is suspected.

Chronic Venous Insufficiency (p. 1294)

• A complete history and clinical examination are ordinarily sufficient to diagnose venous insufficiency and to determine whether it involves the superficial, deep, or perforating veins individually or in combination. Symptoms of chronic venous insufficiency are highly variable and depend on the degree and duration of insufficiency. Patients generally note aching, edema, skin changes, decreased activity tolerance, and progressive leg pain with prolonged standing. If the patient states that the symptoms are unrelieved by leg elevation, especially overnight, the diagnosis of venous insufficiency should be questioned. The earliest sign of chronic venous insufficiency is edema of the lower legs. Early in the disease, intermittent soft pitting edema is present, but fibrosis eventually develops and the skin demonstrates firm induration. Pigmentation develops next, especially in the medial perimalleolar areas. A weepy pruritic dermatitis can develop, and recurrent secondary cellulitis is a fairly common complication. Chronic venous insufficiency results in chronic edema, scarring, obliteration of cutaneous lymphatics, decreased skin integrity, hemosiderin deposition (with brownish discoloration), dermatitis, and ulceration.

Vascular Testing (pp. 1294–1295)

• Although the evaluation of venous disease is accomplished principally with the history and physical examination, noninvasive testing modalities can complement these examinations (Table 56–2).

TABLE 56–2 Noninvasive Vascular Studies Used to Diagnose Venous Disease, Lymphedema, Arteriovenous Fistula, and Arteriovenous Malformation Fistula

Vascular Disease	Anatomic	Hemodynamic/ Functional	Disadvantages
Venous insufficiency	Continuous wave Doppler		Operator dependent
		Exercise venous plethysmography	
Obstruction	Duplex ultrasonography Continuous wave Doppler	Duplex ultrasonography	Expense Operator dependent
		Strain gauge outflow plethysmography	Limited availability
		Impedance plethysmography	Variable accuracy
Lymphedema	Duplex ultrasonography	Duplex ultrasonography Lymphoscintigraphy	Expense
Arteriovenous fistula		Continuous wave Doppler	
Arteriovenous malformation	Magnetic resonance imaging	Pulse volume recording	Poor reproducibility Expense

Impedance Plethysmography (p. 1294)
• Impedance plethysmography assesses volume changes at rest produced by a proximal, pneumatic, veno-occlusive cuff. The normal leg swells when a veno-occlusive tourniquet is placed and rapidly returns to its normal size when the tourniquet is released. In the presence of a proximal lower-extremity DVT, the cuff is inflated, there is little additional increase in venous volume, and after tourniquet release the return to baseline is delayed.

Exercise Venous Plethysmography (p. 1295)
• Lower limb venous function is tested by performing a plethysmographic evaluation of limb volume before, during, and after exercise. In a normal individual, plethysmography shows a progressive decrease in leg volume during exercise followed by a period after exercise when the volume slowly returns to normal. In venous insufficiency, the exercise-induced decrease in venous volume is less than expected. In addition, when venous incompetence is present, the postexercise return in volume will be more rapid than expected. Exercise venous plethysmography provides a quick and relatively inexpensive way to yield quantitative information about the severity of venous insufficiency that is not readily obtained with other noninvasive methods.

Duplex Scanning (p. 1295)
• Duplex scanning is used to diagnose deep or superficial venous thrombosis, assess venous incompetence, and map the superficial veins before surgical harvest for bypass operations. The diagnosis of venous thrombosis can be established by demonstrating noncompressibility of the vein with use of real-time, two-dimensional, B-mode imaging. The pulsed-wave Doppler confirms the lack of venous flow and provides indirect evidence that spontaneous flow through the vein has disappeared (by the absence of phasic changes with respiration or the reduction or absence of augmentation). Duplex scanning can also document the presence of venous incompetence, identify the anatomic sites involved, and quantify the severity.

Treatment (pp. 1295–1296)

Superficial Thrombophlebitis (pp. 1295–1296)
• Superficial thrombophlebitis is treated with elevation and superficial heat. Appropriate compressive stockings, 30 to 40 mm Hg, should be worn when ambulating. Aspirin or nonsteroidal anti-inflammatory medications can be administered for pain relief. If the process extends near the saphenofemoral junction, a duplex examination should clarify the status of the deep veins.

Deep Venous Thrombosis (p. 1296)
• Standard therapy for acute DVT consists of anticoagulation, bed rest, elevation, and support of the extremity (Table 56–3).

Chronic Venous Insufficiency (p. 1296)
PATIENT EDUCATION
• Patient education is important in the management of chronic venous insufficiency. Patients must understand the disease process and the correct use of measures to decrease edema. The first step of treatment should be to reduce the venous pressure. When elevation is used for edema control, the extremity must

TABLE 56–3 Initial Treatment[1] of Acute DVT

Method	Agent	Duration of Rx
Conventional	IV Heparin	5+ days[2]
Outpatient	Subcutaneous low-molecular-weight heparin	5+ days[2]
Lytic	IV: Urokinase	1–3 days
	Streptokinase	
	TPA	

[1]All patients with DVT/PE need to have "Initial Treatment" followed by 3–6 months of coumadin.
[2]Heparin and coumadin must be overlapped a minimum of 5 days.

be elevated above the level of the heart. The optimal duration and frequency of leg elevations are not known but should be tailored to the severity of disease.

COMPRESSION
• Compressive dressings aid venous return by compressing the leg and increasing the interstitial tension. With no history of congestive heart failure and no evidence of venous obstruction on noninvasive studies, lower extremity volume can be stabilized with an intermittent pneumatic compression pump. Compressive wraps should be used between pumping sessions. After the volume stabilizes, the patient can be measured for stockings. Greatest patient compliance is achieved by prescribing knee-length, graduated elastic compression stockings with a pressure gradient of 30 to 40 mm Hg. In patients with concomitant arterial disease, lower compression might be required to avoid further compromise of arterial inflow by the extrinsic compression.

EXERCISE
• The value of exercise in the management of chronic venous insufficiency has not been conclusively demonstrated. Exercises involving the leg musculature (e.g., walking, bicycling, and swimming) promote muscle tone in the calf and enhance venous return. Exercise, however, produces variable reductions in venous hypertension.

MEDICATION
• Pentoxifylline reduces leukocyte adhesiveness and the release of oxygen-free radicals and has been shown to be effective in the treatment of venous leg ulcers in early trials.

SURGERY
• Surgical intervention for chronic venous insufficiency can include ligation of perforators, direct valve repair, vein segment transposition, or axillary valve autotransplantation.

SCLEROTHERAPY
• Sclerotherapy (which uses the injection of an irritant substance into the vein) can also be used to obliterate incompetent veins in certain settings. Sclerotherapy is used for the treatment of spider veins, small distal varicose veins, and venous insufficiency resulting from superficial and perforator incompetence. Elastic compression is suggested for at least 6 weeks after treatment. Complications are rare and usually minor.

LYMPHATIC DISEASE (pp. 1296–1298)

Etiology (pp. 1296–1297)

• Lymphedema is the abnormal accumulation of water and protein in the skin and subcutaneous tissues. Primary lymphedema is caused by aplastic or hypoplastic lymphatic trunks. Secondary lymphedema can occur after recurrent infection; tumor; lymphoproliferative disease; or injury to the lymphatic system stemming from surgical excision, trauma, or irradiation. Without treatment, the protein-rich interstitial fluid is replaced by fibrinoid material. Inflammatory cells accumulate and progressive fibrosis, sclerosis, and (in the final stage) elephantiasis develop. Lymphangiosarcoma, a severe late complication of secondary lymphedema, is rare.

History and Clinical Findings (p. 1297)

• For evaluation of a swollen limb, it is important to determine the underlying diagnosis. Malignancy or metastatic disease must be excluded. Peripheral examination of the limb with lymphedema helps to differentiate it from other causes of peripheral edema. The edema usually involves the dorsal forefoot but spares the metatarsal phalangeal joint. Dark pigmentary changes of the skin, prominent veins, and ulceration are unusual.

Evaluation (p. 1297)

• Lymphoscintigraphy provides a functional assessment of lymph transport capacity and identifies major morphologic abnormalities of the lymphatic system. If venous disease is in question, noninvasive studies of the venous system should be obtained, including impedance plethysmography or duplex scanning. Magnetic resonance or computerized tomographic imaging may be needed to evaluate for malignancy or other problems.

Treatment (pp. 1297–1298)

• The goals of treatment for lymphedema are to preserve skin integrity, soften subcutaneous tissues, avoid lymphangiitis, reduce limb size, and avoid contracture. In severe lymphedema, hospitalization can be required for 2 or 3 days to control limb volume with bed rest and a lymphedema sling.

Compression (p. 1297)

• The use of compression in the management of lymphedema consists of pneumatic single-chamber compression at 60 to 80 mm Hg, or sequential compression at 80 to 130 mm Hg as tolerated, used twice daily for 3 or 4 days until the volume is stabilized.

• Manual decongestive massage and isometric exercises are used to increase venous and lymphatic flow and reduce edema. The patient is instructed in a program of bandaging, elevation, and exercise to be done between treatments.

• After reduction of edema, new fluid will accumulate in the tissue space unless the volume is restricted by external support. This support is commonly supplied by compressive bandages or stockings. Elastic graded-compression stockings are prescribed at 30 to 40 or at 40 to 50 mm Hg. The patient should be supplied

with two pairs to allow cleaning of one pair while wearing the other. Selective refractory patients can benefit from simultaneously using two compressive stockings, 40 to 50 mm Hg and 50 to 60 mm Hg.
• The patient must be instructed in meticulous skin care to avoid fungal infection or injury. Long-sleeved shirts or pants should be worn to avoid insect bites, cuts, or abrasions. Needle sticks or intravenous lines should never be permitted in the lymphedematous extremity. Patients should avoid exposure to extreme temperatures (e.g., a hot tub). A general conditioning program and weight loss are encouraged.

Medications (p. 1298)
• Any evidence of infection needs immediate treatment. The cause of cellulitis is almost always group A streptococci. If the patient has no allergies, penicillin is the drug of choice.
• Benzopyrones can reduce the volume of high-protein edema by stimulating proteolysis, but are not available for use in North America. Flavonoids (benzo-[γ]pyrone) are available and can be beneficial in the treatment of lymphedema, although gastric irritation can be a problem.
• The use of diuretics in the management of lymphedema is controversial. With chronic use, these agents generally become ineffective. Diuretics can be used for temporary relief in severe lymphedema or to provide symptomatic relief for patients with a terminal malignancy.

Surgery (p. 1298)
• Surgery for lymphedema is indicated in only a small percentage of patients. Excisional operations are aimed at removing excess tissue to decrease the volume of the extremity. Physiologic operations consist of lymphatic-to-lymphatic or lymphatic-to-venous anastomosis, which, it is hoped, will improve drainage. None of these operations is considered curative.

ARTERIOVENOUS FISTULAS AND ARTERIOVENOUS MALFORMATION (pp. 1298–1299)

Etiology (p. 1298)

• Vascular malformations are classified as either congenital or acquired. Acquired arteriovenous fistulae result from surgical construction of angioaccess for dialysis, penetrating injuries, infection, neoplasm, and aneurysmal erosion.

History and Clinical Findings (p. 1298)

• A history of penetrating trauma should promote a high index of suspicion of possible acquired arteriovenous fistula. In the acute phase, a pulsating hematoma, palpable thrill, and bruit are present. If pulses are decreased or absent and the distal systolic pressure is low, a large-volume shunt is indicated. In rare instances, the amount of blood siphoned by the fistula can produce heart failure, peripheral ischemia, or gangrene.
• Ischemia can develop after fistula construction for dialysis in a patient with preexisting arterial disease. Clinical findings include pain, paresthesias, and muscular weakness in the affected extremity, which become more prominent during dialysis.

Evaluation (pp. 1298–1299)

• The same diagnostic studies used to evaluate chronic arterial occlusive disease in the extremities, and to a lesser extent venous insufficiency, can provide useful information about the fistula. Continuous-wave Doppler shows a high-flow, low-resistance pattern with loss of endsystolic reversal and considerable flow continuing throughout diastole.

• Magnetic resonance imaging is the best technique to evaluate patients with congenital vascular malformations. It defines hypertrophy of bone, muscle, or subcutaneous tissue and images varicose veins and hemangiomas in the subcutaneous space and muscles.

Treatment (p. 1299)

• Early recognition and management of an acquired arteriovenous fistula are preferred. Management of large, chronic arteriovenous fistulae is complicated. Bleeding can be profuse from multiple arterial and venous collateral vessels in the area. Elastic support is beneficial to treat symptoms of chronic venous insufficiency. Appropriate footwear is important to accommodate limb hypertrophy and compensate for leg-length discrepancy. Physical therapy intervention should maintain mobility and preserve a normal gait pattern. Orthopedic intervention can be beneficial to avoid or correct leg-length discrepancy.

VASCULAR WOUNDS (pp. 1299–1303)

Etiology (p. 1299)

• Nonhealing vascular wounds result from (1) ischemia, (2) venous insufficiency, and (3) neuropathy.

History and Clinical Findings (pp. 1299–1300)

Ischemic (p. 1299)

• Ischemic ulcers typically result from a minor laceration, abrasion, or pressure in a distal limb with compromised blood flow. Ulcers below the ankle with a pale or gray, nongranulating base are usually the result of major arterial insufficiency. Simultaneous appearance of livedo reticularis and cutaneous toe infarcts suggests atheromatous embolization, but these conditions can occur less commonly in periarteritis nodosa, systemic lupus erythematosus, or livedoid vasculitis. Small vessel ischemic ulcers are usually located on the leg and have areas of cutaneous infarction that coalesce and proceed to ulceration.

Venous (p. 1299)

• With a history of chronic venous insufficiency, clinical findings include edema, hyperpigmentation, and soft tissue fibrosis. Ulcers are typically located on the medial perimalleolar area of the lower extremity. Upper extremity ulcerations are not caused by chronic venous insufficiency unless an arteriovenous fistula is present.

Neuropathic (p. 1300)

• In patients with a history of autonomic and peripheral neuropathy, clinical findings can include decreased perspiration, dry skin, dependent rubor, impaired sensation, and denervation of foot intrinsic muscles with associated clawfoot deformity. Charcot changes can be present. Ulcers are typically located at the metatarsal heads, pulp or tip of a rigid great toe, lateral surface of the foot at the base of the metatarsal, heel, or midfoot. Neuropathic ulcers are characteristically painless and rimmed by callus; they can be present for years before the patient seeks medical consultation.

Treatment (pp. 1301–1303)

Debridement (p. 1301)
• Simple sharp debridement using topical lidocaine and occasionally surgical debridement might be necessary. Necrotic debris not only causes a foreign body reaction, but also provides an ideal environment for microorganisms. Wounds with a small amount of superficial necrotic tissue can be mechanically debrided gently using saline moistened coarse mesh gauze. Enzymatic agents can help loosen a large eschar to facilitate sharp debridement. Whirlpool, shower cart, or pulsed-water (Waterpik) debridement can be useful adjuncts for ongoing debridement of large ulcers.
• Indications for surgical debridement include the presence of a draining sinus, an infected nongranulating ulcer, an abscess, osteomyelitis, necrotic abscess formation, exposed nonviable tissue, and exposed nongranulating cartilage or bone surface. Although bone scans are generally used to diagnose osteomyelitis, in some cases magnetic resonance imaging may be more sensitive for detecting the early bone changes of osteomyelitis.
• Caution must be used to limit the debridement to devitalized tissue. It is important to evaluate the arterial supply carefully before sharp debridement. If the blood supply is inadequate, the margin of debridement is at risk for necrosis. With distal ischemia (dry gangrene) in a patient who is not a candidate for debridement or distal amputation, management can include protection of the extremity while awaiting demarcation and subsequent autoamputation in the affected region.

Wound Care Products (pp. 1301–1302)
• Many products are available for the treatment of wounds, but formal protocols are needed to evaluate the efficacy and cost of most. The faster rate of healing observed in wounds that are kept moist has been attributed to the avoidance of tissue injury during dressing removal and the fact that desiccation of the wound inhibits epithelialization. Dressings that promote lysis of necrotic tissue and fibrin can facilitate the release of growth factors and reduce time to healing.
• With any wound care product, the skin surrounding the wound should be monitored for erythema, swelling, pain, or maceration. Erythema, swelling, and pain might be caused by unrelieved pressure or adverse reactions to wound care treatments.

Hyperbaric Oxygen Therapy (p. 1302)
• Although enhanced wound healing is a postulated benefit of adjunctive therapy with hyperbaric oxygen, the paucity of randomized controlled trials makes it difficult to assess the efficacy of hyperbaric oxygen.

Electrical Stimulation (p. 1302)
• Electrical stimulation has been demonstrated to enhance wound healing through effects on blood flow, edema reduction, antibacterial properties, cellu-

lar migration, fibroblast activity, and wound tensile strength. The ideal parameters for clinical use have not yet been fully determined.

Vacuum (p. 1302)
• Polyvinyl foam under negative pressure using a vacuum has recently been shown to facilitate granulation tissue production while maintaining a relatively clean wound bed.

Protective Footwear (p. 1303)
• After the infection has been contained, edema controlled, and necessary revascularization performed, it is important to arrange for proper protective footwear. Total-contact casting has been shown to be beneficial for the treatment of neuropathic ulcers. A custom total-contact, bivalved polypropylene ankle-foot orthosis (AFO) with custom foot bed has been tried recently. It is indicated if patients are unable to return for cast changes, or if the referring physician desires continued access to the wound. When either a total-contact cast or a custom bivalved AFO is used, footwear on the sound side must be adjusted to avoid a leg-length discrepancy. After initial healing, a total-contact sandal with a custom foot bed of moderate density, closed-cell, polyethylene foam and poron (PPT) interface can be fabricated. The patient wears this sandal for approximately 2 weeks until proceeding with definitive footwear. Definitive footwear includes an extra-depth shoe and a moderate-density inlay. A rocker-bottom sole can help to further dissipate the forces of ambulation.

57

Original Chapter by Theresa A. Gillis, M.D., and Fae H. Garden, M.D.

Principles of Cancer Rehabilitation

DEFINING THE NEED FOR CANCER REHABILITATION (p. 1305)

• Cancer survivors often face significant physical and psychosocial problems that adversely influence their quality of life. Significant problems in activities of daily living (ADL) and vocational pursuits were also reported (see Fig. 57–2 in the Textbook). It has been estimated that up to 50% of persons with cancer may meet the diagnostic criteria for clinical depression.

TYPES OF CANCER REHABILITATION (pp. 1305–1306)

• The goal of *preventive rehabilitation therapy* is to achieve maximal function in patients considered to be cured or in remission. For patients whose cancer is progressing, the goals of *supportive rehabilitation therapy* include providing adaptive self-care equipment in an attempt to offset what can be a steady decline in the patient's functional skills. *Palliative rehabilitation therapy* goals are to improve or maintain comfort and function during the terminal stages of the disease.

CAUSES AND MANAGEMENT OF FUNCTIONAL IMPAIRMENT IN CANCER PATIENTS (pp. 1306–1309)

Complications of Disuse and Bed Rest (p. 1306)

• Special issues in the cancer patient include the side effects of chemotherapy, especially from therapy with cardiotoxic drugs. When possible, a conditioning program started prior to cancer treatment is advisable (see Chapter 34).

Nutritional Concerns of Cancer Patients (pp. 1306–1307)

Diet (pp. 1306–1307)
• The value and benefit of nutrition is generally recognized in the medical management and rehabilitation of cancer patients, and many cancer patients place appetite and ability to eat at the top of the list of items determining their sense of physical well-being. The comprehensive cancer treatment team should include a registered dietitian.

• Caloric intake should generally be between 115% and 130% of resting energy expenditure. Protein needs range from 1.5 to 2.5 g/kg/day. The impact of various surgical procedures on the nutritional status of cancer patients is summarized in Table 57–1.

Radiation Effects (p. 1307)
• Treatments to the head and neck area can produce alterations in taste and in saliva production. Distortion of food temperature and texture sensations can occur from radiation changes to the oral mucosa. Swallowing difficulties can result as well (see Chapter 26).
• Radiation treatments delivered to the stomach and intestines often lead acutely to nausea, vomiting, cramps, and diarrhea. Chronic complications include partial or complete intestinal obstruction, intestinal perforation, gastrointestinal bleeding, malabsorption, and enteral fistulas.
• Attempts to feed patients who have sustained radiation damage to the intestines usually begin with lactose-free, low-residue oral diets and progress to enteral feedings or parenteral nutrition in more refractory cases. Parenteral nutrition is recommended for patients who have lost 20% or more of their body weight.

Chemotherapy Effects (p. 1307)
• The rapidly reproducing cells of the bone marrow and gastrointestinal tract are vulnerable to the effects of chemotherapy as well. Nausea, vomiting, and anorexia are common initial gastrointestinal side effects. Severe and recurrent vomiting may cause vitamin B_1 deficiency, with resultant beriberi. The late effects of chemotherapy include stomatitis, mucosal ulceration, cheilosis, glossitis, and pharyngitis.

TABLE 57–1 Potential Adverse Effects of Various Surgical Procedures on Nutrition in Cancer Patients

Procedure	Potential Adverse Effect
Neck dissection/glossectomy	Impaired mastication
	Impaired swallowing
	Impaired taste
	Impaired smell
Esophageal resection with vagotomy	Gastric stasis
	Diarrhea
	Steatorrhea
Pancreatomy	Diabetes mellitus
	Impaired digestion
Bowel resection	Malabsorption (short bowel syndrome)
	Vitamin deficiency (B_{12}, D, A)
Gastrectomy	Impaired digestion
	Malabsorption
	Megaloblastic anemia
	Hypoglycemia

- Numerous nutritional deficiencies can result from the use of antimetabolite drugs such as methotrexate. This drug inhibits folic acid metabolism, which is necessary for the synthesis of DNA. This inhibition causes a folic acid deficiency that results in macrocytic anemia, leukopenia, and an ulcerative stomatitis.
- The antimetabolites 5-fluorouracil and 6-mercaptopurine prevent nucleic acid synthesis by interfering with thiamine in DNA synthesis. Clinical signs of thiamine deficiency can be noted in the lips and oral cavity.
- Vitamin K deficiency results from long-term treatment with antibiotics such as moxalactam disodium, which can result in ecchymosis and a pronounced bleeding tendency.

Learned Food Aversion (p. 1307)
- During the course of cancer treatment, patients often reject specific foods or certain flavors. Although the exact mechanism for learned food aversion is unknown, it has been described as a variant of classical conditioning.
- Aggressive intervention to correct nutrient deficiencies and to maintain good nutritional status should be ongoing throughout the rehabilitation process. The use of appetite-stimulating drugs such as megestrol can improve quality of life in cancer patients with anorexia. When needed, enteral or parenteral feeding supplementation is useful in preventing weight loss, malnutrition, dehydration, and weakness.

Sexual Function in the Cancer Patient (pp. 1307–1308)
- Sexual partners can contribute to sexual dysfunction by fostering dependent role changes or reacting in a negative way to the patient's physical disfigurement. Economic stress caused by the treatment can lead to marital problems that are expressed by avoidance of sexual contact.

Concerns of Women (pp. 1307–1308)
- Although mastectomy has no direct physical effect on a woman's sexual response, the emotional effects of the procedure can have a profound negative impact. Fear of partner rejection can lead to avoidance of sexual intercourse. Encouraging partners to resume sexual activity as early as possible helps break this cycle.
- Women who have undergone pelvic surgery can feel a sense of guilt related to a false belief that sexual intercourse contributed to their disease. Fear of disease recurrence can cause these women to avoid resumption of sexual activity.
- Regardless of a patient's age, the loss of fertility can precipitate a grief reaction. Presurgical preparation and counseling can reduce some of the psychodynamic causes of sexual dysfunction.
- The side effects of chemotherapy and radiation therapy include nausea, fatigue, hair loss, and weight changes. These, along with hormonal depletion, can produce additional psychological and physical impediments to resuming sexual relationships.

Concerns of Men (p. 1308)
- Surgical treatment of prostate cancer can cause damage to the vascular or nerve pathways, resulting in impotence, retrograde ejaculation, or infertility. Orchiectomy has obvious hormonal and reproductive implications. Preoperative

and pretreatment discussions of reproductive concerns should include consideration of sperm banking if permanent sterilization is anticipated.
• Pelvic and abdominal radiation can produce fatigue, diarrhea, and erectile dysfunction. Irradiation of the urethra can cause painful ejaculation. The effects of chemotherapy can adversely affect self-image, libido, and sexual performance. Sexual rehabilitation can include the use of erectile assistive devices and surgical reconstruction of the penis.

Neuropsychological Abnormalities (p. 1308)

• The neurobehavioral abnormalities found in tumor patients range from subtle problems with attention and motivation to frank delirium and clouding of consciousness. These deficits can be either primary, because of the tumor; or secondary, caused by the treatment. They can also result from chronic illness, depression, or immobility.

Primary Tumor Effects (p. 1308)
• Patients with brain tumors can have milder cognitive deficits and greater variability in the nature and extent of these deficits than patients with strokes in similar anatomical sites. Even after extensive surgical resection of brain tissue, patients with slow-growing tumors often do not demonstrate neuropsychological deficits, perhaps because of a reorganization of cognitive functions to other brain regions.
• Patients with rapidly growing tumors (e.g., glioblastoma multiforme) exhibit behavioral and cognitive deficits secondary to rapid destruction of white matter tracts, increased intracranial pressure, and metabolic deficits.
• Improvements in cognitive and physical function have been noted in brain tumor patients receiving 10 mg of methylphenidate twice daily. Patients receiving this dosage showed increased stamina and motivation to perform activities in our center.

Radiation Effects (p. 1308)
• Additional effects on neuropsychological functioning can occur as a result of radiation therapy. The acute effects of radiation (during the time of treatment) are mostly symptomatic (e.g., headache and nausea).
• Subacute effects can occur 1 to 4 months after therapy is completed. At this time a reversible demyelination occurs in approximately 14% of brain tumor patients. It is only by a gradual improvement in functional status during the ensuing 4 months that these symptoms can be distinguished from those caused by early tumor recurrence. Delayed effects of radiation treatment can manifest 6 months to a year after therapy.
• The therapeutic dose of radiation for brain tumors can cause necrosis within 6 months of treatment. Most of these lesions develop within the white matter of the forebrain. In addition to focal necrosis, the delayed effects of brain irradiation can include atrophy, calcification, necrotizing leukoencephalopathy, aneurysms, and the formation of secondary cancers.

Chemotherapy Effects (p. 1308)
• Chemotherapy, once believed to cause only early and reversible effects on cognition, is now recognized to be able to cause marked and prolonged neurobe-

havioral deficits. It is estimated that as many as 18% of neurologically normal cancer patients who have received chemotherapy have cognitive deficits 3 weeks after therapy is discontinued. Deficits include impairments in visual-perceptive abilities, verbal memory, and judgment. Survivors of brain tumors who have received multimodality therapy (chemotherapy plus radiation) can have more profound impairments of intellectual function than those who receive single-modality treatment.

Cancer Pain (pp. 1308–1309)

Defining the Problem (p. 1308)
• The World Health Organization (WHO) estimates that 25% of all cancer patients die with unrelieved pain. Up to 60% of patients at all stages of the disease process experience significant pain. Most of this pain can be adequately relieved by oral analgesics. Unrelieved pain can be a risk factor for suicide in cancer patients.

Etiology (p. 1308)
• Cancer pain can result from direct tumor invasion of pain-sensitive tissues or can be secondary to treatment or diagnostic procedures (Table 57–2). It can also be unrelated to any of these factors.

TABLE 57–2 Causes of Treatment-Related Pain in Cancer Patients

Chemotherapy-related pain
    Oral mucositis
    Peripheral neuropathy
    Acute and chronic herpetic pain
    Osteonecrosis secondary to steroids
    Pseudorheumatism
Radiation-related pain
    Osteoradionecrosis
    Myelopathy
    Brachial plexopathy
    Lumbar plexopathy
    Radiation-induced peripheral nerve tumors
Postsurgical pain
    Postmastectomy
    Postnephrectomy
    Postthoracotomy
    Postradical neck dissection
    Residual limb and phantom limb
Procedure-related pain
    Bone marrow biopsy
    Bone biopsy
    Lumbar puncture and spinal headache
    Venipuncture

From Campa JA, Payne R: Pain syndromes due to cancer treatment. In Patt R (ed): Cancer Pain. Philadelphia, JB Lippincott, 1993, p. 42.

Treatment (pp. 1308–1309)

• Opioid agonists do not exhibit ceiling effects. Dosing is guided by efficacy and is limited by side effects. Long-acting oral preparations, particularly sustained-release morphine, are commonly used. Breakthrough pain can be treated with immediate-release "rescue doses" of morphine. Patients with moderate to severe pain requiring opioid therapy for more than a few days can be treated with a long-acting semisynthetic narcotic such as oxycodone hydrochloride. The recommended initial dose of oxycodone hydrochloride is 10 mg every 12 hours in patients not already taking opioid medications. A 5-mg immediate-release dosage is also available for breakthrough pain. Transdermal fentanyl provides an alternative method of analgesia with a longer duration for a given dose. It takes up to 24 hours for blood concentrations of fentanyl to stabilize after the application of a patch. Although oral administration is preferred, transdermal, rectal, and intravenous routes are indicated in some patients. Spinal routes, both epidural and intrathecal, can be employed with internal delivery systems that allow patients to be fully ambulatory. Children often need larger doses of opioids to achieve adequate pain relief.

• Tolerance to analgesia is an infrequent problem and is usually managed by changing doses or agents. Physical dependence develops with chronic opioid use.

• *Addiction,* defined as a behavioral syndrome of compulsive, harmful use not requiring the existence of physical dependence or tolerance, is not likely to occur in patients without a substance abuse history. The autonomic symptoms of withdrawal can be partly alleviated by the use of transdermal clonidine.

• Adjuvant drugs include antidepressants, anticonvulsants, benzodiazepines, neuroleptics, psychostimulants, antihistamines, corticosteroids, and calcitonin. These medications are chosen to supplement analgesics for their specific secondary effects or to treat side effects.

• Radiation therapy can also be highly effective in treating pain by shrinking the tumor mass.

• A significant number of patients whose pain does not respond to oral therapy might be helped by anesthetic procedures such as nerve blocks. Surgical ablation of nervous structures by procedures such as rhizotomy or cordotomy can also play a role in pain relief for certain patients. There is, however, a risk of developing a delayed pain syndrome following such surgical deafferentation.

• Deafferentation pain can be caused by a loss of normal sensory input when a peripheral nerve is severed or involved by tumor. Transcutaneous electrical nerve stimulation can provide some patients with relief. In addition, carefully selected patients might also benefit from surgical implantation of stimulation devices.

LATE EFFECTS OF CANCER TREATMENT (pp. 1309–1311)

Effects of Radiation Therapy (pp. 1309–1311)

Myelopathy (pp. 1309–1310)

• The most common form of radiation-induced spinal cord injury is a transient myelopathy that occurs in patients being treated for head and neck tumors or lymphoma. The syndrome typically develops after a latent period of 1 to 30 months, with a peak onset at 4 to 6 months. The clinical onset is marked by electrical shock sensations or paresthesias that radiate from the cervical spine to the extremities. The paresthesias are typically symmetrical and do not follow a dermatomal distribution. Myelography and computed tomography (CT) are typically negative, and the syndrome usually resolves in 1 to 9 months. The occurrence of transient radiation myelopathy does not put a person at a higher risk for the development of more severe delayed radiation-induced myelopathy.

• Delayed myelopathy is an irreversible condition with a reported incidence of 1% to 12%. The onset of symptoms usually occurs 9 to 18 months after completion of treatment, with most cases identified within 30 months. The latent period for delayed myelopathy decreases with increased radiation dose and is shortened in children. The onset of symptoms usually begins with lower extremity paresthesias, followed by sphincter dysfunction and weakness. A partial Brown-Séquard syndrome consisting of sensory changes on one side and motor weakness or pyramidal tract signs on the opposite side can develop below the level of the injury. Functional deficits typically occur progressively and depend, for the most part, on the level of neurological injury. A central pain syndrome can be present in up to 20% of patients with radiation myelopathy. Patients typically note pain in their midback region and dysesthetic sensations in their lower extremities. Central pain syndrome may show some clinical response to treatment with tricyclic antidepressant, steroid, or anticonvulsant medications.

Plexopathy (pp. 1310–1311)

• Brachial plexopathy is a well-recognized complication of radiotherapy in patients with breast, lung, and mediastinal tumors, as well as lymphoma and other neoplasms. The latent period between the end of radiotherapy and the appearance of clinical symptoms ranges from 1 month to 15 years. Chemotherapy can enhance the radiation-induced effects on nerve tissue and decrease the latency period for the development of plexopathy. The predominant initial symptoms are paresthesias and pain (Table 57–3). Clinical signs include sensory loss, decreased or absent reflexes, and weakness.

• Lumbosacral plexopathy is reported less commonly than brachial plexopathy but can occur in patients with colorectal and gynecological tumors who undergo

TABLE 57–3   Differential Diagnosis Between Cancerous and Postradiation Brachial Plexopathies

Parameter	Cancerous	Postradiation
Incidence	10 times more common	Dose-related
Initial symptom	Pain 90%	Numbness, paresthesia, pain in less than 20%
Signs	Predominantly lower trunk	Predominantly upper trunk
Progression rate	Slow	Insidious, self-limiting
Latency	Months to over 20 yr; mean: several years	
Tumor progression	CT: focal lesions in over 90%	CT: loss of planes, no focal lesions
EMG		Myokymia

Abbreviations: EMG, electromyography; CT, computed tomography. From Hildebrand J: Lesions of the peripheral nervous system. In Hildebrand J (ed): Management in Neuro-Oncology. Berlin, Springer-Verlag, 1992, p. 80.

radiation therapy. Symptoms often present bilaterally although seldom symmetrically (see Table 57–5 in the Textbook). Pain or paresthesias usually precedes the development of motor symptoms, which include weakness and muscle atrophy.

Effects of Chemotherapy (p. 1311)

• A progressive distal symmetrical sensory neuropathy occurs with cisplatin treatment. Vincristine and cytarabine also have peripheral neuropathy as a principal toxic and dose-limiting side effect (see Chapter 47).

Bleeding Problems (p. 1311)

• Both chemotherapeutic and radiotherapeutic procedures can cause thrombocytopenia. Exercise in the presence of thrombocytopenia can increase the risk of intra-articular bleeding. Bleeding from the lungs or oral and nasal mucosa can also occur. In general, platelet levels below 10,000/mL preclude exercise therapy, and the risk of intracerebral bleeding becomes significant below this level. Some centers allow aerobic but not resistive activities in patients with platelet counts between 10,000 and 20,000/mL.

REHABILITATION ISSUES IN SPECIFIC CANCERS
(pp. 1311–1318)

Breast Cancer (pp. 1311–1313)

• Eighteen percent of all cancer deaths in women are caused by breast cancer, and it remains the leading cause of death for women 40 to 55 years of age.

Surgical Options (pp. 1311–1312)
• Standard treatment has evolved from radical mastectomies to breast conservation strategies. Radical mastectomy requires resection of both the pectoralis major and minor muscles and the axillary lymph nodes. This leads to significant shoulder dysfunction, pain, lymphedema, and emotional trauma. Modified radical mastectomies, which spare the pectoralis major but include axillary dissection, are now more common. Other surgical options include lumpectomy and segmental (partial) or simple (total) mastectomy with or without axillary dissection. A common breast reconstruction procedure is the transverse rectus abdominis muscle (TRAM) flap (see Fig. 57–4 in the Textbook), which leads to a weakened abdominal musculature in some patients. Other reconstruction options include the use of tissue expanders, followed by prosthetic implants; and latissimus dorsi transfers.

Rehabilitation Issues (p. 1312)
• ROM exercise is particularly critical during and after radiation treatment to lessen the likelihood of fibrotic contracture formation.

Lymphedema (p. 1312)
• Lymphedema is a common complication of breast cancer treatment. Arm swelling can occur transiently in the immediate postoperative period, and this early form may resolve spontaneously.

• The onset of lymphedema 2 years or more after treatment can be a sign of recurrent tumor occluding the lymphatic system. Lymphedema is painless but is often accompanied by sensations of tightness or heaviness, and it is associated with neck or shoulder discomfort as the limb grows larger. A gradual progression occurs if left untreated, with an increased risk of cellulitis, further lymphatic damage, and extremity enlargement in a vicious cycle.

• Elevation, manual lymphatic drainage, compressive bandaging and garments, and pneumatic pumps may be employed in treatment. Patients must be taught a lifelong management plan for their lymphedema (see Chapter 56).

Pain *(pp. 1312–1313)*

• Chest wall tenderness is common after radiation treatment and can continue for years after treatment. Allodynia or dysesthesia often occurs in the distribution of the intercostobrachial nerve. Adhesive capsulitis of the shoulder, transient brachial plexus neuritis, and acute and chronic radiation-related plexopathies can also occur. Phantom breast pain has also been described, affecting at least 10% of mastectomy patients. It occurs more commonly in women with premastectomy pain.

Cosmetic Concerns *(p. 1313)*

• A permanent prosthesis can usually be fitted 3 to 8 weeks after surgery, when the chest wall edema has resolved and the tissue is well healed. Both immediate and delayed reconstruction options exist, and irradiated skin in the axilla and chest are not contraindications.

Bone and Soft Tissue Tumors (p. 1313)

• Bone and soft tissue sarcomas are uncommon, accounting for just 0.5% to 1.0% of adult malignancies in the United States, but the rehabilitation concerns of these patients are particularly pertinent. The most common sarcoma in both adults and children is osteosarcoma of the knee or proximal humerus.

• Amputation remains the preferred procedure for most high-grade malignancies of the distal lower extremity.

• Tumor amputees differ from dysvascular and traumatic amputees in several ways. Chemotherapy-induced fatigue, anemia, nausea, and cardiovascular toxic effects can sharply diminish functional capacity. Wound healing is often delayed over irradiated ports, and skin may be less tolerant of prosthesis wear. Anorexia with weight loss, muscle atrophy, and fluid shifts during chemotherapy can delay definitive prosthesis fabrication.

• Criteria for limb salvage procedures include the ability to totally resect the tumor without sacrifice of major nerves and vessels, and the ability of a reconstruction to provide function equal or superior to that of an appropriate prosthesis. Pathological fractures and distant metastases are contraindications to such procedures.

Metastatic Bone Lesions (pp. 1313–1314)

• The most commonly encountered bone tumors are metastatic in origin. Prostate carcinoma accounts for 60% of all bone metastases in men, and carcinomas of the breast account for 70% of all metastatic lesions in women.

• Skeletal metastases appear to arise primarily through hematogenous spread. Batson described a venous system connecting to and bypassing pulmonary, portal, and caval venous flow (see Fig. 57–6 in the Textbook). This network of veins has multidirectional flow determined by external pressure and related to biomechanical action and position. It is commonly believed to be a major hematogenous route for the spread of metastasis.

• Patients with symptomatic bone lesions complain of localized pain that increases in severity and frequency, and is often worse at night than during the day. Patients may develop reduced ROM at involved hips or shoulders, and increased pain with axial loading of involved long bones. Such symptoms in cancer patients should prompt a search for metastases, starting with radiographs for most sites and MRI for spinal complaints. Radionuclide bone scintigraphy is helpful when radiographs are inconclusive but metastasis is suspected. However, in cases of lung tumor, melanoma, and multiple myeloma, bone scans often have false negative results.

Long Bone Involvement (p. 1314)
• Pathological fractures are most common in the long bones, especially the femur and humerus. Cortical destruction makes bone particularly susceptible to torsion and rotation fractures because such forces are no longer transmitted uniformly through the cortex.

• Most guidelines suggest increase fracture risk, and therefore appropriateness for surgical stabilization, when painful lesions are greater than 2.5 cm in diameter, occupy 50% or more of bony cortical diameter, or involve greater than 50% of medullary cross-sectional area or cortex. Determining such involvement may be facilitated by CT coronal views. Surgical fixation usually involves removal of the tumor through curettage, with the use of methyl methacrylate, intramedullary rods, modular prostheses, or other hardware to repair the defect. Radiation treatments create transient softening of bone and theoretically increase the fracture risk for 6 to 8 weeks. Reduced weight bearing may be recommended during this time for patients not treated with surgical fixation.

Vertebral Involvement (p. 1314)
• Metastases to the spine often involve the vertebral body, although they can settle in the paravertebral tissues, and they most commonly occur within the thoracic spine. Pain can arise from epidural or root compression, intraosseous pressure from growing tumor cells, or mechanical instability. Severe neck or back pain or radicular or myelopathic findings require an immediate MRI evaluation and consideration of bolus dosing of methylprednisolone to prevent spinal cord compression.

• Goals of treatment should include pain control, avoidance of neurological compromise by tumor or spinal instability, local tumor control, and maximizing patient function. Pain can respond to external-beam radiation therapy, chemotherapy, bone-seeking radioisotopes, or surgical stabilization, individually or in combination. Management may also include the use of external orthoses and analgesic medications.

Head and Neck Tumors (pp. 1314–1316)
• Head and neck cancers constitute about 5% of all malignancies. The larynx is the most commonly affected site, followed by the oral cavity, pharynx, and salivary gland.

- Malignant disease of the head and neck region can result in profound swallowing and nutritional problems. The sensory functions of vision, hearing, balance, taste, and smell can be altered either by the disease or by its treatment. The goals of treatment, which include (1) eradication of cancer, (2) maintenance of adequate physiological function, and (3) achievement of socially acceptable cosmesis, can only be achieved through a multidisciplinary approach.
- Delayed surgical problems may arise and include deficits in swallowing (see Chapter 26) and speech (see Chapter 3).

Shoulder (pp. 1315–1316)
- Of special concern to the physiatrist are the shoulder impairment and chronic neck pain that can occur following radical neck dissection.
- The spinal accessory nerve is usually sacrificed during radical neck dissection. It can be incised in the lower neck, where it enters the trapezius muscle, and in the upper neck, where it enters the sternocleidomastoid muscle. Postoperative shoulder problems occur with the loss of trapezius muscle function. This causes the scapulae to move laterally, and deepens the axilla.
- Strengthening of the levator scapulae, rhomboids, and serratus anterior, although not capable of completely substituting for trapezius function, can diminish pain and improve scapular stability and shoulder elevation.
- The pectoralis muscle group is the main antagonist of the trapezius. Unopposed pull of the pectoralis muscles following radical neck dissection results in shoulder contracture with the scapulae in a protracted position. Avoiding contracture of this muscle group is a major goal of postoperative rehabilitation.

Neck (p. 1316)
- Unilateral disruption of the sternocleidomastoid, platysma, omohyoid, and diagnostic muscles can lead to asymmetrical neck motion. These patients often need to support their neck and head with their hands when changing from a supine to sitting position. Following bilateral radical neck dissection, a patient is unable to flex the neck against gravity. Scar massage and daily stretching following radiation therapy is essential to maintain mobility.

Spinal Cord Lesions (p. 1316)

- Primary tumors (e.g., meningiomas, neurofibromas, and gliomas) are relatively rare. The majority of tumors affecting the spinal cord are metastatic in origin, and 95% are extradural.
- Most extradural metastases arise from the vertebral body and result in compression of the anterior aspect of the spinal cord. The thoracic spine has a smaller ratio of canal to cord diameter than the lumbar or cervical segments; approximately 70% of diagnosed spinal metastasis occurs in the thoracic spine.
- The clinical presentation of spinal cord compression often involves complaints of pain that becomes worse in the recumbent position. Multiple spinal levels can be simultaneously involved. The development of bowel or bladder dysfunction can indicate spinal cord compromise, yet the onset of such symptoms may be obscured in patients taking opiates or adjuvant analgesics, which may cause constipation and urinary retention. Slowly evolving symptoms are indicative of gradual cord impingement and may respond to corticosteroids and radiotherapy. The rapid evolution of paraparesis over several hours usually signifies arterial compromise by tumor invasion or pressure, with a more guarded prognosis for recovery.

Treatment (p. 1316)

• The optimal surgical approach and stabilization procedures for metastatic spine lesions remain controversial. Stability is of special concern if the tumor involves two or three vertebrae. Halo fixation, although providing the greatest stability to the cervical spine, is often poorly tolerated and unacceptable to many cancer patients. Sternal-occipital-mandibular immobilization is usually better tolerated and provides adequate flexion and extension stability to the lower cervical segments. The Philadelphia and similar hard collars can provide acceptable stability in flexion and extension for higher levels, but do not sufficiently restrict rotation and lateral bending in the lower cervical segments (see Chapter 17).

• The "clamshell"-style thoracic-lumbar-sacral orthosis may be used to provide thoracic and lumbar support; however, its considerable support may not be an option for patients with painful rib or iliac crest metastases, friable or intolerant skin from steroid or radiation therapy, or dyspnea because of lung tumors or restrictive lung disease. Less restrictive devices serve only as proprioceptive cues but may still provide comfort and are more easily tolerated.

Brain Tumors (pp. 1317–1318)

• The rehabilitation of brain tumor patients differs from that for stroke or traumatic brain injury patients because of differences in the patterns of recovery. The location of the lesion determines the resultant neurological deficits, which can be entirely reversed when focal pressure is relieved. Some patients experience dramatic improvement in function within hours after surgical resection.

• More than 90% of the primary malignant tumors of the brain in adults are high-grade astrocytomas, and of these, the most common is glioblastoma multiforme. Low-grade astrocytomas are the most common primary brain tumors in children. Medulloblastomas account for 20% of all intracranial tumors in children and are usually located near the cerebellar vermis.

• Pediatric primary tumors tend to be infratentorial, whereas those in adults are more likely supratentorial. Metastatic lesions comprise roughly 25% to 30% of all intracranial tumors.

• Lung, gastrointestinal, and urinary tract tumors account for the majority of these metastases in men. In women, breast, lung, gastrointestinal, and melanoma primary tumors dominate.

Symptoms and Signs (p. 1317)

• The presenting symptoms and signs of brain tumor involvement can include headache, weakness, seizures, and changes in cognition, with headache being the most common.

Rehabilitation Issues (pp. 1317–1318)

• Efforts directed toward preventing skin breakdown and contractures, progressive mobilization and transfer training, and relearning of activities of daily living are appropriate. Speech therapy is indicated for patients with aphasia, dysarthria, and dysphagia and, together with neuropsychology, can provide compensatory strategies for patients with cognitive impairments.

PEDIATRIC CANCER REHABILITATION (p. 1318)

- The most common childhood cancer is leukemia (30% to 40%), especially acute lymphocytic leukemia (ALL), followed by central nervous system (CNS) tumors (20%), bone cancer (7%), and neuroblastoma (5%).
- Brain irradiation done either as a primary treatment or as a prophylactic method, is associated with cognitive decline, particularly when performed on children less than 7 years old. Significant decreases in visuomotor and fine motor skills, along with attrition in arithmetic skills, spatial memory, and intelligence quotient (IQ) scores, have been reported following CNS irradiation in children. Direct tumor effects and combined therapies also contribute to cognitive function decline.
- Children being treated for brain tumors can experience cerebellar disturbances and hemiparesis. Changes in visual acuity and oculomotor function can occur as well.
- Hearing losses from chemotherapy, particularly vincristine, may also restrict normal childhood activities. Children treated for ALL are at increased risk of falling behind a grade level or needing special education classes.
- Musculoskeletal concerns of the pediatric cancer patient include the development of spinal deformities (kyphosis and scoliosis), especially when radiation is given during periods of rapid skeletal growth. Bone sarcoma and the effects of limb salvage surgery or amputation are discussed above. Childhood growth patterns are commonly abnormal after completion of cancer treatment.
- Most children with cancer experience pain, and in nearly two-thirds of cases the pain is treatment related. Direct effects of tumors, including bone metastases and nerve compression, are also important causes of pain. The pharmacological treatment of cancer pain in children includes narcotics, NSAIDs, tricyclic antidepressants, amphetamines, and topical preparations. Oral meperidine use is avoided in children because its toxic metabolite, normeperidine, can cause seizures. Fentanyl is a short half-life narcotic that is effective for use in acute pain from outpatient surgical procedures.
- Children with cancer have a 17% incidence of developing a second malignancy by 20 years of age. Radiation and chemotherapy are potential carcinogens. Chronic immunodeficiency following treatment and genetic predisposition also play a role in secondary tumor development.

58

Original Chapter by M. Catherine Spires, M.D.

Rehabilitation of Patients with Burns

• More than 70,000 persons are hospitalized each year for burn injury. Men in the 18- to 25-year-old age group are most at risk for sustaining a significant thermal injury. Burn size and the patient's age are the cardinal determinants of survival. Mortality is highest in the very young and the elderly, and is greater in females than in males with comparable injuries. The average person believes that a serious burn injury is the most devastating trauma a person can survive.

THE INTEGUMENT (pp. 1321–1324)

• The skin is the largest organ of the body and serves multiple functions. It is composed of a network of specialized epithelial and dermal cells, collagen, elastic fibers, small blood vessels, and nerve endings. Skin is a complex organ that acts as a mechanical barrier to protect internal organs from chemicals and foreign material. It is essential to fluid homeostasis, thermoregulation, and the body's immunological defense.

Skin Components (pp. 1321–1322)

• Skin consists of two major components, the epidermis and the dermis (Fig. 58–1). The epidermis has four layers—the stratum corneum, stratum granulosum, stratum spinosum, and stratum basale. A fifth layer, the stratum lucidum, is present on the palms of the hands and the soles of the feet. The stratum corneum is the resilient, semitransparent outermost layer that acts as a barrier to water transfer. The deepest layer, the stratum basale, is the major site of cell mitosis. Keratinocytes are the most numerous cells of the epidermis. Originating in the stratum basale, keratinocytes migrate to the stratum corneum, undergoing keratinization. During this process, keratinocytes flatten and become anucleate, and leave a protective protein layer of keratin on the skin surface.
• The epidermis has a number of appendages. Hair follicles are lined by epidermal cells, which are in continuity with the epidermis and serve as a reservoir of epidermal cells in the event of injury. The sebaceous glands produce sebum, which moisturizes the skin. Eccrine glands dissipate heat through production of sweat and are essential in thermoregulation.

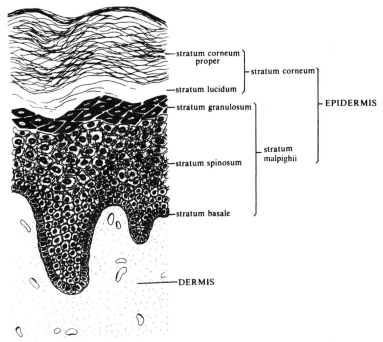

FIGURE 58–1. The histological characteristics of normal skin. Notice that the stratum lucidum is found only on the palms of hands and the soles of feet. (From Borysenko M, Beringer T: Functional Histology, ed 2. Boston, Little, Brown, 1984, p 228.)

• The epidermis is nourished by the underlying dermis. Undulating projections of the dermis, rete pegs, fit intimately with the stratum basale and reduce shear forces during mechanical manipulation. Rete pegs are underdeveloped in children and atrophied in the elderly. The dermis is composed of elastic fibers and loosely arranged collagen, which tend to be oriented in parallel with the epidermis (see Fig. 58–3 in the Textbook).

MEDICAL AND SURGICAL MANAGEMENT OF BURN INJURY (pp. 1324–1328)

• The vast majority of burn injuries are thermal, resulting from flame or hot liquids. Chemical and electrical injuries are less common. The extent of tissue injury depends on the intensity and duration of heat exposure. A significant difference between chemical and thermal injury is the duration of tissue destruction. Heat injury ceases after the source is removed, whereas chemicals continue to destroy tissue until they are inactivated by neutralizing agents or until the chemical reaction with the tissue is complete.

Medical Management (p. 1324)

• The first priorities in medical management are interrupting the burning process and assessing the airways, breathing, and circulation. Further evaluation includes assessment of the total body surface area (TBSA) burned, burn depth, the presence or absence of inhalation injury, and involvement of specialized body regions (e.g., face, hands, perineum). The patient's age, the presence of other injuries, and the patient's premorbid medical condition are also considered. The amount of fluid needed to restore and maintain hemodynamic stability is calculated using the Brooke, Parkland, or other formulas for fluid resuscitation. Clinical response determines further fluid needs. Close monitoring for infection and for cardiopulmonary complications is required on an ongoing basis.

Classification of Burn Severity (pp. 1324–1325)

• The American Burn Association classifies a burn injury as minor, moderate, or severe based on patient age, extent and depth of injury, and associated injuries (Table 58–1). Patients with moderate and severe burns require hospitalization. Major injuries, which include inhalation burns and burns of the eyes, ears, face, feet, or perineum, should be treated in a specialized burn center.

• Burn injury extent is determined by the TBSA injured. The easiest method of calculating TBSA is the rule of nines (Fig. 58–2). Eleven areas of the body are assigned a surface area value of 9%, with a twelfth area, the perineum, assigned a value of 1%. For children, this method is less accurate because the head, particularly during the first year of life, is larger in relation to the body size than is an adult's head. The Lund and Browder chart (Fig. 58–3) accounts for these developmental differences.

• Burn injury depth refers to the extent to which the epidermis and dermis are injured (Fig. 58–4). Superficial burns, also called first-degree burns, cause local erythema and pain. Partial-thickness burns, or second-degree burns, are classified as superficial partial-thickness or deep partial-thickness burns. In superficial partial-thickness injuries, blistering occurs because of microvascular damage and an associated increase in capillary permeability. Sensory nerve endings are exposed, and the wound is painful.

TABLE 58–1 Burn Injury Classification

Type of Injury	Major Burn	Moderate Burn	Minor Burn
Partial-thickness burns			
Children	>20% TBSA	10% to 20% TBSA	<10% TBSA
Adults	>25% TBSA	15% to 25% TBSA	<15% TBSA
Full-thickness burns	>10% TBSA	2% to 10% TBSA	<2% TBSA
Injury to face, eyes, ears, feet, or perineum	+	—	—
Inhalation injury	+	—	—
Electrical injury	+	—	—
Comorbid factors of age, other trauma, or premorbid illness	+	—	—

Abbreviations: TBSA, total body surface area; +, presence of this injury or comorbidity indicates a major burn requiring care at a burn center.

From American Burn Association: Hospital and pre-hospital resources for optimal care of patients with burn injury: Guidelines for development and operation of burn center. J Burn Care Rehabil 1990; 11:98–104.

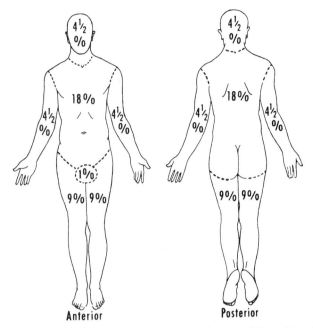

FIGURE 58–2. Rule of nines used to determine body surface area injured. (From Moylan JA: First aid and transportation of burned patients. In Artz CP, Moncrief JA, Pruitt BA (eds): Burns: A Team Approach. Philadelphia, WB Saunders, 1979, p 153.)

• In a deep partial-thickness wound, the dermis and the entire epidermis are injured. Only the skin appendages are spared. Spontaneous healing can occur, but it is associated with significant scarring. Poor cosmesis and function typically result.

• In full-thickness burn injuries, or third-degree burns, the entire thickness of the dermis is devitalized. Because skin appendages are destroyed, the wound cannot heal by re-epithelization. Dermal blood vessels are destroyed, and the wound bed is avascular.

• Even the most experienced clinicians can have difficulty distinguishing a deep partial-thickness injury from a full-thickness injury. In fact, poor wound care, wound infection, or impaired perfusion can convert a deep partial-thickness injury to a full-thickness injury.

Principles of Wound Care (pp. 1325–1327)

• The goals of wound care are to facilitate wound healing, prevent infection, decrease pain, reduce scarring and contracture, and prepare the wound for any necessary grafting. Infection can cause sepsis or convert the wound to a deeper-thickness injury. Burn wounds are covered by an eschar, which is necrotic tissue composed of denatured collagen, elastin, and protein. Because eschar favors wound infection and delays healing, debridement is initiated early. Debridement

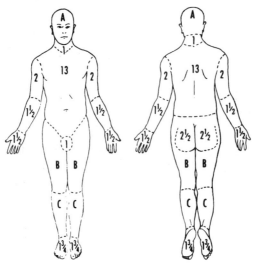

Relative Percentage of Areas Affected by Growth

	Age in Years					
	0	1	5	10	15	Adult
A—½ of head	9½	8½	6½	5½	4½	3½
B—½ of one thigh	2¾	3¼	4	4¼	4½	4¾
C—½ of one leg	2½	2½	2¾	3	3¼	3½

FIGURE 58–3. Lund and Browder method of determining skin surface area; method corrects for differences in percentage of body surface areas by age. (From McManus WF: Immediate emergency department care. In Artz CP, Moncrief JA, Pruitt BA (eds): Burns: A Team Approach. Philadelphia, WB Saunders, 1979, p 154.)

removes devitalized tissue and provides a viable base for wound healing and grafting.
• Debridement is done by several techniques: mechanical, enzymatic, and surgical. Mechanical debridement includes techniques such as hydrotherapy and wet-to-dry dressing techniques. The wet-to-dry dressing technique involves placing saline-soaked gauze over the wound and allowing the dressing to nearly dry. Necrotic tissue adheres to the dressing as the gauze dries and is removed when the dressing is changed. This provides a simple and inexpensive debridement, but it can be painful and can cause local bleeding. Its use is limited by the size of the wound to be debrided. To prevent desiccation of the wound, the dressing requires changing every 6 to 8 hours.
• Hydrotherapy, via immersion or spraying a burn directly, is a reasonably comfortable way to remove dressings and loosen devitalized tissue. It is a time-consuming and labor-intensive procedure. Other disadvantages include hypothermia and bacterial cross-contamination between patients if meticulous care of hydrotherapy equipment is not maintained. Disposable liners are avail-

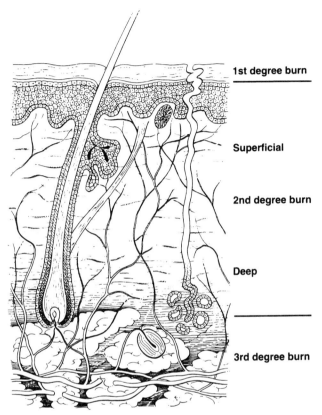

FIGURE 58–4. Normal skin histological characteristics, with depth of burn injury indicated. (From Kucan JO: Burn and trauma. In Ruberg RL, Smith DJ Jr (eds): Plastic Surgery: A Core Curriculum. St Louis, Mosby—Year Book, 1994, p 212.)

able to reduce cross-contamination. Hydrotherapy can be combined with other forms of mechanical debridement.

• Several debriding enzymes (e.g., sutilains) are available for topical application to burn eschar. Enzymatic action includes proteolysis, fibrinolysis, and collagenolysis, with specificity varying from agent to agent. Enzymatic debridement can reduce the need for surgical debridement. Exercise and splinting programs are not contraindicated during enzymatic treatment. Disadvantages include increased pain and fluid loss. The amount of body surface area being enzymatically treated at one time should be limited to less than 20% TBSA. Localized irritation, cellulitis, and elevation in body temperature might also occur. Bleeding can occur at the interface between the eschar and the viable tissue.

• Surgical debridement excises the nonviable tissue by either sequential or fascial excision. The latter removes tissue down to the fascia, which ensures a viable wound bed but leaves a significant tissue defect. Sequential excision consists of sequential removal of thin slices of tissue until bleeding is observed. The bleeding indicates a viable wound bed. Although it is less likely to sacrifice viable tissue, sequential excision causes greater blood loss and requires extensive surgical experience.

• Burn injury can cause massive edema. Compartment syndromes can develop, particularly with circumferential burns, and result in neurovascular compromise and potential limb loss. Escharotomies can be performed to relieve pressure by incising through the burned tissue at specified areas, avoiding flexor surfaces of the upper and lower extremities. Incision is also done over the chest wall if eschar interferes with respiration by preventing chest expansion. Circumferential upper or lower extremity burns require monitoring to ensure that compartment pressures do not exceed 40 mm Hg. If this pressure is reached, fasciotomies are indicated to prevent neurovascular compromise, which can also lead to amputation of the extremity.

Wound Dressings and Grafts (p. 1327)

• Biological dressings (i.e., biological tissue used for covering wounds) provide a means of early burn wound closure. Early closure reduces pain, promotes healing, and decreases bacterial proliferation. Early wound closure reduces evaporative fluid loss and metabolic rate. The primary types of biological dressings include heterografts (such as porcine grafts) and homografts (such as cadaver grafts). Homografts are considered the best biological dressing but are obtained primarily from cadaver donors and can be limited in supply. Biological dressings are often used to achieve early wound closure until an autograft (i.e., the surgical transfer of the patient's skin from one body site to another) is feasible. A biological dressing can also be used as a test graft to see if a wound is ready to accept an autograft.

• Synthetic wound dressings include polyvinyl chlorides, polyurethanes, and other plastic membranes. The advantages of these temporary dressings include water and gas permeability, but they fail to adhere to the wound bed, and fluids accumulate under the dressings. Nylon mesh bonded to silicone (Biobrane) adheres to and successfully covers both partial- and full-thickness wounds. Like biological dressings, however, this type of dressing does not adhere to wounds having high bacterial counts.

• Topical antimicrobials are applied to burns and wounds after debridement and grafting to reduce bacterial proliferation. Sulfadiazine and mafenide acetate are two of the most commonly used topical agents. Mafenide acetate penetrates eschar, but it can cause pain as well as acidosis and leukopenia. Sulfadiazine is also a broad-spectrum topical antibiotic, but it does not penetrate eschar as mafenide acetate does. It has the advantage of causing less pain and is not associated with leukopenia or acidosis.

• Autografting can be performed once the wound is free of devitalized tissue and infection. A split-thickness skin graft can be meshed or applied in sheets. Meshing is a process in which small, staggered, parallel slits are made in the graft to allow it to be expanded 1.5 times or more its original size. The interstices epithelialize, and the pattern of the mesh persists after wound healing. The greater the degree to which the mesh is expanded, the poorer the cosmetic appearance. Mesh grafts are valuable when donor sites are limited and large areas need to be covered. Split-thickness grafts can be applied in sheets without meshing. These grafts are durable, limit contracture formation, and produce better cosmesis for covering the face, neck, and hands. Full-thickness grafts are useful for specialized areas (e.g., the palms of the hands) and are commonly used in reconstructive procedures.

Wound Healing (pp. 1327–1328)

• Wound healing involves three simultaneous processes: (1) epithelization, (2) scar formation (repair of the dermis), and (3) wound contraction. Inflammation begins immediately after injury. This process spans a complex array of events, including initial vasoconstriction followed by vasodilation, marked changes in capillary permeability, and chemotaxis (which attracts neutrophils, macrophages, and lymphocytes). This period is marked by erythema, increased heat, edema, and pain. The inflammatory phase not only controls infection but also heralds the onset of the proliferative stage of healing by attracting fibroblasts.

• Once inflammation is established, epithelium migrates from the edges of the wound or from epidermal appendages. If the burn involves the epidermis and superficial dermis, epithelialization is the primary process. However, with deep partial-thickness injuries and full-thickness injuries, both epithelialization and restoration of the dermis are crucial.

• Fibroblastic activity is the hallmark of the proliferative wound healing phase. During this phase, fibroblasts synthesize collagen, which is the predominant protein found in scar tissue. Collagen gives tensile strength to the wound. Simultaneously, angiogenesis occurs to provide the vascular support needed for the reparative wound activities. Capillary proliferation produces the classic granular appearance of granulation tissue.

• Wound contraction is the active movement of the wound edges toward the center of a wound, shrinking the defect size and aiding closure. The degree of contraction achieved depends on the looseness and redundancy of the surrounding skin. For instance, a wound involving the skin of the buttock results in greater wound contraction and reduction of the wound size than does one involving the less mobile skin of the lateral malleolus. Fibroblasts appear to be the primary cells involved in wound contraction.

• Inflammation and angiogenesis resolve as the scar matures. The tissue becomes paler and flatter. Collagen synthesis is balanced by collagen degradation. The rete pegs do not reappear immediately and require months to form. This contributes to the scarred skin's reduced ability to tolerate applied forces.

ELECTRICAL BURN INJURIES (pp. 1328–1329)

• Electrical burn injuries account for approximately 3% of burn admissions and result in approximately 800 deaths per year. Injuries can be mild or can result in death from cardiac asystole. Electrical injuries are classified as low-tension-line or high-tension-line injuries. High-tension-line injuries result from exposure to greater than 1000 V. In general, the greater the amperage, the greater the injury. Electrical injuries occur predominantly in men younger than 30 years who work with high-voltage equipment or high-tension wires. Low-tension electrical injuries usually occur in residential settings.

• On superficial evaluation, electrical injuries can deceptively appear minor. The entrance site is typically small and charred, whereas the exit wound can be more explosive in appearance. Patients need careful evaluation to ensure that a serious underlying injury is not overlooked. The average TBSA injured in electrical burns is approximately 12%. Electrical injuries can be further compounded if the clothing catches on fire, causing more extensive skin injury.

• The damage of electrical exposure results from the heat produced as the current passes through various tissues. Bone produces the most resistance, resulting in the greatest heat production. Although nerves and blood vessels provide the least resistance, they can sustain significant injury because they are more heat sensitive. As a consequence, the majority of the injuries sustained are in deep tissues.

• The cross-sectional area of the particular body part affects the density of current and the amount of heat generated. Body parts with a small cross-sectional area (e.g., fingers and toes) can sustain massive injury (see Figs. 58–14A and B in the Textbook). Extensive muscle and soft tissue necrosis often results in amputation. One-fourth to nearly one-half of patients hospitalized for electrical burns require limb amputation, and some require multiple limb amputations. The upper extremity is the most common limb amputated. The right upper extremity accounts for two-thirds of these amputations. One-fourth of these patients required shoulder disarticulations.

Neurological Sequelae (p. 1329)

• Immediate neurological problems include loss of consciousness, anoxic encephalopathy, peripheral neuropathies, and spinal cord injury. Persistent coma correlates with a poor prognosis and often results in death. Spinal cord injury, according to some sources the most common permanent neurological sequela of electrical injury, typically occurs when the current travels from one extremity to another. Peripheral neuropathies generally occur in the injured limb but can also be seen in the nonburned limb. Although the pathophysiology of late-appearing neurological deficits is unknown, spinal cord injury and peripheral neuropathies can be observed as late as 2 years postinjury. With electrical injuries to the head and neck, serial eye examinations are required because cataracts can occur up to 3 years after the injury.

REHABILITATION (pp. 1329–1335)

• Rehabilitation from a burn injury continues long after discharge, and in some cases, for life. The overall goal is to assist the individual in achieving the optimal level of functioning. During the acute period, more specific goals include promoting wound healing and preventing complications by preserving joint function, strength, endurance, and functional abilities. Goals are individualized according to the location, depth, and distribution of burn injuries and the individual's previous functional level, and should be continually assessed and modified as the patient improves. The extent of injury correlates with survival as well as with time required to return to independent functioning. Age, previous level of independence, premorbid medical conditions, and other injuries must be considered when assessing the burn patient.

Positioning (p. 1329)

• Proper positioning prevents contracture formation, controls edema, and maintains tissues in an elongated state. Pain causes burn patients to assume a primarily flexed and adducted position that inadvertently favors contracture development; however, body parts should generally be positioned to maintain burned tissues in their elongated state. Typically, limbs should be positioned in extension and abduction (Fig. 58–5). The positioning program must be individualized in accordance with the injury sites. Proper positioning can be achieved using splints, strategically placed pillows, and foam wedges.

Splinting (pp. 1329–1330)

• Splinting should be considered in several circumstances. Contractures can develop quickly during burn healing. Contracture would interfere with joint function when a partial- or full-thickness burn overlies a joint surface or the skin near a joint. Splints are used to maintain proper anticontracture positions and range of motion (ROM) in joints at risk for development of contractures. Serial splinting and serial casting techniques are both nonoperative means of gaining ROM through sustained stretch and pressure.

• Splints are also used to protect newly placed skin grafts and to shield injured anatomical structures (e.g., tendons) from further trauma. Splints can also be designed to prevent scarring in areas in which an important body contour would be lost (e.g., the anterior neck surface).

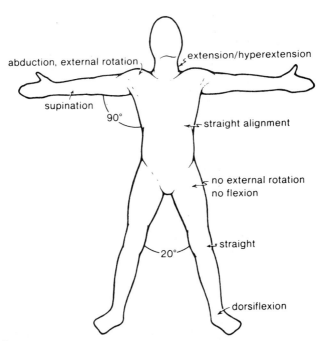

FIGURE 58–5. Suggested positioning guidelines for prevention of burn contractures. (From Helm PA, Kevorkian CG, Lushbaugh M, et al: Burn injury: Rehabilitation management in 1982. Arch Phys Med Rehabil 1982; 63: 8.)

• It is important to consider the benefits and risks of splinting. Splinting is labor intensive and adds significant cost to patient care. Splinting is cost-effective, however, if it reduces the need for surgery or prevents loss of function.

• Not all burned areas require splinting. Areas of superficial partial-thickness burns usually heal without scar contracture formation and do not require splinting. Unburned areas generally do not require splinting unless they are at risk for contracture development secondary to immobilization.

• Splint materials must be compatible with topical medications and wound dressings. Prefabricated or custom splints can be used but require proper fitting. "User-friendly" splints increase the likelihood that they will be used, and the complications of incorrect use will be avoided. Inexpensive and remoldable materials are best suited to accommodate changes as healing occurs.

• The universal burn splint, unfortunately, does not exist. The type of splint used depends on the area burned, the depth of injury, the patient's functional status, and the patient's ability to participate in positioning and exercise programs. A variety of splints can be designed and fabricated. A splinting program should focus on motions at risk as well as ROM that is difficult to regain (e.g., shoulder flexion and abduction, and elbow and knee extension). Splints can be fabricated for virtually any part of the body including the mouth, face, neck, and axilla.

• A resting hand splint maintains the hand in a functional position. The position of function is the hand splinted in full interphalangeal extension, 60 to 80 degrees of metacarpophalangeal flexion, thumb abduction, and wrist extension (Fig. 58–6). This position provides balance between the extensor and flexor tendons and places the ligaments and joint structures under maximum stretch to prevent shortening by inflammation and edema.

• Splints for the upper and lower extremities are among the most common. Lower extremity splints include such devices as the hip abduction splint to limit

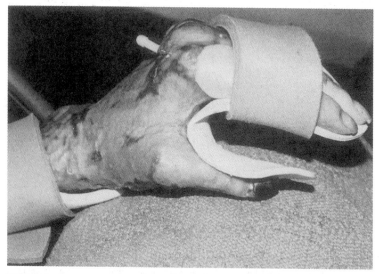

FIGURE 58–6. The left hand splinted in the position of function after skin grafting.

hip adduction, the knee extension splint to prevent knee flexion contractures, and the posterior footdrop splint to maintain the ankle in a neutral position.

- Plantar flexion deformity is a common problem. Prefabricated posterior footdrop splints are commercially available but still require modification to ensure proper fit. These splints can also be readily made by creating a gutter- or trough-shaped splint and attaching a footplate to hold the ankle in a neutral position.

Exercise in Burn Rehabilitation (pp. 1330–1331)

- Exercise is fundamental to maximizing patient function and overall outcome. Factors to consider in prescribing an exercise program include the extent, depth, and location of the injury. In general, the risk of contracture increases with increasing burn depth. The risk of exercise disrupting wound healing requires regular wound inspection, particularly in the case of deep partial-thickness and full-thickness burns over joint surfaces. Stretching can also disrupt already tenuous joint and tendon structures.
- Preexisting medical conditions, such as cardiovascular or pulmonary disease, also affect the type of exercise prescribed. The stress of fluid resuscitation can complicate the recovery of patients with cardiovascular disease. Because deconditioning occurs rapidly in burn patients (see Chapter 34), principles of cardiac rehabilitation are often as important in these situations as burn exercise principles (see Chapter 32).
- The initial exercise program should focus on preserving ROM and maintaining strength. Active forms of exercise are indicated for patients who are alert and able to participate. For obtunded or critically ill patients, the slow, controlled movement of passive ROM exercise is appropriate. While the patient is under anesthesia, passive ROM techniques can be applied to determine true joint ROM and factors limiting motion.
- In the case of the patient who can actively move a joint but who is unable to achieve full ROM, active assistive ROM (AAROM) exercise is appropriate. The patient does as much of the ROM as possible, then a steady prolonged stretch or assistance is applied to complete the ROM. The stretch can be provided manually or by using devices such as pulleys and weights. Pain can limit stretching in some patients, so scheduling exercise shortly after pain medication administration is helpful.
- Applying the principle of skin preconditioning (i.e., stretching the skin several times until phase I of the stress-strain curve stabilizes) can improve the success of a stretching program. Preconditioning can be done by moving a joint to its end ROM several times before applying a sustained stretch. Stretching can be sustained until the stretched tissue blanches. The blanching indicates that dermal capillary flow is impeded and correlates with early phase III of the skin stress-strain relationship. With overstretching beyond phase III, the yield point is reached and passed (i.e., the point in the stress-strain curve at which tissue integrity deteriorates). Once normal joint ROM is achieved, active exercise is preferred.
- Various types of strengthening protocols can be initiated, including progressive resistive exercises and circuit training (see Chapter 20). Endurance training should not be overlooked but requires careful monitoring in the patient with cardiac or pulmonary disease (see Chapters 32 and 33).

Ambulation and Mobility (pp. 1331–1332)

• Early ambulation maintains balance, aids lower extremity function, enhances a sense of well-being, and decreases the risk of deep venous thrombosis. Although ambulation should start as soon as possible after admission, it can be limited by medical status; the presence of new skin grafts; the depth and extent of lower extremity burns; and previous medical conditions, such as peripheral vascular disease. After lower extremity grafting, placing the legs in a dependent position is generally not permitted for up to 5 to 10 days. Although the protocol for the timing of ambulation varies among facilities, the underlying principle is to begin ambulation once competent circulation is established in the graft and the risk of venous pooling, which can cause graft loss, is reduced. Once ambulation is initiated, recent graft and deep tissue injuries of the lower extremities require elastic wraps or stockings. Elastic supports prevent venous stasis, control edema, reduce the risk of local trauma, and decrease pain induced by the dependent position. Before ambulation is begun, it is advisable to have the patient dangle the lower extremities (e.g., sit with the legs hanging over the edge of the bed) to evaluate the predisposition for edema formation. Wounds should be assessed before and after ambulation to note any ill effects.
• Gait deviations are common and reflect the injured areas of the body (see Chapter 5). Reduced trunk and pelvic mobility, decreased weight shifting, and inadequate hip and knee extension are common. Some deviations spontaneously resolve with wound healing, but others require therapeutic intervention. Mirrors can provide feedback to patients for self-correction of posture and gait abnormalities. Assistive devices can optimize gait patterns (see Chapter 25).

Scar Rehabilitation (pp. 1332–1333)

• The appearance of a wound is often satisfactory immediately after closure. However, over the next 1 to 3 months, hypertrophic scarring can occur with deep partial-thickness and full-thickness burn injuries. Hypertrophic scars are characteristically red, raised, and rigid. The significance of these scars varies according to their location, with scarring over joints or on the face having a significant effect on function and appearance. Hypertrophic scars demonstrate random collagen orientation, with fibers arranged in whorls and nodules (see Fig. 58–18 in the Textbook).
• As normal and hypertrophic scars mature, the vascularity is reduced, the redness fades, and hypertrophic scars show a decrease in whorls and nodules on histological examination. With maturity, both types show a predominance of collagen in parallel arrays. Clinically, both scars are soft and pale. A hypertrophic scar requires up to 2 years to reach maturity, whereas a nonhypertrophic scar might mature in weeks to months.
• Mechanical pressure alters the orientation of the collagen fibers found in hypertrophic scarring. The risk of hypertrophic scarring increases with the depth of injury and length of time required for healing. Certain anatomical locations are associated with greater incidence of hypertrophic scarring (e.g., buttocks and chest).
• It is generally accepted that pressure-treated scars have a better functional and cosmetic outcome. The application of continuous pressure through garments, orthoses, and splints is the primary nonsurgical modality used to control hypertrophic scarring. The mechanism by which pressure suppresses hypertrophic

scarring is unclear, but it has been hypothesized that pressure causes decreased capillary perfusion and decreased tissue oxygenation, resulting in reduced cellular activity and collagen synthesis.

• Treatment options for scar suppression include custom-fitted pressure garments (Fig. 58–7), elastic bandages, and custom-made elastic or rigid face masks. Pressure applied to the healing area should be at least 25 mm Hg because it should exceed normal capillary pressure. Pressure is applied at least 23 hours per day. Uneven anatomical areas to which it is difficult to apply pressure (e.g., the web spaces of the hand) often require custom inserts. These pieces of silicone or moldable plastic are placed under pressure garments and orthoses to create a more intimate fit.

• The application of pressure should continue until the scar is mature. Patient education is essential for pressure therapy compliance. Complications of pressure therapy garments include superficial abrasions from the shear forces produced by the garment and local dermatitis. In the young child, pressure effects on skeletal growth require monitoring. Frequent adjustments to accommodate growth spurts are necessary.

Facial Burns (p. 1333)

• Facial burns have a significant impact on a person's appearance and state of well-being. Cosmesis and preservation of facial function are major priorities. Acutely, facial burns should alert the physician to possible inhalation injury. The risk of eye injury is also increased in facial burns. Facial wounds require an experienced wound care physician. Wounds expected to heal in less than 3 weeks often do not require early surgery and are less likely to develop significant scarring.

• Custom-made elastic face masks and transparent orthoses are available for controlling facial scarring. The highly contoured features of the face, especially

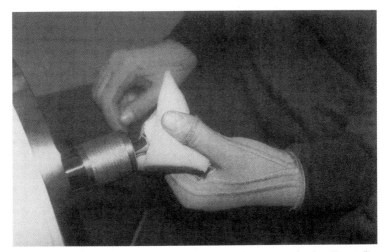

FIGURE 58–7. Custom-fitted pressure garments for scar suppression after hand burns. Fine motor skill training is necessary to maintain hand function and work skills.

the central face, make scar control problematic. The goal is to preserve facial contours, especially the nasal profile and the shape of the mouth and eyes.

• Microstomia orthoses can be fabricated or purchased to maintain the normal mouth aperture (see Fig. 58–21 in the Textbook). Early splinting reduces the need for corrective surgery. Scarring can severely distort the nose, affecting cosmesis and respiratory function.

• Unlike other body regions, pressure is contraindicated during the acute and recovery phase of ear burns. Ears require protection to avoid the development of pressure necrosis and chondritis. Specialized foam protectors and headgear can be designed.

Hand Rehabilitation (pp. 1334–1335)

• Hands are the most common site of burn injury. Treatment goals include edema control, early wound closure, rapid return of hand function, and prevention of hand deformities. Many types of hand deformities can result from deep partial-thickness and full-thickness injuries. The type of deformity relates to the location of the burn injury (e.g., burns of the thenar eminence and first web space cause thumb adduction contracture). Common deformities of the hand include wrist flexion contractures, metacarpophalangeal (MCP) hyperextension contractures, and interphalangeal (IP) flexion contractures. Bands of hypertrophic scarring can develop and limit hand function.

• After the hand is assessed for potential hypertrophic scarring and contracture formation, a well-designed program of exercise, splinting, and hypertrophic scar suppression should be prescribed. Exercise coupled with splint use, when indicated, can prevent hand deformities and restore optimal hand function. When splints are used, they should maintain the hand in an anticontracture position, which prevents the anticipated deformity. The dorsum or the full circumference of the hand is commonly injured. These injuries require that the hand be splinted in the position of function (i.e., IP joint extension, MCP joint flexion, thumb abduction, and wrist extension). This position preserves the maximal length and mobility of the extensor hood mechanism. Splint design should also preserve the transverse arch of the hand. In addition to static splints that hold the hand in a prescribed position, dynamic splints are available to facilitate ROM restoration or to substitute for a particular motion. Dynamic splints provide force in a specific plane, generally through elastic traction, while allowing motion in other planes.

• Exposed tendons and joints of the hand demand specialized treatment. Any exposed tendons require dressings that will keep them moist because dehydration can lead to tendon rupture. Exposed tendons are splinted in a slackened position. Once the wound is covered, passive ROM exercises can be performed judiciously. If the joint capsule is intact, gentle active exercise can be done. This exercise should be done under the supervision of an experienced therapist. The risk of septic arthritis is increased in open or exposed joints.

NEUROMUSCULAR COMPLICATIONS (p. 1335)

• Peripheral nerve injury after burns is common but not well recognized. Neurological involvement includes focal nerve compression, multiple mononeuropathies, and generalized peripheral neuropathies. Focal mononeuropathies commonly occur secondary to positioning, improperly applied splints, or bulky dressings.

• Multiple mononeuropathies can also occur. These have an incidence of about 2%, and are more likely to occur in males than in females (4.3:1). Electrodiagnostic studies show predominantly axonal involvement. The mononeuropathies are typically asymmetrical and more likely to occur in the upper limbs (3:1). They are not always found in burned regions.

• Henderson and colleagues first proposed that burn injuries are intrinsically associated with generalized peripheral neuropathy. Approximately 15% of the inpatients have peripheral neuropathy, which occurred primarily in patients who have injuries on more than 20% of TBSA.

• A generalized peripheral neuropathy with an incidence as high as 52% has been reported. The incidence correlates with the amount of TBSA affected (i.e., neuropathy was more likely to occur in adults with more than 20% TBSA injury and in children with more than 30% TBSA injury). Electrodiagnostic studies show a predominance of motor, rather than sensory, axonal peripheral neuropathy. These findings are consistent with critical care polyneuropathy seen in patients with multiple organ failure. The generalized peripheral neuropathy of the burn patient might be a subset of critical care polyneuropathy. The etiology of the peripheral neuropathy of burns has not been established, but neurotoxicity from antibiotics and the possibility of a circulating neurotoxin from the burn injury itself have been hypothesized.

HETEROTOPIC OSSIFICATION (p. 1335)

• Heterotopic ossification (HO) occurs after serious burns and represents abnormal calcification of soft tissues surrounding a joint. The risk of HO is increased in injuries that affect 20% or more of TBSA. Heterotopic ossification occurs in about 2% of burn patients and is more likely to occur the longer wounds remain open and the patient remains immobile. The most common site is the posterior elbow. The second most common site is the hip in children and the shoulder in adults. The site of ossification does not necessarily correlate with the location of burn injuries and can occur in single or multiple joints.

• HO can cause progressive loss of joint ROM and nerve entrapment mononeuropathies. HO can spontaneously resolve in some cases. If HO significantly interferes with function and is unresponsive to nonsurgical treatment, surgery is indicated. Surgical excision is typically not performed until the bone has matured to reduce the risk of recurrence.

BURN-INDUCED AMPUTATION (pp. 1335–1336)

• Limb amputation can be necessary after severe burn injury, particularly after electrical burns. Electrical injury is the leading cause of amputation in the burn patient population. The basic principles of amputee rehabilitation apply (see Chapters 13 and 14). The preprosthetic problems are similar to those with other amputations, but additional problems can occur (e.g., skin fragility, hypertrophic scarring, burn contractures, and altered skin sensation). The prosthesis might have to be fitted over scar tissue or previous graft sites, which can be less tolerant than normal of the shear forces created by the prosthesis. Blistering and open sores can develop more easily, forcing the patient to temporarily discontinue prosthesis use.

• Painful bony spurs can occur at the distal end of the residual limb, especially with electrical injuries. Bony spurs occur in up to 82% of patients who have electrical injuries and require amputation. The pathophysiological process that causes the bone spur formation is not known.

• Prosthesis fitting and training in burn patients is often complicated by the presence of wounds, multiple amputations, or ongoing medical problems. Successful prosthesis use can be achieved in patients with multiple amputations, but more intensive rehabilitation efforts are required.

• There is a higher rate of successful upper extremity prosthesis use when patients are fitted within 30 days of amputation.

PEDIATRIC BURNS (p. 1336)

• Mortality rates are higher for infants than adolescents or young adults. Children younger than 1 year are at greater risk for mortality than during subsequent preschool and school years. More than half of the 26,000 children hospitalized each year for burns are younger than 5 years. Children aged 6 months to 2 years account for more than half of pediatric burn admissions. This correlates with the developmental stages during which children rapidly acquire motor skills that allow them to get into potentially dangerous situations. Burn treatment of pediatric patients is somewhat different from that of adults. The TBSA-to-body-weight ratio of children is greater than that of adults until adolescence. This predisposes children to even more significant fluid loss from evaporation and injury. Thermoregulation is more easily disturbed because of the relatively large body surface. Fluid resuscitation protocols should be adjusted to the child's weight and height.

• The causes of burns in children are also different from those in adults. Scalding is the most common burn experienced by children. In children 4 years of age and under, 75% of all burns are caused by scalding. Burn injury is a common form of child abuse. Nonaccidental injuries account for approximately 10% to 28% of pediatric burns. Of all nonaccidental injuries experienced by children, 10% are because of burns. The child who experiences a nonaccidental scald injury is typically younger than 2 years. The hospital course for children who sustain nonaccidental scald burns is significantly longer, and their medical course tends to be more complicated.

• The rehabilitation program is based on the child's injury and developmental stage. Children are often unable to cooperate with many aspects of therapy and do not understand long-term goals. Loss of function, such as hand dexterity and ROM, not only interferes with activities appropriate to the child's current developmental level but also can limit future academic and vocational success. Therapeutic success often depends on making therapy fun by incorporating age-appropriate recreation and play activities. Educating the child's family and establishing rapport with the child and family early in the course can improve participation, long-term compliance, and final outcome. Both the child and the family need emotional, social, and medical support to achieve the best rehabilitative outcome.

• A child's size often makes positioning, splinting, and fitting of compression garments challenging. Children's growth makes more frequent modification of splints and custom-fitted pressure garments necessary. Skeletal and dental development can be compromised by compression therapy. For example, it is impor-

tant to monitor jaw development and dental alignment during the use of face masks and orthoses to avoid malocclusion.
• It is fairly common for children to regress emotionally, socially, and developmentally during the acute period of a burn injury. Assessment instruments are available to assess developmental delays if needed (see Chapter 2).

GERIATRIC BURNS (pp. 1336–1337)

• Skin atrophies with age, which results in deeper burn injuries in geriatric patients. Mortality rates are higher because the risk of death increases with age from the middle years onward. The likelihood of survival is markedly decreased by the presence of an inhalation injury in all age groups, but it is accentuated in elderly persons. Cardiopulmonary disease, diabetes mellitus, peripheral vascular disease, and other preexisting medical conditions can complicate burn management in the elderly.
• Geriatric patients often experience an initial drop in independence at discharge because of wound care, deconditioning, and outpatient therapy needs. Early planning for home health care services can prevent or shorten stays in an extended care facility and enable a geriatric patient to return home.
• The elderly appear to have less hypertrophic scarring and tend to experience slower healing than the young. Elderly persons can be less accepting of pressure garments because of difficulty in donning the garments and their high cost. The inclusion of zippers in pressure garments can make donning and doffing more feasible.
• Splinting, positioning, and exercise principles in this population are similar to those of other adults. Splints require careful monitoring because of increased skin fragility and decreased sensation secondary to scarring and preexisting disease. Early mobilization is imperative because the effects of immobility occur more rapidly and are more pronounced in elderly persons. Exercise protocols should emphasize functional activities of ambulation and mobility in addition to ROM and basic strengthening. Functional mobility is a first priority.

PSYCHOLOGICAL ADJUSTMENT (pp. 1337–1338)

• Preinjury psychological status is a strong predictor of a patient's long-term emotional status after a serious burn. Patients who were previously well-adjusted emotionally are likely to continue to demonstrate appropriate emotional adjustment. Burn patients with previous emotional dysfunction are more likely to have medical complications and significantly longer hospital stays.
• The epidemiology of burns shows that alcohol, senility, and psychiatric disease all predispose individuals to burn injuries. Approximately 45% to 69% of patients hospitalized for burns have a premorbid psychiatric history, including alcohol and substance abuse. A history of depression increases the likelihood that patients sustained injury as a consequence of risk-enhancing behaviors.
• Delirium, adjustment disorders, major depression, and post-traumatic stress disorder are the most commonly seen psychiatric disorders during recovery from a burn injury. Delirium, a transient disorder, is the most common, occurring in more than half of hospitalized burn patients. The etiology is often multifactorial, resulting from sepsis, anoxia, anemia, liver and renal dysfunction, and other organic causes. Pediatric and geriatric patients are at greater risk for development of delirium. With correction of the underlying cause, the delirium resolves.

• Adjustment disorder is the second most commonly encountered disorder. It occurs within 3 months of a stressful event and typically resolves within 6 months of termination of the stressor. It can persist longer in the presence of chronic conditions (e.g., a disabling medical condition or financial difficulties resulting from unemployment). Depression and anxiety are commonly present. Anticipatory anxiety (e.g., an exaggerated expectation of pain with dressing changes or ROM exercise) is particularly common among patients with burn injuries. Individualized psychotherapeutic intervention and judiciously prescribed medications are indicated for these problems.

• Major depression and posttraumatic stress disorder are significant complications of burn injury. Serial evaluation and awareness of the potential for these complications can lead to early intervention, which can help prevent loss of function and improve rehabilitative outcome.

OUTPATIENT REHABILITATION (pp. 1338–1339)

• Home treatment programs usually involve a daily exercise regimen of stretching and strengthening, endurance training, use of pressure garments and splints, and wound care. Splints are often used and require that the patient learn the purpose and proper application of the devices. Visiting nurses can help reduce the risk of complications by assisting in wound care, monitoring wound healing and medication administration, and educating the patient about burn injury recovery.

• The need for physical and occupational therapy does not end at discharge. The patient should ideally be referred to therapists with previous experience in treating burn injuries on an outpatient basis. Therapy programs need to continue the focus on ROM, strengthening, endurance, mobility, and gait.

• Skin that has been injured by burns has special needs. Moisturizers are required to control dryness, itching, and cracking. The skin must be protected from ultraviolet light because it is less tolerant and will burn more easily. Protection from sun and other sources of ultraviolet radiation is most critical during the period of scar maturation (i.e., the first 1 to 2 years).

• During the months and years that follow discharge from the hospital, patients often require reconstructive surgery to correct or prevent deformity and loss of function. Reconstructive surgery is typically delayed until scar maturation is achieved. An immature scar is more vascular, and local tissue response to the trauma of surgery is greater than in the mature scar. As a result, surgical outcomes are less favorable. However, if severe deformity is developing, surgery can be performed early to prevent irreversible loss of function (e.g., ectropion of the eyelid, which can lead to corneal damage and loss of vision). Serial procedures are often required to address cosmesis, function, or impaired physical maturation (e.g., female breast development). Because scar tissue does not expand with growth, children might need multiple operations during their growing years to correct and prevent loss of function and to improve cosmetic outcome.

• Determining the timing of surgical releases and other reconstructive procedures requires consideration of the body region burned as well as the patient's age, lifestyle, occupation, and medical and psychological well-being. Though restoration of function is typically the first priority, cosmesis can be more important in cases of severe facial burns. The function and appearance of the hands and face generally are given the highest priority. After consideration of all factors, an overall surgical plan needs to be established that reflects the identified priorities and needs of the patient.

• After discharge, the patient faces the task of family and community reintegration. Self-esteem can be significantly altered by changes in appearance and functional abilities. After a burn injury, women and girls have lower self-esteem than men and boys who experience comparable injuries. Physical attractiveness is known to be more important for self-esteem in females than in males. Persons with burn scars often do not experience the empathy from others that is typically seen with other disabilities. Burn patients can be seen as unattractive. Children with facial, buttocks, or genital injuries are at increased risk of depression and poor self-esteem.

• The greater the patient's perception of social support from family and friends, the more positive is the body image and the higher the sense of self-esteem. Symptoms of depression occur less commonly in this group of patients as well. Social support appears to be a key factor in a person's psychological adaptation to a burn injury.

WORK ISSUES (p. 1339)

• Returning to work is an issue of major importance to many burn patients. The TBSA injured, followed by the percentage of full-thickness and partial-thickness burns, correlates most strongly with the time needed to return to work. The presence of hand burns, the type of employment, and age are also significant factors. Overemphasis on ROM without adequate attention to the importance of endurance, strength, and power required in work settings can delay return to employment.

• Special problems affecting return to work include pruritus, skin fragility, heat and cold intolerance, altered sensation, and impaired coordination and dexterity. Burn injuries often occur at work, and affected individuals can have difficulty returning to the site of their injury. In the case of severe injury, approximately 20% to 50% of patients require a change in occupation.

• Work hardening is a highly structured work program that focuses on the tasks that a patient needs to be able to perform a given job (see Chapter 45). Individualized programs of training are developed after the individual's current level of function has been determined.

• Medical reports supporting impairment ratings should also address the unique long-term impairments in mobility, including standing and walking tolerance, hand function, skin fragility, sensitivity to ultraviolet light and chemicals, chronic pain and pruritus, heat and cold intolerance, impaired strength and sensation, and cardiopulmonary limitations.

59

Original Chapter by Gerald Felsenthal, M.D., Jeffrey A. Lehman, M.D., and
Barry D. Stein, M.D.

Principles of Geriatric Rehabilitation

DEMOGRAPHICS (p. 1343)

• In 1990, more than 30 million Americans, or 12.7% of the U.S. population, were 65 years of age or older. This is expected to increase to 17.3% by 2020 and to 21.8% by 2050. The greatest increase will be the oldest-old age group of 85 years and older, which is forecast to grow from approximately 3.3 million to 7.0 million between 1990 and 2020. The greatest functional decline is in this oldest-old age group, as compared to the young-old (65 to 74 years) and the old-old (75 to 84 years).

• As age increases, there is an increase in the prevalence of chronic conditions and activity limitations. Some 70% to 80% of the elderly live in the community.

ETIOLOGY OF FUNCTIONAL PROBLEMS (pp. 1343–1344)

• See Figure 59–1 for a list of age-related etiology of functional problems.

GERIATRIC REHABILITATION (pp. 1344–1346)

• *Geriatric rehabilitation* can be defined as medical treatment plus prevention, restoration plus accommodation, and education.

• One component of geriatric rehabilitation is accommodation is to the irreversible effects of aging; this requires education of the patient and family. A second component is the prevention of disability and the restoration of function. Exercise can be used to prevent or reverse the effects of disuse caused by inactivity. Functional loss may be reversible. Medical treatment of impairment is the third integral part. Treatment is needed to cure or to stabilize the disease process.

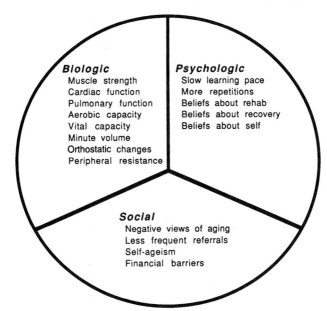

FIGURE 59–1. Age-related factors that may affect rehabilitation. (From Brummel-Smith K: Rehabilitation. In Ham RJ, Sloane PD (eds): Primary Care Geriatrics: A case-based approach. St. Louis, CV Mosby, 1992, p. 141.)

BIOLOGY AND PHYSIOLOGY OF AGING (pp. 1346–1349)

Body Composition (p. 1346)

• The loss of lean tissue reflects loss of muscle mass. Body fat increases to 30% of body weight at age 80 years, as compared to 15% at age 30 years. Peak bone density occurs in the 30s and 40s and gradually declines thereafter.

Postural Changes of Aging (p. 1346)

• Figure 59–2 shows the anterior thrust of the head and extension of the cervical spine, accentuated thoracic kyphosis, and straightening of the lumbar spine. Increased extension of the arms and scapular protraction at the shoulders is associated with flexion of the elbows, ulnar deviation at the wrists, and finger flexion. In the lower extremity, there is an increase in hip and knee flexion and a decrease in ankle dorsiflexion. During ambulation, there is diminished arm swing and a shorter step length.

• Additional changes with aging include widening of the bony pelvis. The angle of the femoral neck to the shaft increases, resulting in a valgus deformity of the hips. Widening of the standing base is noted. Women commonly develop varus deformities of the knees with narrowing of the standing base.

• There is a shift of the center of gravity so that it no longer favors extension of the lower extremity joints. The patient shifts the center of gravity behind the hips by flexing the knees. This may require the use of ambulatory aids.

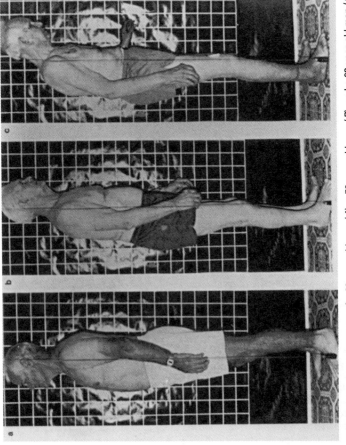

FIGURE 59-2. Lateral posture of a 60-year-old man (*A*), a 78-year-old man (*B*), and a 93-year-old man (*C*).

• Increased postural sway occurs. The ability to balance on one leg decreases. Righting reflexes decrease and reaction time increases.

Normal Neurological Changes of Aging (pp. 1346–1348)

• Table 59–1 lists neurological changes in elderly patients. Absent ankle jerks and diminished vibratory sense in the legs are not uncommon. Just because a physical finding is normal for an elderly patient doesn't mean that has no functional significance. For instance, loss of upward gaze is often seen in elderly patients. Mechanical neck problems are also common in the elderly, and this combination of restricted cervical motion and vertical gaze can make it difficult to see orienting information. To compensate for this, the patient might lean backward, contributing to a fall.

• Diminished muscle strength occurs, with the lower limbs more involved and with more weakness proximally. Exercise, along with accommodation and education, is necessary to limit loss of strength. Diminished strength leads to the common complaint of difficulty arising from a chair or toilet seat. Patients are more functional if seated in chairs with firm seats, hips and knees at 90-degree angles, and feet flat on the floor. The chairs should have armrests. The patient should move his or her buttocks to the front of the chair and flex the knees to

TABLE 59–1 Common Neurological Changes in Elderly Patients

Eye signs
    Small, irregular pupils
    Diminished reaction to light and near reflex
    Diminished range of movement on convergence and upward gaze
    Slowed pursuit movements with cogwheeling
Motor signs
    Tendency to tremor (>69 yr, 43% have hand tremor, 7% have head tremor [titubation])
    Gait: short-stepped or broad-based with diminished associated movements
    Dysmetria (in all >65 yr)
    Dysdiadochokinesia
    Atrophy of interossei (thenar wasting in 66%, anterior tibial wasting in 25%)
    Increased muscle tone: legs more than arms, proximal more than distal
    Diminished muscle strength: legs more than arms, proximal more than distal
Sensory signs
    Diminished vibratory sense distally, legs much more than arms
    Possible change in proprioception
    Mildly increased threshold for light touch, pain, and temperature
    Impaired double simultaneous stimulation
Reflex signs
    Diminished or absent ankle jerks
    Some reduction in knee, biceps, and triceps reflexes
    Abdominal reflex sometimes lost
    Babinski's sign may not occur (when it would in younger patients)
    Primitive reflexes occur in 20% to 25% (palmomental, snout, and nuchocephalic [doll's eyes])

From Ham RJ: Assessment. In Ham RJ, Sloane PD (eds): Primary Care Geriatrics: A Case-Based Approach. St Louis, Mosby—Year Book, 1992, p. 87.

bring the feet under the front edge of the chair. Many patients will also need to use their arms.
• Decline in cognitive function with normal aging tends to be minor. Mentation changes in the elderly are more likely to be associated with pathological conditions such as dementia, depression, or delirium.

Skin (p. 1348)

• Aging changes in the skin include decreases in moisture content, epidermal renewal, elasticity, and blood supply; and decreased sensitivity to touch, pain, and temperature. The effect of these changes is to make the patient more susceptible to injury or infection.

Cardiopulmonary Changes (p. 1348)

• Cardiac changes that occur with aging include decreased cardiac reserve, contractile function, heart rate, and response to exercise. Blood pressure tends to rise with aging. Pulmonary function mildly decreases. The main functional deficits are secondary to disease and not just to aging alone.

Urological Changes (p. 1348)

• Frequency, hesitancy, retention, and nocturia are common. Bladder capacity is reduced and residual volume increased. Prostatic hypertrophy is almost universal among elderly men. A reduction in creatinine clearance can predispose the elderly to toxic drug effects.

Hydration (pp. 1348–1349)

• The elderly have approximately a 25% decrease in thirst perception. This, along with medication side effects, increases the risk of dehydration. Many diseases common in the elderly and many drugs commonly used by the elderly can cause the syndrome of inappropriate antidiuretic hormone secretion and lead to water retention and hyponatremia.

Temperature (p. 1349)

• Elderly people have impairment of their thermoregulatory mechanisms and are more susceptible to hyperthermia and hypothermia. The febrile response to infection and other inflammatory diseases can fail to develop.

EXERCISE (p. 1349)

• Decrease in physiological functioning is also because of inactivity. Exercise can improve the physiological age of inactive patients as measured by maximum oxygen consumption (see Fig. 59–6 in the Textbook). Table 59–4 in the Textbook summarizes the adaptations to strength conditioning, and Table 59–5 in the Textbook summarizes the adaptations to aerobic conditioning. It is important to note that the elderly are capable of improving fitness and strength with activity. For example, strength has been reported to improve from 7% to 29% on isokinetic studies.

- ROM should be maintained in the major joints.
- Precautions and contraindications have to be considered before initiating an exercise program in the elderly. Limited ROM and arthritic joint involvement might require modification of the exercise program. Any co-existing medical conditions should be under optimal management. The possible impact of medications on the exercise program must be considered. High temperature and humidity might necessitate modification.

PHARMACOLOGY AND SUBSTANCE ABUSE
(pp. 1349–1350)

- Because of physiological changes affecting liver and kidney function, and the absorption and distribution of drugs, the elderly are more sensitive to medication. Table 59–2 lists drugs causing functional impairments. Elderly individuals take an average of five medications, and the incidence of adverse reactions increases with the number of medications. Elderly patients admitted to a rehabilitation service often show improvement in function after their medication regimens have been modified.
- Substance abuse, usually with alcohol, is common among the elderly. A mnemonic for screening for alcoholism is CAGE: "Have you tried to *C*ut down on your drinking?"; "Have others *A*nnoyed or *A*ngered you by criticizing your drinking?"; "Have you ever felt *G*uilty about your drinking?"; *E*ye-opener, "Have you used alcohol to steady your nerves or to reduce the effects of a hangover?".
- An acronym for drug therapy in the elderly is MASTER: *m*inimize number of drugs; *a*lternatives should be considered; *s*tart low and go slow; *t*itrate; *e*ducate; *r*eview.

FUNCTIONAL ASSESSMENT (pp. 1350–1352)

- In the elderly, assessment tools measuring ADL and instrumental ADL have particular significance. Accurate comparison can lead to early diagnosis and intervention.
- The *Mini-Mental State Examination* is a screening tool that can be used to detect and assess dementia and delirium (Table 59–3). There are a number of depression scales that can be used in the elderly, including the *Geriatric Depression Scale* in Table 59–9 in the Textbook.
- Gait and balance instruments are also useful functional assessment instruments. An assessment that reproduces mobility maneuvers is a better method than neuromuscular findings on physical examination. Some of these are noted in Table 59–10 in the Textbook.
- Impairment of driving limits ability to function independently. Factors for adverse driving events include near vision acuity worse than 20/40, limited neck rotation, and poor performance on a test of visual attention.

Balance (p. 1352)

- Balance depends on the interaction of multiple systems—the peripheral nervous system, proprioception, vestibular and cerebellar function, and visual acuity. Adequate muscle strength in the extensors of the hips and knees and

TABLE 59-2 Drug-Induced Impairment

Drug	Impairment
Antiepileptics	
Phenytoin	Osteoporosis, osteomalacia, neuropathy, sedation, cerebellar dysfunction, delirium, skin disorders
Barbiturates	Sedation, ataxia, skin disorders, behavior changes, respiratory depression, hypotension
Carbamazepine	Dizziness, sedation, ataxia, anemia, water retention, cardiac arrhythmias, vision disorders
Clonazepam	Sedation, respiratory depression, hypotension
Ethosuximide	Sedation, movement disorders, skin disorders
Valproate	Sedation, tremor, ataxia
Psychiatric	
Neuroleptics	Extrapyramidal symptoms, orthostatic hypotension, impaired balance, incontinence (central inhibition), dementia, constipation
Sedative hypnotics	Sedation, incontinence (oversedation), dementia
Lithium	Arthralgias, myopathies, polyuria, behavior changes, drowsiness, ataxia, impaired memory, skin disorders, confusion
Antidepressants	
Tricyclics	Sedation, delirium, constipation, urine retention, cardiac arrhythmias, orthostatic hypotension
Monoamine oxidase inhibitors	Irritability, agitation, tremor, urine retention, hypertension
Serotonin uptake inhibitors	Varies in sedative vs. stimulant effects
Other cyclics	Varies in sedative vs. stimulant effects

Parkinsonian Agents

Dopamine Agonists — Postural hypotension, delirium

Anticholinergic — Delirium, constipation, urine retention

Amantadine — Orthostatic hypotension, delirium, depression, skin disorders

Analgesics

Aspirin — Hypertension, impaired hearing, tinnitus, edema

Other nonsteroidal anti-inflammatory agents — Hypertension, edema

Narcotics (opioid) — Delirium, sedation, constipation, respiratory depression

Autonomic-Cardiovascular

Cholinergics — Bronchoconstriction, bradycardia

Anticholinergics (antimuscarinics) — Blurred vision, urine retention, constipation, tachycardias, delirium

Alpha-2 agonists (central) — Sedation, bradycardia, depression

Adrenergic agonists — Restlessness, tremors, hypertension, tachycardia

Beta-receptor blockers — Bronchoconstriction, bradycardia, cardiac failure, orthostatic hypotension, depression, lethargy, sleep disorders, behavior changes

Calcium channel blockers — Hypotension, peripheral edema, muscle weakness, bradycardia

Diuretics — Hypotension, weakness, electrolyte imbalance, glucose abnormalities

Alpha antagonists (peripheral) — Hypotension, incontinence (stress)

Other

Corticosteroids — Arthralgias, myopathies, osteoporosis, osteomalacia, glucose levels, behavior changes, depression, electrolyte abnormalities

Antihistamines — Sedation, urine retention, behavior changes

TABLE 59–3 Mini-Mental State Examination

I. Orientation (Ask the following questions)

What is today's date?	Date (e.g., Jan. 21)
What is the year?	Year
What is the month?	Month
What day is today?	Day (e.g., Monday)
Can you also tell me what season it is?	Season
Can you also tell me the name of this hospital (clinic)?	Hospital (clinic)
What floor are we on?	Floor
What town or city are we in?	Town or city
What county are we in?	County
What state are we in?	State

□□□□□□□□□

II. Immediate Recall

Ask the subject if you may test his/her memory. Then say "ball, flag, tree" clearly and slowly, about 1 sec for each. After you have said all three, ask him/her to repeat them. This first repetition determines his/her score (0–3), but keep saying them until he/she can repeat all three, up to six tries. If he/she does not eventually learn all three, recall cannot be meaningfully tested.

"Ball" □
"Flag" □
"Tree" □

Number of trials: _____

III. Attention and Calculation

Ask the subject to begin with 100 and count backward by 7. Stop after five subtracts (93, 86, 79, 72, 65). Score the total number of correct answers.

"93"
"86"
"79"
"72"
"65"

If the subject cannot or will not perform "the count backward test "task", ask him/her to spell the word "world" backward. The score is the number of letters in correct order. For example, *dlrow* is 5, *dlorw* is 3.

D
L
R
O
W

□□□□□□□□□

IV. Recall

Ask the subject to recall the 3 words you previously asked him/her to remember. Score 0–3.

☐ ☐ ☐   "Ball"
            "Flag"
            "Tree"

V. Language

NAMING
Show the subject a wrist watch and ask him/her what it is. Repeat for pencil.

☐ ☐   Watch
       Pencil

REPETITION
Ask the subject to repeat, "No ifs, ands, or buts."

3-STAGE COMMAND
Give the subject a piece of plain blank paper and say, "Take the paper in your right hand, fold it in half and put it on the floor."

☐ ☐ ☐ ☐   Repetition
             Takes paper in right hand
             Folds paper in half
             Puts paper on floor

READING
On a blank piece of paper print this sentence "Close your eyes," in letters large enough for the subject to see clearly. Ask him/her to read it and do what it says. Score correct only if he/she actually closes his/her eyes.

☐   Closes eyes

WRITING
Give the subject a blank piece of paper and ask him/her to write a sentence. It is to be written spontaneously. It must contain a subject and a verb and be sensible. Correct grammar and punctuation are not necessary.

☐   Writes sentence

COPYING
On a clean piece of paper, draw intersecting pentagons, each side about 1 inch, and ask subject to copy it exactly as it is. All 10 angles must be present and two must intersect to score one point. Tremor and rotation are ignored.

☐   Draws pentagons

e.g.

Deriving Total Score

Sum the number of correct replies to the test items. If item "world spelled backward" was used then add the number of correct letters given in proper sequence (one to five). The maximum score is 30 for this test.

TOTAL SCORE ☐

Reproduced with permission from Folstein MF, Folstein SE, McHugh PR: Mini-Mental State: A practical method for grading the cognitive state of patients for the clinician. J Psychiatr Res 1975; 12:189–198; and Kewas CH: Evaluation of cognition in the elderly rehabilitation patient. In Felsenthal G, Garrison SJ, Steinberg FU (eds): Rehabilitation of the Aging and Elderly Patient. Baltimore, Williams & Wilkins, 1994, pp. 289–294.

normal ankle muscles are also necessary. When more than one component is affected, balance is often impaired.

Gait (p. 1352)

• Men typically develop a pattern of small steps with a wide base. Women typically develop a waddling gait with a narrow base. The swing phase decreases and the period of double support increases. These changes increase the energy of ambulation.

• Pathological gait patterns can be caused by neurological or musculoskeletal causes. Examples include circumduction (hemiparesis); scissoring (upper motor neuron disease); festinating (Parkinson's disease); ataxia (vitamin deficiency, cervical spondylosis, and cerebellar dysfunction); apraxia (normal pressure hydrocephalus); senility (arterial degeneration); and waddling (muscle weakness). Other musculoskeletal causes of pathological gait include problems of the feet, hip, knee, and lumbar spine.

FALLS (pp. 1352–1356)

• Falls and near falls occur in about one-third of the elderly. Some 90% of fractures of the hip, pelvis, and forearm are the result of falls. Normal aging changes that contribute to falls are listed in Tables 59–1 and 59–4. Tables 59–5 and 59–6 also list risk factors for falls and strategies/guidelines for prevention. One of the significant consequences of falling is the fear of another fall.

COMMON IMPAIRMENTS (pp. 1356–1363)

Pain (pp. 1356–1359)

• Musculoskeletal pain is the most common: consider secondary gain or hidden agendas. Hearing loss, dementia, pseudodementia, and underreporting of symptoms by the patient all influence the accuracy of information. The physical examination has several potential findings (Table 59–7). Physical measures should be the cornerstone of treatment.

• Spinal problems are common. Spondylitic changes are present in up to 82% of persons in their sixth decade. Cervical disk degeneration presents most commonly at C5 to C6, followed by C6 to C7 and C4 to C5. Cervical spondylitic myelopathy is the most common reason for spinal cord dysfunction in patients over the age of 55 years. Lumbosacral spinal stenosis typically produces bilateral symptoms that are worse with standing or walking. Sitting down or flexing the spine while standing usually relieves these symptoms.

• At least 25% of the elderly have shoulder pain. Elbow, wrist, and hand pain occur commonly because of C7 radiculopathy, epicondylitis, nerve entrapment, de Quervain's tenosynovitis, or generalized arthritis. Hip pain is commonly caused by arthritis, trochanteric bursitis, or radiculopathy. Arthritis and trauma are major reasons for knee pain. Atrophic fat pads, bony deformities in the foot, and ill-fitting shoes can cause tendinitis, nerve entrapments, and tenosynovitis.

Dysphagia (p. 1359)

• Motor function of the lips, tongue, and masticatory muscles slows with aging. The latency from entry of the bolus into the pharynx until the elevation of the

TABLE 59–4 Normal Aging Changes That Predispose to Falls and Injuries

Visual impairments
 Presbyopia and decreases in accommodative capacity, visual acuity, night vision, peripheral
  vision, glare tolerance, impaired blue-green discrimination, and contrast sensitivity
Nervous system impairments
 Reduced righting reflexes, proprioceptive input, and cerebral function; increased reaction time;
  lessened awareness of vibration, touch, and temperature; increased distractibility
Musculoskeletal impairments
 Osteopenia; musculoskeletal stiffness; reduced or uncoordinated muscle control
Cardiovascular impairments
 Postural hypotension
Gait changes
 Women: waddling gait, narrow walking and standing base
 Men: Small-stepped gait, wide walking and standing base
Auditory impairments
 Reduced speech discrimination
 Increased high-frequency threshold
 Wax accumulation

Adapted from Tideiksaar R: Falls in the elderly: An approach to management. Phys Assistant 1988; 10:114–132;
and Barclay AM: Falls in the elderly: Is prevention possible? Postgrad Med 1988; 83:241–248.

TABLE 59–5 Some Factors Implicated in Traumatic Fractures in the Elderly

Aspects of aging
 Primary osteoporosis
 Impaired balance/vision
 Alteration in gait
 Loss in muscle/fat "padding" at hip
 Falls forward (Colles' fracture/humerus) vs.
  falls down (hip/pelvic)
Environment
 Outdoor
  Cracked walkway
  Poor lighting
  Poor weather
  Uneven ground
  Crime (assault and battery)
 Indoor
  Throw rugs
  Wires across path
  Slippery tub
  Poor lighting
  Stairs/railings
  Pet causing a fall
Genetic
 Sex (females > males)
 Race (white > black)

Illnesses
 Cerebrovascular accident
 Syncopal episodes
 Hypotensive illnesses
 Secondary osteoporosis
  Hyperthyroidism
  Hypoparathyroidism, etc.
 Osteomalacia
 Parkinson's disease
 Dementia
 Arthritis
 Paraparesis
 Previous fracture
Lifestyle
 Exercise/nutrition
 Alcoholism/other abused drugs
 Bed rest/immobilization
 Shoe style
Medications
 Benzodiazepines
 Tricyclic antidepressants
 Antipsychotic medications
 Corticosteroids (secondary osteoporosis)
 Barbiturates

From Stein BD, Felsenthal G: Rehabilitation of fractures in the geriatric population. In Felsenthal G, Garrison SJ,
Steinberg FU (eds): Rehabilitation of the Aging and Elderly Patient. Baltimore, Williams & Wilkins, 1994, p. 123.

TABLE 59-6 Guidelines for Home Safety

Problem Area	Risk Potential for Falls	Modifications to Recommend
Floors	High polish or wet surfaces may cause slipping	In bathrooms, use nonslip tiles, nonslip adhesive strips on floor next to tub, sink, and toilet, or indoor-outdoor carpeting; on linoleum floors, use slip-resistant floor wax with minimal buffing; use nonskid floor mat by kitchen sink to guard against wet floor
Carpets	Thick pile and carpet borders may cause tripping	Suggest carpets of low pile
Area rugs and mats	Rugs and mats may slide out from under person	Use rugs and mats with nonskid backing, or apply double-faced adhesive tape as backing
Lighting	Low or uneven lighting may obscure hazards	Increase lighting in high-risk areas (e.g., stairs, bathroom, bedroom)
Glare	Visual impairment and distraction may be produced by glare from bright lights (especially sunlight) on polished floors and from unshielded light bulbs	Use polarized window glass, or apply tinted material to windows to eliminate glare without reducing light; reduce flood glare by repositioning light sources
Stairs	Poor lighting may contribute to tripping on stairway	Place light switches at top and bottom of stairway to avoid traveling up and down in the dark, or place night-lights by top and bottom step to provide visual cuing of steps; apply colored nonskid adhesive strips to stair edges; set maximum step rise at 6 in.
Handrails	Lack of support may result from missing or improper handrails	Place cylindrical rails 1-2 in. away from wall on both sides, with ends turned in and extending beyond top and bottom steps to provide easy grasping and signal top and bottom step
Sink edge and towel bar	Weak towel bar or wet, slippery sink edge may not provide adequate support	Replace towel bars with nonslip grab bars

	Problem	Recommendation
Toilet seat	Transfer falls often occur because seat is too low	Advise use of elevated toilet with grab bars placed on wall next to toilet
Wet bathtub and shower floor surfaces	Slipping and falling are common on wet surfaces	Place nonslip adhesive rubber strips or suction-cup mat on tub floor; install nonslip grab bars in and around tub and shower; advise use of shower chair and flexible handheld shower hose for patients with balance impairment
Bed height	Transfer falls are more common if height is not optimal	Adjust bed height distance from patella to floor (18in. from top of mattress to floor allows for safest transfer by most persons)
Soft bed mattress	Poor sitting balance and support may lead to falls from bed	Bed mattress edges should be firm enough to support a seated person without sagging
Chair height	Transfer falls from low chairs are common	Replace low chairs with more suitable ones (chair height should be 14–16in. from seat edge to floor; armrests should be present 7in. above the seat and extend 1–2in. beyond the seat edge for maximal leverage)
Shelf height	Reaching or bending to retrieve objects from high or low shelves leads to imbalance and falling	Rearrange frequently used kitchen and closet items to avoid excessive reaching and bending; encourage use of handheld reach tools
Gas range	Difficult-to-see dial may not be turned off and may cause gas leak; fall may be first sign of gas asphyxiation with impaired smell	Mark on and off dial positions clearly
Temperature	Low room temperature may cause hypothermia; falls may be secondary to hypothermia	Maintain indoor temperature at 72°F in winter

Adapted from Tideiksaar R: Falls in the elderly: An approach to management: Phys Assistant 1988; 10:114–132; and Christiansen J, et al: The prevention of falls in later life: A report of the Kellogg International Work Group on the Prevention of Falls in the Elderly. Dan Med Bull 1987; 34:1–24.

TABLE 59–7 Examples of Geriatric Physical Examination Issues for the Pain Patient

Clinical Problem	Functional Consequence	Pain, Other Consequences
Hamstring and back extensor muscle contractures, decreased range of motion of heel cords (from high heels)	Excess knee and hip flexion and abnormal spinal postures to avoid falling from a heel cord contracture	Pain at multiple sites from fatigue and muscle overuse; give attention to heel cords
Restriction of upward gaze	Compensation by neck extension and lordosis, with foraminal narrowing, facet compression, and alterations in balance	Radicular compression at foramen with pain; increased risk of dizziness and falls
Orthostatic hypotension	Alterations in balance and gait	Differentiate from other neuromusculoskeletal reasons for altered gait

larynx increases with age. The amplitude of esophageal contractions decreases with age.

Arthritis (p. 1359)

• Arthritis is more common and may present differently.
• The tendons, ligaments, and joint capsules lose elasticity resulting in decreased ROM and a sense of stiffness. ROM exercises should start at a few degrees and should be done gently.
• Joint replacement surgery may be appropriate in medically intractable joint dysfunction.

Osteoporosis and Paget's Disease (p. 1359)

• Acute symptomatic vertebral fractures from osteoporosis can be treated with bed rest and physical measures. Flank pain can be caused by kyphoscoliosis with the rib cage rubbing the pelvic rim. Back-strengthening exercises contribute to good posture and skeletal support, but flexion exercises of the spine are not recommended owing to the possibility of anterior wedge fractures. Paget's disease in the elderly can lead to fractures, rare cancerous changes, total joint replacement, and paraplegia.

Fractures (pp. 1359–1360)

• Osteoporosis and falls are the major contributing factors. Weight bearing and ROM are important issues. Restrictions are dependent on the fracture and repair. Concomitant deep venous thrombosis, stroke, pain, and peripheral neuropathy may be present.
• Pelvic fractures may require prolonged bed rest. Colles' fractures can be disabling and may result in carpal tunnel syndrome.

Stroke (pp. 1360–1361)

• Older persons are at greater risk of being institutionalized after a stroke. Multi-infarct dementia can be a confounding problem (see Chapter 50).

Traumatic Brain Injury (p. 1361)

• Falling is the most common cause of TBI in those older than 65 years. Pedestrian accidents yield the most fatalities. Advancing medical and neurological illnesses often increase the severity of the injury as well as its mortality. Protection from a second fall is a major goal to prevent further TBI and fractures (see Chapter 49).

Motor Neuron Disease and Parkinson's Disease (pp. 1361–1362)

• Attention to dysphagia, respiratory problems, self-care, balance and mobility, nutrition, and psychotherapy is important (see Chapters 46 and 51).

Peripheral Nervous System Impairments (p. 1362)

• Elderly persons have decreased vibratory sense and ankle muscle stretch reflexes. Drug-related and toxic neuropathies; nutritional and alcoholic neuropathies; and postherpetic, diabetic, entrapment, rheumatic, carcinomatous, and paraproteinemic neuropathies are common in the elderly. Neuromuscular junction changes and muscle atrophy are commonly seen. Carefully timed exercises and energy conservation are important with myasthenia gravis.

Visual Impairments (pp. 1362–1363)

• Vision is a factor contributing to balance. Visual impairment is especially challenging when combined with mobility impairment. Poor vision often results in social isolation, impaired morale, and a decreased sense of well-being. Cataracts, age-related macular degeneration, glaucoma, and diabetic retinopathy are amenable in varying degrees to visual rehabilitative services.

Hearing Loss (p. 1363)

• The incidence of significant hearing loss appears to be 25% to 50% in those more than 65 years of age. The varying types of sensorineural hearing loss can be clarified by audiometric evaluation. Often patients refuse to wear hearing aids because of sound distortion, impaired dexterity in their use or adjustment, uncomfortable fit, or vanity.

Peripheral Vascular Disease and Ischemic Skin Ulceration (p. 1363)

• Intermittent claudication should be distinguished from similar complaints of discomfort in the aged caused by other conditions. Foot care is important. Chronic venous insufficiency and lymphedema can be helped with compression garments. Skin ulceration needs careful, aggressive treatment (see Chapter 56).

Foot Disorders (p. 1363)

• The geriatric ankle and foot has decreased shock absorption and spring abilities as a result of problems such as bony disfigurement, joint disorders, and muscular imbalances. Aging can result in insensitive feet with potential for ulceration and decreased ability to heal. Strengthening and other physical therapies, foot care, proper shoe selection, and appropriate podiatric treatment are important.

Sexual Function (p. 1363)

• Sexual activity is affected by age-related changes in hormonal levels; alterations in vision, hearing, and smell; negative social attitudes; erectile and ejaculatory changes; vaginal dryness and dyspareunia; urinary stress incontinence; decreases in muscle strength and endurance; and limitations in movement from osteoarthritis. Additional problems in sexual functioning can arise from medical illnesses and drugs. Treatment may include counseling and medication (see Chapter 30).

AGING WITH A DISABILITY (pp. 1363–1364)

Poliomyelitis (p. 1363)

• Of the more than 640,000 living people in the United States who have experienced paralytic poliomyelitis, more than 50% report having excessive fatigue, progressive weakness, pain, loss of function, and occasional muscle atrophy 30 to 40 years after the acute episode. The diagnosis of the *post-polio syndrome* requires evidence of a prior episode of poliomyelitis, a characteristic pattern of recovery from that episode, and exclusion of other conditions that could cause new symptoms. Management includes careful strengthening, pain treatment with emphasis on physical medicine techniques, orthoses, referral to a pulmonologist if needed, and attention to psychological issues. (See Chapter 46.)

Spinal Cord Injury (p. 1363)

• Motor function is the predominant limiting factor in attainment of goals. Age is associated with a lower statistical chance of achieving some of the functional goals (e.g., dressing, bathing, stair climbing, and complex transfers). The aging family also poses care issues for the newly injured geriatric patient as well as the aging patient with a chronic spinal cord injury (see Chapter 55).

Multiple Sclerosis (p. 1363)

• Weakness and fatigue in multiple sclerosis is compounded by age-related peripheral nerve changes, muscle atrophy, and diminished cardiopulmonary reserve. Exercise is important to promote fitness. Elderly MS patients often have problems such as hyperthermia, decreased skin sensation, diminished special senses, impairments of the genitourinary and gastrointestinal systems, cognitive dysfunctions, and affective disorders (see Chapter 52).

Aging with Pediatric-Onset Disabilities (pp. 1363–1364)

• Chronic back pain, scoliosis, cervical spine pain, the sequelae of hip dislocation, and spastic deformities of the feet and toes have been reported in adults with *cerebral palsy*. A high incidence of bowel, bladder, skin, cognitive, and dystonic problems is found.

• Epilepsy in adulthood is more common in those with *Down's syndrome*. Pathological findings of neurofibrillary tangles and neuritic plaques suggest a link between Down's syndrome and Alzheimer's disease and raise the question as to whether this is associated with an observed cognitive deterioration. Atlantoaxial instability, commonly with pain, is reported in 9% to 12% of Down's syndrome patients.

• Persons with *spina bifida* can have late sequelae from hydromyelia, tethered cord, symptomatic Arnold-Chiari malformation, inclusion dermoid, shunt failure, urinary and renal system dysfunction, arthritis, rotator cuff injury, and entrapment neuropathies.

REHABILITATION (p. 1364)

• The goals for each patient must be functionally significant and achievable within a reasonable time. Three factors that interact to determine whether a patient can be discharged to a noninstitutional setting are ADL status; cognitive, judgment, and safety status; and the social support system.

TREATMENT SITE (p. 1365)

• The elderly rehabilitation patient can be treated in multiple sites ranging from a geriatric program in a nursing home to a comprehensive rehabilitation center. Each site must be modified for the special needs of the elderly. These modifications can be both architectural and programmatic.

• Architectural and environmental factors that should be considered in living areas for the elderly are listed in Tables 59–7, 59–8, and 59–9.

• Reality orientation should be emphasized. Clocks and calendars should be placed in patient areas. Daily schedules should be posted and patients given the responsibility of learning and following a schedule. Holidays, birthdays, news, and scheduled events should be part of the daily routine. Patients should be taken outside to reorient to external factors such as the weather, day versus night, and the season of year.

MOTIVATION (p. 1365)

• Abstract goals such as improving strength, balance, dexterity, and ambulation distance are often insufficient to ensure cooperation. Concrete goals such as getting to the toilet or to a meal are more realistic and more likely to get patient cooperation.

PRINCIPLES OF MANAGEMENT (p. 1365)

• Table 59–8 is a summary of the principles of geriatric rehabilitation.

PRESCRIPTION MODIFICATION (p. 1365)

• The environment in which elderly patients exercise should be neither too hot nor too cold. Monitoring for dehydration is a necessity. Transient circulatory insufficiency (e.g., postural hypotension) can occur and lead to falls and

TABLE 59–8 Principles of Rehabilitation Management of the Elderly Patient

1. Ascertain level of function (functional assessment)
2. Ascertain available resources and options
3. Avoid immobilization
4. Be aware of altered physiological reactions
5. Determine patient's significant goals, motivation
6. Determine family expectations (psychosocial issues)
7. Differentiate between delirium, dementia, and depression
8. Emphasize function; management not diagnosis; cure
9. Emphasize task-specific exercise; simplify program
10. Encourage socialization and stimulation
11. Minimize medications
12. Realize that function may not be regained
13. Recognize that patients have multiple interacting impairments
14. Understand that improvement occurs in slow increments

syncope. Postural instability can also lead to falls. Cardiopulmonary impairments are common and require appropriate precautions. Similarly, medications can affect the ability to participate in therapy and increase the risk involved in therapy.

DISCHARGE PLANNING (pp. 1365–1366)

• Discharge planning should begin with the rehabilitation referral. The goals of the patient and the support system should be ascertained. The bottom-line functional abilities required for the family to be able or willing to take a patient home should be determined.

LEGAL AND ETHICAL ISSUES (p. 1366)

• The rehabilitation of the elderly is made more complicated by the fact that laws dealing with the elderly differ among jurisdictions.
• The ethical dilemma in determining how much to do and whether to do it involves the wishes of the patient and the family and the laws pertaining to each jurisdiction.

OUTCOME (p. 1366)

• Most elderly patients can be kept in the community. With the application of methodologies discussed in this chapter, their quality of life can be maintained or improved. Most elderly patients live in the community, and even among those aged 85 years and above, only 15% of men and 25% of women live in a nursing home. Our challenge as rehabilitation professionals is not to give in to the biases of ageism, but to employ our abilities in assisting our elderly patients to maintain the quality and dignity of their lives.

60

Original Chapter by Michael W. O'Dell, M.D., Mary E. Dillon, M.D., and Anthony A. Oreste, M.D.

Rehabilitation Management in Persons with AIDS and HIV Infection

OVERVIEW OF AIDS AND HIV INFECTION
(pp. 1369–1372)

Epidemiology (p. 1369)

• As of June 1998, over 665,000 AIDS cases and 401,000 deaths of AIDS had been reported in the United States. After exponential increases through the 1980s, the epidemic plateaued, and actual decreases were reported in 1995. These decreases have continued through 1997. Groups hardest hit in recent years (i.e., those infected through heterosexual transmission, IV drug users, and women) experienced less impressive declines. The least decreases were observed among African-Americans (9%) and among those infected by heterosexual transmission (6% for women and 3% for men). The AIDS epidemic continues to claim a disproportionate number of ethnic minorities.

• HIV has limited modes of transmission (i.e., intimate sexual contact, blood product exposure, and perinatal transmission). There are actually no risk groups for HIV infection, only risk behaviors. Rehabilitation professionals should adhere to universal precautions for all patient encounters.

Biology, Natural History, and Treatment (pp. 1369–1372)

• HIV, a human retrovirus, has unique tendencies (i.e., nervous system invasion, long latency period, and failure to elicit a neutralizing response). HIV has primary and secondary destructive effects.

• AIDS is the end-stage manifestation of chronic HIV infection. Within a few weeks of initial infection, symptoms occur that are typical of an acute viral syndrome. Antibodies can usually be detected within 1 to 3 months after infection. The acute infection is followed by a period of relative clinical latency. The time from infection to symptom development varies from 2 to 15 years. There is a steady decline of immune function during this "asymptomatic" phase.

TABLE 60–1 Common Organ System Involvement for Selected Pathogens in AIDS

Pathogen and Class	Typical Site of Involvement
Parasites	
Toxoplasma gondii	Brain
Cryptosporidium	Gastrointestinal (GI) tract
Pneumocystis carinii	Lung
Fungi	
Candida albicans	Mouth, esophagus, vulva, and vagina
Cryptococcus neoformans	Meninges, lung
Viruses	
Cytomegalovirus	Retina, lungs, nervous system, GI tract
Herpes simplex, varicella-zoster	Cutaneous, esophagus, brain
JC virus	Brain—white matter
Mycobacteria	
Mycobacterium tuberculosis	Lungs, meninges, disseminated
Mycobacterium avium-intracellulare	GI tract, bone marrow, disseminated

- Familiar manifestations generally occur late in the course of HIV infection. Examples are listed in Table 60–1. Kaposi's sarcoma is the most common presenting cancer, followed by CNS lymphoma. Other late manifestations related to a direct effect of HIV include constitutional symptoms ("HIV wasting syndrome"), cytopenias, and neurological disease.

- The rapid replication of HIV causes progressive damage to immune function. The error-prone nature of replication also results in very high levels of genetic mutations. The combination of rapid rates of replication and mutation rate leads to rapid development of drug resistance.

- Plasma HIV RNA assay is the most sensitive and reliable measurement of plasma viral load. The extent of immune system damage that has already occurred in an HIV-infected person is indicated by the CD4+ count, which when combined with RNA levels, provides the most accurate assessment of the relative risk of disease progression and time to death.

- Since 1995, two or three new antiretroviral agents have been approved yearly (see Table 60–3 in the Textbook). These agents are reverse transcriptase inhibitors. Additionally, protease inhibitors are available. Their main antiviral action of HIV is to block the infectivity of nascent virons and to prevent subsequent waves of infection. These agents have no effect on infected cells with integrated viral DNA. Commonly used drugs and associated side effects are listed in Table 60–2.

- Antiretroviral monotherapy is no longer recommended for treatment, except possibly to suppress perinatal transmission. Choices for initiating therapy are expanding; however, the current recommended standard for initial therapy consists of a protease inhibitor combined with two reverse transcriptase inhibitors.

- Plasma RNA levels are the best measure of the effectiveness of antiretroviral therapy. The goal of combination antiretroviral therapy is to suppress plasma RNA levels below the limit of detection, but this does not mean the infection has been eradicated or that the risk of transmission has been eliminated. Most,

TABLE 60–2 Summary of Antiretroviral Medications

Medication Class	Generic Name	Trade Name	Side Effects
NRTI	Zidovudine	Retrovir	Bone marrow suppression, anemia, neutropenia, GI intolerance, headache, insomnia, asthenia
NRTI	Didanosine (ddI)	Videx	Pancreatitis, peripheral neuropathy, nausea, diarrhea
NRTI	Zalcitabine (ddC)	Hivid	Peripheral neuropathy, stomatitis
NRTI	Stavudine (d4T)	Zerit	Peripheral neuropathy
NRTI	Lamivudine (3TC)	Epivir	Minimal toxicity
NNRTI	Nevirapine	Viramune	Rash, increased transaminase levels, hepatitis
NNRTI	Delavirdine	Rescriptor	Rash, headache
PI	Indinavir	Crixivan	Nephrolithiasis, GI intolerance, nausea, indirect bilirubinemia (inconsequential), headache, asthenia, blurred vision, dizziness, rash, metallic taste, thrombocytopenia, hyperglycemia
PI	Ritonavir	Norvir	GI intolerance, nausea, vomiting, diarrhea, paresthesias, hepatitis, asthenia, taste perversion, increased triglycerides (up to 200%), transaminase, uric acid, and CPK elevation, hyperglycemia
PI	Saquinavir	Invirase	GI intolerance, nausea, diarrhea, headache, increased transaminase enzymes, hyperglycemia
PI	Saquinavir	Fortovase	GI intolerance, nausea, diarrhea, abdominal pain, dyspepsia, headache, increased transaminase enzymes, hyperglycemia
PI	Nelfinavir	Viracept	Diarrhea, hyperglycemia

Abbreviations: NRTI, nucleoside reverse transcriptase inhibitor; NNRTI, non-nucleoside reverse transcriptase inhibitor; PI, protease inhibitor; GI, gastrointestinal.
Adapted from Centers for Disease Control: Guidelines for the use of antiretroviral agents in HIV-infected adults and adolescents. MMWR 1998; 47:43–82.

if not all, infected patients have a small amount of virus in long-lived cellular reservoirs, where it is no longer detected. The future challenges include inactivating these latently infected reservoirs.

REHABILITATION MEDICINE AND HIV INFECTION (pp. 1372–1373)

• The epidemiology of functional deficits throughout the spectrum of HIV infection has been delineated over the past few years. Functional limitations are uncommon early, becoming more pronounced as the disease progresses.

• HIV disease remains a moving target in terms of planning for rehabilitation services. There is a strong association between symptoms in HIV infection and functional deficits. Disabling symptoms can persist among persons living longer. New, more disabling symptoms could arise as a result of improved treatments, as well as secondary disability as a result of those treatments. On the other hand, better primary anti-HIV treatments might decrease the use of prophylactic medications and subsequent side effects. Recent evidence suggests that rehabilitation physicians are providing more care to persons with HIV. Access to rehabilitation services might well be among the most important factors in the provision of rehabilitation services to persons with HIV infection.

• Many kinds of rehabilitation interventions are appropriate in persons with HIV infection. Examples included therapeutic exercise, gait aids, bathroom and safety equipment, orthoses, vocational counseling, pain management, and whirlpool treatment.

CLINICAL MANIFESTATIONS OF HIV INFECTION AND THE REHABILITATION APPROACH (pp. 1373–1377)

• For the sake of simplicity, the clinical manifestations of HIV infection are grouped as neurological and nonneurological. Single impairments rarely lead to a specific disability. Fluctuating, multiple impairments are the rule, especially in late HIV disease. The approach to rehabilitation is discussed after the description of each complication.

Neurological Manifestations (p. 1373)

• Because multiple pathogens infecting multiple levels of the nervous system are common, a few principles regarding the neurological manifestations of HIV infection bear review. First, certain neurological processes tend to occur during certain clinical disease stages. For example, demyelinating neuropathies tend to occur early, whereas cerebral infections occur late. Second, it is common for central and peripheral nervous system processes to occur simultaneously. Third, the potential effects of systemic disease and of medication side effects must be considered in the differential diagnosis. Finally, the clinician should not fail to consider more common causes of nervous system dysfunction in appropriate circumstances.

Central Nervous System Complications (p. 1373)

• Typical CNS diseases in HIV infection are outlined in Table 60–3. Diffuse processes in HIV-related CNS disease can be broadly viewed within the

TABLE 60-3 Causes of CNS Dysfunction in HIV-Related Disease

Cause	Frequency	Cognitive Deficits	Focal CNS Deficits	Blindness	Myelopathy	Rehabilitation Prognosis
Viruses						
Primary HIV encephalitis	65%–90%	+++	–	–	++	Good early Poor late
CMV encephalitis	Up to 90%	++	±	–	+	Fair
CMV retinitis	20%–25%	–	–	+++	–	Good
PML (JC virus)	Up to 3.8%	++	+++	±	–	Very poor
Herpes simplex	Rare	+	++	±	+	Generally good
Varicella-zoster	Rare	+	±	–	+	Good
Epstein-Barr virus	Common	±	±	–	±	Generally good
Others	Rare	±	±	±	±	Variable
Bacteria						
Mycobacterium tuberculosis	Rare	+	+	–	±	Good except drug-resistant
Mycobacterium avium-intracellulare	Rare	+	–	–	–	Poor when disseminated
Others	Very rare	±	±	±	±	Variable
Fungi						
Cryptococcal meningitis	9%	+++	+	±	±	Variable (40% mortality)
Others	Very rare	±	±	±	±	Variable
Protozoa						
Toxoplasmosis	>2%	+	+++	±	±	Excellent with medical treatment
Malignancies						
Primary CNS lymphoma	1.5%	+	+++	±	–	Poor
Metastatic (Kaposi's sarcoma)	Rare	+	+++	±	±	Fair-poor
Cerebrovascular	Rare	++	+++	±	±	Poor
Multiple sclerosis	Unknown	+	+++	+	+++	

Abbreviations: CNS, central nervous system; CMV, cytomegalovirus; PML, progressive multifocal leukoencephalopathy; +++, usually present; ++, very common; +, common; ±, occasionally present; –, not found.

From Levinson SF, Merritt L: Disability due to CNS impairment. Phys Med Rehabil 1993; 7:S101–S118.

traumatic brain injury model in terms of intervention; focal processes within the stroke model; and myelopathies, similar to SCI rehabilitation (see Table 60–7 in the Textbook). The general approach to managing functional deficits in AIDS is no different from that used for corresponding non-HIV processes. In this sense, HIV rehabilitation directly parallels the philosophy of cancer rehabilitation (see Chapter 57).

Diffuse Processes (pp. 1374–1375)

Presentation (pp. 1374–1375)

• The most common diffuse CNS processes are AIDS-dementia complex (ADC) and cryptococcal meningitis. Less common processes include viral encephalopathies, bacterial and lymphomatous meningitis, and metabolic abnormalities. It is important to consider mood disorders and medication side effects. Mild cognitive dysfunction is also common in patients with focal neurological presentations.

• ADC is a relentlessly progressive encephalopathy characterized by cognitive, motor, and behavioral impairment. As opposed to Alzheimer's disease, ADC is classified as a subcortical dementia characterized by slowness of thought, inattention, and forgetfulness. It resembles the cognitive and motor presentation of Parkinson's disease. Arousal and insight are well preserved until quite late. Motor deficits include lower extremity weakness, gait abnormalities, ataxia, cogwheel rigidity, and tremor. Behavioral manifestations include apathy and even frank psychoses. ADC is almost always a late complication of AIDS. It is a diagnosis of exclusion. Neuroimaging typically shows brain atrophy. Evidence is gradually accumulating showing that treatment can prevent, slow, or reverse ADC.

• Cryptococcal meningitis is seen in about 5% to 10% of persons with AIDS. Symptoms generally occur for less than 3 weeks prior to diagnosis and include headache, fever, and mental status changes. The diagnosis is confirmed by laboratory analysis of CSF or blood. Neuroimaging studies are usually normal. Treatment consists of initiation and lifetime maintenance with fluconazole. Other possible fungal infections include aspergillosis, candidiasis, and histoplasmosis.

Rehabilitation Approach (p. 1375)

• Rehabilitation professionals can adapt an approach similar to traumatic brain injury. The progressive nature of the late manifestations of AIDS necessitates an emphasis on relatively short-term, functionally based goals. Cognitive deficits can limit the rehabilitation potential of persons.

• Early in the course of cognitive attrition, performance can be enhanced with compensatory strategies. Although the patient should be the focus of intervention, caretakers should be involved when ADC is diagnosed. Neuropsychological testing may be indicated.

• Psychosocial interventions are paramount. Counseling for patients, partners, family, and caretakers can facilitate adjustment to disability. Legal matters (e.g., living wills, power of attorney, and guardianship) should be addressed early while the patient is mentally competent.

Focal Processes (pp. 1375–1376)

Presentation (pp. 1375–1376)

• Prophylactic antibiotics have dramatically decreased the incidence of cerebral toxoplasmosis. Progressive multifocal leukoencephalopathy (PML) may also be occurring with greater relative frequency. Cranial MRI is more sensitive than CT in demonstrating small lesions and in determining lesion age.

- *Toxoplasma gondii* usually manifests with focal signs. The typical presentation occurs over 1 to 2 weeks with fatigue, fever, and progressive hemiparesis and/or aphasia. CT usually shows multiple, ring-enhancing lesions with a propensity for the basal ganglia and frontoparietal lobes. MRI might show lesions in the absence of CT findings. Although empirical treatment with pyrimethamine and sulfadiazine has been the standard of care, the dramatic drop in the incidence of toxoplasmosis has called this practice into question. A clinical response with drug therapy requires lifetime maintenance. The prognosis is favorable for patients with CNS opportunistic infections, with survival of a year not uncommon.

- Cerebrovascular disease is seen clinically with HIV infection; however, whether it is because of HIV remains unclear. Ischemic infarctions are more common than hemorrhagic strokes. As in strokes in young persons in general, often no specific cause is found. Survival usually ranges from a few days to 2 years.

- Progressive multifocal leukoencephalopathy (PML) is a CNS demyelinating disorder seen in about 4% to 5% of persons with AIDS and results from infection with papovavirus. Cognitive and visual complaints and weakness in the absence of fever are the most common clinical presentations. Brain CT demonstrates nonenhancing, multiple low-density white matter lesions. Brain biopsy confirms the diagnosis. Prognosis is poor for most patients. There is also very preliminary evidence that the clinical course of PML can be altered with the use of highly active antiretroviral therapies.

- Primary CNS lymphoma is seen in 1% to 3% of persons with AIDS. The presentation is variable, including solitary or multiple intracerebral masses, lymphomatous meningitis, and localized intradural spinal masses. Lymphoma appears on radiographs as single or multiple discrete lesions, with some degree of surrounding edema and contrast enhancement. SPECT can be helpful in differentiating lymphoma from toxoplasmosis. Treatment consists primarily of radiotherapy, with chemotherapy in selected patients. Survival is usually measured in months, with most patients often succumbing to other complications.

- Uncommon neurological presentations include a fulminant variant of multiple sclerosis and parkinsonian symptoms.

Rehabilitation Approach (p. 1376)

- The approach in focal CNS disease is similar to stroke rehabilitation. Interventions include providing appropriate orthoses, assistive devices, and therapeutic exercise; treating spasticity; and enhancing communication abilities. Because of parallel tracking, clinicians should check carefully for concomitant peripheral neuropathy before prescribing orthoses. Basic rehabilitation concerns such as preventing skin compromise and contractures, maintaining bowel and bladder function, and ensuring safety of swallowing are no different from routine rehabilitation practice. Painful sequelae such as complex regional pain syndrome, musculoskeletal shoulder pain, and central pain syndrome are also seen. The team should be aware of mild to moderate cognitive deficits that can affect new learning and the teaching of compensatory strategies. Education of family members or significant others should be initiated in nearly all cases.

Myelopathy (pp. 1376–1377)

Presentation (p. 1376)
• Spinal cord involvement is found in 20% to 50% of persons at autopsy. HIV-associated myelopathy, termed *vacuolar myelopathy,* tends to affect the dorso-lateral portion of the thoracic and cervical spinal cord, almost always in very advanced disease. The resulting clinical picture is one of ataxia and mild to moderate weakness with spasticity progressing over 1 to 4 months. Other causes of spinal cord impairment include infection, lymphoma, and vitamin deficiency. Neuroimaging is critical to rule out treatable causes.
• High-dose antiretroviral medication has been suggested as treatment. Recent reports of some improvement in impairment associated with HIV myelopathy are encouraging. The prognosis is variable.

Rehabilitation Approach (pp. 1376–1377)
• As in rehabilitation for non-HIV myelopathy, aggressive management of bladder dysfunction is a high priority. Options include urological medications and intermittent catheterization. Because of the multiple enteric pathogens seen in the setting of HIV infection, constipation is unusual.
• Orthotic devices and adaptive equipment should be prescribed with clear functional goals in mind. Evaluation for concomitant peripheral neuropathy should accompany any orthotic prescription. In many cases, fatigue and overall debilitation preclude all but household mobility.

NEUROMUSCULAR COMPLICATIONS (pp. 1377–1378)

• Abnormalities at virtually every level of the peripheral neuromuscular system have been implicated in HIV infection. Peripheral neuropathy and myopathy are far more common.

Peripheral Neuropathic Pain (p. 1377)

• There are several types of peripheral neuropathy associated with HIV infection. The most common is distal symmetrical polyneuropathy (DSP). DSP presents with distal pain, paresthesias, hyporeflexia, and relatively normal strength. Symptoms tend to manifest late, develop over weeks to months, and persist once present. Another painful neuropathy is a necrotizing vasculitis. This condition occurs relatively early in infection, has a more rapid onset, and had asymmetrical clinical features. DSP is treated similarly to other painful neuropathies. Inadequate control of symptoms is a common problem. With vasculitic neuropathy, corticosteroid treatment can lead to rapid relief, followed by arrest of the neuropathic process.
• Iatrogenic neuropathies present in a similar manner but over a shorter time. The most likely sources are the antiretroviral treatments ddI, d4T, and ddC. In the case of ddC treatment, peripheral neuropathy is the most common dose-limiting adverse effect and is generally reversible upon discontinuation. Other potential sources include the antituberculous drugs, vincristine, and dapsone. Progressive polyradiculomyelopathy (PPR) is a severe, usually fatal infection of nerve roots and the cauda equina. This infection is commonly caused by cytomegalovirus and less often by *M. tuberculosis.* Symptoms include lower extremity pain and weakness with urine retention. Rapid diagnosis is important

because treatment can arrest or partly reverse this otherwise fatal infection. Lastly, depending on the cranial, spinal, or peripheral nerve involved, mononeuropathies may be a cause of neuromuscular pain. Although in some cases the symptoms progress, the prognosis in mononeuropathy is generally good.

Neuromuscular Weakness (pp. 1377–1378)

• Causes of neuromuscular weakness include acute and chronic inflammatory demyelinating polyneuropathies (AIDP and CIDP) and myopathy, as well as PPR and mononeuropathy simplex or multiplex (Table 60–4). True neuromuscular weakness should be distinguished from weakness associated with deconditioning and HIV-related fatigue. AIDP and CIDP both present primarily with weakness. The acute form is similar to Guillain-Barré syndrome. Generally, AIDP and CIDP tend to occur earlier in the disease course. Plasmapheresis generally improves the symptoms.

• Skeletal muscle disorders can be classified into (1) HIV-associated myopathies, (2) zidovudine myopathy, (3) HIV wasting syndrome, and (4) opportunistic infections and tumoral infiltration of muscle. Myopathy associated with HIV infection has no particular predilection for a given disease stage. AZT myopathy is usually seen after greater than 9 months of use, with severe myal-

TABLE 60–4 Etiologies and Classification of Neuromuscular Weakness in HIV Infection

Diagnosis	Etiology	CDC Clinical Category	Clinical Presentation
AIDP	Immune-mediated	A, B	Proximal and distal weakness, areflexia, mild sensory signs, onset over days, autonomic dysfunction
CIDP	Immune-mediated	A, B	Proximal and distal weakness, areflexia, mild sensory signs, onset over weeks, relative lack of autonomic dysfunction
Myopathy	Likely immune-mediated	A, B, C	Gradual onset, proximal weakness, myalgia in lower extremities, "wasting syndrome" a possible variant
Progressive polyradiculomyelopathy	Cytomegalovirus, TB	C	Rapid-onset paraparesis/paraplegia, decreased ankle jerk reflex and patellar reflex, urinary retention
Mononeuropathy multiplex/simplex	Immune-mediated, vasculitis	C	Variable, depending on the nerve affected

Abbreviations: AIDP, CIDP, acute and chronic inflammatory demyelinating polyneuropathies; TB, tuberculosis.
From O'Dell MW: Rehabilitation management of HIV neuromuscular disease. Phys Med Rehabil 1993; 7:S83–S99.

gias a more prominent symptom. HIV wasting syndrome is unintentional weight loss plus either chronic diarrhea or chronic weakness and documented fever. This syndrome is likely caused by metabolic and/or nutritional factors. Oral anabolic steroids have shown a positive impact on the weight and well-being.

Autonomic Neuropathy (p. 1378)

• Autonomic neuropathy is fairly common, but its functional significance is unclear. There is a variable relationship between autonomic neuropathy and disease stage or presence of peripheral neuropathy. Implications include orthostasis and bladder function.

NONNEUROLOGICAL MANIFESTATIONS (pp. 1378–1380)

• Single, isolated medical complications can be seen early in the course of HIV infection, but are unusual in AIDS. The more common medical conditions, or those that substantially affect a rehabilitation effort, are addressed here.

Pulmonary Manifestations (pp. 1378–1379)

Presentation (p. 1378)
• Pulmonary disease is one of the most common and most disabling manifestations. Not only are primary functional limitations related to lung pathological changes, but poor endurance can substantially limit rehabilitation interventions.
• The most common pulmonary process is bacterial pneumonia, although PCP is more often a cause of death. TB and CMV are also common. Drug-resistant strains of TB complicate management. MAI does not often cause pneumonia in isolation, but it is common at extrapulmonary sites and is difficult to treat. Fungal infections usually occur in the setting of fungicemia. Viral pneumonias and MAI infections usually occur in conjunction with other pathogens. Non-Hodgkin's lymphoma and Kaposi's sarcoma are the most common lung malignancies. In addition, upper respiratory tract infections, sinusitis, and bronchitis are seen commonly.

Rehabilitation Approach (pp. 1378–1379)
• Goals include symptom control and improvement in quality of life. Although any patient may be a candidate for rehabilitation, the best results are obtained early. Options include smoking cessation, oxygen therapy, exercise conditioning, breathing techniques, chest physiotherapy, nutritional evaluation, and psychological support. A modified 6-minute walking test can be used as both an evaluatory and outcome measure tool. At a minimum, the ability to perform ADLs should improve following intervention (see Chapter 33).

Cardiac Manifestations (p. 1379)

Presentation (p. 1379)
• Cardiac disease can occur as a direct result of HIV infection, from a secondary process, or as a side effect of treatment. The most common cardiac manifestations in HIV infection are myocarditis, pericardial effusions, and cardiomyopthy. Less common are valvular abnormalities. It is unclear whether hyperlipidemia associated with antiretroviral therapies and longer survival will result in more ischemic disease.

• Most HIV cardiac disease is asymptomatic. Abnormalities tend to be seen more with advanced disease and in IV drug abusers. Although both cardiac and pulmonary disease can cause fatigue and shortness of breath, pulmonary abnormalities are far more common. Cardiac disease should be considered in patients whose symptoms are out of proportion to the demonstrated pulmonary abnormalities.

Rehabilitation Approach (p. 1379)
• The approach resembles that used with patients with congestive heart failure. The benefits are more likely because of peripheral adaptations rather than changes in actual cardiac function. The end-points of exercise training are fatigue and dyspnea rather than pain, arrhythmias, or hypotension seen in ischemic disease. Programs should be designed around "long-duration, low-intensity" exercise. Fatigue rather than dyspnea signals the need for rest breaks. Although there is uncertainty about the long-term impact of exercise, short-term increases in quality of life and functional performance have been documented (see Chapter 32).

Rheumatological Manifestations (p. 1379)

Presentation (p. 1379)
• There are multiple rheumatological manifestations including myopathies, vasculitides, sicca syndrome, arthralgias, arthritis, and fibromyalgia. Rheumatological complications may occur more commonly in the homosexual than in the IV drug user risk behavior group. Knees, shoulders, and elbows are the joints most often affected.
• HIV-related arthritis tends to affect the lower extremities, especially the ankles and knees. The etiology of HIV-associated arthritis is probably multifactorial. The myalgias and arthralgias seen in HIV infection can be an independent manifestation or components of fibromyalgia. The prevalence of fibromyalgia is 11% to 29%.

Rehabilitation Approach (p. 1379)
• In the acute phase of rheumatic disease, rest, isometric exercise, and immobilization are the mainstays of treatment. Orthotic devices help provide pain relief acutely and support unstable joints chronically. Progressive resistance exercise and further joint mobilization can begin as the acute synovitis revolves. NSAIDs and other analgesics, intra-articular steroids, low-dose cyclosporin, and possibly AZT are all options. For fibromyalgia, treatment includes NSAIDs, trigger point injections, medications, and aerobic exercise (see Chapter 19).

Fatigue (pp. 1379–1380)

• Fatigue is one of the most functionally limiting aspects of chronic HIV infection. Fatigue might be the single most common symptom in persons with HIV infection. The cause of HIV-related fatigue is undoubtedly multifactorial, with contributions from both physical and psychological sources. Although fatigue can be seen as an isolated symptom, especially early in the disease course, it is more common later in the course and can be the primary limitation in the rehabilitation of other impairments.

Rehabilitation Approach *(pp. 1379–1380)*

• Identification and treatment of correctable causes should be the first step in evaluation. Despite the number of medications required by many persons with HIV infection, fatigue as a medication side effect appears to be relatively unusual. In most cases, no specific cause is found for fatigue.

• Behavioral modification (energy conservation and work simplification) is the intervention with the least risk. There are no well-researched medications for specific use in HIV-associated fatigue. Dextroamphetamine, amantadine, and methylphenidate are possible options. Dietary supplementation with fatty acids has been found useful in patients with chronic fatigue syndrome.

PSYCHOSOCIAL AND REHABILITATION TEAM ISSUES (pp. 1380–1382)

• Persons with HIV infection must face the psychologically devastating reality of the need for physical care, financial assistance, and changing social worth. Individuals also face unequaled social stigma, discrimination, loss of mental acuity, and difficulty accessing health care, while confronting spiritual questions and their own mortality. Addressing wide-ranging disabilities and handicaps is fundamental to rehabilitation medicine, making it a medical specialty uniquely qualified to address the many needs for the patient.

Emotional Sequelae (p. 1380)

• The significant emotional trauma confronts persons with HIV infection. Challenges include a progressive disease, poor prognosis and losses of bodily function, vocational abilities, and significant relationships. Stressors are numerous. In addition, there are major decisions to be made regarding putting one's affairs in order, sharing the diagnosis, and disclosure of sexual orientation.

• The caregivers must deal with bereavement stemming from the eerie sense of watching their own future unfold. Women face the additional stressors of parenting, pregnancy, and child custody.

• Literature from other conditions supports the theory that psychosocial factors can reduce morbidity and improve survival. Those who successfully cope with the diagnosis often develop new psychological skills. An increased use of active coping strategies, relaxation exercises, elicitation of social supports, and the decreased use of denial or avoidance can be key to longer-term functioning.

Discrimination (p. 1380)

• Persons with HIV can face discrimination in the form of loss of confidentiality and employment, denial of insurance, limited access to health care, and denial of public services. Confronted with homophobia, prejudice against IV drug users, and unfounded fear of contagion, patients face the adverse effects of legislation placing constraints on homosexual behavior, requiring mandatory HIV screening, and restricting jobs. Such misconceptions have served to misinform large segments of society, leading to fear and prejudices and causing barriers that prevent persons with HIV from receiving life-care services. The widespread AIDS awareness movement has helped lessen such attitudes.

Legislation and Access to Health Care (pp. 1380–1381)

• Access to health care and financial support is a significant problem. As the disease progresses, many develop a work disability. The legislative response to AIDS has been limited. The Supreme Court considered AIDS a handicap. The rules governing Social Security as they apply to persons with AIDS have been liberalized.

• Public health insurance plays a large role in financing the health care of people. Medicare coverage remains limited because only a percentage of AIDS patients live long enough to qualify for benefits. State-sponsored programs often do not cover many of the expenses incurred. These gaps have been spanned by the tremendous array of volunteer services.

Unique Rehabilitation Team Issues (p. 1381)

• Rehabilitation teams are faced with several unique issues. The team must be comfortable with alternative lifestyles and nontraditional family dynamics. Often rehabilitation becomes an arena of confrontation between nontraditional significant others and biological family members. Learning to understand these emotionally charged dynamics and counseling all parties involved are essential to achieving the patient's wishes. Other important issues include establishing who will be the primary caregivers, assigning power of attorney, establishing a legal guardian for the patient, and addressing preparations for death.

Women and Children with HIV Infection or AIDS (p. 1381)

• The number of children orphaned by mothers with AIDS is growing rapidly. Children with HIV and those orphaned by AIDS have unique needs. FACE (For AIDS Children Everywhere) provides a host of services for HIV-positive families.

Vocational Rehabilitation (pp. 1381–1382)

• A nationwide survey of people with HIV and AIDS indicated that their most important concern was having enough money. Approximately one-half of the respondents noted minor or major problems funding basic necessities, food, rent, and health care.

• There are many barriers to working for those with HIV infection. Many persons lack education, job skills, transportation, and options for job accommodations. Women with HIV infection are more likely to be minority or uneducated. A major disincentive is the need to declare inability to work to be eligible for federal disability benefits. Many end up preferring the guaranteed income and federal medical insurance. Other options like volunteer work can provide the therapeutic benefits of being in the workforce without endangering private or public disability benefits.

• In 1990, the Rehabilitation Services Administration published its first policy statement on serving clients with HIV. The policy recognizes HIV infection as a physical disability-qualifying clients for vocational rehabilitation services.

61

Original Chapter by Mark A. Young, M.D., and Steven A. Stiens, M.D.

Rehabilitation Aspects of Organ Transplantation

• The goal of rehabilitation of the transplantation patient is to improve functional outcome and speed the return to a lifestyle as near to normal as possible.

ORGAN TRANSPLANTATION EPIDEMIOLOGY AND TRENDS (pp. 1385–1386)

• There is considerable competition for donor organs. One current federal policy change likely to result in an increasing number of transplant survivors requiring rehabilitation services is the effort to change organ allocation methodology. The new organ allocation system chooses recipients on the basis of medical criteria rather than geography.

THE PHYSIATRIST'S ROLE IN ORGAN TRANSPLANT REHABILITATION (pp. 1386–1388)

• The physiatric baseline evaluation should be performed *prior* to surgery. The physiatrist should conduct a thorough musculoskeletal, neurological, and functional assessment of the patient. Emphasis should be placed on the maintenance of bodily systems that are likely to be adversely affected by immobilization. This includes contracture prevention, deep vein thrombosis and pulmonary embolism preventive measures, skin maintenance, and preservation of bowel and bladder function. The prevention of disuse atrophy of major muscle groups can be addressed through bedside isometric exercise protocols.

• A therapeutic plan emphasizing exercise and remobilization should be generated that takes into account the patient's presurgical functional status. After transplantation, close ongoing daily surveillance is needed to ensure adequate immune system suppression, to prevent opportunistic infection, and to maintain rehabilitation goals. Emphasis should be placed on the underlying functional, medical, socioeconomic, and psychological needs of the patient.

REHABILITATION OF THE CARDIAC TRANSPLANTATION PATIENT (pp. 1388–1393)

Epidemiology of Cardiac Transplantation (p. 1388)

- The current cardiac transplant survival rates are 81% for 1 year and 78% for 5 years. It is estimated that survival rates after heart transplantation will continue to improve because of improved rejection prevention, better surgical techniques, and enhancement of antirejection methodology.

Pretransplant Considerations (p. 1388)

- There are several criteria for cardiac transplant candidate selection, as outlined in Table 61–1. Congestive heart failure is the leading indication for heart transplantation. Less common indications for cardiac transplantation include idiopathic cardiomyopathy and postpartum cardiomyopathy.

Post-Transplant Complications (pp. 1388–1389)

- Among post-transplant complications, the most dreaded are allograft failure from rejection; and immunosuppression complications including infection, neurological deficits, and physiological complications. One study of cardiac transplant recipients on an inpatient rehabilitation unit reported multiple secondary complications including hypertension, nutritional limitations, neuromuscular deficits, and compression fractures. Stress fractures of the weight-bearing extremities have also been described, most likely because of steroid-induced osteoporosis.
- One of the most immediate problems during the early postoperative period is the inability of the transplanted right ventricle to cope with preexisting pulmonary hypertension. Pulmonary hypertension can be associated with chronic left-sided heart failure. Often the heart requires ionotrophic support during the period immediately following transplant. The physiatrist is usually seeing the patient in an intensive care unit at this stage of the postoperative course, and typically prescribes low-intensity bedside exercises.
- Many patients develop cyclosporine-related hypertension because of cyclosporine-induced renal vasoconstriction superimposed on chronic renal hypoperfusion, third spacing of fluids, and an abnormal distribution of blood flow. Blood pressures should be closely monitored with morning blood pressure values used as a guide to antihypertensive therapy. Alternative cyclosporine dosing regimens, calcium channel antagonists, and angiotensin-converting

TABLE 61–1 Indications for Cardiac Transplantation

Having life-threatening recurrent arrhythmia uncontrolled by medicine or electrophysiologic means
Reduced VO$_2$ max less than 14/mL/kg/min and severe limitations in life activity
Having severe angina without successful revascularization
Heart failure/CHF consistently uncontrollable by medical therapy

From Tayler A, Bergin J: Cardiac transplantation for the cardiologist not trained in transplantation. Am Heart J 1995; 129:578–592.

enzyme inhibitors are preferred therapies to promote arteriolar dilation and can help facilitate full participation in the rehabilitative process.
• Cardiac transplantation can lead to neurologic complications including metabolic encephalopathy, stroke, central nervous system infection, seizures, and psychosis. The mechanism of stroke includes particulate embolism, air embolism, or inadequacy of perfusion during the transplantative process.
• The cardiac transplant recipient is generally less immunologically depressed than the renal transplant patient. This is because of the prolonged uremia associated with kidney failure. Table 61–2 lists the monitoring parameters for immunosuppressive medication.
• Acute rejection in cardiac transplantation is a major complication that can be heralded by fulminant exacerbation of congestive heart failure (CHF), development of peripheral edema, premature atrial contractions, and/or by diastolic gallop and sudden marked reduction in exercise capacity. Chronic rejection can manifest itself as accelerated graft atherosclerosis. Ultimately this type of coronary artery disease is a key barrier to the long-term survival of cardiac transplant patients; however, recent studies suggest that this condition can be improved with calcium channel blockers.
• Beyond the postoperative complications just outlined, the leading cause of death in postcardiac transplant patients is infection. The types of infections include mediastinitis, pneumonia, urinary tract infections, or intravenous catheter-induced sepsis.

Exercise Considerations in Cardiac Transplantation
(pp. 1389–1391)

• New research suggests a vitally important role for the initiation of exercise therapy beginning within a month after transplant surgery. Benefits that accrue from this include improved strength, enhancement of aerobic capacity, and improved physical work capability.
• Although almost every cardiac transplant patient will face episodes of graft rejection, it is rarely necessary to curtail the patient's exercise workout during episodes of moderate rejection. However, when the patient shows signs of new arrhythmias, hypotension, or fever, the physiatrist should adjust the exercise

TABLE 61–2 Immunosuppressive Medication Monitoring for Physiatrists

Side Effects	Monitor
Prednisone	
GI irritability	Stool occult blood, Hct
Water, fluid retention	Daily weight
Diabetes mellitus	Fasting, urine glucose
Cyclosporine	
Nephrotoxicity	BUN, creat. (lavender tube)
Hepatotoxicity	LFTs
Drug toxicity	Cyclosporine level
Azathioprine	
Pancytopenia	CBC
Hepatotoxicity	LFTs

regimen to balance medical management with restorative rehabilitative services. The patient's long-term prognosis generally becomes poorer as rejection episodes increase in frequency and severity.

Physiology of the Transplanted Heart (pp. 1391–1393)

• The normal heart is innervated and hence affected by the sympathetic nervous system, which activates chronotropic and ionotrophic effects. The sympathetic nervous system enhances venous return, cardiac output, and stroke volume.

• When orthotopic heart transplant is performed, the complete denervation of the heart leads to a loss of the autonomic nervous system control mechanism. Reliance is then placed on circulating catecholamines for adjustment of heart rate during exercise activity. The denervated heart has a higher than normal resting heart rate, and is typically affected by carotid massage, Valsalva's maneuver, and body inclination. The most widely accepted explanation for this higher than normal heart rate is the loss of vagal tone associated with denervation.

• When the patient begins to exercise, heart rate can increase slightly as a result of either the Bainbridge reflex or the increased rate of ventricular work. There is usually a delay of 3 to 5 minutes in the onset of cardiac acceleration. The gradual heart rate increase can continue into the recovery period, and the patient might also experience a slower than normal return to preexercise heart rate. The peak heart rate achieved during maximal exercise is considerably lower in cardiac transplant recipients than in age-matched control subjects. (See Table 61–5 in the Textbook for a summary of cardiac transplant on various cardiovascular parameters.)

• Because heart transplant patients display this unusual cardioacceleratory response to exercise, exercise prescriptions based on target heart rates have limited utility and are not recommended. More beneficial measures of exercise intensity may be blood pressure reserve, perceived exertion, or the dyspnea index. Blood pressure reserve is the difference between the maximal systolic (or diastolic) blood pressure and the resting systolic (or diastolic) blood pressure.

• The resting stroke volume of patients with transplanted hearts is less than that of individuals without transplantation. Despite this, cardiac output is virtually normal. Most patients experience a rapid increase in stroke volume of about 20% when they begin their exercise regimens. Subsequent increases in stroke volume or cardiac output during prolonged submaximal exercise are mediated by inotropic responses to circulating catecholamines.

• The effect of transplantation on blood pressure is that both systolic and diastolic blood pressures are higher than expected; however, pulse pressure is essentially normal at rest. Diastolic blood pressure can decline early in submaximal exercise because of reduced peripheral resistance. The peak systolic blood pressure is less than that of individuals without cardiac transplants, but diastolic blood pressure is not much different.

PULMONARY TRANSPLANT REHABILITATION
(pp. 1393–1395)

• Indications for lung transplant include chronic obstructive pulmonary disease (COPD), pulmonary hypertension, cystic fibrosis, alpha-1 antitrypsin deficiency, and sarcoidosis. Not all patients with decreased heart and lung function are candidates for transplantation, and common contraindications are noted in Table 61–3.

Rehabilitation, Exercise, and Complications in the Preoperative Period (pp. 1393–1394)

• To optimize the patient's physical condition, physiatrists typically prescribe exercise that improves ventilation, mucociliary clearance, aerobic conditioning, strength, and flexibility. Compared to education alone, pulmonary rehabilitation has been shown to increase exercise performance and to decrease muscle fatigue and shortness of breath. Increased tolerance of exercise also reduces morbidity after thoracotomies. The exercise prescription typically includes the use of either a cycle ergometer or treadmill. Some patients with higher exercise capacity can eventually use a stair climber apparatus. Upper limb exercise should be approached with caution prior to transplantation.

• Interval rather than continuous training is often more appropriate for patients with end-stage lung disease because it puts less stress on ventilatory demand. Rest periods can be gradually decreased so that the patient advances toward periods of continuous exercise.

• Diaphragmatic and segmental breathing exercises can increase lung volume and gas exchange. Exercise training of inspiratory muscles can improve their function and might help improve overall function of the pulmonary system. Energy conservation exercises can help the patient adjust to the low functional capacity caused by advanced pulmonary disease.

• Target heart rates have been applied to patients with lung disease. Exercise regimens using 60% of peak heart rate as a target, as determined by an exercise test, have been demonstrated to increase exercise tolerance.

• To prescribe and monitor exercise intensity in patients with dyspnea, one helpful tool is the "dyspnea index," which evaluates the number of breaths a patient needs to take while counting out loud from 1 to 15. An alternative measure is the dyspnea scale in which the patient rates the degree of dyspnea

TABLE 61–3 Most Common Primary Diagnosis in Pulmonary Transplant Rehabilitation Patients

Pulmonary vascular disease
    Primary pulmonary hypertension
    Eisenmenger's syndrome
    Cardiomyopathy with pulmonary hypertension
Obstructive lung disease
    Emphysema—idiopathic
    Emphysema—alpha-antitrypsin deficiency
    Cystic fibrosis
    Bronchiectasis
    Post-transplant obliterative bronchiolitis
Rejection
    Acute, chronic
Side effects of immunosuppressive therapy
Psychosocial issues

during exercise. A third alternative is the Borg Rating Scale of Perceived Exertion (RPE), which provides a rating of the overall effort needed during an activity or at rest. This scale asks the patient to evaluate all bodily sensations that indicate the effort of exercise.

Acute Postoperative Rehabilitation (p. 1394)

• The transplanted lung is denervated, which leads to an impaired cough reflex. This can result in ineffective clearance of airway secretions, necessitating chest physical therapy (PT). Diaphragmatic dysfunction can also be present in lung transplant recipients, which can be evaluated with electrodiagnostic studies. The problems associated with the transplant procedure itself are often compounded by intubation and mechanical ventilation, prolonged static positioning during surgery, immunosuppression, pain, recumbency, and restricted mobility.

• Bed rest in these patients can cause orthostatic intolerance, reduced ventilation, increased resting heart rate, and decreased oxygen uptake. Altering the patient's position from supine to side-lying or upright can increase drainage from chest tubes as well as promote drainage of pulmonary secretions. The decreased mucociliary clearance associated with denervated lungs can contribute to increased susceptibility to infection in the early postoperative period. The patient should be assisted with airway clearance beginning on the first postoperative day if the patient is stable. Patients who are mechanically ventilated can benefit from a combination of shaking and hyperinflation with a manual ventilation bag.

• Following extubation, the patient can use the active-cycle-of-breathing technique or a Flutter valve device. Positive expiratory pressure therapy has been used in the post-transplant period. Removing secretions requires an effective cough, but patients find it difficult to cough because of incisional pain and decreased sensation in the transplanted airway because of lung denervation. The patient should be encouraged to sit upright during coughing because this produces the greatest expiratory flow rates.

• Huff coughing, performed without closing the glottis, has been demonstrated to produce a larger volume of expired air at a higher flow rate than conventional coughing. For patients unable to generate substantial airflow, the technique of stacking breaths before the expulsion phase can increase the effectiveness of a cough. Splinted coughing, with a pillow against the incision, can help reduce the pain. Patients may complain of pain originating from the chest tube sites and from the abdomen (if an omental wrap is used). Epidural analgesia can help in pain management and allows the patient to participate more enthusiastically in rehabilitation.

Exercise Considerations (pp. 1394–1395)

• Progressive activity should be initiated on the first postoperative day, beginning with range of motion exercises. These can be advanced to transfers out of bed to a chair and then to ambulation. After the patient leaves the intensive care unit, rehabilitation should continue to focus on alveolar ventilation, mucociliary transport, and ventilation perfusion matching to optimize the efficiency of oxygen transport. Thoracic mobility might be improved by instructing the patient in chest and upper extremity mobilization exercises. Breathing exercises should be included in the thoracic mobility and cardiovascular exercise programs, coughing and airway clearance, and general activities.

- As the patient progresses, a treadmill and cycle ergometer can be introduced in the isolation exercise room, allowing the patient to improve cardiovascular endurance and strength without coming into contact with other patients. Denervation of the lungs does not impair the ability to increase ventilation during physical exertion, and most studies show that physical training results in an improved endurance and strength.
- Before discharge from the hospital the patient should progress to stair climbing, which is the hallmark of recovery because advanced pulmonary disease typically has made it impossible for most patients to do this for a period of weeks to years.
- Aerobic capacity, judged by maximal oxygen uptake, typically remains reduced at 32% to 60% of the predicted value. This reduction in aerobic capacity is thought to underlie the exercise limitations in lung transplant patients. Abnormalities of gas exchange and ventilation-perfusion are not thought to play a major role in the reduced exercise capacity of single lung transplant patients. Many other factors may contribute to reduced exercise reserve, including chronic deconditioning and muscle atrophy. Peripheral muscle work capacity is reduced following lung transplant and is predominantly responsible for exercise performance limitation.

Medical Complications (p. 1395)

- To prevent acute and chronic rejection, patients are placed on triple drug immunosuppressant regimens consisting of cyclosporine, azathioprine, and prednisone. Recently a new generation of immunosuppressant medications has emerged including FK 506 (Tacrolimus), rapamycin (Sirolimus), and leflunomide. A majority of acute rejection episodes occur during the initial 3 months following transplantation. Chronic rejection can also occur and can manifest as a sudden decrease in the 1-second forced expiratory ventilation (FEV-1). This is produced histologically as bronchiolitis obliterans.
- Infection is the most common complication in lung transplantation and can lead to premature death if not properly recognized and treated. Cytomegalovirus is a common viral pathogen and generally appears 14 to 100 days postoperatively. The diagnosis of its infection can be made with a bronchoscopic lavage and biopsy. Fungal pathogens include Candida, Aspergillus, and Pneumocystis.

RENAL TRANSPLANT REHABILITATION (pp. 1395–1396)

- Many renal failure patients seek a kidney transplant because they are unable to perform even the most basic tasks of everyday life. Postsurgical complications include bleeding, infection, and rejection. Kidney rejection is often heralded by malaise, anorexia, fever, hypertension, blood urea nitrogen (BUN) elevation, kidney enlargement with localized tenderness, and leucocytosis.
- Immunosuppressant medications typically include prednisone, azathioprine, and cyclosporine. (See Table 61–8 in the Textbook for a complete list of the signs associated with kidney transplant rejection.)

Rehabilitation Considerations in Renal Transplant
(pp. 1395–1396)

- Patients with compromised renal function who engage in aerobic exercise may diminish renal perfusion and in so doing reduce the glomerular filtration rate.

This can lead to a compromised ability to conserve water. Because patients with kidney disease often have anemia, they might not have the energy to tolerate much exercise. However, there are several ways to increase the patient's ability to exercise, including exercise training and treatment with recombinant human erythropoietin. A successful kidney transplant can increase a patient's exercise capacity to near normal values for sedentary healthy individuals.

• Exercise training after transplant further increases exercise capacity and counteracts some of the negative side effects of glucocorticoid therapy, such as muscle wasting and excessive weight gain.

• Often, kidney transplants are performed in conjunction with pancreas transplants for patients with severe end-organ damage resulting from diabetes mellitus.

LIVER TRANSPLANT REHABILITATION (pp. 1396–1397)

• The current 1-year survival rate postliver transplant is approximately 80% to 90%, whereas the 5-year patient survival rate is about 70%. There are many patients awaiting liver transplantation, representing an extreme shortage of human livers. Quality of life issues following liver transplantation are heightening in importance as survival rates continue to improve.

Indications for Liver Transplant and Presurgical Considerations (pp. 1396–1397)

• One of the most common reasons for liver transplantation is the development of hepatic failure. In general, patients with liver failure fall into two major categories:

1. *Fulminant hepatic failure.* These patients develop liver failure after a toxic episode or secondary to viral hepatitis. This type of liver failure characteristically occurs acutely and without warning in otherwise healthy patients. Although fulminant liver failure patients are markedly deconditioned and fatigued, they seldom require immediate urgent transplantation after presentation of their disease. By virtue of their prior good health, fulminant hepatic failure patients tend to be well-nourished and have limited functional deficits.

2. *Chronic liver failure.* This group includes patients with autoimmune disease, chronic hepatitis C, alcoholic cirrhosis, sclerosing cholangitis, inborn errors of metabolism such as alpha I antitrypsinase deficiency, and primary biliary cirrhosis.

• A common denominator seen in the liver failure population is the presence of hepatocellular dysfunction. Laboratory abnormalities commonly associated with hepatocellular dysfunction include thrombocytopenia, prothrombin time elevations, leukopenia secondary to splenomegaly, and anemia. Other major medical issues associated with hepatocellular damage and liver failure include portal hypertension and ascites. Patients with portal hypertension can require frequent endoscopic procedures and blood transfusions.

• Other features associated with the disease include neurologic dysfunction, fatigue, and forgetfulness. Neurologic complications are commonly the result of the therapeutic interventions required to maintain function of the transplanted liver.

• Metabolic abnormalities such as hyperbilirubinemia can induce nausea and anorexia. The presence of ascites can promote excessive protein loss and worsen the nitrogen balance. Protein losses through ascites can exacerbate negative nitrogen balance, which can lead to muscle atrophy and skin fragility. Chronic fatigue in this population is also a concern. The enzymes typically used to track graft function following liver transplant are specified in Table 61–10 in the Textbook.

Rehabilitation Concerns in the Liver Transplant Patient
(p. 1397)

• A special emphasis must be placed on sustaining the patient's nutritional status. Priorities should include restoration of muscle mass and strength through graded isometric exercises, as well as enhancement of aerobic endurance. Early mobilization postoperatively should be achieved.

INDEX

Note: Page numbers followed by the letter f refer to figures and those followed by t refer to tables.